TOXICOLOGIC PATHOLOGY

NONCLINICAL SAFETY ASSESSMENT

TOXICOLOGIC PATHOLOGY

NONCLINICAL SAFETY ASSESSMENT

edited by
Pritam S. Sahota
James A. Popp
Jerry F. Hardisty
Chirukandath Gopinath

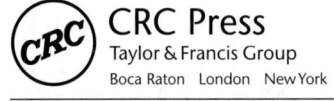

CRC Press
Taylor & Francis Group
Boca Raton London New York

CRC Press is an imprint of the
Taylor & Francis Group, an **informa** business

CRC Press
Taylor & Francis Group
6000 Broken Sound Parkway NW, Suite 300
Boca Raton, FL 33487-2742

© 2013 by Taylor & Francis Group, LLC
CRC Press is an imprint of Taylor & Francis Group, an Informa business

No claim to original U.S. Government works

Printed and bound in India by Replika Press Pvt. Ltd.
Version Date: 20121003

International Standard Book Number: 978-1-4398-7210-9 (Hardback)

Library of Congress Cataloging-in-Publication Data

Toxicologic pathology : nonclinical safety assessment / edited by Pritam S. Sahota ... [et al.].
    p. ; cm.
   Includes bibliographical references and index.
   ISBN 978-1-4398-7210-9 (hardcover : alk. paper)
   I. Sahota, Pritam S.
   [DNLM: 1. Drug Evaluation, Preclinical. 2. Risk Assessment. QV 771]

   615.9'07--dc23   2012039723

**Visit the Taylor & Francis Web site at
http://www.taylorandfrancis.com**

**and the CRC Press Web site at
http://www.crcpress.com**

Contents

SECTION I   Concepts in Drug Development

SECTION II   Organ Systems

Preface

Toxicologic Pathology: Nonclinical Safety Assessment is the result of careful planning and diligence by the editors and authors. When entering the field of toxicologic pathology related to drug development, the authors recognize the currently limited and scattered resources available to assist the toxicologic pathologist, despite the best of basic diagnostic training and committed mentorship. The editors have each served as mentors to toxicologic pathologists entering the arena of drug development over the years and were struck by these shortcomings. Therefore, the current text has been specifically designed to assist the students/residents and toxicologic pathologists in the early phase of their careers by serving as a resource that can effectively be used as a ready reference next to the microscope. Of course, even the most experienced pathologist in drug development has not "seen it all," as areas of drug emphasis shift over time and more targeted therapies are developed, resulting in previously unseen, exaggerated pharmacologic or off-target effects. Since the initiation of this book, toxicologists have expressed great interest in such a resource to better appreciate the gravity of pathological lesions and processes described by the pathologist in toxicology reports and to promote a much more fruitful dialog with pathologists toward a common understanding.

Toward these ends, the editors have organized this volume into two major sections, each composed of multiple chapters. Since it is critical that the toxicologic pathologist has a basic understanding of areas beyond diagnostic pathology to function effectively in an ever-increasing, integrated approach to drug development, eight concept chapters are included. While numerous concept chapters are possible, the current book includes those eight topics that have been judiciously selected to orient the pathologist in areas that are important for effective interaction with other pathologists as well as the many nonpathologists involved in drug development. The second major section is composed of 13 chapters oriented by organ system. While this approach is generally used in pathology texts, the limitation of presenting material on a multiorgan pathologic entity (e.g., phospholipidosis) presented across several chapters is recognized. In such instances, information in various sections should be identifiable from the index.

Any book of this nature is only as good as the authors who prepare the specific sections, thus their selection was given very careful consideration. They were obviously chosen for their knowledge, expertise, and focused interest on a topic. While multiple potential authors may be able to develop a solid treatise on a topic based on literature review, we also know that extensive knowledge and expertise based on the experience of working through toxicologic pathology issues that often do not appear in the literature add a critical dimension. Therefore, the book was designed to present important information, both published and unpublished, as gained through personal experience, so this knowledge can be used by others to improve the quality of drug safety evaluation and, as importantly, to expedite and improve the efficiency of the process. The editors and the future readers are indebted to the authors for sharing such personal knowledge in addition to organizing and summarizing the latest information available in the literature.

While extensive care has been taken by the authors to identify the most important topics and effectively address them within the constraints of this book, there will inevitably be topics that have been missed or have not been given enough space, and there will certainly be unforeseen topics that will need to be added in the future. Therefore, the editors solicit input from readers as they use the text. The goal is to continually upgrade and update the book at reasonable intervals so it can be of even greater value to future users. Creators and users of future revisions will surely benefit from the contributions made by the readers and users of this initial edition of *Toxicologic Pathology: Nonclinical Safety Assessment.*

Acknowledgments

The editors wish to acknowledge and thank the many individuals who made valuable contributions toward the completion of this book. Their efforts not only ensured the quality of the text and photographs but also contributed to its timely completion.

We acknowledge Robert H. Spaet for reviewing each chapter in detail for consistency, completeness, and overall harmonization. His contributions are especially appreciated as they come from the viewpoint of a bench toxicologic pathologist, the individual for whom this book is primarily written. Robert has over 35 years of experience as a toxicologic pathologist in the pharmaceutical industry. He has also served as an international project team representative for a number of successfully marketed pharmaceuticals. This level of experience in toxicologic and regulatory pathology and an appreciation for the questions that are most often asked by the bench toxicologic pathologist made him the perfect individual to review this work to keep it focused on the needs of the prospective reader and thereby ensure its use as a practical reference next to the microscope.

We would like to thank Gregory Argentieri and Diane Gunson for their contributions toward the postprocessing of images, photocomposition, photo layout, and review of the chapter figures and legends. We appreciate their willingness to devote considerable expertise and time to this project as it was only after long hours of such dedication that it was successfully completed. We would also like to thank Gregory Argentieri and David Sabio for helping create the cover of this book. In addition, we express our gratitude to Cathy Cummins for reformatting the text and references before submitting the final drafts of all chapters to the publisher and to Robert Stull for spot verification of literature references as a quality control check.

The editors also wish to acknowledge those individuals who provided additional scientific review of selected chapters: David Beckman, Philip Bentley, Dominique Brees, Kristin Henson, Daher Ibrahim Aibo, William Kluwe, Vito Sasseville, and Spencer Tripp. We also want to thank Page Bouchard for his continued support that helped us to achieve the highest-quality input and optimum timelines for submission of the final draft to the publisher.

Lastly, the editors wish to acknowledge the excellent working relationship with the Taylor & Francis staff, especially Jill Jurgensen, Sara Svendsen, Sharlene Glassman, Amor Nanas, Ed Curtis and Barbara Norwitz, that resulted in expert advice and timely responses to their many inquiries.

Editors

Pritam S. Sahota, Novartis, East Hanover, New Jersey, has extensive experience in toxicologic pathology and drug development within the framework of nonclinical safety assessment of pharmaceuticals and is Executive Director, Preclinical Safety, at Novartis Pharmaceuticals. Dr. Sahota obtained his veterinary medicine (BVSc) and veterinary pathology degrees (MSc and PhD under Dr. Balwant Singh) from Punjab Agricultural University, India. He is a Diplomate of the American Board of Toxicology.

After receiving his PhD, Dr. Sahota emigrated to the United States in 1976 and began working as a toxicologic pathologist for Dawson Research Corporation (DRC) in Orlando, Florida, a contract research organization involved in the preclinical safety evaluation of drugs and chemicals. Under the leadership of Dr. Thomas E. Murchison, he accepted roles of increasing responsibility over the next 10 years. As scientific director, he was responsible for the scientific aspects of pathology and toxicology at DRC. While working briefly for Dynamac Corporation in North Carolina, Dr. Sahota conducted retrospective scientific audits of over 20 NTP rodent carcinogenicity studies and participated in discussions with the representatives of NTP, FDA, and EPA to summarize the results of scientific audits of over 200 carcinogenicity studies. In 1987, Dr. Sahota joined Ciba-Geigy Pharmaceuticals in New Jersey as head of pathologists in preclinical safety and was responsible for establishing pathology peer review and quality control systems. He continued to work primarily in this position with increasing responsibility at Ciba-Geigy and then Novartis (Ciba/Sandoz merger in 1997) to become director and eventually executive director of pathology. During this time, he also served as an international project team representative for a number of successfully marketed CNS, immunosuppression, diabetes, and cardiovascular drugs, including Diovan, a widely used antihypertensive.

Dr. Sahota additionally held an adjunct academic appointment at the University of Medicine and Dentistry, New Jersey, for 8 years. Recently, he has successfully led the global preclinical safety initiatives at Novartis, including patient centricity (patient in the lab), review of best practices in cardiotoxicity and ocular toxicity safety assessment, and evaluation of rodent carcinogenicity potential based on noncarcinogenicity studies to minimize future delays in regulatory submissions.

James A. Popp, Stratoxon LLC, Lancaster, Pennsylvania, is widely recognized for his research and leadership contributions in toxicologic pathology and toxicology with special emphasis on nonclinical safety assessment of pharmaceuticals. He is an independent consultant at Stratoxon LLC. Dr. Popp received a doctor of veterinary medicine followed by a PhD in comparative pathology and is a Diplomate of the American College of Veterinary Pathologists. Following postdoctoral training in biochemical pathology and chemical carcinogenesis, he served on the faculty of the Division of Comparative Pathology in the College of Veterinary Medicine and Department of Pathology in the College of Medicine at the University of Florida before joining the Chemical Industry Institute of Toxicology (CIIT) shortly after the institute was founded. Over the ensuing 15 years, Dr. Popp developed and directed a productive research program in hepatotoxicity and hepatocarcinogenesis with emphasis on liver tumor promotion using stereologic approaches for assessing morphological development of tumors. During part of his tenure at CIIT, he served as a department head of the Department of Experimental Pathology and Toxicology and vice president of the institute. He has held several vice president positions overseeing safety assessment programs in the pharmaceutical industry for 11 years before initiating consulting activities in safety assessment at Stratoxon LLC.

Dr. Popp has served in the leadership of several professional societies including the positions of president of the Society of Toxicologic Pathology, president of the Academy of Toxicological

Sciences, and president of the Society of Toxicology. Dr. Popp has been a frequent contributor to governmental toxicologic pathology and toxicology efforts including participation in numerous pathology working groups at the National Toxicology Program (NTP). He has completed a 3-year term on the NTP Board of Scientific Counselors and the report on carcinogens subcommittee. Dr. Popp has also served as chair of NTP special workshops and served as chair of the board of scientific advisors for the FDA National Center for Toxicological Research.

Jerry F. Hardisty, Experimental Pathology Laboratories, Sterling, Virginia, has extensive expertise in nonclinical safety assessment of pharmaceuticals through his direct microscopic evaluation of tissues and contribution to resolution of toxicologic pathology issues related to drug development. He is the CEO and President of Experimental Pathology Laboratories, Inc. (EPL). He graduated from Iowa State University College of Veterinary Medicine and received his pathology training in the US Army Preceptorship Program. He has been a Diplomate of the American College of Veterinary Pathologists since 1976.

Dr. Hardisty is an adjunct assistant professor with the North Carolina State University College of Veterinary Medicine. He has worked with the NCI/NTP Carcinogenesis Testing Program closely for over 25 years. He has participated in the publication and presentation of significant results of the NCI/NTP Pathology Quality Assessment Program and of several specific carcinogenesis bioassay tests. He has coauthored several publications in experimental pathology, pathology quality assessment, and pathology peer review.

Dr. Hardisty has served on the editorial board for Toxicologic Sciences, Toxicologic Pathology, and Experimental and Toxicologic Pathology. He specializes in the conduct of Pathology Peer Review of subchronic and carcinogenicity nonclinical toxicology studies. Dr. Hardisty also organizes and chairs pathology working groups and scientific advisory panels in the United States, Japan, and Europe. He is active in the Society of Toxicologic Pathologists (STP) as a member of the Executive Committee, Standard Systematized Nomenclature and Diagnostic Criteria Committee (SSNDC), liaison with the American College of Toxicology, and as president (2001–2002). He has also served as the chair of the STP nominating and fundraising committees. He is a member of the International Academy of Toxicologic Pathologists and served as the North American director of the IATP.

Chirukandath Gopinath, Alconbury, Cambridgeshire, UK, has expertise in toxicologic pathology related to safety assessment of pharmaceuticals based on a distinguished career as a bench pathologist, supervisor of other toxicologic pathologists, and author of publications relevant to drug development. He is an independent consultant in toxicological pathology in the United Kingdom. He has worked as director of pathology at Huntingdon Research Center, Cambridgeshire, UK. His other work positions include head of pathology at Organon International, the Netherlands; Lecturer at the Department of Veterinary Pathology, University of Liverpool, UK; Veterinary Officer, British Guyana; lecturer of veterinary pathology, University of Kerala, India; and veterinary surgeon, Kerala, India.

Dr. Gopinath received his veterinary degree from the University of Kerala, India, and did his postgraduate training at the University of Liverpool, UK, where he obtained his master's and PhD. He gained his membership with the Royal College of Pathologists, London, in 1977 and was awarded an honorary fellowship of the International Academy of Toxicological Pathologists in 2004. Dr. Gopinath has held several positions in various professional societies including past president of BSTP and IFSTP. He has published extensively in scientific journals and many books on toxicological pathology. Dr. Gopinath has organized and operated several educational modules on the topics of toxicological pathology in different countries including India, China, and Brazil.

Contributors

Daher Ibrahim Aibo
Novartis
East Hanover, New Jersey

Richard A. Altschuler
Kresge Hearing Research Institute
Ann Arbor, Michigan

Lydia Andrews-Jones
Allergan
Irvine, California

Graham R. Betton
Betton ToxPath Consulting
Macclesfield, United Kingdom

Page R. Bouchard
Novartis
Cambridge, Massachusetts

Alys Bradley
Charles River Laboratories
Edinburgh, United Kingdom

David Brott
AstraZeneca Pharmaceuticals
Wilmington, Delaware

Jeanine L. Bussiere
Amgen
Thousand Oaks, California

Mark T. Butt
Tox Path Specialists LLC
Frederick, Maryland

Russell C. Cattley
Auburn University
Auburn, Alabama

Sundeep Chandra
GlaxoSmithKline
Research Triangle Park, North Carolina

David D. Christ
SNC Partners LLC
Newark, Delaware

Christopher J. Clarke
Amgen
Thousand Oaks, California

Karyn Colman
Novartis
East Hanover, New Jersey

Dianne M. Creasy
Huntingdon Life Sciences
East Millstone, New Jersey

Robert Dunstan
Biogen Idec
Cambridge, Massachusetts

Glenn Elliott
Charles River Laboratories
Reno, Nevada

Jeffery A. Engelhardt
Experimental Pathology Laboratories
Sterling, Virginia

Heinrich Ernst
Fraunhofer Institute of Toxicology and
    Experimental Medicine (ITEM)
Hanover, Germany

Kendall S. Frazier
GlaxoSmithKline
King of Prussia, Pennsylvania

Patrick J. Haley
Incyte Corporation
Wilmington, Delaware

D. Greg Hall
Lilly Research Laboratories
Indianapolis, Indiana

Robert L. Hall
Covance
Madison, Wisconsin

Kristin Henson
Novartis
East Hanover, New Jersey

Mark J. Hoenerhoff
National Institute of Environmental Health
    Sciences
Research Triangle Park, North Carolina

Robert C. Johnson
Novartis
East Hanover, New Jersey

Joel R. Leininger
WIL Research
Hillsborough, North Carolina

David J. Lewis
GlaxoSmithKline
Ware, United Kingdom

Philip H. Long
Vet Path Services, Inc.
Mason, Ohio

Calvert Louden
Drug Safety Sciences
Janssen Pharmaceuticals
Raritan, New Jersey

David E. Malarkey
National Institute of Environmental Health
    Sciences
Research Triangle Park, North Carolina

Peter C. Mann
Experimental Pathology Laboratories
Seattle, Washington

Judit E. Markovits
Novartis
Cambridge, Massachusetts

Tom P. McKevitt
GlaxoSmithKline
Ware, United Kingdom

Donald N. McMartin
PathTox Consulting LLC
Flemington, New Jersey

Michael L. Mirsky
Pfizer
Groton, Connecticut

Thomas M. Monticello
Amgen
Thousand Oaks, California

Daniel J. Patrick
MPI Research
Mattawan, Michigan

Richard Peterson
GlaxoSmithKline
Research Triangle Park, North Carolina

James A. Popp
Stratoxon LLC
Lancaster, Pennsylvania

Daniel L. Potenta
Novartis
East Hanover, New Jersey

James A. Render
NAMSA
Northwood, Ohio

Kenneth A. Schafer
Vet Path Services, Inc.
Mason, Ohio

John Curtis Seely
Experimental Pathology Laboratories, Inc.
Research Triangle Park, North Carolina

Robert Sills
National Institute of Environmental Health
    Sciences
Research Triangle Park, North Carolina

Robert H. Spaet
Novartis
East Hanover, New Jersey

Gregory S. Travlos
National Institute of Environmental Health
    Sciences
Research Triangle Park, North Carolina

Oliver C. Turner
Novartis
East Hanover, New Jersey

John L. Vahle
Lilly Research Laboratories
Indianapolis, Indiana

Justin D. Vidal
GlaxoSmithKline
King of Prussia, Pennsylvania

Steven L. Vonderfecht
Beckman Research Institute
City of Hope National Medical Center
Duarte, California

Katharine M. Whitney
Abbott Laboratories
Abbott Park, Illinois

Zbigniew W. Wojcinski
Drug Development Preclinical Services LLC
Ann Arbor, Michigan

Section I

Concepts in Drug Development

1 Overview of Drug Development

James A. Popp and Jeffery A. Engelhardt

CONTENTS

1.1 SCIENTIFIC HISTORY

1.1.1 ORIGIN OF MODERN THERAPEUTIC AGENTS

As with all other endeavors in human progress, the identification and use of therapeutic agents to treat disease and alleviate pain and suffering have changed dramatically over time (Rubin 2007; Scheindlin 2001; Tsinopoulos and McCarthy 2002). The origin of the use of potential therapeutic agents is lost in antiquity but certainly dates back several millennia. The use of presumed therapeutic agents was described in written records from ancient Greece and Egypt, as well as other areas of the world. While a detailed history of drug discovery of pharmacologic agents is available (Sneader 2005), only a brief overview is provided here.

As might be expected, the origin of the use of various agents for therapy apparently began through trial and error, though probably influenced by significant levels of superstition. From ancient times until the nineteenth century, agents of reputed therapeutic value were primarily, although not exclusively, "botanicals" but also included selected metals and, in some cases, various animal parts. The collection of various plant materials including leaves and roots provided the primary resources of the "pharmacy" for several millennia. To enhance the possibility of therapeutic success, concoctions made from several dozen sources were sometimes prepared, providing an early approach to "polypharmacy." While some material had varying therapeutic value, the specter of toxicity stalked the use of these agents. In the highly developed world of today, the use of relatively crude botanical products in native, dried, or extracted form has been largely supplanted by much purer products made by synthetic processes. While we may at first think of botanical products as being associated with less developed cultures, it is important to recognize that the use of botanicals has continued to this day for marketed drugs, an example being the senna-based laxatives that are currently on the market. Indeed, in the last several decades, we have seen a resurgence of the use of many crude plant-based agents with reputed therapeutic effects, which have been collectively referred to as herbal products or "nutraceuticals." It is important to note that these products do not fall under the review of the Food and Drug Administration (FDA) in the United States as long as no therapeutic claim is made. However, anyone can peruse the local drugstore or "natural products" store and find innumerable products that appear to be making therapeutic claims. These agents have generally not been subjected to modern toxicological evaluation and, in most cases, not subjected to even rudimentary toxicity testing. Toxicologic pathologists rarely see the results of these products unless they participate in government programs such as the National Toxicology Program.

The identification of the action of naturally derived agents such as curare that was used in poison arrows, and the subsequent study of the action of chloroform in the latter half of the nineteenth century, set the basis for the future of pharmacology. In the later part of the nineteenth century and the early decades of the twentieth century, the population of the Western world became more health conscious and interested in disease remediation. This led to the rather bleak period of "patent medicines" where numerous manufacturers produced a wide assortment of products for sale with wide disease prevention and disease curative claims. It should be noted that patent medicines during this era do not suggest that they were legally patented as occurs under current legal processes. Indeed, "patent medicines" in the earlier era were not legally patented. These products were widely marketed through extensive advertising campaigns using print medium. Claims for cures ranged from the improvement of normal bodily functions to a cure for cancer; most impressively, or perhaps unimpressively, diverse curative capacities were claimed for a single product. During this period, there was no regulatory control over claims of either efficacy or toxicity, with the United States lagging several other Western countries in developing a modicum of control. As one can well imagine, the efficacy claims could not be substantiated. On the basis of knowledge of the ingredients, it is apparent today that they would have most likely not had any therapeutic value. While the use of these products undoubtedly prevented or delayed the patient's efforts to seek medical attention for real medical conditions, an equal if not greater issue was the fact that a number of these products were toxic. Multiple incidences of life-threatening toxicity occurred in adults as well as in children, either through the administration of toxic "medicines" of the day or through adulterated foods. The attention to these issues through the effort of government officials such as Harvey Wiley and a newly interested press resulted in the first laws addressing the safety of foods and drugs, which occurred in the first decade of the twentieth century. This effort provided a basis for a very nascent activity to evaluate safety, and later efficacy, although progress on this front was relatively slow.

Giant strides toward the scientific development of therapeutic agents occurred in the middle of the twentieth century with the advent of what some have referred to as the antibiotic era (Tsinopoulos and McCarthy 2002). Along with the identification of the first sulfa drugs, the identification of penicillin in 1928 was a landmark event resulting from an interesting combination of serendipity, careful scientific observation, and pursuit of the scientific process. The use of these new antibiotics, after the development of production techniques, resulted in a dramatic change in survival of battlefield combatants in World War II, setting the basis for wider acceptance and use throughout the general population in the postwar period. The value of these early antibiotics stimulated the scientific quest for additional antibiotic drugs, resulting in substantial success. It should be noted that penicillin is a "natural product," that is, produced by a living organism and adding emphasis for the search for new drugs via the collection of biota from around the world. Indeed this effort resulted in the identification of a number of useful therapeutic agents, particularly during the middle and later half of the twentieth century. While the identification of the therapeutic agent may have been derived from natural sources, many of the resultant drugs were soon being produced through chemical synthesis of the identified active agent, resulting in marketed products that were cheaper and of higher purity.

Fortunately, the development of the scientific process with the resultant increase in scientific knowledge led to the modern era of drug discovery and drug development. In addition to continuing progress in combating infectious diseases, scientific expertise was increasingly devoted to developing pharmaceuticals for noninfectious conditions. In regard to drug discovery, "targets" known or believed to be associated with specific diseases were identified as potential sites for therapeutic intervention as the result of progress in basic medical research. The attempts (in many cases, highly successful) in chemically developing molecules to directly interact with specific targets have been referred to as "rational design" of drugs in contrast to screening or serendipitous identification of drugs (Scheindlin 2001). Success in rational drug design was substantial beginning in the 1970s, one excellent example being the antihypertensive drugs. In this case, a molecule was developed to fit into the active site of the angiotensin-converting enzyme, resulting in the blockage of formation of angiotensin, thereby preventing its hypertensive effects. A second area of rational drug design was related to the specific targeting of drugs against cellular receptors in an attempt to block key steps in the pathogenic process of a specific or related set of diseases. Early progress in the development of receptor-blocking agents (receptor antagonists) occurred with the development of adrenergic receptor active agents (Rubin 2007). While receptor biology is complex owing in part to the plethora of receptor types, this approach opened the opportunity for development of numerous receptor active agents that continue to be the basis for extensive drug development efforts today. In the last several decades, increasing numbers of biologically derived (as opposed to chemistry derived) compounds have been developed as therapeutic agents, again based on advanced understanding of disease processes provided through basic medical research. Despite this progress in the understanding of the basic biology of disease, it is increasingly clear that drug development is often stymied by a lack of an adequate understanding of disease pathogenesis at the cellular and molecular level. The 1990s was recognized as the decade of neuroscience, with official designation by the US Congress as the "Decade of the Brain." Efforts during this and the subsequent decade resulted in astounding progress in neurobiology, with the results pursued in attempts to develop new therapies. While new therapies have been identified and marketed in the last several years, numerous pharmaceutical companies have had great difficulty in utilizing this knowledge to advance the treatment of neurological-based diseases, particularly neurodegenerative diseases. Indeed, toward the end of the first decade of the twenty-first century, multiple pharmaceutical companies are retrenching by reducing efforts to develop therapies for dreaded neurological diseases such as Alzheimer's that will become more prevalent with an aging population.

Despite the enhancement of the scientific basis for drug development that has been important in the last several decades, everyone in drug development should be cognizant that serendipity still plays an important role in drug identification and development. It is not uncommon for a potential therapeutic agent to be under development for a specified therapeutic use, but for it to be finally marketed for a different indication based on observations noted during development. Several specific examples include the marketing of minoxidil to treat male baldness of specified types when the drug was originally being developed as an antihypertensive. Likewise, the development of sildenafil for erectile dysfunction resulted from observations made during development of this drug for a different therapeutic effect. Such happenstance observations are likely to occur in the future. Therefore, it is important that everyone in drug development, including the toxicologic pathologist, make careful observations and give full considerations for the potential mechanisms that may be related to the observations noted during performance of toxicity studies. Such attention may result in the serendipitous finding of a potential therapeutic use that was not previously considered.

Until the last several decades, nearly all drugs (or potential drugs) were chemicals, whether created through natural synthesis by a living object or through the expertise of a synthetic chemist. The well-known exceptions to this generalization include the early isolation and subsequent therapeutic use of insulin and several of the steroids. The last several decades have seen a dramatic increase in the successful development and production of peptides and proteins of natural origin as effective therapeutic agents (biologics). It is important for a toxicologic pathologist to note that the evaluation and development of these more complex agents have resulted in new and different issues to be addressed during safety evaluation of potential therapeutic agents.

The toxicologic pathologist's role in the scientific development of drugs has slowly but progressively evolved, such that the pathologist now plays a central role in drug development efforts. While pathology may or may not have been included in the rudimentary evaluation of toxicity in the early part of the twentieth century, the mandated evaluation of safety in 1938 (see discussion below) set the stage for the development of modern toxicologic pathology. In the middle of the twentieth century, pathology was included in toxicity studies on a sporadic basis, generally with evaluation of a very restricted tissue list compared to today. The advent of the NCI Bioassay Program in the United States and, very importantly, its successor, the National Toxicology Program, resulted in great advancements in the standardization of pathology evaluation in toxicity studies that have affected all aspects of diagnostic toxicological pathology, including the safety evaluation of drugs. Just as importantly, the inclusion of more modern technologies into the evaluation of drug effects on organisms, tissues, and cells continues to provide the basis for current and future scientific contributions of the toxicologic pathologist.

1.2 REGULATORY HISTORY

1.2.1 REGULATORY ASPECTS OF DRUG DEVELOPMENT

The development of new medicines around the globe is highly regulated by a wide variety of governmental agencies. But three major regions set the tone for much of what follows in the rest of the world, namely, the United States, the European Union (EU), and Japan. Legislation and guidelines are shaped continuously by emerging adverse events and the evolution of science. To understand global drug development and the role that the toxicologic pathologist must play in the development of new medicinal and biopharmaceutical agents, a basic understanding of the history of the genesis of regulatory drug laws in the different regions and the basic framework of their pharmaceutical legislation is necessary.

1.2.2 US FOOD AND DRUG LAW

The US FDA had its beginnings in 1906 with the passage of the Pure Food and Drugs Act (also see FDA web site: http://www.fda.gov). Until that time, the only federal controls on drugs in place involved the inspection of imported drugs, which started in 1848, and the production of reliable smallpox vaccine (the Vaccine Act) in 1813. Around 1848, the United States Patent Office established a unit to conduct analyses on agricultural products, which was passed on to the Department of Agriculture in 1862 as the Bureau of Chemistry. Chief Chemist, Dr. Harvey Washington Wiley, arrived at the Bureau of Chemistry in 1883 and changed the course of how the government handled adulteration and misbranding of food and drugs. In 1927, the Bureau of Chemistry was divided and the Food, Drug, and Insecticide Administration was established to oversee regulatory functions. In 1930, the name was shortened to what we know today, the FDA. In 1940, the FDA was transferred from the Department of Agriculture to the Federal Security Agency, which became the Department of Health, Education, and Welfare in 1953. Though the function has passed from department to department over the years, the core public health mission of the agency has never changed.

Dr. Wiley's concern regarding chemical preservatives as adulterants led to the formation of his much publicized "poison squad" lunches where volunteers consumed different quantities of food additives of questionable value to determine any ill effects. As Dr. Wiley continued to pursue the enactment of a law to protect consumers, the publication of "The Jungle" by Upton Sinclair caused a stirring public outcry for action. Finally, on June 30, 1906, President Theodore Roosevelt signed the Pure Food and Drugs Act, known simply as the Wiley Act. The act prohibited the interstate shipment of unlawful food and drugs and enforced truth in product labeling. After Dr. Wiley resigned in 1912, the bureau continued the campaign for drug regulation. It was not for another two decades that the issue regarding false claims for products would come to a head.

A new bill intended to replace the 1906 Act wandered aimlessly through Congress for 5 years until a major therapeutic disaster occurred, the result of which was to increase momentum. In 1937, a production batch of elixir sulfanilamide containing an untested solvent, propylene glycol, was released. Over 100 people died, many of them children, after consumption of the drug. The incident prompted Congress to move quickly and President Franklin Roosevelt signed the Food, Drug, and Cosmetic Act on June 25, 1938. The new law added cosmetics and medical devices to the regulatory listing and required that drugs be labeled with adequate information for safe use. Importantly, the act mandated premarketing approval for all new drugs where the manufacturer was obligated to demonstrate safety of the drug before it could be sold. Amendments to the law occurred over the years to address regulatory issues as they arose. One of the most important amendments, the Kefauver–Harris Amendment, came about as a result of a near-therapeutic catastrophe in the United States in 1962 after the introduction of thalidomide. It is notable that the approval of thalidomide was delayed by the FDA in the early 1960s by Frances Kelsey, who had concern for the drug's safety. Thalidomide, though, was approved and marketed in approximately 20 countries and resulted in serious malformations in children. The response to crisis again changed the oversight of drug development. The new law mandated demonstration of efficacy as well as safety before a drug could be sold and instituted the concept of informed consent to be part of all clinical studies. It also went further in mandating that clinical studies must be based on animal investigations to ensure safety. Other amendments addressed the presence of pesticide residues in food, food additives, and color additives culminating in 1958 with the Delaney Clause, which banned any carcinogenic additive in foods, but did not apply to drugs. The Delaney Clause did, however, permit the use of possible carcinogens in food-producing animals as long as the residues of the product did not remain in any edible tissues. This allowed diethylstilbestrol to continue to be used in beef cattle as a growth-promoting agent. In 1962, the Good Manufacturing Practice regulations went into effect. The Good Laboratory Practice regulations were established in 1978.

The regulation of biologics has followed a similar route of maturation. The Biologics Control Act was passed in 1902 to ensure the purity and safety of vaccines and serums to prevent or treat diseases in humans after administration of tetanus-contaminated diphtheria vaccine derived from horses. The Hygienic Laboratory of the Public Health and Marine Hospital Service was the home of the regulatory group. The Hygienic Laboratory was renamed the National Institute of Health in 1930, and the National Institutes of Health (NIH) in 1948. In 1955, the Laboratory of Biologics Control was made an independent regulatory organization within the NIH after the release of a faulty polio vaccine from Cutter Laboratories. Oversight for biologics, including serum, vaccines, and blood products, was transferred from NIH to FDA in 1972 as the Center for Biologics Evaluation and Research (CBER). CBER was assimilated by Center for Drug Evaluation and Research (CDER) in 2008; however, the independent biologics review continues within the respective review divisions.

The major components of the FDA include the CDER, the Center for Veterinary Medicine, the Center for Devices and Radiological Health, the Center for Food Safety and Applied Nutrition, and the National Center for Toxicological Research (NCTR). The centers that are based in the Washington, DC, metropolitan area have regulatory responsibility and interact directly with pharmaceutical companies on specific drug development issues and drug approvals. In contrast, NCTR, located in central Arkansas, has a primary research function to address toxicology issues that are important to the decision-making activities of the centers.

The legislation governing drug development is located in Part 21 of the Code of Federal Regulations. Specifics for the investigation of new drugs are covered in Section 312 (Investigational New Drug [IND]) and outline the necessary data to initiate human studies, including expectations for pharmacology and toxicology information. Guidance documents have been periodically issued by the FDA to help clarify the regulations and lay out the expectations of drug developers. There is a key distinction here: the regulation specifies what the law mandates, whereas a guidance or guideline describes performance that will satisfy legal requirements.

1.2.3 EUROPEAN DRUG LAW

The current regulatory framework in the EU arose from a harmonization of national drug laws to form the European Medicines Agency (EMA) in 1995 (see EMEA web site: http://www.ema.europa .eu). Much of the basis for the national laws stemmed from adulteration of foodstuffs and then spread into the area of medicines. Similar to the FDA, the EMA is responsible to protect and promote public and animal health through the evaluation and supervision of medicines for human and veterinary use. The agency is responsible for the scientific evaluation of marketing applications for both human (Committee for Human Medicinal Products [CHMP]) and veterinary (Committee for Veterinary Medicinal Products [CVMP]) therapeutic and prophylactic agents. There are six scientific committees that carry out the functions of the EMA: CHMP, CVMP, the Committee for Orphan Medicinal Products, the Committee on Herbal Medicinal Products, the Pediatric Committee, and the Committee for Advanced Therapies. All the committees are composed of representatives from all EU member states and European Economic Area–European Free Trade Association states. The agency also works with a network of more than 4500 European experts that serve on the scientific committees, working parties, or scientific assessment teams.

The EMA is responsible for coordinating the existing scientific resources provided by the member states for the evaluation, supervision, and pharmacovigilance of medicinal products. The agency also provides advice relating to the evaluation of the quality, safety, and efficacy of medicinal products for human or veterinary use, in accordance with the provisions stated in the EU governing legislation. The primary pharmaceutical legislation is Regulation 2309/93 and Directives 2001/82/ EC and 2001/83/EC that lay out the requirements for the content of a marketing application and approval criteria and establish the Clinical Trials Directive that governs the Investigative Medicinal Product Dossier (IMPD). The IMPD is used for initial data review prior to beginning human studies in the EU in the same manner that the IND is used in the United States. As with the FDA, the EMA issues guidelines, position papers, and points to consider to clarify the legislation, or to provide advice to applicants.

Another key role of the EMA is to provide scientific advice and protocol assistance to drug developers [EMEA-H-4260-01 (Rev. 4) 2007; EMEA (382712) 2006]. This centralized procedure ensures consistency of advice across applicants and provides a broad involvement of internal and external European experts. It is important that the applicant knows that only the question asked will be answered. The advice is also not legally binding, but an applicant must justify any deviations in the marketing application.

1.2.4 JAPANESE DRUG LAW

The Japanese Pharmaceutical Affairs Law was first enacted in 1948 and revised several times between 1961 and 2005 (also see the Pharmaceutical and Medical Devices Agency [PMDA] web site: http://www.pmda.go.jp/english/index.html). The legislation provides the basic organization for regulation and guidance, and the requirements for clinical trials and marketing approval. The Ministry of Health, Labor, and Welfare (MHLW) is the cabinet-level office of the Japanese parliament and is known as the "Korosho" or "Koseirodosho" in Japanese. The PMDA is the MHLW section, analogous to the FDA and EMA. The Japanese name for the PMDA is "Iyakuhin Iryokiki

Sogo Kiko" or "Kiko" for short. The group relies heavily on the guidelines put forward by the International Conference on Harmonization of Technical Requirements for the Registration of Pharmaceuticals for Human Use (ICH), which will be discussed later.

Unlike its previous structure, one team now handles a clinical candidate from initial clinical trial stage through marketing approval. The first interaction of the Kiko team with a drug developer is at the submission of a clinical trial notification (CTN) [PMDA Notification (0307001–0307007) 2007; MHLW (No. 0331003) 2005]. This document is very similar in structure to the IMPD of the EU and IND in the United States and is an explanatory document that presents the rationale of the clinical study. The marketing application process follows a very stepwise fashion from receipt of the CTN to when a recommendation is made to the MHLW.

1.2.5 INTERNATIONAL HARMONIZATION

Until the early 1990s, drug development was governed by several sets of regulations that often varied widely in requirements across the different regions of the globe. Differences in regional regulations and expectations resulted in the conduct of repetitive studies or inclusion of more animals in dose groups than was necessary. As a result, the ICH was convened to bring the key stakeholders from the three major regions together. The six parties to the ICH represented the pharmaceutical manufacturers and regulatory authorities from the United States, the EU, and Japan. The result of these discussions was agreement on the acceptable standards and requirements for the development and registration of pharmaceutical agents in these regions.

The agreed upon guidelines can be found on the web site of each of the central regulatory authorities or from the ICH directorate (www.ich.org). The guidance documents cover key topics in nonclinical, manufacturing, and clinical development and are the basis for the studies that are evaluated by the toxicologic pathologist. The nonclinical section covers the broad areas of carcinogenicity testing, genotoxicity, drug exposure, single and repeated dose toxicity studies, developmental and reproductive toxicity studies, preclinical development of biotechnology-derived pharmaceuticals, safety pharmacology studies, immunotoxicity studies, preclinical evaluation of anticancer drugs, and general guidance on safety studies necessary to conduct human clinical trials and marketing authorizations. As new topics arise, the ICH Steering Committee decides whether or not a new guidance is needed. If so, it follows the same procedure that was used to develop the existing guidance documents and any follow-on revisions (see the ICH web site for the most current versions of each guidance).

One additional area of harmonization was in the format and content of the marketing application called the Common Technical Document (CTD). The CTD is the dossier containing all critical and supportive information on the nonclinical, manufacturing, and clinical development of the candidate drug presented in such a way as to facilitate the assessment of the data by the reviewing health authorities. Full details of the CTD can also be found on the ICH web site (www.ich.org/products/ctd.html). With respect to the nonclinical portion of the CTD, there are three main sections where the data are housed and summarized. Briefly, Module 4 (Safety) contains the individual study reports, including all individual animal data. Module 2.6 contains the textual and tabular summaries for the individual reports, and Module 2.4 contains the integrated nonclinical overview. Each of the modules builds an integrated and interpretive data pyramid that, hopefully, facilitates the review, understanding, and assessment of the data contained in the in vitro and in vivo studies.

1.2.6 CURRENT REGIONAL REGULATORY DIFFERENCES

Despite the ICH process and guidelines, regional differences in requirements for drug development and market authorization still exist (Wang et al. 2010). Most countries around the globe use ICH requirements as a primary basis, but differences in timing of nonclinical studies or need for additional studies can and do occur. The toxicologic pathologist needs to be aware of these differences and determine how the pathology evaluation can aid in obviating the need for additional animal studies. For instance, local irritation of parental drug products can be assessed by the pathologist as part of the general toxicity studies by describing not only what was present but also what was not present at the injection site. This small addition can preemptively prevent a question from a regulator or a request for a specific local tolerance study. This is where awareness by the pathologist of the regulatory environment and registration expectations can reduce the number of animal studies conducted and aid the drug development timeline.

1.2.7 REGULATORY REVIEW PROCESS

Even with the harmonized format, each region still has specific ways that data are reviewed. For example, the marketing application in Japan looks for more of a scientific story than do other regions and typifies the regional differences in data review (Figure 1.1). In the review of the Japan New Drug Application (NDA), the linear development of the candidate drug is of most interest. In this way, the rationale for each study must be justified by the results of previous studies; dose selection is based on previous results and not solely on dose multiples or maximum tolerated dose (MTD). As a result, the entire thought process in the preclinical development of the drug is laid out for the reviewer in such a way that this development continuum, from early pharmacology to carcinogenicity testing, is evident in the data presentation.

The European system, on the other hand, begins with the critical review presented by the company in the integrated nonclinical overview (Figure 1.2). This summary is also known as "Module 2.4." The "expert opinion" presented in the summary is the initial basis of review by the rapporteur and co-rapporteur for assessment of the preclinical dossier. If further detail is required to make an assessment, the more detailed study summaries are then referred to, which also contain tabular summaries of each study. Finally, the individual study reports may be used to answer more specific questions about results presented in the integrated overview.

The system followed in the United States tends to begin with the individual data from each study where the assessment is built from the bottom up (Figure 1.3). It is in this style of review that variations in nomenclature used in the pathology evaluation or clinical observations in individual studies can create confusion for the reviewer. Utilization of standardized diagnostic criteria and nomenclature, such as the Standardized System of Nomenclature and Diagnostic Criteria guideline or the International Harmonization of Nomenclature and Diagnostic Criteria for Lesions in Rats and Mice (Society of Toxicologic Pathology web site: https://www.toxpath.org/ssndc.asp), hopefully minimizes this confusion.

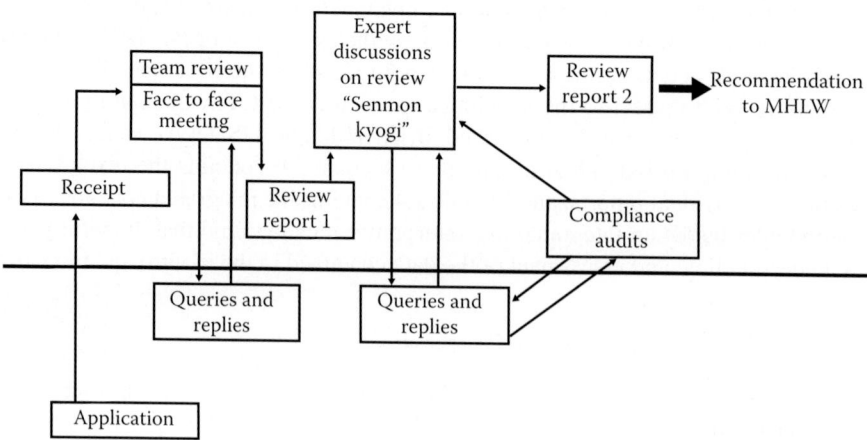

FIGURE 1.1 Stylized review process used by the PMDA for evaluation of new drug applications in Japan.

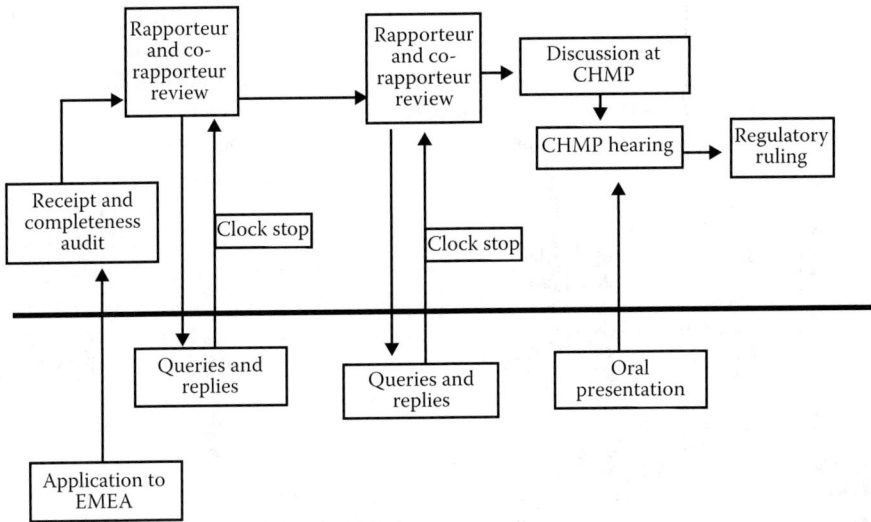

FIGURE 1.2 Stylized review process used by the CHMP for evaluation of new marketing authorization applications in Europe.

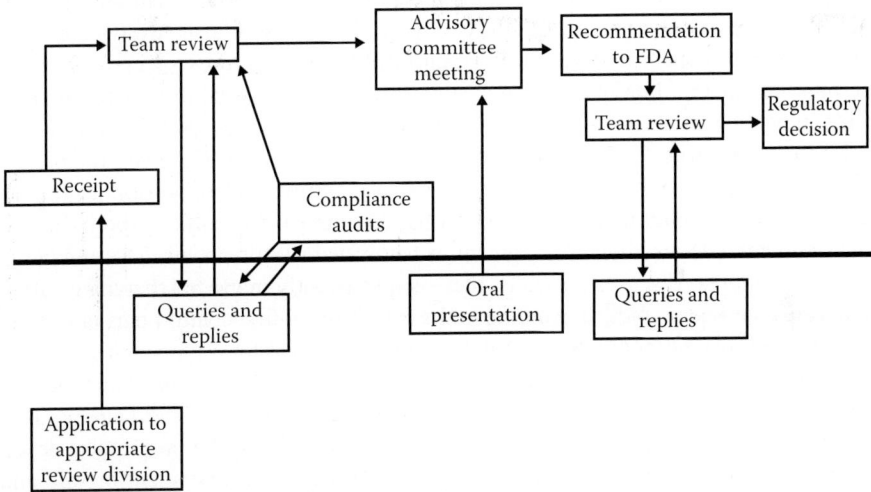

FIGURE 1.3 Stylized review process used by the FDA review divisions for evaluation of new drug applications in the United States.

1.3 SEQUENCE OF SMALL-MOLECULE DRUG DEVELOPMENT

It is valuable for the toxicologic pathologist to have a basic understanding of the drug development process to understand how the pathology data are used. The drug development process is very complex with essential contributions from multiple groups with specialty scientific expertise and administrative capabilities. The following provides generalized descriptions of activities, responsibilities, and interactions that lead to successful drug development. Obviously, there is no single approach to drug development, and the experience of a toxicologic pathologist will vary depending on the company and the therapeutic area(s) of interest to the company. As an example, the drug development process tends to be shorter and more limited for anticancer drugs than for drugs intended for extended (perhaps lifetime administration) use to treat a chronic disease such as hypertension or diabetes. The development of an antibiotic requires special consideration in the drug development process for various reasons, including the short periods of intended use in most cases, and the potential to alter normal bacterial flora in animals used in toxicity evaluation. While the size of the drug development program influences the processes and structure in various companies, basic differences in organizational and management philosophy are also important factors in the drug development process, irrespective of the size of the company. The interactions between areas of varying scientific expertise tend to be more fluid and informal in smaller organizations than in the very large organizations. Likewise, the breadth of responsibilities is frequently greater in very small companies in contrast to large companies.

The drug discovery and development sequence is generally divided into several major steps, each consisting of important intermediate steps that ultimately contribute to successful development. The major steps include Drug Discovery, Nonclinical Development, and Clinical Development, which is in turn subdivided into Phase I, Phase II, and Phase III (Tonkens 2005). The toxicological pathologist may be involved during most, if not all, of the steps in drug discovery and development, though the type of involvement may be very different depending on the stage.

1.3.1 Selection of Areas for Drug Development

Medical needs are too diverse for any one company to have active efforts to develop drugs for all disease processes; thus, decisions as to which areas to develop an expertise and specialization must be made. This decision is based on broad corporate input and may follow many different scenarios. However, there are a few basic points that are always considered in the selection of a therapeutic area or disease process for potential drug intervention. Sales potential is always considered in a decision to enter into a specific drug development effort. This requires specialized expertise to determine multiple factors. Foremost is the current or near-term availability of competitive drugs for the same indication. If a very effective medication is on the market with limited safety issues, the potential for a new drug to enter this commercial area is reduced. However, the presence of a commercially successful drug certainly does not preclude future sales opportunities if a new drug can be developed that is either more efficacious or has a better safety profile, or both. Indeed, much of drug development is focused on development of better therapeutic agents. The number of drugs in development to address diseases for which there is no currently marketed therapy is rather small, although this area has been rapidly expanding in the early twenty-first century particularly for drugs with relatively small patient populations. A drug being developed for a therapeutic application for which a current drug exists can include a potential drug that acts through the same mechanism as the marketed drug or may act through a new or novel biological mechanism to ameliorate the disease or disease symptoms. Both approaches can be very important to the progressive development of more effective drugs. Indeed, medical research, including the development of safe and effective drugs, generally progresses through steady improvement of existing knowledge and experience rather than on totally new or novel approaches.

The determination of market potential may result in the development of a required product profile for success. In other words, the commercial section of a company may determine that a drug will be useful and can be successfully marketed if a certain profile can be achieved. This profile could specify a certain reduction in symptoms, frequency of required administration, or an acceptable versus unacceptable side-effect profile. In some cases, a significantly improved side-effect profile compared to a marketed drug may be an important factor in deciding to pursue a drug development effort. The process for making the determination of need from a commercial perspective is based on input from prescribing physicians, patients (including patient advocacy groups), and experience and expertise of the individual or group making the assessment. While sales potential must always be considered in identifying research objectives, there are a number of equally important considerations as noted below.

"Unmet medical need" is a very important determinant in selecting an area for current and future drug development. It should be recognized that there are various degrees of unmet medical need. Obviously, if there is no therapy marketed for a specific indication and the indication is a significant medical entity in terms of the disease impact on patients, there is an unmet medical need. However, an unmet medical need may also occur when there is a currently marketed therapy, but there is general agreement that this therapy is far from adequate to cure or control the disease or ameliorate symptoms. As noted above, progress in human therapy is generally incremental rather than through *de novo* identification of the perfect therapeutic agent entering the market first.

Scientific opportunity is an important requirement for modern drug development and is determined by the scientific basis for the rational interference or alteration of a disease process or symptoms. Scientific opportunity is generally identified through progress in basic biomedical research, which continually evolves through the intricate interaction of basic science investigation and, subsequently, tied to a proposed hypothetical clinical application. Scientific opportunities generally come from research in academia and government laboratories, most notably the NIH in the United States, from counterpart laboratories in the developed world, and, more recently, from expanding laboratories in emerging markets. Therefore, it is imperative that individuals in drug discovery be up to date on advances in biomedical research so that possible scientific opportunities are not missed. Likewise, pathologists supporting or working in drug discovery must be familiar with the basic medical advancements in the areas of interest to the company so that they may fully interface in the early assessment of toxicity. For the toxicologic pathologist, it is also important to be up to date on the scientific opportunities to assess toxicity through new or novel technologies and approaches (see Chapters 4 and 7). Certainly, the advancements in the last decade in toxicogenomics and metabolomics and the role they have in identifying safety biomarkers are a recent example of the need for the toxicologic pathologist to be knowledgeable of new approaches for assessing toxicity.

Expertise of staff is another important criterion in the selection of areas for drug development by a company. Expertise must be assured in at least two different arenas. First, the company must have staff that are scientifically and technically competent and have a superior knowledge of the area being pursued. There is no substitute for understanding the basic science supporting a drug development initiative. The company may not have staff with basic scientific knowledge in a given area and the staff, in turn, must have the ability to retool to address a new scientific opportunity. However, in some cases, the company may need to seek additional scientific expertise if it is choosing to enter into a specialized area of drug discovery/development wherein the staff lacks the needed experience and background. The second arena regarding scientific expertise is the ability to take basic knowledge and expertise and apply them to successfully determine how they can be utilized to address a basic medical issue or disease process. While this point may seem self-evident, it is not always so easy to achieve in practice. There are many well-trained, highly skilled scientists in the world that have excellent skills to address basic biological and biomedical processes, and yet lack the ability or, in some cases, the interest to apply that expertise to create solutions to medical issues. The expertise and efforts of these basic biomedical researchers are very important for medical advancement since an understanding of fundamental biological processes underlies the entire drug discovery and drug development efforts in the world, but such expertise alone is inadequate to result in lifesaving therapies.

1.3.2 Scientific Expertise Required for Drug Development

Expertise in multiple scientific disciplines is required for effective drug development. The expertise of the toxicologist and toxicologic pathologist is an essential component of the drug development process to meet the responsibilities as outlined in Chapter 2 ("Nonclinical Safety Assessment of Drugs"). Drug metabolism and pharmacokinetics (DMPK) expertise is essential to meet the responsibilities as outlined in Chapter 3 ("Drug Metabolism and Pharmacokinetics") and is particularly important for the toxicologist and toxicologic pathologist since the interpretation and understanding of toxic effects are frequently dependent on information generated by this scientific group. Since these areas are covered in separate chapters, they are not further discussed here. However, the role of several other areas of scientific expertise will be briefly mentioned since they are not addressed in other chapters.

Synthetic chemistry expertise is obviously essential for the development of small-molecule drugs, but the diversity of required expertise may not be readily apparent. Chemistry expertise is essential in the early phases of the discovery process to produce the myriad of small molecules that enter into evaluation by the discovery biologists. Indeed, a very close collaboration between the discovery biologist and chemist is essential for success. The chemist has the expertise to produce molecules that are subtle variations to a basic chemical structure but maintain the ability to interact with the pharmacologic target, whether it is an enzyme, a receptor, or a gene product. Simply stated, the drug discovery process for small molecules cannot be initiated in the laboratory until a chemist provides material for assessment, first by the discovery biologist and, subsequently, by the toxicologist for evaluation of early toxicity assessment. The amount of material required is substantially increased as a molecule progresses in the drug discovery and development process. Larger-scale batches of drug are required for safety assessment than was required for discovery support, but this amount is very small as compared to the requirement for human clinical trials. In clinical trials, the amount of drug required progressively increases as the number of humans receiving the potential drug increases from perhaps a handful of individuals receiving the drug for short periods in Phase I studies to thousands of individuals receiving the drug for prolonged periods in Phase III studies. Obviously, the chemistry expertise and the facilities used by that expertise are very different for the support of the various phases of drug discovery and development.

Analytical chemistry expertise is also essential in drug development. Once the molecule has been produced, the material must be characterized. While purity is determined using batches of drug in the early stages of development, such as the material used in early and all subsequent toxicity studies, progressive development of a molecule requires progressively more detailed evaluation of the batch of material used. Identification of impurities must be made for material used in later development phases and must conform to the ICH guidelines.

Pharmaceutical science expertise is also essential. This group is frequently involved in the selection, development, and evaluation of the pharmaceutical characteristics of salt forms of a new molecular entity, which has implications for material used in nonclinical safety evaluation. Pharmaceutical science expertise is utilized to determine stability of drug substance and drug product, particularly for the support of clinical trials and, subsequently, for the commercial form of the drug to be marketed. This group develops the final marketed product formulation, which requires careful compounding of the drug with the appropriate and acceptable excipients.

Physicians are obviously required to evaluate and oversee the administration of the potential pharmaceutical to humans at all phases of clinical development. They are ultimately responsible for the safety of the clinical trial subjects, from the volunteers involved in Phase I trials to patients receiving the drug to assess efficacy in Phase III trials. Physicians overseeing the clinical trials generally have specialty expertise in the diseases for which the drug is being developed and would frequently have specialty medical certification in the relevant area. However, the physician must also be knowledgeable of the rules, regulations, and acceptable approaches regarding the design, performance, and monitoring of clinical trials.

Project management can play various roles across different organizations, but this group generally ensures that the drug development program progresses according to earlier defined objectives and timelines. Project management leads and supports the interaction of the various project team members, which generally represent the multiple scientific disciplines that are involved in the development process at any given stage of development, including nonclinical safety.

1.3.3 STAGES OF DRUG DEVELOPMENT

Drug development is typically divided into three steps or areas: discovery, nonclinical development, and clinical development. While this categorization is still useful to gain a basic understanding of the various areas of drug development, it is also misleading for modern drug development where the three areas are, or should be, very interactive and integrated rather than being viewed as separate steps as was common in the past. For example, the results of early toxicity studies may result in modification of the molecular structure in the discovery area. Likewise, specific adverse event findings such as elevated serum ALT in a clinical study may result in assessment of liver toxicity in specially designed toxicity studies. For the purpose of the present discussion, the three areas of drug development are maintained, but their interrelationship will be stressed. In addition, it is important to recognize that the division of these activities across administrative departments may be very different from one company to another.

1.3.4 DRUG DISCOVERY

Once a decision has been made to pursue a therapeutic indication and a target has been identified in the disease process, the drug discovery activities start in earnest in the laboratory. While there are no standardized steps taken depending on the target selected and the approaches preferred by the specific company, the following would not be unusual. The discovery support chemists and the discovery biologists work together to identify a molecular structure that has the potential to interact with a target. Typically, a large number of molecules are synthesized using one or several chemical structures sometimes referred to as "scaffolds." Binding assays may be used to determine the interaction with the target, as well as in vitro functional assays to assess the effect(s) of the molecule on the target. Once a molecular structure or a small number of molecular structures show the potential for interaction with the target, the functional activity of the molecule on the disease process is assessed typically using in vitro cellular-based assays followed by in vivo animal efficacy model(s). This is frequently a major challenge since animal models of the disease process may be limited or incompletely correlate to the human disease process. In addition, the marker for clinically relevant action with a disease process may not be apparent. Despite these deficiencies and challenges, the in vivo assessment of the molecule is a very important step before proceeding further in the selection of molecules for drug development where resource requirements are much greater.

Either prior to, in conjunction with, or immediately after the evaluation of the molecule in in vivo efficacy models, basic pharmacokinetic characteristics of the molecule are established. In vitro cell systems may be first used to determine if the molecule can cross intact cells. It is very important to know that the drug has been absorbed in vivo to interpret the presence, or lack of an effect, in the efficacy model. During this discovery step, chemical synthesis pathways to provide a greater quantity of material for the next stage in development or may need to be refined to provide material of greater purity.

Early toxicity evaluation generally occurs during the discovery step in most organizations today. This is in contrast to approaches of several decades ago where toxicity evaluation rarely occurred in the discovery phase. This previous approach has been largely abandoned since a molecule, fully evaluated for pharmacologic characteristics but not for toxicity potential, frequently resulted in rapid termination due to severe toxicity in the initial toxicity studies, resulting in a substantial waste of resources. There is no standard approach for limited assessment of toxicity in discovery, with wide variation depending on the philosophy and approaches of the individual company and previous knowledge of toxicity, and with pharmacologically related molecules or chemical scaffolding. However, in vitro cytotoxicity assays would be commonly used in conjunction with assessment of receptor binding specificity followed by short-term animal studies, again dependent on the preferred approach of the organization. Such studies would be more common where a previous and related molecule may have failed in toxicity evaluation after progressing into development.

Again, it is stressed that there is no uniform approach across companies as to which activities are included in discovery versus the early nonclinical development phase. In addition, the activities included in discovery may be altered based on experience with the molecules of the chemical class or molecules that are chemically unrelated, but designed for interaction at the same target. This lack of uniformity, based on experience, should be viewed positively since decisions are being made on scientific knowledge and judgment, and not based on a standard "cookie cutter" approach.

1.3.5   NONCLINICAL DEVELOPMENT

Nonclinical development begins once a molecule has been accepted or approved for entry into the drug development program. This is generally a very important decision requiring formal review, since the decision to progress a molecule from discovery to development results in a substantially increased resource requirement. Therefore, a company must frequently make priority decisions on the use of development resources since there may be multiple competing molecules available to enter into development.

Toxicology and, therefore, the toxicologic pathologist have a very central role in this step of drug development. The toxicology profile, as well as the related pharmacokinetic and an initial drug metabolism profile developed at this step, is the primary basis for progressing a molecule into humans in the first phase of clinical development. While nonclinical development must, by necessity, precede clinical assessment where humans are given the molecule, nonclinical development activities continue to support the next stage of clinical development.

For additional details on nonclinical development activities related to safety assessment as well as DMPK, the reader is referred to Chapters 2 and 3.

1.3.6   CLINICAL DEVELOPMENT

Clinical development starts with the first administration of drug to humans and continues until the drug is submitted to regulatory agencies for approval or is removed from clinical development for any one of various reasons, but most often owing to a lack of efficacy or unacceptable side-effect profile. The clinical development program is divided into three phases that are relatively distinct. While these phases will be different based on disease indication, the following assumes a therapeutic drug for long-term use. The approach for an anticancer drug would be substantially different. It is also important to realize that the following phases generally consist of multiple studies and not a single one.

Phase I clinical trials will be initiated in the United States after submission of an IND submission to the FDA, with comparable submissions preceding human studies in other parts of the world. The initial study in Phase I is frequently referred to as First-in-Human studies. Typically, this phase involves administration of drug to small numbers of volunteers, frequently several dozen, in a controlled setting where the effects can be readily monitored under appropriate medical supervision. The objective of Phase I is to determine safety, including the identification of adverse events, obtain the first human pharmacokinetic data, and determine pharmacodynamic effects, when possible. Volunteers initially receive single or multiple administrations of the drug over a few days, though follow-up is often for longer periods to ensure safety. The dose of drug will generally be progressively increased to obtain dose-related data on safety, pharmacokinetics, and pharmacodynamics, which provide the crucial information for selecting doses for subsequent phases of evaluation. The highest dose administered in the first segment of a Phase I study may be determined in advance of the study based on toxicity data, including the data generated by the toxicologic pathologist. This highest dose prior to study start may be exceeded, based on careful assessment of initial human data at lower doses. The availability of accepted, sensitive biomarkers for both pharmacological activity and toxicity provides an important resource for determining the acceptable, and potentially efficacious, dose for subsequent human studies. Therefore, the role of the toxicologic pathologist in the development and validation of biomarkers in laboratory animals can have important, direct implications on the clinical development program at all three phases of clinical development. Multiple Phase I studies may be required to generate the data necessary to proceed to the next phase of clinical investigation. As noted earlier, this phase may be different, depending on the therapeutic indication, such as for anticancer drugs where Phase I consists of administration of the drug to cancer patients in place of volunteers.

Phase II clinical studies are frequently divided into two steps designated as Phase IIa and Phase IIb. Phase IIa studies are primarily designed to determine preliminary dose range that would be most appropriate for later clinical studies and generally include a relatively small number of patients with uncomplicated forms of the disease for which the drug is being developed. In this case, more extensive pharmacokinetic, pharmacodynamic, and adverse event data are generated, usually with multiple administrations of the molecule as compared to a more limited number of administrations investigated in Phase I. These data may be similar to or significantly different from the data generated in Phase I since the pharmacokinetics, pharmacodynamics, and adverse events may be modified by the disease process. Phase IIb studies, also performed in patients, are definitive dose-range response studies and generally provide the first substantial proof of efficacy, though preliminary evidence for efficacy may be noted in the Phase IIa studies. These studies are well controlled to provide critical information to support the progression to Phase III studies.

Phase III studies are definitive and provide proof of efficacy and safety in a population with the targeted disease. This patient population has fewer restrictions for entry in the study than may occur with Phase IIb studies. These studies are substantially larger than previous ones and would include hundreds to thousands of patients, with some studies having more than 10,000 subjects. The size and complexity of these studies make them very expensive, frequently in the range of several hundred million dollars per study. Two Phase III studies are generally required, in part to demonstrate reproducibility of results though, under unusual circumstances, a single positive Phase III study may be accepted for marketing approval.

In addition to the basic studies in the three phases described, additional special human studies may be required for regulatory approval and are generally performed concurrent with the Phase IIb and Phase III studies. The specific studies required can be based on a variety of factors and are not uniform from one development program to the next. Drug interaction studies are, however, very important and generally if not always included. First, an interaction with food is very important and must be known prior to the pivotal studies. The presence or absence of food in the gastrointestinal tract can substantially alter drug absorption and thereby alter plasma drug levels and efficacy. The potential for interference of drug metabolism (drug–drug interaction) is another important aspect to be addressed, particularly for interactions with commonly used drugs, notably those that may be taken as concomitant medications with the drug under development. Special studies to address ethnic and gender sensitivities and cardiac liabilities, particularly effects on the electrocardiogram QT interval, have been increasingly required in recent years. Other specialty human studies that may be required could include evaluations in special populations, including those with renal or hepatic insufficiency, and particularly where these routes are the major excretory routes of the drug. Other special studies may focus on evaluation of potential toxicity endpoints noted or suspected in either preclinical or clinical studies.

1.3.7 POSTMARKETING

Ideally, all relevant studies would be successfully completed prior to marketing approval. However, it is not uncommon for a drug to be approved contingent on postmarketing (Phase IV) studies that generally focus on special human populations or to further address potential human adverse effects. In rare cases, toxicology studies may be required after marketing approval. However, a postmarketing requirement most frequently pertains to the completion of carcinogenicity studies that are in progress but not completed prior to NDA submission.

1.3.8 DECISION PROCESS FOR ADVANCEMENT OR TERMINATION DURING DRUG DEVELOPMENT

Most molecules that enter any stage of drug discovery or development do not become marketed drugs for many different reasons, though toxicity (in animals or humans) and lack of efficacy, either in preclinical discovery models or subsequently in human trials, are the major reasons for their attrition. The process for making the decision on advancement or termination of a drug from development is very different from one company to another, but there are several basic points of which toxicologic pathologists should be aware.

As with other aspects of drug development, the process is affected by the size of the company. In small companies, the final decision is generally made by the head of research and development or the chief scientific officer. However, in large organizations, the sheer number of molecules being addressed requires evaluation of the possibility of success at other levels, as delegated by management, though those decisions may be reviewed at a higher level.

Project Teams generally have the responsibility to successfully develop a drug candidate and are generally not given the sole responsibility for determining the future fate of a given development compound. Indeed, in practice, the Project Team frequently becomes the advocate for advancing the molecule. Given this responsibility, it is not surprising to see the Project Team strongly advocating for moving a molecule forward in development because of faith in future success and a sense of ownership, both of which may lead to bias in assessment.

Project Teams are not the only potential source of advocacy. Clearly, the drug discovery team that was the origin of the molecule in question expends much effort, in some cases leading to emotional attachment to the potential drug candidate. This group has seen the very positive aspects of the molecule that allowed it to progress into clinical development but is generally less aware of shortcomings identified further into development. In some cases, other groups will have the same attachment to a molecule if the group was instrumental in recommending the in-licensing or purchase of a molecule after due diligence efforts. In addition, it is not rare for a molecule to have an internal advocate when the basis of such advocacy is not obvious. Whether Project Teams, in-licensing due diligence teams, or other advocacy groups, it is always hard to accept failure when members of these teams have spent much time and given their best efforts in advancing a potential drug candidate. However, failure of a potential drug is inherent in the world of drug development and must ultimately be accepted as part of the drug development process. All advocacies for progression of a molecule must be taken seriously and treated with respect, but ultimately should not alter the final decision on the basis of a full and comprehensive assessment of the attributes and deficiencies of a molecule, based on the information available at the time the decision is being made.

Irrespective of the person or group responsibility for determining the future fate of a molecule in development, there are basic and multiple criteria that must be considered. Obviously, the newest data from nonclinical and clinical investigations must be of primary consideration. While severe toxicity with minimal safety margin or lack of efficacy would be obvious criteria for ending development, most decisions are not that simple. Nearly every molecule that becomes a successful drug has had toxicity identified in nonclinical studies (perhaps at high multiples of exposure compared to human exposure at therapeutic doses) or in clinical studies as adverse events. Therefore, considerable judgment is required to make a decision of the importance of each type of toxicity/adverse event. On the other side, lack of efficacy may appear to be a sure predictor of imminent termination of development and usually is. However, it is not uncommon to see a molecule progress in clinical development, perhaps using a higher dose or altered clinical protocol. Again, judgment is of the essence. It is also interesting that a molecule that lacks efficacy in clinical trials for the primary indication may continue in development for another potential indication.

In addition to evaluation of the most recent data developed from company research, other factors are important in the consideration of whether to promote a given molecule. Scientific data may dampen the perceived potential that a molecule will actually be effective therapy. It is not uncommon for basic medical research to identify a mechanism of the disease process that could be altered by drug intervention but then later be disproven. Therefore, it is important to reassess whether such changes have occurred before committing to continuation of development. Commercial and competitive status of a potential drug continually changes. It is indeed very rare that a single company will be working on a new approach for drug intervention of a disease. In most cases, multiple companies will have become aware of the scientific opportunity about the same time and will have initiated drug discovery efforts at roughly the same time. This creates a very competitive atmosphere where excellent progress may be occurring in one company while another company may be having technical problems in their program. If a molecule is slipping behind the development of competitors, particularly if there is more than one competitor, the financial value of the future drug may be seriously impaired. While this may seem reasonable and obvious, it is again not as easy as portrayed since the competitors are not sharing status information.

In summary, evaluation of a molecule at a given stage of development may result in one of several different decisions. Development could be continued along the original development plan, it could change, or be altogether terminated. However, other decisions such as altering the indication may also occur. It is important to note that drugs terminated from development are not necessarily permanently terminated. "Terminated" molecules are sometimes reconsidered at a later stage when more information is available, such as information on the basic biology of a disease process, including diseases other than the original indication. This point is more important than it first appears, particularly to those outside the pharmaceutical industry, as there is a belief that any molecule in which development has been stopped should be made available for investigation by anyone who might request the molecule. However, this attitude is based on a lack of understanding of how frequently a molecule that is terminated from clinical development may come back with substantial commercial success at a later point in time.

1.3.9 Role and Responsibility of Toxicologic Pathologist in Drug Development

While very diverse scientific and administrative expertise is required to achieve successful drug development as noted above, it is very obvious that the toxicological pathologist has a significant and central role to play in the drug development process. The toxicological pathologist must be astute in the identification of tissue components altered by administration of the drug to animals. However, this expertise and contribution does not fulfill the responsibility and, especially, the opportunities offered to the toxicologic pathologist. First interpretation of the lesion is essential. This includes being able to outline potential mechanisms that have led to the development of the lesion and suggestions for approaches to support the hypothetical mechanism. This responsibility may be initially accomplished by interactions with colleagues in the safety assessment group, particularly the Study Director and, ultimately, the leadership of the safety assessment group. Interaction with the discovery group is very important, particularly when the toxicity may be related to the pharmacologic effect(s) of the drug or where the discovery group may be aware of a potential drug effect on a nontarget site causing what is referred to as an off-target effect.

Another major responsibility of the toxicologic pathologist is effective communication, an essential attribute that is often not adequately considered or practiced. Communication should never rely solely on the preparation and distribution of the pathology narrative report and summary tables but also upon interpretation of lesions relative to the biological mechanisms and pharmacology of the development compound. The pathologist may also need to demonstrate the lesions through the use of selected photomicrographs, in some cases in conjunction with simplified diagrams. The pathologist is successful only when the other members of the drug development team, irrespective of the scientific background, can understand the effects caused by the drug and the potential implications. The lesions should be put into the context of the clinical pathology observations and basic concepts of lesion pathogenesis. Once communication has been effectively achieved with regard to the pathology findings, the toxicologic pathologist should be willing and able to participate in the discussion of future actions to address the issues identified.

1.4   APPROACHES TO DRUG DEVELOPMENT OF BIOTHERAPEUTICS

The development of biotherapeutics has become increasingly important over the last several decades. While there are a number of similarities between the development of small molecules and biotherapeutics, there are also a number of distinct differences. Some general differences in approach to the development of a biotherapeutic compared to small molecules should be understood and are discussed here and presented in Table 1.1. While the toxicity of a small molecule is most often, though not always, related to the chemical structure of the parent molecule or metabolite, or a result of creating reactive metabolites, the toxicity of a biotherapeutic is more often related to the intended pharmacodynamics of the molecule than with small-molecule pharmaceuticals. The innate toxicity of small molecules allows dose selection to follow a predictable pattern to achieve an MTD. As the biotherapeutic rarely establishes an MTD, dose selection becomes much more problematic. Often, the maximum feasible dose that can be administered is used, but this results in exposures many hundreds or even a thousand-fold greater than that necessary for saturation of the target receptor or to achieve a maximum pharmacologic response. As such, the ICH process specifically addresses the topic of dose selection, indicating that a multiple above the clinical exposure may be used as the highest dose in the nonclinical animal studies (ref ICH S6).

Owing to the protein nature of most biotherapeutics, immunogenicity in animals is also an issue that must be addressed. It is well recognized that immunogenicity in animals is not predictive of effects in humans, but it does limit the exposure of the animals to the drug candidate. In this instance, several methods are available to increase exposure for the necessary duration of the study.

The protein base of the biotherapeutic also creates another divergence from small-molecule development. Small molecules most often are removed from the body via metabolic conversion in the liver and excretion though the bile or urine. Biologics, on the other hand, are metabolized by the patient in the same manner as an endogenous protein where it undergoes catabolism by peptidases and reincorporation of the amino acids into new proteins. Therefore, the traditional radioactive molecule studies for small molecules that examine routes of metabolism and metabolic products and distribution to host tissues are not required or expected for biotherapeutics.

For monoclonal antibodies, a tissue binding study evaluating the potential for off-target binding and toxicity in animal and human tissues is presently required. As the monoclonal antibodies intended to be therapeutics have been optimized to bind to specific human receptors, and often have modified Fc regions as a part of their structure, these molecules make poor reagents for what is, in essence, an immunohistochemical screen for target distribution. As such, the value of this assay is questionable when a full toxicity profile in animals can be determined to establish potential risks for patients.

Beyond these high-level differences, the number and types of toxicity studies conducted with a biotherapeutic to support clinical studies in humans and marketing authorization are also divergent from small molecules. Specifics of these differences are discussed in Chapter 2.

TABLE 1.1

Typical Drug Safety Tests Conducted with Biomolecules Relative to Small Molecules

Biomolecule Development	Small-Molecule Development
• Range-finding studies	• Safety pharmacology
• 1-, 3-, and 6-month studies	• Acute studies
• Safety pharmacology	• Range-finding studies
• Developmental toxicity studies	• 1-, 3-, and 6-month studies
• Irritation/Tolerance	• 1 year non-rodent
• Others as needed	• Genotoxicity studies
• Linear time: 2–2.5 years	• Carcinogenicity studies
	• Developmental toxicity studies
	• Route-specific studies
	• Industrial toxicology
	• Linear time: 4.5–5 years

1.5 TIME AND RESOURCE UTILIZATION IN DRUG DEVELOPMENT

Drug development is a high-risk and high-cost endeavor. This simple statement has broad implications for toxicologic pathologists that choose to work in the pharmaceutical industry. The high risk provides not only a level of excitement but also a level of instability for the employees in the business compared to other employment opportunities. The nature of the business provides an opportunity for those with a more entrepreneurial outlook. However, it must be recognized that the degree of stability and opportunity for entrepreneurial applications is very different from one company to another. While the large companies have been viewed as having greater employment stability compared to small companies, largely due to a greater stability of revenue, this fact has changed in the past decade as downsizing and altered career paths have affected many individuals. To provide a better understanding of the stability (or lack thereof), and to understand the opportunity for contributions by the toxicologic pathologist, a few basic facts of the economics of pharmaceutical companies must be understood. Additional details are available through multiple sources, but notably through the efforts of the Tufts Center for the Study for Drug Development (TCSDD). Their web site (http://csdd.tufts.edu/) gives a full listing of publications and other publicly available information. The "Outlook 2010" report from the TCSDD provides specific and up-to-date information on various topics, including R&D efficiency, the regulatory environment, biotechnology trends, and prescription drug policy (Outlook 2010).

To those outside of the pharmaceutical industry, the public announcement of a new drug may appear to be the culmination of a rather straightforward, albeit protracted, effort by the company; however, this is far from the truth. The retention rate of molecules under various stages of development is very low. Estimates generally indicate that only 1 in 10,000 molecules that are considered in early drug discovery actually make it to the market. While molecule attrition occurs in the drug discovery phase, significant losses occur even after a very thorough analysis of the potential of the molecule to become a drug and the probability of success that occurs before the molecule moves from discovery to drug development. In nonclinical development prior to first administration to humans, approximately 1 in 3 molecules progress from first safety and pharmacokinetic studies to human administration. The loss may occur because of unexpected safety concerns arising in the toxicology studies, most often when a toxicologic pathologist has identified the specific target organ toxicity of concern. However, significant loss may also occur because of the unacceptable absorption, distribution, or metabolism characteristics of the molecule. It should, however, be noted that there is a serious attempt to reduce loss of molecules at the nonclinical phase of development through closer scrutiny for potential toxicity, as well as better characterization of pharmacokinetic parameters, prior to the decision to commit the major resources that are necessary in drug development.

Despite the attrition of many molecules prior to human administration, the loss of molecules in subsequent drug development is still substantial. Unacceptable characteristics of a molecule may still be identified in nonclinical studies after human administration has begun. For example, toxicities may be identified after more chronic animal treatment (e.g., 3 or 6 months) that was not noted after administration for shorter periods. Such late-appearing toxicity may occur because of the nature of the toxicity, or toxicity at a later time point may first become apparent because greater numbers of animals are generally used in chronic versus short-term studies. Identification of reproductive and carcinogenic effects are rarely, if ever, noted early since these studies are not completed until the molecule has progressed into the intermediate or later stages of clinical development.

Since toxicities and pharmacokinetic characteristics of a molecule are not always similar between species, it is no surprise that molecules may have unexpected characteristics in humans compared to the effects in nonclinical in vitro and whole animal models. Only 1 in 6 molecules that enter clinical development become marketed drugs (Outlook 2010). This lack of success is due to a variety of reasons, including unanticipated safety issues, unacceptable pharmacokinetic characteristics, and lack of efficacy. Safety issues may be unique to humans. Alternatively, a molecule may be progressed into humans with knowledge of a nonclinical toxicity at substantially higher drug exposures than anticipated in the human but greater human exposure is required for efficacy obviating the safety margin. Pharmacokinetic characteristics are a very important point of evaluation in early clinical trials where the drug plasma profile may not be acceptable owing to various reasons, including an unacceptable short half-life in plasma. However, the greatest reason for attrition in the clinical program is a lack of efficacy despite the best of efforts during the drug discovery stage. Unfortunately, lack of efficacy cannot be determined until late Phase II or, more usually, in late Phase III after substantial expenditures during clinical evaluation.

Drug development is very expensive and is becoming more expensive with time. The TCSDD (Outlook 2010) estimated a cost of $54 million to develop a new drug in 1979. By 1991, the cost was estimated to be $231 million, and by 2001, $802 million. In 2010, the estimate had increased to $1 billion per successful drug. The advent of biotherapeutics in the last several decades has also incurred comparable increases in cost estimates for each successful drug, resulting in an estimate of $1.2 billion per marketed drug by 2006. This cost is, in part, related to the resources used for unsuccessful molecules prior to the termination of development. The increasing cost with time is multifactorial, and the basis of considerable disagreement. Factors that purportedly have driven the increase in cost with time include more difficult disease processes being addressed, enhanced expectations of physicians, more stringent requirements of regulatory agencies, and perhaps increased demands for greater efficacy.

Drug development time increased over several decades until the average time was over 9 years by the 1990s (Outlook 2010). This included not only the actual time for development by the company prior to submission to the regulatory agencies for consideration for marketing approval but also the time required for review by the regulatory agencies. Subsequent to the early 1990s, serious attempts have been made to reduce development time. Foremost has been the reduction in time during the approval phase when the health authorities review data for consideration of approval. This reduction followed the passage of The Prescription Drug User Fee Act of 1992 that established user fee charges to the submitting pharmaceutical company. These fees were designated to increase the staffing of the FDA to allow more rapid review, but the act also established time targets for completion of the review process. During the 1990s, many pharmaceutical companies went through "reengineering" reviews in an attempt to identify and eliminate unnecessary steps or management practices that were hindering rapid drug development. The activities taken by the reviewing agencies and the pharmaceutical companies have generally resulted in progress in reducing the drug development time to approximately 7 years, even though clinical trials continue to increase in complexity.

Irrespective of the specific causes for the enormous expenditures required for successful drug development, the current projection of cost versus successful marketed drug is not sustainable. While costs for clinical development have approximately doubled from 2001 to 2009 (Outlook 2010), the number of approved drugs each year has remained the same or decreased over this same period, though there is now an indication that the number of US drug approvals is rebounding in 2011. These basic economic realities are driving the current changes in the drug development arena, resulting in mergers, acquisitions, and partnerships and downsizing activities in the last several years. The toxicologic pathologist should be cognizant of these changes and monitor them in the future since they are likely to have an important impact on the toxicologic pathologist's role in drug development in the years to come.

1.6 FUTURE CHANGES IN DRUG DEVELOPMENT

Drug development is a continually changing and evolving process. Numerous changes have occurred in the past and are currently ongoing. Additional changes will occur in the future. While it is impossible to comprehensively predict the future, there are certain changes in drug development occurring today that are affecting the process, though the magnitude of these changes may not be universally agreed upon by various players in the field.

"Personalized medicine" has become a buzzword in the pharmaceutical field and has extended into the lay press. In its most simplistic form, personalized medicine simply indicates that medical developments, but more specifically drugs in the future, will be tailored to the individual with a given disease rather than be focused on use by all or at least most individuals with that disease. The need for drugs that better control a disease process in a given individual has been evident for some time as documented by the variable efficacy of a given drug within a diseased population. While such variability has long been appreciated, the basis for variability in efficacy from one individual to another was generally not clear in the past. With the extensive advancements in our under-standing of genetics in the last one to two decades, the basis for the difference in response is now better appreciated for some diseases, most notably in cancer where treatment of an individual is now being determined based on the genetic and related receptor characteristics of the tumor. This approach has a very positive outcome since the efficacy rate has been increased in many defined populations. However, several obstacles must be overcome before such personalized approaches will become common in drug therapy. First, the genetic basis of disease processes that might guide personalized approaches to therapy is unclear in many diseases, particularly the common chronic diseases where the genetic basis is likely to be multifactorial. Second, developing drugs for personalized medicine has a significant economic barrier. If a developed drug is appropriate for only a subset of individuals with a disease, the market is reduced, resulting in the necessity of recouping the development cost from a smaller number of treated patients translating into higher costs per treated patient. However, this higher cost must be considered in relation to effective treat-ment rather than simply the number of individuals treated. The toxicologic pathologist must be aware of and monitor this trend since there is likely to be an impact on drug toxicity evaluation. Simply stated, the advent of developing drugs for defined patient populations through personalized medicine should remind the toxicologist and toxicologic pathologist of the potential for "personal-ized toxicity." While this term has not been generally used, the concept of personalized toxicity is well known in medicine and in drug development through the occurrence of rare, adverse events in treated patients that have generally been referred to as "idiosyncratic" events. In summary, personalized medicine approaches may drive greater concern for understanding and avoiding the idiosyncratic events in humans, thereby putting greater pressure on toxicologists and toxicologic pathologists to refine toxicity assessment approaches to identify and prevent such personalized toxicity in humans in the future.

Expanding globalization of business, including the business of research and development, has already had dramatic effects on how they operate and how responsibilities are distributed globally. The globalization trend will surely continue although the impact over the next decade is difficult to predict. The impact on the toxicologic pathologist is that responsibilities are likely to change concurrent with changes in employer expectations. While globalization in the past has been gener-ally business—and not science—based, the rising scientific expertise around the world will likely change this situation. Whether globalization continues on the basis of business acumen or scientific skill, globalization will surely continue and will alter how scientists, including toxicologic patholo-gists, participate in the scientific process.

Technical advancements and advancements in the basic understanding of disease processes have provided the opportunity to develop therapeutics that could never have been predicted in the not-too-distant past. Likewise, continuing technical and scientific advancements will set the basis for new approaches and opportunities in drug development in the future, even though the specifics cannot be predicted today.

In summary, drug development is not and never has been static. The changes in the future will likely be much greater than those in the past because of the persistent increase in the rate of change. Toxicologic pathologists have a great opportunity to participate in this exciting future, but only if they remain adaptable and scientifically current.

REFERENCES

EMEA guidance for companies requesting scientific advice or protocol assistance. EMEA-H-4260-01-Rev. 4, 2007.

EMEA guidance on pre-submission meetings for initial marketing authorisation applications for human medicinal products in the centralised procedure. EMEA/382712, 2006.

European Medicines Agency (EMEA) Web site: http://www.ema.europa.eu.

FDA Web site: http://www.fda.gov/.

Improvement in clinical trial consultations regarding new medicinal products. PMDA Notification 0307001–0307007. 30 Mar 2007.

Incorporated Administrative Agency–Pharmaceuticals and Medical Devices Agency (PMDA): Midterm plan. MHLW No. 0331003. 31 Mar 2005.

Outlook 2010, Tufts Center for the Study of Drug Development. Tufts University. http://csdd.tufts.edu/_documents/www/Outlook2010.pdf.

PMDA Web site http://www.pmda.go.jp/english/index.html.

Rubin, R.P. 2007. A brief history of great discoveries in pharmacology: In celebration of the centennial anniversary of the founding of the American Society of Pharmacology and Experimental Therapeutics. *Pharmacological Reviews* 289–359.

Scheindlin, S. 2001. A brief history of pharmacology. *Modern Drug Discovery* 4:87–88.

Sneader, W. 2005. *Drug Discovery: A History*. Chichester, West Sussex, John Wiley & Sons Ltd.

Society of Toxicologic Pathology Web site. https://www.toxpath.org/ssndc.asp.

Tonkens, R. 2005. An overview of the drug development process. *The Physician Executive* May–June: 48–52.

Tsinopoulos, C. and McCarthy, I. P. 2002. An evolutionary classification of the strategy for drug discovery, Tackling industrial complexity: the ideas that make the difference. G. Fizelle and H. Richards. Cambridge, Institute for Manufacturing: 373–386.

Wang, T., Jacobson-Kram, D., Pilaro, A.M., Lapadula, D., Jacobs, A., Brown, P., Lipscomb, J., and McGuinn, W.D. 2010. ICH guidelines: Inception, revision, and implications for drug development. *Toxicological Sciences* 118:356–367.

2 Nonclinical Safety Evaluation of Drugs

Thomas M. Monticello and Jeanine L. Bussiere

CONTENTS

2.1 INTRODUCTION

Drug development is often divided into three distinct areas composed of (1) drug discovery with subsequent lead optimization, (2) nonclinical drug development, and, finally, (3) testing of the potential drug in clinical trials (Figure 2.1). The transition between these areas is a continuum and forms the basis of translational research and medicine. Importantly, the development of new drugs involves the evaluation of both animal model (nonclinical) and human (clinical) safety information. The drug development process is a highly regulated process in which specific regulatory agency criteria, including Good Laboratory Practice (GLP) regulations, must be followed (OECD 1998). GLPs apply to nonclinical studies conducted for the assessment of the safety or efficacy of chemicals (including pharmaceuticals) to man, animals, and the environment. GLPs help assure regulatory authorities and sponsors that the data submitted are a true reflection of the results obtained during the study and can therefore be relied upon when making risk/safety assessments.

The regulatory authority for pharmaceutical development and marketing approval in the United States is the Food and Drug Administration (FDA: http://www.fda.gov); in the European Union, the European Medicines Agency (EMA: http://www.ema.europa.eu); and in Japan, the Ministry of Health, Labor, and Welfare (MHLW: http://www.mhlw.go.jp/english). The reader is encouraged to visit these and other regulatory web sites for more detailed information (http://www.ich.org).

A major milestone in pharmaceutical development is the transition from nonclinical safety studies to the first-in-human (FIH) clinical trial. Goals of the nonclinical safety evaluation program include characterizing possible toxic effects in the animal model with identification of potential target organs, mechanism of action and biomarkers of organ injury that could be monitored in the

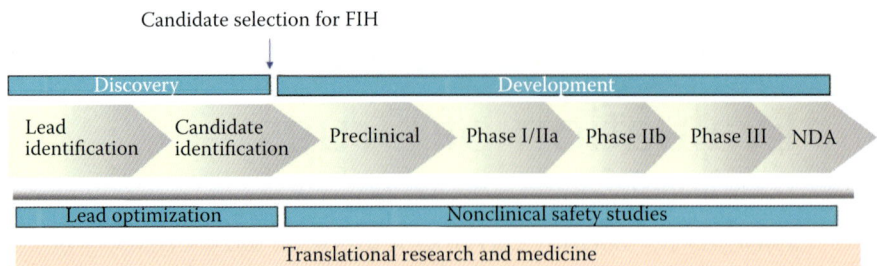

FIGURE 2.1   Stages of drug development and the role of translational research and medicine.

clinic, and determining the relationship of the toxicity to systemic exposure (i.e., toxicokinetics)—the margin of safety.

An important aspect of interpreting the results of nonclinical safety studies is assessing the risk/benefit relationship, which is based on the effects observed in the nonclinical animal studies that may be predictive of adverse events in the clinic. Traditionally, in toxicology, compound-related effects would be expected to follow a dose–response pattern in regard to incidence and severity, so a dose level could be identified where the effects do not occur or are interpreted as not being adverse. To be effective, this requires an evaluation of whether or not the effects observed in the animal model are important or even relevant to human risk assessment (Dorato 2007).

The toxicologic pathologist needs to identify, assess, and interpret the impact of the histopathological observations from the nonclinical animal safety study and determine if there is a real difference between control and treated groups and if the effects observed are adverse or translatable to humans. It would not be expected that all nonclinical "adverse" effects have equal impact in assessing potential human risk. Factors to consider regarding the translation of a potential adverse event in the clinic include the possibility of patient monitoring via an assessable biomarker and if the effect is expected to be reversible. Goals of nonclinical safety studies consist of the identification of potential target organs of toxicity, potential for reversibility of the toxicity, and determination of a no-observed-effect level (NOEL), the dose that did not result in any changes to the animal, or a no-observed-adverse-effect level (NOAEL).

The NOAEL is identified as the dose that produced no significant adverse effect in the animal in that specific nonclinical toxicology study. All of the parameters evaluated in a toxicology study such as clinical signs, body weight, clinical pathology endpoints, macroscopic observations obtained at the necropsy, and histopathology data contribute to the identification of the NOAEL. The abundant and complex nature of the toxicology study data combined with the lack of precision in the scientific process often creates difficulty in identifying the NOAEL (Black 2007). A NOAEL has been defined as the highest dose (or exposure) that does not cause biologically important or toxicologically relevant increases in the frequency or severity of adverse effects. Minimal toxic effects could still be observed at the NOAEL, but they would not be expected to endanger human health or be precursors of serious events. For pharmaceutical development, the lower of the two NOAELs identified in the rodent and non-rodent repeat-dose nonclinical toxicology studies is used to help calculate the starting dose in the clinic. The identification of the NOAEL provides a basis for moving forward into clinical trials; however, it is understood that this approach is not risk free (Dorato 2007).

As the majority of relevant data in establishing the NOAEL is determined by histopathology results, the toxicologic pathologist plays a vital role in nonclinical drug safety data generation, interpretation, and risk assessment. Toxicologic pathologists with a clinical pathology specialty are also involved in the interpretation of biomarkers of organ injury (e.g., liver enzymes) that may be identified from the animal toxicology studies (Schultze et al. 2008). Biomarkers of organ injury help enable clinical monitoring for potential adverse effects. Although toxicology data are limited in the early stages of clinical drug development (e.g., Phase I), the animal toxicology studies must be adequately designed to characterize potential toxic effects under the conditions of the supported clinical trial as per guidelines provided by the International Conference on Harmonization (ICH M3 [R2] 2009).

In general, the nonclinical safety assessment for marketing approval of a pharmaceutical includes general toxicology studies, development and reproductive toxicology (DART) studies, safety pharmacology studies, and genotoxicity studies. For drugs that are intended for a long duration of use or have special cause for a cancer concern, an assessment of carcinogenic potential is also conducted. Specialized nonclinical studies such as a phototoxicity study, an immunotoxicity study, a juvenile animal toxicology study in support of a pediatric indication, an abuse liability animal study for central nervous system (CNS) drugs, or a toxicology study investigating the effects of an intended marketing of combination of drugs may also be necessary based on specific need or regulatory agency recommendation.

2.2 LEAD OPTIMIZATION SAFETY ASSESSMENT

Over the past decade, the importance of discovery toxicology, responsible for facilitating the selection of the best quality candidate with the fewest safety liabilities, has become a mainstream practice in the pharmaceutical industry. Years before a possible drug candidate is nominated to move forward into development and clinical trials, researchers identify and investigate a putative biologic target believed to be critical for modifying the disease of interest. Scientists then begin the process of screening a series of compounds, by use of many different technologies (e.g., computational analysis, high-throughput screens, and *in vitro* models) with the goal of identifying a short list of molecules that possess the desired biological properties, target engagement, and specificity. Lead optimization can be defined as the drug discovery period where a "short list" of lead molecules are "optimized" to improve a variety of attributes such as target specificity, potency, pharmaceutical properties, pharmacokinetic (PK) properties, and reduced safety liabilities. The goal of lead optimization is to rank-order this shorter list of candidate molecules and select the top candidate with the best profile that would then move into more formal nonclinical drug development.

Toxicity is not only a safety concern but also a common cause of attrition in drug development. Productivity in the pharmaceutical industry is at an all-time low, while time and costs to develop a new drug are continually rising (Stevens and Baker 2008). Much of the attrition due to toxicity can be identified preclinically, indicating that screening for more predictive toxicity earlier in drug development could avoid later drug development attrition due to safety concerns (Kramer et al. 2007).

Prior to initiation of exploratory animal toxicology studies during lead optimization, other safety liabilities are oftentimes first assessed and screened *in silico* and *in vitro* owing to the ease, throughput, and minimal compound requirements. *In vitro* screening assays include those to detect mutagenicity, clastogenicity, and a specific cardiac arrhythmia biomarker (e.g., human ether-a-go-go-related gene [hERG] channel binding and inhibition). Variations of the "abbreviated" or "miniaturized" or "mini-Ames" assay are commonly utilized, owing to very small compound requirements, as an early screen to detect compounds that are mutagens (i.e., cause DNA damage), since a positive result indicates that the chemical may also act as a carcinogen (Ames et al. 1973). These mutagenicity tests use multiple strains of *Salmonella typhimurium* engineered to be histidine deficient (*his⁻*), necessitating histidine in the culture media for growth. The bacteria are plated and, over time, only those that have mutated back to *his⁺* survive; revertants indicate that the molecule is Ames positive. An additional genotoxicity test, often conducted during lead optimization, is an *in vitro* clastogenicity assay (Fenech 2000). A positive clastogen is an agent that can cause structural damage to the chromosome or induces aneugenic aberrations resulting in the loss or gain of chromosomes. In general, a genotoxic molecule would not be a good candidate to move forward into drug development because of the increased risk of the molecule being a carcinogen in humans.

Torsades de pointes (TdP) is a specific and rare variety of ventricular tachycardia that can progress to ventricular fibrillation. Prolongation of the QT interval, observed on an electrocardiogram (ECG), precedes the onset of this serious and often life-threatening arrhythmia. A common cause of long QT syndrome is a block of the hERG potassium ion channel. The hERG ion channel is a major contributor to cardiac repolarization. Several marketed drugs have been reported to block the hERG channel, resulting in acquired long QT syndrome and TdP (Redfern et al. 2002; Roden 1998). The potential for drug-induced hERG binding, therefore, is now routinely evaluated and screened in a high-throughput assay during lead optimization (Bowlby et al. 2008).

In vitro screening to identify other possible safety liabilities during lead optimization is a growing and evolving field. Assays to screen for possible interference with bile salt export pump function, which may affect human liver injury (Morgan et al. 2010), are becoming more common, in addition to those used to identify mitochondrial function and impairment (Dykens and Will 2007).

Nonclinical safety evaluation is starting earlier in drug discovery. Exploratory pathology (non-GLP-based studies) approaches are now utilized to determine potential toxicities that could be limiting for progression into drug development and clinical trials. Identifying both exaggerated pharmacology (i.e., on-target) and chemically based (i.e., off-target) toxicities can contribute to the intelligent design and modification of the molecule of interest.

Genetically engineered mouse models that either overexpress the target of interest or specifically have the target of interest gene "knocked-out" (KO) are utilized in drug discovery to obtain information on the intended target that is to be investigated (Boverhof et al. 2011). Utilization of such models has become routine in the pharmaceutical industry (Bolon et al. 2000; Bolon and Galbreath 2002; Rudman and Durham 1999). The evaluation of KO mice in the literature, or histopathological evaluation to phenotype the model, can identify possible safety liability concerns that may need further investigation. Phenotyping of transgenic mice serves as one approach to elucidate putative safety liabilities associated with a specific target of interest and is proving to be helpful in furthering our understanding of disease processes (Cohen 2004a).

Evaluation of phenotypic differences between genetically modified mice and their wild-type controls includes a wide range of endpoints such as clinical signs of behavior, macroscopic observations at necropsy, and clinical and anatomic pathology parameters (Kramer et al. 2007). Combining phenotypic data from the genetically modified animal model with target organ toxicities identified in more routine toxicology studies can aid in the understanding of the pathogenesis of potential safety findings. Moreover, the effect of novel pharmaceutical candidates on certain safety endpoints can be estimated in KO mice. For example, the generation of viable and fertile animals with null mutations for a potential target protein implies that pharmacological inhibition of the molecule *in vivo* would elicit no major developmental adverse effects. KO and other genetically engineered mice, however, are often structurally normal, even if functional abnormalities are apparent; in other cases, these mice have both structural and functional defects. Subtle phenotypes may sometimes be unmasked using pharmacological challenges or other physiological stressors (Bolon and Galbreath 2002; Doetschman 1999). Genetically engineered mouse models have been used to assess drug specificity, investigate mechanisms of toxicity, and screen for mutagenic and carcinogenic activities of therapeutic candidates (Boverhof et al. 2011).

Toxicologic pathologists, collaborating with their discovery colleagues, are able to provide early toxicology data that have the potential to facilitate the selection of a lead compound. During the testing of compounds for efficacy in the specific animal model of human disease, additional valuable information may be gained from these studies to help inform on possible toxicities (Bass et al. 2009; Fielden and Kolaja 2008; Sasseville et al. 2004). A complement of toxicological endpoints, including clinical pathology, macroscopic assessment, and light microscopic evaluation, can be incorporated into these efficacy studies. If there is an adequate supply of test compound, a cohort of animals that are administered a higher dose (i.e., 10-fold above the proposed efficacious dose) could be added to the study to facilitate the identification of possible target organs of toxicity. The goal of this early screening is to provide toxicology data to support the selection of the molecule with the highest "probability of success" regarding safety concerns in later stages of development.

Other approaches to improve candidate selection are to conduct dedicated exploratory toxicology studies prior to candidate nomination. The value of conducting these studies is to identify unwanted toxicities evident after repeat administration for a short duration (e.g., 14 days), as well as to identify putative toxicities based on a known cause of concern (e.g., prior knowledge based on class of compound or the literature). Clinical pathology data and histopathological evaluation of tissues provide important information during lead optimization in drug development. While the approach of conducting short-term exploratory toxicology studies is to mitigate the risk of identifying a safety liability later in development, it is important to recognize that toxicities may still arise after long-term exposure (e.g., 4 weeks or greater) that were not identified in the shorter-term studies. Different strategies in study conduct and design (e.g., rising-dose approach in the beagle dog, single gender, limited group size) are utilized by pharmaceutical companies with the availability of drug substance often being the critical component of the exploratory study design.

The benefits of conducting exploratory safety studies are many. Results of these studies can provide the data to move the best candidate forward, allow to test for a specific cause of concern, and can also provide data to help understand both on-target and off-target toxicity (Bass et al. 2009). Toxicologic pathologists play an important role in these exploratory studies in the generation and interpretation of pathology data that can influence decisions on moving candidates forward or terminating them owing to an unwanted safety concern.

2.3 NONCLINICAL ANIMAL TOXICOLOGY STUDIES FOR SMALL MOLECULES

In the 1920s, J.W. Trevan proposed an experiment in mice to determine the dose of a chemical that would cause a 50% death rate, termed the median lethal dose (LD_{50}). Pharmacologists branching into toxicology subsequently proposed acute testing in several species, on the basis of observations regarding species differences in responsiveness to both the pharmacological and acute toxic effects of chemicals. When the guidelines for repeat-dose toxicity experiments were developed in the early 1940s, the concept of using more than one species was automatically included. In response to demands from the US FDA and other national and international regulatory bodies in the 1960s, the protocols for toxicology testing became highly formalized with requirements to conduct all studies in a rodent and non-rodent species (Zbinden 1993). Because of advances in animal toxicology study designs and endpoints, the LD_{50} approach is no longer utilized as we no longer need to depend on crude estimates of achieving lethality.

Because of the larger size as compared to the mouse, the default rodent species is the rat, which permits easier manipulation (e.g., oral gavage dosing, blood collection) and greater blood volumes. The purpose-bred beagle is the default non-rodent owing to the domesticated nature of the dog, the consistent quality of health, and the lack of background pathologies that could confound results of a toxicology study. Today, there is a wealth of historical toxicology and pathology data on the rodent (mouse and rat) and purpose-bred beagle dog. The historical database on the cynomolgus monkey and minipig, other non-rodent species, continues to expand.

An internationally agreed upon guidance, ICH M3 (R2) (2009), is the standard reference for nonclinical safety programs that are needed to support both human clinical trials and the eventual marketing authorization of small molecular new chemical entities (NCEs). A global guidance decreases the likelihood of interregional differences in nonclinical safety requirements, promotes the timely conduct of clinical trials, decreases overall development costs, and reduces animal use according to the 3R initiative of reduce, refine, and replace (Goldberg and Locke 2004). For small molecules, the nonclinical safety studies need to be conducted in both a rodent model and a non-rodent with assurance that major human metabolites and the parent molecule are present and, therefore, qualified by at least one or both of the nonclinical safety species.

Standard animal toxicology studies should include assessment of drug exposure, primarily parent drug plasma concentration. In general, the drug plasma concentrations obtained in the nonclinical studies help guide both exposure limits and safety monitoring in the clinic. This approach is sufficient when the metabolic profile in humans is similar to at least one of the animal species used in the nonclinical safety studies. Metabolic profiles across species can differ both quantitatively and qualitatively, however, and there are cases when clinically relevant metabolites have not been adequately evaluated in the nonclinical safety studies (CDER 2008). If the metabolite is active, for example, and binds to the therapeutic target or other unintended targets, it could result in an unanticipated safety liability; however, this phenomenon is very rare.

The identification of potential differences in drug metabolites between the animal species used in the nonclinical safety assessment program and humans should be conducted early in the drug development process (Baillie et al. 2002). For example, if the nonhuman primate (NHP) has a more similar metabolic profile to humans as compared to the beagle dog, then the NHP may be selected as the non-rodent test species for that drug candidate. Metabolites identified only in human plasma or metabolites present at disproportionately higher levels in humans than in any of the animal test species may need to be qualified and evaluated in a dedicated animal toxicology study with the specific metabolite as the test article. Human metabolites that can raise a safety concern are those formed at greater than 10% of total drug-related exposure and at much greater levels in humans than the maximum exposure achieved in the toxicology studies (ICH M3 [R2] 2009).

An important part of the nonclinical safety evaluation program is determining the relevance of drug-related toxicities in animals to humans. Certain toxicological findings often occur more frequently in some animal species but not others. An animal species that has a drug profile similar to the human in terms of pharmacology and PK would be considered to be more relevant such that the drug-related findings may be given more consideration. Data from the nonclinical safety studies are used to determine the margin of safety of a drug, defined as the multiple (in doses or exposure) between the NOAEL defined from the most sensitive nonclinical animal toxicology study (rodent versus non-rodent) and the targeted maximum clinical efficacious dose in humans.

For both small and large molecules, the repeat-dose toxicology studies follow the principles outlined in ICH M3 (R2) (2009) with regard to timing of nonclinical studies relative to clinical development. In principle, the duration of the nonclinical animal toxicology studies should be equal to or exceed the duration of the proposed human clinical trial (Table 2.1). Approval and market authorization of small-molecule drugs (non-oncology indication) require longer-term testing of a 6-month study in the rodent and a 9-month study in the non-rodent. Examples of study design and group size numbers for a standard toxicology study are presented in Table 2.2.

It is important for the pathologist to know the age of the animals on a toxicology study if reproductive organs will be evaluated in order to differentiate between immature sexual organs versus compound-related toxicity. To properly evaluate effects on spermatogenesis, for example, animals should be sexually mature by at least the termination of the study. Rats are sexually mature at 9 weeks, whereas mice, at 7 weeks. Beagle dogs should be 9–12 months of age to minimize

---

TABLE 2.1

Recommended Durations of Repeat-Dose Toxicology Studies to Support the Conduct of Clinical Trials (Non-Oncology Products)

Duration	Rodent	Non-Rodent
Up to 2 weeks	2 weeks	2 weeks
2 weeks to 6 months	Same as clinical trial	Same as clinical trial
Greater than 6 months	6 months	9 months

Source: ICH M3 (R2), Guidance on Non-Clinical Safety Studies for the Conduct of Human Clinical Trials and Marketing Authorization for Biopharmaceuticals. June 2009. Retrieved June 2011 from http://www.ich.org. With permission.

TABLE 2.2
Study Design Examples for Standard Toxicology Studies

		Rodent		Non-Rodent	
Study Duration	Dose Groups	Main Study Animals	Recovery (Control and High-Dose Groups Only)	Main Study Animals	Recovery (Control and High-Dose Groups Only)
		n/Sex/Group		*n*/Sex/Group	
4 or 13 weeks	Control, low, intermediate, high	10	5	3	2
26 weeks or greater	Control, low, intermediate, high	20	5	4	2

confounding aspects of immaturity (Lanning et al. 2002). Male cynomolgus monkeys are more likely to be sexually mature at greater than 5 years of age and greater than 5 kg of body weight (Smedley et al. 2002).

2.4 NONCLINICAL ANIMAL TOXICOLOGY STUDIES FOR BIOPHARMACEUTICALS

The regulatory review processes applied to biopharmaceuticals are the same as those applied to an NCE (small molecules). Regulatory guidelines specific to issues and challenges associated with the unique properties of biopharmaceuticals have been generated to harmonize the nonclinical testing required for the development and worldwide approval of these large molecules. The primary nonclinical guidance document for biopharmaceuticals is the ICH S6, "Preclinical Safety Evaluation of Biotechnology-Derived Biopharmaceuticals" (1997). General principles addressed in this guidance include selection of a relevant animal model, dosing route and frequency, and the specification of the test material. A recent addendum further clarifies the topics of species selection, study design, immunogenicity, reproductive and developmental toxicity, and assessment of carcinogenic potential (ICH S6 [R1] 2011).

Biopharmaceuticals (or large molecules) are defined as products in which the active substance is produced by, or extracted from, a biological source. Since the first FDA biologic approval of insulin in 1982, there have been more than 250 additional biopharmaceutical approvals, including recombinant and monoclonal antibody (mAb)-based products, and recombinant vaccines (Shankar et al. 2006). Recently, biopharmaceuticals have represented over 20% of all new and approved drugs (Walsh 2006), some of which have had safety-related regulatory actions post-approval, such as a notification letter sent to healthcare professionals, a modification to the drug insert label, or an added "black box" warning to the label (Giezen et al. 2008). Such safety warnings have included general disorders, administration side effects, infections, immune system disorders, and tumor risk.

Regulatory guidance from the ICH S6 outlines special considerations in the design and conduct of toxicology studies for biopharmaceuticals. Unique properties of biopharmaceuticals can create various challenges in conducting nonclinical safety assessment studies owing to their complex structural and biological nature. The goals for conducting a nonclinical safety program for a biopharmaceutical are similar to those for a small molecule, including identification of potential adverse effects and target organs of toxicity and determination of potential safety biomarkers that can be monitored in clinical trials.

Toxicology studies of up to 6 months in duration are needed for regulatory approval and marketing of a biopharmaceutical intended for chronic use (ICH S6 [R1] 2011). On the basis of a retrospective analysis of nonclinical and clinical safety data for approved biopharmaceuticals, the 6-month toxicology testing paradigm was determined to be adequate for predicting human safety with biopharmaceuticals (Clarke et al. 2008). When there are two pharmacologically relevant species for the biopharmaceutical candidate (one rodent and one non-rodent), then both species are used for the short-term (<6 months) general toxicology studies in support of FIH clinical trials. If the toxicity profile of the biopharmaceutical is similar between the rodent and non-rodent from the short-term studies, or if the toxicity profile is understood from the mechanism of action, then only one species is needed for the 6-month study. Applying the 3Rs of animal research, the rodent species should be considered for the longer-duration toxicology study.

The complex nature of biopharmaceutical drug products gives rise to their distinctive properties, making these molecules fundamentally different from more traditional, small-molecule pharmaceuticals. Biopharmaceuticals have diverse characteristics; therefore, critical points such as selection of a relevant animal species and the immunogenic potential of the drug must be considered in the design and interpretation of nonclinical safety studies. Additionally, since each biopharmaceutical has novel properties, each one must be considered individually.

2.5 REVERSIBILITY/RECOVERY OF DRUG-INDUCED PATHOLOGY IN NONCLINICAL SAFETY STUDIES

The ICH M3 (R2) and ICH S6 (R1) discuss reversibility in nonclinical toxicology studies. Goals of the nonclinical safety evaluation generally include a characterization of toxic effects with respect to target organs, dose dependence, relationship to exposure, and, when appropriate, potential reversibility. Recovery from pharmacological and toxicological effects with potential adverse clinical impact should be understood when they occur at clinically relevant exposures. The purpose of the non-dosing (recovery) period is to examine reversibility of compound-related effects, not to assess delayed toxicity.

Evaluation of the potential for reversibility of toxicity, defined as a return to the original or normal condition, should be provided when there is severe toxicity in a nonclinical study that would have potential adverse clinical impact. The evaluation can be based on a study of reversibility (e.g., recovery period from the toxicology study) or can be based on a scientific assessment. Thus, a subset of animals designated for recovery on a standard toxicology study is not always needed. The scientific assessment of reversibility would include the extent and severity of the pathologic lesion, the regenerative capacity of the affected organ system, and knowledge of other drugs that induce a similar toxicity. Toxicologic pathologists are best suited to make an interpretation as to reversibility based on scientific justification owing to their extensive knowledge in the pathogenesis of disease processes. Evidence of partial or incomplete reversibility, such as a decrease in the incidence or severity of the finding and scientific assessment that the recovery would eventually progress to full reversibility given sufficient time, are generally sufficient. A toxicology study that includes a terminal non-dosing recovery period could be warranted if the scientific assessment cannot predict whether the toxicity will be reversible or if there is a severe toxicity at clinically relevant exposures. Providing evidence of reversibility for species-specific target organs, such as the rodent Harderian gland, would not be needed, as the effect in rodents would not translate to the clinic since humans lack this rodent-specific organ.

2.6 COMPARING BIOPHARMACEUTICALS TO TRADITIONAL SMALL-MOLECULE DRUGS

It is useful to examine some key differences in the nonclinical safety assessment of biopharmaceuticals versus that of traditional small-molecule drugs (Table 2.3). Similar to small-molecule nonclinical safety studies, two species (rodent and non-rodent) are needed for the toxicology studies with a

TABLE 2.3

Generalized Comparisons of Small-Molecule Drugs and Large-Molecule Drugs

Attribute	Small Molecule	Large Molecule
Molecular weight	Less than 1 kDa	Greater than 30 kDa
Composition	High purity, homogeneous	Heterogeneous mixture
Dose selection	Achieve target organ toxicity	Optimal biologic dose (10-fold)
Safety animal model	Rodent, dog	Species specific, often NHP
Half-life	Short, usually <24 h	Long, weeks
Metabolism	Cytochrome P450	Proteolytic degradation
Nonclinical immunogenicity	Rare	Common
Route of administration	Oral usually	Parenteral (IV, SC)
Toxicities	Often off-target	Exaggerated pharmacology
Dosing interval	Usually daily	Weekly to monthly

biopharmaceutical, unless it is pharmacologically active in only one species. A pharmacologically relevant species is the one in which the target receptor or epitope (in the case of mAbs) is expressed and functionally active in the nonclinical test species. Considerations for species selection include activity/affinity of the test material, cross-reactivity of the test material with the target, and, most importantly, functional activity of the test material at the target. Human proteins may not be pharmacologically active in rodents, as the target may not be expressed, or there is so much difference in homology that the human protein does not recognize or cross-react with the rodent target. Comparison of the sequence homology among various species, as compared to the human, can help establish the relevance of nonclinical test animals. Toxicology studies in nonrelevant species may be misleading and are discouraged (ICH S6 1997).

Often a biopharmaceutical is pharmacologically active in only one species, which is especially common with mAbs; thus, the nonclinical program should be conducted in that single species. In the majority of nonclinical safety programs for biopharmaceuticals, the NHP is oftentimes the only relevant animal model (Bussiere 2008a). Alternate models such as the minipig are presently being investigated (Bode et al. 2010).

Biopharmaceuticals have to be administered by the parenteral route (IV, SC, IM) or by inhalation because of the large size and lability of the molecule, in contrast to small-molecule drugs that are designed for oral bioavailability after administration of a tablet or capsule. Since biopharmaceuticals are designed to act on highly specific targets and bind extracellularly, off-target activity and toxicity are considered to be uncommon (Haller et al. 2008). Thus, with biopharmaceuticals, adverse reactions are often a result of exaggerated pharmacology or nonspecific anti-drug antibody (ADA)-mediated responses. In contrast, small-molecule drugs may have direct intracellular effects and frequently exhibit off-target activities that are distinct from the desired target.

The PK terminal half-life ($t_{1/2}$) of small molecules is, in general, short lived (minutes to hours), while for large molecules, the $t_{1/2}$ is often hours for small peptides and up to multiple weeks for mAbs. Small molecules gain rapid entry through blood capillaries, distribute to many organs/tissues, and can be metabolized to active and non-active metabolites, primarily by the cytochrome P450 system of the liver. The distribution of mAbs is based on size and is limited to only the plasma and extracellular fluid compartments.

Large molecules are metabolized by the same catabolic pathways as endogenous proteins and are degraded to amino acid fragments excreted via the kidney (Mahmood and Green 2007). In general, the metabolic products of large molecules are not considered a safety risk. Drug–drug interactions, which can be significant for small molecules, are less of a concern for biopharmaceuticals and limited to interactions related to additive or synergistic pharmacological activity. Clinical drug–drug interaction studies are conducted with small-molecule drugs during development, but very few drug interaction studies have been performed with biopharmaceuticals since they are not metabolized by the cytochrome P450 system. It has been shown, however, that cytokine biopharmaceuticals such as interferons, given in combination with a small-molecule drug, can have an impact on transcription of the cytochrome P450 system that could then alter the PK and pharmacodynamics (PD) of the co-administered small-molecule drug (Mahmood and Green 2007). The PD effects of biopharmaceuticals typically do not correlate with PK parameters of concentration or time of maximal exposure (C_{max} or T_{max}), as PD tend to lag in clinical activity and have a prolonged duration of action (Haller et al. 2008). Area under the plasma concentration time curve is a better predictor of PD response. In contrast, small-molecule drugs usually manifest concentration-dependent therapeutic activity and toxicity-based events.

Immunogenicity is an inherent property of biopharmaceuticals that distinguishes these molecules from traditional small-molecule drugs and is often a confounding factor when testing a human protein in an animal model. ADAs that can neutralize the activity of the biopharmaceutical and reduce exposure as well as possibly elicit ADA-mediated toxicities in the animal model may develop. Immune responses against a biopharmaceutical, identified as an ADA response, often occur in the animal toxicology studies but occur only at a low incidence in the clinic (Chamberlain and Mire-Sluis 2003; Frost 2005; Kessler et al. 2006; Koren et al. 2002; Mire-Sluis et al. 2004; Niebecker and Kloft 2010; Schellekens 2002; Wierda et al. 2001). Most biopharmaceuticals are human proteins that are highly targeted to a human receptor or are antibodies specific for a human target protein. Thus, it is not unexpected that the administration of a biopharmaceutical to animals may result in the production of antibodies against the biopharmaceutical (Cavagnaro 2002; Dempster 1995; Working 1992). As a general rule, the greater the dissimilarity between the sequence of the human protein and the sequence of the animal protein, the more likely it is that the immune system of that animal will produce an antibody response to the biopharmaceutical (Bugelski and Treacy 2004; Wierda et al. 2001).

Antibody responses can affect the outcome of nonclinical toxicology studies by altering the PK, tissue distribution, or pharmacological activity of the biopharmaceutical, and may consequentially result in a misleading interpretation of the toxicology data (Koren et al. 2002; Serabian and Pilaro 1999; Terrell and Green 1994; Wierda et al. 2001; Working 1992). During nonclinical safety testing of a biopharmaceutical, it may be important to determine and measure the presence of ADAs and then determine any potential correlation with the pharmacology, PD, PK, or immune-mediated toxicity response (ICH S6 1997; Shankar et al. 2006).

Immunogenicity assessments are conducted to assist in the interpretation of the study results and design of subsequent studies. Such analyses in nonclinical animal studies, however, are not relevant in terms of predicting potential immunogenicity of human or humanized proteins in the clinic (ICH S6 [R1] 2011). Measurement of ADAs in nonclinical studies should be conducted when there is evidence of altered PD activity, there are unexpected changes in exposure in the absence of a PD marker, or there is evidence of immune-mediated toxicity (ICH S6 [R1] 2011). Since it is difficult to predict whether analysis of ADA samples will be needed prior to completion of the in-life phase of the study and evaluation of histopathology data, it is appropriate to obtain serum samples during the course of the study, which can then be analyzed, if necessary, to aid in interpretation of the study results. When ADAs are detected, their impact on the study results should be assessed, which could include a direct individual animal correlation with toxicokinetics (TK) and the histopathology data.

The various types of antibody responses that can develop in animal toxicology studies, which can potentially alter interpretation, include cross-linking antibodies that result in either accelerated clearance of the molecule or prolongation of exposure, cross-linking antibodies that neutralize the pharmacological activity of the biopharmaceutical, and cross-linking antibodies that neutralize the natural, endogenous counterpart protein (Dempster 1995; Koren et al. 2002; Wierda et al. 2001). Clearing and neutralizing antibodies are most likely to influence nonclinical safety studies. Clearing antibodies bind to the biopharmaceutical, resulting in increased plasma clearance of the drug (Gunn 1997; Wang et al. 2001). Increased plasma clearance ultimately results in a decrease in the distribution and exposure of the biopharmaceutical to the target organ of interest (Working

1992). Neutralizing antibodies can bind at or near the target-binding domain of the biopharmaceutical and interfere with its ability to bind to its target receptor, thus resulting in a partial or complete reduction in the intended pharmacological activity (Dempster 1995; Gunn 1997). When conducting nonclinical toxicology studies with biopharmaceuticals, the primary concern for the development of clearing or neutralizing antibodies in animals is the potential for lower exposure of the pharmacologically active drug, resulting in an underestimation of the potential for human toxicity (ICH S6 1997). Assessment of ADAs can help determine if a decrease in a PD response is due to the development of neutralizing antibodies or whether there is the development of tolerance to the effect. Altered PK could be due to redistribution of the biotherapeutic from the circulation to target organs or due to the presence of neutralizing/clearing antibodies. It is important to determine the impact of ADAs and how they may confound the interpretation of nonclinical toxicology studies.

Another issue with development of ADAs in nonclinical toxicology studies is the potential for the binding of antigens with antibodies to form systemic circulating immune complexes (CICs) that may deposit in certain organs. Usually, CICs are eliminated by the reticuloendothelial system without development of pathological changes. However, when antigen–antibody complexes induce an inflammatory reaction or deposit in tissues with subsequent inflammatory changes, toxicity can result (e.g., immune complex disease, vasculitis). Assessment of ADAs can help determine if the toxicity is a result of immunogenicity of the human protein in animals (which is not relevant to humans) or whether it is a true toxicity of the biotherapeutic.

Immunogenicity remains a challenge with biopharmaceuticals when conducting repeat-dose toxicity studies in animals, particularly in terms of maintaining exposure of pharmacologically active drug throughout the duration of the study. There are some approaches to manage and mitigate the development of clearing and neutralizing antibodies in toxicology studies. For example, increasing the dose levels administered in the toxicology study to saturate or "dose through" the ADA response may allow exposure of free (unbound) drug throughout the study. More frequent dosing (e.g., twice weekly rather than once weekly) is another approach to overwhelm the antibody response and maintain systemic drug exposure. Immunogenicity testing strategies should be adapted to the specific needs of each therapeutic development program, and data generated from such analyses should be integrated with available clinical and anatomic pathology, PK, and PD data to properly interpret nonclinical study results (Ponce et al. 2009).

Similar to a small-molecule drug safety program, the route of administration used in the toxicology studies should be similar to the intended clinical use, which, for biopharmaceuticals, is the parenteral route. The frequency of test article administration used in the toxicology studies should be as close as possible to that intended for clinical use. A more frequent dosing schedule might be scientifically appropriate in certain situations, such as to compensate for a biopharmaceutical having a shorter half-life in the animal model as compared to the human or when immunogenicity occurs with increased drug clearance.

A standard toxicology study design consists of three dose groups: low, intermediate, and high, in addition to a vehicle control group. As in designing a toxicology study with a small molecule, the high dose should produce clear evidence of toxicity and identification of target organs. The low dose should produce no toxicity, to allow for clear definition of a NOAEL, with an intermediate dose somewhere between the high and low dose. This paradigm, however, cannot be readily applied to biopharmaceuticals that typically result in only expected pharmacology with limited or no toxicity. In these cases, regulatory guidance suggests that dose selection be based upon the expected pharmacological and physiological effects of the product, availability of suitable test material, and the intended clinical use (ICH S6 1997; ICH S6 [R1] 2011).

Since the pharmacological action of biopharmaceuticals often occurs at very low doses, a NOEL may not be established in repeat-dose toxicology studies. Evaluating the biopharmaceutical at doses lower than the clinical range to achieve a NOEL would not add value to the nonclinical safety program. Therefore, the goal of the nonclinical safety study is typically to identify a NOAEL rather than a NOEL. PK–PD modeling, the application of nonclinical PK data, and its integration with the pharmacologic response can assist in selecting the high dose (Tibbetts et al. 2010). Regulatory guidance states that the high dose should provide the maximum intended pharmacological effect in the nonclinical animal model, or the dose that provides an approximately 10-fold exposure multiple over the targeted maximum exposure to be achieved in the clinic. The higher of these two doses should be selected for the nonclinical toxicology study (ICH S6 [R1] 2011). It can be difficult for the pathologist to determine which histopathological changes in a toxicology study are due to exaggerated pharmacological activity and when these findings become adverse toxicological effects.

Many biopharmaceuticals are highly specific for a human target. Therefore, oftentimes the only relevant nonclinical animal model is the NHP, such as the cynomolgus macaque monkey (Chapman et al. 2007, 2009). It is not unusual for the entire nonclinical safety program to be conducted in a single species such as the cynomolgus monkey. When the biopharmaceutical is so human species specific that it will only cross-react with the chimpanzee, alternative approaches are utilized since the use of the chimpanzee as an animal model is not favored because of ethical reasons (Bettauer 2011; IOM 2011). Alternative approaches include safety testing of a surrogate molecule. Surrogate molecules (or homologous proteins) are proteins that recognize the target in an animal model that is analogous to the human target recognized by the clinical product. The use of a surrogate molecule allows for hazard detection related to the pharmacologic activity of the biopharmaceutical but does not allow for safety testing of the clinical candidate itself or quantitative risk assessment. Another approach to consider for the nonclinical safety program is to use transgenic or KO mice that either overexpress or have a deletion of the targeted protein (Bussiere et al. 2009).

Tissue cross-reactivity (TCR) studies are conducted to support FIH trials and are recommended for antibody and antibody-like molecules that contain a complementarity-determining region. TCR studies involve immunohistochemical staining using the labeled test article (Leach et al. 2010) on a panel of human tissues. The purpose of the TCR is to identify potential sites of tissue binding but tissue binding does not necessarily indicate biological activity *in vivo*. There is variable correlation with TCR tissue binding results and toxicity or efficacy, and the results usually do not affect the nonclinical safety plan strategy (Bussiere et al. 2011). Any TCR findings of concern should be further evaluated and interpreted in the context of the entire pharmacology and safety assessment data package. The overall design, implementation, and interpretation of TCR studies should follow a case-by-case approach (Leach et al. 2010).

2.7 IMMUNOTOXICOLOGY

Immunotoxicity testing guidelines exist (ICH S8 2004) for small molecules where the toxicity is often unexpected or off-target and rodent species are typically used. A tiered approach is utilized for small molecules in that additional immunotoxicity testing is based on results of the standard toxicology studies. Indicators of possible immunotoxicity from a general toxicology study include hematological changes such as decreased neutrophil or lymphocyte counts; changes in weight or histopathology of immune organs such as the thymus, spleen, or lymph node; or evidence of increased infection (Haley et al. 2005). If the weight of evidence in general toxicity testing suggests an impact on the immune system, additional testing could be conducted such as the T-dependent antibody response (TDAR) or immunophenotyping of leukocyte populations. Despite the lack of a specific guidance on immunotoxicity evaluation for biopharmaceuticals, similar approaches can be taken as for small molecules (Brennan et al. 2004). As the immune system is often the intended target of therapy for biopharmaceuticals, the immunomodulation observed may represent exaggerated pharmacology. It is important to distinguish between immunopharmacology, where the immune system is the target of the therapeutic effect, and immunotoxicity, where nontarget immune effects may be observed (e.g., immunosuppression), and to distinguish both of these from immunogenicity, which represents an immune response to the drug (Bussiere and Mounho 2008).

A commonly used *in vivo* assay to assess immune competence is the TDAR. The ability to mount an antigen-specific antibody response requires a fully functioning immune system (e.g., T cells,

B cells, antigen-presenting cells, cytokine production). For the TDAR methodology, the animal model is immunized with keyhole limpet hemocyanin or tetanus toxoid, and circulating antigen-specific antibody levels are subsequently measured by an enzyme-linked immunosorbent assay (ELISA) or by other methods (Bussiere 2008b). Although immunomodulation via the TDAR can be assessed in the NHP, the circulating antigen-specific antibody assays are not as well characterized as those for the rodent. Moreover, there is wide interanimal variability in the TDAR response in the NHP. Additional TDAR historical control data are needed in the NHP (Lebrec et al. 2011).

A major hurdle for the development and early clinical investigation of many of the immuno-modulatory mAbs is the inherent risk for adverse immune-mediated drug reactions in humans, such as infusion reactions, cytokine storm, immunosuppression, or autoimmunity. A thorough understanding of the immunopharmacology of the mAb in the animal model and human is required to anticipate the clinical risk of adverse immunotoxicological events and to select a safe starting dose for FIH clinical studies. One approach in selecting a safe starting dose with immunomodulatory mAbs is based on the minimum anticipated biological effect level (MABEL) and its consideration in the selection of a safe maximum recommended starting dose (MRSD). The MABEL represents the lowest animal dose or concentration required to produce pharmacological activity in an *in vivo* or *in vitro* cell system (Muller and Brennan 2009). The MRSD should be selected based on demonstration of an adequate safety margin, compared with a dose that produces toxicity, or the NOAEL, as well as consideration of the MABEL. A tiered approach is recommended to assess effects on immune status, immune function, and risk of infection and cancer, governed by the mechanism of action and structural features of the mAb (Brennan et al. 2010). In general, toxicities arising from the use of pharmacologic immunostimulation can be mechanistically interpreted as imbalances in cytokine signaling due to supraphysiologic cytokine concentrations or to secondary events resulting in exaggerated production of endogenous cytokines. Cytokines function in both a cascade and network fashion, and their dysregulation can lead to a number of clinically significant syndromes (Gribble et al. 2007). Methods to evaluate nonclinical cytokine release include *in vitro* human or NHP blood cell cytokine release assays and *in vivo* assessments (ELISA multiplex).

2.8 SAFETY PHARMACOLOGY

The ICH S7A (2000) and ICH S7B (2005) guidance documents provide the general principles and recommendations for safety pharmacology studies. Safety pharmacology studies are defined as those studies that investigate the potential undesirable effects on physiological functions in relation to the exposure in the clinical therapeutic range and above. The core battery of safety pharmacology studies consists of the assessment of effects on the cardiovascular system, the CNS, and the respiratory system. In accordance with ICH S7A and S7B, the core battery of studies should be completed prior to FIH clinical trials.

During lead optimization for small molecules, screening studies are conducted to identify potential liabilities on direct hERG channel block and QT interval prolongation. During stages of development, additional *in vitro* studies may be conducted to assess the effect of the test article on action potential and cardiac ion channels; these studies are usually conducted in accordance with GLP standards according to ICH S7B. Because of the very large size of a biopharmaceutical molecule, the risk for QT-mediated proarrhythmia resulting from direct hERG channel blockade is generally not a concern and specific hERG channel assays are not typically conducted (Vargas et al. 2008).

In vivo electrophysiologic studies are conducted for both small and large molecules in support of FIH studies. ECGs, which provide information on electrophysiological function and rhythm of the heart, are also performed as part of a general toxicology study in the non-rodent and can also be obtained from stand-alone specialized safety pharmacology telemetry ECG studies. Additional endpoints in the telemetry study may include blood pressure, heart rate, respiratory rate, and body temperature. Recently, it has been demonstrated that body core temperature can influence QT intervals and that corrections for body temperature may be needed (Van der Linde et al. 2008). Study designs that utilize implanted telemetry to assess QT prolongation risk for small molecules are typically single dose and are conducted in animals housed in stock colony facilities. After an adequate "washout" period in which systemic exposure of the test article is no longer detected, the telemetry stock colony can be used again to assess a different small molecule. The protracted washout period due to the extended half-life of a mAb, in addition to the potential to induce ADAs, makes the stock colony telemetry approach with large molecules not practical. External jacketed, noninvasive telemetry methodologies to obtain ECG parameters may be more appropriate for biopharmaceutical assessment and can be performed as part of a general toxicology study (McMahon et al. 2010). In contrast to small molecules, the overall risk of QT prolongation is low for biopharmaceuticals (Mascelli et al. 2007; Piccini et al. 2009).

A functional observational battery or modified Irwin test may be used to evaluate the effects of a small molecule on the CNS, which would include parameters of motor activity, behavioral changes, coordination, sensory and motor reflex, and body temperature. Respiratory function endpoints should include quantitative measurement of respiratory rate and tidal volume. The ICH S7A guidance is applicable to small molecules and to biopharmaceuticals but states that in the case of a highly targeted biopharmaceutical, safety pharmacology parameters can be included as endpoints in general toxicology studies, which reduces or eliminates the need for stand-alone safety pharmacology studies. Often, the only relevant animal model for safety evaluation of a biopharmaceutical is the NHP in which cardiovascular and respiratory endpoints would then be assessed during the general toxicology study (McMahon et al. 2010). CNS evaluation in the NHP is conducted primarily by cage-side observation and veterinary physical examination since more formal CNS evaluation, such as the modified Irwin evaluation in the rodent, is not routinely available.

2.9   DEVELOPMENT AND REPRODUCTIVE TOXICOLOGY

It is desirable to use the same rodent strain for the DART studies as was utilized in general toxicology studies for a small-molecule safety assessment program. Reasons to use the rat are ease of use and the large amount of reproductive background knowledge accumulated in this animal model. The purpose of DART studies is to determine if the test article or metabolite has any deleterious effect on specific stages of mammalian reproduction. Data obtained from these studies are considered in addition to results from repeat-dose general toxicology studies that provide histopathological data for both male and female reproductive organs. The specific stages of embryo–fetal development covered by the DART studies are presented in Figure 2.2.

A study of fertility and early embryonic development (Figure 2.3) evaluates test article–related changes starting before mating of males and females through the mating process and implantation. This approach detects effects on the estrus cycle, tubal transport, implantation, and development of preimplantation stages of the embryo (ICH S5 [R2] 2005). In males, endpoints like libido and sperm maturation that cannot be detected from routine histopathology of the male sex organs from repeat-dose toxicology studies are evaluated.

Studies for effects on embryo–fetal development (Figure 2.4) address possible adverse effects on the pregnant female and effects on embryo to fetal development (up to closure of the hard palate). Specific to embryo–fetal toxicity studies, a second mammalian species is required, with the rabbit being the preferred choice owing to a large and extensive background knowledge base (ICH S5 [R2] 2005). Usually, preliminary studies are first conducted in the rabbit to obtain data on dose and early teratogenic potential of the test article, prior to the conduct of the definitive embryo–fetal rabbit study. A preliminary study in the rat may not be necessary since data from the rat general toxicology study can oftentimes be used to help select the doses.

Finally, studies to evaluate the effect of the test article on prenatal and postnatal development (Figure 2.5), including maternal function, are needed. A goal of this study is to determine adverse effects on the pregnant/lactating female. In addition, data from these studies help determine potential

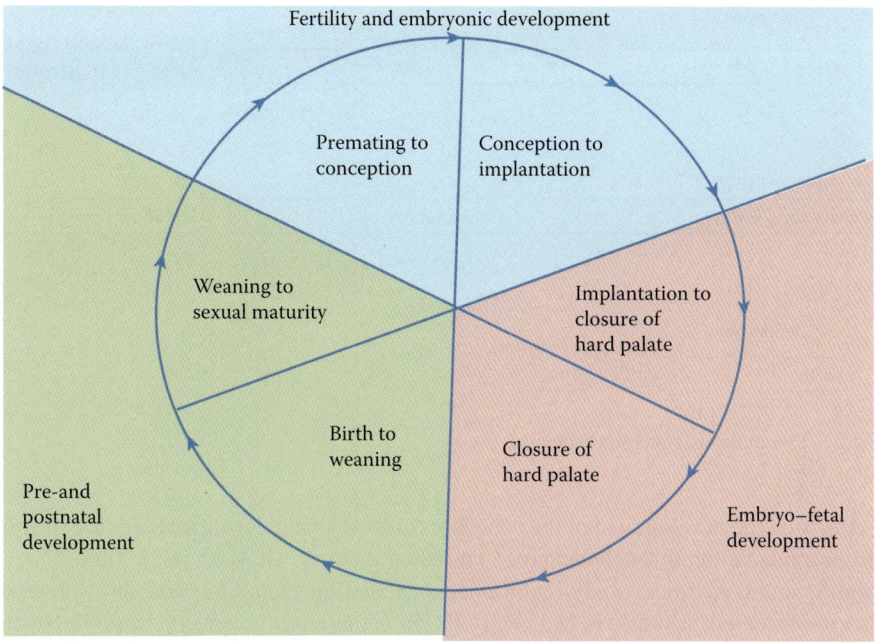

FIGURE 2.2 Stages of reproductive development and DART studies supporting nonclinical safety of pharmaceuticals.

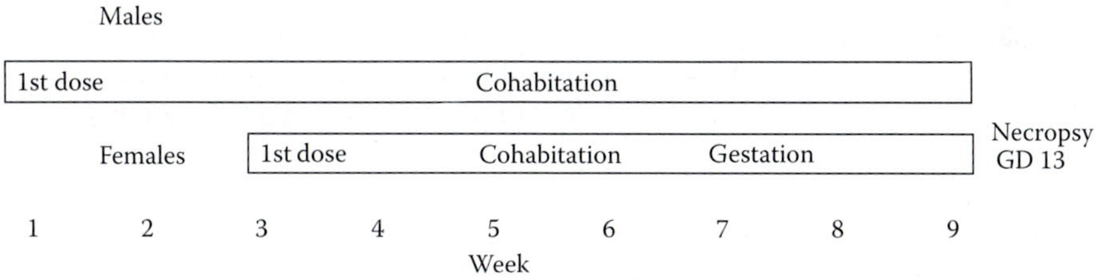

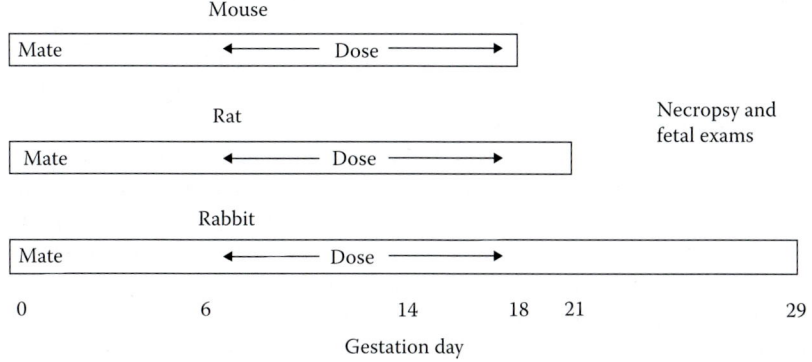

FIGURE 2.3 Generalized fertility and early embryonic development study design.

FIGURE 2.4 Generalized embryo–fetal toxicity/teratogenicity study design.

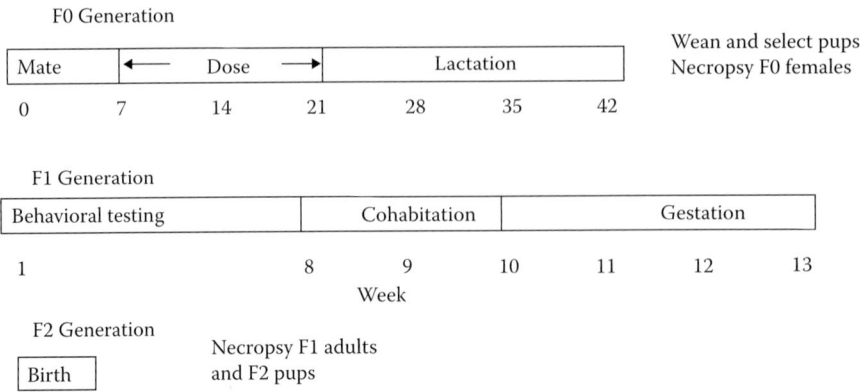

FIGURE 2.5   Prenatal/postnatal study design.

adverse effects on the development of the conceptus and offspring during test article exposure of the female from implantation through weaning and sexual maturity (ICH S5 [R2] 2005).

The timing and nonclinical study requirements needed for including men and women on clinical trials are presented in the ICH M3 (R2) (2009). Generally, the specific reproductive toxicology study needed is determined by the population to be exposed in the clinical trial. Men can be included in Phase I and II trials before a male fertility study is completed because histopathological data from male reproductive organs are obtained from the general repeat-dose toxicology studies. Women that are not of childbearing potential (e.g., sterilized or postmenopausal) can be included in clinical trials since histopathological data from female reproductive organs are also obtained from the repeat-dose toxicology studies. When the appropriate preliminary embryo–fetal toxicology studies have been completed in two species, and where precautions to prevent pregnancy in the clinical trial are employed, inclusion of a limited number (e.g., 150) of women of childbearing potential may be appropriate in a clinical trial of short duration (e.g., up to 3 months) as per regulatory guidance (ICH M3 [R2] 2009).

ICH S6 (R1) (2010) provides some regulatory guidance for reproductive testing of biopharmaceuticals. Because of the unique properties of biopharmaceuticals, a case-by-case approach is needed for reproductive toxicology evaluation, which requires consideration of specific product attributes (including biochemical and biophysical characteristics that can affect placental transfer), pharmacological activity, and intended clinical indication (Martin et al. 2009). The range of studies defined in ICH S5 is most applicable to products that are being tested in rats and rabbits, the primary species used for DART testing. If a biopharmaceutical is pharmacologically active in rats and rabbits, then ICH S5-recommended studies can be conducted unless immunogenicity, with reduction in systemic exposure, limits the duration of testing. In many cases, however, biopharmaceuticals are cross-reactive only in the NHP, which presents a number of challenges in the conduct of reproductive toxicology studies. The cynomolgus monkey is preferred over the rhesus monkey for reproductive toxicology studies since the rhesus monkey is a seasonal breeder, which would complicate the study design.

Surrogate molecules that cross-react with the more traditional rodent species may need to be developed and used for reproductive testing for those biopharmaceuticals that are uniquely specific and only active on the intended human target. Alternatively, genetically modified transgenic animals may also need to be considered. To reduce the use of NHPs, a surrogate molecule or a transgenic animal model could be considered for reproductive toxicology testing when the biopharmaceutical is active only in the NHP (Bussiere et al. 2009).

Study designs that use the monkey are available for developmental and reproductive toxicology endpoints, such as fertility, embryo–fetal development, prenatal/postnatal development, and enhanced prenatal/postnatal development (Chellman et al. 2009). Variations on these study designs

TABLE 2.4
Species Comparison of Embryonic and Fetal Development Gestation Time (Days)

Species	Preimplantation	Organogenesis	Fetal Maturation
Mouse	0–6	6–15	~19
Rat	0–9	9–17	~21
Rabbit	0–6	6–18	~29
Cynomolgus monkey	0–15	15–50	~155
Human	0–18	18–57	~270

to address reproductive toxicity concerns have been used in the development of biopharmaceuticals (Martin et al. 2007, 2010). New study designs that consolidate multiple aspects of the reproductive assessment, and thereby conserve animal use, are continually being evaluated.

Conducting reproductive toxicology studies in the NHP when scientifically necessary for the biopharmaceutical does offer some advantages. There are good similarities between humans and the cynomolgus monkey (Table 2.4) with respect to the endocrine system and duration of the menstrual cycle and early pregnancy (Weinbauer et al. 2008). Other similarities include placental morphology and physiology, timing of implantation and subsequent rates of embryonic development, spermatogenesis, placental transfer of IgG, and response to known teratogens (Elger 2000; Weinbauer 2002).

Utilizing the cynomolgus monkey for reproductive toxicity testing also has several disadvantages as compared to the use of the rat and rabbit. Because of animal welfare and support of the 3Rs, only a small number of monkeys are used in such studies. The cynomolgus monkey has a smaller number of offspring (generally 1 fetus per dam), which limits the number of fetuses to evaluate in the study. Other disadvantages include a much longer duration of study (e.g., 150-day gestation period), low conception rate coupled with a high abortion rate, a limited historical database, and a paucity of contract research organizations that are able to conduct such specialized studies.

When the NHP is the only scientifically relevant species, the potential for test article effects on male and female fertility may be assessed by evaluation of the reproductive tract (organ weight and histopathological evaluation) from a repeat-dose toxicity study of 3 months or greater in duration, using sexually mature males and females. If there is a specific cause for concern on the basis of pharmacological activity or previous toxicological observations, specialized assessments can be evaluated in the context of the repeat-dose toxicology study, or as a stand-alone fertility study. A stand-alone male fertility study can be conducted to evaluate testicular volume and weight, sperm parameters (e.g., sperm count, morphology, motility), hormone analysis, or histopathological evaluation of testicular biopsies to evaluate spermatogenesis (Vogel 2000; Weinbauer and Cooper 2000). A stand-alone female fertility study generally consists of three pretreatment observation cycles, three treatment cycles, and one or more recovery cycles. Changes in menstrual cycling are measured as well as cycle-related hormone analysis. Mating is not evaluated in fertility studies in the NHP owing to the low conception rate.

2.10   GENETIC TOXICOLOGY

Genetic toxicity screens for mutagenicity and clastogenicity may be conducted during lead optimization for small-molecule candidates. For clinical trials, a tiered approach for a standard genotoxicity test battery needs to be completed following GLP guidelines (ICH S2A 1995; ICH S2B 1997; ICH M3 [R2] 2009). In general, an *in vitro* test for mutations and chromosomal damage is required prior to first human exposure. An *in vivo* test for chromosomal damage using rodent hematopoietic cells completes the standard genotoxicity package, which is needed prior to start of Phase II clinical trials. The range and type of genotoxicity studies routinely conducted for small-molecule drugs are not applicable to biopharmaceuticals (ICH S6 1997). Biopharmaceuticals are not expected to interact directly with DNA or other chromosomal material and are degraded by proteolysis to amino acids or peptides, which are also believed not to have any genotoxic potential. With the exception of some anticancer small molecules with a cytotoxic mechanism of action, small-molecule candidates are usually terminated from development if they are positive genotoxicants. A genotoxic molecule would not be a good candidate to move forward into drug development owing to the increased risk of the molecule being carcinogenic in humans.

2.11 CARCINOGENICITY TESTING

An important aspect of the nonclinical safety package for an NCE is assessing if the test article has the potential to increase the risk of cancer in the intended patient population. Carcinogenicity testing guidelines are covered by a wide range of ICH documents (ICH M3 [R2] 2009; ICH S1A 1995; ICH S1B 1997; ICH S1C 1994; ICH S2A 1995; ICH S2B 1997; ICH S6 [R1] 2011). A 2-year carcinogenicity study in both the rat and mouse is required for marketing approval of a small-molecule drug that would be prescribed as a long-term treatment (6-month duration or longer, or in a frequent but intermittent basis with cumulative lifetime exposure over 6 months). Since small-molecule drug candidates would not be genotoxic (positive genotoxicants would be removed from development), any tumor response observed in the rodent carcinogenicity study attributed to the test article would have to occur through nongenotoxic mechanisms, such as tumor promotion or immunosuppression (Hernandez et al. 2009).

A traditional 2-year rodent carcinogenicity study involves hundreds of animals; takes up to 3 years to plan, execute, and report; and is costly. The scientific limitations of the rodent bioassay for determining cancer risk assessment in humans have been widely debated (Alden et al. 1996; Boobis et al. 2009; Cohen 2004b; Monro and MacDonald 1998; Ward 2007). Rodent carcinogenicity study designs usually consist of a control group and three dose groups (low, intermediate, and high) composed of 50–60 rodents per gender per group. In designing the rodent carcinogenicity experiment, it is important that a biostatistician be consulted prior to the start of the study to avoid misuse of statistics both in the design and in the interpretation of the results (Gad and Rousseaux 2002). Comparison of the histopathological observations between groups, with an emphasis on proliferative changes and tumor characterization and incidence, provides the basis for assessing the carcinogenic potential of the test article. As histopathologic diagnoses form the foundation of the rodent carcinogenesis assay, toxicologic pathologists are intimately involved in data generation and interpretation.

The Society of Toxicologic Pathology (STP) has provided position papers that can help guide the pathologist in the study design and interpretation of histopathology data from rodent carcinogenicity studies. These guidance papers include the recommended tissue list for light microscopic evaluation (Bregman et al. 2003), assessment of hyperplastic lesions (Boorman et al. 2003), and recommendations on statistical analysis (Morton et al. 2002a). For the practicing toxicologic pathologist involved in the interpretation of rodent carcinogenicity studies, applying globally harmonized nomenclature and diagnostic criteria is vital, as data from these studies are reviewed by regulatory agencies around the world in support of global marketing authorization. The International Harmonization of Nomenclature and Diagnostic Criteria for Lesions in Rats and Mice (INHAND) was created as a framework to standardize terminology globally. INHAND is a joint initiative between the Societies of Toxicologic Pathology from the United States (STP), Great Britain (BSTP), Japan (JSTP), and European countries (ESTP) (Mann et al. 2012). The goal of INHAND is to harmonize nomenclature and diagnostic criteria for proliferative lesions of the various organ systems of the rodent. INHAND serves as a valuable resource for pathologists involved in rodent carcinogenicity studies (Renne et al. 2009; Thoolen et al. 2010).

Over a decade ago, ICH guidelines allowed for an alternative approach to the traditional 2-year mouse carcinogenicity assay, that is, the conduct of a 6-month carcinogenicity assay in genetically engineered mice (ICH S1B 1997). On the basis of scientific rationale, the 2-year mouse study can be substituted with a 6-month transgenic mouse carcinogenicity study. The rasH2 and p53 trans-genic mouse models are the most widely used alternative models in the pharmaceutical industry. Transgenic rasH2 mice are hemizygous, carrying three copies of the prototype human c-Ha-ras oncogene with its own promoter (Tamaoki 2001). The ras protein has the potential to act as a potent carcinogen when expressed by the ras gene that has undergone mutations in certain critical domains. Overexpression of the normal ras gene also induces cell transformation. The rasH2 trans-genic mouse model is responsive to both genotoxic and nongenotoxic chemicals. The general study design of the rasH2 carcinogenicity assay includes treatment groups of mice (e.g., 25/sex/group) with several different doses of the test agent and a negative vehicle control group. A positive control group may also be added, if scientifically necessary, to demonstrate the responsiveness of the rasH2 model to a known positive reference carcinogen (Long et al. 2010). In the validation process for this model, results of 6-month carcinogenicity studies demonstrated the rasH2 model to be equivalent or superior to the conventional 2-year mouse bioassay (Morton et al. 2002b; Storer et al. 2011).

The p53[def] transgenic mouse model has one functional wild-type p53 allele and one inactivated allele. The p53 gene is critical to cell cycle control and DNA repair and is often found to be mutated or lost in human and rodent tumors. Transgenic p53 mice with a single copy of the wild-type allele (p53[+/−] heterozygote) would increase the probability for either loss of the p53 tumor suppressor function or gain of transforming activity, by requiring only a single mutation. The utility of the p53 model is primarily in identifying mutagenic carcinogens and may be the preferred transgenic model for those pharmaceutical agents that are equivocal or positive for *in vitro* genotoxic activity (Jacobson-Kram et al. 2004).

Biopharmaceuticals do not produce direct genotoxicity and would not be expected to form active or genotoxic metabolites. Because of a lack of direct genotoxic effects and because of the specific and selective effect on the target of interest, the potential cancer concern for biopharmaceuticals is not that the agent is a direct-acting carcinogen. Rather, the concern is that the biopharmaceutical agent could affect epigenetic mechanisms, such as enhancement of cell proliferation, mechanism-based influence on a specific tumor type, or altered immune function (Vahle et al. 2010). For most biotechnology-derived biopharmaceuticals (e.g., mAbs or fusion proteins), the 2-year rodent car-cinogenicity bioassay is not feasible owing to a lack of appropriate rodent pharmacology, that is, lack of cross-reactivity in the rodent. In addition, even if there is cross-reactivity in the rodent, a feasibility concern exists from immunogenicity resulting in neutralizing antibodies and accelerated clearance of the test article. When the biopharmaceutical only cross-reacts in the NHP, a lifetime or carcinogenicity study in the NHP is neither feasible nor practical, and inconsistent with the 3Rs.

In those cases where the biopharmaceutical product is biologically active and nonimmunogenic in the rodent model, and where other ancillary studies have not provided sufficient information to allow an assessment of carcinogenic potential, additional experimentation is warranted, which should be hypothesis driven and could include a variety of experimental approaches. Alternatives to evaluation of carcinogenicity are continually being explored. Ultimately, it is important that the nonclinical car-cinogenic data obtained provide useful guidance in product labeling (Vahle et al. 2010).

Because of these limitations, the guidelines propose alternate approaches to assessing the car-cinogenic potential of a biopharmaceutical (ICH S6 [R1] 2011). For example, a biopharmaceutical that might have the potential to support or induce proliferation of transformed cells and clonal expansion, potentially leading to neoplasia, could be evaluated for cell proliferation endpoints in an appropriate *in vitro* system. Appropriately designed *in vivo* studies might be needed if *in vitro* studies identify cause for concern. To date, putative carcinogenicity that might be associated with immunosuppressive products has not been routinely addressed by conducting a rodent bioassay, primarily due to a lack of pharmacological activity of the biopharmaceutical in rodents. Overall, determining appropriate methods to assess the clinical relevance of theoretical risks for biopharma-ceuticals is challenging.

In a retrospective review of 80 marketed biopharmaceuticals (on the basis of publicly available data), no assessments related to investigating carcinogenic potential or tumor growth promotion were conducted for 51 of the test articles, while in the other 29, various experimental approaches were employed to assess potential carcinogenic concerns (Vahle et al. 2010). Alternative approaches scientifically directed to the specific type of biopharmaceutical (e.g., insulin analog, mAb, growth factors, peptide hormones, interferons) included the following: *in vitro* assays for mitogenesis, growth stimulation or cell proliferation assays, rodent toxicology studies of 1–2 years in duration, and the use of rodent-specific homologue protein studies in the mouse (Vahle et al. 2010). Therefore, for carcinogenicity risk assessment for biopharmaceuticals, the most appropriate approach is one in which the biology of the proposed therapy is carefully considered, and a weight of evidence approach is used to characterize carcinogenic or tumor growth potential. This weight of evidence approach can include review of published data (e.g., transgenic mice, animal disease models, human genetic diseases), information on class effects and target biology, data from chronic toxicology studies, and clinical data. As the discovery and development process continues, additional nonclinical pharmacology and toxicology data could also be generated to aid in characterizing carcinogenic risk.

Key principles to aid in the assessment of carcinogenic potential include consideration of the mechanism of action to identify theoretical risks, detailed review of existing data for indications of proliferative or immunosuppressive potential, and characterization of any proliferative or immunosuppressive signals detected in the nonclinical safety studies. The interest in evaluating immunosuppressive activity is related to the putative protective role of the immune system in the development of cancer. The relationship between immunosuppression and cancer is not completely understood, however, and currently, the association with neoplasia is mostly related to specific infectious agents, for example, the Epstein–Barr virus.

2.12   SAFETY ASSESSMENT OF ONCOLOGY PRODUCTS

Results from nonclinical toxicology studies help establish a safe starting dose for FIH studies and define potential toxicities. Both the US FDA and the EMA recommend that anticancer agents be evaluated in both the rodent and non-rodent animal models to support dose selection for Phase I cancer clinical trials. Because of the unique considerations for the safety assessment of oncology products, a separate ICH guideline covering both small and large molecules has been issued (ICH S9 2009). The scope of this guidance is to assist in the design of an appropriate program of nonclinical studies for the development of anticancer drug candidates for the treatment of patients with advanced cancer or who have limited therapeutic options. These patients are defined as those who have failed standard care or have progressive disease and limited life expectancy. The intent of ICH S9 is to provide an outlined approach of the minimal nonclinical safety package required to start a Phase I clinical trial in the appropriate cancer population. ICH S9 also presents the additional nonclinical safety studies needed for later stage development and marketing authorization. Vaccines, gene therapy, treatment of symptoms, or side effects of chemotherapeutics and candidates for cancer prevention are not covered under the ICH S9 guideline. As in other therapeutic areas for biopharmaceuticals, if there is only one pharmacologically relevant species, then the nonclinical safety program is directed toward evaluating only in that relevant species. The duration of the nonclinical animal toxicology studies should support the FIH trial.

An objective of the Phase I clinical trial for traditional cytotoxic small-molecule therapies is to define the MTD. The MTD is often utilized for Phase II efficacy trials under the assumption that the higher the dose, the greater the antitumor activity. A clinical MTD for oncology is defined as the dose that causes a specific clinical toxicity such as bone marrow suppression (Kummar et al. 2006). More recently introduced targeted therapies (e.g., selective estrogen receptor modulator, antibody drug conjugates, and growth factor receptors) are being evaluated with the expectation of achieving optimal clinical efficacy at doses much below the MTD. Clinical trials in the advanced cancer population are to provide patients with novel and potentially beneficial therapy, and as such, clinical oncologists attempt to start with a dose that can achieve the highest possible exposure without compromising patient safety. It is also a goal to specify a starting dose that is high enough to reduce the number of dose escalation steps needed to reach the clinical MTD.

Results from general toxicology studies identifying more standard endpoints such as the NOEL and NOAEL are usually not applicable with cytotoxic oncology agents, and these endpoints are not considered essential to determine a starting dose in the clinic. Oncologists rarely use anticancer agents at or below the NOAEL. The more common approach in determining the starting dose in the clinic for anticancer agents is to conduct the nonclinical FIH–enabling package and identify the dose that causes severe toxicity in 10% of the rodents (STD10) in a repeat-dose toxicology study, and then also determine if that dose is tolerated in the non-rodent species, as scaled by body surface area (ICH S9 2009). If the rodent STD10 is not tolerated in the non-rodent species, or if the toxicology studies in the dog or monkey demonstrate significant toxicity, then the starting dose in the clinic can be calculated by using the highest non-severely toxic dose (HNSTD) in the non-rodent. By definition, the HNSTD is the dose above which lethality, life-threatening toxicities, or irreversible toxicities occur in the non-rodent toxicology study. A retrospective analysis of the STD10 and HNSTD approach for anticancer agents generated from the toxicology studies indicates that the resulting FIH starting dose selection is generally considered safe (Le Tourneau et al. 2010; Tomaszewski 2004).

Another ICH S9 principle is that the dosing regimen for the toxicology studies should reflect the intended clinical dosing schedule. The inclusion of a recovery group (non-dosing period) at the end of the in-life portion of a toxicology study is currently a common practice. It is important to assess the potential for recovery when the toxicity is serious and observed at the approximate (equivalent) intended targeted clinical exposure. The design of nonclinical studies should be appropriately chosen to accommodate different dosing schedules that might be utilized in initial clinical trials (Table 2.5). It is not expected that the exact clinical schedule always will be followed in the toxicology study, but the information provided from these studies should be sufficient to support the clinical dose and schedule and to identify potential toxicity. In support of continued development of an anticancer agent for patients with advanced cancer, results from a 3-month repeat-dose toxicology study, following the intended clinical schedule, should be completed prior to initiating Phase III studies. Nonclinical toxicology studies of 3 months' duration are also considered sufficient to support market authorization.

Safety pharmacology studies to assess vital organ functions (including the cardiovascular system, respiratory system, and CNS) for anticancer agents should be completed in the FIH nonclinical safety package. Specific safety pharmacology endpoints can be included in the general toxicology studies. Detailed clinical observations following dosing and appropriate ECG measurements in the

---

TABLE 2.5

Examples of Treatment Schedules for Anticancer Drugs to Support the First-in-Human Clinical Trials

Clinical Schedule	Nonclinical Schedule
Once every 3–4 weeks	Single-dose study
Daily for 5 days every 3 weeks	Daily for 5 days
Daily for 5–7 days on alternating weeks	Daily for 5–7 days on alternating weeks for 2 dose cycles
Once weekly for 3 weeks with 1 week off	Once weekly for 3 weeks
Two or three times per week	Two or three times per week for 4 weeks
Daily	Daily for 4 weeks
Weekly	Once weekly for 4–5 doses

Source: ICH S9, Nonclinical Evaluation for Anticancer Biopharmaceuticals. October 2009. Retrieved June 2011 from http://www.ich.org. With permission.

non-rodent study are generally considered sufficient. In cases where specific safety pharmacology concerns that could be a potential risk to patients have been identified, appropriate follow-up safety pharmacology studies should be considered (ICH S7A 2000; ICH S7B 2005).

The nonclinical DART package for anticancer agents is abbreviated. Embryo–fetal toxicology studies are needed for marketing application but are not considered essential to support clinical trials intended for the treatment of patients with advanced cancer. Embryo–fetal toxicology studies are typically conducted in two species as described by ICH S5 (R2) (2005) except where an embryo–fetal developmental toxicity study in one species/the first species tested is positive for lethality or teratogenicity; in this case, a confirmatory study in a second species is usually not warranted. A reproductive toxicity assessment in one pharmacologically relevant species is sufficient for oncology biopharmaceuticals. Embryo–fetal toxicology studies are not needed for a cytotoxic drug candidate that is genotoxic and targets rapidly dividing cells (e.g., intestinal crypt cells, bone marrow) or one that belongs to a class of drugs that has been well characterized as causing developmental toxicity. Toxicologic injury to male and female reproductive organs is assessed during the general toxicology studies; thus, a separate fertility study is not needed. Moreover, peri- and postnatal toxicology studies are usually not needed to support clinical trials or market authorization, since the therapeutic is intended for the treatment of patients with advanced cancer.

Genotoxicity studies are not considered essential to support clinical trials for therapeutics intended to treat patients with advanced cancer. In general, these studies need to be completed to support marketing approval (ICH S2A 1995; ICH S2B 1997). The principles outlined in ICH S6 (1997) should be followed for biopharmaceuticals.

2.13 CHALLENGES WITH NONCLINICAL SAFETY ASSESSMENT IN THE NHP

The NHP is an important animal model utilized in the safety assessment of therapeutics. The use of this animal model has increased in recent years because of the increase in the development of biopharmaceuticals and the evaluation of these products in specific disease states. For example, NHPs are used to study geriatric diseases and osteoporosis (Jerome 2002) and for the study of many ocular indications including macular degeneration and retinopathy (Dayhaw-Barker 2000; Goralczyk 2000). NHP models are also being developed to evaluate the effects of biopharmaceuticals on the reproductive and the immune systems in order to better understand potential translational effects that could be observed in humans.

The cynomolgus monkey (*Macaca fascicularis*) is the most commonly used NHP species for nonclinical safety assessment programs to determine potential toxicities of biopharmaceuticals, although rhesus monkeys (*Macaca mulatta*) are also used. A historical database exists for cynomolgus monkeys for clinical and anatomic pathology, in addition to specialized endpoints (i.e., flow cytometric analysis of lymphocyte subtypes) that may be measured in repeat-dose toxicology studies.

The cynomolgus monkey can harbor a variety of pathogenic and potentially opportunistic organisms that may result in overt infectious disease during the conduct of a toxicology study (Olivier et al. 2010). Several viral, bacterial, and parasitic pathogens are endemic in certain cynomolgus colonies, which can remain subclinical or result in a mild and self-limiting disease state in the immunocompetent animal. However, for both small- and large-molecule drug candidates that are intended to be immunomodulatory, these spontaneous subclinical infections may no longer be self-limiting and lead to a florid outbreak of disease, complicating the interpretation of the toxicology study. A clinical disease outbreak in one or more animals on a toxicology study may be useful in identifying a potential effect on host resistance, or a spontaneous occurrence of infection may inappropriately suggest a test article effect (Evans and Kawabata 2010).

To assess possible compound-related effects in safety assessment toxicology studies utilizing the cynomolgus macaque, it is essential that toxicologic pathologists have detailed knowledge of common spontaneous infections, opportunistic infections, and background lesions (Sasseville and Mansfield

2010). Viral infections can include measles, hepatitis A, and simian type D retrovirus. Primary bacterial infections that often interfere with toxicology study interpretation include *Shigella*, *Campylobacter*, *Helicobacter*, and *Moraxella catarrhalis* (Sasseville and Mansfield 2010). Opportunistic infections, such as adenovirus, cytomegalovirus, and *pneumocystis carinii* may occur in the macaque infected with an immunosuppressive retrovirus, or as a result of intended immune modulation from a targeted biopharmaceutical.

Several types of opportunistic infections have occurred in NHP toxicology studies potentially complicating the interpretation of the results. For example, gamma herpes virus–mediated B-lymphocyte proliferation associated with a T-lymphocyte depleting fusion protein test article was reported on a toxicology study, as was an increased *Plasmodium* burden that was associated with a mAb inhibitory to T-lymphocyte trafficking and macrophage function (Hutto 2010). Confounding toxicological endpoints as a result of subclinical and undetected retrovirus infections have included NHP mortality, virus-induced clinical pathology abnormalities, histopathologic lesions, alteration of physiologic parameters, and interference with *in vitro* assays (Lerche 2010; Lerche and Osborn 2003). Small-molecule development of a class of immunomodulatory compounds resulted in skin, upper respiratory tract, and gastrointestinal tract infections that often progressed to bacteremia and mortality (Price 2010). The NHP may also be infected by a rich flora of herpes viruses that cause persistent and latent, lifelong infections. Periodic and frequent asymptomatic viral recurrences can occur from latency throughout the lifetime of the animal. With immune modulation or suppression, however, immune control of herpes virus infections can be lost, resulting in significant disease and even death of the affected animal (Simmons 2010). These examples all demonstrate the importance of understanding the health status of the NHP used on the toxicology study and being able to accurately differentiate between a spontaneous infection from a true test article–related toxicity. Country of origin of the NHP is also important, as disease status and background disease incidence in monkeys obtained from different locales, such as China and Southeast Asia, can differ (Taylor 2010).

Other considerations for the use of the NHP on toxicology studies are the age and body weight of the animal. Generally, cynomolgus monkeys should be greater than 2 kg in body weight at study start, as the use of smaller animals limits the blood volume available for sampling during the study. Smaller animals are also more vulnerable to stress associated with various procedures encountered during the study and may be more prone to develop diarrhea. Because of their size, these smaller animals may be more sensitive to the secondary effects of diarrhea like dehydration, which can progress to an overall condition of poor health, unrelated to the test article.

For biopharmaceuticals, the potential for effects on male and female fertility can be assessed by light microscopic evaluation of the reproductive organs from animals on a 3-month or longer repeat-dose toxicity study using sexually mature NHPs. A sexually mature female cynomolgus monkey has been reported to be 4–5 years of age and 2.5–5.0 kg in body weight (Smedley et al. 2002; Weinbauer et al. 2008). Male cynomolgus monkeys are more likely to be sexually mature at greater than 5 years of age and greater than 5 kg of body weight (Smedley et al. 2002).

2.14 REPORTING PATHOLOGY DATA FOR THE REGULATORY SCIENTIST AND CLINICIAN

Pathology data from nonclinical toxicology studies, consisting of both clinical pathology endpoints and light microscopic evaluations, compose an essential part of the nonclinical safety data set that supports both clinical development and subsequent new drug application and approval. Toxicologic pathology encompasses the study of changes in tissue morphology that help define potential safety risk to humans (Wolf and Mann 2005). The interpretation of these pathology data, in addition to other nonclinical data, forms the basis for judgment about the safety of the product. Therefore, the scientific generation and interpretation of pathology data must be unimpeachable (Dua and Jackson 1988).

Histopathology is the study of the structural manifestation of disease at the light microscopic level. Histopathology is necessarily a largely descriptive and interpretive science. The trained and experienced toxicologic pathologist must be able to distinguish normal variation and spontaneous disease processes from those changes resulting from the administration of a test article (Crissman et al. 2004). Histopathology results are one of the most important parts of the nonclinical safety assessment process. In toxicologic pathology, the goal is to determine if the test article produces changes through a comparison of treated animals with control animal data (both concurrent and historical controls). It is important, therefore, that microscopic observations be recorded in a consistent, objective manner that readily allows tabulation and comparison of group effects. In this setting, the use of descriptive, rather than diagnostic, terminology is preferred (Mann et al. 2012). A disease or etiologic diagnosis implies a particular pathogenesis or impact on organ function on the basis of what is known about that disease process; this would be misleading in the experimental setting of a toxicity study. Consistently using descriptive rather than diagnostic terminology in tabulating anatomic pathology data will decrease confusion and misconceptions (Mann et al. 2012).

The pathology report must be complete, must be accurate, and must communicate the relative importance of various findings in a study. The quality of the report is determined by three major categories: thoroughness, accuracy, and consistency (Shackelford et al. 2002). All lesions need to be recorded, including those frequently observed, such as spontaneous incidental background changes. It is important for the toxicologic pathologist to realize that "normal" is in reality an array of individual variations within an accepted reference range. Both qualitative and quantitative (i.e., tabulated format of descriptors) components of the pathology report convey to the reader that the data were reported to the highest standards of diligence and consistency. When appropriate, the pathology report and discussion should be integrated with other endpoints of the study such as TK, PD, and impact of ADAs.

A pathology peer review ensures consistency and accuracy of the diagnostic terminology and confirms the target tissues, which increases the quality of the pathology data set (Gosselin et al. 2011). While formal pathology peer review is not a regulatory requirement, both sponsors and regulatory agencies acknowledge that collaborative review by more than one pathologist increases confidence in the accuracy of the descriptions and the quality of the interpretations. Objectives of a formal histopathology peer review include determining accuracy and consistency of nomenclature, determining completeness, and confirming the appropriateness of the NOEL or NOAEL. The pathology peer review also ensures the correctness of the textual interpretation derived from the pathology data. Overall, the intention of the peer review is to ensure that test article–related findings are properly and consistently identified and correctly interpreted (Crissman et al. 2004; Morton et al. 2010).

A problem often encountered by regulators reviewing pathology data is a lack of adequate morphologic description of the change. It is difficult to interpret the impact of a test article–related lesion with only a minimal description of the morphological characteristics. This is a particular problem when terminology for a lesion is poorly defined or controversial, which is compounded by inconsistency of applying diagnostic terminology within a study (Dua and Jackson 1988). The use of several different terms without explanation is also a problem for the regulatory reviewer. Morphologic diagnoses should represent currently accepted criteria. The INHAND was created as a framework to standardize terminology globally (Mann et al. 2012; Thoolen et al. 2010).

Sufficient information needs to be presented to support both the strength and quality of the pathology data (Dua and Jackson 1988). If the pathology results are presented as an individual contributing scientist report that is appended to the full toxicology report, it is important that background information is provided regarding experimental design and methodology. Changes to the original study protocol need to be indicated and adequately explained, such as when a full set of tissues are evaluated from a lower-dose group or when a special stain is used to better characterize a light microscopic finding.

Following the pathology result section in the report, the pathologist should provide a summary narrative giving an overview of the findings from the study pathologist's perspective. Discussion on pathogenesis, supported by scientific literature, is critical as it provides information on significant events that may have occurred in the study, such as incidental disease outbreaks that may complicate study interpretation. Strictly utilizing incidence tables to convey the results is not recommended. If incidence or severity differences are not interpreted as being test article related, then the basis for this conclusion must be provided (Zbinden 1976). The final report represents the pathologist's best professional judgment regarding the relevant tissue changes and their interpretation in the context of the study (Crissman et al. 2004).

When pathology data are well written, organized, and presented in a clear fashion, the regulatory review is likely to be more reliable with less chance of misinterpretation. Unclear language; inappropriate, misleading, or unexplained terminology; conclusions not justified by data; and any discrepancy between text and tables may all raise unnecessary questions (Mann et al. 2012). Discerning the difference between control and treatment groups and effectively communicating these differences and their impact on safety risk to humans in a manner that the larger audience of non-pathologists (e.g., regulators, clinical pharmacologists, clinicians) can readily understand are the fundamental responsibility of the toxicologic pathologist. The safety evaluation of pathology data submitted to regulatory agencies deserves paramount efforts by both industry and regulatory scientists to ensure patient safety and the expeditious development of novel therapies for diseases with unmet medical needs.

REFERENCES

Alden, C.L., Smith, P.F., Piper, C.E. et al. 1996. A critical appraisal of the value of the mouse cancer bioassay in safety assessment. *Toxicol Pathol* 24:722–25.

Ames, B.N., Lee, D.F., and W.E. Durston. 1973. An improved bacterial test system for the detection and classification of mutagens and carcinogens. *Proc Natl Acad Sci USA* 70:782–86.

Baillie, T.A., Cayen, M.N., Fouda, H. et al. 2002. Drug metabolites in safety testing. *Toxicol Appl Pharmacol* 182:188–96.

Bass, A.S., Cartwright, M.E., Mahon, C. et al. 2009. Exploratory drug safety: A discovery strategy to reduce attrition in development. *J Pharm Toxicol Methods* 60:69–78.

Bettauer, R.H. 2011. Systemic review of chimpanzee use in monoclonal antibody research and drug development: 1981–2010. *ALTEX* 28(2):103–16.

Black, H.E. 2007. Establishing the NOAEL in repeat dose toxicity studies for a new medicine: Issues that may arise. *Foods Food Ingredients J Jpn* 212(6):460–64.

Bode, G., Clausing P., Gervals, F. et al. 2010. The utility of the minipig as an animal model in regulatory toxicology. *J Pharmacol Toxicol Methods* 62:196–220.

Bolon, B., Galbreath, E., Sargent, L. et al. 2000. Genetic engineering and molecular technology. In: *The Laboratory Rat* (G. Krinke, ed.). Academic Press, London, pp. 603–34.

Bolon, B. and E.J. Galbreath. 2002. Use of genetically engineered mice in drug discovery and development: Wielding Occam's razor to prune the product portfolio. *Int J Toxicol* 21:55–64.

Boobis, A.R., Cohen, S.M., Doerrer, N.G. et al. 2009. A data-based assessment of alternative strategies for identification of potential human cancer hazards. *Toxicol Pathol* 37:714–32.

Boorman, G., Dixon, D., Elwell, M. et al. 2003. Assessment of hyperplastic lesions in rodent carcinogenicity studies. *Toxicol Pathol* 31:709–10.

Boverhof, D.R., Chamberlain, M.P., Elcombeet, C.R. et al. 2011. Transgenic animal models in toxicology: Historical perspectives and future outlook. *Toxicol Sci* 121(2):207–33.

Bowlby, M.R., Peri, R., Zheng, H. et al. 2008. hERG (KCNH2 of Kv11.1) K+ channels: Screening for cardiac arrhythmia risk. *Curr Drug Metab* 9:965–70.

Bregman, C.L., Adler, R.R., Moron, D.G. et al. 2003. Recommended tissue list for histopathological examination in repeat-dose toxicity and carcinogenicity studies: A proposal of the Society of Toxicologic Pathologists (STP). *Toxicol Pathol* 31:252–53.

Brennan, F.R., Morton, L.D., Spindeldreher, S. et al. 2010. Safety and immunotoxicity assessment of immunomodulatory monoclonal antibodies. *mAbs* 2(3):233–55.

Brennan F.R., Shaw, L., Wing, M.G. et al. 2004. Preclinical safety testing of biotechnology-derived biopharmaceuticals. *Mol Biotechnol* 27:59–74.

Bugelski, P.J. and G. Treacy. 2004. Predictive power of preclinical studies in animals for the immunogenicity of recombinant therapeutic proteins in humans. *Curr Opin Mol Ther* 6:10–6.

Bussiere, J.L. 2008a. Species selection considerations for preclinical toxicology studies for biopharmaceuticals. *Expert Opin Drug Metab Toxicol* 4(7):871–7.

Bussiere, J.L. 2008b. General toxicity testing and immunotoxicity testing for biopharmaceuticals. In: *Preclinical Safety Testing of Biopharmaceuticals: A Science Based Approach to Facilitating Clinical Trials* (J.A. Cavagnaro, ed.). John Wiley & Sons, Inc., New Jersey, pp. 343–56.

Bussiere, J.L., Martin, P., Horner, M. et al. 2009. Alternative strategies for toxicity testing of species-specific biopharmaceuticals. *Int J Toxicol* 28(3):230–53.

Bussiere, J.L. and B. Mounho. 2008. Differentiating between desired immunomodulation and potential immunotoxicity. In: *Immunotoxicology Strategies for Biopharmaceutical Safety Assessment* (D. Herzyk and J.L. Bussiere, eds.). John Wiley & Sons, Inc., New Jersey, pp. 191–8.

Bussiere, J.L., Leach, M.W., Price, K.D. et al. 2011. Survey results on the use of the tissue cross-reactivity immunohistochemistry assay. *Reg Toxicol Pharmacol* 59:493–502.

Cavagnaro, J.A. 2002. Preclinical safety evaluation of biotechnology-derived biopharmaceuticals. *Nat Rev Drug Discov* 1:469–75.

Center for Drug Evaluation and Research (CDER). 2008. Guidance for industry: Safety testing of drug metabolites. http://www.fda.gov/cder/guidance/index.htm.

Chamberlain, P. and A.R. Mire-Sluis. 2003. An overview of scientific and regulatory issues for the immunogenicity of biological products. In: *Immunogenicity of Therapeutic Biological Products* (F. Brown and A. Mire-Sluis, eds.). Karger AG, Basil, Switzerland, pp. 3–11.

Chapman, K., Pullen, N., Coney, L. et al. 2009. Preclinical development of monoclonal antibodies: Considerations for the use of non-human primates. *mAbs* 1(5):505–16.

Chapman, K., Pullen, N., Graham, M. et al. 2007. Preclinical safety testing of monoclonal antibodies: The significance of species relevance. *Nature Rev* 6:120–126.

Chellman, G.J., Bussiere, J.L., Makori, N. et al. 2009. Developmental and reproductive toxicology studies in nonhuman primates. *Birth Defects Res (Part B)* 86:446–62.

Clarke, J., Hurst, C., Martin, P. et al. 2008. Duration of chronic toxicity studies for biotechnology-derived biopharmaceuticals: Is 6 months still appropriate? *Reg Toxicol Pharmacol* 50:2–22.

Cohen, S.M. 2004a. Risk assessment in the genomic era. *Toxicol Pathol* 32(Suppl 1):3–8.

Cohen, S.M. 2004b. Human carcinogenic risk evaluation: An alternative approach to the two-year rodent bioassay. *Toxicol Sci* 80:225–29.

Crissman, J.W., Goodman, D.G., Hildebrandt, P.K. et al. 2004. Best practices guideline: Toxicologic histopathology. *Toxicol Pathol* 32:126–31.

Dayhaw-Barker, P., 2000. The eye as a unique target for toxic and phototoxic effects. In: *Towards New Horizons in Primate Toxicology* (R. Korte and G.F. Weinbauer, eds.). Waxmann, Munster, pp. 145–58.

Dempster, A.M. 1995. Pharmacological testing of recombinant human erythropoietin: Implications for other biotechnology products. *Drug Dev Res*. 35:173–8.

Doetschman, T. 1999. Interpretation of phenotype in genetically engineered mice. *Lab Anim Sci* 49:137–43.

Dorato, M.A. 2007. The No-Observed-Adverse-Effect-Level (NOAEL) in drug safety evaluations. *Foods Food Ingredients J Jpn* 212(6):436–47.

Dua, P.N. and B.J. Jackson. 1988. Review of pathology data for regulatory purposes. *Toxicol Pathol* 16: 443–50.

Dykens, J.A. and Y. Will. 2007. The significance of mitochondrial toxicity testing in drug development. *Drug Discovery Today* 12(17/18):777–85.

Elger, W. 2000. The role of primate models for reproductive pharmacology. In: *Towards New Horizons in Primate Toxicology* (R. Korte and G. F. Weinbauer, eds.). Waxmann, Munster, 65–82.

Evans, E.W. and T.T. Kawabata. 2010. Workshop on naturally occurring infections in non-human primates and immunotoxicity implications: Introduction. *J Immunotoxicol* 7(2):77–8.

Fenech, M. 2000. The in vitro micronucleus technique. *Mutat Res* 455:81–95.

Fielden, M.R. and K.L. Kolaja. 2008. The role of early in vivo toxicity testing in drug discovery toxicology. *Expert Opin Drug Saf* 7(2):107–10.

Frost, H. 2005. Antibody-mediated side effects of recombinant proteins. *Toxicol* 209:155–60.

Gad, S.C. and C.G. Rousseaux. 2002. Use and misuse of statistics in the design and interpretation of studies. In: *Handbook of Toxicologic Pathology*, 2nd Edition (W.M. Haschek, C.G. Rousseaux, and M.A. Wallig, eds.). Elsevier Inc., Oxford, UK, pp. 327–417.

Giezen, T.J., Mantel-Teeuwisse, A.K., Straus, S.M. et al. 2008. Safety-related regulatory actions for biologicals approved in the United States and the European Union. *JAMA* 300:1887–96.

Goldberg, A.M and P.A. Locke. 2004. To 3R is humane. *Environ Forum* July/August.

Goralczyk, R. 2000. Histological aspects of primate ocular toxicity with special emphasis on canthaxanthin-induced retinopathy in the cynomolgus monkey model. In: *Towards New Horizons in Primate Toxicology* (R. Korte and G.F. Weinbauer, eds.). Waxmann, Munster, pp. 159–74.

Gosselin, S.J., Palate, D., Parker, G.A. et al. 2011. Industry–contract research organization pathology interactions: A perspective of contract research organizations in producing the best quality pathology report. *Toxicol Pathol* 39:422–8.

Gribble, E.J., Sivakumar, P.V., Ponce, R.A. et al. 2007. Toxicity as a result of immunostimulation by biologics. *Expert Opin Drug Metab Toxicol* 3(2):209–34.

Gunn, H. 1997. Immunogenicity of recombinant human interleukin-3. *Clin Immunol Immunopathol* 83:5–7.

Haley, P., Perry, R., Ennulat, D. et al. 2005. STP position paper: Best practice guideline for the routine pathology evaluation of the immune system. *Toxicol Pathol* 33:404–7.

Haller, C.A., Cosenza, M.E., and J.T. Sullivan. 2008. Safety issues specific to clinical development of protein therapeutics. *Clin Pharmacol Therapeutics* 84(5):624–7.

Hernandez, L.G., van Steeg, H., Luijten, M. et al. 2009. Mechanisms of non-genotoxic carcinogens and importance of a weight of evidence approach. *Mutat Res* 682:94–109.

Hutto, D.L. 2010. Opportunistic infections in non-human primates exposed to immunomodulatory biotherapeutics: Considerations and case studies. *J Immunotoxicol* 7(2):120–7.

ICH M3 (R2), Guidance on Non-Clinical Safety Studies for the Conduct of Human Clinical Trials and Marketing Authorization for Biopharmaceuticals. June 2009. Retrieved June 2011 from http://www.ich.org.

ICH S1A, Guideline on the Need for Carcinogenicity Studies of Biopharmaceuticals, November 1995. Retrieved June 2011 from http://www.ich.org.

ICH S1B, Testing for Carcinogenicity of Biopharmaceuticals. July 1997. Retrieved June 2011 from http://www.ich.org.

ICH S1C, Dose Selection for Carcinogenicity Studies of Biopharmaceuticals. October, 1994. Retrieved June 2011 from http://www.ich.org.

ICH S2A, Specific Aspects of Regulatory Genotoxicity Tests for Biopharmaceuticals. July 1995. Retrieved June 2011 from http://www.ich.org.

ICH S2B, Genotoxicity: A Standard Battery for Genotoxicity Testing of Biopharmaceuticals, July 1997. Retrieved June 2011 from http://www.ich.org.

ICH S5 (R2), Detection of toxicity to reproduction for medicinal products & toxicity to male fertility. November 2005. Retrieved June 2011 from http://www.ich.org.

ICH S6, Preclinical Safety Evaluation of Biotechnology-Derived Biopharmaceuticals. July 1997. Retrieved June 2011 from http://www.ich.org.

ICH S6 (R1), Addendum to ICH S6 guideline: Preclinical Safety Evaluation of Biotechnology-Derived Biopharmaceuticals. Guideline May 19, 2011. Retrieved June 2011 from http://www.ich.org.

ICH S7A, Safety Pharmacology Studies for Human Biopharmaceuticals, November 2000. Retrieved June 2011 from http://www.ich.org.

ICH S7B, The Nonclinical Evaluation of the Potential for Delayed Ventricular Repolarization (QT interval prolongation) by Human Biopharmaceuticals. May 2005. Retrieved June 2011 from http://www.ich.org.

ICH S8, Immunotoxicology Studies for Human Biopharmaceuticals. November 2004. Retrieved June 2011 from http://www.ich.org.

ICH S9, Nonclinical Evaluation for Anticancer Biopharmaceuticals. October 2009. Retrieved June 2011 from http://www.ich.org.

IOM, Institute of Medicine December 2011. Report Brief. www.iom.edu/chimpstudy.

Jacobson-Kram, D., Sistare, F.D. and A.C. Jacobs. 2004. Use of transgenic mice in carcinogenicity hazard assessment. *Toxicol Pathol* 32:1:49–52.

Jerome, C. 2002. Osteoporosis and aging: the nonhuman primate model. In: *Primate Models in Biopharmaceutical Drug Development* (R. Korte, F. Vogel and G.F. Weinbauer, eds.). Waxmann, Munster, pp. 85–92.

Kessler, M., Goldsmith D., and H. Schellekens. 2006. Immunogenicity of biopharmaceuticals. *Nephrol Dial Transplant* 21(5):9–12.

Koren, E., Zuckerman L.A., and A.R. Mire-Sluis. 2002. Immune responses to therapeutic proteins in humans—clinical significance, assessment and prediction. *Curr Pharm Biotechnol* 3:349–60.

Kramer, J.A., Sagartz, J.E., and D.L. Morris. 2007. *Nature Rev Drug Discov* 6:636–49.

Kummar, S., Gutierrez, M., Doroshow, J.H. et al. 2006. Drug development in oncology: Classic cytotoxics and molecularly targeted agents. *Br J Clin Pharmacol* 62:15–26.

Lanning, L.L., Creasy, D.M., Chapin, R.E. et al. 2002. Recommended approaches for the evaluation of testicular and epididymal toxicity. *Toxicol Pathol* 30:507–20.

Le Tourneau, C., Stathis, A., Vidal, L. et al. 2010. Choice of starting dose for molecularly targeted agents evaluated in first-in-human phase I cancer clinical trials. *J Clin Oncol* 28:1401–7.

Leach, M.W., Halpern, W.G., Johnson, C.W. et al. 2010. Use of tissue cross-reactivity studies in the development of antibody-based biopharmaceuticals: History, experience, methodology, and future directions. *Toxicol Pathol* 38:1138–66.

Lebrec, H., Cowan, L., Lagrou, M. et al. 2011. An inter-laboratory retrospective analysis of immunotoxicological endpoints in non-human primates: T-cell-dependent antibody responses. *J Immunotoxicol* 8(3):238–50.

Lerche, N.W. and K.G. Osborne. 2003. Simian retrovirus infections: Potential confounding variables in primate toxicology studies. *Toxicol Pathol* 31:103–10.

Lerche, N.W. 2010. Simian retroviruses: Infections and disease—implications for immunotoxicology research in primates. *J Immunotoxicol* 7(2):93–101.

Long, G.G., Morton, D., Peters, T. et al. 2010. Alternative mouse models for carcinogenicity assessment: Industry use and issues with pathology interpretation. *Toxicol Pathol* 38:43–50.

Mahmood, I. and M.D. Green. 2007. Drug interaction studies of therapeutic proteins or monoclonal antibodies. *J Clin Pharmacol* 47:1540–54.

Mann, P.C., Kennan, C., and J. Vahle. 2012. International harmonization of toxicologic pathology nomenclature: An overview and review of basic principles. *Toxicol Pathol* (in press).

Martin, P.L., Breslin, W., Rocca, M. et al. 2009. Considerations in assessing the developmental and reproductive toxicity potential of biopharmaceuticals. *Birth Defects Res (Part B)* 86:176–203.

Martin, P.L., Oneda S., and G. Treacy. 2007. Effects of an anti-TNF-α monoclonal antibody, administered throughout pregnancy and lactation, on the development of the macaque immune system. *Am J Reprod Immunol* 58:138–49.

Martin, P.L., Sachs, C., Imai, N. et al. 2010. Development in the cynomolgus macaque following administration of ustekinumab, a human anti-il-12/23p40 monoclonal antibody, during pregnancy and lactation. *Birth Defects Res (Part B)* 89(5):351–63.

Mascelli, M.A., Zhou, H., and R. Sweet. 2007. Molecular, biologic, and pharmacokinetic properties of monoclonal antibodies: Impact of these parameters on early clinical development. *J Clin Pharmacol* 47: 553–65.

McMahon, C., Mitchell, A.Z., Klein, J.L. et al. 2010. Evaluation of blood pressure measurement using a miniature blood pressure transmitter with jacketed external telemetry in cynomolgus monkeys. *J Pharmacol Toxicol Methods* 62:127–35.

Mire-Sluis, A.R., Barrett, Y.C., Devanarayanet, V. et al. 2004. Recommendations for the design and optimization of immunoassays used in the detection of host antibodies against biotechnology products. *J Immunol Methods* 289:1–16.

Monro, A.M. and J.S. MacDonald. 1998. Evaluation of the carcinogenic potential of biopharmaceuticals: Opportunities arising from the International Conference on Harmonization. *Drug Saf* 18(5):309–19.

Morgan, R.E., Trauner, M., van Staden, T. et al. 2010. Interference with bile salt export pump function is a susceptibility factor for human liver injury in drug development. *Toxicol Sci* 118(2):485–500.

Morton, D., Alden, C.L., Roth, A.J. et al. 2002b. The Tg rasH2 mouse in cancer hazard identification. *Toxicol Pathol* 30:139–146.

Morton, D., Elwell, M., Fairweather, W. et al. 2002a. The STP's recommendations on statistical analysis of rodent carcinogenicity studies. *Toxicol Pathol* 30:415–8.

Morton, D., Seller, R.W., Barale-Thomas, E. et al. 2010. Recommendations for pathology peer review. *Toxicol Pathol* 38(7):1118–27.

Muller, P.Y. and F.R. Brennan. 2009. Election for first-in-human clinical trials with immunomodulatory monoclonal antibodies. *Clin Pharmacol Therapeutics* 85:247–58.

Niebecker, R. and C. Kloft. 2010. Safety of therapeutic monoclonal antibodies. *Curr Drug Saf* 5:275–86.

OECD Principles of Good Laboratory Practice. 1998. OECD Environmental Health and Safety Publications (OECD) 1.

Olivier, K.J., Price, K.D., Hutto, D.L. et al. 2010. Naturally occurring infections in non-human primates (NHP) and immunotoxicity implications: Discussion sessions. *J Immunotoxicol* 7(2):138–46.

Piccini, J.P., Whellan, D.J., Berridge, B.R. et al. 2009. Current challenges in the evaluation of cardiac safety during drug development: Translational medicine meets the Critical Path Initiative. *Am Heart J* 158:317–26.

Ponce, R., Abad, L., Amaravadi, L. et al. 2009. Immunogenicity of biologically-derived therapeutics: Assessment and interpretation of nonclinical safety studies. *Reg Toxicol Pharmacol* 54:164–82.

Price, K.D. 2010. Bacterial infections in cynomolgus monkeys given small molecule immunomodulatory antagonists. *J Immunotoxicol* 7(2):128–37.

Redfern, W.S., Carlson, L., Davis A.S. et al. 2002. Relationships between preclinical cardiac electrophysiology, clinical QT interval prolongation and torsade de pointes for a broad range of drugs: evidence for a provisional safety margin in drug development. *Cardiovasc Res* 58:32–45.

Renne, R., Brix, A., Harkema, J. et al. 2009. Proliferative and nonproliferative lesions of the rat and mouse respiratory tract. *Toxicol Pathol* 37:5S.

Roden, D.M. 1998. Mechanisms and management of proarrhythmia. *Am J Cardiol* 82:491–571.

Rudman, D.R. and S.K. Durham. 1999. Utilization of genetically altered animals in the biopharmaceutical industry. *Toxicol Pathol* 27:111–4.

Sasseville, V.G., Lane, J.H., Kadambi, V.J. et al. 2004. Testing paradigm for prediction of development-limiting barriers and human drug toxicity. *Chem-Biol Interact* 50:9–25.

Sasseville, V.G. and K.G. Mansfield. 2010. Overview of known non-human primate pathogens with potential to affect colonies used for toxicity testing. *J Immunotoxicol* 7(2):79–92.

Schellekens, H. 2002. Immunogenicity of therapeutic proteins: Clinical implications and future prospects. *Clin Ther* 24:1720–40.

Schultze, A.E., Bounous, D.I., and A.P. Bolliger. 2008. Veterinary clinical pathology in the biopharmaceutical industry. *Vet Clin Pathol* 37/2:146–58.

Serabian, M.A. and A.M. Pilaro. 1999. Safety assessment of biotechnology-derived biopharmaceuticals: ICH and beyond. *Toxicol Pathol* 27:27–31.

Shackelford, C., Long, G., Wolf. J. et al. 2002. Qualitative and quantitative analysis of nonneoplastic lesions in toxicology studies. *Toxicol Pathol* 30:93–6.

Shankar, G., Shores, E., Wagner, C. et al. 2006. Scientific and regulatory considerations on the immunogenicity of biologics. *Trends Biotechnol* 24:274–80.

Simmons, J.H. 2010. Herpesvirus infections of laboratory macaques. *J Immunotoxicol* 7(2):102–13.

Smedley, J.V., Bailey, S.A., Perry, R.W. et al. 2002. Methods for predicting sexual maturity in male cynomolgus macaques on the basis of age, body weight, and histologic evaluation of the testes. *Contemp Top Lab Anim Sci* 14(5):18–20.

Stevens, J.L and T.K. Baker. 2008. The future of drug safety testing: Expanding the view and narrowing the focus. *Drug Discov Today* 14:162–7.

Storer, R.D., Sistare, F.D., Reddy, V. et al. 2011. An industry perspective on the utility of short-term carcinogenicity testing in transgenic mice in pharmaceutical development. *Toxicol Pathol* 38:51–61.

Tamaoki, N. 2001. The rasH2 transgenic mouse: Nature of the model and mechanistic studies on tumorigenesis. *Toxicol Pathol* 29(1):81–9.

Taylor, K. 2010. Clinical veterinarian's perspective of non-human primate (NHP) use in drug safety studies. *J Immunotoxicol* 7(2):114–9.

Terrell, T.G. and J.D. Green. 1994. Issues with biotechnology products in toxicologic pathology. *Toxicol Pathol* 22:187–93.

Thoolen, B., Maronpot, R.R., Harada, T. et al. 2010. Proliferative and nonproliferative lesions of the rat and mouse hepatobiliary system. *Toxicol Pathol* 38:5S–81S.

Tibbetts, J., Cavagnaro, J.A., Haller, A. et al. 2010. Practical approaches to dose selection for first-in-human clinical trials with novel biopharmaceuticals. *Reg Toxicol Pharmacol* 58:243–251.

Tomaszewski, J.E. 2004. Multi-specie approaches for oncology drugs: The US perspective. *Eur J Cancer* 40:907–13.

Vahle, J.L., Finch, G.L., Heidel, S.M. et al. 2010. Carcinogenicity assessments of biotechnology-derived biopharmaceuticals: A review of approved molecules and best practice recommendations. *Toxicol Pathol* 38:522–53.

Van der Linde, H.J., Van Deuren, B., Teisman, A. et al. 2008. The effect of changes in core body temperature on the QT interval in beagle dogs: a previously ignored phenomenon, with a method for correction. *Br J Pharmacol* 154(7):1474–81.

Vargas, H.M., Bass, A.S., Breidenbach, A. et al. 2008. Scientific review and recommendations on preclinical cardiovascular safety evaluation of biologics. *J Pharmacol Toxicol Methods* 58:72–6.

Vogel, F. 2000. How to design male fertility investigations in the cynomolgus monkey. In: *Towards New Horizons in Primate Toxicology* (R. Korte and G.F. Weinbauer, eds.). Waxmann, Munster, pp. 43–52.

Walsh, G. 2006. Biopharmaceutical benchmarks. 2006. *Nat Biotechnol* 24(7):769–76.

Wang, D.S., Ohdo, S., Koyanagi, S. et al. 2001. Effect of dosing schedule on pharmacokinetics on alpha interferon and anti-alpha interferon neutralizing antibody in mice. *Antimicrob Agents Chemother* 45:176–80.

Ward, J.M. 2007. The two-year rodent carcinogenesis bioassay—will it survive? *Toxicol Pathol* 20:13–9.

Weinbauer, G.F. 2002. The nonhuman primate as a model in developmental and reproductive toxicology. In: *Primate Models in Biopharmaceutical Drug Development* (R. Korte and G.F. Weinbauer, eds.). Waxmann, Munster, pp. 49–66.

Weinbauer, G.F. and T.G. Cooper. 2000. Assessment of male fertility impairment in the macaque model. In: *Primate Models in Biopharmaceutical Drug Development* (R. Korte and G.F. Weinbauer, eds.). Waxmann, Munster, pp. 13–42.

Weinbauer, G.F., Niehoff, M., Niehaus, M. et al. 2008. Physiology and endocrinology of the ovarian cycle in macaques. *Toxicol Pathol* 36:7–23.

Wierda, D., Smith, H.W., and Zwickl, C.M. 2001. Immunogenicity of biopharmaceuticals in laboratory animals. *Toxicol* 158:71–4.

Wolf, D.C. and P.C. Mann. 2005. Confounders in interpreting pathology data for safety and risk assessment. *Toxicol Appl Pharmacol* 202:302–8.

Working, P.K. 1992. Potential effects of antibody induction by protein drugs. In: *Protein Pharmacokinetics and Metabolism* (B.L. Ferraiolo, M.A. Mohler, and C.A. Gloff, eds.). Plenum Press, New York, pp. 73–92.

Zbinden, G. 1976. Formal toxicology: The role of pathology in toxicity testing. In: *Progress in Toxicology—Special Topics. Vol. 2*. Springer-Verlag, Berlin, pp. 8–18.

Zbinden, G. 1993. The concept of multispecies testing in industrial toxicology. *Reg Toxicol Pharmacol* 17:85–94.

3 Toxicokinetics and Drug Disposition

David D. Christ

CONTENTS

3.1 INTRODUCTION AND OBJECTIVE

The goals of drug metabolism and pharmacokinetics (PK) as they apply to toxicology in general and pathology in particular are simple; place the biological observations (toxicity, tissue damage, species differences) in a chemical, physiological, and quantitative context. While many of the drug development and regulatory conclusions are still based on dosage (e.g., NOAEL), it is the concentration of parent or metabolite at the site of toxicity (or its surrogate, plasma or serum) and the time course of drug appearance and elimination that provide a scientifically rigorous interpretation of the observations and enable the formation of hypotheses. The objectives of this chapter are to provide the reader with a working understanding of the critical toxicokinetic (TK) parameters, how they are derived and applied, and what they mean. While distinctions have been drawn between the use of "toxicokinetics" or TK and "pharmacokinetics" or PK, the concepts and mathematics underlying the parameters used to describe the time course of a molecule's fate in a biological system are the same, whether the molecule is a toxin or a potential therapeutic. This chapter will refer to TK parameters as those calculated for a molecule or metabolite after high dosages in a toxicology study, ignoring the characterization of the molecule's biological activity. In practice, most of these data are presented and discussed in a team setting; therefore, understanding the design, limitations, and realistic interpretation of TK and metabolism data will be highlighted, so the pathologist can participate in the critical evaluation of these data. Additionally, important concepts in the biochemistry and physiology of absorption, distribution, metabolism, and excretion that are responsible for the TK will be reviewed briefly. While the focus of this chapter will be primarily on the study of small, organic molecules rather than biologically derived peptides, antibodies, siRNA, etc., the concepts and assumptions are generally applicable to studies of these larger molecules. Often these biological molecules, especially those that are "humanized," are cleared rapidly from the circulation in animals by processes that are not similar to the human disposition of these molecules. Importantly, this chapter cannot cover all the important metabolic reactions, nor will this chapter focus on the mathematical derivations of the key kinetic parameters since excellent reviews of these derivations have been published (Benet 1984; Wilkinson 1987).

3.2   IMPORTANCE OF EXPOSURE-BASED INTERPRETATION

It is now universally accepted that measures of systemic exposure to chemicals are more relevant parameters than dosage for the evaluation of biological effects produced by direct and reversible interactions with a molecular target. One of the earliest examples illustrating the importance of blood or tissue concentration, dose, and response comes from the observations made in the 1940s that the antimalarial effect of quinine could not be related to dose, but rather could be explained by blood concentrations (Shannon et al. 1948). It is also commonly accepted that species differences or sex differences in toxicity at the same dosage can be explained by differences in TK, in addition to species or gender-specific biological responses.

One of the fundamental assumptions in interpreting biological response after administration of endogenous or exogenous chemicals is that the response is related to the concentration of the chemical at the site of action, either directly or indirectly. This is critically distinct from relating effect to the total amount of chemical introduced into the system, typically referred to as the dose. But some additional definition is in order. While many scientists conversationally equate dose to the actual amount given (in absolute mass or mass normalized to body weight or surface area), dosage is the more precise description of "how much" while dose is most appropriately used to describe the act of administration, or "how many." This distinction is usually not critical, except when considering that exposure, that is, the systemic (blood, plasma, or serum) concentrations of the chemical of interest, can vary little with different dosage in the same species, vary markedly at the same dosage (e.g., between male and female animals), or vary markedly from dose to dose at the same dosage (e.g., after multiple doses of a chemical that induces its own metabolism and elimination). While many regulatory decisions are still based on dosage i.e., selection of the maximum starting dose for clinical trials using the NOAEL as described in the FDA Guidance (2005), more sophisticated interpretation of response is concentration based.

One of the tenets of biological response to chemicals is that the effects produced are related, either directly or indirectly, to their combination with effector molecules. While advances in sampling and imaging technologies have provided better ways to measure concentrations at the site of action, most often measurement of the chemical concentrations in the peripheral circulation or other fluid is assumed to relate to the concentration at the effector site. In the absence of diffusional barriers or active transport processes that would skew this relationship (and which are discussed in greater detail below), the fundamental assumption is that distribution from the bloodstream is rapid and extensive such that concentrations measured in plasma are a surrogate for concentrations at the site of action. This assumption is most valid after repeated dosing to steady state but is often made after acute dosing too. Conceptually, the simplest relationship is one where the direct combination of drug and target produces a graded response that is directly proportional to the concentration of free or unbound drug. Responses are then quantified by relating an effective concentration or inhibitory concentration calculated from the sigmoidal relationship between concentration and response, analogous to receptor binding or enzyme kinetics. Indirect effects are often produced by molecules interacting with cellular targets but whose ultimate response depends on the production of subsequent cascading biological responses, and therefore, the relationships between concentration and effect are more complex. Binding to a target is still necessary, but relating concentration to response, especially with respect to time, may show delays because of distinct temporal phases associated with subsequent intracellular interactions involving translocation, stimulation, or repression of regulatory elements, or protein synthesis (Mager et al. 2003). Good examples of indirect models are the biology of corticosteroids or the vitamin K–dependent anticoagulants like warfarin, where relating the plasma concentrations to biological effects must account for multiple, discrete interactions between receptors and downstream regulatory elements (Jusko and Ko 1994). Understanding the biological target and chemical mechanism are therefore critical elements for interpreting the concentration effects seen and relating the TK to the biology, especially when the time course for biological response does not mirror plasma concentration.

Measurement of parent drug or metabolites forms the basis for all TK calculations and subsequent conclusions, and the development and application of robust, sensitive, and selective assays using whole blood or, most often, plasma or serum are critical. Most often, these assays combine the separation capacity of HPLC with the exquisite sensitivity and selectivity of mass spectrometry and are adapted from assays developed to investigate the PK of much lower doses. Defining the appropriate concentration range for the assay with respect to accuracy (i.e., the agreement between the theoretical and measured concentration) and precision (i.e., the variability of replicate measurements of the same concentration) is key since the assay must be able to measure concentrations spanning the time course for drug action and the dosing interval. While high sensitivity, that is, nanogram or sub-nanogram per milliliter concentration limits, is often not required (since the dosages used are relatively high), the ability to dilute samples and still maintain accuracy and precision is necessary. For those molecules with inherent chemical or metabolic instability because of oxidation or hydrolysis, establishing appropriate collection and storage conditions is key to ensuring accurate measurements. Species differences in potential matrix effects (suppression or enhancement of the mass spectral response), produced by endogenous components in plasma, must also be evaluated. Important matrix effects can also be produced by excipients in the dosing vehicles, or by hemolysis of samples, and must be eliminated. Detailed requirements for the successful validation of chemical assays according to international regulatory standards can be found in ICH and FDA Guidance documents and industry-FDA workshop reports (Viswanathan et al. 2007).

3.3 TK OR PK PARAMETERS: WHAT THEY ARE, HOW THEY ARE DERIVED, AND WHAT THEY MEAN

The two most critical questions about drug disposition in blood or tissue are "how much" and "how fast." This section will focus on those raw and transformed data generally derived from measurements of drug or metabolite in plasma or serum that are used to answer these two questions. The goal of this section is not to provide the reader with the mathematical derivation of these parameters or the ability to calculate them, but rather to understand their definition, application, and limitations. The most commonly reported TK parameters are defined in Table 3.1 and will be discussed subsequently in greater detail.

The critical application of drug disposition in the interpretation of toxicology and pathology is based on (1) raw data derived from the study design, sampling scheme, and the subsequent determination of plasma or serum concentrations; and (2) transformed data, the expression of TK parameters using the relationships between concentration and time. This chapter will refer to plasma concentrations, recognizing that serum and rarely whole blood concentrations can be measured and used in the calculations, and we will assume that the calculation of the TK parameters is by non-compartmental analysis. "Compartments" are simply kinetically (mathematically) distinguishable phases, which may or may not have any relevance to real biological spaces or processes, but which

TABLE 3.1

TK Parameters and Their Definition

1. C_{max}: The maximum (systemic, e.g., plasma) concentration observed.
2. T_{max}: The time at which C_{max} is observed (reported as the median).
3. AUC: Area under the concentration–time curve, generally integrated by trapezoidal approximations, from 0 to the last measureable sample (AUC_{0-last}), over a specified interval (i.e., $AUC_{0-24\,h}$), or extrapolated from 0 to infinity (AUC_{0-inf}).
4. AUMC: Area under the first moment curve. AUMC is most often calculated using the AUC and time and is used in the calculation of mean residence time (MRT).
5. MRT: Mean residence time. Another measure of compound elimination, expressed as the average time the compound stays in the body (such that the greater the MRT, the longer the residence and, hence, the slower the elimination).
6. k_{el}: Typically the first-order rate constant for the apparent terminal elimination phase (also known as β).
7. $T_{1/2}$: The apparent terminal elimination half-life. The terminal elimination most importantly reflects drug clearance; however, it is often confused with the last, slowest phase of drug disappearance from plasma (which often does not reflect drug clearance, as discussed later in greater detail).
8. CP_0: The concentration after an IV bolus dose extrapolated to time 0. (Note that this is not the same as C_{max}, which is dependent upon the sampling scheme).
9. CL_s: Systemic or total body clearance. This is the sum of all processes irreversibly removing drug from the body.
10. V_d: The apparent volume of distribution calculated for steady state (V_{dss}) or using the terminal elimination phase (V_z or $V_{d\beta}$).
11. F: The bioavailability or fraction of the non-parenteral dose that reaches the systemic circulation intact.
12. R: The accumulation factor calculated after multiple dosing. Often expressed for C_{max} and AUC.

are often used in the construction of the equations describing plasma concentration–time relationships and drug transfer. The analysis of concentration–time data by noncompartmental methods, typically using commercially available computer programs like WinNonlin, is preferred because no assumptions need to be made about the number of compartments or phases, or whether the sampling scheme was adequate to provide enough experimental data to accurately describe each compartment. It cannot be overemphasized (and will be discussed in greater detail subsequently) that appropriate experimental design (collecting enough samples at the right times) is the foundation for reliable TK.

There are obvious differences in the appearance of the concentration–time curves for different routes of drug administration and fundamental differences in the meaning of the raw and transformed concentration data obtained after parenteral (typically IV), oral, or other routes with an absorption element. While the TK parameters derived to quantitate these processes and form the basis for interpreting differences between species, dosages, genders, and responses are identical (e.g., area under the curve [AUC] or $T_{1/2}$), their interpretation must account for important differences in the route of administration and the physiological or biochemical processes underlying the numbers.

3.3.1 PLASMA CONCENTRATION–TIME CURVES: WHERE THE NUMBERS COME FROM

Typical concentration–time curves, and the processes reflected by each portion of the curve, are described below.

Concentration–time curves are depicted in both rectilinear and log-linear plots of concentration (ordinate) versus time (abscissa), and the reason for this and the advantages of each depiction requires a brief note about rates and their order. When the rate, defined as a change in some variable (like concentration) over time, is constant, the reaction is called zero order with respect to the concentration of drug and the rectilinear graph is a straight line. The rate of elimination can be independent of concentration if, for example, the elimination is saturated above a certain threshold concentration, and this is obviously important in toxicology studies where very high dosages are often given and may saturate the mechanisms for clearance. In contrast to a zero-order reaction, the rate of most biological processes changes with concentration, that is, the rate is first order with respect to concentration, with a constant fraction eliminated per unit time. A rectilinear graph of a first-order reaction will curve, slowing down as concentrations diminish, while a log-linear graph of a first-order reaction reveals a straight line. The advantage of depicting concentration–time data for drugs in a log-linear plot is the ease in visually estimating the half-life for elimination (Figure 3.1).

After an oral dose, there are usually three distinct phases in the concentration–time profile that represent the processes of absorption, distribution, and elimination (Figure 3.1). In the early phase where concentrations are rising, the process of absorption is faster than the processes of distribution and elimination, although the latter are still occurring. Under the simplest conditions, when the rate of elimination equals the rate of absorption, concentrations are neither rising nor falling, and a peak (C_{max}) is observed. As the rate of absorption diminishes and the rate of elimination predominates, concentrations fall with time. These phases are also observed after other routes of dosing where absorption occurs, that is, intraperitoneal, intramuscular, or subcutaneous. If subsequent doses are given before the entire preceding dose is eliminated, plasma concentrations accumulate and eventually reach steady state, where the rate of input equals the rate of elimination.

After a constant-rate IV infusion, plasma concentrations also rise as the rate of input (analogous to absorption) exceeds the rate of exit (i.e., elimination) and plateau as the rate of input (infusion rate) equals elimination (clearance). When the infusion is turned off, plasma concentrations decline as elimination occurs. By definition, the plateau concentration is the steady-state concentration, and as long as the clearance stays constant, a change in the infusion rate will produce a proportional change in the steady-state concentration. One key experimental advantage to conducting investigative toxicology studies at steady state is the ability to produce and hold concentrations at a desired level and know that in the absence of any transporter-mediated disequilibria, the concentrations of free or unbound drug are the same in plasma and the target site of action.

Bolus IV doses often produce plasma concentration–time curves with distinct phases having different slopes. Since there is no absorption component, these phases most often represent the decline in concentrations as distribution is faster than elimination, the transition between distribution and elimination, and the terminal elimination of drug. Additional phases in the plasma concentration–time curves, especially at longer periods postdose where concentrations are very low, can sometimes be seen if the assay is very sensitive. These phases are often interpreted as the redistribution of drug from deep tissue (i.e., fat) and elimination, and should not be confused with the clearance of the drug.

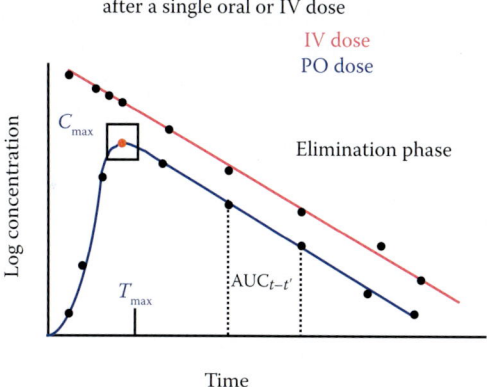

FIGURE 3.1   Typical plasma concentration–time curves for an oral dose and an IV bolus dose.

3.3.2 TK PARAMETERS DERIVED FROM RAW DATA

One critical measure of drug exposure is the maximum plasma concentration produced by a given dosage, or C_{max}. This parameter is taken directly from the measured plasma concentrations in each animal and is therefore critically dependent on the study design. As noted earlier, C_{max} occurs when the rates of absorption and elimination are equal; therefore, the absolute value of C_{max} (for a given dosage) can reflect changes in both processes. Increasing the rate of absorption (e.g., by enhancing solubility through formulation, without changing the rate of elimination or drug distribution) will produce a higher C_{max}. C_{max} may be decreased if the elimination is enhanced, for example, by enzyme induction and more rapid metabolism. C_{max} is also a function of the dosage, bioavailability, and volume of distribution. Often, "C_{max}" is reported for IV bolus studies, but this is likely not the maximum plasma concentration produced by the dose but rather the concentration at the first sampling time. For those drugs with an extensive distribution phase, the true maximum plasma concentrations produced by the bolus dose may be greatly underestimated by a study design using delayed and infrequent blood sampling. The maximum concentration extrapolated after an IV bolus, CP_0, can only be obtained by extrapolation and curve fitting.

T_{max} is the other important parameter taken directly from the raw data. While T_{max} is often used to judge the rate of absorption, this parameter can also reflect biopharmaceutical properties like disintegration of solid dosage forms, dissolution rates, and gastric emptying, in addition to the balance between absorption and elimination rates mentioned earlier. For example, a delay in gastric emptying may produce a lag phase in the appearance of the plasma concentration–time curve (shifting the entire curve to later times) but may ultimately produce the same C_{max} at a later time (T_{max}). Important physiological factors influencing both the rate and extent of absorption and hence C_{max} and T_{max} are discussed in a subsequent section.

3.3.3 TK PARAMETERS DERIVED FROM TRANSFORMED DATA

The simplest transformation of the raw plasma concentration–time data is the calculation of the AUC. This is a key value since it serves as an important exposure parameter *per se* and is the foundation for the calculation of other TK parameters such as clearance (CL), volume of distribution (V_d), bioavailability (F), and mean residence time (MRT). AUC is most often calculated by the summation of distinct trapezoids representing the individual areas for each change in concentration over time or by computer algorithms integrating the function describing the concentration–time curve. The accurate calculation of AUC depends intimately on the sampling scheme, because taking few samples spaced widely results in large trapezoids with the potential to significantly under- or overestimate the AUC, or insufficient points needed to construct the mathematical equation describing the curve. It is important to recognize that while AUC provides a number for the time-averaged exposure to a compound, differently shaped concentration–time curves can produce the same AUC, so the graph of the concentration–time curves must be examined when comparing two drugs with the same AUC. While the importance of this concept is often recognized in therapeutic areas such as infectious disease, where antiviral or antibiotic efficacy is dependent upon maintaining concentrations above a threshold value for a certain period, it is obviously applicable for toxicities. The AUC over the sampling interval can be calculated directly from the data, but extrapolating the AUC to infinity requires the rate constant for the terminal slope (k_{el}) and the last measureable concentration (C_{last}) so that the last wedge of area can be calculated according to Equation 3.1:

$$\text{AUC}_{last-inf} = C_{last}/k_{el}. \tag{3.1}$$

There are two important relationships between the AUC after single and multiple doses: (1) the AUC_{0-inf} is equal to the AUC over the dosing interval at steady state, and (2) the AUC over the dosing interval at steady state divided by the AUC over the first dosing interval defines the accumulation (R) of the drug.

Because these relationships only hold true if the factors governing the AUC remain constant during repeated dosing, deviations from these relationships indicate a change in those factors responsible for AUC, that is, clearance, distribution, or both.

Clearance, typically expressed in units of volume per unit of time, is the sum of all processes removing drug from the sampling site (assumed to represent the body) and is independent of any other factors. Clearance is an independent parameter and is the critical measure of a drug's elimination. Clearance is calculated as the ratio of the administered dose and the resultant AUC (calculated as $Dose/AUC_{0-inf}$ for an IV dose or $Dose \cdot F/AUC_{0-inf}$ for an oral dose, where F is the bioavailability) and is an additive parameter of all processes (Equation 3.2).

$$CL \text{ total} = CL \text{ metabolism} + CL \text{ renal} + CL \text{ biliary} + CL \text{ other}. \qquad (3.2)$$

Total body clearance or systemic clearance is most rigorously determined after an IV dose, since no assumptions need to be made about the fraction of the given dose that reaches the circulation and is therefore available for elimination. Clearance can be determined after extravascular dosing, but unless the fraction reaching systemic circulation (F) is 100% or is known, this clearance term must be defined as "apparent" and is much less useful in relating the value to physiological variables, since F could also be changing. Many drugs are cleared by saturable hepatic mechanisms such as enzymatic metabolism or active transport into the bile, and their extraction from perfusing blood can be classified as either "high" or "low," depending upon the efficiency of the clearance mechanism. When, for example, intrinsic hepatic metabolism and hence extraction is high, clearance after an IV dose will be dependent upon drug delivery to the liver (i.e., hepatic blood flow), while for drugs that are not extracted efficiently, but are still totally metabolized, clearance will depend on the enzymatic activity of the liver (Wilkinson and Shand 1975). These two categories for drug clearance are important to consider, since changes in the extraction by the liver, for example, by enzyme induction, can produce differing effects on apparent half-life, as well as clearance. Clearance can often be saturated at high concentrations, leading to a disproportionate increase in the AUC and a nonlinear relationship between dosage and AUC. Saturation may also be observed after a single dose and is often evident as a change in the slope of the curve, as the elimination goes from a first-order to a zero-order reaction. Clearance can also be accelerated with repeated dosing, most often because of enzyme induction. For compounds that are highly extracted, changes in enzyme activity have little effect on the AUC after IV doses, since clearance is already high and depends on drug delivery to the clearing organ, while the AUC after oral doses would be changed (lowered) in proportion to the change in enzymatic activity. The effects of changing extraction on the AUC of an oral dose for a highly extracted compound differs from the effects on the IV dose because the small fraction of the dose escaping extraction after oral absorption is exquisitely sensitive to any additional change in the efficiency of the elimination of that small fraction. The reader is referred to the seminal paper by Wilkinson and Shand (1975) for a detailed discussion of the equations, their derivation, and the biochemical and physiological interpretation of clearance.

Plasma or serum concentrations are most often measured, but blood is the perfusate *in vivo*. A fundamental assumption in the physiological interpretation of PK or TK parameters is that concentrations in plasma (or serum) and blood are equivalent or that plasma concentrations are corrected to reflect blood concentrations using the blood/plasma partition ratio (B/P). This is easily done experimentally and is especially important when drugs may selectively partition into erythrocytes and bind to intracellular targets like carbonic anhydrase.

Another important PK or TK variable is the volume of distribution (V_d). Like clearance, V_d is most rigorously determined and most commonly reported for drugs given intravenously. V_d is not a physiological volume but is a proportionality constant that relates the *amount* of drug in the body to the *concentration* in plasma. The V_d can be calculated several ways from different data, and it is important to appreciate the differences because the resulting number reflects the experimental design and the sources of variability, as well as fundamental differences in assumptions and interpretation. The simplest but most inaccurate method of calculating the apparent V_d is done by dividing the IV dose (amount in milligrams) by the experimentally determined initial plasma concentration, CP_0 (in milligrams per milliliter). This method depends critically on the time chosen for the initial sample collection and the extrapolation to CP_0. The apparent $V_{d\beta}$ is calculated using the terminal rate constant for elimination (k_{el} or β) and is therefore critically dependent on the accurate determination of the "terminal" elimination phase and is influenced by the rates of distribution. Both of these calculations assume that drug is in rapid equilibrium between plasma and tissue and that elimination occurs from the systemic circulation. The most accurate estimate of the distribution volume is determined after infusion to steady state or after a bolus IV dose and calculation of V_{dss} from the plasma AUC and AUMC using statistical moment analysis. Often, the V_d for a drug is interpreted in the context of physiological volumes such as total body water, extracellular water, or total blood volume, to place the number in perspective relative to biological and chemical characteristics. Drug distribution is governed by chemical factors (e.g., lipophilicity, polarity, size, and ionization) and biological factors (e.g., permeability and plasma and tissue protein binding). For drugs that are un-ionized, moderately lipophilic, freely permeable across biological membranes, and negligibly bound to plasma proteins, V_d will be high and typically exceed total body water. Examples of drugs or toxins with V_d that exceed any physiological volumes are chloroquine (132–261 L/kg) or chlorpromazine (21 L/g), while compounds such as the sugar inulin (0.16 L/kg) or urea (0.67 L/kg) are confined to extracellular water (0.26 L/kg) or total body water (0.6 L/kg), respectively. It is important to emphasize that while V_d is often interpreted in physiological and physicochemical terms, and V_d for some molecules are markers of distinct anatomical space, this interpretation must be made cautiously. Moreover, the tissue expression of biochemical transporters such as the P-glycoprotein transporter (P-gp), especially those in liver and kidney, can affect the actual distribution of molecules and the calculated V_d (Grover and Benet 2009).

Depictions of log plasma concentration–time curves, most notably after IV doses, are often multiphasic, with different linear phases representing apparent distribution and elimination. While half-life is the most visible parameter associated with the terminal phase of drug elimination, it is often the most misunderstood PK or TK parameter. Unlike clearance or volume, two independent parameters, half-life is entirely *dependent* upon clearance and volume, and half-life cannot be changed without a change in one or both of these two fundamental parameters. The relationship between clearance, volume, and half-life is illustrated in Equation 3.3:

$$T_{1/2} = 0.693 \cdot V/CL_s. \tag{3.3}$$

For compounds whose clearance is relatively low and dependent on the intrinsic rate of enzyme metabolism, half-life can be lengthened when clearance is decreased (e.g., by saturation of metabolism at high concentrations), and conversely half-life can be shortened by increased clearance (e.g., via enzyme induction) (Wilkinson and Shand 1975). Changes in distribution can also affect the apparent half-life, with increasing V_d producing a longer half-life and decreasing V_d shortening the half-life. While half-life is most accurately determined after IV administration, especially after an infusion to steady state is stopped, most TK experiments are not designed to accurately capture half-life, especially after repeated oral dosing, and this parameter must be interpreted cautiously.

As discussed previously, the shape of the concentration–time curve after oral (or intramuscular or dermal application) is a composite of absorption and elimination phases (Figure 3.1), and in some cases, absorption can be enhanced or prolonged, especially after the administration of high dosages of freely permeable compounds or when co-solvents or depot formulations are used. When the rate of absorption exceeds the rate of elimination, disappearance of compound after C_{max} is prolonged, and the *apparent* elimination half-life is lengthened (especially if the sampling interval is short). This phenomenon of prolonged, rapid absorption contaminating the apparent elimination of concentrations at later time points is referred to as "flip-flop pharmacokinetics" (because the usual interpretation of the rates controlling the appearance of the concentration–time curve are flipped, i.e., the disappearance of drug actually reflects the rate of absorption rather than the rate of elimination). This phenomenon can have a profound effect on the apparent elimination phase and estimated half-life, in addition to the appearance of a broad C_{max} (Yanez et al. 2011). The magnitude of this effect and the degree to which the apparent elimination half-life is overestimated depend on the relative differences between the rate constants for absorption (k_a) and elimination (k_{el}) and physiological factors such as the gastrointestinal (GI) segments participating in drug absorption and GI transit times. This phenomenon should not be confused with enterohepatic circulation of drugs (Roberts et al. 2002), the process by which drugs or their conjugates are excreted efficiently in the bile and then into the intestine and are reabsorbed intact or after enzymatic deconjugation by GI flora, therefore also prolonging the apparent absorption of the dose. Flip-flop kinetics are often uncovered or demonstrated by experiments that alter oral absorption rate (e.g., a different formulation) or after comparison with the half-life determined after IV dosing. Enterohepatic circulation is most often demonstrated using bile duct–cannulated rats or dogs, where the diversion of bile prevents bile release into the lumen and subsequent hydrolysis of conjugates and reabsorption of intact drug.

3.4 IMPORTANCE OF EXPERIMENTAL DESIGN AND DATA PRESENTATION

Providing an accurate and complete collection of plasma concentrations from which the TK parameters are calculated is *the* essential foundation upon which accurate conclusions are built. But drawing the blood samples for analysis is a compromise between the desire to provide accurate data and the practical limits and logistics of technician time, blood volume allowances, assay sensitivity, and cost. Preliminary TK or PK is essential in defining the sampling scheme for pivotal GLP studies, in determining the relationship between dosage and exposure, and in providing the best choice for the limited sampling scheme necessary, especially for rodent studies. While blood volume is not often limiting in dog and nonhuman primate studies, the potential need for restraint, either chemical (sedation or anesthesia) or physical (chairs or squeeze cages), must also be considered in the design of studies using these species.

The design of rodent TK studies depends on the plasma volume needed for the analytical method, knowledge from dose-range finding studies, and the potential variability of the drug. Typically, a staggered, overlapping composite sampling scheme will be used where different groups of animals are bled at different times, and a composite concentration–time curve is constructed from the mean data at each time point. Table 3.2 illustrates a typical design.

TABLE 3.2
Typical Staggered Sampling Scheme for Repeated Oral Dose Rat TK Studies

Time (h)	Animal Number											
	1	2	3	4	5	6	7	8	9	10	11	12
Predose	X	X	X									
1				X	X	X						
2							X	X	X			
4										X	X	X
8	X	X	X									
24[a]				X	X	X						

[a] Predose for the next daily dose.

Typically the same animal can provide a maximum of three samples over a 24 h period, assuming a 1 ml total blood sample (to provide approximately 0.4 ml of plasma). Terminal blood samples are usually provided from mice, and the number of animals per group per sampling time must be adjusted accordingly.

Plasma concentrations from each animal are measured, and the mean and standard deviation for each sampling time are calculated. Group C_{max} and AUC values are then calculated using the mean concentration at each time, generating a composite plasma concentration–time curve. These composite parameters are then used to determine linearity of exposure with dosage, sex differences in exposure at each dosage, and differences after repeated dosing in comparison with Day 1 C_{max} and AUC (i.e., unexpected accumulation or decreased exposure). Typically, differences of less than twofold between sexes or after repeated dosing are not considered biologically meaningful, since the small sample size, variability inherent in the composite study design, and the biological variability in drug disposition preclude a more precise characterization. A more rigorous study design (i.e., more individual animals and greater sampling frequency) or different route of administration (i.e., IV infusion to steady state, eliminating variability in oral absorption) would be required if significant biological differences were suspected, and a precise TK toxicity evaluation was needed.

Tabular data can often be misleading, and individual as well as mean concentration–time curves must always be available for review. When few samples are drawn, typically four to six time points from 0 to 24 h postdose from satellite TK groups, the accuracy of T_{max} and C_{max} values is often compromised, especially when the highest dosages produce either saturation of metabolism or prolonged absorption. The accurate estimation of half-life also requires an adequate number of samples (minimally 3) to define the elimination phase, and this is often difficult to satisfy when the concentration–time curves are broad and few or no samples are taken between 8 and 24 h postdose. The other pivotal exposure parameter, AUC, is also dependent upon the experimental design and sampling scheme. Longer intervals between samples create larger trapezoids, whose shape can obviously be skewed if the plasma concentrations (e.g., at higher dosages) are shifted. The AUC can also be determined from the analysis of a single plasma sample, created by pooling different volumes corresponding to the different collection intervals (Hamilton et al. 1981). The premise of this method is that the concentration in the sample (e.g., in micrograms per milliliter), multiplied by the overall time interval for sample collection (in hours), equals the AUC (in microgram-hour per milliliter). While this method is theoretically valid and can be technically attractive, especially for determining the AUC of metabolites across different studies with many samples, it obviously eliminates any possibility to examine the shape of the concentration–time curves.

3.5 IMPORTANT CHEMICAL AND BIOLOGICAL FACTORS GOVERNING TK: ABSORPTION, DISTRIBUTION, METABOLISM, EXCRETION, TRANSPORT

3.5.1 Factors Governing Oral Absorption

The appearance of drug in the systemic circulation is the end result of many biological and physicochemical processes, including absorption and metabolism. To be absorbed, a molecule must be in solution, and while many studies administer drug as solutions, higher dosages can often be suspensions *per se*, or drug may precipitate out of solution *in vivo* where different pH environments can be encountered. Occasionally, neat drug in capsules is dosed, introducing additional steps (i.e., capsule wetting and disintegration, then powder wetting and dispersion) that can affect both the rate and the extent of absorption. The biology of the GI tract, in both the fed and fasted state, also regulates absorption and contributes to the variability in TK. Overall, absorption depends on the sequential events of dissolution, solubility at a given pH, GI transit times, intrinsic membrane permeability, and the concentration gradient between free drug in solution in the lumen and bloodstream at the site of absorption. Producing high concentrations of drug molecules in solution is essential for maximizing absorption, in the absence of permeability barriers. While the subsequent discussion will focus on oral absorption, most of the physicochemical and biological concepts also apply to absorption from depot sites.

The rate and extent of absorption depend on the fundamental chemical properties of the molecule (i.e., pH-dependent ionization, polar surface area, polarity, lipophilicity), the drug substance properties, and the biological milieu. Drug absorption of highly permeable compounds is typically characterized as dissolution rate limited or solubility rate limited (Sugano et al. 2007), and while these two processes are linked, the distinction between dissolution and solubility is critical for understanding those drug characteristics that enhance or limit absorption. Dissolution is a time-dependent event and is the process of breaking apart the molecular forces holding together chemical solids and producing molecules that can be surrounded by solvent, that is, in solution. Solubility is a fundamental property of chemical structure and can be defined as the concentration of molecules that exist in a specified solvent (e.g., water, or gastric or intestinal fluid at a given pH) under specified conditions (e.g., at equilibrium with undissolved powder). These are important distinctions since large doses of relatively insoluble compounds are often administered in toxicology studies, where maximizing systemic exposure is critical, and the success of different approaches to increasing absorption and exposure depends on defining the rate-limiting step.

Dissolution is a surface phenomenon, most often increased experimentally by decreasing the particle size of drugs, thus providing more surface area for solvent interactions, and by increasing solubility by the addition of excipients such as detergents or buffers to modify the solvent environment. Dissolution rate may vary in different fluids (e.g., simulated gastric or intestinal fluid), *in vitro* surrogates for physiological milieu (Klein 2010). For drugs that dissolve rapidly and extensively, increasing the mass (dosage) will increase the rate and amount absorbed, and thus, the C_{max} and AUC would be proportional to dosage. Decreasing particle size and increasing the mass (dosage) will have little or no effect on the oral absorption of solubility-limited drugs, since the driving force is the concentration of molecules in solution, a process that depends on inherent chemical properties (lipophilicity, polarity, ionization) and chemical form (e.g., crystalline versus amorphous drug, salt versus free base or acid). Once maximum solubility (saturation) in the fluid is reached, adding more mass (dosage) would not produce a higher concentration in solution, and thus, C_{max} and AUC would not be proportional to an increase in dosage for solubility-limited drugs. At the molecular level, there is an unstirred solvent layer surrounding the solid drug that must be traversed before a molecule can be considered in solution in the bulk fluid (i.e., gastric or intestinal fluid), but the effects of this unstirred layer (and that of the unstirred layer surrounding the epithelial cells of the intestine) are outside the scope of this discussion. The other likely cause of poor absorption, permeability, will be discussed below in the context of biological factors controlling absorption.

pH plays a critical role in the solubility and oral absorption and TK of ionizable drugs, whether given as free acids or bases, or as salts. Because there may be dramatic differences in the solubility of salts and free acids or bases, the solubility of both must be determined to understand potential discrepancies between *in vitro* and *in vivo* behavior. The species-dependent differences in gastric and intestinal pH, and the effects on oral drug absorption, are discussed in a subsequent section.

The basic processes of intestinal absorption at the cellular level are depicted in Figure 3.2. Once in solution, drug absorption most often occurs passively, either by transcellular flux across the lipid membranes of the epithelial cells or by paracellular flow through the junctions between cells. Active influx transporters can also facilitate drug absorption in a structure- and species-dependent manner (International Transporter Consortium 2010; Shugarts and Benet 2009). Active transport can occur at either the apical or basolateral membrane and can serve to facilitate or limit drug absorption or remove drug from circulation into the intestinal lumen (which ultimately appears as intestinal secretion).

Conceptually, those factors regulating passive, transcellular absorption are described by Fick's law, where

$$\text{Rate} = P \cdot A \cdot (C_{lumen} - C_{blood})/t,$$

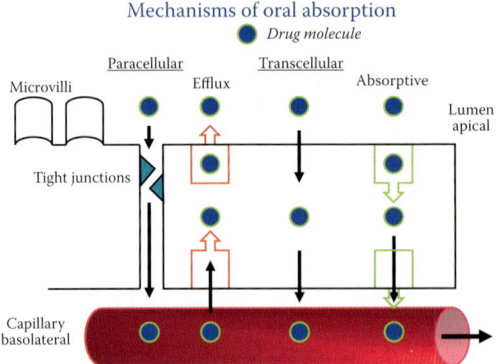

FIGURE 3.2   Schematic representation of oral absorption mechanisms.

where P is the permeability coefficient (including a diffusion and partitioning term related to chemical structure), A is the surface area over which the absorption will occur, $(C_{lumen} - C_{blood})$ is the concentration gradient of the drug in solution in the GI lumen and blood, and t is the thickness or path length across which the molecule must move. This equation clearly shows that the rate of passive flux is directly proportional to the concentration gradient, the area available for absorption, and the intrinsic permeability of the molecule and is indirectly proportional to the thickness of the barrier. The importance of manipulating dissolution and solubility to establish the maximum concentration gradient has been discussed previously.

The intrinsic permeability of a molecule to cross lipid membranes, expressed as flux and often measured *in vitro* using artificial membrane assays such as PAMPA (which stands for parallel artificial membrane permeation assay) (Avdeef 2005) or cell-based assays such as the Caco-2 or MDCK systems (Volpe 2011), is a fundamental property of the molecule and must reflect a balance between aqueous solubility and lipophilicity. In general, poorly permeable molecules are poorly absorbed passively, and exposure is variable and not proportional to an increase in dosage. Poorly permeable and poorly soluble drugs often present the greatest challenge to achieving high systemic exposure and reliable TK because little can be done to experimentally manipulate transcellular permeability, even in the face of enhanced solubility.

Although most lipophilic, low-molecular-weight drugs are absorbed transcellularly, absorption may also occur paracellularly, through the tight junctions between epithelial cells. This route may be important for polar, hydrophilic chemicals and is governed by both size and charge restrictions (Knipp et al. 1997). Paracellular absorption is an important consideration for toxicologists because of the pronounced species dependence for this pathway in dogs. For example, the oral absorption of polyethylene glycol mixtures, which are markers for paracellular passage, was greater in dogs than in rats, apparently because of larger pore sizes and greater paracellular capacity (He et al. 1998). Thus, dogs may have greater systemic exposure to molecules absorbed by this route than other species, including humans. As will be discussed subsequently, rats and macaques have other similarities to humans with respect to GI physiology that suggest that oral absorption in these species, in contrast to the dog, more closely reflects absorption in humans.

Absorption *in vivo* must also include a time element, since the administered dose and drug in solution passes through several finite anatomical regions, each associated with its own segment length, transit time, pH, and effective surface area characteristics. In general, gastric emptying of liquids is faster than that of solids (Camilleri 2006), and smaller-sized particles are also emptied more rapidly in animals such as dogs and monkeys (Ikegami et al. 2003; Kaniwa et al. 1988). Changes in gastric emptying times can affect absorption (e.g., by introducing lag phases until the drug is introduced to the small intestine) and prolong T_{max} and possibly lower C_{max}.

3.5.2 Species Differences in GI Physiology

Species differences in GI pH may have dramatic effects on drug solubility for acids or bases, while differences in gastric emptying and intestinal transit times may affect the time course for drug presentation to portions of the intestines with the greatest surface area and from which absorption is most likely to occur. Additionally, the presence of bile salts acting as detergents may aid in the solubilization of molecules with inherently low aqueous solubility. As discussed previously, absorption by dogs may be greater than by rodents or monkeys because of the pronounced paracellular capacity in dogs. Important species differences in GI physiology are listed in Table 3.3, and the processes of pH-dependent absorption and gastric emptying are discussed in greater detail subsequently.

There is often a marked difference in exposure (AUC or C_{max}) between fasted rats and dogs given the same dosage of permeable compounds absorbed transcellularly. In rats, a species with good basal acid secretion, fasted pH is low and stable throughout the day, including the evening period when feeding occurs (Rudholm et al. 2008). This is in contrast to the dog where the fasting gastric pH can be low but has been measured experimentally in gastric aspirates or using an *in vivo* telemeterized capsule to vary widely from 2.05 or 2.7 to 8.3 (Akimoto et al. 2000; Sagawa et al. 2009). This profound species difference and variability in dogs are most often observed when basic molecules are dosed because weak bases are most soluble in acidic solutions. The pH-dependent absorption of the HIV protease inhibitor indinavir (Crixivan) is an excellent example of the importance of pH for the absorption of weak bases and the potential magnitude of the species difference between dogs and rats. Lin et al. found a statistically significant 4.2-fold increase in the mean AUC of indinavir in dogs when the drug was given orally in a citric acid vehicle versus methylcellulose,

TABLE 3.3
Important Species Differences in GI Physiology That Affect TK

Parameter	Units	SD Rat	Beagle Dog	Cynomolgus Monkey	Human
Gallbladder		No	Yes	Yes	Yes
Bile Flow	ml/day	12–23	190–360	95–160	350
Gastric Emptying	h, fasted	1	1.5 ± 0.5	2.6	~1
	h, fed	>6	9–20	7.3 (slurry)	3–4
			6–11	11.6 (biscuit)	
Small Intestine Transit Time	h	ND	1.9 (variable)	2.2–4.2 (fasted) 2.2–3.2 (fed)	5–7 (fasted)
Oral–Cecal Transit Time	h	4 (fasted) >6 (fed)	ND	ND	ND
Gastric pH	Fasted	2.3	1.8–6.8	1.9 (chair) 2.0–2.2 (cage)	1.8 2.9 ± 2.0
	Fed	2.3	1.1–1.3	4.8 (slurry) 4.9 (biscuit)	6.4 → 2.7
Duodenal pH		ND	7.3 ± 0.1	ND	6.2 6.6 → 5.2
Jejunal pH		ND		ND	7.1 ± 0.6 7.2

Source: The data are mean, median, or range values compiled from the following literature: Davies and Morris (1993), DeSesso and Jacobsen (2001), Karali (1995), Rudholm et al. (2008), Kimura and Higaki (2002), Boillat et al. (2010), Sagawa et al. (2009), Akimoto et al. (2000), Lui et al. (1986), Chen et al. (2008), Dressman (1986), Willmann et al. (2007), Ikegami et al. (2003), Kalantzi et al. (*Pharm Res*, 23:165–176, 2006), Lindahl et al. (1997), and Russell et al. (1993).

Note: SD, Sprague–Dawley rat; ND, no data available.

while the AUC in rats was not significantly different (Lin et al. 1995). Mean C_{max} was similarly increased in dogs by 3-fold but was unchanged in rats. In addition to buffered dosing vehicles, gastric pH can be manipulated experimentally *in vivo* using the acid secretagogue pentagastrin to lower pH and H2 antagonists like famotidine to raise gastric pH. The AUC of the weak base ketoconazole was increased 30-fold in dogs given pentagastrin versus control or those given famotidine (Zhou et al. 2005), again emphasizing the importance of maximizing solubility and the concentration gradient for absorption.

Cynomolgus monkeys have a lower and more consistently acidic fasting gastric pH, similar to rats and humans, and this pH is the same in monkeys held in chairs or cages, approximately 1.9–2.2 (Table 3.2; Chen et al. 2008). Feeding raises gastric pH in macaques to a peak of 6.1–6.6 and an elevated pH (mean of 4.8–4.9) is maintained 60 min after the meal (Chen et al. 2008). This is similar to the response in humans, likely because of the buffering capacity of the meal, but different from the response in dogs, where pH is unchanged or actually decreased, likely because of the increased acid production stimulated by the meal. The effects of food and feeding on TK can be complex and may be different for molecules with differing solubility and permeability, since feeding may change gastric pH and emptying time, bile secretion, and intestinal pH (via pancreatic stimulation and bicarbonate secretion).

Feeding slows gastric emptying in all species (Table 3.3), thus delaying entry of the dose into the region with the most absorptive surface area and favorable pH for weak bases. In fasted rats, gastric emptying of an unabsorbable marker was rapid and essentially complete within 1 h but could be prolonged for up to 6 h in some animals (Haruta et al. 2001). Kimura and Higaki (2002) combined data from several literature sources to develop an integrated model of GI transit and absorption in rats, and this model also projected segmental transit rates for individual segments of the small intestine. The average gastric emptying time for a solid Bravo pH-sensing capsule in fasted dogs ($n = 16$) was 1.4 h, while after a 10 or 200 g solid food meal, the mean time was increased to 9.4 and 20 h, respectively (Sagawa et al. 2009). In addition to their role in toxicology, dogs are often used to predict potential food effects on drug disposition in humans (Lentz 2008), although the important differences in physiology and anatomy must be recognized. The gastric residence time for fasted or fed cynomolgus monkeys was highly variable, ranging from 31 to 294 min (fasted), from 192 to 950 min (after a slurry meal), and from 406 to 932 min (after a meal of biscuits), and was significantly ($p < 0.05$) prolonged after either meal (Chen et al. 2008). Feeding also prolonged the mean absorption time of acetaminophen given as an oral solution, enteric-coated granules, or enteric-coated tablets to cynomolgus monkeys by approximately twofold, and high variability was also observed in this PK surrogate for gastric emptying regardless of feeding status (Ikegami et al. 2003). While mean T_{max} was also increased approximately twofold after feeding, the effects on C_{max} and AUC were mixed, with a twofold reduction in C_{max} observed after feeding for the solution and granules, with negligible changes in AUC. These data emphasize that gastric emptying in macaques can vary widely, and while feeding may prolong emptying, the effects on TK parameters may be complex.

3.5.3 Drug Distribution, Protein Binding, and the Importance of Free (Unbound) Drug and Regulation of Concentrations in Privileged Sites

Drug molecules circulate in the bloodstream and reside in tissues in equilibrium between the free (unbound) form and drug reversibly bound to proteins, most often albumin and alpha-1-acid glycoprotein. Concentrations of the free drug are most important, since it is the free drug that crosses membranes and interacts with receptors, enzymes, channels, and transporters to produce desired and undesired effects. The critical concept to emphasize is that the free fraction (typically expressed as percentage) is the value to use when calculating and comparing the exposure to active drug at different dosages and plasma concentrations, in different animal species, for different molecules, and against *in vitro* potency or affinity data. Many *in vitro* assays contain little additional protein other than the target receptor, and the potency for ligand binding, expressed in concentration units, most often reflects the assumption that the added drug is all unbound (free). The critical role of the free fraction is illustrated by considering two drugs having the same potency against a critical receptor or channel and the same total plasma concentrations, but with differing protein binding. If drug A is 96% bound to plasma proteins while drug B is 99% bound, it may appear that systemic exposure to the active molecule is similar for both compounds, but in fact, the exposure for drug A is fourfold greater than that for drug B, since the free fraction is four times larger (4% versus 1%). As reviewed by Trainor (2007), plasma protein binding acts as a buffer, and unless the binding is saturable, free drug concentrations will remain a constant percentage of total drug concentrations. To ensure that the free fraction is known and constant, protein binding should be done in all toxicology species at both high and low plasma concentrations.

In the absence of diffusion barriers or carrier-mediated transport, free drug concentrations at steady state will be the same in plasma and in extracellular tissue water. Many tissues, however, have evolved mechanisms to restrict drug distribution or to facilitate elimination and alter the balance of free drug. As reviewed extensively by Grover and Benet (2009), the activity of transporters may change the calculated volume of distribution, especially for compounds excreted actively by the kidney or liver, as well as tissue distribution. This change in V_d may or may not be accompanied by a change in clearance or half-life, depending on the magnitude of the effect, and the mechanism for drug clearance, and are most rigorously determined after IV dosing.

The relationship between free drug concentrations in plasma and tissue is often complicated to construct when toxicity is produced in privileged sites such as the CNS, testes, eye, or fetus because of the potential effects of transporters. The exquisite sensitivity to the neurotoxicity of the antiparasitic avermectins by animals deficient in P-gp is a classic example of the importance of transporter effects and species or breed differences in drug distribution in the brain. Mice and a subpopulation of collie dogs deficient in the mdr1 gene coding for P-gp were shown to be sensitive to the neurotoxicity produced by ivermectin in the absence of differences in systemic exposure (Kwei et al. 1999; Mealey et al. 2001; Umbenhauer et al. 1997). Transporters and their effects on the disposition of drugs in the brain have been reviewed extensively (Lee et al. 2001). Similar to the brain, there are anatomical barriers (tight junctions) and transporters separating free drug in blood from the testes, retina, and fetus (via the placenta). Impairment of male fertility or testicular toxicity, uncovered during repeat-dose toxicology or reproductive toxicology studies, can be an important and often dire observation in drug development. Testicular exposure to drugs and environmental toxins (e.g., heavy metals) may be modified by drug transporters, producing species- or strain-dependent toxicity (Augustine et al. 2005; Melaine et al. 2002). While the mechanism for the testicular necrosis produced by cadmium is complex, one key element in the marked sensitivity of certain mouse strains is the expression of *Slc39a8*, which codes for a ZN^{2+}/HCO_3^- transporter found on testicular vascular endothelial cells of Cd-sensitive strains, and which mediates cadmium uptake and participates in the toxicity observed (Dalton et al. 2005; He et al. 2009). Similarly, drug transporters expressed at the blood–retinal barrier may also modulate drug concentrations in this important anatomical space (Hosoya et al. 2011; Tomi and Hosoya 2010). Transporter effects on drug distribution may also be important in development and reproductive studies, regulating drug exposure to the developing fetus in animals and humans (Eshkoli et al. 2011; Myllynen et al. 2010; Ni and Mao 2011).

3.5.4   DETERMINING TISSUE DISTRIBUTION: QUANTITATIVE WHOLE-BODY AUTORADIOGRAPHY (QWBA) AND MICROAUTORADIOGRAPHY (MARG)

Pathologists are keenly interested in the relationship between the tissue- or cell-specific lesion and chemical disposition, and the concepts and parameters discussed thus far have assumed that unbound or total plasma or serum concentrations are a direct reflection of tissue concentrations.

While this assumption is often an appropriate start, the ability to measure drug disposition directly at the tissue and cellular level may often be needed. The imaging techniques of QWBA and MARG provide the ability to localize and quantitate the distribution of drug and metabolites in different tissues and cells within tissues after the administration of radiolabeled compounds. Cellular localization using MARG provides a powerful tool for defining substructure localization, but unlike QWBA, it cannot be considered quantitative because of current technical limitations (as reviewed by Solon et al. 2010). Moreover, these techniques can be combined with mass spectrometry to identify the chemical structures of the localized radioactivity, thus providing a powerful tool to relate histopathology, cellular disposition, and chemical identity (Solon et al. 2010).

An important prerequisite for QWBA or MARG studies is the synthesis of radiolabeled drug, incorporating a beta particle emitter such as ^{14}C, ^3H, ^{125}I, or ^{35}S in a chemically and metabolically stable position, with maximum specific activity. Incorporating the label in an unstable position or with low specific activity decreases the ability to localize drug-related material and diminishes the sensitivity of detection. For a typical QWBA study, the animals are dosed and killed at different times, and the carcass is immediately snap frozen. The frozen carcass is embedded in a matrix, and 30–50 μm sections are cut using a cryotome and collected on tape. After drying, these sections are placed against phosphor-imaging plates or X-ray film (together with a set of quantitative standards) and exposed for different lengths of time (e.g., 3–4 days). Digital images are then collected and used to construct standard curves for quantitation and photographs for depiction of tissue deposition. Concentrations of radioactivity in tissues are then typically expressed in units of radioactivity (i.e., microcurie per gram) or converted to concentration units using the specific activity and recognizing that concentration reflects both parent and metabolite (i.e., nanogram equivalents per gram). While rodents (typically pigmented rats) are most often used for QWBA studies, larger animals including dogs and macaques can also be sectioned and imaged with the proper equipment. The regulatory aspects of QWBA, as well as case studies in drug discovery and development, including the use of QWBA in maternal–fetal (placental) and milk transfer studies, have recently been reviewed by Solon (2012).

MARG studies, similar to QWBA, also require dosing with radioactivity and cryosectioning of tissues but differ in that the imaging of the thinner (4–10 μm) tissue slides uses the direct application of emulsion to the slides, followed by exposure, development, any further staining, and final examination microscopically (Solon et al. 2010). Because of the difficulty in controlling slide thickness and emulsion uniformity, the data from MARG studies are generally considered semiquantitative. This deficiency is often inconsequential when considering the ability to localize drug-related material to individual cell types in juxtaposition with traditional histological and immunochemical examination. This technique, however, is highly dependent upon the skill and experience of the investigator and is difficult to control experimentally. While technical innovation may overcome some of these limitations, it is likely that MARG studies will remain a sophisticated research tool, rather than a routine imaging screen.

3.5.5 EXAMPLES OF SEX AND SPECIES DIFFERENCES IN DRUG METABOLISM

Plasma concentrations and TK for small organic molecules are most often governed by metabolism, primarily in the liver, as well as in the GI epithelium and sometimes lung. The most important drug metabolism reactions are typically oxidation/reduction, primarily via the cytochromes P450 (CYP) superfamily, hydrolysis by blood and tissue esterases, and conjugation by glucuronidation, sulfation, and glutathione addition. Many of these enzymes are regulated and expressed in a sex- and species-dependent manner. Moreover, the tissue content of many of these enzymes can be increased (induced) in a species-selective fashion by exogenous chemicals acting via specific intracellular transcription factors, and enzyme or transporter induction is often a major mechanism responsible for the time-dependent changes in TK observed with repeated dosing.

3.5.5.1   Sex Differences in CYP Metabolism in Rodents

Sex differences in TK for drugs cleared by CYP-mediated oxidation in rats and mice are not uncommon because of the sex-dependent expression and regulation of CYP isozymes (Waxman and Holloway 2009). These differences in metabolism can occur because sex-specific CYP isozymes are expressed in the liver in response to hormonal factors, primarily the pulsatile secretion of growth hormone by the rodent pituitary (Waxman et al., 1991; Yamazoe et al. 1986). In rats, CYP2C11 is male specific while CYP2C12, considered to be female specific under normal conditions, can be induced in male rats with continuous (unphysiological) GH exposure (Waxman and O'Connor 2006). *In vitro*, CYP2C11 metabolizes the monoterpenes limonene and carvone much more avidly (up to 38-fold faster) than CYP2C12 (Miyazawa et al. 2002; Shimada et al. 2002) and is much more active in the formation of the 5′-hydroxy and 5,6-dihydroxy metabolites of thalidomide (Ando et al. 2002). Growth hormone similarly regulates some hepatic mouse CYPs in a sex-dependent manner (Waxman and Holloway 2009). While sex differences in enzyme expression and activity have been documented for other species (see Waxman and Holloway 2009 and references therein), these are generally less pronounced than for rodents and less likely to be manifested as material (i.e., >2-fold) differences in TK.

3.5.5.2   Species Differences in Metabolic Enzymes and Induction

The CYP mixed-function oxidases are responsible for the metabolism of a diverse spectrum of endogenous and exogenous substrates (Guengerich and Cheng 2011) and together with the UDP-glucuronosyltransferases are often the biological determinant of systemic exposure and TK, especially after oral dosing. While species differences in CYP metabolism and glucuronidation are commonly responsible for differences in TK, differences in other metabolic reactions such as skin esterases (Prusakiewicz et al. 2006) can also be important in regulating systemic concentrations after environmental exposure or dermal application. Species differences in metabolism are not uncommon and may be manifested in both magnitude (i.e., more extensive metabolism) and selectivity (i.e., different metabolites formed by the same pathway, or different pathways of metabolism) and produce changes in TK or toxicity. The rat-specific nephrotoxicity produced by the non-nucleoside reverse transcriptase inhibitor efavirenz is an excellent example of a species-specific tissue lesion produced by species-specific metabolism. Proximal tubular cell necrosis is observed in rats but not in cynomolgus monkeys given high oral doses of efavirenz, and this necrosis appears to be produced by formation and subsequent renal processing of a rat-specific glutathione conjugate (Mutlib et al. 2000).

There are many reports of species-dependent metabolic reactions, and while a comprehensive review is outside the scope of this chapter, some examples are useful to consider. Sharer et al. (1995) reported key differences in the *in vitro* metabolism of marker substrates by hepatic subcellular fractions from human, beagle, and rhesus and cynomolgus monkeys, including the lack of isoniazid acetylation by dog liver cytosol. In addition to species differences, there may also be strain differences in the expression of both CYP and other enzymes, for example, the relative lack of CYP2D2 expression in the female Dark Agouti versus Sprague–Dawley rat (Schulz-Utermoehl et al. 1999) and the well-characterized deficiency in the glucuronidation of bilirubin, thyroxine, and other substrates by Gunn rats, which are derived from the Wistar strain and are deficient in Ugt1a enzymes (Coughtrie et al. 1987; Richardson and Klaassen 2010). In general, all seven major CYP subfamilies responsible for xenobiotic metabolism (1A, 2A, 2B, 2C, 2D, 2E, and 3A) are represented in all species, including beagle dogs (Shou et al. 2003) and cynomolgus monkeys (Uno et al. 2011). While many of these enzymes are orthologous, additional species-selective isozymes with important substrate selectivity may be present, for example, the expression of CYP2C76 in cynomolgus monkeys (Uno et al. 2010), which is responsible for the metabolism of pitavastatin (Uno et al. 2007). Polymorphic expression of some CYP isozymes has been observed for CYP1A2 and 2C41 in beagle dogs (Blaisdell et al. 1998; Kamimura 2006) and may contribute to the variability observed within and between species. Additional physiological and biochemical differences between dog breeds have been summarized by Fleischer et al. (2008), although purpose-bred beagles are almost exclusively used for toxicology studies. These examples illustrate another level of complexity that must be considered in the interpretation of TK parameters from different species.

Pivotal toxicology studies most often use multiple doses, and changes in systemic exposure and TK can occur after repeated dosing because of induction, that is, an increase in protein content and hence activity of important drug-metabolizing enzymes and transporters like P-gp (Graham and Lake 2008; Lin 2006). These changes in TK can be large; after 28 days of dietary dosing, the plasma $AUC_{0-24\,h}$ for the cognitive enhancer linopiridine was decreased from 20.6 µg·h/ml (Day 1) to 1.8 µg·h/ml and was accompanied by increased hepatic metabolism via induction of CYP2B and 3A enzymes (Diamond et al. 1994). Induction most often occurs by increased gene transcription, initiated by the intracellular binding of xenobiotics with the nuclear regulatory factors AhR (aryl hydrocarbon receptor), PXR (pregnane X receptor), and CAR (constitutive androstane receptor) followed by heterodimerization with Arnt (Ahr nuclear translocator) or RXR (retinoid X receptor). Binding to and activation of PXR are important since this receptor mediates induction of the key CYP 2B, 2C, and 3A subfamilies; glucuronosyltransferases 1A; sulfotransferases; and the P-gp and MRP2 transporters (Gao and Xie 2010). These receptors have distinct species-selective ligand binding domains, and species selectivity in xenobiotic binding and induction, especially for PXR, is common (Ekins et al. 2008; LeCluyse 2001). While avoiding the potential for enzyme induction and changes in TK with multiple dosing may not be possible because of critical elements in the chemical structure, this potential can be easily determined *in vitro* using reporter gene transactivation or cultured hepatocyte assays (Sinz et al. 2008).

3.6   SUMMARY

Relating pathology and toxicity to the systemic exposure of xenobiotics is essential for interpreting data, evaluating risk, and forming hypotheses. While the magnitude of the TK parameters is critical, the experimental limitations in obtaining them and the assumptions underlying their derivation must be considered. The calculated TK parameters can only be as sound as the concentration data supporting them, and a robust and reliable bioanalytical method is an essential first step. Plasma or serum are often analyzed, but relating TK parameters to physiological blood flows or tissue volumes requires that the analogous concentrations in blood are calculated using the blood/plasma partition ratio. After dosing, the maximum concentrations produced (C_{max}) and the time-averaged exposure (AUC) are important parameters describing the extent of exposure. The rates of compound transfer into the system after non-parenteral dosing or out of the tissues and body after absorption is complete are also important TK parameters to determine but are composite values reflecting the contribution of different processes. Both clearance and distribution are independent parameters, reflecting fundamental biological and chemical properties, while the terminal half-life, often widely used as an indicator of drug removal, is a dependent parameter, reflecting the balance between clearance and distribution. These TK parameters result from differences in sex- and species-dependent GI physiology and anatomy, binding to plasma and tissue protein, and expression and activity of enzymes and transporters. The importance of TK parameters lies in the ability to describe changes or consistency in these important underlying biochemical and physiological determinants and to provide a quantitative measure of the relationship between systemic exposure and toxicity.

REFERENCES

Akimoto, M., Nagahata, N., Furaya, A., Fukushima, K. et al. (2000) Gastric pH profiles of beagle dogs and their use as an alternative to human testing. *Eur J Pharm Biopharm* 49:99–102.
Ando, Y, Fuse, E., and Figg, W.D. (2002) Thalidomide metabolism by the CYP2C subfamily. *Clin Cancer Res* 8:1964–1973.

Augustine, L.M., Markelewicz, R.J., Boekelheide, K., and Cherrington, N.J. (2005) Xenobiotic and endobiotic transporter mRNA expression in the blood–testis barrier. *Drug Metab Dispos* 33:182–189.

Avdeef, A. (2005) The rise of PAMPA. *Expert Opin Drug Metab Toxicol* 1:325–342.

Benet, L.Z. (1984) Pharmacokinetic parameters: which are necessary to define a drug substance? *Eur J Resp Dis* 65:45–61.

Blaisdell, J., Goldstein, J.A., and Bai, S.A. (1998) Isolation of a new canine cytochrome P450 cDNA from the cytochrome P450 2C subfamily (CYP2C41) and evidence for polymorphic differences in its expression. *Drug Metab Dispos* 26:278–283.

Boillat, C.S., Gaschen, F.P., Gaschen, L., Stout, R.W., and Hosgood, G.L. (2010) Variability associated with repeated measurements of gastrointestinal tract motility in dogs obtained by use of wireless motility capsule system and scintigraphy. *Am J Vet Res* 71:903–908.

Camilleri, M. (2006) Integrated upper gastrointestinal response to food intake. *Gastroenterology* 131:640–658.

Chen, E.P., Mahar Doan, K.M., Portelli, S., Coatney, R. et al. (2008) Gastric pH and gastric residence time in fasted and fed conscious cynomolgus monkeys using he Bravo pH system. *Pharm Res* 25:123–134.

Coughtrie, M.W., Burchell, B., Shepherd, I.M., and Bend, J.R. (1987) Defective induction of phenol glucuronidation by 3-methylcholanthrene in Gunn rats is due to the absence of a specific UDP-glucuronosyltransferase isoenzyme. *Mol Pharmacol* 31:585–591.

Dalton, T.P., He, L., Wang, B., Miller, M.L. et al. (2005) Identification of mouse SLC39A8 as the transporter responsible for cadmium-induced toxicity in the testis. *Proc Natl Acad Sci USA* 102:3401–3406.

Davies, B. and Morris, T. (1993) Physiological parameters in laboratory animals and humans. *Pharm Res* 10:1093–1095.

DeSesso, J.M. and Jacobsen, C.F. (2001) Anatomical and physiological parameters affecting gastrointestinal absorption in humans and rats. *Food Chem Toxicol* 39:209–228.

Diamond, S., Rakestraw, D., O'Neil, J., Lam, G.N., and Christ, D.D. (1994) Induction of cytochromes P-450 2B and 3A in mice following the dietary administration of the novel cognitive enhancer linopiridine. *Drug Metab Dispos* 22:65–73.

Dressman, J.B. (1986) Comparison of canine and human gastrointestinal physiology. *Pharm Res* 3:123–131.

Ekins, S., Reschly, E.J., Hagey, L.R., and Krasowski, M.D. (2008) Evolution of pharmacologic specificity in the pregnane X receptor. *BMC Evol Biol* 8:103.

Eshkoli, T., Sheiner, E., Ben-Zvi, Z., and Holcberg, G. (2011) Drug transport across the placenta. *Curr Pharm Biotechnol* 12:707–714.

Fleischer, S., Sharkey, M., Mealy, K., Ostrander, E.A., and Martinez, M. (2008) Pharmacogenetic and metabolic differences between dog breeds; their impact on canine medicine and the use of the dog as a preclinical anima model. *AAPS J* 10:110–119.

Gao, J. and Xie, W. (2010) Pregnane X receptor and constitutive androstane receptor at the crossroads of drug metabolism and energy metabolism. *Drug Metab Dispos* 38:2091–2095.

Graham, M.J. and Lake, B.G. (2008) Induction of drug metabolism: species differences and toxicological relevance. *Toxicology* 254:184–191.

Grover, A. and Benet, L.Z. (2009) Effects of drug transporters on volume of distribution. *AAPS J* 11:250–261.

Guengerich, F.P. and Cheng, Q. (2011) Orphans in the human cytochrome P450 superfamily: approaches to discovering functions and relevance to pharmacology. *Pharmacol Rev* 63:684–699.

Hamilton, R.A., Garnett, W.R., and Kline, B.J. (1981) Determination of mean valproic acid serum level by assay of a single pooled sample. *Clin Pharmacol Ther* 29:408–413.

Haruta, S., Kawai, K., Jinnochi, S., Ogawara, K.I. et al. (2001) Evaluation of absorption kinetics of orally administered theophylline in rats based on gastrointestinal transit monitoring by gamma scintigraphy. *J Pharm Sci* 90:464–473.

He, L., Wang, B., Hay, E.B., and Nebert, D.W. (2009) Discovery of ZIP transporters that participate in cadmium damage to testis and kidney. *Toxicol Appl Pharmacol* 238:250–257.

He, Y.L., Murby, S., Warhurst, G., Gifford, L. et al. (1998) Species differences in size discrimination in the paracellular pathway reflected in oral bioavailability of poly(ethylene glycol) and D-peptides. *J Pharm Sci* 87:626–633.

Hosoya, K., Tomi, M., and Tachikawa, M. (2011) Strategies for therapy of retinal diseases using systemic drug delivery: relevance of transporters at the blood:retinal barrier. *Expert Opin Drug Deliv* 8:1571–1587.

Ikegami, K., Tagawa, K., Narisawa, S., and Osawa, T. (2003) Suitability of the cynomolgus monkey as an animal model for drug absorption studies of oral dosage forms from the viewpoint of gastrointestinal physiology. *Biol Pharm Bull* 26:1442–1447.

International Transporter Consortium. (2010) Membrane transporters in drug development. *Nat Rev Drug Discov* 9:215–236.

Jusko, W.J. and Ko, H.C. (1994) Physiologic indirect response models characterize diverse types of pharmaco-dynamics effects. *Clin Pharmacol Ther* 56:406–419.

Kalantzi, L., Goumas, K., Kalioras, V., Abrahamsson, B. et al. (2006) Characterization of the human upper gastrointestinal contents under conditions simulating bioavailability/bioequivalence studies. *Pharm Res* 23:165–176.

Kamimura, H. (2006) Genetic polymorphism of cytochrome P450s in beagles: possible influence of CYP1A2 deficiency on toxicological evaluations. *Arch Toxicol* 80:732–738.

Kaniwa, N., Aoyagi, N., Ogata, H., and Ejima, A. (1988) Gastric emptying rates of drug preparations. I. Effects of size of dosage forms, food and species on gastric emptying rates. *J Pharmacobiodyn* 11:563–570.

Karali, T.T. (1995) Comparison of the gastrointestinal anatomy, physiology, and biochemistry of humans and commonly used laboratory animals. *Biopharm Drug Dispos* 16:351–380.

Kimura, T. and Higaki, K. (2002) Gastrointestinal transit and drug absorption. *Biol Pharm Bull* 25:149–164.

Klein, S. (2010) The use of biorelevant dissolution media to forecast in vivo performance of a drug. *AAPS J* 12:397–406.

Knipp, G.T., Ho, N.F., Barsuhn, C.L., and Borchardt, R.T. (1997) Paracellular diffusion in Caco-2 cell mono-layers: effect of perturbation on the transport of hydrophilic compounds that vary in change and size. *J Pharm Sci* 86:1105–1110.

Kwei, G.Y., Alvaro, R.F., Chen, Q., Jenkins, H.J. et al. (1999) Disposition of ivermectin and cyclosporine A in CF-1 mice deficient in MDR1A P-glycoprotein. *Drug Metab Dispos* 27:581–587.

LeCluyse, E.L. (2001) Pregnane X receptor: molecular basis for species differences in CYP3A induction by xenobiotics. *Chem Biol Interact* 16:283–289.

Lee, G., Dallas, S., Hong, M., and Bendayan, R. (2001) Drug transporters in the central nervous system: brain barriers and brain parenchyma considerations. *Pharmacol Rev* 53:569–596.

Lentz, K.L. (2008) Current methods for predicting human food effect. *AAPS J* 10:282–288.

Lin, J.H. (2006) CYP induction-mediated drug interactions: in vitro assessment and clinical implications. *Pharm Res* 23:1089–1116.

Lin, J.H., Chen, I.-W., Vastag, K.J., and Ostovic, D. (1995) pH-dependent oral absorption of L-753,524, a potent HIV protease inhibitor, in rats and dogs. *Drug Metab Dispos* 23:730–735.

Lindahl, A., Ungell, A-L, Knutson, L, and Lennarnas, H. (1997) Characterization of fluids from the stomach and proximal jejunum in men and women. *Pharm Res* 14:497–502.

Lui, C.Y., Amidon, G.L., Berardi, R.R., Fleisher, D. et al. (1986) Comparison of gastrointestinal pH in dogs and humans: implications on the use of the beagle dog as a model for oral absorption in humans. *J Pharm Sci* 75:271–274.

Mager, D.E., Wyska, E., and Jusko W.J. (2003) Diversity of mechanism-based pharmacodynamics models. *Drug Metab Dispos* 31:510–519.

Mealey, K.L., Bentjen, S.A., Gay, J.M., and Cantor, G.H. (2001) Ivermectin sensitivity in collies is associated with a deletion mutation of the mdr1 gene. *Pharmacogenetics* 11:727–733.

Melaine, N., Lienard, M.O., Dorval, I., Le Goascogne, C. et al. (2002) Multidrug resistance genes and p-glyco-protein in the testis of the rat, mouse, guinea pig, and human. *Biol Reprod* 67:1699–1707.

Miyazawa, M., Shindo, M., and Shimada, T. (2002) Sex differences in the metabolism of (+) and (−)-limonene enantiomers to carveol and perillyl alcohol derivatives by cytochrome P450 enzymes in rat liver micro-somes. *Chem Res Toxicol* 15:15–20.

Mutlib, A.E., Gerson, R.J., Meunier, P.C., Haley, P.J. et al. (2000) The species-dependent metabolism of efavirenz produces a nephrotoxic glutathione conjugate in rats. *Toxicol Appl Pharmacol* 169:102–113.

Myllynen, P., Kummu, M., and Sieppi, E. (2010) ABCB1 and ABCB2 expression in the placenta and fetus; an interspecies comparison. *Expert Opin Drug Metab Toxicol* 6:1385–1398.

Ni, Z. and Mao, Q. (2011) ATP-binding cassette efflux transporters in human placenta. *Curr Pharm Biotechnol* 12:674–685.

Prusakiewicz, J.J., Ackermann, C. and Voorman, R. (2006) Comparison of skin esterase activities from differ-ent species. *Pharm Res* 23:1517–1524.

Richardson, T.A. and Klaassen, C.D. (2010) Disruption of thyroid hormone homeostasis in Ugt1a-deficient Gunn rats by microsomal enzyme inducers is not due to enhanced thyroxine glucuronidation. *Toxicol Appl Pharmacol* 248:38–44.

Roberts, M.S., Magnusson, B.M., Burczynski, F.J., and Weiss, M. (2002) Enterohepatic circulation. Physiological, pharmacokinetic and clinical implications. *Clin Pharmacokinet* 41:751–790.

Rudholm, T., Hellstrom, M.H., Theodorsson, E., Campbell, C.A. et al. (2008) Bravo capsule system optimizes intragastric pH monitoring over prolonged time: effects of ghrelin on gastric acid and hormone secretion in the rat. *World J Gastroenterol* 14:6180–6187.

Russell, T.L., Berardi, R.R., Barnett, J.L., Dermentoglou, L.S. et al. (1993) Upper gastrointestinal pH in seventy nine healthy, elderly, North American men and women. *Pharm Res* 10:187–196.

Sagawa, K., Li, F., Liese, R., and Sutton, S.C. (2009) Fed and fasted gastric pH and gastric residence time in conscious beagle dogs. *J Pharm Sci* 98:2494–2500.

Schulz-Utermoehl, T., Bennet, A.J., Ellis, S.W., Tucker, G.T. et al. (1999) Polymorphic debrisoquine 4-hydroxylase activity in the rat is due to differences in CYP2D2 expression. *Pharmacogenetics* 9:357–366.

Shannon, J.A., Earle, D.P. Jr., Berliner, R.W., and Taggart, J.V. (1948) Studies on the chemotherapy of the human malarias. I. Method for the quantitative assay of suppressive antimalarial action in vivax malaria. *J Clin Invest* 27:66–74.

Sharer, J.E., Shipley, L.A., Vandenbranden, M.R., Binkley, S.N. and Wrighton, S.A. (1995) Comparison of phase I and phase II in vitro hepatic enzyme activities of human, dog, rhesus monkey, and cynomolgus monkey. *Drug Metab Dispos* 23:1231–1241.

Shimada, T., Shindo, M., and Miyazawa, M. (2002) Species differences in the metabolism of (+) and (−)-limonenes and their metabolites, carveols and carvones, by cytochrome P450 enzymes in liver microsomes of mice, rats, guinea pigs, rabbits, dogs, monkeys and humans. *Drug Metab Pharmacokinet* 17:507–515.

Shou, M., Norcross, R., Sandig, G., Lu, P. et al. (2003) Substrate specificity and kinetic properties of seven heterologously expressed dog cytochromes P450. *Drug Metab Dispos* 31:1161–1169.

Shugarts, S. and Benet, L.Z. (2009) The role of transporters in the pharmacokinetics of orally administered drugs. *Pharm Res* 26:2039–2054.

Sinz, M., Wallace, G., and Sahi, J. (2008) Current industrial practices in assessing CYP enzyme induction: preclinical and clinical. *AAPS J* 10:391–400.

Solon, E.G. (2012) Use of radioactive compounds and autoradiography to determine drug tissue distribution. *Chem Res Toxicol* 25:543–555.

Solon, E.G., Schweitzer, A., Stoeckli, M., and Prideaux, B. (2010) Autoradiography, MALDI-MS, and SIMS-MS imaging in pharmaceutical discovery and development. *AAPS J* 12:11–26.

Sugano, K., Okazaki, A., Sugimoto, S., Tavornvipas, S. et al. (2007) Solubility and dissolution profile assessment in drug discovery. *Drug Metab Pharmacokinet* 22:225–254.

Tomi, M. and Hosoya, K. (2010) The role of blood:ocular barrier transporters in retinal drug disposition. *Expert Opin Drug Metab Toxicol* 6:1111–1124.

Trainor, G.L. (2007) The importance of plasma protein binding in drug discovery. *Expert Opin Drug Discov* 2:51–64.

Umbenhauer, D.M., Lankas, G.R., Pippert, T.R., Wise, L.D. et al. (1997) Identification of a P-glycoprotein-deficient subpopulation in the CF-1 mouse strain using a restriction fragment length polymorphism. *Toxicol Appl Pharmacol* 146:88–94.

Uno, Y., Fujino, H., Iwasaki, K., and Utoh, M. (2010) Macaque CYP2C76 encodes cytochrome P450 enzyme not orthologous to any human isoenzymes. *Curr Drug Metab* 11:142–152.

Uno, Y., Iwasaki, K., Yamazaki, H., and Nelson, D.R. (2011) Macaque cytochromes P450: nomenclature, transcript, gene, genomic structure, and function. *Drug Metab Rev* 43:346–361.

Uno, Y., Kumano, T., Kito, G., Nagata, R. et al. (2007) CYP2C76-mediated species difference in drug metabolism: a comparison of pitavastatin metabolism between monkeys and humans. *Xenobiotica* 37:30–43.

Viswanathan, C.T., Bansal, S., Booth, B., DeStefano, A.J. et al. (2007) Quantitative bioanalytical methods validation and implementation: best practices for chromatographic and ligand binding assays. *Pharm Res* 24:1962–1973.

Volpe, D.A. (2011) Drug-permeability and transporter assays in Caco-2 and MDCK cell lines. *Future Med Chem* 3:2063–2077.

Waxman, D.J. and Holloway, M.G. (2009) Sex differences in the expression of hepatic drug metabolizing enzymes. *Mol Pharmacol* 76:215–228.

Waxman, D.J., and O'Connor, C. (2006) Growth hormone regulation of sex-dependent liver gene expression. *Mol Endocrinol* 20:2613–2629.

Waxman, D.J., Pampori, N.A., Ram, P.A., Agrawal, A.K. and Shapiro, B.H. (1991) Interpulse interval in circulating growth hormone patterns regulates sexually dimorphic expression of hepatic cytochrome P450. *Proc Natl Acad Sci USA* 88:6868–6872.

Wilkinson, G.R. (1987) Clearance approaches in pharmacology. *Pharmacol Rev* 39:1–47.

Wilkinson, G.R. and Shand, D.G. (1975) A physiological approach to drug clearance. *Clin Pharmacol Ther* 18:377–390.

Willmann, S., Edginton, A.N., and Dressman, J.B. (2007) Development and validation of a physiology-based model for the prediction of oral absorption in monkeys. *Pharm Res* 24:1275–1282.

Yamazoe, Y., Shimada, M., Murayama, N., Kawano, S., and Kato, R. (1986) The regulation by growth hormone of microsomal testosterone 6 beta-hydroxylase in male rat livers. *J Biochem* 100:1095–1097.
Yanez, J.A., Remsberg, C.M., Sayre, C.L., Forrest, M.L., and Davies, N.M. (2011) Flip-flop pharmacokinetics—delivering a reversal of disposition: challenges and opportunities in drug development. *Ther Deliv* 2:643–672.
Zhou, R., Moench, P., Heran, C., Lu, X. et al. (2005) pH-dependent dissolution in vitro and absorption in vivo of weakly basic drugs: development of a canine model. *Pharm Res* 22:188–192.

4 Introduction to Toxicologic Pathology

Judit E. Markovits, Page R. Bouchard,
Christopher J. Clarke, and Donald N. McMartin

CONTENTS

4.1 INTRODUCTION

Pathology is the medical discipline that studies the nature of diseases, especially the changes in body tissues and organs to determine their pathogenesis and consequences. Clinical pathology is a branch of pathology that uses laboratory methods to characterize diseases by analyzing body fluids. Pathologists typically have a medical or veterinary medical background with an understanding of basic biochemistry, physiologic processes, familiarity with diseases, and their impact on the subject. A pathologist studies naturally occurring diseases or changes produced in experimental models of diseases. Toxicologic pathologists (in the context of this paper) in turn deal with characterizing the toxicity to organisms when exposed to chemical or biological agents intentionally, such as a drug for medical purposes, or unintentionally, such as through environmental exposure. This review will focus on the practice of toxicological pathology in the context of intentional exposure under controlled laboratory conditions. In this circumstance, the toxicologic pathologist needs to be able to accurately describe the produced effects, understand the pathogenesis of the observed findings, and understand the biologic significance produced by the test article in nonclinical studies. Additionally, the pathologist needs to draw conclusions about the relevance of the nonclinical findings for human relevance and, in most cases, the potential risks associated with the controlled clinical use of the test article.

A major event in standardization of the discipline of toxicologic pathology, at least in the United States, was the establishment of the National Cancer Institute and its subsequent initiation of carcinogenicity testing in the early 1970s (Squire 1997). In the United States, physicians and veterinarians working in academic pathology with an interest in toxicity and veterinarians working primarily in the pharmaceutical industry had, in the mid-twentieth century, organized a society that, in 1971, became the Society of Toxicologic Pathologists (STP) (Iatropoulos and Williams

2011). Sister organizations to STP were formed in many countries in the following decades along with increasing informal and formal global collaboration of individual pathologists and peer organizations. The globalization was also driven by changes in pharmaceutical industry, the establishment of multinational companies, and international collaborations of regulators in different regions of the world. The newly formed discipline of toxicologic pathology initially was limited to studies that are often referred to as developmental or regulatory studies. However, over time, the discipline broadened from the initial diagnoses of changes owing to low-molecular-weight drug candidates to include biologics as well as medical devices and nonclinical samples from regenerative medicine and tissue engineering. These new areas resulted in new regulations as well as specialized studies requiring additional expertise from pathologists. Most toxicologic pathologists have a veterinary or medical degree followed by specialization in pathology and many are certified in pathology but, with the exception of Japan and the United Kingdom, are not certified in toxicologic pathology (Ettlin et al. 2008). Moreover, on the basis of cultural differences and traditions in different regions in the world, practitioners of toxicologic pathology may have alternative educational background from the conventional medical or veterinary training and, hence, do not hold a general pathology certification. In recent years, however, with increasing globalization of the pharmaceutical industry and markets, along with increasing harmonization of toxicologic pathology practice, recommendations were made and accepted by members of the International Societies of Toxicologic Pathologists concerning scientific curriculum and formal or on-the-job training in the specialty of pathology (Bolon 2011; Bolon et al. 2010).

The practitioner of pathology, including that of toxicologic pathology, in the early days was often thought of as the lonely scientist sitting at his or her microscope. However, more recently, this picture changed, especially for toxicologic pathologists working in the biopharmaceutical industry. In response to new demands in medicine for safer drugs with innovative approaches, and the desire to shorten the drug development process and reduce attrition due to safety, nonclinical studies became more complex and increasingly bring together teams with diverse expertise. This chapter will provide an overview of modern toxicologic pathology in a multidisciplinary setting.

4.2   GENERAL CONSIDERATIONS

This chapter introduces the discipline of toxicologic pathology while emphasizing the role of the pathologist in drug development. Earlier chapters (Chapters 1 and 2) provide overviews of the drug development process and the nonclinical safety assessment of drugs. Additionally, Chapter 5 provides more details on the technical aspects of toxicologic pathology.

A drug was defined by the WHO Scientific Group as "any substance or product that is used or intended to be used to modify or explore physiological systems or pathological states for the benefit of the recipient" (Dorato et al. 2008). Hence, the primary focus of drug development is the patient, and nonclinical safety testing based on animal models is used to predict how patients may react to drug candidates, a process that is referred to as risk assessment. In order to effectively function as a toxicologic pathologist, one needs to be aware of the broader picture of drug research and development and the regulatory environment. A survey of new molecular entities (NMEs) or biologics approved by the US Food and Drug Administration (FDA) the last 60 years indicated an essentially constant rate of new drug introductions despite the ever-changing landscape of pharmaceutical industry. During these 60 years, the formation of international conglomerates resulted either from mergers of large companies or by the acquisition of small or large companies (Munos 2009) without an apparent effect on innovation as indicated by the total number of approved drugs. In another recent review, the impact of the genomic era of the last 20 years was surveyed by examining the molecular mode of action (MMOA) of NMEs for drugs approved between 1999 and 2008 (Swinney and Anthony 2011). In this data set, there were a few serendipitous discoveries during phenotypic screening, but the vast majority of NMEs resulted from intentional screening followed by optimization of molecules targeting a specific molecular target. The reviewers emphasized the significance of MMOA when the change from "first in class" to "best in class" was evaluated. When toxicity was not associated with the pharmacologic mechanism, improvement was made by changing the chemical behavior, such as decreased dissociation rate from target with antihistamines and angiotensin receptor blockers. Similarly, when toxicity was based on MMOA, an improved therapeutic index was achieved as illustrated by selective estrogen receptor modulators (SERMs) such as raloxifene. On the basis of the above, familiarity of targets and understanding of mode of action are imperative for members of research and development teams (including pathologists) in today's pharmaceutical industry. One of the most common and important contribution of toxicologic pathologists is to determine if the observed toxicity is on- or off-target (i.e., is or is not due to the pharmacological action of the drug). Data available for 2010 confirmed that very few truly novel drugs were approved and the number of biologics also lagged behind expectations (Mullard 2011). It is often stated that much of biomedical research is a long process coming to fruition through novel treatment modalities after decades of careful investigations. This is true for the tyrosine kinase inhibitor Gleevec that seemingly revolutionized oncology by being the first cancer therapy targeted toward a specific mutant molecular target in a defined cancer procuring pathway but was also the culmination of multidisciplinary research performed over decades. The biggest trend recognized during the review of FDA approvals for 2010 was the emerging emphasis on specialty medicine (including orphan drugs) rather than primary care (Mullard 2011).

Regardless of the focus of research and development in the biopharmaceutical industry, there is an ever-increasing collaboration of scientists and physicians from many disciplines in the discovery and development of new drugs. It is no longer sufficient for scientists from different disciplines to "hand off" to one another in this process, but rather to be in intense collaboration where scientists and physicians complement each other in an interdisciplinary team environment. In a new approach building on such collaboration, rather than a traditional approach of focusing on individual "drug-gable" targets, teams of scientists use a variety of molecular and genetic tools to probe whole molecular pathways potentially providing novel targets for diseases that were not clearly associated in the past (Fishman and Porter 2005). In this paradigm, unique defects within a defined molecular pathway may result in different diseases. For example, specific defects in the hedgehog signaling pathway are associated with diverse disease outcomes such as basal cell carcinoma, medulloblastoma, and a proliferative skin disease, called Gorlin's syndrome, when Patched (Ptcl) is affected and glioblastoma when Gli1 is affected. Furthermore, more common diseases may have perturbations of the same molecular pathway and could benefit from drugs developed for specific diseases (prostate and gastrointestinal tumors are examples for smoothened [Smo] involvement). In order to recognize potential downstream events and distinguish those from off-target changes, pathologists need to develop a deep understanding of the molecular pathways that is being modulated by any particular drug candidate. Pathologists may also contribute to the selection/development of appropriate disease models and their standardized interpretation (Ward 2010).

The majority of toxicologic pathologists contribute to studies testing drug candidates in somewhat advanced stages of development. Studies conducted under Good Laboratory Practice (GLP) regulations form the basis of filing for permits in order to test the drug candidate in humans. A typical study design in nonclinical testing includes healthy, young animals that serve as controls (when receiving the vehicle as treatment) and animals exposed to different doses of the drug candidate. Alternative study designs, especially in Europe in keeping with the 3Rs (refine, reduce, replace) of animal use, may reduce or even eliminate concurrent controls in certain studies or phases of studies (especially for large-animal recovery groups). The primary role of the pathologist for regulatory studies is to recognize differences produced by the test article among the cohorts (groups) of the study and separate those changes from background lesions that may develop spontaneously, unrelated to treatment. In this context, the practice of pathology is quite different from most diagnostic settings, and the way most pathologists are generally trained, where changes in individual animals are characterized in great detail and diagnoses are made either to facilitate treatment (as with biopsy or clinical pathology samples from clinical cases) or (in the case of postmortem examinations) to resolve clinical questions that could be informational for the future. The same holds true for retrospective studies of a series of diagnostic cases over time. In contrast, toxicologic pathologists review material from multiple animals in order to recognize trends in changes related to the test article. In this setting, while individual animals are important, decisions are being made based on changes in groups of animals; depending on study design, the groups may be only a few animals or, in the case of rodent carcinogenicity studies, 50 or more. Therefore, uniform handling of samples, including awareness of and compensation for circadian changes in some parameters, is essential. In order to accomplish this, pathologists should have input to study design and need to have an understanding of the experimental system being used from animal species and strain, through the general toxicokinetic profile of the drug to other factors.

4.3 STUDY DESIGN

According to general guidelines concerning the length of a nonclinical study needed to support human studies, animal studies should be at least as long as the intended clinical study, with some exceptions made for oncology indications. Chapter 2 describes the length and general study design of studies for both small molecules and biologics in order to support first-in-human (FIH) testing and marketing. Prior to initiating single-dose studies in humans, typical testing program would include two or four week-long animal studies in a rodent (usually rat), large-animal species (often dog). Depending on the developmental phase of the drug candidate, 1-month human trials are supported by 1- to 3-month-long rodent and non-rodent studies. Clinical trials requiring 6 months' or longer treatment of patients are supported by 6-month rodent and 6- to 12-month non-rodent studies. In the case of non-oncology indications, the purpose of the initial short-term rodent and non-rodent studies is to gain enough information about the general safety of the product that human volunteers may be tested for initial safety in Phase I studies. Phase II clinical trials expose a larger number of patients to assess efficacy whereas Phase III trials confirm efficacy and safety in even larger patient populations. Oncology products by contrast are typically tested in patients rather than healthy volunteers and have different safety requirements. In general, 3-month-long studies are sufficient to support oncology clinical trials of any duration and have an appropriate recovery phase to demonstrate that the toxicologic changes are reversible. Carcinogenicity studies in general are not required for oncology products when the patient population has a limited life expectancy of 3 years or less.

In the early days of pharmaceutical development, nonclinical studies and activities were spread over years with predictable and quite uniform designs. Much has changed in the last couple of decades because of technical and scientific advances and changed regulatory environment. The scientific community (industry and regulatory bodies) for example concluded that chronic studies for rodents should be 6 months long rather than 12 months as was the standard until the early 1990s. In the past, most GLP studies included recovery groups; however, a more modern approach instead includes study designs appropriate to the clinical program in keeping with the 3Rs of animal use (Pandher et al. 2012). In this newer paradigm, the demonstration of complete recovery for anticancer drug candidates is not necessary, but nonclinical studies should indicate if the severe toxicity could be reversible in the clinical setting. The recovery phase (or non-dosing period) for small molecules with indications other than oncology depends on the specifics of the developmental program and at least one of the nonclinical studies should include recovery, although a recovery arm may be included in more than one nonclinical study. The primary purpose of the non-dosing phase is to demonstrate reversibility of toxicity. The assessment of delayed toxicity is often misinterpreted for antibody-based therapeutics because toxicity observed with drug candidates with a long circulating half-life and duration of action may be due to an extended exposure rather than a truly delayed effect. The length of the non-dosing "recover" period is frequently 2 to 4 weeks for small molecules with short half-life and limited duration of action, whereas maybe up to several months for a biologics with long half-life and duration of action. The length of the recovery period for a biotherapeutic is generally dictated by the time required for the plasma drug concentration to fall below pharmacologically active concentrations.

While it has been recognized that life span (i.e., carcinogenicity) rodent studies are suboptimal because of differences between humans and rodents and because these studies lack mechanistic information, a reliable alternative has not been identified or endorsed to date. Carcinogenicity studies are generally the longest, largest, hence most expensive studies in a nonclinical safety program. Additionally, taking approximately 3 years from start to completion, they can often be on the critical path to a product approval document submission. Because of extensive resource requirements (including the use of several hundred animals and the time it takes to finalize the report), carcinogenicity studies are limited to promising late-stage products with typical timing close to new drug application (NDA) submission. Pathologists are key contributors to data generation and interpretation of carcinogenicity studies since the primary objective of these studies is the morphological characterization of proliferative changes diagnosed by the study pathologist. Pathologists have long been and continue to be opinion leaders on reassessing carcinogenicity testing. To that end, over 200 marketed pharmaceuticals based on the *1994 Physician Desk Reference* were surveyed for carcinogenicity in rodents (Davies and Monro 1995). Approximately half of these compounds showed some evidence of producing tumors in rodent 2-year tests, indicating that for these drugs, the human benefits were considered to outweigh the risks. The survey identified certain factors for positivity in rodent bioassays, including genotoxicity, immunosuppression, and chronic irritation leading to increased cell turnover or causing hormonal perturbations. Two surveys of the results of nearly 200 rat studies probed the predictability of carcinogenic potential based on chronic rat studies up to 12 months. The results indicated that if a compound resulted in certain histology findings, including hyperplasia, cellular hypertrophy, or atypical cellular foci in 6- or 12-month rat studies, then the compound would probably cause neoplasia in a rat carcinogenicity study, but not necessarily in the same tissue as indicated in the shorter study. Conversely, if the 6- or 12-month study was negative for proliferative signals, then there would be a high, but not 100%, probability that the compound would not produce neoplasms in a rat carcinogenicity study (Reddy et al. 2010; Sistare et al. 2011).

There is now substantial experience with short-term alternatives of carcinogenicity testing in genetically engineered mouse (GEM) strains having either insertion or deletion of genes relevant in human cancer. On the basis of this experience, the use of mouse strains heterozygous for p53 tumor suppressor genes (for genotoxic compounds) and the TgrasH2 strain that carries the human c-Ha-ras oncogene in addition to the murine Ha-ras oncogene (for non-genotoxic as well as genotoxic compounds) in 6-month studies is accepted as a replacement for the traditional 2-year mouse study. The study design for these GEM studies usually includes an appropriate positive reference compound and wild-type animals in order to confirm genotype and the potential mechanism of tumorigenesis. Substantial experience has been gained with the use of these transgenic models over the past decade and they are now commonly used as an alternative to the traditional 2-year mouse study.

4.4   GROSS CHANGES AND ORGAN WEIGHTS

Although a long list of tissues is routinely examined microscopically from safety studies, the recognition of gross abnormalities and their correlation with in-life (clinical) observations remains important. Pathologists rely on well-trained technical staff to identify the gross lesions and bring those to their attention. This is especially true for rodent studies that require simultaneous necropsy of several animals. The well-trained staff needs to be aware of anatomy and what is the normal appearance of tissues and organs for the given species, strain, age, and sex of animals. Fresh tissues, especially those of the endocrine organs, must be handled with care in order to prevent the introduction of artifact that may interfere with the detailed microscopic evaluation of tissues. In general, the pathologist provides leadership in recognition and naming of gross lesions. Computer systems and standard operating procedures (SOPs) may assist in assuring that similar gross changes are identified with the same term, using a limited lexicon and constructing diagnoses uniformly (Frame and Mann 2008). Details of necropsy procedures are addressed in Chapter 5 of this book.

Organ weight changes may occur and could be meaningful indicators of test article–related changes with or without corresponding microscopic findings in repeat-dose rodent studies up to 6 months of duration and in subchronic and chronic studies of large animals. Only a brief discussion is provided as the reader is referred to the regulatory forum series of STP (Michael et al. 2007; Sellers et al. 2007) as well as the next chapter of this book. Organ weights are typically collected in conventional toxicity studies, but less frequently in discovery studies. The STP recommendations are in keeping with general practice in the US pharmaceutical industry by including minimally liver, kidney, heart, brain, adrenal gland, and testis from all multidose studies from 7 days to 1 year duration in all species. By contrast, collection of organ weights is not recommended from carcinogenicity studies, including alternatives of the 2-year life span studies. The recommendations also include special suggestions concerning tissues notoriously presenting with interpretation challenges (primarily large-animal lymphoid and reproductive tissues). Customized organ weight collection may include lung in the case of inhalation studies or any tissue that might be affected by the test article. Nonroutine tissues should be weighed only, however, if tissues can be prepared for weighing uniformly and if weight changes would contribute to interpretation.

4.5 MICROSCOPIC EVALUATION

The successful performance of toxicologic histopathology is a complex process and requires a qualified pathologist with access to detailed study information and familiarity with the product tested as well as results of previous studies (Crissman et al. 2004). Toxicologic pathology studies are performed in close collaboration with other investigators having a wide range of expertise and working together as a team following appropriate SOPs and using checks and balances to assure high-quality data collection and interpretation. Detailed information on study design (including protocol and amendments), access to in-life observation provided by colleagues in toxicology, access to clinical pathology parameters, and general understanding of the drug metabolism and pharmacokinetic (PK) profile of the product all provide background information to the pathologist that is often essential for the microscopic examination and interpretation of study findings. Within the pathology group, attention must be paid to sample processing and quality control in order to assure unbiased, uniform representation of samples from each animal. The standardized list of tissues has been recommended for 28-day and carcinogenicity studies by the appropriate committees of the European Medicines Agency (EMEA 2000). Further comments were made by STP concerning best practices of histological evaluation and other considerations (Bregman et al. 2003). This list included a core list of tissues for repeat-dose GLP studies, regardless of the route of administration and provided further guidance for additional tissues for inhalation studies. However, some tissues recommended by different regulatory agencies such as three different salivary glands, Zymbal glands, and oviducts (among others) were not included in the STP proposal because these tissues seldom have morphological changes suggestive of toxicity or carcinogenicity. A valuable guide for rodent tissue sampling and for comparative regulatory considerations is available at the RENI web site (RENI 2012), and these guidelines have also been published (Kittel et al. 2004; Morawietz et al. 2004; Ruehl-Fehlert et al. 2003).

Microscopic examination is traditionally a qualitative assessment of changes by bright field microscopy using routine slide preparations stained with hematoxylin and eosin (HE). Many nonpathologists are surprised how much trained eyes can recognize with the combination of the purple blue nuclear stain of hematoxylin and the pink eosin stain for cytoplasmic and other tissue components. As Finch described in his review of recent developments in toxicological pathology, our practice of pathology is closely linked with the history of the Americas going back to the sixteenth century by way of hematoxylin (today used in the form of either iron or alum salt), the extract of the indigenous logwood tree (*Haematoxylon campechianum*) in the Campeche and Yucatan regions

(Finch 2005). Even during deforestation around 1970, when hematoxylin shortage developed, a search for a better alternative was not rewarding. The discovery of the red dye, eosin (from the Greek word *Eos*, meaning dawn), along with the ability of early histologists in the nineteenth century to produce relatively thin sections after embedding the samples in wax (and rehydrating the samples in order to take on the aqueous stains) provided the histological preparations that are still the "bread and butter" of pathologists. To round out this brief history of histology, the discovery of early permanent mounting media allowed permanent preparations that could be archived for many years. The nonaqueous mounting medium was originally extracted from a Canadian fir (*Abies balsamea*) and over the years has been replaced by synthetic media.

Staining methods other than HE may be requested by the pathologist in order to assist the characterization of test article–related changes or facilitate the diagnostic process in cases of opportunistic infections or in carcinogenicity studies. Histochemical stains may be required for detailed evaluation of tissues, such as periodic acid–Schiff (PAS) for the assessment of testis. PAS is a versatile stain that may be used for the evaluation of intracellular glycogen, the diagnosis of renal glomerular changes, or opportunistic fungal infections. Detailed description of special stains is beyond the scope of this chapter and the reader is referred to Chapter 5 for details. In addition to histochemical stains, immunohistochemical (IHC) methods are now used routinely to further characterize tissue changes. In contrast to histochemical reactions, the basis of IHC is the recognition of epitopes by antibodies and the visualization of the complexes being formed. Some of the most commonly used antibodies are directed to intermediate filaments within the cells in order to identify them, against cell surface antigens especially for phenotyping mononuclear cells and against intracellular products such as insulin, or may identify specific stages of cell cycle (Hall and Rojko 1996; Painter et al. 2010; Ward et al. 2006). In situ hybridization is used less frequently in toxicologic pathology and is employed mainly to detect specific RNA by hybridization with different length of nucleic acid sequences either for diagnosis of opportunistic infections (LCV in primates for example), if a protein cannot be detected, or most commonly to associate morphologic results with gene expression profiling.

Electron microscopy can be used in selected instances to identify the subcellular structure involved in a change seen by the light microscopy. However, electron microscopy uses sample sizes that are too small and processing is too labor intensive to be routinely used on most studies. The best results are obtained when it is known what to sample at necropsy based on previous light microscopic findings. For example, peroxisome proliferation could be verified as the explanation for drug-induced hepatocellular hypertrophy (Maronpot et al. 2010). Less satisfactory samples that are still interpretable can sometimes be processed from residual formalin-fixed tissues if deemed useful following light microscopic examination of histology slides.

Microscopic evaluations in toxicologic pathology need to be reproducible in order to assure that the incidence of test article–related changes could be compared across studies. Diagnostic pathologists are generally trained during their formal education to provide detailed descriptions of changes as well as specific diagnoses for the purposes of informing treatment or disease control. In contrast, toxicologic pathologists need to use succinct descriptive terms for microscopic changes (rather than morphologic diagnoses) using standardized nomenclature and reproducible diagnostic criteria (SSNDC guides). To that end, international organizations including the STPs in Europe, Asia, and the United States and the Registry of Industrial Toxicology Animal data (RITA) database group in Europe issued standardized nomenclature for rodents initially for rat proliferative changes and are currently developing similar standardized nomenclature for nonproliferative changes. A new global initiative as a collaboration of the European Society of Toxicologic Pathology with RITA, STP in the United States, and the Japanese Society of Toxicologic Pathology (JSTP) combining diagnostic criteria for lesions of rats and mice is in the process of being published in print and on the web (Kaufman et al. 2005). This effort is the INHAND Nomenclature Project (International Harmonization of Nomenclature and Diagnostic Criteria for Lesions in Rats and Mice) and can be accessed at the web site www.goreni.com. The new diagnostic criteria will have a more holistic approach across organ systems than previous nomenclatures. Guidance is being provided for grading and general constructs of diagnoses as well as special considerations are being given in order to make the new nomenclature computer friendly to use. The organ working groups followed a general concept for the nonproliferative changes and also produced criteria for proliferative lesions. Furthermore, the new nomenclature will provide examples of generalized changes regardless of specific tissues or organs, will allow for combination of terms such as degeneration/regeneration, and will identify lesions that could be accounted for as present, but would not require grading. The nomenclature will also suggest modifiers to be used to clarify either distribution or topography of lesions. Careful consideration of seemingly subtle changes cannot be overemphasized since these changes may reflect differences in metabolic activity (such as enzyme induction in the liver causing decreased hepatocellular vacuolation) due to test article (Shackelford et al. 2002). Additionally, reproducible grading of lesions within a study and across studies is important when determining no-observed-effect level (NOEL), and a simple grading using only a few categories is recommended for the purpose of consistency. Grading of lesions is not strictly required by regulatory agencies but is nonetheless often critically important and the subject of questions from regulators from time to time (Ward and Thoolen 2011). Grading of findings is often important in discovery pathology in assessing efficacy across studies. A good grading scheme should be defined, reproducible, and meaningful.

The actual method for tissue evaluation in toxicity studies (either by animal or by tissue) is mostly a personal preference. Tissue-wise evaluation may provide greater control for consistent grading of severity whereas evaluation of tissues by animal assures that each animal is evaluated as a whole (useful for the determination of cause of death/moribundity and a must when examining carcinogenicity studies). So-called blind unbiased reading (when the pathologist is not aware of the treatment the animal received) is typically not used as an initial evaluation but often has utility in case of subtle changes, for example, hepatocellular hypertrophy or thyroid follicular epithelial changes. Recently, some publications favor the more extensive use of unbiased histopathological evaluation in keeping with some other investigative (and mostly quantitative) tests that are typically done in a blinded fashion (Holland and Holland 2011a,b), although this approach is not widely accepted or recommended. The reader is referred to the article by Holland and Holland (2011a) for examination strategies (such as an ordering method and a pair-contrast method) that are used by pathologists for the common problem of determining if a subtle microscopic change is due to treatment.

In addition to standardized nomenclature, increased use of proliferation assessment using IHC methods combined with computer-assisted morphometric evaluation is commonly used to provide quantitative assessment of the degree of proliferation. The prototype publication (based on bromodeoxyuridine [BrdU] labeling as the gold standard) provides details on considerations for the administration of BrdU, the concepts of sampling specific tissues, and image analysis strategies for the generation of labeling index as an indicator of proliferation (Nolte et al. 2005). This and other frequently used methods rely on standardized sampling of the tissue based on optimal tissue sections. A thought-provoking publication argues that such an assumption-based approach may lead to incorrect conclusions and offers some details on the design-based (unbiased) stereological methods (J. T. Boyce et al. 2010). As an illustration of unwanted (incorrect) conclusions, the evaluation of testicular changes is presented using both the assumption-based design and the design-based methods. In this example, degenerate testes had greater tissue shrinkage than concurrent normal controls and thus differences should not be measured by conventional two-dimensional (2D) assessment of cellular density, which resulted in an inaccurate interpretation of interstitial cell numbers. Additional details on sampling methods, some practical approaches for the selection of 2D- or three-dimensional (3D)-based quantitative assessment, and associated statistical methods are beyond the scope of this chapter and the reader is referred to the review by R. W. Boyce et al. (2010).

Pathology data from regulatory toxicologic studies are presented in reports either as part of an integrated toxicologic report or as freestanding scientific contribution. During the finalization of pathology data, most organizations rely on peer review by another pathologist. The peer review process is a nonadversarial examination that assures quality and accuracy of data for diagnostic criteria used, confirms target tissues, and confirms doses with adverse findings. The resulting data and the interpretation of data are the reflection of consensus rather than the opinion of an individual contributor. A memo is typically issued by the peer review pathologist describing the process and confirming that the study report reflects the pathology data (Morton et al. 2010). There are no regulatory requirements within the United States or Europe for peer review (with the exception of some recommendations for the peer review of carcinogenicity studies by ICH). According to FDA and EPA, pathology raw data are the signed pathology report since pathology results may be recreated by the review of the archived histological slides. In Japan, where data locking is required prior to sponsor peer review and unlike in the United States and Europe, findings that are changed during the peer review process must be listed in the final report (McKay et al. 2010). The JSTP is pursuing the revision of these guidelines in order to be aligned with the United States and Europe. The issue of peer review in the United States is currently under review by the Office of Compliance at FDA, and there are many ongoing opinions and discussion about how the process is to be handled. It is expected that the FDA will soon issue a clear directive to those submitting study data and most laboratories will modify their procedures to comply with the regulatory agency. A special type of peer review is conducted by pathology working groups (PWGs) when issues arise concerning the diagnosis and interpretation of morphologic changes. Recently published examples included the review upon the request of Health and Environmental Science Institute (HESI) Peroxisome proliferator-activated receptor (PPAR) Agonist Project Committee on hemangiosarcomas in mice and hamsters, liposarcomas/fibrosarcomas in rats, and pathological changes of the urinary bladders in cynomolgus monkeys after treatment with PPAR agonists (Hardisty et al. 2007, 2008). PWGs are composed of pathologists with special experience in the subject (such as extensive experience with nonhuman primates or MD pathologists with comparative pathology experience). Slides are randomized and blinded as to treatment group (or in case of the PPAR PWG, the originating sponsor of slides was not known), and each participant reviews either all the slides for a target organ or a representative selection of the slides that demonstrate the range of change present and illustrate the question addressed by the PWG. Each slide is then discussed and the diagnosis is agreed upon by confirming specific features of criteria being used.

4.6 INTEGRATION OF EXPOSURE, DRUG METABOLISM, AND HISTOPATHOLOGY FINDINGS

Toxicologic pathology findings must be put into context in relation to drug and metabolite plasma levels; hence, pathologists need to have a basic understanding of how toxicokinetic data could be used in nonclinical safety assessment (Ploemen et al. 2007). Detailed discussion of the subject is beyond the scope of this chapter and the reader is referred to Chapter 3 of this book. In practical terms, pathologists can focus on the major PK parameters (AUC, C_{max}, T_{max}, half-life), major metabolites, and tissue distribution. Understanding toxicokinetic data is useful when morphological changes do not clearly correspond to the administered dose levels. For example, supraproportional or subproportional changes in plasma levels may be observed and are often explained by either saturation of elimination or absorption, respectively. Toxicodynamic responses may change after longer-term dosing and pathologists must take these changes into account in order to carefully assess organs of clearance. Another common finding is gender-related differences in the expression of enzymes involved in biotransformation; one well-known example is P450 expression being higher in male rats than in females. Variability of individual response and plasma exposure is especially frequently encountered in large-animal studies because of smaller animal number of less homogenous population than that of rodent studies. In fact, intractable vomiting in dogs resulting in limited exposure is commonly a reason to use another non-rodent test species such as the minipig or monkey. Finally, variation in toxicokinetic data across studies may result from indicated differences between batches of test substance, changes in formulation, and differences related to the study animals (e.g., change in suppliers).

Integration of toxicokinetic data with toxicologic pathology changes provides a better interpretation of test article–related findings than viewing these changes only on the basis of doses administered. Ultimately, for an integrated risk assessment, the safety margin or therapeutic index is determined on the basis of comparative exposure rather than dose (except in oncology indications). With small molecules for which there may be serum protein binding and variation in the degree of protein binding across species, one should always consider the percentage of drug that is not protein bound or the "free fraction." In principle, only the free fraction is pharmacologically available to interact with targets and therefore free-fraction exposure calculations can be an important way to express therapeutic index. For large molecules (monoclonal antibodies), pathologists should be aware that the half-life and duration of action of the molecule in the plasma can extend into months and therefore provide continuous exposure levels well beyond the end of dosing. Alternatively, exposure to biologics may be greatly reduced if the generation of anti-drug antibody responses accelerates clearance of the test article. Because of these unique considerations with biologics, the study pathologist must consider individual animal exposure and immunogenicity data when evaluating histopathology findings.

4.7   REPORTING AND RISK ASSESSMENT

The toxicologic pathology report provides an important summary to a wide range of potential readers/reviewers who will use it to make critical decisions about the scientific, strategic, and medical risks. Clinical and anatomic pathology findings are typically the central findings used during the review process by health authorities. The report therefore must be written clearly without ambiguity, using appropriate and consistent terminology and offering accurate and transparent interpretation (Black 1994, 1997; Wolf and Mann 2005). The report must be structured in a logical and consistent manner and reflect the protocol (and its amendments) and the work done. Materials and methods therefore need to be appropriately detailed and results need to identify all treatment-related target tissues, doses, incidence, and severity of lesions, and when studied, reversibility of findings. Terminology used needs to be in keeping with current standards (reflecting accepted nomenclature) and must be consistent within the study and across studies with the given xenobiotic. Finally, the discussion and conclusion should provide an integrated picture of all the pathology findings, correlating those findings with the clinical observations, body weight changes, dose response, exposure levels, etc. The study interpretation should also represent how these changes relate to any known mechanism of action of the test article.

The conclusion for each study report should contain a statement of either a NOEL or a no-observable-adverse-effect level (NOAEL), maximum tolerated dose, or other appropriate conclusion about the toxicological dose response for that specific study when treated animals are compared to controls. NOEL refers to a level where no changes distinguish dosed animals from controls. For non-life-threatening clinical indications, NOAEL is generally the focus of the conclusion and this dose and the associated test article exposure will then be used for determining a safe starting dose for clinical trials, and potential exposure cannot generally be exceeded (Lewis et al. 2002, Ochoa and Rousseaux 2009), although exceptions are noted, especially in oncology and neurology indications. While determination of NOAEL may appear to be a simple definition, there is considerable judgment involved in this decision. Such a dose is not considered to endanger human health or be a precursor of serious events. In contrast to non-oncologic therapeutics, different criteria are used for establishing the clinical starting dose for small-molecule oncology products administered to patients in late-stage disease. Because these agents are frequently cytotoxic, they are expected to produce severe toxicity in humans. The goal of FIH dose selection is to identify a dose that could be managed clinically with a tolerable toxicity profile in human but while still potentially offering some pharmacological benefit to the patient. The intent for dose selection is to identify a pharmacologically active dose that is not severely toxic by selecting either one-tenth of the severely toxic dose in 10% of rodents (STD10) or, in case the large animal cannot tolerate this dose, one-sixth of the highest non-severely toxic dose (HNSTD) in non-rodents based on body surface calculations for both rodents and large animals (Maziasz et al. 2010; Ponce 2011). Some additional principles for FIH dose selection have been introduced for biologics because they often have significant differences in potency across species, can sometimes exert potent agonist properties, and often have a long duration of action, even after a single dose. As a result, the concept of the minimum anticipated biological effect level has been introduced as a method to determine a safe stating dose for clinical trials. This concept involves an integrated assessment of the in vitro pharmacology and in vivo pharmacology and toxicity data to predict a starting dose that when administered to humans will produce a minimal pharmacological effect in humans (Muller et al. 2009).

While there is an ongoing dialogue if rodent 2-year studies are appropriate to predict human cancer risk, there are general guidelines on when and how they should be performed and on the evaluation of data generated from the studies. In general, an important aspect of toxicologic pathology is not only to recognize differences between concurrent controls and dosed animals but also to recognize if those changes are test article related. Familiarity with the spectrum of background lesions and historical data are important for all types of studies, but especially carcinogenicity studies. There are several sources for historical data, including the test facility, peer organizations that share the data from several sponsor organizations (RITA 2012), and published literature (Keenan et al. 2009). Published literature is especially useful in settings with a limited number of studies in a given test facility such as primate studies that are not collected by peer organizations; for example, RITA only collects rodent data (Chamanza et al. 2010). When considering if the observed tumor incidence was treatment related, the most appropriate comparison is with concurrent controls. However, comparison from historical data ideally from the same test facility and typically from the last 5 years is often necessary. Such comparison may be needed for rare tumors or tumors with variable incidence. FDA guidelines (2001) state, for statistical interpretation of tumor incidences, that a lower P value may be used for rare tumors than for common tumors. Another important tool for the weight of evidence approach of carcinogenicity assessment includes the combination of appropriate neoplasms from the same cell lineage, for example, hemangiomas and hemangiosarcomas from different locations and the possible use of hyperplasia of the same tissue as supporting evidence for tumorigenicity (McConnell et al. 1986). Statistical tests for tumor analysis studies have been created to deal with differences between rate of survival between control and dosed groups having an effect on tumor incidences. It is beyond the scope of this manuscript which test to use or to discuss the dispute (Morton et al. 2002) concerning use of cause-of-death designations used in the Peto et al. (1980) statistical analysis. Elmore and Peddada (2009) discussed the use of historical controls when analyzing carcinogenicity data.

The majority of biologics presently on the market were not tested in carcinogenicity studies, either because the clinical use and indication did not require it or because of the lack of cross-reactivity with rodents or immunogenicity that causes rapid drug clearance in rodents making it impossible to maintain exposure. An approach that has been commonly used is to make an integrated assessment of the cancer risk associated with a particular biologic based on knowledge of the target biology, human and animal genetic knock-out (KO) or overexpression of the target, and findings from general toxicity studies to estimate potential carcinogenicity risk. On the basis of scientific rationale, potential risk may be identified by a biologics' mechanism of action such as immune suppression or mitogenic activity (growth factor), which may imply a carcinogenic risk. Some growth factors for example have been tested in cell proliferation assays, but others received warning labels without nonclinical testing (Vahle et al. 2010). Clinical experience with some of the immune-suppressive agents indicated an increased risk of certain patient populations for the development of posttransplantation lymphoproliferative disorder due to Epstein–Barr virus. A carcinogenicity testing strategy for biologicals and decisions concerning modeling of the theoretical risk needs to be made on a case-by-case basis in discussion with health authorities.

4.8   DRUG DISCOVERY

The purpose of nonclinical safety testing is to predict human toxicity. An industry-wide survey of outcomes indicated that conventional nonclinical testing strategies established decades ago predicted 70% of human toxicities on an organ-by-organ basis (Olson et al. 2000). This number may be misleading because some drug candidates with marked toxicity in animals are generally never tested in humans. Because of the time and increasing expense required to identify the dose/development-limiting toxicities, there is an increased industry-wide emphasis on earlier identification of toxicity by shifting the conventional nonclinical developmental paradigm (Kramer et al. 2007). There are several points to consider in shortening the nonclinical phase of drug development and improving its success rate. These approaches include (not necessarily in order of feasibility) the improved safety profile of drugs for known targets by improving efficacy while decreasing known liabilities, identification/decrease of idiosyncratic toxicities in human, and reducing the time it takes to identify the dose-limiting toxicities referred to above. In an effort to overcome toxicity-related failures during drug development in recent years the apparent divide between research activities and safety assessment blurred. In this setting, multiple parallel activities involve the comprehensive *in silico* and in vitro characterization of small molecules in order to optimize ADMET (absorption, distribution, metabolism, excretion, toxicity) profiles. These characteristics can be predicted by using a wide range of bioinformatics tools (C2-ADME, TOPKAT, CLOGP, Gastroplus, etc.) in addition to being measured in the laboratory. The computational *in silico* tests include construction of drug target interactions, virtual screening and prediction of key characteristics, and determination of protein–ligand binding. In vitro high-throughput testing requires small amounts of compound (Wang et al. 2007). These tests include kinetic solubility, estimation of permeability metabolic stability across several relevant species, and assessing the potential for drug–drug interactions. Additional early testing using in vitro systems include targets/mechanisms that caused past failures of drug candidates such as genotoxicity, cardiotoxicity (hERG), hepatotoxicity, myelotoxicity, and adverse events associated with well-characterized targets (5HT2B). Cellular imaging techniques using a different type of fluorescence microscopy may be useful in the early phase of drug development for specific applications by imaging entire cell populations for migration or angiogenesis (cardiology or oncology indication) or for neurite outgrowth (Lang et al. 2006). Several laser technologies are available including flow cytometry, laser scanning cytometry, and confocal scanning microscopy for immunophenotyping, apoptosis assessment, cell cycle analysis, or quantification of dopaminergic fibers in brain and 3D reconstruction of the sample (Roman et al. 2002). The early profiling of drugs gives an indication of toxicity and pharmacological promiscuity that is useful in decision making and improves the quality of drug candidates. At this early phase of development, medicinal chemists modify structures of compounds in order to diminish or overcome the initially identified liabilities. Early efficacy testing also primarily uses in vitro systems of human and other key species of origin, requiring small amounts of the compound. During early in vivo efficacy studies, discovery pathologists contribute to lead optimization by identifying potential liability in the animal model or in satellite groups using higher doses (10× the high efficacious dose) (Sasseville et al. 2004). Even earlier in the drug discovery process, pathologists and safety scientists can discern potential liabilities based on past experience and careful review of the literature around drug targets to understand the consequences of target perturbation via stimulation or inhibition of particular pathways. Mapping out potential safety issues at an early stage can allow the focused interrogation of systems or tissues to gather decision-making data at an early timepoint, or develop appropriate mitigation strategies. Knowledge of the target expression profile across tissues is key component that can aid the understanding of target biology. Focused analyses using appropriate methodologies (ISH, qPCR, IHC) can determine the detailed pattern of mRNA and protein expression across tissues and cells, and can be helpful in determining the suitability of a target as well as potential safety liabilities.

As another parallel activity in the development paradigm, KO or transgenic models using conditional or unconditional systems often prove informative of on-target toxicity. Phenotyping of GEMs includes comparison with the wild-type strain, by behavioral, clinical, and anatomic pathology evaluations. Results from GEM studies may not be completely in synchrony with compound-related changes because of metabolism, alternative signaling (developmental redundancy), different levels of expression, or other reasons. Conditional GEM strains are especially useful if the unconditional strain is developmentally lethal. One of the classic examples of on-target toxicity due to primary pharmacology is the effect angiotensin-converting enzyme (ACE) inhibitors have during prenatal development that is also present in ACE-KO mice (Kramer et al. 2007). Because of this finding, the use of ACE inhibitors is excluded from specific patient populations. More often, however, on-target toxicity can be managed by careful monitoring of patient's exposure. An increasing industry-wide awareness is developing toward unintended secondary pharmacology causing toxicity. The classic example for secondary pharmacology is the diet drug fen-fen and associated valvulopathy resulting in postmarketing withdrawal. The adverse events in this case are thought to be due to interactions with the 5HT2B receptor, whereas the primary and intended pharmacology (efficacy) most likely is due to 5HT2C receptor activity. The use of structurally unrelated compound or inactive enantiomers may contribute to the identification of chemically mediated toxicity versus on-target toxicity. Chemically mediated toxicity may be due to the characteristics of a specific scaffold or a specific functional group. Most of the time, chemically mediated toxicity can be designed out of the drug candidate during lead optimization. An example of commonly occurring chemically mediated (and predictable) toxicity is phospholipidosis due to cationic amphiphilic xenobiotics (many of them marketed products) that interact with cellular membranes and lysosomes. In addition to early in vivo studies in efficacy models, short-term non-GLP repeat-dose studies in rats often predict dose-limiting toxicity in 4-week GLP studies. The short-term studies can also be used as dose range finders for the longer-term studies in non-rodent species as well and may further contribute to lead optimization. The pathologist's role during the discovery phase of development has a different emphasis from regulatory toxicologic pathology because it calls for close interaction with pharmacology and medicinal chemistry and is often experimental in nature. Pathologists working in this earlier "discovery" phase are called upon to assess efficacy when there is a morphologic endpoint to the efficacy study. These evaluations may include image analysis of different cell types (e.g., islet cell quantitation in diabetes models), proliferation or apoptosis (e.g., xenografts of oncology models), or semiquantitative scoring of lesions in models of inflammation. Pathologists may collaborate with imaging groups by histologically validating novel imaging methods that are often antibody or metabolic activity based or by further characterizing measurements made by imaging (histological characterization of computed tomography scans for example). These imaging technologies include micro-positron emission tomography and single-photon emission computed tomography imaging indicating tissue perfusion, glucose, or oxygen metabolism (Ying and Monticello 2006). Another role for pathologists in the discovery and then the development of antibody therapeutics is tissue cross-reactivity studies using human and animal tissue sections (Leach et al. 2010). Tool antibody(ies) to the therapeutic target can be used to understand the distribution of the target in normal or diseased human and animal tissues for the purpose of target validation. The tissue cross-reactivity study on human tissues is a required component of the safety assessment package to support clinical dosing, although some limitations of the assay are recognized. Tissue cross-reactivity studies on tissues of preclinical species are often performed as well, though they are generally viewed as useful to help in interpreting the results of *in vivo* toxicologic studies when findings are observed, rather than for species selection (Bussiere et al. 2011). As with all IHC validation, the most sensitive and practical detection system should be selected and applied with either no or only minor modification to all tissues (the methods may be modified for tissues with high endogenous levels of components of the detection system). However, just because an antibody is effective and specific in vivo, it may not be a good reagent for IHC; hence, the outcomes of tissue cross-reactivity studies need to be carefully evaluated.

Pathologists are also heavily involved in mechanistic studies to investigate pathogenesis of potential liabilities and to identify biomarkers that could be used both in a nonclinical and clinical setting. In these studies, gene expression profiling and data mining using bioinformatics tools are commonly applied molecular pathology tools. It is essential that the interpretation of tissue-based gene expression data be grounded and interpreted in the context of clearly defined morphological changes in the tissues (Boorman et al. 2002). Gene expression profiling is now a commonly used tool to bring a deeper understanding of the molecular pathogenesis of toxicity. Collating the different types of histological, molecular data along with conventional and special clinical pathology parameters and relevant exposure data provides the complete picture that is needed for making the appropriate recommendations concerning the fate of the project. This critical analysis of the integrated various data sets to generate a comprehensive and balanced interpretation of the pattern of changes is fundamental to the high-quality risk assessment expected of a pathologist in the biopharmaceutical industry.

In summary, the key contributions to safety assessment in early discovery are to identify important target organs, identify on- and off-target toxicity and their potential for reversibility, facilitate decision making on the basis of chemical structure (scaffold), and improve safety margins (therapeutic index) for short-term studies, up to 4 weeks (Stevens and Baker 2009). Other aspects of discovery pathology include using molecular pathology tools in order to identify targets across species and to contribute to the understanding of disease models and processes by studying human and animal samples and by providing a bridge with translational medicine through these activities.

4.9   CLINICAL PATHOLOGY AND BIOMARKERS

General guidelines dictate clinical pathology testing of animals on toxicity studies to include hematology, coagulation, clinical chemistry, and urine analysis. The individual who interprets these routine tests (and supervises the laboratories that perform the analyses) very much depends on traditions for the region and the type of institution. The ideal approach is that clinical pathologists interpret these data, as suggested in a harmonization communication from some 10 global scientific organizations, and their membership with a broad background was involved globally (Weingand et al. 1996). This harmonization document provides guidelines for most of the clinical pathology testing conducted in subchronic and chronic studies. Recent best practices recommendations limit clinical pathology testing to the collection of blood smears during carcinogenicity studies (Young et al. 2011). The number of veterinary clinical pathologists in the pharmaceutical industry remains low, although the industry in general has recently become a more attractive career choice than in the past (Schultze et al. 2008). One of the reasons for the greater interest may be some of the new directions clinical pathology is exploring especially in identification and validation of novel biomarkers as an extension of the role of clinical pathology (Dieterle et al. 2010; Ennulat et al. 2010b; Harpur et al. 2011; Sistare et al. 2010). Clinical pathologists are uniquely qualified to lead efforts in the validation of biomarkers for the use in both nonclinical and clinical settings, although collaboration with anatomic pathologists, toxicologists, and other scientists in the interpretation of changes in routine studies remains a focus of toxicologic clinical pathologists. The first international effort for the identification and qualification of urinary biomarkers for renal safety brought together experts from industry, academia, and regulatory agencies (Dieterle et al. 2010; Sistare et al. 2010). The outcome of this effort was the nomination of 7 biomarkers (from the 23 potential biomarkers identified) that may allow the specific localization of renal damage within the nephron using noninvasive methods. As a follow-up, additional urinary markers were tested in male rats using the same approach as the previous studies, albeit relying on smaller cohorts, resulting in an additional marker indicating collecting duct damage (Harpur et al. 2011). Another area of interest is the identification of biomarkers indicating a wide range of hepatic changes encountered during toxicity studies, including drug-metabolizing enzyme induction (often resulting in hepatocellular hypertrophy) and lipidosis, just to name a few. These changes to date have not confirmed the utility of traditional biomarkers studied (Ennulat et al. 2010a,b). Drug-induced vascular injury is another area of interest for both the industry and regulatory agencies because animals typically do not show clinical signs and conventional biomarkers did not prove to be predictive of vascular damage. A review by the expert working group on drug-induced vascular injury outlined a holistic approach proposing the use of a wide range of technologies, including gene expression profiling, proteomics, and metabonomics in order to understand the underlying mechanisms of vascular injury (Kerns et al. 2004). Follow-up publications confirmed that on the basis of complex mechanisms at play, a panel of markers needs to be evaluated in each specific situation (Brott et al. 2005a,b; Louden et al. 2006; Tesfamariam and DeFelice 2007). In particular, components of the coagulation pathway, secretory elements, and constituents of endothelial and smooth muscle cells and inflammatory cytokines are of interest as potential biomarkers.

An emerging field in the search of biomarkers is the identification of tissue-specific micro-RNAs (miRNAs) whose blood levels have been linked to a number of pathological conditions from cancer to liver injury (Chen 2009; Laterza et al. 2009; Wang et al. 2009). MiRNAs are small, non-coding RNAs that regulate gene expression at the posttranscriptional level and are concurrently being explored as clinical and nonclinical biomarkers because of their presumed function to regulate all aspects of cell activities. Toxicologic pathologists will be able to contribute to further our understanding of miRNA function by the characterization of transgenic or KO models of tissue-specific miRNAs as well as the qualification of specific miRNAs as biomarkers of toxicity. It is fairly well established that miRNA122 is associated with liver damage in rats whereas miRNA133 was recently proposed as a marker of muscle injury and miRNA124 was associated with ischemic brain injury 8 h after induction (Laterza et al. 2009).

Metabonomics is another technology that has held promise but is also associated with technical difficulties; hence, its utilization is limited. Metabonomics refers to a primarily nuclear magnetic resonance (NMR)-based method to analyze endogenous metabolite profiles in body fluids, most commonly urine. Because of urine collection, animals need to be in metabolism cages, making this technology cumbersome to use. Furthermore, interpretation of data requires complex pattern recognition methods such as principal component analysis (Liebler and Guengerich 2005). The advantage of metabonomics is that recognized signal patterns may indicate temporal development of toxicity (that can be correlated with morphological changes) as well as organ specificity. NMR-based metabolic profiling of urine after naproxen-induced injury in rats indicated that the method may be used to evaluate gastrointestinal injury by noninvasive methods—an unmet diagnostic need (Jung et al. 2011).

Another emerging technology that toxicologic pathologists must be aware of is proteomics using a number of different technology platforms. The most widely known approach used 2D gel electrophoresis mass spectroscopy (2D-MS), which is flexible and requires relatively small volumes of any type of sample. In contrast, antibody- or aptamer-based arrays are not as widely used today (and need greater amounts of sample), but these types of technologies offer huge promise in terms of superior sensitivity and ability to directly identify protein compared to 2D-MS. It is expected that surveys of low abundance serum proteins will lead to markers of tissue-specific toxicity (Wetmore and Merrick 2004). The caveat for using proteomics in the near future for assessment of toxicity is that no one proteomic platform can yet distinguish the many forms of proteins, including posttranslational modifications and different phosphorylation states. Future development of these technologies should allow their routine application to assaying tissue samples and, in association with complementary techniques such as laser-capture microdissection, offer the promise of defining specific molecular changes within highly selected tissue or cell types.

Safety biomarker qualification relies on morphological characterization of specific changes in a reproducible way by a toxicologic pathologist in order to identify the pathological process associated with the biomarker of interest. In response to questions raised by consortia and working groups that are in the process of qualifying novel biomarkers for specific disease processes, the STP provided recommendations for this purpose (Burkhardt et al. 2011). During the careful consideration of some of the special challenges of biomarker qualification, great similarities were recognized to the best practices for conduct of toxicological histopathological evaluation (Crissman et al. 2004). The importance of a tiered approach was emphasized, which allowed for both open and blinded review of changes by pathologists and called for the involvement of pathologists during the meta-analysis of data. Comments were solicited recently to the draft recommendations published by the FDA for the histopathological qualification of biomarkers (FDA 2011).

Up until now, the focus has been on safety biomarkers that identify either nonclinical or clinical liabilities. In the last two decades, however, biomarkers have been introduced as means of measuring efficacy and, in the age of personalized medicine, a way to stratify patient populations. Tissue-based expression of biomarkers that the general public is familiar with include Her2/neu positivity of breast cancer for treatment with trastuzumab (Herceptin) and estrogen receptor or progesterone receptor positivity of breast cancer as a prerequisite for treatment with tamoxifen or aromatase inhibitors such as letrozole (Femara). Increasingly, in this age of rational hypothesis-driven drug development, scientists including toxicologic pathologists are asked to advise on and assess PK and pharmacodynamic (PD) markers that could be used nonclinically during lead optimization and ultimately clinically to indicate efficacy. Measurement of PD markers often involves non-morphological approaches, such as gene expression microarrays or mass spectrometry (Rojas et al. 2011; Ross and Ginsburg 2003; Sarker et al. 2007). The PD biomarker data will be correlated with the pharmacokinetic (PK) parameters as an aid in decision making. In general, biomarker validation has been considered in different technical levels from definitely quantitative, relative quantitative, quasiquantitative, to qualitative assays. The highest level of quantitative assay included methods expressed in continuous numeric units of a definitive standard (mass spectrometry), whereas IHC using grades of low, medium, and high was considered as qualitative (Sarker et al. 2007). Since assays that are quantitative do not provide the same insight as IHC does, introduction of a value-based IHC would contribute to greater biologic precision than what is available today (Dunstan et al. 2011). The complex problems around the standardization of IHC in this context open up new opportunities for toxicologic pathology in the digital age.

4.10   NOVEL MODELS

Earlier, we discussed the increased acceptance of GEM strains as alternatives to carcinogenicity testing. In addition to these fairly widely used models, other strains may be used for mechanistic evaluation of potential liabilities by probing perturbations of pathways. Broadly, these strains may be divided into categories such as *evaluation of cell injury* from cytokines (TNF) and enzymes (SOD, MMP) or death factors (APP), *metabolism* (P450), *signal transduction* (PPAR, cyclins), or *mutagenesis* (lacZ) (Bolon and Galbreath 2002; Boverhof et al. 2011). The increased utilization of GEM was presented in an issue of *Veterinary Pathology* dedicated to different aspects of phenotyping of GEMs (*Vet Pathol* 2012). Furthermore, during an international workshop on high-throughput phenotyping efforts of the International Mouse Phenotyping Project, some compromises and harmonization efforts were presented including physiologic screens along with a streamlined pathology phenotyping by working up only two animals per sex for a single gene mutation (Schofield et al. 2011).

Zebrafish are another animal model that is being used by several laboratories both in academia and in the pharmaceutical industry for the study of genes and signaling pathways, modeling human development and diseases as well as toxicity. Genetic manipulations resulted in models of several human diseases including Parkinson's and Alzheimer's and heart disease as well as drug-induced liver injury (Cheng et al. 2011; Hill et al. 2012; Menke et al. 2011). One hurdle for the use of the zebrafish in biomedical research is that few pathologists are familiar with the normal histology. To that end, Menke's paper fills a gap by providing detailed and well-illustrated description of normal zebrafish histology.

In recognition that approximately 95% of cancer drugs fail in clinical testing, new directions are emerging in search of predictable nonclinical models with opportunities for toxicologic pathologists to contribute (Caponigro and Sellers 2011; Zhou et al. 2010). Traditionally, the most commonly used strategy involves tumor cell lines xenografted into immune-compromised mice, potentially creating two difficulties. Laboratory cell lines may not be representative of clinical populations; this may be a reason for failure of some Phase III trials especially for drugs that have efficacy on cell lines but not in the clinic when there is not the deep biologic understanding of interactions between these novel drug candidates and specific cancers. Second, therapeutic index determinations are difficult since little nonclinical testing is usually done in mice. Strategic use of immunodeficient nude rats in efficacy studies with toxicology endpoints to be cross referenced with toxicity studies in immune-competent rats will assist in decision making. Another emerging trend is the use of primary human tumor fragments in the establishment of new xenograft models perhaps presenting new opportunities and also pitfalls. When initially established, these tumors may represent tumor heterogeneity and contain human stromal elements in addition to the primary tumor. Upon passage of these cells, however, in order to produce enough tumors to be tested in efficacy studies, human stromal elements are typically lost; such loss however, also opens a window of opportunity to test changes in pathway components of murine and human origin. These new approaches provide opportunities for toxicologic pathologists to contribute to the assessment of murine and human tumor components and molecular events resulting in drug treatment. Finally, genetically engineered models using stem cells carrying specific genetic alterations with predictable tissue distribution of tumors resulted in chimeric mouse models that allowed the investigation of interactions between murine tumor and murine stromal elements.

REFERENCES

Black, H. E. 1994. Design and writing of the preclinical safety report. *Toxicol Pathol* 22:202–5.

Black, H. E. 1997. The pebble in the pond. *Toxicol Pathol* 25:80–1.

Bolon, B. 2011. The world weighs in on optimal toxicologic pathology training practices: it's unanimous! *Toxicol Pathol* 39:294.

Bolon, B., Barale-Thomas, E., Bradley, A. et al. 2010. International recommendations for future toxicologic pathologists participating in regulatory-type, non-clinical toxicity studies. *Toxicol Pathol* 38:984–92.

Bolon, B. and Galbreath, E. 2002. Use of genetically engineered mice in drug discovery and development: wielding Occam's razor to prune the product portfolio. *Intern J Toxicol* 21:55–64.

Boorman, G. A., Anderson, S. P., Casey, W. M. et al. 2002. Toxicogenomics, drug discovery and the pathologist. *Toxicol Pathol* 30:15–27.

Boverhof, D. R., Chamberlain, M. P., Elcombe, C. R. et al. 2011. Transgenic animal models in toxicology: historical perspectives and future outlook. *Toxicol Sci* 121:207–33.

Boyce, J. T., Boyce, R. W., and Gundersen, J. 2010. Choice of morphometric methods and consequences in the regulatory environment. *Toxicol Pathol* 38:1128–33.

Boyce, R. W., Dorph-Petersen, K. A., Lyck, L. et al. 2010. Design-based stereology: introduction to basic concepts and practical approaches for estimation of cell number. *Toxicol Pathol* 38:1011–25.

Bregman, C. L., Adler, R. R., Morton, D. G. et al. 2003. Recommended tissue list for histopathological examination in repeat-dose toxicity and carcinogenicity studies: a proposal of the Society of Toxicologic Pathology (STP). *Toxicol Pathol* 31:252–3.

Brott, D. A., Gold, S., Jones, H. 2005a. Biomarkers of drug-induced vascular injury. *Toxicol Appl Pharmacol* 207:S441–5.

Brott, D. A., Jones H. B., and Gould, S. 2005b. Current status and future directions for diagnostic markers of drug-induced vascular injury. *Cancer Biomarkers* 1:15–28.

Burkhardt, J. E., Pandher, K., Solter, P. F. et al. 2011. Recommendations for the evaluation of pathology data in nonclinical safety biomarker qualification studies. *Toxicol Pathol* 39:1129–37.

Bussiere, J., Leach, M. W., Price, K. D. et al. 2011. Survey results on the use of the tissue cross-reactivity immunohistochemistry assay. *Reg Toxicol Pharmacol* 59:493–502.

Caponigro, G. and Sellers, W. R. 2011. Advances in the preclinical testing of cancer therapeutic hypothesis. *Nature Rev Drug Discov* 10:179–87.

Chamanza, R., Marxfeld, H. A., Blanco, A. I. et al. 2010. Incidences and range of spontaneous findings in control cynomolgus monkeys (*Macaca fascicularis*) used in toxicity studies. *Toxicol Pathol* 38:642–57.

Chen, X. M. 2009. MicroRNA signatures in liver disease. *World J Gastroenterol* 15:1665–72.

Cheng, H., Kari, G., Dicker, A. P. et al. 2011. A novel preclinical strategy for identifying cardiotoxic kinase inhibitors and mechanisms of cardiotoxicity. *Circ Res* 109:1401–9.

Crissman, J. W., Goodman, D. G., Hildebrandt, P. K. et al. 2004. Best practices guideline: toxicologic histopathology. *Toxicol Pathol* 32:126–31.

Davies, T. S. and Monro, A. 1995. Marketed human pharmaceuticals reported to be tumorigenic in rodents. *Toxicol Pathol* 14:90–107.

Dieterle, F., Sistare, F., Goodsaid, F. et al. 2010. Renal biomarker qualification submission: a dialog between the FDA-EMEA and Predictive Safety Testing Consortium. *Nat Biotechnol* 28:455–62.

Dorato, M. A., McMillan, C. L., and Vodicnik, M. J. 2008. The toxicologic assessment of pharmaceuticals and biotechnology products. In: *Principles and Methods in Toxicology* (A. Wallace Hayes, editor). Fifth Edition. CRC Press, Boca Raton, FL, pp. 325–68.

Dunstan, R. W., Wharton, K. A., Quigley, C. et al. 2011. The use of immunohistochemistry for biomarker assessment—can it compete with other technologies? *Toxicol Pathol* 39:988–1002.

Elmore, S. A. and Peddada, S. D. 2009. Points to consider on the statistical analysis of rodent cancer bioassay data when incorporating historical control data. *Toxicol Pathol* 37:672–6.

EMEA. 2000. The European Agency for the Evaluation of Medicinal Products Committee for Proprietary Medicinal Products. Note for guidance on repeated dose toxicity. http://www.eu/docs/en_GB/document_library/Scientific_guideline/2009/09/WC500003102.pdf. (accessed March 2012).

Ennulat, D., Magid-Slav, M., and Rehm, S. 2010a. Diagnostic performance of traditional hepatobiliary bio-markers of drug-induced liver injury in the rat. *Toxicol Sci* 116:397–412.

Ennulat, D., Walker, D., Cierno, F. et al. 2010b. Effects of hepatic drug-metabolizing enzyme induction on clinical pathology parameters in animals and man. *Toxicol Pathol* 38:810–28.

Ettlin, R. A., Bolon, B., Pyrah, I. et al. 2008. Global recognition of qualified toxicologic pathologists: where we are now and where we need to go. *Toxicol Pathol* 36:753–9.

FDA. 2011. Draft guidance. Guidance for industry: Use of histology in biomarker qualification studies. Washington, DC. USDHEW.

Finch, J. M. 2005. Recent developments in preclinical toxicological pathology. *Toxicol Appl Pharmacol* 207:S209–13.

Fishman, M. C. and Porter, J. A. 2005. A new grammar for drug discovery. *Nature* 437:491–3.

Frame, S. and Mann, P. 2008. Principles of pathology for toxicology studies In: *Principles and Methods in Toxicology* (A. Wallace Hayes, editor). Fifth Edition. CRC Press, Boca Raton, FL, pp. 591–610.

Hall, W. C. and Rojko, J. L. 1996. The use of immunohistochemistry for the evaluation the liver. *Toxicol Pathol* 24:4–12.

Hardisty, J. F., Anderson, D. C., Brodie, S. et al. 2008. Histopathology of the urinary bladders of cynomolgus monkeys treated with PPAR agonists. *Toxicol Pathol* 36:769–76.

Hardisty, J. F., Elwell, M. R., Ernst, H. et al. 2007. Histopathology of hemangiosarcomas in mice and hamsters and liposarcomas/fibrosarcomas in rats associated with PPAR agonists. *Toxicol Pathol* 35:928–41.

Harpur, E., Ennulat, D., Hoffman, D. et al. 2011. Biological qualification of biomarkers of chemical-induced renal toxicity in two strains of male rat. *Toxicol Sci* 122:235–52.

Hill, A., Mesens, N., Steeemans, M. et al. 2012. Comparisons between in vitro whole cell imaging and in vivo zebrafish-based approaches for identifying potential human hepatotoxicants earlier in pharmaceutical development. *Drug Metab Rev* 44:127–40.

Holland, T. and Holland, C. 2011a. Analysis of unbiased histopathology data from rodent toxicity studies (or, are these groups different enough to ascribe it to treatment?). *Toxicol Pathol* 39:569–75.

Holland, T. and Holland, C. 2011b. Unbiased histological examinations in toxicological experiments (or, the informed leading the blinded examination). *Toxicol Pathol* 39:711–4.

Iatropoulos, M. J. and Williams, G. M. 2011. Toxicologic pathology. Society of Toxicology Historical perspective. 11-2. http://www.toxicology.org/AI/MEET/AM2011/FAST_HistoricalPerspectives.pdf (accessed March 2012).

Jung, J., Park, M., Park, H. J. et al. 2011. ^{1}H NMR-based metabolic profiling of naproxen-induced toxicity in rats. *Toxicol Lett* 200:1–7.

Kaufmann, W., Nolte, T., Rittinghausen, S. et al. 2005. INHAND International Harmonization of nomenclature and diagnostic criteria for lesions in rats and mice. http://www.toxpath.org/inhand_112105.pdf (accessed March 2012).

Keenan, C., Elmore, S., Francke-Carroll, S. et al. 2009. Best practices for use of historical control data of pro-liferative rodent lesions. *Toxicol Pathol* 37:679–93.

Kerns, W., Schwartz, L., Blanchard, K. et al. 2004. Drug-induced vascular injury—a quest for biomarkers. *Toxicol Appl Pharmacol* 203:62–87.

Kittel, B., Ruehl-Fehlert, C., Morawietz, G. et al. 2004. Revised guides for organ sampling and trimming in rats and mice—part 2. A joint publication of the RITA and NACAD groups. *Exp Toxicol Pathol* 55:413–31.

Kramer, J. A., Sagartz, J. E., and Morris, D. L. 2007. The application of discovery toxicology and pathology towards the design of safer pharmaceutical lead candidates. *Nat Rev Drug Discov* 6:636–49.

Lang, P., Yeow, K., and Nichols, A. 2006. Cellular imaging in drug discovery. *Nat Rev Drug Discov* 5:343–56.

Laterza, O. F., Lim, L., Garrett-Engele, P. W. et al. 2009. Plasma microRNAs as diagnostically sensitive and specific biomarkers of tissue injury. *Clin Chem* 55:1977–83.

Leach, M. W., Halpern, W. G., Johnson, C. W. et al. 2010. Use of tissue cross-reactivity studies in the development of antibody-based biopharmaceuticals: history, experience, methodology and future directions. *Toxicol Pathol* 38: 1138–66.

Lewis, R. W., Billington, R., Debryune, E. et al. 2002. Recognition of adverse and nonadverse effects in toxicity studies. *Toxicol Pathol* 30:66–74.

Liebler, D. C. and Guengerich, F. P. 2005. Elucidating mechanisms of drug-induced toxicity. *Nat Rev Drug Discov* 4:410–20.

Louden, C., Brott, D., Katein, A. et al. 2006. Biomarkers and mechanisms of drug-induced vascular injury in non-rodents. *Toxicol Pathol* 34:19–26.

Maronpot, R. R., Yoshizawa, K., Nyska, A. et al. 2010. Hepatic enzyme induction: histopathology. *Toxicol Pathol* 38: 776–795.

Maziasz, T., Kadambi, V. J., Silverman, L. et al. 2010. Predictive toxicology approaches for small molecule oncology drugs. *Toxicol Pathol* 38:148–64.

McConnell, E. E., Solleveld, H. A., Swenberg, J. A. et al. 1986. Guidelines for combining neoplasms for evaluation of rodent carcinogenesis studies. *J Natl Cancer Inst* 76:283–9.

McKay, J. S., Barale-Thomas. E., Bolon, B. et al. 2010. A commentary on the process of peer review and pathology data locking. *Toxicol Pathol* 38:508–10.

Menke, A. L., Spitsbergen, J. M., Wolterbeek, A. P. M. et al. 2011. Normal anatomy and histology of the adult zebrafish. *Toxicol Pathol* 39:759–775.

Michael, B., Yano, B., Sellers, R. S. et al. 2007. Evaluation of organ weights for rodent and non-rodent toxicity studies: a review of regulatory guidelines and survey of current practices. *Toxicol Pathol* 35:742–50.

Morawietz, G., Ruehl-Fehlert, C., Kittel, B. et al. 2004. Revised guides for organ sampling and trimming in rats and mice—part 2. A joint publication of the RITA and NACAD groups. *Exp Toxicol Pathol* 55:433–49.

Morton, D., Elwell, M., Fairweather, W. et al. 2002. The Society of Toxicologic Pathology's recommendations on statistical analysis of rodent carcinogenicity studies. *Toxicol Pathol* 30:415–8.

Morton, D., Sellers, R. S., Barale-Thomas, E. et al. 2010. Recommendations for pathology peer review. *Toxicol Pathol* 38:1118–27.

Mullard, A. 2011. 2010 FDA drug approvals. *Nat Rev Drug Discov.* 10:82–5.

Muller, P. Y., Milton, M., Lloyd, P. et al. 2009. The minimum anticipated biological effect level (MABEL) for selection of first in human dose in clinical trials with monoclonal antibodies. *Curr Opin Biotechnol* 20:1–8.

Munos, B. 2009. Lessons from 60 years of pharmaceutical innovation. *Nat Rev Drug Discov* 8:965–8.

Nolte, T., Kaufman, W., Schorsh, F. et al. 2005. Standardized assessment of cell proliferation: the approach of RITA-CEPA working group. *Exp Toxicol Pathol* 57:91–103.

Ochoa, R. and Rousseaux, C. 2009. The role of toxicologic pathologist in risk management. *Toxicol Pathol* 37:705–6.

Olson, H., Betton, G., Robinson, D. et al. 2000. Concordance of the toxicity of pharmaceuticals in humans and in animals. *Regul Toxicol Pharmacol* 32:56–67.

Painter, J. T., Clayton, N. P., and Herbert, R. A. 2010. Useful immunohistochemistry markers of tumor differentiation. *Toxicol Pathol* 38:131–41.

Pandher, K., Leach, M. W., Burns-Naas, L. A. 2012. Appropriate use of recovery groups in nonclinical toxicity studies: value in a science-driven case-by-case approach. *Vet Pathol* 49:357–61.

Peto, R., Pike, M. C., Day, N. E. et al. 1980. Guidelines for simple sensitive significance tests for carcinogenic effects in long-term animal experiments. In: IARC Monographs on the Evaluation of the Carcinogenic Risk of Chemicals to Humans, upplement 2: Long-term and Short-term Screening Assays for Carcinogens: A Critical Appraisal. Lyon: International Agency for Research on Cancer, pp. 311–346

Ploemen, J. P. H. T. M., Kramer, H., Krajnc, E. I. et al. 2007. The use of toxicokinetic data in preclinical safety assessment: a toxicologic pathologist perspective. *Toxicol Pathol* 35:834–7.

Ponce, R. 2011. ICH S9: developing anticancer drugs, one year later. *Toxicol Pathol* 39:913–5.

Reddy, M. V., Sistare, F. D., Christensen, J. S. et al. 2010. An evaluation of chronic 6- and 12-month rat toxicology studies as predictors of 2-year tumor outcome. *Toxicol Pathol* 47:614–29.

Revised guides for organ sampling and trimming in rats and mice. http://reni.item.fraunhofer.de/reni/trimming/index.php (accessed January 2012).

RITA. http://reni.item.fraunhofer.de/reni/public/rita/ (accessed January 2012).

Rojas, C., Stathis, M., Polydefkis, M. et al. 2011. Glutamate carboxypeptidase activity in human skin biopsies as a pharmacodynamic marker for clinical studies. *J Transl Med* 9:27–34.

Roman, D., Greiner, B., Ibrahim, M. et al. 2002. Laser technologies in toxicopathology. *Toxicol Pathol* 30:11–14.

Ross, J. S. and Ginsburg, G. S. 2003. The integration of molecular diagnostics with therapeutics. Implication for drug development and pathology practice. *Am J Clin Pathol* 119:26–36.

Ruehl-Fehlert, C., Kittel, B., Morawietz, G. et al. 2003. Revised guides for organ sampling and trimming in rats and mice—part 1. *Exp Toxicol Pathol* 55:91–106.

Sarker, D., Pacey, S., and Workman, P. 2007. Use of pharmacokinetic/pharmacodynamic biomarkers to support rational cancer drug development. *Biomarkers Med* 1:399–417.

Sasseville, V. G., Lane, J. H., Kadambi, V. J. et al. 2004. Testing paradigm for prediction of development-limiting barriers and human drug toxicity. *Chem Biol Interact* 150:9–25.

Schofield, P. N., Dubus, P., Klein, L. et al. 2011. Pathology of the laboratory mouse: an international workshop on challenges for high throughput phenotyping. *Toxicol Pathol* 39:559–62.

Schultze, A. E., Bounous, D. I., and Provencher Bollinger, A. 2008. Veterinary clinical pathologists in the biopharmaceutical industry. *Vet Clin Pathol* 37:146–58.

Sellers, R. S., Morton, D., Michael, B. et al. 2007. Society of Toxicologic Pathology position paper: organ weight recommendations for toxicology studies. *Toxicol Pathol* 35:751–5.

Shackelford, C., Long, G., Wolf, J. et al. 2002. Qualitative and quantitative analysis of nonneoplastic lesions in toxicology studies. *Toxicol Pathol* 30:93–6.

Sistare, F., Dieterle, F., Troth, S. et al. 2010. Toward consensus practices to qualify safety biomarkers for use in early drug development. *Nat Biotechnol* 28:446–454.

Sistare, F. D., Morton, D., Alden, C. et al. 2011. An analysis of pharmaceutical experience with decades of rat carcinogenicity testing: support for a proposal to modify current regulatory guidelines.

Squire, R. A. 1997. A quarter century of toxicologic pathology: a personal perspective. *Toxicol Pathol* 25:423–5.

Standardized system of nomenclature and diagnostic criteria (SSNDC) guides. http://www.toxpath.org/ssndc.asp (accessed January 2012).

Stevens, J. L. and Baker, T. K. 2009. The future of drug safety testing: expanding the view and narrowing the focus. *Drug Discov Today* 14:162–7.

Swinney, D. C. and Anthony, J. 2011. How were new medicines discovered? *Nat Rev Drug Discov* 10:507–19.

Tesfamariam, B. and DeFelice, A. F. 2007. Endothelial injury in the initiation and progression of vascular disorders. *Vasc Pharmacol* 46:229–37.

Vahle, J. L., Finch, G. L., Heidel, S. M. et al. 2010. Carcinogenicity assessments of biotechnology-derived pharmaceuticals: a review of approved molecules and best practice recommendations. *Toxicol Pathol* 38:522–53.

Vet Pathol 2012. Special focus: phenotyping of genetically engineered mice. 49(1):4–235.

Wang, J., Urban, L., and Bojanic, D. 2007. Maximising use of in vitro ADMET tools to predict in vivo bioavailability and safety. *Expert Opin Drug Metab Toxicol* 3:641–65.

Wang, K., Zhang, S., Marzolf, B. et al. 2009. Circulating microRNAs, potential biomarkers for drug-induced liver injury. *Proc Natl Acad Sci USA* 106:4402–7.

Ward, J. M. 2010. The roles of the toxicologic pathologist in cancer research. *Toxicol Pathol* 38:39–42.

Ward, J. M., Erexson, C. R., Faucette, L. J. et al. 2006. Immunohistochemical markers for the rodent immune system. *Toxicol Pathol* 34:616–30.

Ward, J. M. and Thoolen, B. 2011. Grading of lesions. *Toxicol Pathol* 39:745–6.

Weingand, K., Brown, G., Hall, R. et al. 1996. Harmonization of animal clinical pathology testing in toxicity and safety studies. *Fundam Appl Toxicol* 29:198–201

Wetmore, B. A. and Merrick, B. A. 2004. Invited review: toxicoproteomics: proteomics applied to toxicology and pathology. *Toxicol Pathol* 32:619–42.

Wolf, D. C. and Mann, P. 2005. Confounders in interpreting pathology for safety and risk assessment. *Toxicol Appl Pharmacol* 202:302–8.

Ying, X. and Monticello, T. 2006. Modern imaging technologies in toxicologic pathology: an overview. *Toxicol Pathol* 34:815–26.

Young, J., Hall, R. L., O'Brien, P. et al. 2011. Best practices for clinical pathology testing in carcinogenicity studies. *Toxicol Pathol* 39:429–34.

Zhou, Y., Rideout, W. M., Zi, T. et al. 2010. Chimeric mouse tumor models reveal differences in pathway activation between ERBB family- and KRAS-dependent lung adenocarcinomas. *Nat Biotechnol* 28:71–8.

5 Routine and Special Techniques in Toxicologic Pathology

Daniel J. Patrick and Peter C. Mann

CONTENTS

5.1   INTRODUCTION

Pathologists have been involved in the evaluation of specimens from toxicology studies over the last two centuries. The primary or "routine" responsibility of the pathologist in nonclinical safety assessment is the necropsy of the test animals at the end of the studies and microscopic evaluation of hematoxylin and eosin (H&E)–stained tissue sections on glass slides. Today's digital and molecular technologies offer an almost limitless possibility of new techniques (many of which are discussed in this chapter) for more sensitive assessment of compound-induced changes. Even so, standard histopathology is still the most commonly used method to assess compound-induced toxicity. This evaluation relies heavily on the extensive anatomical pathology training of pathologists and his or her ability to recognize often subtle microscopic changes, distinguish them from spontaneous (background) changes, and accurately communicate them to non-pathologists. As part of this communication, it is important for pathologists to attempt to describe these changes within the context of pathogenesis, biological and toxicological significance, and adversity. In addition to the tissue section, the pathologist must be provided with accurate macroscopic observations and organ weights collected at necropsy, to correlate any compound-related macroscopic or organ weight findings with the microscopic findings. It is no wonder anatomical pathology is often regarded as a subjective art, and a specialty that is extremely difficult to master.

This chapter will provide a generalized overview of some of the more common routine and special procedures, with a focus on those that are most commonly used in nonclinical safety assessment by toxicologic pathologists. The first part of the chapter will focus on routine techniques such as necropsy, organ weights, and histology. The second part of the chapter will focus on some of the special techniques that are occasionally used such as *in situ* protein, RNA, and DNA evaluations and imaging methods outside of bright-field microscopy. Technical details have been published extensively elsewhere for each procedure, so the reader is encouraged to review the list of references at the end of this chapter. It is important to stress that, at least for the immediate future, routine light microscopy of repeat-dose *in vivo* studies will continue to be the foundation of nonclinical safety assessment and the primary determinants of safety margins or dose-limiting toxicity, and special techniques should continue to be used to supplement, further understand, and assess the human risk of the microscopic findings.

5.2   ROUTINE TECHNIQUES

5.2.1   Necropsy Procedures

The necropsy is one of the most critical points in a toxicology study. Since the necropsy straddles the in-life and postmortem segments of the study, extreme care must be taken to accurately complete each step of the necropsy procedure (Frame and Mann 2008; Mann et al. 2002). Any information or samples that are lost, inadvertently not recorded, or misplaced *cannot* be reproduced. For these reasons, it is essential that the necropsy process be thoroughly planned prior to the day of necropsy. Technicians must be trained (and their training documented) for the prosection of the specific species being necropsied. Laboratory standard operating procedures (SOPs) for all aspects of the necropsy must be reviewed and understood. Finally, the particular study protocol must be reviewed, understood, and followed. This is especially true in contract research organizations (CROs), where different sponsors' requirements may be unique to their study or program.

It is recommended that animals be euthanized and necropsied in a replicate or "round robin" method. For example, an animal from the control group is followed by an animal from the high-dose group, followed by an animal from the mid-dose group, followed by an animal from the low-dose group, followed by a control, and so forth. There are several advantages to following this pattern, rather than all controls followed by all high-dose animals. First, the probability of group apparent artifacts, such as differences in the amount of glycogen in the liver due to fasting time, or increases in sodium values due to time from blood collection until analysis, is reduced. Also, there will be animals from different groups being necropsied at the same time, allowing the pathologist to compare control and treated animals to ascertain subtle differences in the gross appearance of potential target tissues.

The roles of the technicians are to complete the prosection of the animal, weigh required tissues, place the tissues into appropriate fixatives, and complete any special requirements for the particular study. Depending on the number of prosectors available and the type of animal and study, there may be one or more prosectors for each animal. When several prosectors are involved, one should perform the initial incisions and remove the major organ systems. These systems can then be split among the prosectors for final prosection and tissue preparation. In this manner, the putative target organs, as well as those that autolyze most rapidly, can be processed in a rapid and efficient manner. Multiple prosectors are typically involved when larger animal species (e.g., dogs, nonhuman primates) are being necropsied, or when there are complicated special procedures, such as freezing tissue for nucleic acid analyses.

The role of the pathologist in the necropsy room is twofold. The first is to be the responsible scientist for this phase of the study and to ensure that the entire necropsy procedure is conducted according to SOPs and protocol. Should deviations occur, it is the necropsy pathologist, together with the study director, who must decide how to proceed and make immediate decisions to preserve as much of the protocol-driven necropsy as possible.

The necropsy pathologist's second responsibility is to ensure that gross changes are accurately described. Experienced prosectors generally do an excellent job at dissection and the prosector (by virtue of having observed many hundreds of normal tissues) is generally an excellent judge of when a tissue does not appear "normal"; however, it is the role of the necropsy pathologist to describe the gross changes, on the basis of his or her medical training as well as changes seen in previous studies with the same compound, or with similar compounds in the same class. For this reason, the prosector should call the necropsy pathologist to the necropsy table whenever there is an apparent abnormal tissue, and the pathologist should decide how to describe the change and record it.

Necropsy observations may be entered manually on a necropsy form, or they may be entered into a computer, along with the organ weights, tissue lists, and so forth, as required by SOPs. Standard glossary lists should be used. One pathologist can handle observations from multiple necropsy stations, even for studies with numerous gross changes. The necropsy pathologist may be the pathologist assigned to microscopically evaluate the study slides. In some organizations, especially busy CROs, there is a pathologist dedicated to the necropsy room and the findings are entered into the database and passed along to the study pathologist.

Organ weights are also collected from a subset of the protocol-required tissues. It is important to remove all the extraneous fat and tissue in a consistent manner for all animals. Each necropsy station may have a digital scale, or there may be a technician that is dedicated to the collection of organ weights from several necropsy stations at the same time. In the latter arrangement, the prosectors "hand over" the tissues (covered in saline to prevent tissue dehydration) to the weigher. After all the required tissue samples have been removed, they are placed in a fixative. The necropsy form contains a listing of each tissue required for the animal, and the technicians should check each individual tissue as it is placed into the fixative. One technician should verbally announce the individual tissue as it is placed in the fixative, while a second technician should check the appropriate box on the form. Occasionally, tissues are lost during the necropsy process; this information should also be registered on the necropsy forms.

After all the required tissues have been placed in the appropriately labeled container and the carcass has been disposed of, the work station can be cleaned, and the next animal euthanized and brought to the station. At no time should there be more than one animal at a station.

The time interval between euthanasia and the placement of tissues into the fixative is critical to prevent autolysis and provide quality tissues for microscopic examination. For example, liver samples that are delayed in fixation may have increased liver weights and develop postmortem artifactual vacuolization that can be difficult to differentiate from treatment-related effects. Tissues that have been removed from the animal but not yet put in the fixative should be placed in a tray and covered with normal saline to prevent excessive drying. A properly trained technician should be able to complete a rodent necropsy in approximately 20 min; a dog or a nonhuman primate could take longer. Necropsy times longer than 30 min may allow autolytic changes to develop in tissues that could make microscopic evaluation more difficult.

5.2.1.1 Terminal Procedures

5.2.1.1.1 Euthanasia

A number of different methods of euthanasia are used in laboratories. The choice depends on local legal requirements, availability of euthanasia agents, and training of technical staff to ensure that euthanasia is quick and provides the maximum amount of anesthesia to the animal to minimize unnecessary suffering (AVMA guidelines on euthanasia 2007; Frame and Mann 2008).

5.2.1.1.1.1 Sodium Pentobarbital Anesthesia followed by Exsanguination   An overdose of this injectable anesthetic agent will provide rapid euthanasia. After the animal is no longer responsive to the external stimuli (gauged by toe pinch response, etc.), the chest and abdominal cavities should be quickly opened. The diaphragm should be cut to prevent further respiratory attempts, and the animal should be exsanguinated via the abdominal aorta/vena cava or femoral/axillary vein. If required, large amounts of blood can be collected from the heart and aorta before exsanguination.

5.2.1.1.1.2 Methoxyflurane or Isoflurane   Methoxyflurane and isoflurane are both inhalation anesthetic agents; overdose will provide euthanasia. As with sodium pentobarbital, euthanasia should be followed by exsanguination. Methoxyflurane or isoflurane may be administered either via nose cone or in a euthanasia box with a sliding lid to prevent the escape of gases when the lid is lifted.

5.2.1.1.1.3 Carbon Dioxide Asphyxiation   Exposure to high concentrations of carbon dioxide followed by exsanguination is a commonly used euthanasia agent for rodents, since it is inexpensive and easy to use. It has rapid depressant, analgesic, and anesthetic effects. Induction of loss of consciousness at lower concentrations (<80%) may produce pulmonary and upper respiratory tract lesions. Carbon dioxide should not be used alone in animals under 16 weeks of age except to induce loss of consciousness followed by death by some other means such as exsanguination. Since many more humane methods of euthanasia are readily available today, carbon dioxide asphyxiation should not be the first choice for euthanasia.

5.2.1.1.1.4 Other Methods of Euthanasia   Specialized studies may require alternative methods of euthanasia. Cervical dislocation and decapitation are both used in some cases. Both of these methods require extensive training to ensure that the method of euthanasia is rapidly and humanely conducted.

5.2.1.1.2 Blood and Urine Collection

As mentioned, if terminal blood collection is required by protocol, it can be easily achieved when the animal is anesthetized just prior to the beginning of the necropsy. Similarly, terminal urine samples can be obtained from the urinary bladder using a syringe and needle before the necropsy begins.

5.2.1.2 Dissection and Gross Examination

The process of dissection (prosection) and gross examination of the animals in a study is one of the key events in the entire study. Careful attention to detail is essential. It cannot be emphasized enough that data lost at necropsy are data lost forever. A systematic approach ensures that all protocol-required tissues and gross observations will be recorded and saved. The quality of the necropsy determines the quality of the slides, which in turn affects the overall quality of the study (Bono and Elwell 2000; Bucci 2002; Frame and Mann 2008; Mann et al. 2002).

5.2.1.2.1   External Examination

Before the dissection begins, the state of anesthesia must be determined. This is accomplished by pinching the toe or touching the eye to verify that the animal no longer responds to these stimuli. The dorsal and ventral surfaces of the animal should be examined for any masses or other changes (ulcers, scabs, etc.). All of the body orifices are examined for blood, mucus, or other abnormalities. The ears and eyes are examined for exudate and corneal or lens opacities. The nose and oral cavity are examined for excess mucus, misaligned teeth, or soft tissue changes. The presence or absence of any masses tracked during the in-life portion of the study should be correlated.

5.2.1.2.2   Internal Examination

Several different methods for examination of the internal organs of a test animal are available. The method used does not matter so much as the use of a fixed routine so that all required organs are examined and collected in the same manner from each animal in the study. The following descriptions of order and flow are the methods that have worked well in our experience.

5.2.1.2.3   Eyes, Optic Nerves, Harderian/Lacrimal Glands

Since these organs are on the surface of the animal, are generally delicate, and must be removed to provide access to the brain, they are removed first. In rodents, they can be removed as one block of tissue, and the Harderian and lacrimal glands can be left attached to the eyes for fixation, if desired.

5.2.1.2.4   Brain

In order to remove the brain, the calvarium must be first removed using bone clippers or a saw. After the brain is exposed, a small spatula is used to sever the brain from the cervical spinal cord and the olfactory bulbs and to elevate the brain so that it can be placed in the fixative. When elevating the brain, care should be taken not to disturb the pituitary, which lies under the brain.

5.2.1.2.5   Pituitary

After the brain has been removed, the pituitary can be seen in the sella turcica (the term means Turkish saddle, so called for its resemblance to a saddle) at the base of the skull. The pituitary is very fragile and is usually fixed *in situ* in the skull. Since there is little difference in the density of formalin compared to water, the pituitary weight will not be affected by fixation, and the pituitary is much easier to handle when fixed.

5.2.1.2.6   Nasal Turbinates and Zymbal's Glands

Remove the skull from the cervical spinal column. In order to ensure that the internal surfaces of the nasal cavity fix properly, the fixative should be injected into the nasopharyngeal opening at the back of the oral cavity until the fixative flows out of the nares. Zymbal's glands are located at the base of the ear below the ear canal. They are left attached to the head for fixation.

5.2.1.2.7   Skin and Mammary Gland

Prior to opening the body cavities, the ventral skin is peeled back, and any masses noted during the external examination are collected. The routine sections of skin and mammary gland are from the ventral midline area. Since rodents have mammary glands that extend from the inguinal to the cervical areas, large sections may be collected from either the thoracic or inguinal skin. A commonly used technique for fixation of the skin/mammary tissue is to place the section gland-side down on a piece of cardboard (staples can be used). This keeps the skin from folding onto itself, which can create microtoming artifacts.

5.2.1.2.8   Thoracic Cavity

The salivary glands and submandibular lymph nodes, which are located in the ventral cervical area under the skin, are collected before the thorax is opened. The ribs and sternum are collected together by cutting the ribs on either side of the sternum. After the ribs have been removed, the thoracic pluck can be removed *en masse*.

5.2.1.2.9   Thoracic Pluck

The pluck consists of the heart, thymus, lungs, aorta, thyroid glands, parathyroid glands, tongue, larynx, trachea, and esophagus. The lungs and trachea should be removed from the rest of the organs and the lungs fixed by inflation with formalin through the trachea. The remaining tissues can be fixed intact or removed for weighing as directed by protocol.

5.2.1.2.10   Abdominal Cavity

The abdominal tissues are usually examined and removed in a standard order. The spleen and pancreas are removed first, followed by the kidneys and adrenals, taking care to locate the ureters if required before the kidneys are removed. The liver and diaphragm are then removed together.

The entire gastrointestinal tract is removed as a single unit. The stomach is separated from the intestines just below the pylorus. The stomach is generally opened along the greater curvature and the mucosal surfaces are examined for changes. The gastric mucosa is gently rinsed with saline to aid in the identification of changes. The stomach can then be pinned to a small corkboard or stapled to a card to keep it from curling during fixation. In some cases, the stomach may be infused with the fixative and opened for examination after it has fixed.

The following sections of the intestinal tract should be collected: duodenum, jejunum, ileum, cecum, colon, and (often) rectum. In rodents, the cecum will be opened and rinsed before collection; the other sections will not. Some laboratories will inject formalin into the entire intact intestinal tract before taking samples. In the case of large animals, it is often advantageous to open the entire length of the intestinal tract before samples are collected. The mesenteric lymph node and associated vessels can be collected along with the cecum, colon, and ileum (with Peyer's patches/ gut-associated lymphoid tissue).

5.2.1.2.11   Urogenital Tract

In females, the vagina, uterus, urinary bladder, and ovaries are removed as a block. In males, the testes and epididymides are removed from the scrotal sac, and the prostate, seminal vesicles, and urinary bladder are removed together.

5.2.1.2.12   Skeletal Muscle and Sciatic Nerve

A section of the biceps femoris muscle and the attached sciatic nerve are removed together.

5.2.1.2.13   Spinal Cord

The spinal cord may be left in place until after fixation, removed using bone clippers (generally restricted to large animals), or it may be blown out of the vertebral column with a blast of air from a syringe. After fixation, sections of cervical, thoracic, and lumbar spinal cord may be processed.

5.2.1.3   Description of Gross Lesions

All changes noted during the necropsy should be described using simple, clear, concise terminology (Frame and Mann 2008). Descriptions should be recorded at the time of necropsy. Diagnostic terms such as neoplasm or atrophy should not be used since they indicate a specific pathologic change, the entirety of which cannot be assessed by gross examination alone. Rather, the terms for gross changes should be descriptive, using general criteria such as location, number, size, distribution, color, characteristics, and consistency.

Location: The general location refers to the organ, body cavity, or body region where a lesion is located. A specific location refers to more localized regions such as subcutaneous, right or left, or a specific lobe (caudal) or region (cortex or medulla) of an organ.

Number: Numbers are used to map out masses and correlate them to masses tracked during the in-life phase of the study. All masses and abnormalities observed at necropsy should be recorded and sampled. When multiple masses occur within an organ such as liver or lung, each mass should receive a separate number so that they can be identified and tracked.

Size: A decrease or increase in the size of a normal structure can be described with actual measurements or by using generally qualitative terms such as slight, minimal, moderate, or marked. For example, measurements should be provided for readily quantifiable lesions, that is, white focus (2 mm diameter) on the liver capsule. Tissue masses should be individually described with three measurements (length, height, width). However, in some instances, more general descriptive terms are preferable, that is, pinpoint red foci on the gastric mucosa.

Distribution: Some of the more common terms for distribution of a lesion include bilateral, unilateral, focal, and diffuse.

Color: Color description is self-explanatory. Straightforward terms such as tan, red, black, white, and so forth should be used.

Characteristics: The characteristics of a lesion describe the nature and conformation of the change. In addition, the demarcation between normal and abnormal may be either poorly or well circumscribed. Modifiers such as pedunculated, umbilicated, or thickened (i.e., gastric mucosa diffusely thickened) may be used to describe the characteristics of a lesion.

Consistency: Nodules and masses may be soft or firm and fluids may be gelatinous or watery. Changes in the consistency of normal structures should be noted, such as scaliness of the skin or the irregular, roughened surface of an organ.

When used consistently and appropriately, these terms will allow for comparison of changes across animals and studies. In addition, they will allow a future reader or reviewer to "visualize" the appearance and potential significance of the gross changes noted at necropsy.

5.2.1.4 Organ Weights

Organ weights can be an extremely sensitive indicator of treatment effects, often showing increases before any changes can be appreciated with the microscope. In the case of livers with cytochrome P450 induction, it is possible to see up to a 20% weight increase before any histologic evidence of centrilobular hypertrophy can be reliably observed microscopically. Organs should be consistently trimmed of all extraneous tissue (connective tissue, fat) before they are weighed to ensure accurate comparison between groups. Some tissues such as thymus require special care, since it is not always possible to separate thymic tissue from surrounding thoracic tissues. In order to minimize individual variation, organ weights can be compared relative to body weight or brain weight. The reasoning is that as body weight increases or decreases, so would individual organ weights. Similarly, brain weight is conserved until an animal is extremely cachexic. It has been suggested that organ-to-body weight ratios are predictive for liver and thyroid, while organ-to-brain weight ratios are predictive for ovaries and adrenal glands (Bailey et al. 2004). When evaluating organ weight changes, it is useful to calculate the percentage increase of a treatment group compared to controls. Generally speaking, absolute and relative percentages should be at least 10% increased (or decreased) from controls, should both trend in the same direction, and should show a dose relationship before the organ weight data are considered biologically relevant.

5.2.1.5 Tissue Fixation

At the moment of death, the heart stops beating, oxygenation of tissues ceases, all active biological processes are halted, and the process of autolysis begins. In order to preserve tissue samples so that they can be processed and examined under the microscope, tissues must be placed into a fixative solution as soon as possible to arrest the process of autolysis and to preserve the tissues until they can be further processed (Bono and Elwell 2000; Frame and Mann 2008; Mann et al. 2002). A number of fixatives are available for both routine and specialized uses. Tissue fixation can be achieved by immersion, inflation, or perfusion.

5.2.1.5.1 Neutral Buffered Formalin

Ten percent neutral buffered formalin (NBF) is the most common immersion fixative used in routine studies. It consists of 10% of "strong" formalin (which is 37%–40% formaldehyde), giving a final percentage of approximately 4% formaldehyde. NBF is easy to use, is inexpensive, and achieves rapid penetration of tissues. Although it can be made in the laboratory, the most economical and consistent method is to purchase premade buffered formalin. The phosphate buffers bring the formalin solution to a pH of ~7.0. This pH avoids the formation of formalin pigments (acid hematin) in preserved tissues. Tissue preservation in NBF is good, and tissues can be kept in formalin for long periods without adverse effects, except for excessive cross-linking of antigenic sites if immunohistochemistry (IHC) is later elected (this is covered in Section 5.3). Tissue should be kept in formalin for at least 24–48 h, in order to achieve complete fixation, and before they can be trimmed for histology. Any residual tissues should remain in NBF for long-term "wet tissue" storage.

Negative aspects of NBF include the fact that it is highly toxic and a known mutagen, as well as an inhalation carcinogen in rodents. For this reason, it requires special handling and adequate ventilation. Occupational Safety and Health Administration regulations require regular monitoring of exposure for workers exposed to formalin.

Other disadvantages of NBF include excessive tissue shrinkage, poor cellular detail (especially in eyes and testes), retinal detachment, and loss of certain staining characteristics. In addition, NBF will cause staples, pins, and metal identification tags to rust and degrade over long periods. To some degree, these disadvantages can be overcome by post-fixation in picric acid fixatives or by different processing. If the disadvantages present significant problems, a primary fixative other than formalin should be used.

5.2.1.5.2 Bouin's Fluid

There are a number of fixatives that use picric acid along with primary fixatives such as formaldehyde. Bouin's fluid is the most widely used of these. It is good for the fixation of eyes, pancreas, ovaries, testes, thyroids, adrenals, fetuses, and fish (where it aids in decalcification). There is less shrinkage than with 10% NBF.

On the other hand, Bouin's fluid has a number of distinct disadvantages: Picric acid in its dry state is explosive. Bouin's fluid will stain tissues bright yellow, and the color will carry through to processing solutions. Fixation in Bouin's for more than 24 h will cause excessive shrinkage and dryness of tissues, but this can be avoided by transferring the tissues to NBF after 24 h of fixation in Bouin's. There is an overall increase in eosinophilia with H&E stain in tissues fixed in Bouin's. Finally, Bouin's fluid must be treated as a hazardous substance for disposal.

Although Bouin's has been used in the past for fixation, especially of eyes and testes, the disadvantages outweigh the advantages of using this fixative and is used much less frequently these days since there are better alternatives available.

5.2.1.5.3 Modified Davidson's Fluid

As noted above, there are disadvantages to using either NBF or Bouin's fluid (e.g., loss of cellular detail, excessive tissue shrinkage). These issues are especially problematic for the fixation of eyes and testes. Since eyes contain tissues of markedly differing hardness (lens and retina), it is extremely difficult to produce sections in which both are optimally prepared. For the testes, fixatives that cause shrinkage (NBF or Bouin's) cause differential shrinkage of the tubules away from the interstitial tissue, making interpretation of testicular changes difficult. Modified Davidson's fluid has been shown to provide excellent cellular detail for both eyes and testes and does not have the disposal or safety hazards of either NBF or Bouin's fluid (Latendresse et al. 2002). Many laboratories now routinely use Modified Davidson's fluid for fixation of eyes and testes.

5.2.1.5.4   McDowell's and Trump's 4F:1G Fixative

The fixatives listed above are sufficient for light microscopic examination. Different fixatives, using glutaraldehyde rather than formaldehyde, are required for tissues that will be examined by transmission electron microscopy (TEM). McDowell's and Trump's 4F:1G fixative contains both formaldehyde and glutaraldehyde (in a 4:1 ratio). This fixative produces tissues that can be examined using either light microscopy or TEM. In addition, studies have shown that tissues fixed in McDowell's and Trump's can be maintained for several years at 4°C without noticeable loss of ultrastructural integrity (Dykstra et al. 2002).

5.2.1.5.5   Alcohol Fixation

Formalin and other aldehyde fixatives preserve tissues by cross-linking proteins. For the purposes of many of the newer technologies (IHC, RNA analysis, etc.), this cross-linking makes molecular profiling much more difficult. Although there are post-fixation methods to improve protein availability for tissues fixed with an aldehyde fixative (covered in Section 5.3), the use of alcohol-based fixatives does not involve cross-linking of proteins and may be recommended for these types of studies. Different authors have recommended slightly different protocols, ranging from 70% ethanol to modified methacarn, which consists of 8 parts methanol:1 part glacial acetic acid. Another option is to fix tissue in formalin for no more than 24 h and then transfer them to 70% alcohol. This method provides for the more rapid fixation of an aldehyde fixative but prevents excessive cross-linking of proteins and has proved to be acceptable for many immunohistochemical stains (Cox et al. 2006; Gillespie et al. 2002).

5.2.1.5.6   Fixation Techniques

Regardless of the type of fixative chosen for a particular tissue, there are several methods for delivering the fixative to the tissue—immersion, inflation, and perfusion (Frame and Mann 2008).

5.2.1.5.7   Immersion

Fixation by immersion is the most common method used in routine toxicology studies. Since fixatives penetrate from the outer surfaces inward, it is essential that the pieces of tissues be appropriately thin. It is far better to have a long thin piece of tissue than a short thick one. Tissues should be trimmed to no greater than 5 mm thick. Organs (liver and kidney) that are thicker than this should be "bread loafed" (a number of parallel cuts into but not through the organ, so as to maintain the gross integrity of the organ prior to trimming) before they are immersed in fixative. The volume of the fixative is important: most texts recommend a 10:1 fixative-to-tissue volume ratio, although in practice, the ratio can be as low as 5:1 without loss of tissue integrity. The smaller ratio can be used if organs are cut to allow fixative penetration into multiple surfaces. Tissues should be fixed for at least 24 to 48 h. If the tissues are to be kept in the fixative for any length of time before processing, or if there is excessive blood or other fluids in the container, the fixative should be changed after the initial period of fixation.

5.2.1.5.8   Inflation

Certain tissues are normally expanded in-life by fluids (e.g., urinary bladder) or air (e.g., lungs). If these tissues are simply immersed in fixative, they will not maintain their in-life orientation, and microscopic interpretation could be problematic. Inflation with fixative before immersion will alleviate these problems. It is important that the amount of pressure applied during the inflation process be very gentle, so that the organs inflate to no more than their normal in-life diameter. This is especially true for lungs, where overenthusiastic inflation can cause artifactual changes that resemble perivascular edema. After the lungs have been inflated, the trachea should be tied off to prevent the backflow of the fixative along with surfactant.

5.2.1.5.9 Perfusion

For certain studies, it is essential that the fixative reach the critical tissues as soon after death as possible. For example, in some studies involving the central nervous system as a target, the delay involved in a normal necropsy procedure might cause artifacts in the target tissues. In these cases, perfusion provides the solution. The animal is euthanized using an intravenous agent. The body cavity is then opened, and vessels are secured for both inflow (arterial) and outflow (venous) of the perfusion fixative. The euthanasia solution is then followed by isotonic saline, which is used to clear the blood from the vascular system. As soon as the blood has been removed from the body (fluids run clear), the fixative is applied. Depending on the vessels chosen, the perfusion fixation can be for the entire body, or for a particular organ or set of organs.

5.2.2 HISTOLOGY PROCEDURES

After the necropsy, the collected tissues go through a series of defined steps in order to produce slides for the pathologist to examine. The primary goal is to produce high-quality slides that are free from avoidable artifacts. By adhering to a set of laboratory-specific SOPs, each step of each process will be performed in the same way every time, and there is tissue accountability at every point. This method removes most of the variability that might be introduced by using random, nonstandardized methods in the laboratory.

5.2.2.1 Trimming

Following proper fixation, the first step in producing slides is trimming (Bono and Elwell 2000). The primary goal is to produce tissue sections that will fit into the appropriate cassettes for further processing, so that the maximum surface area of tissue will be available for examination. In order to standardize the sections that will be examined, it is essential that each piece of tissue be trimmed in exactly the same manner from all animals in a study. For example, if two lobes of liver are to be processed, the trimmer must take the sections from the same two lobes from every animal. The tissue surface to be examined microscopically should be placed face down in the cassette. If necessary, the cut surface may be identified by notching, or marking the opposite surface with tissue-marking ink. It is essential that the cassette be permanently identified, either by an automated stamping machine, with pencil or an indelible marker. The ink in many pens will be removed during standard processing, leaving unmarked, unidentifiable cassettes. For further security, a paper identification label can be placed in the cassette on top of the tissue, which will end up embedded in the paraffin block on top of the tissue. Multiple sections should be trimmed of tissue masses that are large or variable. In addition, a portion of adjacent normal tissue should be included if possible. Sections should be trimmed no thicker than 0.3 cm thick for processing. Tissues less than 0.3 cm may be left intact. Cassettes with a fine mesh or sponges are available for small tissues to ensure that they remain in the cassette during processing. Tissue trimming should be done by technicians who have received training in gross anatomy, who are familiar with medical terminology, and who understand the meaning of the gross observation made at necropsy. Specific trimming instructions for all tissues should be included in the SOPs for trimming. In addition to the tissues that are specified by the study protocol, all gross lesions identified at the time of necropsy must be trimmed in as well. In addition to gross lesions noted at necropsy, the trimmer may identify gross changes seen at the time of trimming. These lesions identified at trimming should be recorded and added to the protocol-required tissues for the particular animal. For most routine toxicology studies, multiple tissues are embedded in a single cassette. The tissues should be selected on the basis of organ-system groupings when possible, keeping in mind that certain tissues should not be grouped since differences in tissue hardness would cause problems when the blocks are microtomed. It is important to note that, similar to necropsy, tissues lost or damaged during trimming are likely lost forever.

5.2.2.2 Processing

After the tissues have been trimmed and placed in cassettes, they go through a series of steps that include dehydration and impregnation with paraffin to produce blocks. Since paraffin is not miscible with water, tissue must be dehydrated and then cleared in solutions miscible with paraffin before impregnation. The paraffin keeps the tissue firm and in the proper orientation so that uniform thin sections of tissue can be cut using a microtome.

5.2.2.2.1 Dehydration

Dehydration is the removal of all extractable water from the tissue samples. A series of graded alcohols is the most commonly used method of dehydration, starting with 70%–80% alcohol and progressing to absolute (100%) alcohol. Enough time must be allowed at each step for complete infiltration of the tissue. Generally, processing schedules are developed by species, that is, longer dehydration times for larger animal species.

5.2.2.2.2 Clearing

Clearing is the step after dehydration. The alcohol remaining from the dehydration step is removed and the tissue clears, becoming translucent. Clearing reagents must be miscible with both the dehydrant (alcohol) and paraffin. Xylene is the most widely used clearing agent. Other clearing agents include toluene and D-limonene. Clearing time must be carefully regulated to avoid excessive hardening of the tissue, which will cause problems later in the process.

5.2.2.2.3 Infiltration

After clearing, the tissue is infiltrated with paraffin. Infiltration is the complete removal of the clearing reagents, by substitution with paraffin. The tissue is placed in a paraffin bath, where liquid paraffin penetrates the tissue. The temperature of the paraffin bath is critical. The melting point of most paraffin is 56°C–58°C. Temperatures >5°C above the melting point will cause excessive shrinkage and hardening of tissue samples. After infiltration, the cassettes are exposed to a vacuum that removes air, gases, and any remaining clearing reagent and at the same time will aid in drawing paraffin into all areas of the tissue.

5.2.2.3 Embedding

While most of the previous processes are generally automated, embedding is a hands-on process. The paraffin-impregnated tissue samples are placed into molds along with additional molten paraffin. The technician assures that the tissues are properly placed in the mold when the paraffin is still melted. The molds are then chilled to produce tissue blocks. The solid paraffin provides a firm medium for keeping all parts of the tissue in the proper orientation when sections are made. The tissues should be transferred from the processing cassette to the mold so that the correct surface is embedded face down in the mold. The orientation and location of tissue in the paraffin block must be consistent from animal to animal, according to the laboratory's SOPs. Care must be taken to ensure that all processed tissue is placed in the block. If utilized, the paper label from the cassette should be placed in the paraffin on the upper surface of the paraffin block (above the tissue sample). After the paraffin has been chilled and solidified, the paraffin block is removed from the mold and is ready for the microtome.

5.2.2.4 Sectioning (Microtomy)

In microtomy, tissue sections are prepared from the paraffin blocks and mounted on glass slides. The sections are generally prepared using a rotary microtome, an instrument that produces uniformly thick sections from paraffin blocks. The block is placed in a chuck in the microtome. As the wheel on the microtome is turned, the block comes into contact with a steel knife advancing 4–6 µm with each turn of the wheel, producing ribbons of paraffin-embedded tissue. The blocks are routinely microtomed to produce 4–6 µm sections for most tissues. Thinner sections (2–4 µm) are desirable for some tissues, especially lung and kidney. Thicker sections (8–12 μm) are often taken from brain and spinal cord. Before the tissue sections are cut, the surface of the block is placed on ice to harden the paraffin and moisten the tissue. The first few sections produced from a block (facing) are discarded, so as to avoid a "moth-eaten" artifact in sections. The ribbons of paraffin sections are carefully removed from the edge of the knife blade and floated on the surface of a warm water bath, which may have adhesive added to prevent the tissue from washing off the slide during later staining processes. Glass slides are dipped in the water bath under the tissue sections and lifted out with the tissue sections attached. Care must be taken to avoid inaccuracies in slide identification. Glass slides with unstained tissues must be identified by one of the following methods: automated slide markers, lead pencil, indelible ink, or hand etching with a diamond pen.

After the tissue sections have been placed on the glass slides, the slides are placed in a warming oven or dried overnight at room temperature, so that the paraffin melts and only the tissue section remains adhered to the glass slide. At this point, the slide is ready for staining.

5.2.2.5 Staining

The slides produced by the foregoing process contain translucent tissue sections, with no contrast between various parts of organs, tissues, or cells; thus, microscopic interpretation of these sections would be impossible. Over time, a number of stains that enable the pathologist to make accurate interpretations of tissue changes have been developed (Bancroft and Gamble 2007; Kiernan 2008; Prophet et al. 1992). It should be stated that all stains are artifacts, since tissues do not "naturally" contain these colors. However, they are controlled artifacts, which allow the pathologist to determine changes on a cellular level.

5.2.2.5.1 Routine H&E

The most commonly used stain for routine studies is H&E. Hematoxylin is a basic dye that stains nuclei blue (basophilic) because of an affinity for the nucleic acids in the cell nucleus. Eosin is an acidic dye that stains the cytoplasm of cells pink to red (eosinophilia). This stain has been the "workhorse" for tissue staining for decades, since it produces slides where the nucleus and cytoplasm can be clearly differentiated, and changes in both are clearly appreciated.

5.2.2.5.2 Special Stains

There are certain cases where a stain is needed to understand specific changes in a cell or organ. For these purposes, a number of "special stains" have been developed. Each of these histochemical stains illustrates a particular property of tissues or cells, intracellular structures, or microorganisms. As such, they are not useful for routine evaluation and should only be used when required to help elucidate the presence or absence of the specific change being investigated. Some of the more commonly used special stains are described below.

5.2.2.5.2.1 Periodic Acid–Schiff

Periodic acid–Schiff (PAS) is a staining method most often used to identify the presence of glycogen in tissue sections. The periodic acid oxidizes glucose residues in tissue, creating aldehydes that then react with the Schiff reagent, creating a magenta color. A blue counterstain is often added to make interpretation easier. PAS is used to identify structures that have a high proportion of carbohydrate macromolecules (glycogen, glycoproteins, and proteoglycans) typically found in connective tissue, mucus, and basal laminate. PAS is often used to elucidate changes in basement membranes. It also selectively stains most protozoa organisms as well as many fungal organisms. The presence of glycogen can be confirmed by using diastase to remove the glycogen. A PAS with diastase slide (glycogen digested) will not show any magenta staining, while a PAS without diastase negative slide will show magenta staining. The PAS staining for glycogen will depend on preservation of glycogen in the organs as it is subject to leeching out into the normal fixatives.

5.2.2.5.2.2 Toluidine Blue   Toluidine blue (T-blue) is a cationic (basic) stain that stains the granules in mast cells violet red. T-blue interacts with the acidic heparin in the mast cell granules to produce the characteristic violet red color.

5.2.2.5.2.3 Oil Red O   Oil Red O is used to demonstrate the presence of neutral lipids in tissue sections. This technique can only be used on unprocessed (unfixed frozen or formalin-fixed) tissue samples. If the tissue has undergone processing, the stain will not work, since the dehydration step will remove the lipid from the tissue. Oil Red O stains neutral lipids red.

5.2.2.5.2.4 Trichrome   Many trichrome stains (trichrome means three colors) are available for the differential staining of tissues, with Masson's trichrome being one of the most commonly used. Masson's trichrome stains collagen blue, muscle red, and erythrocytes orange. Trichrome stains can be very helpful in estimating the amount of collagen in a tissue sample.

5.2.2.5.2.5 Perls' Iron/Perls' Prussian Blue   Perls' iron is the classic stain for demonstrating the presence of hemosiderin (ferric iron) in tissue. The iron granules in hemosiderin, as well as other iron deposits (e.g., hemochromatosis), react to form a bright blue insoluble compound known as Prussian blue, which is readily identifiable within the section.

5.2.2.5.2.6 Von Kossa's Method   Von Kossa's method is used to visualize calcium deposits in tissue sections. Using this method, calcium stains brown to black.

5.2.2.5.2.7 Luxol Fast Blue   A number of specialized stains are used in neuropathology. The luxol fast blue stain for the myelin sheath is one of the most commonly used. The stain reacts with the lipoprotein in myelin. With this stain, myelinated nerve fibers appear blue, neutrophils appear pink, and neurons appear purple.

5.2.2.6 Coverslipping

In the final stage of preparation, a glass coverslip is placed over the tissue section on the slide, using mounting medium to keep the coverslip in place as well as to seal the section, so that the tissue section is protected from the environment (air, etc.), which will cause loss of quality of the staining. Coverslipping can be done by hand, or using a robotic coverslipping machine. The latter method is preferred, since it frees a histology technician for more appropriate tasks.

5.2.2.7 Histotechnique Quality Assessment

After a slide has been made, stained, and coverslipped, but before it is given to the pathologist for examination, a Histotechnique Quality Assessment should be performed. This process is also known as Slide Checkout or Slide Review and should typically consist of the following: making sure that all of the gross lesion observations and all of the protocol-required tissues for the study are present, assuring that all blocks and slides are correctly labeled, ensuring that each tissue is an adequate section, and making sure that the overall stain quality is satisfactory. A number of artifacts can occur during the slide-making and staining procedures. These artifacts can obscure the tissue or make it impossible to evaluate. Some examples of potential artifacts include the following: excessive or inadequate mounting media, air bubbles, knife marks, tissue folds, tissue holes, excessively thick and shattered sections, tissue floaters, and adhesive residue and processing artifacts.

Recuts should be requested for any missing tissues, as well as for those artifacts that might interfere with tissue examination and evaluation. Finally, the slides should be organized for the pathologist's examination, ideally in the laboratory's standard order. This final check will enable the pathologist to efficiently examine all the tissues from a study and minimize recut requests.

5.3 SPECIAL TECHNIQUES

5.3.1 Introduction

The four most critical questions that the toxicologic pathologist must answer after identifying a particular microscopic change are as follows: (1) What is the best descriptive term? (2) Is the change compound induced (versus iatrogenic, spontaneous, stress related)? (3) What is the magnitude of the compound effect, especially in relation to dose? (4) What does the change mean? Answering questions 1 and 2 relies heavily on the extensive veterinary medical training, anatomical pathology training, and experience of the pathologist, as well as on knowledge of the compound's mechanism of action. Histochemical staining, immunohistochemical staining, and electron microscopy can also greatly assist the toxicologic pathologist in choosing and recording the most accurate diagnosis for the change. Answering question 3 regarding the magnitude of the change, pathologists can provide semiquantitative grade estimates, but when more detailed quantification is needed, special procedures such as histomorphometry or stereology are needed. Answering the fourth question (what does the identified change mean?), especially in terms of human risk, is often where special techniques such as IHC, electron microscopy, *in situ* hybridization (ISH), confocal microscopy, *in vivo* imaging, and so forth come into play and where mechanistic risk assessments of the change should be investigated.

Determining the mechanism of a light microscopic change, if possible, is essential in nonclinical safety assessment, as it helps prevent harm to human subjects in clinical trials, helps in the selection of first dose in humans, and helps prevent the unnecessary removal of a drug that had potential for human benefit. Investigating the mechanism of a particular nonclinical study change also allows investigators to refine the compound and possibly make it safer. It is important for toxicologic pathologists to be up to date and familiar with some of the more common special procedures with applications in nonclinical pathology assessment. A basic understanding of these techniques allows a pathologist to recognize when they can (or, sometimes more importantly, cannot!) be used for a particular application, communicate intelligently with other scientists, and contribute as a valuable member of the nonclinical research team. Often, a variety of these techniques must be used in conjunction with light microscopic findings to answer a particular question or understand the pathogenesis in greater depth.

5.3.2 Imaging Methods

The foundation of the practice of anatomical pathology is the interpretation of images. Traditionally, this has consisted of a pathologist being physically seated at the microscope viewing transmitted light images through the eyepieces of a light (bright-field) microscope. However, this scenario is rapidly evolving, and it is important for pathologists to be aware of other imaging modalities outside of bright-field microscopy. These include fluorescent microscopy (there are many new and improved fluorochromes now available) or those that use imaging signals other than visible light, such as electrons (electron microscopy), radiofrequency (magnetic resonance imaging [MRI]), x-ray (computed tomography [CT]), and gamma rays (positron emission tomography [PET] and single-photon emission computed tomography [SPECT]). This section will provide a brief overview of the various types of imaging methods outside of traditional bright-field microscopy. Many of these methods can provide additional information and answer questions outside the scope of traditional light microscopy, which potentially can lead to a much greater understanding of pathological processes and risk assessment.

5.3.2.1 Electron Microscopy

There are two major types of electron microscopies, TEM, which produces a two-dimensional micrograph of a thin slice of tissue, and scanning electron microscopy (SEM), which produces a three-dimensional micrograph of the surface topography of a tissue. TEM provides visualization of extracellular material such as collagen and amyloid, cell membranes, and cellular organelles including nuclei, mitochondria, smooth endoplasmic reticulum, rough endoplasmic reticulum, lysosomes, and peroxisomes. SEM is more frequently used for implanted device studies than in pharmaceutical studies. It provides visualization of surface topography and allows for the assessment of changes, an example of which would be the degree of endothelialization within an implanted coronary artery stent.

TEM allows for an examination of subcellular structures that can help elucidate mechanisms of toxicity, evaluate various organelles for morphological changes, and detect signals not detectable by light microscopy. This is because TEM can markedly increase resolution through the use of a beam of accelerated electrons that have a much shorter wavelength than photons, since resolution is inversely proportional to wavelength. Disadvantages of TEM include the need for special fixatives for optimal results, resin rather than paraffin embedding, and the extended number of steps and time to produce electron micrographs. These factors, in combination with the evolution of newer techniques and applications such as IHC, confocal microscopy, and reverse transcriptase polymerase chain reaction (RT-PCR), have limited the use of electron microscopy in nonclinical research. Also, despite TEM's ability to provide detailed ultrastructural information, this technique still relies on the skill and experience of a pathologist in recognizing and interpreting the morphological changes.

TEM in nonclinical safety evaluation is most commonly utilized prospectively, when the test article belongs to a class of compounds with a known ultrastructural effect, or retrospectively, when there is a well-defined question related to a light microscopic finding. The two most common light microscopic findings that lead to retrospective TEM are the presence of inclusions or vacuoles in cells. Electron microscopy is not (and should not be) routinely performed on nonclinical studies since this would be very labor intensive, time consuming, and likely unhelpful as significant ultrastructural changes are rarely present in a cell without the presence of light microscopic tissue changes. Regulatory requirements can also mandate the inclusion of TEM evaluations of particular tissues within nonclinical studies. Care must be taken to follow Good Laboratory Practices (GLPs) in the nonclinical safety assessment of GLP-compliant studies. TEM can further characterize the following: ultrastructural changes related to light microscopic changes (e.g., cellular hypertrophy, phospholipid-induced vacuolation, inclusions, thickened glomeruli, corneal changes, and changes in spermatozoa), ultrastructural changes responsible for biomarker changes in the absence of light microscopic changes (e.g., podocyte damage-induced proteinuria), and animal disease models (e.g., myelin presence and character in myelopathy models).

Typically, the main steps in TEM consist of sample collection containing the cells or structures of interest, glutaraldehyde fixation, buffer wash, osmium tetroxide post-fixation for lipid/phospholipid preservation, buffer wash (± uranyl acetate staining), ethanol or acetone dehydration, epoxy or acrylic resin embedding, preparation and examination of T-blue-stained semithin (0.5–1.0 μm) sections, preparation of ultrathin (~80 nm) sections mounted on specimen grids, staining with heavy metal atoms, and imaging via film or charge-coupled device (CCD) sensor. Electron microscopy is optimized when the tissue samples are preserved in an electron microscopy–type glutaraldehyde-based fixative such as McDowell's and Trump's 4F:1G fixative (Dykstra et al. 2002); however, routine formalin fixation may be adequate and is often all that is available when TEM is added after light microscopy. Autolytic changes, especially in mitochondria and endoplasmic reticulum, can be visible by TEM within a few postmortem minutes, so it is important to immerse the tissue sample in cooled fixative as quickly as possible and then trim the section down to roughly 1 mm^3 with a scalpel or razor blade. Perfusion fixation can aid in the fixation of some tissues of interest. Since nonclinical safety evaluations typically deal with effects of treatment in comparison to control animals, it is important to collect and examine samples from the same anatomical locations, both at necropsy and through the use of semithin plastic sections to identify the same areas of interest for the ultrathin sections.

5.3.2.2 Fluorescence Microscopy

The term "fluorescence" refers to the property of some substances (fluorophores) to absorb light of a certain wavelength called excitation light and simultaneously reemit it at a longer wavelength referred to as emission light. The difference in wavelength between excitation and emission is known as Stokes' shift and is fundamental to fluorescence labeling (Lichtman and Conchello 2005). Some substances (e.g., vitamin A and porphyrins) fluoresce naturally under ultraviolet excitation, which is primary or autofluorescence. Structures within tissues can also be made to fluoresce by the addition of a fluorochrome, termed secondary fluorescence. Each fluorochrome will fluoresce under light within a range of wavelengths, but optimal fluorescence occurs at a particular wavelength called the excitation peak. Fluorochrome labeling can identify cells, subcellular components, and other materials with a high degree of specificity and a high degree of sensitivity since only an extremely small number of fluorescent molecules are needed for detection by the human eye or digital sensor.

Traditional fluorochromes that are commonly used include fluorescein isothiocyanate (FITC, green color), 4',6-diamidino-2-phenylindole (DAPI, blue color, binds to DNA in nuclei), and Texas Red (red color). Today, there are hundreds of fluorochromes available with various excitation peak and emission wavelengths. Desirable features of fluorochromes include a large extinction coefficient (likelihood of absorption of the excitation light), high quantum yield (ratio of light emitted to light absorbed, higher = brighter fluorescence), narrow emission spectrum (to minimize overlapping emissions when using multiple fluorochromes in a specimen), and good resistance to photobleaching (the irreversible decomposition of the fluorochrome by light excitation). Newer fluorochromes that possess more of these desirable features include cyanine dyes, Alexa Fluor dyes, DyLight fluorescent dyes, and Oyster fluorescent dyes.

Quantum dots are a new type of fluorochrome composed of inorganic nanocrystals (Resch-Genger et al. 2008). They emit light similar to light-emitting diodes, but instead of activation by an electrical stimulus, they are activated by the absorption of a photon. Advantages include exceptional photostability, increased fluorescence intensity, and excitation over a broad range of wavelengths with emission of a very narrow and particular band of light based on the composition and size of the nanocrystal. This allows for the excitation of multiple quantum dot sizes (and colors) in the same specimen with a single excitation wavelength, making them especially useful for multiple labeling studies.

Naturally occurring fluorescent proteins (such as green fluorescent protein) and mutated derivatives allow for the labeling of a wide spectrum of intracellular processes in living organisms in addition to *in vitro* applications (Lang et al. 2006). These proteins can be fused to virtually any protein in living cells using recombinant complementary DNA cloning technology. Advantages of fluorescent proteins over the traditional organic and inorganic fluorochromes described above include a response to a wider variety of biological events and signals, an ability to specifically target fluorescent probes in subcellular compartments, an extremely low or absent photodynamic toxicity, and widespread compatibility with tissues and intact organisms.

There are two major types of fluorescent microscopes: conventional wide field and confocal. Wide-field fluorescent microscopes pass excited light onto the specimen field and visualize the emitted light from all of the fluorophores that are illuminated. Confocal fluorescent microscopes differ from wide field in that the excited light is focused onto just one spot in the plane of focus in the specimen and the detected emission light is also only collected from another focal point. This elimination of out-of-focus light greatly decreases background and increases contrast, and by scanning the entire specimen, highly detailed two-dimensional and three-dimensional fluorescent images can be generated (Conchello and Lichtman 2005).

5.3.2.2.1 Conventional Wide-Field Fluorescence Microscopy

Conventional wide-field fluorescence microscopy is also referred to as reflected light fluorescence microscopy, incident light fluorescence, episcopic fluorescence, or simply epifluorescence.

Epifluorescent microscopes generate an image much different than traditional (bright-field) microscopes where light from below the specimen is transmitted up through the specimen and objective lens. Instead, epifluorescent microscopes pass excited light from above down through the objective and onto the specimen, where the objective then magnifies and transmits the image back up to the viewer. Typical epifluorescent microscope components include two illumination sources (tungsten–halogen for transmitted light and mercury arc discharge for episcopic observations), excitation filter, dichroic mirror, and an emission (or barrier) filter (Lichtman and Conchello 2005). A microscope of this design can combine or alternate reflected light fluorescence with transmitted light microscopy duties. This setup allows for excitation of the specimen with selectively filtered illumination followed by isolation of the much weaker fluorescence emission using a second filter. Different dichroic mirrors (designed for particular fluorochromes) are able to selectively reflect wavelengths of a certain range (the excited light) onto the specimen, while simultaneously transmitting the longer light wavelengths emitted by the particular fluorochrome to the observer. Special filter blocks (or fluorescence filter sets) that fit into a revolving turret on the epifluorescent microscope consist of the excitation filter, dichroic mirror, and emission filter, all of which are optimized for the particular fluorochrome (e.g., FITC). Multiple fluorescence filter sets allow for simultaneous excitation and observation of emission by more than one fluorochrome. Disadvantages of multiple filter sets include expense and background, which can decrease image contrast. Because of this, some individuals prefer to image each fluorochrome separately with optimized filter sets and later combine these images to create a composite image of the multiple fluorochromes. Dummy blocks, which do not contain any filters, block any excitation emission while allowing light to pass unimpeded from the objective to the observer, allowing for bright-field microscopy.

Fluorescent microscopy finds numerous applications in nonclinical safety assessment. Examples include immunofluorescent antigen labeling, fluorescent *in situ* hybridization (FISH), tetracycline labeling of bone growth, propidium iodide staining of necrotic cells, and Fluoro-Jade (FJ) staining of degenerate neurons. Some of the potential advantages of examining FJ-stained brain sections in addition to routine H&E-stained sections include the highlighting of degenerate neuronal processes, faster identification of degenerate neurons, and differentiation of degenerate neurons from dark neuron artifacts. However, these potential benefits do not warrant the addition of FJ staining to all studies since degenerate neurons, when present, are usually identifiable in routine H&E-stained sections (Houle 2011).

5.3.2.2.2 Confocal Microscopy

Confocal microscopy, or confocal laser scanning microscopy, is a type of optical sectioning microscopy that provides high-resolution images. It shares many of the same principles of conventional wide-field fluorescent microscopy except that excitation and detection are both in focus. To achieve this, the excited light comes from a laser beam and is focused to one point in the specimen (the illumination spot, or Airy disk), the return emitted light from that spot is also focused, and a small pinhole over the detector screens out almost all of the undesirable emitted light outside the plane of focus. Use of these two focal points for illumination (excited light) and detection (emitted light) almost completely eliminates background fluorescence, which markedly increases contrast (Conchello and Lichtman 2005). Typically, to create an image, the illumination spot is moved in a raster fashion (like reading a book) over a thin focal plane section of the specimen and the two-dimensional image is generated by adding all of the information together. Three-dimensional images can be generated by computationally combining the image data from a stack of two-dimensional images. Extremely fine detail of fluorescently labeled structures near or below the limit of resolution can be visualized, such as cytoskeletal microtubules, organelles, inorganic metallic ions, and receptors.

5.3.2.3 Digital Microscopy

Digital microscopy makes use of digital cameras that convert an optical image (photons) into an electronic signal by use of either a CCD or a complementary metal-oxide semiconductor image sensor. Digital cameras used in pathology need to have large color dynamic ranges, high spatial resolutions, and high image acquisition and data transfer rates. Other key components include an optical connector for the digital camera to the microscope, a computer with imaging software, and a high-definition color monitor for viewing the digitized images (Ying and Monticello 2006). Digital images of particular fields (digital photomicrographs) can be manually captured, or digital images of the entire slide (virtual slides) can be captured by automated slide scanning technology.

Radiology adopted digital media years ago, and there is a growing interest in digital media in pathology. Advantages of digitization in pathology include easier archiving and retrieval, multi-slide integrated viewing, remote viewing, and image analysis. Digital images can be stored in various image file formats, and currently there is no standard. Two types of image file compression algorithms exist, lossless and lossy (Tengowski 2004). Lossless methods reduce file size without losing image quality; however, these files are very large. Lossy methods discard information that are less visible to the human eye and still meet the requirements of the particular application. JPEG2000 is a lossy compression image format for digital microscopy that uses wavelet encoding and generally results in similar or even higher-quality images with higher compression ratios than JPEG. Another potential file format for pathology image storage is Digital Imaging and Communications in Medicine (DICOM), a format currently used for storing radiology images (x-ray, MRI, and CT).

Digital pathology has greatly advanced the current and potential status of "telepathology," which is broadly defined as the practice of pathology at a distance. Telepathology allows a pathologist to evaluate microscopic images without being physically stationed at a microscope looking at tissue sections mounted on glass slides. This is especially promising for multisite institutions, including those that are international, and has the potential to improve cross-institutional communication, collaboration, consultation, and consistency. There are three major types of telepathology systems: static, dynamic (or real time), and virtual slide systems (McCullough et al. 2004). Static image systems involve the digital capture of microscopic image fields (photomicrographs) that are stored and then forwarded (usually by e-mail) for off-site access. Dynamic telepathology systems allow for online digital image exchange in real time. This can occur either by an off-site pathologist actively operating a robotically controlled motorized microscope or by viewing a live digital video feed controlled by a host pathologist. Static and dynamic telepathology systems are rapidly being replaced by virtual slides, which represent all of the information on an entire glass microscopic slide.

5.3.2.3.1 Virtual Slides

Whole-slide imaging (WSI), or "virtual" microscopy, involves the scanning of glass slides to produce "digital slides" or "virtual slides." Virtual slides allow a pathologist to view different magnifications, move the slide in any direction, save screenshots as image files, and annotate specific areas if desired. Virtual microscopy utilizes digital slide scanners and stitching software that create a whole-slide digital image file. The two most important criteria in digital slide scanners is speed of acquisition and resolution. Virtual slides are stored on large servers with massive capacities and can be viewed using a browser.

Interpretations of virtual slides have been shown to be as accurate as interpreting glass slides (Furness 2007). At this time, retrieval and evaluation of virtual slides over the Internet are significantly slower than evaluating glass slides. It is anticipated that advances in technology will eliminate this difference in the future.

5.3.2.3.2 Quantitative Image Analysis

Anatomical pathologists traditionally evaluate tissue morphologies in a descriptive fashion and record qualitative observations that are semiquantitatively graded (e.g., minimal, mild, moderate, severe). This approach is subjective, but it has and continues to work well for assessing tissue changes since the human visual system has a tremendous capability for pattern recognition. However, the human visual system does not have the same aptitude for detection of spatial or density changes, especially if the changes are subtle or far apart. Quantitative tissue assessments provide an objective approach for the detection of subtle changes in tissue morphologies, intensities, and percentages. The quantification of tissue changes also allows for statistical analysis and greatly facilitates the study of structural and functional relationships since much of the functional data (e.g., biomarkers) are already in a numerical format. Quantification can also increase the sensitivity, precision, and repeatability of data for pathologists. Recent advances in digital imaging and analysis software have greatly improved the speed, practicality, and utility of tissue measurements in nonclinical safety assessment settings. Quantification can be applied to almost any type of image (bright-field micros-copy of histochemical or immunohistochemical-stained sections, wide-field fluorescent microscopy, confocal microscopy, electron microscopy, *in vivo* imaging, etc.). There are many commercial, as well as some "freeware" or "shareware," image analysis software packages available.

Image analysis can generally quantitate changes in cell size, cell numbers, tissue infiltrates, or other morphological changes. Image analysis can also be used to quantitate histochemical, immu-nohistochemical, immunofluorescent (Hashiguchi et al. 2010), or ISH labeling, usually by measur-ing area and intensity. Regarding IHC, when some pathologists desire to provide more than just a binary positive–negative end point, they provide an "H-score," which is calculated by summing the percentages of cells staining at each intensity, multiplied by the weighted intensity of stain-ing (H-score = 3 × percentage of strongly staining nuclei + 2 × percentage of moderately staining nuclei + percentage of weakly staining nuclei, giving a range of 0 to 300). This calculation can be performed by the pathologist; however, the assignments of labeling intensity and percentage of cells for each intensity are highly subjective, with high levels of intraobserver and interobserver vari-ability. Automated image analysis significantly reduces the variability of pathologist-based scoring and may also increase the sensitivity and dynamic range of IHC quantification (Cregger et al. 2006; Taylor and Levenson 2006; Walker 2006).

When using image analysis for quantification of particular changes, it is important to be as consistent as possible in necropsy sampling, sample fixation, trimming, and staining of the tis-sue samples of interest. It is also important to locate sample areas within tissue sections similarly between animals, and the sample areas should be similar in size (pixel count).

Histomorphometry can simply be defined as any quantitative measurement or count of morpho-logical structures in a digital image of a tissue section. The statistical derivation of three-dimensional quantitative measurement data (number, length, surface area, or volume) based on measurements of two-dimensional tissue sections (also usually digital images) is referred to as stereology.

5.3.2.3.2.1 Histomorphometry The first step in histomorphometry is to segment the objects of interest from the rest of the specimen. Common measurements include length, perimeter, area, intensity, and number. Some examples include the following: counts of cells with immunohisto-chemical labeling (Ki67, caspase-3, proliferating cell nuclear antigen [PCNA], bromodeoxyuridine [BrdU]), stented coronary arteries (lumen area, stent area, strut inner surface-to-luminal border distance), liver (hepatocyte hypertrophy, bile duct hyperplasia, lipidosis, fibrosis, necrosis, glyco-gen accumulation), small intestine (villus length, crypt depth, villus/crypt ratios), spleen (lymphoid hyperplasia or depletion), heart (infarct, fibrosis), pancreas (islet size and number), thyroid gland (follicle size, follicular epithelial height and numbers), adrenal gland (cortical hypertrophy), skin (angiogenesis, epidermal hyperplasia), and microvessel analysis of implants and tumors.

5.3.2.3.2.2 Stereology Stereology refers to the statistical derivation of three-dimensional data based on measurements of two-dimensional tissue sections (Weibel et al. 1966). Stereological assessments require planning prior to necropsy since the entire organ of interest must be available for sampling. Traditional stereological methods required assumptions about the size and shape of the particles being measured, which was considered a biased method. The benefits of current stereo-logical methods include unbiased random sampling and increased statistical accuracy, sensitivity, and precision (reproducibility). Various stereological methods in use today rely only on sampling designs and allow for the counting and sizing of particles without the introduction of bias owing to assumptions on size and shape. These methods are often referred to as "design-based" or "unbiased" stereological methods (R. W. Boyce et al. 2010). Design-based stereological methods are the most sensitive and accurate methods to obtain quantitative data about tissues and are preferred over two-dimensional morphometric methods when critical decisions need to be made in the drug development or risk assessment process. Today, stereological methods are becoming much more efficient and practical because of advances in stereological theory, stereological software, sampling techniques, and imaging devices including automated WSI. One of the most common applications of stereological methods in nonclinical safety assessments is in neurotoxicity evaluations.

Stereology in nonclinical pathology is often used to count cells or structures, which is possible through the use of a disector. A disector is a stereological probe for counting or selecting objects using two parallel planes of section. These planes can be from two separate thin sections (physical disector) or from a stack of optical sections created by moving a focal plane through a known distance within a thick section (optical disector). The volume of tissue can be calculated by multiplying the area of the section by the disector height. Only structures of interest appearing in one section and absent in the other are counted, so that the structures are counted only once and height and size bias are removed. Another key stereology tool is the two-dimensional rectangular counting frame. It is typically displayed using the colors red and green, where objects that touch the green lines are considered within the counting frame and are counted and objects that touch the red exclusion lines are outside and not counted. These counting rules prevent a single cell or structure from being counted more than once and also result in all cells or structures having an equal probability of being selected regardless of shape, size, orientation, or distribution. The disector is combined with a fractionator, which is a systematic random (unbiased) sampling method that selects a portion of a region of interest. Stereology software using thin section digital image pairs that can be aligned and automated fractionator sampling have greatly increased the feasibility of stereological assessments in nonclinical pathology. Further gains in efficiency can be realized through the use of proportionator sampling. Documentation and archiving of digital stereological assessments allow for reconstruction for auditing or verification purposes, which is needed in a GLP setting.

Stereological principles are validated by mathematical proofs, similar to other statistical principles, rather than experimental data (R. W. Boyce et al. 2010). The validation of the stereology software system needs to be in compliance with the internal SOPs for computerized systems (documented system installation and verification of function by the vendor and the generation of installation-, operational-, or performance-qualification documentation). Archiving of a pair of disector sections, scanned images of those sections, and the sampling process for cells in those sections along with data collected from several replicates of the sampling protocol are also required (J. T. Boyce et al. 2010).

5.3.2.4 Noninvasive (*In Vivo*) Imaging

Noninvasive *in vivo* assessments provide information on tissues by penetrating the body by physical phenomena (e.g., x-rays, gamma rays, radiofrequency waves, and high frequency sound waves) rather than by scalpel or bone saw. Since these assessments are antemortem, they allow for repeated evaluations of the same animal over a period. This section will provide a brief overview of some of the more common *in vivo* imaging used in nonclinical research, including MRI, magnetic resonance spectroscopy (MRS), optical imaging, CT, ultrasound (US), PET, and SPECT (see Figure 5.1a and b). For a more extensive review of molecular imaging in the context of drug development, the reader is referred to Peterson et al. (2011), Willmann et al. (2008), and Ying and Monticello (2006). Like serum biomarkers (e.g., cardiac troponin or alanine aminotransferase), much of the nonclinical data generated by noninvasive imaging techniques can serve as valuable translational biomarkers since they have the potential for translation to patients in clinical phases of drug development. The use of noninvasive imaging can provide evidence of biological activity, confirm on-target activity, and identify patients that would be more likely to benefit from the treatment. Gathering of this information during the nonclinical phases of drug development can be highly valuable in the selection of

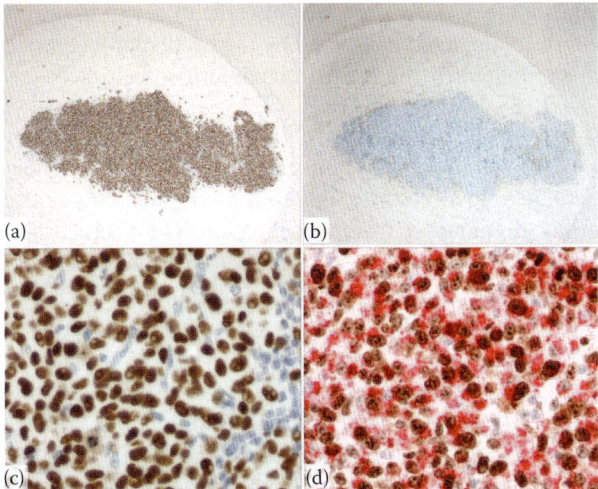

FIGURE 5.1 (a–c) The images shown are formalin-fixed paraffin-embedded rat brain that has been injected with human glioblastoma cells. The tissue has been stained with an antihuman nuclear matrix antibody and counterstained with hematoxylin. A serial control section stained with the same procedure, minus the primary antibody. (d) The image shown is formalin-fixed paraffin-embedded rat brain that has been injected with human glioblastoma cells, with a dual IHC stain. Cells with granular red cytoplasmic staining are positive for human mitochondrial antibody; blue nuclei are normal rat brain cells counterstained with hematoxylin. Brown nuclei are positive for proliferation marker Ki-67. (Photos a–d courtesy of Kristi Bailey, MPI Research Discovery Center Core Laboratory.)

promising drug candidates and termination of those that are not, leading to a conservation of time and resources overall and a potential reduction in the compound attrition rates during initial clinical phases.

MRI, CT, SPECT, and PET all generate sectional images called tomograms, some of which can be reconstructed into three-dimensional images. For nonclinical evaluations, the imaging technique must have spatial resolution that is adequate for small animals and sensitivity to detect biochemical events and small, clinically relevant changes over time. Noninvasive imaging techniques can be broadly divided into those that provide primarily morphological information (MRI, CT, and US) and those that provide functional information on biological processes (PET, SPECT, MRS, and optical imaging). Each technique has certain advantages and limitations, and usage should depend on which techniques can provide the greatest complementary information toward answering a particular nonclinical question. Combining the strengths of morphological/anatomical and functional imaging modalities (i.e., PET and CT or PET and MRI) can detect and provide information on pathophysiological changes early in the disease process. By repeating these techniques over time, temporal information such as development of structural changes, progression, and resolution can be gathered. Noninvasive imaging data can be correlated with histopathology and clinical pathology findings to provide an integrated data set. Also, compound-related changes can be longitudinally monitored before the treatment interval, during treatment, and after removal of treatment in the same animal; in this sense, the animal can act as its own control. Multiple evaluations of the same animal over time also have the potential of increasing the amount of information gathered from each animal and reducing the overall numbers of animals used (Willmann et al. 2008).

5.3.2.4.1 *Morphological/Anatomical Imaging Techniques (MRI, CT, and US)*

The noninvasive imaging techniques that provide primarily morphological information include MRI, CT, and US. These techniques can provide detailed images of tissue structures and morphological changes; however, they do not provide specific information on the various biochemical alterations that led to the changes. Also, they are only able to detect tissue changes after the structural changes become large enough to be detected by the particular technique. A summary of each morphological/anatomical imaging technique will be described below.

5.3.2.4.1.1 Magnetic Resonance Imaging MRI utilizes nuclear magnetic resonance, and the signal is primarily derived from the hydrogen nuclei (protons) of water molecules. The technique uses a powerful magnetic field to align the magnetization of atoms in the organism and a pulse of radiofrequency to alter the alignment of this magnetization. The scanner then detects the magnetic field to produce an image of the scanned area. Unlike radiography or CT, no ionizing radiation is used. Intravenous contrast agents are used to enhance signal and help delineate vessels or tumors (Pathak et al. 2010). MRI is most useful for imaging soft tissues, especially those with little density contrast such as the liver or brain, and is most frequently used to provide anatomical images and delineate lesions such as tumors or areas of necrosis. Magnetic resonance microscopy is MRI with resolutions of better than 100 µm³. Advantages of this technique include high resolution (roughly 10–100 µm with no limit of depth) and high soft tissue contrast; disadvantages include limited molecular applications and long scanning times (Ying and Monticello 2006). Functional information can be gathered in a related technique known as MRS, which provides information on particular endogenous biochemicals (metabolites) since a specific pattern of metabolites can be associated with certain diseases and tumors or on the concentration and distribution of magnetic nuclear isotope–labeled drugs in tissues (Willmann et al. 2008).

5.3.2.4.1.2 Computed Tomography In CT, x-rays are emitted from an x-ray source rotating around the subject placed in the center. A detector opposite the x-ray source detects the amount of x-rays that are not absorbed by the tissue, and this absorption is inversely related to the density of the tissue structures. The x-ray absorption profile is then used to reconstruct high-resolution (roughly 6–50 µm with no depth limit) tomographic anatomical images. CT can be used for bone studies (arthritis, osteoporosis, bone healing), developmental and reproductive toxicology studies to evaluate potential fetal skeletal variations (instead of macroscopic evaluation after Alizarin Red S staining), oncology studies (tumor volumes, orthotopic models, and anticancer therapeutic responses), vascular studies, and lung studies. Disadvantages of CT include low soft tissue contrast, use of radiation, and limited molecular applications (Ying and Monticello 2006). CT is able to provide a high-quality anatomical framework for functional imaging techniques, particularly PET.

5.3.2.4.1.3 Ultrasound US utilizes high-frequency sound waves emitted from a transducer and analyzes the returning echoes from the tissue to provide an image of the plane being scanned. With higher frequencies, resolution improves but penetration decreases. In nonclinical settings, high frequencies can be used on small animals and a resolution of 40–80 µm is achievable (Ying and Monticello 2006). Contrast agents such as microbubbles can improve image quality. US is highly translatable to clinical studies and can be used for the assessment of the cardiovascular system, tumor vascularity, response to antiangiogenic therapy, and real-time functional intravascular information when contrast agents such as microbubbles are functionalized with specific molecules such as monoclonal antibodies, peptides, or proteins. Disadvantages include a high dependence on operator skills, restriction of targeted imaging to the intravascular compartment, partial rather than whole-body assessments, and exclusion of imaging of osseous structures or gas containing organs such as the lungs.

5.3.2.4.2 Functional/Biochemical/Molecular Imaging Techniques
*   (Optical Imaging, PET, and SPECT)*

The noninvasive imaging techniques that are able to characterize and quantify biological processes or functional changes at the cellular and subcellular level include optical imaging, SPECT, and PET. MRS, related to MRI, can also provide functional information. These imaging techniques usually use specific molecular probes and intrinsic tissue characteristics as the source of image contrast, providing sufficient spatial and temporal resolution for studying biological processes in the living animal.

5.3.2.4.2.1   Optical Imaging   In vivo optical imaging includes fluorescence and biolumines-cence imaging. Both techniques are highly sensitive (picomolar) at limited depths of a few millimeters, quick and easy to perform (with a high-throughput capability), and in general do not require costly instrumentation. This makes them particularly suited to the drug development and validation process. Fluorescence imaging utilizes the ability of traditional or quantum dot fluorochromes (Papagiannaros et al. 2010) to absorb external excitation light of one wavelength and reemit light of a longer wavelength, which can be detected as discussed previously. In bioluminescence imaging, an enzyme (i.e., luciferase from the North American firefly *Photinus pyralis* or from the sea pansy *Renilla*) that is capable of generating light in the presence of a substrate (i.e., D-luciferin or coel-enterazine, respectively) is used as a reporter to assess the transcriptional activity in cells that are transfected with a genetic construct containing the enzyme's gene under the control of a promoter of interest. The enzymes can also be used to detect the level of cellular ATP (cell viability or kinase activity assays), tumor growth (Hawes and Reilly 2010), or other enzyme activity (i.e., caspase, cytochrome P450). Thus, the externally detected light is an indicator of biological/molecular processes. The imaging process involves anesthesia of the animal, injection of the respective substrate, and placement of the animal in a dark chamber with a thermoelectrically cooled CCD camera, which is extremely sensitive to even weak luminescence. The light emitted can then be semiquan-titatively analyzed. Disadvantages of optical imaging include low depth of penetration and limited clinical translation (Ying and Monticello 2006).

5.3.2.4.2.2   Positron Emission Tomography   In PET imaging, a compound (natural biological molecule or drug) labeled with a positron emitting radioisotope, which generally does not affect the physical or biochemical behavior of the compound, is injected into the animal in nonphar-macological trace quantities. A positron ejected by a radionuclide combines with an electron in adjacent tissue to emit a pair of photons resulting from annihilation of a positron–electron pair. The PET scanner uses the annihilation coincidence detection method to obtain projection images of the localization and quantification of the radiolabeled compound in the living animal. PET can be used for drug distribution (*in vivo* absorption, distribution, metabolism, and excretion studies), organ per-fusion (cerebral blood flow), cell labeling (bacteria, T-cells, stem cells), radiolabeling (antibodies, peptides, nucleotides, and nanoparticles), tumor models (xenograft, orthotopic, metastasis), tumor metabolism, tumor proliferation, tumor angiogenesis, tumor hypoxia, tumor apoptosis, disease models (CNS, autoimmune), and bone growth/healing. Advantages of this technique include high molecular sensitivity (nanomolar) with unlimited depth penetration. Disadvantages of PET include low spatial resolution (1–2.5 mm), radiation, and high cost (Ying and Monticello 2006). PET func-tional imaging is often combined with either CT or animal MRI.

5.3.2.4.2.3   Single-Photon Emission Computed Tomography   SPECT imaging detects mainly gamma rays emitted from a radionuclide in the living animal and shares many of the same fea-tures as PET imaging, such as the ability to localize and quantify radiolabeled compounds, high molecular sensitivity, and unlimited depth penetration (Ying and Monticello 2006). In preclinical SPECT imaging, the most recently developed multi-pinhole collimator technology achieves submil-limeter high resolution in small animals. In contrast to PET imaging, SPECT allows two or more compounds with different labeled SPECT radioisotopes to be distinguished within the same study. However, SPECT isotopes require chelating moieties (except for iodine) that have the potential to modify the physical or biochemical properties of a small molecule and may also limit determining specific binding of a small compound to its target. Although the molecular sensitivity of SPECT is one to two orders of magnitude lower than that of PET in general, SPECT imaging continues to be widely used in both clinical practice and preclinical research because of its advantages of lower cost, dual-labeled compounds, and relatively long half-life radionuclides that allow monitoring longer *in vivo* biological process compared to PET.

The gap between postmortem evaluations (i.e., bright-field microscopy, IHC, etc.) and in-life evaluations offered by noninvasive imaging is closing rapidly. By understanding the strengths and limitations of each, they can be used together (multi-modality imaging) to maximize the understanding of concurrent morphological and functional compound-induced changes.

5.3.2.5 Digital Image Data and Compliance with GLP Regulations

In 2007, the Society of Toxicologic Pathology published the following recommendations for the use of pathology images in compliance with the Code of Federal Regulations (CFR), Volume 21, Part 58 (GLP) and Part 11 (Electronic Records/Signatures) in the journal *Toxicologic Pathology* (Tuomari et al. 2007):

1. On the basis of current technologies and practices, pathology images (printed, electronic, or digital) used for data generation (e.g., to make a diagnosis or for morphometric analysis) are raw data that must be authenticated and archived.
2. Authentication of an image may be done either by initialing and dating a print of the image or by specifically annotating the electronic image file in compliance with Part 11 regulations.
3. Images used for raw data are subject to GLP procedures and controls in order to ensure data integrity including written SOPs, testing/validation of equipment, and training of personnel.
4. Validation or performance qualification of imaging systems used to support GLP studies must be documented and any exceptions to full validation/qualification must be described in the GLP Compliance Statement for the study.
5. Images that are not used for data generation are illustrative images, are not raw data, and generally do not have to be archived.
6. Illustrative images should not be used to reevaluate or supersede the pathologist's diagnosis.

5.3.3 *In Situ* Protein, DNA, and RNA Assays

In nonclinical safety assessment, morphological changes in cells are often accompanied by alterations in DNA, RNA, or protein molecules. A further understanding of these molecular changes can be extremely helpful in the elucidation of pathogenesis and determination of mechanistic risk assessments of toxicity or carcinogenicity. There are numerous molecular biology techniques, some of which involve tissue homogenization (*in vitro* or solution-based techniques) and others that preserve tissue architecture (*in situ* or slide-based techniques). Advantages of *in situ* techniques include the ability to preserve cellular identification and morphology and provide spatial localization/distribution information about DNA, RNA, or protein within a tissue. *In situ* techniques are the techniques that most commonly involve and necessitate the need for pathologists that are trained in the assessment of tissue morphology and morphological alterations. Target proteins can be detected using antibodies (immunolabeling), and specific nucleic acid (DNA and RNA) sequences can be detected using complementary nucleic acid sequences known as probes. These probes hybridize (bind) to the nucleic acid sequence of interest. Visualization is usually accomplished through the use of chromogenic or fluorescent labels. Both immunolabeling and nucleic acid hybridization labeling will be discussed in the following sections.

5.3.3.1 Immunolabeling (IHC and Immunofluorescence)

Immunolabeling is one of the most useful and utilized special techniques available to nonclinical pathologists. Because immunolabeling uses antibodies to distinguish particular antigens on the surface or within cells, it is a highly specific method for identifying particular cells, cell components, or molecules of interest beyond what routine H&E or histochemical (special) staining can (see Figures 5.1c and d and 5.2a–c). Although antibodies usually target structural proteins, antibodies can also be generated against soluble proteins such as enzymes, hormones, and neurotransmitters. This extremely sensitive and specific identification method can provide important information about test article effects and pathogenesis in nonclinical safety assessment. IHC can also be used to

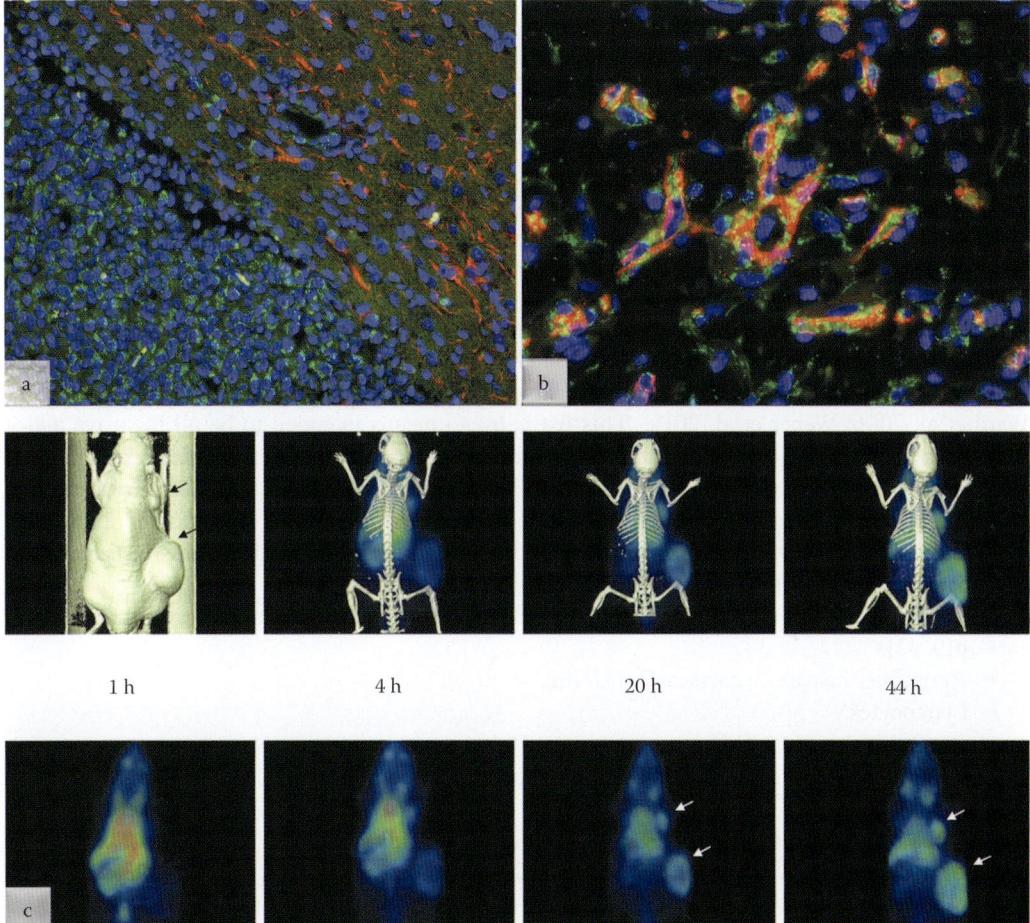

1 h   4 h   20 h   44 h

FIGURE 5.2 (a) The fluorescent image shown is formalin-fixed paraffin-embedded rat brain that has been injected with human glioblastoma cells. Cells with green granular cytoplasmic staining are positive for Alexa Fluor 488–labeled human mitochondrial antibody and can be seen in the cell injection area. Cells with red staining are positive for Alexa Fluor 594–labeled glial fibrillary acidic protein (GFAP), which is an astrocyte marker and can be seen in the surrounding normal rat brain tissue. Blue nuclei have been counterstained with DAPI. (b) The fluorescent image shown is formalin-fixed paraffin-embedded rat heart that has been injected with human stem cells. Cells with green granular cytoplasmic staining are positive for human mitochondrial antibody labeled with Alexa Fluor 488. Cells with red staining are positive for Alexa Fluor 594–labeled CD31, which is an endothelial cell marker. Blue nuclei have been counterstained with DAPI. (Photos a and b courtesy of Kristi Bailey, MPI Research Discovery Center Core Laboratory.) (c) This figure shows microPET/CT fused images acquired at 1 h, 4 h, 20 h, and 44 h postinjection of 200 µCi/40 µg ^{64}Cu-bevacizumab in a MIAPaCa-2 pancreatic xenograft tumor model. The dynamic imaging data show whole-body distribution of ^{64}Cu-bevacizumab in a tumor animal model in which the tumor sites are pointed by arrows. (Photo courtesy of Zheng Wang, MPI Research Radiochemistry and Molecular Imaging.)

help classify poorly differentiated neoplasms and diagnose metastases of uncertain origin. IHC is best utilized to further characterize or refine an H&E morphological diagnosis and should include proper controls and utilize panels instead of single antibodies whenever possible.

Once the primary antibody binds to the particular antigen of interest, a secondary antibody against the primary antibody is usually applied and visualization is possible owing to development of a colored histochemical reaction (IHC) or with fluorochromes under light of a particular wavelength (immunofluorescence). In contrast to the two commonly used chromogenic colors (brown or red) in IHC, immunofluorescence provides five or more different colors and is more suitable for quantification and multiple labeling (especially of the same structure) applications. Other types of immunolabels such as colloidal gold-conjugated antibodies can be used to identify antigens in electron microscopy.

Some potential uses for immunolabeling in nonclinical pathology include the following: identification of particular cells (e.g., beta cells in the pancreatic islets, macrophages within a mixed inflammatory reaction, endothelial cells, and proliferating cells), localization of the test article, determination of whether a protein is a good target for a drug (i.e., expressed in diseased tissue) and where the target is localized (subcellular compartments or extracellular locations), evaluation for any test article–related changes in the expression of targets in animal models (oncology xenografts), and explaining or predicting different toxicity profiles in different laboratory animal species (differential expression and inducibility of COX2 in the kidney between species). Below is a brief list of some of the common antibodies used in nonclinical toxicologic pathology (Galluzzi et al. 2009; Kepp et al. 2011; Kunder et al. 2007; Mikaelian et al. 2004; Obert et al. 2007; Painter et al. 2010; Ward et al. 2006; Weber et al. 2011). This list is by no means intended to be all inclusive and it is important to note that the antibodies listed may not be applicable for all species and fixation methods.

- Angiogenesis: CD31 (PECAM-1), VEGF, CD105 (endoglin), CD106 (VCAM-1), Factor VIII (vWf), CD141 (thrombomodulin)
- Cell proliferation: PCNA, Ki-67 (MIB-1), BrdU,* other cell cycle proteins (cyclin D1, p15, p19, p21)
- Apoptosis: caspase-3, caspase-7, TUNEL[†]
- Leukocytes:
  - Pan leukocyte: CD45
  - T-cells: CD3 (pan T-cells), CD4 (T-helper), CD8 (thymocytes and natural killer [NK] cells)
  - B-cells: CD79a, CD20, Pax5
  - Macrophages: F4/80, CD163 (ED2), CD68 (ED1)
- Neuroendocrine: synaptophysin, chromogranin A, neuron-specific enolase (NSE)
- Undifferentiated tumor differentiation: alpha smooth muscle actin or a-SMA (smooth muscle), desmin (skeletal, cardiac, smooth muscle), vimentin (mesenchymal), pancytokeratin (epithelial), S100 (melanomas, Schwannomas, astrocytomas, ependymomas)
- Nervous system: glial fibrillary acidic protein or GFAP (glial cells such as astrocytes and ependymal cells in the CNS, Schwann cells in the PNS), MAP2 (neurons), NeuN (neurons), neurofilament (neurons, ganglia, neuroendocrine), O4 (oligodendrocyte), S100 (Schwannomas, ependymomas, astrocytomas, melanomas), NSE (neuroendocrine)
- Human cell detection: human mitochondria, human immunoglobulin G (IgG), human nuclear antigen, human nuclear matrix
- Immune complexes: endogenous IgA, IgM, IgG

---

* Detects the S phase of the cell cycle and requires antemortem exogenous administration.
† Terminal deoxynucleotidyl transferase dUTP nick end labeling. Utilizes biotin conjugated to dUTP primary labeling of free 3′-OH terminal with streptavidin-HRP or avidin-FITC secondary labeling.

- Cytochrome P450 induction: CYP1A2, 2B1, 2D1, 2E1, and 3A1
- Complement: C3, C1q, C5b-C9
- Hepatic phospholipidosis: LAMP-2(+), adipophilin(−)
- Amyloid: amyloid P (pan-amyloid), amyloid A, beta amyloid
- Hormones: estrogen receptor (alpha and beta), prolactin, insulin, glucagon, LH

Buchwalow and Bocker (2010), Kumar and Rudbeck (2009), and Ramos-Vara (2005) are three excellent references on IHC from which the following principles and technical aspects are summarized from.

5.3.3.1.1 Antibodies

A basic understanding of antibody structure is important in the understanding of the basic technical aspects of IHC. Antibodies are bivalent "Y"-shaped proteins of the Ig family, where the "tail" of the "Y" is the Fc (crystalline fragment) portion and the identical "arms" of the "Y" are the Fab (antigen-binding fragment) portions. Hypervariable regions within the Fab portions of the primary antibody bind to particular epitopes of an antigen, and the secondary antibody binds to the Fc portion of the primary antibody. IgG is the most common type of antibody used in IHC.

Immunohistochemical evaluations in nonclinical safety studies involving various test system species can be challenging, especially when an SOP for the particular antibody and application (in a particular species or tissue) has not been developed. Also, many of the commercially available antibodies are generated against human antigens ("antihuman antibodies"). Fortunately, there is a growing number of commercial antibodies generated against rodent antigens ("antimouse" and "antirat" antibodies), and a large number of antihuman antibodies cross-react with laboratory animal antigens ("cross-species cross-reactivity"). Cross-species cross-reactivity is more likely to occur with less evolutionary divergent species. Human antigens are more likely to contain homologous epitopes in nonhuman primates and less likely in rodents. This principle also applies at the protein level. More evolutionarily conserved proteins like GFAP and S100 are more likely to cross-react between species than a highly divergent cluster of differentiation proteins (CDs). Whenever there is a need for an IHC assay involving a novel antibody or species, adequate time should be allotted for method development consisting of literature searches, trial-and-error experimentation (especially various pretreatment and antibody dilutions), and validation of the antibody within the particular species of interest if the study is being conducted under GLP guidance. Antibody selection should take into account the host species in which the antibody was generated and any knowledge of cross-species cross-reactivity. If the sample tissue is from the same species as the host species in which the antibody was generated, background staining occurs owing to binding of the secondary antibody to endogenous Igs and other components in the tissue. This situation is most often encountered in mouse studies in which IHC labeling of a particular antigen utilizes a mouse monoclonal primary antibody. There are various methods, including commercially available "mouse on mouse" kits, to minimize this background staining so that monoclonal antibodies can still be used on mouse tissues. Whenever possible, it is best to select a primary antibody from a host species that is different from the study species.

Antibodies may be polyclonal or monoclonal, each with their own advantages and disadvantages. Regarding the particular antigen of interest, polyclonal antibodies bind various different epitopes of an antigen, whereas monoclonal antibodies only bind a single epitope. Epitopes are regions of antigens that antibodies bind to and are usually 5–21 amino acids long. Antigens can have different structures (isoforms) due to alternative splicing of the primary gene transcript and posttranslational modifications. Because polyclonal antibodies are able to bind various different epitopes, they usually have higher antigen sensitivity, can identify various antigen isoforms, can often bind the same antigen in multiple species, and usually have a higher tolerance to the effects of fixation and processing. However, this robust reactivity can also be associated with lower antigen specificity (antibody cross-reactivity) and higher irrelevant Ig content that can lead to false positives. Polyclonal antibodies are generated by different B-lymphocyte clones ("polyclonal") within an animal and are most frequently produced by immunizing rabbits against a purified antigen of interest; however, other species such as goats, pigs, guinea pigs, and cattle may be used as hosts. At the end of the immunization period, the serum from the host is collected for use as a heterogeneous mixture of antibodies or further purified. Monoclonal antibodies are most frequently produced by immunizing mice (or, less commonly, rabbits or rats) against the purified antigen, removing a single ("mono-clonal") splenic B-lymphocyte clone from the host that produces the specific Ig, and fusing it with immortal myeloma cells to create a hybridoma cell line. These hybridoma cell lines are usually either maintained in tissue culture, where the antibody is present in the culture supernatant, or injected into the abdominal cavity of an animal (usually mouse) where the antibody is present in ascites fluid. Collected ascites fluid has a very high concentration of the antibody of interest, but it also contains small amounts of irrelevant antibodies and other proteins that are not present in tissue culture supernatant. The primary advantage of using monoclonal antibodies is high antigen speci-ficity. Since monoclonal antibodies bind only a specific epitope, the chance for cross-reactivity with other antigens is greatly reduced. Disadvantages of monoclonal antibodies are that they are mostly of mouse origin, limit their use in mouse studies, and have a lower antigen sensitivity and tolerance to the effects of fixation and processing.

Antibody titer and dilutions, incubation time, and temperature are all important consider-ations when optimizing the desired antigen–antibody binding and minimizing cross-reactivity. Immunohistochemical laboratory technicians that are experienced with various immunohistochemi-cal techniques and are skilled at problem solving are invaluable.

IHC throughput can be increased by the use of either tissue microarrays, where an antibody is applied to many different tissue specimens on a single slide, or the multiplex immunostaining chip, where many different antibodies are applied to different regions of a single tissue specimen (Furuya et al. 2004).

5.3.3.1.2 *Fixation and Antigen Retrieval (Demasking)*

Immunohistochemical evaluations may be planned or added after routine H&E microscopic exami-nation generates a question. Even when planned, tissue preparation typically involves formalin fixation using 10% NBF and embedding in paraffin. Fixation is necessary to preserve tissue mor-phology and prevent antigen degradation or diffusion. When planned, greater success with IHC can be achieved if the tissues are not stored in formalin for long periods prior to paraffin or plastic embedding. In the fast-paced world of nonclinical safety assessment, this is usually not a prob-lem, and particular tissue samples can be removed from formalin at 24 h if immunohistochemical evaluations are planned. Prolonged fixation (greater than 24 h) can result in excessive protein cross-linking and antigen masking, which can lead to false negatives. This is due to blockage of binding of primary antibodies to epitopes or by the alteration of the tertiary structure (folding) of the epitope, which can greatly hinder primary antibody recognition. If long-term storage of tissues is needed, and there is a chance for IHC, it is best to remove the tissue from formalin after 24 h fixation and to store in 70% ethanol at 4°C.

Epitope masking by formalin protein cross-linking can mostly be removed by the use of heat-induced epitope retrieval (HIER). HIER was one of the most revolutionary technical advances in the evolution of IHC as it greatly increased the ability to detect antigens in formalin-fixed tissues. HIER has decreased the need for frozen sections or coagulating (non-cross-linking) fixatives such as etha-nol. Microwave oven, pressure cooker, and steam are the most common heating methods; autoclave and water bath are also sometimes used. HIER can also be modified by varying the types of buffers used and varying the pH of the buffers. Antigen retrieval can also be achieved by enzymes (e.g., proteinase K, trypsin, pepsin), alone or more commonly as a pretreatment before HIER. Certain methods can be harsher than others, and overall, there is no best retrieval method for every antigen. The degree of background staining increases proportionally to the intensity of antigen retrieval. Since fixation times are often short in nonclinical studies, HIER is sometimes unnecessary. HIER can also be used to unmask antigens in semithin sections of tissue that have been embedded in methyl methacrylate (MMA) after thorough deplasticization, which allows for various immunohistochemical evaluations of MMA plastic-embedded tissue (Hand and Church 1998).

5.3.3.1.3   Antibody Labeling Methods (Detection Systems)

Immunohistochemical labels utilize histochemical enzymes such as horseradish peroxidase (HRP) or calf intestine alkaline phosphatase (AP) to which chromogenic substrates (i.e., diaminobenzidine [DAB]) are applied, followed by a hematoxylin counterstain. Immunofluorescence labeling utilizes fluorochromes such as FITC, which are visible when illuminated by light of a certain wavelength. Paraffin and plastic sections can exhibit autofluorescence, which is why frozen sections are often preferred for fluorescent labeling. Particulate labels such as electron opaque colloidal gold can be used for electron microscopy.

There are two types of antibody-labeling methods, direct and indirect. Direct methods employ a one-step process where the primary antibody with label is applied to the tissue of interest. Direct labeling is most commonly used in immunofluorescence, especially in dual- and triple-labeling procedures where there are multiple antibodies raised in the same species. With IHC, direct methods usually do not result in enough labeling for detection by light microscopy and have largely been replaced by indirect labeling owing to amplified antigen sensitivity. This increased sensitivity of indirect labeling occurs because the activity of the primary antibody is not impeded by having a label being directly attached to it, and there is amplification of the visualization owing to increased numbers of labels per primary antibody. Indirect methods employ a two-step process where a secondary antibody with multiple, often polymeric, labels binds to the Fc portion of the primary antibody. There are various indirect methods in use today, one of which is the avidin–biotin complex (ABC), which takes advantage of the strong affinity of avidin for the vitamin biotin. In the ABC method, the Fab portions of biotinylated secondary antibodies bind the Fc portion of the primary antibody, and then the biotin on the secondary antibody serves as the binding site for unbound biotin binding sites on avidin–biotin label complexes. A related indirect method utilizing streptavidin instead of avidin is the labeled streptavidin–biotin (LSAB) method, which has greater sensitivity and less background staining than the ABC method. Commercially available, biotin-free polymer-based labels, consisting of a polymer backbone and multiple secondary antibodies and enzymes, are now popular since they offer the advantages of greater sensitivity and lower background staining, especially in tissues rich in endogenous biotin or avidin, such as in liver and kidney. Greater sensitivity can also be achieved by tyramide amplification methods, where application of biotinyl tyramide to primary antibodies indirectly labeled with peroxidase via ABC or LSAB methods results in the deposition of numerous biotin signals in the immediate vicinity of the primary antibody. Visualization then occurs through the application of avidin bound to HRP. The drawback of this method is a greater potential for nonspecific staining. Even greater sensitivity and less background staining is possible by rolling circle amplification, where an oligonucleotide primer is coupled to the primary or secondary antibody and amplification is achieved through the addition of DNA by polymerases that can be visualized by hybridization with labeled complementary oligonucleotide probes.

Labeling of more than one antigen within a tissue section can be an extremely useful technique in providing spatial and associative information about various cells, cell components, or molecules. Multiple labeling utilizes different primary antibodies linked to different chromogen or fluorescent labels. Particular steps must be taken to avoid false-positive staining, especially when the primary antibodies are from the same host species.

5.3.3.1.4   Controls

Use of controls, both positive and negative, is required for accurate immunohistochemical interpretations. Positive tissue controls are tissue sections that have been previously determined to contain the target epitope, ideally with areas of weak to strong reactivity. Negative controls should include both negative reagent controls and a negative tissue control section. The negative reagent controls involve staining the test tissue with all of the same steps except that the primary antibody is omitted and/or replaced with 1) an antibody of the same class which does not exhibit reactivity to the epitope of interest (monoclonal antibodies), or 2) normal/nonimmune serum (polyclonal antibodies). Negative tissue controls are additional sections that are devoid of the target of interest and are included in the staining run. Both positive and negative controls can be present within the tissue section, referred to as internal controls. Positive and negative controls allow for assessment of labeling specificity and are invaluable in troubleshooting and avoiding false-positive or false-negative results.

5.3.3.1.5 Tissue Cross-Reactivity Studies

Tissue cross-reactivity (TCR) studies are screening assays recommended for monoclonal antibody and antibody-like molecules that contain a complementarity-determining region (Leach et al. 2010). This assay is primarily used to identify off-target antigen binding (cross-reactivity) and, secondarily, to assess sites of on-target antigen binding in unexpected cells/tissues. These studies involve immunolabeling, using the candidate antibody as the primary antibody, of a panel of frozen tissues from humans and animals. Tissue labeling can be helpful in the assessment of potential target organs in both nonclinical research animals and human subjects in clinical trials. Demonstration of tissue reactivity in a particular laboratory species comparable to human reactivity is not utilized in the selection of a relevant species in a nonclinical safety assessment study, but it often serves to confirm or further support the species selection. In addition, differences in which tissues show reactivity between a particular laboratory species and humans can be used to explain differences between animal and human *in vivo* tissue effects or why a particular laboratory species did not predict effects or toxicities in humans. TCR studies can also be used to determine off-target antigen binding effects in humans and help predict possible unexpected clinical effects or toxicities (Bussiere et al. 2011). As with all special procedures, TCR studies are not perfect and cannot always predict off-target antigen binding effects in humans, optimal animal species for testing, or human or laboratory animal *in vivo* toxicity.

5.3.3.2 Probe Hybridization Labeling (Chromogenic *In Situ* Hybridization and FISH)

Whereas IHC and immunofluorescence utilize antibodies to detect particular proteins, ISH techniques utilize probes to detect particular DNA or RNA sequences. A probe consists of a labeled nucleic acid sequence that is complementary to a DNA or RNA sequence of interest. Probes may consist of double-stranded DNA, single-stranded DNA, RNA (riboprobes), or synthetic oligonucleotides. Riboprobes and oligonucleotide probes are most commonly used, with riboprobes being larger (~100–500 base pairs) and containing more labels, resulting in greater sensitivity than smaller oligonucleotide probes (~20–50 base pairs). Similar to immunolabeling of proteins, detection of the probe can be through labeling of the probe with a fluorochrome, referred to as FISH, or a chromogen, referred to as chromogenic *in situ* hybridization, or CISH. Chromogen labeling consists of probes containing biotin- or digoxigenin-conjugated nucleic acid, to which enzyme-conjugated (HRP or AP) antibodies bind to and react with chromogenic substrates (e.g., DAB) to produce a color that can be detected with a bright-field microscope. CISH is a newer technique than FISH and has the advantages of utilizing a bright-field microscope and counterstains, such as hematoxylin, so that the cells of interest and surrounding tissue architecture are easily visualized. As a result, the chromogenic reaction is much more stable over time than fluorescent labels, and IHC can easily be performed on additional tissue sample sections and compared with CISH labeling to gain a greater understanding of both gene expression and proteins together (Halling and Wendel 2009). Commercial kits that allow for the conversion of FISH to CISH are available. Advantages of FISH over CISH include direct labeling of the specific nucleic acid sequence and the greater number of color labels available.

Prior to chromogenic or fluorescent visualization, the probe needs to hybridize to the target nucleic acid sequence. Generally, these steps include formaldehyde-based fixation, paraffin embedding, sectioning onto slides, deparaffinization, proteolytic digestion, prehybridization (application of all reagents except the probe to reduce nonspecific binding), and heating the probe and target together followed by cooling to allow for hybridization. The proteolytic digestion step unmasks the nucleic acid sequences and increases cell permeability to facilitate probe penetration. The term "stringency" refers to the conditions that affect the specificity of the probe binding. Higher stringency results in more on-target complementary binding and lower stringency results in probe binding to sequences outside of the target sequence (Sterchi 2010).

ISH is particularly useful when the protein product of interest is rapidly degraded or transported out of the target cell, limiting the usefulness of protein immunolabeling (IHC). ISH can also be a valuable adjunct technique to protein immunolabeling in that it can provide clues about genes (DNA) or gene expression (mRNA) and provide upstream information regarding toxicity or carcinogenicity. In contrast to protein immunolabeling, where there can be a lack of cross-reactivity of the antibody between species, ISH probes often work in various animal species as well as in humans because small regions of mRNA are often conserved across species (Gillett et al. 2002). This aspect of ISH makes this technique particularly useful when studying animal models of human disease processes and determining mechanistic risk. ISH has great potential in assessing the efficacy and safety of gene therapy. It can determine if the inserted therapeutic DNA is present within the target host cells, if the desired mRNA of interest has been transcribed, if any tissue lesions are associated with the sites of DNA transfer, or if DNA has been transferred to unintended target cells. ISH also provides a sensitive method to identify and assess the distribution and accumulation of antisense oligonucleotides in tissues (Goebl et al. 2007).

Small quantities of DNA or mRNA can sometimes be below the sensitivity of ISH methods. In these instances, *in situ* PCR and *in situ* RT-PCR can be used to first amplify the DNA or mRNA, respectively (Malarkey and Maronpot 1996).

5.3.4 Laser Microdissection

Laser microdissection allows for the isolation and collection of particular cells, even single cells, from solid tissue sections for subsequent various DNA, RNA, or protein analyses. This technique can also be used on samples such as cytologies and blood smears. Both frozen and formalin-fixed paraffin-embedded tissue may be used; however, frozen sections (cryosections) provide optimal recovery. The tissue sections can be unstained, stained (such as with T-blue), or immunostained with fluorochromes or chromogens, which allows for even greater distinction of particular cell types by phenotype rather than just cellular morphological features. The process involves visualization of the tissue section with a laser microdissection microscope to identify cells of interest, using a laser to isolate (capture or cut) these cells and remove them by a variety of methods and, subsequently, inspecting the isolated cells or the tissue from which they were removed to verify that the correct cells were collected. Capture isolation methods involve placing the tissue section in contact with a thermoplastic membrane mounted to the inside of a microcentrifuge cap that can be melted by a laser beam aimed at the cells of interest, so that only these cells are pulled from the adjacent unbound cells when the cap is lifted from the section. Cutting isolation methods involve using a smaller-diameter laser beam to trace around and cut out the cells of interest, but instead of relying on a thermoplastic membrane in contact with the cells, it utilizes a variety of techniques to transport the excised cells from slide to collection container (Murray 2008). Because laser microdissection techniques allow for the collection of specific cells within a larger mixture of cells within a tissue section, they offer a way to acquire a pure sample of cells of interest and avoid contamination by other cells, which occurs in traditional homogenization techniques. This is particularly useful in nonclinical safety assessment in that focused evaluations, such as on the gene or protein expression of particular cells exhibiting a compound-related change, can be performed to better understand the pathogenesis of the change (Dalmas et al. 2008).

5.3.5 FLOW CYTOMETRY AND FLUORESCENCE-ACTIVATED CELL SORTING

Flow cytometry allows for the rapid counting, lineage and phenotypic characterization, and sorting of heterogeneous cell populations suspended in a stream of fluid. Possible parameters that can be evaluated include physical (size, granularity, or amount of DNA), antigenic (membrane, cytoplasmic, or nuclear antigen expression), and functional (NK cell activity, neutrophil oxidative burst) parameters. An extension of flow cytometry, fluorescence-activated cell sorting, allows for the separation and collection of subpopulations of cells from the heterogeneous sample. Charged deflector plates divert any cells that meet the criteria for selection into a separate tube that can be used for further evaluations, including *in vitro* cytokine production, cell-based assays, or as reagents in other assay protocols. Contemporary flow cytometers are capable of simultaneous measurements of multiple parameters. Some of the more common applications of flow cytometry in nonclinical research include immunophenotyping of peripheral blood leukocytes, assessment of cell membrane integrity (viability), cell-based pharmacodynamics, detection of DNA/RNA content (cell cycle analysis), diagnosis of hematopoietic/lymphoid disorders and neoplasia, assessment of apoptosis, and assessment of cell proliferation. Functional assessments are also possible via assays that measure activation state, intracellular signal transduction events, cytokine production, and other cell activities. Flow cytometry is especially valuable in that it allows for multiple specific cell evaluations during the course of a study, and it may also be used during human clinical trials to assess and monitor for compound-related specific cell changes (Hedley et al. 2008). Advantages of flow cytometry over IHC include simultaneous multiparametric analysis of individual cells, less interpretational subjectivity, improved quantification, small sample size requirements, rapid turnaround, and digital results. Key factors affecting the predictive power of flow cytometry are sample type and condition, timing of sample collection, parameters evaluated, granularity, and the abundance or rarity of the population being measured.

Flow cytometry requires cells in suspension, such as whole blood or bone marrow, or cells from solid tissue fine-needle aspirates or biopsies (e.g., lymph node, spleen, or thymus) in which the cells are mechanically or enzymatically dissociated. These cells are passed through a fluid sheath sleeve to create laminar flow, and by hydrodynamic focusing, a column of single cells that are passed through a laser beam (or beams) is created. At the point of intersection between the cells and the laser beam, known as the interrogation point, forward scatter light and side scatter light from each cell are collected by detectors. Side scatter light also passes through a number of dichroic mirrors with fluorescent detectors so that multiple wavelengths of emitted fluorescent light can be simultaneously detected. Care must be taken to make sure that the correct excitation sources with wavelengths compatible with particular fluorescent probes are used to avoid spectral overlap and reduce potential compensation issues. The detected light can then be digitized, analyzed, and graphically displayed by a computer. The data can be plotted in a single dimension to produce a histogram or in two-dimensional dot plots. The distribution regions representing populations of cells on these plots can be isolated by applying an electronic "gate" to isolate the cell populations of interest, which can simplify and increase the relevance of the statistical analysis. Once a cell population has been classified, statistical analysis to determine test article–related effects can be accomplished by various statistical methods. Critical controls include unstained cells, matching isotype controls, compensation controls, and biological controls, including a known positive, if available.

One of the most common applications of flow cytometry in nonclinical safety assessment is immunophenotyping, which allows for the quantification of subtypes of cells with similar morphologies but different functions, by utilizing the differential antigen expression of each cell subtype. When immunophenotyping of leukocytes in peripheral blood is performed, relative and absolute changes in the cellular components of the immune system (i.e., B-cells, mature T-cells, CD4+

T-cells, CD8+ T-cells, NK cells) can be quantified, which can help determine possible alterations in the immune system. It is important to note that changes in the relative number of immune cells do not always correlate to functional or anatomical alterations in the immune system. Flow cytometry used in conjunction with standard immunotoxicology measurements provides a more thorough assessment for potential immunomodulatory effects. An excellent review of the use of flow cytometry and IHC in the identification and characterization of immunotoxicity is presented by Lappin and Black (2003).

Although flow cytometry can provide a great deal of information regarding cells, it cannot assess cellular morphological details and alterations, does not allow for imaging of the cell or tissue so that areas of interest can be localized and studied further, and does not allow for physical sample reanalysis (only data reanalysis). One flow cytometry technology that provides morphological details is the imaging of each cell in the stream (Amnis ImageStream) so that individual cells can later be selected and inspected. For additional details on the principles and technical aspects of flow cytometry, the reader is referred to Dimmick (2009), Gossett et al. (1999), Hannon-Fletcher and Maxwell (2009), Mach et al. (2010), Narayanan et al. (2008), Petrausch et al. (2006), and Zu et al. (2009).

5.3.6 Laser Scanning Cytometry

Laser scanning cytometry (LSC) is a newer technology that allows for the qualitative and quantitative analysis of cells within paraffin-embedded or frozen tissue sections on a microscopic slide. It has been referred to as microscope-based flow cytometry since it shares many of the same features of flow cytometry, with additional advantages of allowing for repeated sample analyses, detailed morphological evaluations, and image analysis (Peterson et al. 2008). It utilizes automated slide scanning in combination with many of the similar components of flow cytometry (i.e., lasers, optics, detectors, computer) to make highly precise measurements on individual cells within the section. The analysis can be based on immunolabeling (fluorescent or chromogenic) or routine histochemical staining of cells, and the data generated can be displayed in various forms, including scatter plots, histograms, distribution plots, and tables with statistical analysis. LSC also allows for the correlation of cellular phenotype (biochemical or morphological) with patterns of tissue change, since the morphological features of the tissue section are maintained (Pruimboom-Brees et al. 2005). Also, in instances when the expression of a marker is confined to small numbers of cells, LSC is more sensitive than protein or gene expression profiling, using whole tissue levels in which many of the cells do not exhibit the change. The position of each cell is recorded, allowing for relocation/visual confirmation, correlation of biochemical and morphometric measurements, and digital imaging of the cells of interest. Quantitative measurements can include cell to nuclei counts, cell area, stromal elements, and labeling intensity, which correlate well with traditional quantification methods (Peterson et al. 2008).

REFERENCES

Routine Techniques

AVMA guidelines on euthanasia June 2007. Available from http://www.avma.org/issues/animal_welfare/euthanasia.pdf (accessed 9-15-11).

Bailey, S. A., R. H. Zidell, and R. W. Perry. 2004. Relationships between organ weight and body/brain weight in the rat: What is the best analytical endpoint? *Toxicol Pathol* 32: 448–466.

Bancroft, J. D. and M. Gamble, eds. 2007. *Theory and Practice of Histologic Techniques*, 6th edition. Edinburgh: Churchill and Livingston.

Bono, C. D. and M. R. Elwell. 2000. Necropsy techniques with standard collection and trimming of tissues. In *The Handbook of Experimental Animals (The Laboratory Rat)*. ed. G. Krinke, 569–600. San Diego: Academic Press.

Bucci, T. J. 2002. Basic techniques. In *Handbook of Toxicologic Pathology*, 2nd edition. ed. W. M. Haschek, C. G. Rousseaux, and M. A. Wallig, 171–85. San Diego: Academic Press.

Cox, M. L., C. L. Schray, C. N. Luster et al. 2006. Assessment of fixatives, fixation, and tissue processing on morphology and RNA integrity. *Exp Mol Pathol* 80: 183–91.

Dykstra, M. J., P. C. Mann, M. R. Elwell, and S. V. Ching. 2002. Suggested standard operating procedures (SOPs) for the preparation of electron microscopy samples for toxicology/pathology studies in a GLP environment. *Toxicol Pathol* 30: 735–43.

Frame, S. R. and P. C. Mann. 2008. Principles of pathology for toxicology studies. In *Principles and Methods of Toxicology*, 5th edition. ed. A. W. Hayes, 591–609. Boca Raton: CRC Press.

Gillespie, J. W., C. J. M. Best, V. E. Bischel et al. 2002. Evaluation of non-formalin tissue fixation for molecular profiling studies. *Am J Pathol* 160: 449–57.

Kiernan J. 2008. *Histological and Histochemical Methods: Theory and Practice*, 4th edition. Cold Spring Harbor: Cold Spring Harbor Laboratory Press.

Latendresse, J. R., A. R. Warbrittion, H. Jonassen, and D. M. Creasy. 2002. Fixation of testes and eyes using a modified Davidson's fluid: Comparison with Bouin's fluid and conventional Davidson's fluid. *Toxicol Pathol* 30: 524–33.

Mann, P. C., J. F. Hardisty, and M. D. Parker. 2002. Managing pitfalls in toxicologic pathology. In *Handbook of Toxicologic Pathology*, 2nd edition. ed. W. M. Haschek, C. G. Rousseaux, and M. A. Wallig, 187–206. San Diego: Academic Press.

Prophet, E. B., B. Mills, J. B. Arrington, and L. H. Sobin, eds. 1992. *Laboratory Methods in Histotechnology*. Washington, DC: American Registry of Pathology.

SPECIAL TECHNIQUES

Boyce, J. T., R. W. Boyce, and H. J. Gundersen. 2010. Choice of morphometric methods and consequences in the regulatory environment. *Toxicol Pathol* 38 (7): 1128–33.

Boyce, R. W., K. A. Dorph-Petersen, L. Lyck, and H. J. Gundersen. 2010. Design-based stereology: Introduction to basic concepts and practical approaches for estimation of cell number. *Toxicol Pathol* 38 (7): 1011–25.

Buchwalow, I. B., and W. Bocker. 2010. Immunohistochemistry: Basics and methods. Berlin Heidelberg: Springer-Verlag.

Bussiere, J. L., M. W. Leach, K. D. Price, B. J. Mounho, and R. Lightfoot-Dunn. 2011. Survey results on the use of the tissue cross-reactivity immunohistochemistry assay. *Regul Toxicol Pharmacol* 59 (3) (Apr): 493–502.

Conchello, J. A. and J. W. Lichtman. 2005. Optical sectioning microscopy. *Nature Methods* 2 (12) (Dec): 920–31.

Cregger, M., A. J. Berger, and D. L. Rimm. 2006. Immunohistochemistry and quantitative analysis of protein expression. *Arch Pathol Lab Med* 130 (7) (Jul): 1026–30.

Dalmas, D. A., M. S. Scicchitano, Y. Chen et al. 2008. Transcriptional profiling of laser capture microdissected rat arterial elements: Fenoldopam-induced vascular toxicity as a model system. *Toxicol Pathol* 36 (3): 496–519.

Dimmick, I. 2009. Flow cytometry. In *Advanced Techniques in Diagnostic Cellular Pathology*, eds. M. Hannon-Fletcher and P. Maxwell. Hoboken: John Wiley & Sons, Ltd.

Dykstra, M. J., P. C. Mann, M. R. Elwell, and S. V. Ching. 2002. Suggested standard operating procedures (SOPs) for the preparation of electron microscopy samples for toxicology/pathology studies in a GLP environment. *Toxicol Pathol* 30: 735–43.

Furness, P. 2007. A randomized controlled trial of the diagnostic accuracy of Internet-based telepathology compared with conventional microscopy. *Histopathology* 50 (2) (Jan): 266–73.

Furuya, T., K. Ikemoto, S. Kawauchi et al. 2004. A novel technology allowing immunohistochemical staining of a tissue section with 50 different antibodies in a single experiment. *J Histochem Cytochem* 52 (2) (Feb): 205–10.

Galluzzi, L., S. A. Aaronson, J. Abrams et al. 2009. Guidelines for the use and interpretation of assays for monitoring cell death in higher eukaryotes. *Cell Death Differ* 16 (8) (Aug): 1093–107.

Gillett, N. A., C. Chan, C. Farman, and P. Lappin. 2002. Special techniques in toxicologic pathology. In *Handbook of Toxicologic Pathology*, 2nd edition. ed. W. M. Haschek, C. G. Rousseaux, and M. A. Wallig, 207–42. San Diego: Academic Press.

Goebl, N., B. Berridge, V. J. Wroblewski, and P. L. Brown-Augsburger. 2007. Development of a sensitive and specific in situ hybridization technique for the cellular localization of antisense oligodeoxynucleotide drugs in tissue sections. *Toxicol Pathol* 35 (4): 541–8.

Gossett, K. A., P. K. Narayanan, D. M. Williams et al. 1999. Flow cytometry in the preclinical development of biopharmaceuticals. *Toxicol Pathol* 27 (1) (Jan–Feb): 32–7.

Halling, K. C. and A. J. Wendel. 2009. In situ hybridization: Principles and applications. In *Basic Concepts of Molecular Pathology*. eds. P. T. Cagle and T. C. Allen. New York: Springer.

Hand, N. M. and R. J. Church. 1998. Superheating using pressure cooking: its use and application in unmasking antigens embedded in methyl methacrylate. *J Histotechnol* 21 (3) (Sept): 231–6.

Hannon-Fletcher, M. and P. Maxwell. 2009. Advanced techniques in diagnostic cellular pathology. In *Flow Cytometry*. ed. I. Dimmick. Hoboken: John Wiley & Sons.

Hashiguchi, A., Y. Hashimoto, H. Suzuki, and M. Sakamoto. 2010. Using immunofluorescent digital slide technology to quantify protein expression in archival paraffin-embedded tissue sections. *Pathol Int* 60 (11) (Nov): 720–5.

Hawes, J. J. and K. M. Reilly. 2010. Bioluminescent approaches for measuring tumor growth in a mouse model of neurofibromatosis. *Toxicol Pathol* 38 (1): 123–30.

Hedley, D. W., S. Chow, C. Goolsby, and T. V. Shankey. 2008. Pharmacodynamic monitoring of molecular-targeted agents in the peripheral blood of leukemia patients using flow cytometry. *Toxicol Pathol* 36 (1): 133–9.

Houle, C. D. 2011. Neuropathology standards: What constitutes an optimal histomorphologic evaluation of the nervous system in general toxicity studies. *Toxicol Pathol* 39 (6): 1010–12.

Kepp, O., L. Galluzzi, M. Lipinski, J. Yuan, and G. Kroemer. 2011. Cell death assays for drug discovery. *Nature Rev Drug Discov* 10 (3) (Mar): 221–37.

Kumar, G. L. and L. Rudbeck, eds. 2009. *Immunohistochemical (IHC) Staining Methods*. 5th edition. Carpinteria: Dako North America.

Kunder, S., J. Calzada-Wack, G. Holzlwimmer et al. 2007. A comprehensive antibody panel for immunohistochemical analysis of formalin-fixed, paraffin-embedded hematopoietic neoplasms of mice: Analysis of mouse specific and human antibodies cross-reactive with murine tissue. *Toxicol Pathol* 35 (3): 366–75.

Lang, P., K. Yeow, A. Nichols, and A. Scheer. 2006. Cellular imaging in drug discovery. *Nature Rev Drug Discov* 5 (4) (Apr): 343–56.

Lappin, P. B. and L. E. Black. 2003. Immune modulator studies in primates: The utility of flow cytometry and immunohistochemistry in the identification and characterization of immunotoxicity. *Toxicol Pathol* 31 Suppl (Jan–Feb): 111–8.

Leach, M. W., W. G. Halpern, C. W. Johnson et al. 2010. Use of tissue cross-reactivity studies in the development of antibody-based biopharmaceuticals: History, experience, methodology, and future directions. *Toxicol Pathol* 38 (7): 1138–66.

Lichtman, J. W. and J. A. Conchello. 2005. Fluorescence microscopy. *Nature Methods* 2 (12) (Dec): 910–9.

Liebler, D. C. and F. P. Guengerich. 2005. Elucidating mechanisms of drug-induced toxicity. *Nature Rev Drug Discov* 4 (5) (May): 410–20.

Mach, W. J., A. R. Thimmesch, J. A. Orr, J. G. Slusser, and J. D. Pierce. 2010. Flow cytometry and laser scanning cytometry, a comparison of techniques. *J Clin Monit Comput* 24 (4) (Aug): 251–9.

Malarkey, D. E. and R. R. Maronpot. 1996. Polymerase chain reaction and in situ hybridization: Applications in toxicological pathology. *Toxicol Pathol* 24 (1) (Jan–Feb): 13–23.

McCullough, B., X. Ying, T. Monticello, and M. Bonnefoi. 2004. Digital microscopy imaging and new approaches in toxicologic pathology. *Toxicol Pathol* 32 Suppl 2 (Jul–Aug): 49–58.

Mikaelian, I., L. B. Nanney, K. S. Parman et al. 2004. Antibodies that label paraffin-embedded mouse tissues: A collaborative endeavor. *Toxicol Pathol* 32 (2) (Mar–Apr): 181–91.

Murray, G. I. 2008. Laser microdissection. In *Molecular Biomethods Handbook*. eds. J. M. Walker and R. Rapley. 2nd edition. Totowa: Humana Press.

Narayanan, P., R. J. Capocasale, N. Li, and P. J. Bugelski. 2008. Application of flow cytometry in drug development. In *Immunotoxicology Strategies for Pharmaceutical Safety Assessment*. eds. D. J. Hersyk and J. L. Bussiere. 1st ed. pp. 141–61. Hoboken: John Wiley & Sons Inc.

Obert, L. A., G. P. Sobocinski, W. F. Bobrowski et al. 2007. An immunohistochemical approach to differentiate hepatic lipidosis from hepatic phospholipidosis in rats. *Toxicol Pathol* 35 (5): 728–34.

Painter, J. T., N. P. Clayton, and R. A. Herbert. 2010. Useful immunohistochemical markers of tumor differentiation. *Toxicol Pathol* 38 (1): 131–41.

Papagiannaros, A., J. Upponi, W. Hartner, D. Mongayt, T. Levchenko, and V. Torchilin. 2010. Quantum dot loaded immunomicelles for tumor imaging. *BMC Med Imaging* 10 (Oct 18): 22.

Pathak, A. P., M. F. Penet, and Z. M. Bhujwalla. 2010. MR molecular imaging of tumor vasculature and vascular targets. *Adv Genet* 69: 1–30.

Peterson, R. A., K. L. Gabrielson, G. Allan Johnson, M. G. Pomper, R. W. Coatney, and C. T. Winkelmann. 2011. Continuing education course #1: Non-invasive imaging as a problem-solving tool and translational biomarker strategy in toxicologic pathology. *Toxicol Pathol* 39 (1) (Jan): 267–72.

Peterson, R. A., D. L. Krull, and L. Butler. 2008. Applications of laser scanning cytometry in immunohistochemistry and routine histopathology. *Toxicol Pathol* 36 (1): 117–32.

Petrausch, U., D. Haley, W. Miller, K. Floyd, W. J. Urba, and E. Walker. 2006. Polychromatic flow cytometry: A rapid method for the reduction and analysis of complex multiparameter data. Cytometry. Part A: *J Int Soc Anal Cytol* 69 (12) (Dec 1): 1162–73.

Pruimboom-Brees, I. M., D. J. Brees, A. C. Shen et al. 2005. Using laser scanning cytometry to measure PPAR-mediated peroxisome proliferation and beta oxidation. *Toxicol Pathol* 33 (1): 86–91.

Ramos-Vara, J. A. 2005. Technical aspects of immunohistochemistry. *Vet Pathol* 42 (4) (Jul): 405–26.

Resch-Genger, U., M. Grabolle, S. Cavaliere-Jaricot, R. Nitschke, and T. Nann. 2008. Quantum dots versus organic dyes as fluorescent labels. *Nature Methods* 5 (9) (Sep): 763–75.

Sterchi, D. L. 2010. Molecular pathology—in situ hybridization. In *Theory and Practice of Histological Techniques*. eds. J. D. Bancroft and M. Gamble. 6th ed. pp. 537–58. China: Churchill Livingstone.

Taylor, C. R. and R. M. Levenson. 2006. Quantification of immunohistochemistry—issues concerning methods, utility and semiquantitative assessment II. *Histopathology* 49 (4) (Oct): 411–24.

Tengowski, M. W. 2004. Image compression in morphometry studies requiring 21 CFR part 11 compliance: Procedure is key with TIFFs and various JPEG compression strengths. *Toxicol Pathol* 32 (2) (Mar–Apr): 258–63.

Tuomari, D. L., R. K. Kemp, R. Sellers, J. T. Yarrington, F. J. Geoly, X. L. Fouillet, N. Dybdal, R. Perry, and Society of Toxicologic Pathology. 2007. Society of toxicologic pathology position paper on pathology image data: Compliance with 21 CFR parts 58 and 11. *Toxicol Pathol* 35 (3): 450–5.

Walker, R. A. 2006. Quantification of immunohistochemistry—issues concerning methods, utility and semiquantitative assessment I. *Histopathology* 49 (4) (Oct): 406–10.

Ward, J. M., C. R. Erexson, L. J. Faucette, J. F. Foley, C. Dijkstra, and G. Cattoretti. 2006. Immunohistochemical markers for the rodent immune system. *Toxicol Pathol* 34 (5): 616–30.

Weber, K., R. H. Garman, P. G. Germann et al. 2011. Classification of neural tumors in laboratory rodents, emphasizing the rat. *Toxicol Pathol* 39 (1) (Jan): 129–51.

Weibel, E. R., G. S. Kistler, and W. F. Scherle. 1966. Practical stereological methods for morphometric cytology. *J Cell Biol* 30 (1) (Jul): 23–38.

Willmann, J. K., N. van Bruggen, L. M. Dinkelborg, and S. S. Gambhir. 2008. Molecular imaging in drug development. *Nature Rev Drug Discov* 7 (7) (Jul): 591–607.

Ying, X. and T. M. Monticello. 2006. Modern imaging technologies in toxicologic pathology: An overview. *Toxicol Pathol* 34 (7): 815–26.

Zu, Y., M. Shahjahan, and C. Chung-Che. 2009. Basic principles of flow cytometry. In *Basic Concepts of Molecular Pathology*. eds. P. T. Cagle and T. C. Allen. New York: Springer.

6 Principles of Clinical Pathology

Robert L. Hall

CONTENTS

6.1   INTRODUCTION

Clinical pathology is a standard element of nonclinical safety assessment studies and typically consists of routine hematology, coagulation, clinical chemistry, and urinalysis tests. Test results provide a broad screen of important tissues and organ systems, metabolic functions, and pathophysiologic responses. Test article–related effects on these results help identify target organs, establish dose responses, corroborate other study findings, assess severity of toxic effects, and quantify certain pharmacodynamic effects. Clinical pathology findings also serve to meet regulatory needs and, most importantly, provide clinicians with important monitoring information prior to clinical trials.

   Test selection, frequency, and timing are dependent on several factors, including study objectives and duration, dosing regimen, test article characteristics, regulatory requirements, and the laboratory animal species studied. Interpretation of results requires an understanding of the purpose and limitations of each test, the many variables that can affect tests, unique species differences, and correlative findings among other toxicity endpoints. While nonclinical studies are generally similar in basic design, small differences in event schedules, procedures, and performance can significantly affect data interpretation. Relative to interpretation of clinical pathology data from an individual sick animal, interpretation of data from a nonclinical study has several advantages: multiple animals per group at increasing dose levels, a concurrent control group, baseline data for larger species, detailed clinical observations, comprehensive anatomic pathology evaluations, and at least some knowledge of potential test article effects based on pharmacologic activity or drug class. However, these advantages can be a double-edged sword, and identification of subtle clinical pathology effects is common. Placing subtle effects into proper context can be not only challenging but also very important to the future development of the test article.

   This chapter addresses study design factors that influence clinical pathology test selection, timing, and frequency; sources of variability that confound data interpretation; general principles of data interpretation; and common patterns and correlative findings for standard hematology, coagulation, clinical chemistry, urinalysis, and urine chemistry tests.

6.2   STUDY DESIGN FACTORS

6.2.1   Test Selection

Test selection is ultimately dependent on study objective but is influenced by the animal model and regulatory expectations. Early investigational-type studies may focus on specific toxicity concerns associated with similar test articles, such as liver toxicity or hemolysis, or assess desired efficacy endpoints of a test article, such as glucose metabolism or red blood cell (RBC) production. In these studies, selection of clinical pathology tests can be limited and targeted to specific needs or interests. On the other hand, if a study is part of the nonclinical package to support regulatory approval, several tests are required or recommended in guidances published by the various regulatory agencies. Unfortunately, guidances are not uniform and are sometimes ambiguous; in a few instances, guidances recommend or require inappropriate tests (Hall 1992). In 1996, an international committee composed of representatives from several professional organizations with scientific expertise in animal clinical pathology published "core" recommended tests for regulated safety assessment and toxicity studies in an effort to provide more standard recommendations (Weingand et al. 1996). More recently, papers have been published specifically addressing clinical pathology testing recommendations to assess liver toxicity (Boone et al. 2005) and for carcinogenicity studies

(Young et al. 2011). The following paragraphs describe clinical pathology tests most commonly assessed in standard nonclinical studies.

Hematology parameters routinely measured include RBC count, hemoglobin concentration, hematocrit, mean cell or corpuscular volume (MCV), mean cell or corpuscular hemoglobin (MCH), mean cell or corpuscular hemoglobin concentration (MCHC), red cell distribution width (RDW), absolute reticulocyte count, platelet count, mean platelet volume (MPV), total white blood cell (WBC) count, and absolute differential WBC count (at minimum, includes neutrophils, lymphocytes, monocytes, eosinophils, and basophils). All these tests can be performed by hematology analyzers with species-specific software currently used in industry. A blood smear should always be made. Some companies routinely examine all or a subset of smears (e.g., control and high-dose animals) microscopically to assess cell morphology characteristics, while others evaluate data generated by the hematology analyzer to determine if microscopic examination of blood smears is warranted. State-of-the-art hematology analyzers can generate a great number of additional measurements about different cell populations that may be beneficial for very specific needs and investigational interests, but their value for standard toxicity screening is limited at this time by lack of experience with interpretation in various laboratory animal species under different conditions.

Routine evaluation of bone marrow smears (e.g., myeloid-to-erythroid [M:E] ratio, cytologic examination, or differential cell count) is not recommended or warranted. Although it may be prudent to prepare bone marrow smears at necropsy for possible future use, indications for microscopic examination of bone marrow smears in standard toxicity studies are limited (Reagan et al. 2011). In contrast to a patient with *unexplained* nonregenerative anemia, leukopenia, thrombocytopenia, or pancytopenia, the cause of these findings in animals being administered a test article is not unexplained. The combination of serial peripheral blood findings that reflect bone marrow function and microscopic findings in bone marrow sections (e.g., sternum and femur) is sufficient to generally understand test article effects on bone marrow. Actual M:E ratios have little or no value and can usually be predicted by the peripheral blood findings or estimated by examination of bone marrow sections. Detailed examinations of bone marrow smears should only be undertaken to answer specific questions about bone marrow effects and may require a study designed specifically for that purpose. For example, bone marrow findings can vary greatly from one day to the next after an acute toxic insult, as reflected in peripheral blood counts that fall sharply and then rebound. Examination of bone marrow smears from a single point in time can result in incorrect assumptions about the nature of the toxic effect. Evaluation of different bone marrow cell populations by flow cytometric techniques has the potential to provide better quantitative information than obtained manually, but technological challenges and practicality limit the use of flow cytometry to specific investigational work.

Coagulation tests routinely performed include prothrombin time (PT), activated partial thromboplastin time (APTT), and fibrinogen. Toxicologically important effects on coagulation are relatively infrequent, and these tests are sometimes eliminated or delayed until terminal sacrifice if blood volume limitations are an issue because of animal size and the number of blood samples required for other assessments (e.g., toxicokinetics, pharmacodynamics, and antidrug antibody). Although part of the coagulation test profile, fibrinogen is an acute phase protein and useful as a marker of inflammation.

Clinical chemistry parameters routinely measured or calculated include glucose, urea nitrogen (or urea), creatinine, total protein, albumin, globulin (calculated from total protein and albumin), albumin-to-globulin ratio (calculated), cholesterol, triglycerides, total bilirubin, alanine aminotransferase (ALT), aspartate aminotransferase (AST), glutamate dehydrogenase (GLDH), alkaline phosphatase (ALP), gamma glutamyltransferase (GGT), creatine kinase (CK), calcium, inorganic phosphorus, sodium, potassium, and chloride. These tests are typically performed on serum, but plasma is occasionally used for mice because the sample yield can be slightly better. If plasma is used for analysis, lithium heparin is the recommended anticoagulant. While GLDH is commonly analyzed in Europe, its use in the United States is limited, in part because of reagent availability.

Most routine clinical chemistry assays developed for human testing require no modification for animals. A notable exception is overestimation of rabbit albumin concentration by dye-binding assays such as bromocresol green (BCG). Rabbit albumin concentrations using BCG can sometimes exceed that of total protein. Use of a rabbit albumin standard for calibration improves accuracy.

Urinalysis parameters routinely evaluated include volume (if collected over a period [e.g., overnight]), color and clarity, pH, specific gravity or osmolality, reagent strip tests, and urine sediment microscopy.

Many other clinical pathology tests are available and may be indicated for assessment of specific test articles. Hematology tests, such as methemoglobin or enumeration of Heinz bodies, could be indicated for test articles causing oxidative injury. Platelet function tests may be appropriate for test articles targeting platelets. If exocrine pancreatic injury is a concern, measurement of amylase or lipase activity may be warranted. Various hormones can be measured to assess possible endocrine dysfunction, and urine chemistry tests (e.g., electrolytes, enzymes, and new biomarkers) may help assess renal function and integrity. Cardiac troponin I or T may be indicated for test articles suspected of causing cardiac toxicity, and biomarkers to detect bone formation or resorption may be useful for test articles targeting bone. The list of possible tests is long and will continue to increase as the search for more specific and sensitive tests continues. Understanding when and how to use these new tests will take time and experience.

The test species influences test selection, most often because of sample volume limitations. Test selection for a mouse study must be carefully considered because an adult mouse has a blood volume of only approximately 2 mL, and collecting even half that volume cleanly is unlikely. However, it is usually possible to obtain enough blood from one mouse for standard hematology tests and a small subset of clinical chemistry tests that provides a broad screen of major organs and overall health status (e.g., urea nitrogen, ALT, total protein, albumin, and globulin). Another option is to designate one subset of animals in each group for hematology tests and a second subset of animals for clinical chemistry tests. Coagulation tests are typically not performed in mouse studies, but if they are indicated by the test article and study objectives, coagulation test sample requirements necessitate inclusion of a subset of animals specifically for that purpose. Similar issues concerning sample volume and test selection can arise in a rat study, especially if interim clinical pathology intervals are desired. It may be necessary to limit the tests done at interim intervals or to perform terminal blood collections under anesthesia prior to sacrifice and necropsy. Blood volume limitations that affect test selection and frequency in monkey (nonhuman primate; refers to cynomolgus monkey unless otherwise stated) studies are due to the combination of their relatively small size, especially young females, and the use of each animal for other tests requiring blood (e.g., pharmacokinetic analyses, antidrug antibody screens, and pharmacodynamic markers). In addition to the obvious effect on test selection and frequency, these multiple blood collections can and do significantly affect the results of many clinical pathology tests. Dogs are much less affected by multiple blood collections because of their size and ease of handling. Clinical pathology testing is rarely limited and data interpretation is rarely compromised in nonclinical dog studies.

A few clinical pathology tests, such as lactate dehydrogenase (LDH), uric acid, serum protein electrophoresis, and M:E ratio, have been used commonly in the past for different reasons (e.g., ambiguous regulatory guidances and use in human medicine) but offer little if any value, and their routine use for nonclinical safety assessment is discouraged.

6.2.2 Test Frequency and Timing

Frequency and timing of clinical pathology testing are dependent on several factors. Blood collection from mice for clinical pathology tests is usually a terminal procedure and can only be done at the time of sacrifice (e.g., end of the dosing or recovery phase). While predose or baseline data are critical for interpretation of clinical pathology results in studies with larger species (i.e., rabbit, dog, and monkey), they offer no advantages in rat studies, and blood collection prior to initiation of dosing in rats can actually be harmful to animals and complicate data interpretation. Baseline data for the larger species serve two purposes. First, data can be used to screen and remove animals with potential health concerns or outlier values that might complicate future data interpretation. Evidence of a potential health concern includes findings such as low hematocrit or albumin concentration and high absolute neutrophil count, fibrinogen concentration, or liver enzyme activity. Examples of outlier values that could complicate future data interpretation include a high cholesterol concentration in a study of a drug indicated for treating hypercholesterolemia or low absolute neutrophil count in a study of a chemotherapeutic agent. Second, data are critical for interpretation of postdose results. Because the number of animals used in a dog or monkey study is small and interanimal variability can be relatively large, especially for monkeys, baseline data provide essential perspectives concerning apparent differences between control and treated animals after dosing. Many range-finding studies in large animals have no control group, so each animal serves as its own control. The optimal number of predose or baseline intervals depends on a few factors, including species, number of animals in the study, and study duration. For rabbit studies, a single baseline collection is usually sufficient. For monkey studies, two baseline collections, at least 5 days apart, are recommended. Not only do they provide more data for perspective concerning inter- and intra-animal variability and preexisting group differences, two collections help animals become accustomed to the blood collection procedure, which serves to reduce variability caused by excitement or fear. For dog studies, two baseline collections are preferred, especially when relatively few animals are on study (e.g., one to three dogs/sex/group). However, if several animals are in each group and the study duration is relatively long (e.g., ≥13 weeks), a single baseline collection is adequate.

As a general rule, clinical pathology testing in a single-dose study is best done approximately 48 to 72 h postdose. The objective is to allow enough time for important toxic effects to be manifested but not reverse. Testing 24 h postdose is often too soon for many changes to occur or reach their peak after toxic injury. Serum liver enzyme activities, tests of kidney function, and peripheral blood cell counts typically are not clearly affected the day after a single significant toxic insult to the liver, kidneys, and bone marrow, respectively. Another reason to avoid an assessment only 24 h postdose is variability caused by study-related procedures that occur on the day of dosing, such as multiple blood collections for toxicokinetics and handling for various procedures. The effects of these procedures, along with effects of transient test article–related events, such as vomiting, diarrhea, and anorexia, can result in variable data that are more difficult to interpret and that increase the likelihood of identifying transient changes (e.g., decreased chloride due to vomiting) not indicative of significant target organ toxicity. Conversely, early data collection is occasionally desirable for certain tests or study objectives. Some tests peak quickly after tissue injury (e.g., urinary enzymes and cardiac troponin) and waiting 48 or 72 h postdose before testing may be too long. If the objective is to follow a specific pharmacodynamic marker (e.g., glucose after insulin treatment), then optimal timing of testing for that marker will be dependent on systemic exposure and test article activity and may be within minutes or hours of dosing. Serial sampling over a period is also occasionally valuable. Peripheral blood effects of chemotherapeutic agents do not all occur simultaneously. In order to assess cell count nadirs and recovery of different blood cell types, it is necessary to collect blood for hematology tests on multiple days postdose (e.g., Days 3, 5, 7, 10, and 14).

For repeat-dose studies of 2 or 4 weeks' duration, there is generally little advantage to interim clinical pathology intervals (e.g., at the end of Week 1), especially for rat studies. For repeat-dose studies of longer duration (e.g., 13, 26, 39, and 52 weeks), one or two interim clinical pathology intervals are valuable for data interpretation, especially for dog and monkey studies. The need for an interim clinical pathology interval in a longer-duration rat study depends in large part on findings from previous studies with the test article. There may be no need to include an interim interval if prior studies provided relatively definitive answers at dose levels relevant to the longer-duration study. Clinical pathology testing is not recommended for rodent toxicity studies longer than 52 weeks because of naturally occurring disease conditions that cause excessive variability in results (Weingand et al. 1996). Clinical pathology testing should be very limited in rodent carcinogenicity studies. The most current recommendation, based on a survey of many companies and clinical pathologists working in industry, is limited to preparation of blood smears from all sacrificed animals (scheduled or unscheduled). Blood smears are then available for examination if necessary as an adjunct for confirmation of potential hematopoietic neoplasia (Young et al. 2011).

When dose administration is intermittent (e.g., once weekly) or cyclical (e.g., five consecutive days of dosing once monthly), timing of sample collection should preferably be consistent with respect to dosing. For example, if dosing occurs once weekly for 13 weeks, interim and terminal clinical pathology samples might be taken either 1 day or 3 days after the 6th and 13th doses as long as the interval between dosing and sample collection is the same. Similarly, if dosing occurs for five consecutive days once each month for 3 months, samples might be taken 1, 3, or 5 days after the first and last dosing cycle as long as the interval is the same. If the interval is not the same (e.g., interim samples collected 1 day after dosing and terminal samples collected 5 days after dosing), interpretation loses the advantage of consistency, and the difference in timing must be considered during data evaluation.

Timing and frequency of clinical pathology sample collection during a recovery phase depend on study needs. If the objective is to simply determine whether effects are reversible, then collection at the end of the recovery phase should suffice. If the objective is to determine the speed of reversibility, then multiple recovery intervals would be necessary, and timing would depend on the nature of the test article (e.g., short versus long half-life) and expected effects. Some effects, such as those on RBC indices (e.g., MCV and RDW), typically take longer to recover than others (e.g., high liver enzyme activities).

6.2.3 Sources of Variability

Nonclinical studies are usually designed and conducted in a tightly controlled manner in order to minimize variability of measured endpoints and more confidently determine effects of test article administration. Understanding sources of variability allows better study design and conduct. Understanding the effects of variability allows better data interpretation because variability unrelated to the test article is present in all studies. Sources of variability can be preanalytical (i.e., before the endpoint is measured) or analytical (i.e., a function of assay characteristics). The most common sources of significant variability are preanalytical and can be loosely divided into three categories: artifact, physiological, and procedural.

Artifact typically results from poor sample quality. Hematology samples with small clots result in low cell counts, especially platelet count. Hemolyzed clinical chemistry samples and delayed separation of serum from clotted blood can result in high values for analytes normally present within red cells (e.g., AST). Hemolysis has the potential to cause interference errors in some assays, and delayed separation of serum can result in low serum glucose concentration as a result of ongoing RBC metabolism. Excess anticoagulant in coagulation test samples results in prolonged PT and APTT. Accidental contamination of blood collected for serum tests with anticoagulant results in changes that depend on the contaminating anticoagulant (e.g., reduction of calcium concentration by sodium citrate or potassium ethylenediaminetetraacetic acid). Exposure of small-volume serum samples (e.g., from mice) to air for a prolonged period results in increased analyte concentrations because of evaporation. Changes in sodium and chloride concentration are most apparent. Prolonged or inappropriate sample storage prior to analysis of unstable analytes results in low concentrations or activities. Sample quality issues often arise because of inexperienced blood collection or blood handling personnel but can also occur as a result of attempting new procedures without adequate training. Another relatively common cause of poor sample quality is difficult blood collection as a result of poor animal health. Blood collection from a moribund animal is often complicated by dehydration and low blood pressure. Collection of blood from moribund mice and rats is particularly difficult, and results acquired from these species are often compromised by sample quality issues. When combined with changes secondary to the animal's poor condition (e.g., prerenal azotemia, stress-induced lymphopenia, and agonal hyperglycemia), clinical pathology results from moribund rodents, especially mice, infrequently contribute to understanding direct toxic effects of a test article.

Physiological sources of variation include factors such as age, sex, strain, diet, fasted condition, time of sample collection, excitement/fear, and stress.

Results for several hematology and clinical chemistry parameters undergo significant changes in early stages of rodent and dog studies because initiation of dosing typically begins during a period of rapid growth and change. Common changes as animals mature include increases in red cell mass (i.e., RBC count, hemoglobin concentration, and hematocrit), absolute neutrophil count, total protein and globulin concentrations and decreases in absolute reticulocyte count, MCV, MCH, absolute lymphocyte count, ALP activity, and inorganic phosphorus concentration. In the absence of age-matched controls, it would be easy to misinterpret these changes, even in a study as short as 2 to 4 weeks. Interanimal variability for many clinical pathology parameters increases in older animals because of spontaneous conditions, and interpretation of data can be more difficult at the end of chronic studies (e.g., 26 to 52 weeks) or in monkey studies using animals of different ages (e.g., 2 to 7 years of age). Examples of relatively obvious differences between males and females include lower absolute neutrophil count for female rats, higher albumin concentration for female rats, and higher ALP for males of most species. These and other differences are reasons to avoid pooling data from both sexes. Mice and rats of different strains, beagle dogs from different suppliers, and cynomolgus monkeys from different countries of origin all exhibit differences in clinical pathology results, as well as other toxicity endpoints. Unless taken into consideration, these differences can affect the understanding of findings between studies in a development program. Although most nonclinical studies use common standard laboratory animal diets, unusual or supplemented diets are occasionally used to create an abnormality (e.g., an atherogenic diet) or prevent one (e.g., iron supplementation for test articles that chelate iron). In addition to feeding the same altered diet to control animals, it is often advantageous to include a control group fed a normal diet to fully understand changes that may occur because of the diet.

Fasting animals prior to sample collection is a common practice in most laboratories. The purpose of fasting is often thought to be avoidance of postprandial spikes in analytes like serum glucose, but more importantly, fasting prior to sample collection standardizes conditions for all animals. If the test article affects food consumption or alters the eating pattern of treated animals compared with concurrent controls, then clinical pathology testing of nonfasted animals has the potential to identify differences simply owing to eating patterns. For example, fasted rats (or, by extension, animals that are anorexic) tend to have lower WBC counts; serum concentrations of urea nitrogen, cholesterol, triglycerides, calcium, and bilirubin; and serum activities of ALT and ALP (Kimball et al. 1995; Matsuzawa and Sakazume 1994). Fasting mice can be problematic as mice tend to become dehydrated quickly when not eating, and dehydration alters several test results, in addition to increasing the difficulty of blood collection. However, because blood collection from mice is usually a terminal procedure done just prior to necropsy, fasting is often desirable to reduce glycogen in hepatocytes and improve microscopic detection of subtle hepatocellular effects. Fasting mice for a limited time (e.g., 4 h) is sometimes done as a compromise to these conflicting interests. If this is done, care must be taken to adjust or stagger the start time for fasting animals on the basis of their projected time of necropsy. Terminal necropsy for a large mouse study may take several hours, and animals at the end of the necropsy period should not be fasted significantly longer than those at the beginning. The length of necropsy procedures presents another source of variability, circadian effects. While circadian effects would be difficult to avoid in this situation, timing of multiple blood collections over the course of a study should be scheduled as uniformly as possible (e.g., always in the early morning or always in the late morning) in order to decrease variability and facilitate data interpretation.

Study-related procedures, including the act of blood collection, have the potential to increase variability as a result of endogenous catecholamine release due to excitement or fear (the *fight or flight* response). This is especially true for monkeys and excitable dogs. The response occurs rapidly but is short lived. In addition to physical effects, such as increased heart rate and blood pressure, common clinical pathology changes include increased red cell mass due to splenic contraction, increased leukocyte counts due to movement from the marginal to circulating pool, and increased glucose due to glycogenolysis. The potential for misinterpreting changes from baseline results is greater when a monkey or dog study includes only a single baseline clinical pathology interval because this response is more common during the early part of a study before animals have become accustomed to handling or blood collection. Effects of stress, or endogenous corticosteroid release, can also increase variability, but these changes take longer to develop and last longer. In addition to stress associated with significant toxicity, study-related activities, such as shipping, surgery, and repeated anesthesia, can cause a stress response. The most common findings associated with stress are decreased absolute lymphocyte and eosinophil counts. If absolute lymphocyte counts are decreased but absolute eosinophil counts are not, the finding for absolute lymphocyte count is less likely stress-related because eosinophils are extremely sensitive to corticosteroids.

Procedural sources of variation include blood collection technique/site, order of sample collection and analysis, and study design factors and events, such as vehicle characteristics, route of administration, surgical manipulations and other procedures requiring anesthesia, and toxicokinetics sample collection.

The most important aspects of blood collection technique/site are proficiency and consistency. Several studies have been done comparing test results using different techniques and sites of collection, especially for rodents (Bennett et al. 1992; Dameron et al. 1992; Khan et al. 1996; Kimball et al. 1995; Matsuzawa et al. 1993, 1994; Millis et al. 1995; Nemzek et al. 2001; Neptun et al. 1985; Roncaglioni et al. 1982; Schnell et al. 2002; Smith et al. 1986; Stringer and Seligmann 1996; Suber and Kodell 1985; Upton and Morgan 1975). Although clear differences for some tests exist on the basis of technique/site (e.g., WBC counts from retro-orbital venous plexus are higher than those from large abdominal vessels), differences should not affect data interpretation as long as blood collection personnel are proficient and the technique used is consistent throughout the course of a study. For example, it would unnecessarily complicate data interpretation to collect blood from anesthetized monkeys at some test intervals and conscious monkeys at others or to collect blood from the jugular vein of rats at an interim collection interval and the vena cava at the terminal collection. Requiring blood collection personnel to use a technique/site to which they are unaccustomed, for any reason, without proper training and sufficient, results-proven practice simply increases the likelihood of variability that can mask test article–related effects.

The order of sample collection and analysis should always be planned to avoid effects of time bias. Collecting and analyzing samples in group order, beginning with the control group and ending with the high-dose group, is scientifically inappropriate because it can result in differences between control and treated groups that have no relationship to the test article. These differences can be reduced or eliminated by collecting samples in random order or round-robin order (i.e., one animal from each group in each collection *round*) and then analyzing samples in the order of collection. This minimizes effects of preanalytical variables at the time of sample collection (e.g., the time serum remains in contact with blood cells) and analytical drift during analysis. If sample collection by group cannot be avoided (e.g., because of timed postdose sample collections), then alter the order of dosing so the control and high-dose groups are dosed and bled consecutively (e.g., mid-dose, control, high-dose, and low-dose groups) and process the samples quickly. If the size or complexity of a study requires a staggered start and staggered procedures over 2 days, effects of day-to-day variability can be minimized by starting and testing males on one day and females on the next.

Certain vehicles or vehicle constituents, such as corn oil or polyethylene glycol, can increase variability of specific tests, and markers of inflammation in particular will be more variable when the route of administration is intravenous infusion via indwelling catheter. Animals surgically manipulated in some other way (e.g., telemetry instrumentation or bile duct cannulation) can also have more variable data. Intramuscular ketamine anesthesia used for many in-life procedures in monkeys is very irritating to muscle, causes marked acute increases in serum activity of muscle enzymes like CK, and can also increase variability of tests, such as acute phase protein concentrations.

A major procedural cause of increased variability is multiple blood sample collections for toxicokinetic analyses and, less frequently, antidrug antibody analysis and pharmacodynamic markers. This is especially problematic in monkey studies. Although the exact amount of blood taken can be calculated, that does not account for rebleeding that may occur when animals are returned to their cages. Animals bled six or eight times within 24 h on Day 1 of a study will often lose more blood than the calculated volume (e.g., 6 or 8 mL). Ultimately, some animals have much larger reductions in red cell mass and serum proteins than others, and a robust regenerative response occurs for some but not others. These differences can easily result in misinterpretation of data because of relatively few animals in each group. If multiple toxicokinetic samples are collected on the final day of dosing in a repeat-dose study (e.g., Day 28 of a 4-week study), then terminal clinical pathology sample collection would best occur with the predose toxicokinetic sample collection on that final day and not before necropsy on the following day.

Although it seems intuitive that all study-related procedures should be identical for control and treated animals, economic pressures and the desire to limit animal use can result in practices that ultimately reduce the power of studies to identify test article–related effects and lead to misinterpretation of test results. Some of these practices include collecting fewer blood samples from control animals than treated animals, collecting multiple toxicokinetic samples from rats used for toxicity endpoints, using different routes of administration or dosing regimens in a single study without an appropriate control for each route or dosing regimen, using different vehicle formulations in a single study without an appropriate control for each, and comparing animals that have been surgically manipulated (e.g., instrumented for telemetry) with those that have not. As some of these practices and others will no doubt continue, it is imperative that these compromises to optimal science be understood and considered during data interpretation.

6.3   DATA INTERPRETATION

Interpretation of clinical pathology data from a nonclinical study is generally no different than that for any other toxicity endpoints. If there are differences between control and treated animal test results, do those differences reflect true or *real* effects of the test article? And if those differences do reflect real effects of the test article, are the effects toxicologically important or adverse? These judgments require considering many factors and using a weight-of-evidence approach. Factors considered include all sources of variability previously described, species and number of animals tested, in-life observations, anatomic pathology findings, characteristics of each clinical pathology test, and the test article itself.

The first step is to identify differences between control and treated animal results at the intervals tested and differences between baseline and postdose results for large animal species. This can be done by subjectively examining the data for each group and for individuals within each group or with the aid of statistical analysis. Whether or not statistics are used, group and individual results must always be examined. Statistics are a tool and never the only interpretive consideration (Carakostas and Banerjee 1990; Chanter et al. 1987). When statistical comparisons are made between multiple groups and sometimes at multiple testing intervals for 40+ clinical pathology tests, it is nearly certain that statistically significant differences between control and treated groups that do not represent real effects will be identified. It is also common that some real effects will not be statistically significant.

Once a difference between control and treated animals has been identified, the decision concerning its relationship to the test article (i.e., is it real?) is based on many factors. For large animals, was there a similar difference present in baseline data before initiation of dosing? If so, the difference is much less likely real. What was the magnitude of the difference with respect to the affected parameter? A 20% difference is virtually meaningless for absolute neutrophil count or ALT activity, quite substantial for hematocrit or calcium concentration, and enormous for sodium or chloride concentration. Was the difference dose dependent, consistent over time, and consistent between sexes? Dose dependency and consistency are not absolutely necessary for a difference to be real, especially with biologics, but they add to the weight of evidence. When did the difference occur with respect to dosing? A difference 2 days postdose is more likely to be real than a difference 14 days postdose for the great majority of test articles. Were there correlative in-life observations or anatomic pathology findings? These clearly add to the weight of evidence. What is known about the test article or drug class? In other words, are questionable differences more or less reasonable given expected or suspected effects based on previous work? Study design factors to consider include the test species, age, number of animals per group, and unique study conditions, such as route of administration, vehicle, multiple or excessive blood collections, and other study-related procedures. The same difference for a given test is more likely to be real in a study with 15 animals/group than a study with 5 animals/group. A small difference for ALT activity is more likely to be real in a rat or dog study than in a mouse or monkey study. In general, clinical pathology data for mice and monkeys are more variable than those for rats and dogs. For mice, this is due, at least in part, to the difficulties associated with sample collection. For monkeys, this is partly due to their relatively small size compared with dogs and differences in their ages, the way they were raised, and their reaction to handling. A small difference for ALT is more likely to be real in a 2-week rat or dog study than a 52-week study because of increased variability in older animals, but a small difference in ALP is more likely to be real in the 52-week study because the bone isoform of ALP has less influence in older animals. A small difference for absolute neutrophil count or fibrinogen is more likely to be real in an oral gavage study than a chronic intravenous infusion study. A small difference for cholesterol is more likely to be real if the vehicle is reverse osmosis water and not corn oil. Small differences for red cell mass and absolute reticulocyte count at Day 4 of a single-dose study are more likely to be real in a dog study than a monkey study because the effect of multiple toxicokinetic sample collections has less impact in dogs. Small differences for AST and CK are more likely to be real in monkeys that have not recently been anesthetized with intramuscular ketamine.

Once a difference has been determined to be test article related, the decision concerning its toxicologic relevance is also based on many factors, but it is rare to consider a clinical pathology effect toxicologically important or adverse without correlative in-life observations or anatomic pathology findings that reflect the significance of the effect. Clinical pathology parameters can be divided into those that are critical to health and those that are simply markers for organ function, tissue integrity, or a process. Some parameters are both. Hemoglobin, glucose, calcium, and potassium are examples of analytes critical to health. Too little of these in blood will have serious negative consequences and be considered adverse. They would be accompanied by clinical observations, such as lethargy, weakness, muscle tremors, or arrhythmias. In contrast, creatinine, liver enzymes, and cardiac troponins are analytes in blood that have no intrinsic effect on health but can certainly be markers of adverse effects. High plasma concentrations of cardiac troponin I and high plasma activities of ALT do not negatively affect health, but these findings are markers for myocardial and hepatocellular necrosis, respectively, that would be identified microscopically in most cases and are considered adverse. Neutrophils and fibrinogen are examples of analytes that are both critical to health and markers for a process. Too few neutrophils increases susceptibility to infection, and too little fibrinogen increases the likelihood of hemorrhage. On the other hand, high absolute neutrophil count and fibrinogen concentration typically have no negative health effects, but they can certainly be markers for an adverse inflammatory process.

Unfortunately, clinical pathology parameters have no well-defined critical values or "magic numbers" that above or below which are certain to indicate a toxicologically important or adverse effect. A weight-of-evidence approach is again needed. Were there correlative findings indicating that the clinical pathology effect was associated with a deleterious effect on organ function, tissue integrity, overall health, or survival? Was the effect reversible? What was the mechanism for the effect? A small increase in urea nitrogen concentration could reflect mild dehydration (i.e., prerenal azotemia) due to transient test article–related emesis or early stages of renal failure due to test article–related proximal tubular necrosis. A small test article–related decrease in red cell mass (e.g., 10% lower hematocrit) is not likely to affect the overall health and performance of an animal, but if present after a single dose and correlated with microscopic evidence of erythroid cell depletion in bone marrow sections, that small change in red cell mass is a marker for an adverse effect. If the test article is a chemotherapeutic agent, and the effect reverses when dosing is discontinued, then the corresponding dose level would normally be described as "not severely toxic," even though the effect on bone marrow integrity and function was clearly adverse. Determining whether a clinical pathology effect is adverse or a marker for an adverse effect is not a simple process and, as with many decisions concerning *adverseness*, often subjective and open to debate with diverse interpretations each having merit.

6.3.1 REVERSIBILITY

Reversibility is always a consideration regarding the importance of test article–related effects. The optimal means of assessing reversibility is to obtain and examine data for individual recovery animals at the end of the dosing and recovery phases. This is typically not possible for mice but recommended for rats and routine for larger species. If only group means are examined, relatively small clinical pathology effects often appear unchanged after the recovery phase because of the limited number of recovery animals evaluated. However, it is unrealistic to expect mean values for an affected group to exactly match or even closely approximate mean values for the control group after recovery. It is imperative that data for individual control and treated animals be assessed with respect to how they change from the end of dosing to the end of recovery. Do individual recovery animals in the affected group exhibit evidence that the effect is in the process of reversing? Do individual recovery animals in the affected group even exhibit the effect at the end of the dosing phase? Is it realistic to expect, on the basis of characteristics of the affected test, clear evidence of reversibility in the time allowed by the length of the recovery phase? Once more, determination of reversibility requires a weight-of-evidence approach. It is unlikely that results for recovery animals at the end of the dosing phase will perfectly represent the effect on their entire group, and it is not unusual for results of one or more recovery animals in an affected group to not exhibit the same evidence of reversibility present in the majority of recovery animals. The term "completely reversed" is often inappropriate for clinical pathology effects and should be avoided. In most studies, the best that can be demonstrated is evidence of reversibility, not complete reversal or recovery.

6.3.2 REFERENCE INTERVALS

Reference intervals (historically referred to as reference ranges or normal ranges) for clinical pathology tests typically define the central 95% of expected results from a specific laboratory and assay method in a reference population defined by specific criteria (e.g., species, strain, sex, age). Reference intervals, like statistics, can be used as a tool for data interpretation but should never be relied upon to determine whether differences between control and treated groups are real effects or whether real effects are adverse. Reference intervals can and do provide perspective but also have important limitations. Reference intervals are perhaps most valuable for assessing possible effects in early investigational or discovery-type studies that lack control animals or baseline data. In those situations, however, it is critical that animals and conditions used to establish the reference intervals match the animals and conditions of studies in question. Reference intervals provide perspective concerning expected interanimal variability for different analytes. For example, reference intervals for urea nitrogen concentration and ALT activity are quite narrow in young rats and dogs compared with those for mice and monkeys. Reference intervals can also serve as nonspecific measures of quality control. Results that fall too far from established reference intervals might signal changes in the assay, changes in husbandry or other preanalytical variables, or even genetic drift in the animals.

With respect to data interpretation in most nonclinical studies, reference intervals have limited value (Hall 1997; Waner et al. 1991; Weil and Carpenter 1969), in large part because animals used to establish reference intervals (the reference population sample group) are rarely an appropriate representation of animals used in a given study. Reference intervals are defined by the criteria or partitioning factors used when constructing them. Examples of general partitioning factors include species, strain, age, sex, supplier, site of blood collection, diet, fasting status, time of sample collection (e.g., a.m. or p.m.), sample matrix (e.g., serum or plasma), and sample handling (e.g., fresh or frozen). Reference intervals are specific to the instruments, reagents, and laboratory from which the data were generated. If control animals from different studies are used to construct references intervals, then additional partitioning factors include route of administration, vehicle control article, previous blood collections, anesthesia, and surgical manipulations. Given these various factors, it is extremely unlikely that reference intervals can be established with enough animals (ideally 120; Horowitz et al. 2008) to appropriately match the conditions of more than a small number of studies. Concurrent control groups and baseline data for large animals provide much better approximations of expected results than reference intervals established from animals under different conditions. More importantly, even if appropriate reference intervals existed for a given study, they would not be sufficient to determine whether apparent differences between control and treated groups were real or if real effects were adverse. Results from unaffected animals can easily reside outside the reference interval (most reference intervals are constructed such that 1 of 20 results from *normal* individuals are outside the interval), and results from affected animals (even those with adverse conditions) can easily reside within the reference interval. Although often applied, it is faulty and dangerous reasoning to conclude differences between control and treated groups *are not* real or adverse simply because values for the treated group fall within a reference interval. It is just as inappropriate to conclude differences between control and treated groups *are* real or adverse when values for the treated group fall outside a reference interval.

6.4 INTERPRETATION OF HEMATOLOGY DATA

Like all clinical pathology data, hematology data cannot be interpreted in isolation. Although the focus of this section is hematology, all types of data are used for pattern recognition and correlations to help determine the cause of findings and whether they are test article related and toxicologically important.

6.4.1 ERYTHROCYTES, LEUKOCYTES, AND PLATELETS

RBC count, hemoglobin concentration, and hematocrit are measures of red cell mass and usually increase or decrease in unison unless there are substantial changes in red cell size and hemoglobin content. Red cell mass represents a balance between erythrocyte production and loss or destruction but is also affected by plasma volume. Changes in red cell mass are frequently observed in nonclinical studies, and absolute reticulocyte count, red cell indices (i.e., MCV, MCH, MCHC, RDW, and others less frequently used), and other test results help determine the cause. The toxicologic importance of effects on red cell mass is related to both magnitude and mechanism. Large reductions, accompanied by clinical signs or tissue damage related to hypoxia, are clearly adverse. Small reductions, not clinically relevant in terms of oxygen delivery to tissues, may still be markers of an adverse effect (e.g., bone marrow toxicity).

Total WBC count and absolute differential cell counts represent a balance between production and peripheral distribution of the different cell types. Production of too few cells clearly can adversely affect health. In contrast, production of increased cell numbers is typically just a marker for a process that may or may not affect health. Neutrophils and lymphocytes are the most numerous peripheral blood leukocytes and are the cells usually affected when leukocyte counts change owing to toxicity. Indirect effects are often observed in response to study-related procedures or test article effects on other tissues. Direct effects are less common (Weiss 1993). However, changes in peripheral distribution of cells, particularly lymphocytes, is becoming a more frequent finding as immunomodulatory drugs that target cell trafficking are developed. With respect to differential cell counts, only absolute cell counts (i.e., cells/unit of volume) need be reported and interpreted. Relative counts (i.e., percentage of total) have little value and are easily misinterpreted.

Platelet count is a product of the balance between production and consumption. Platelet indices, like MPV, are sometimes useful in determining whether production is enhanced. Too few platelets have obvious implications with respect to hemostasis, but most test article–related reductions in platelet count do not reach a level that causes spontaneous hemorrhages (e.g., petechia, epistaxis, melena, or hematochezia). Mildly to moderately increased platelet count is a common finding that does not present a threat of thromboembolic events.

Unless effects on hematology results are severe or the mechanism of an effect is certain, diagnostic terms, such as anemia, neutrophilia, and thrombocytopenia, should be avoided. Test article–related effects are often relatively subtle, and use of these terms implies more significance than warranted.

6.4.2 INCREASED RED CELL MASS

Unless the test article is intended to promote erythropoiesis (e.g., erythropoietin or hypoxia-inducible factor), test article–related increases in red cell mass are usually due to dehydration (decreased plasma volume) of the treated group relative to the control group. Detectable effects on red cell mass are often small enough that affected groups do not exhibit clinical signs of dehydration, but corroborative data, such as increased serum urea nitrogen and protein concentrations, decreased urine volume, and increased urine specific gravity, can be good additional evidence of its presence. Increased red cell mass is a frequent finding in moribund animals and is usually due to dehydration, especially when the onset of clinical signs is not acute. Increased red cell mass in animals that become acutely ill may also be associated with shock and increased vascular permeability or splenic contraction from catecholamine release. Toxicologic relevance of increased red cell mass is a function of cause. Unless the test article produces marked polycythemia (e.g., hematocrit > 65%) because of pharmacologic activity, increased red cell mass is unlikely to be harmful. However, as a marker for causes of dehydration, such as vomiting, diarrhea, or excessive diuresis, increased red cell mass adds to the weight of evidence concerning toxicologic importance of those findings.

6.4.3 DECREASED RED CELL MASS

Decreased red cell mass is first characterized by the animal's response to it. In simple terms, if the absolute reticulocyte count is increased, the response is *regenerative*. If the absolute reticulocyte count is unchanged or decreased, the response is *nonregenerative*. An *appropriate* regenerative response is one that is consistent with the magnitude of the decrease in red cell mass. In other words, if red cell mass is reduced by 50% and the bone marrow is able to respond appropriately, then absolute reticulocyte count should exhibit much more than a small increase. If reduced red cell mass is accompanied by an appropriate regenerative response, then the cause of the reduction is hemorrhage or hemolysis. It usually takes 3 or 4 days for absolute reticulocyte count to notably increase after acute blood loss or destruction. In most species, increased absolute reticulocyte count is accompanied by increased MCV and RDW; MCHC may or may not be decreased. If blood smears are examined, increases in polychromasia and anisocytosis are common, and increases in nucleated RBCs and Howell–Jolly bodies are possible. In contrast to dogs and monkeys, rodents occasionally exhibit decreased MCV in the presence of increased absolute reticulocyte count. Robust regenerative erythroid responses are often accompanied by increased platelet count as a nonspecific effect of bone marrow stimulation. If reduced red cell mass of more than 3 or 4 days is not accompanied by an appropriate regenerative response, then at least part of the cause is something that has negatively affected erythropoiesis, either directly or indirectly. Red cells in nonregenerative conditions usually appear normocytic (normal size) and normochromic (normal color) microscopically.

6.4.3.1 Blood Loss

In addition to decreased red cell mass and increased absolute reticulocyte count, animals suffering blood loss will usually exhibit decreased serum total protein concentration. Dehydration or increased globulin production secondary to inflammation can negate a correlative effect on serum proteins, but with uncomplicated blood loss, albumin, and globulin decrease proportionally. The most common example of uncomplicated blood loss in nonclinical studies occurs in monkeys bled extensively for toxicokinetic and other analyses prior to collection of hematology samples. It is not unusual for red cell mass to drop as much as 20% (e.g., hematocrit decreased from 45% to 36%) in the first week of a study because of iatrogenic blood loss. Other sources or causes of blood loss may be identified by clinical signs (e.g., dermal ulceration, epistaxis, melena, prolonged bleeding from venipuncture sites, or hematoma), other laboratory tests (e.g., fecal or urine occult blood), or at necropsy (e.g., gastrointestinal ulceration or urinary calculi). Bleeding associated with test articles developed as anticoagulant agents is often variable among treated individuals and may not always reflect a clear dose response. Some causes of blood loss, especially those that are chronic and have an inflammatory component, may indirectly affect erythropoiesis and reduce the expected reticulocyte response. Although chronic blood loss can ultimately result in iron deficiency and production of microcytic, hypochromic red cells, iron deficiency is rare in nonclinical studies.

6.4.3.2 Hemolysis

Hemolytic conditions are categorized as intravascular or extravascular. Intravascular hemolysis occurs when red cells lyse directly within circulation. Extravascular hemolysis occurs when red cells, usually damaged in some manner, are phagocytized prematurely by macrophages. Extravascular hemolysis is more common and is associated with increased spleen weight, bone marrow hypercellularity, and extramedullary hematopoiesis (especially in rodents). Pigment from breakdown of hemoglobin may be present, especially in splenic macrophages. Relatively extensive hemolysis may result in increased serum and urine bilirubin concentrations. Extensive intravascular hemolysis is characterized by free hemoglobin in plasma or urine. Most hemolytic conditions result in a mild inflammatory response with increased absolute neutrophil or monocyte counts.

Extravascular hemolysis can occur whenever red cells have structural or surface membrane changes recognized as abnormal by the mononuclear phagocyte system. These changes might occur because of alterations in red cell membrane lipids and proteins, intercalation of test article into the cell membrane bilayer, and effects on RBC metabolic processes. Heinz body and immune-mediated hemolysis are two of the more commonly recognized mechanisms for extravascular hemolysis.

Heinz body formation within red cells is caused by test articles with oxidative properties. Heinz bodies are irreversibly denatured clumps of hemoglobin that attach to the inner surface of the red cell membrane. Macrophages phagocytize affected red cells completely or produce morphologically distinct red cells (e.g., ghost and blister cells) by selective removal of Heinz bodies. If large enough, Heinz bodies can be seen in blood smears using standard Romanowsky-type stains, but even small Heinz bodies stain prominently with supravital stains (e.g., methylene blue, crystal violet, or brilliant cresyl blue). Heinz body size and number are dependent on the causative agent, dose, and time after exposure. A high dose of a potent oxidative agent can cause acute anemia characterized by many red cells with a single large Heinz body (or less frequently multiple small Heinz bodies) and the presence of ghost cells, blister cells, and other morphologic abnormalities. Chronic exposure to a less potent oxidative agent may be associated with notably increased absolute reticulocyte count but only minimally decreased red cell mass because the regenerative process is able to match the increased red cell turnover.

Test articles causing Heinz body hemolysis may also cause methemoglobinemia and vice versa (McGrath et al. 1993). Methemoglobin is hemoglobin with reversibly oxidized iron that cannot transport oxygen. High concentrations of methemoglobin cause blood to appear brown and result in clinical signs of hypoxia (Mansouri and Luri 1993). Methemoglobin concentration is measured with instruments called hemoximeters or co-oximeters, but blood samples must be analyzed quickly because methemoglobin is rapidly reduced to hemoglobin by the red cell enzyme, methemoglobin reductase. Methemoglobinemia is least likely to be observed in mice because their red cells have very high methemoglobin reductase activity (Stolk and Smith 1966).

Many drugs have been associated with immune-mediated hemolysis (Packman and Leddy 1995), but drug-induced immune-mediated hemolysis is usually an idiosyncratic phenomenon and difficult to predict. When observed in a nonclinical study, the finding is usually limited to one or two animals and may not be dose-dependent. Immune-mediated hemolysis is typically not observed until a test article has been administered multiple times, and enough time has passed for antibody production to occur. A test article may act as a hapten bound to red cell membrane, or it may elicit an antibody response to itself with resulting antigen-antibody complexes binding to red cell membrane. It is also possible for a test article to alter the ability of the immune system to recognize self, and true autoantibodies may be produced. Complement-mediated intravascular hemolysis is possible, but immune-mediated hemolysis is usually extravascular. Macrophages may engulf the entire affected red cell or remove just the antibody-coated portion of its membrane to produce morphologically distinct spherocytes readily identified in blood smears. Spherocytes and, less commonly, autoagglutination are the predominant morphologic features of immune-mediated hemolysis. Although a direct antiglobulin test (Coombs' test) may be attempted to confirm the presence of antibody or complement on red cells, species-specific reagents must be used (Wardrop 2005), and false negatives are not uncommon. With repeated test article administration, immune-mediated hemolytic anemia usually causes severe anemia. However, the regenerative response is robust, and recovery nearly always occurs when dosing is stopped. Rechallenging the animal after recovery is a simple means of confirming the immune-mediated mechanism. Hemolysis and spherocytosis should be evident within 1 or 2 days, with or without autoagglutination. Immune-mediated hemolytic anemia is commonly observed in association with large granular lymphocyte leukemia in older Fischer 344 rats (Stromberg 1985).

Intravascular hemolysis due to red cell swelling or direct damage to red cell membrane is typically associated with intravenous administration of a test article. When administered rapidly or in high volumes, hypotonic solutions and test articles with detergent-like properties can cause immediate cell lysis. If released hemoglobin exceeds the carrying capacity of circulating haptoglobin, hemoglobinuria can be observed. Hemoglobin pigment may be observed within renal tubular epithelial cells, and hemoglobinuric nephrosis is possible with severe intravascular hemolysis. Test articles causing extensive intravascular hemolysis when administered intravenously almost always cause local endothelial damage as well.

Many monkeys are subclinically infected with the hemotropic parasite *Plasmodium* sp. (Ameri 2010; Donovan et al. 1983; Riley 2005), and hemolysis secondary to this organism should be considered whenever regenerative anemia is identified in a monkey study. Although these intracellular organisms are frequently observed in blood smears from healthy animals with no evidence of hemolysis, parasitemia is inconsistent and subclinical infection cannot be ruled out on the basis of prestudy blood smear examinations. Rarely, stress of shipment, study-related procedures, or test article–induced toxicity precipitates a parasitemic hemolytic crisis that is easily identified by blood smear examination. In the experience of this author, recrudescence of subclinical infections and significant hemolysis occurs infrequently with administration of immunomodulatory drugs.

Mechanical fragmentation or microangiopathic hemolysis is a rare cause of significant hemolysis in nonclinical studies but can occur with test articles that cause vasculitis or otherwise negatively affect endothelial integrity. Fragmented red cells (schistocytes or helmet cells) can be identified microscopically. Although disseminated intravascular coagulation may be the best known example of a condition causing significant microangiopathic hemolysis, it is rarely encountered in nonclinical studies. Some fragmentation likely occurs with extensive injury to any highly vascular tissue, but under those conditions, any reduction in red cell mass is likely multifactorial and may not exhibit a regenerative response.

6.4.3.3 Bone Marrow Toxicity

Most drug-induced bone marrow toxicities (e.g., cytotoxic chemotherapeutic agents) negatively affect production of all three cell lines produced in the marrow. Because of their short circulating life spans, peripheral blood count reductions are first observed in absolute reticulocyte and neutrophil counts, followed by a reduction in platelet count. If the toxic insult is brief, rebound increases in these cells typically occur quickly and in the same order, and red cell mass is minimally affected or unaffected. If animals do not succumb to secondary effects of bone marrow toxicity (e.g., opportunistic infections) or other concurrent toxic effects (e.g., gastrointestinal damage), prolonged inhibition of hematopoiesis eventually results in severe anemia. Rodents become anemic faster than dogs or monkeys because their red cells have shorter circulating life spans. Decreased absolute neutrophil count is the best early evidence of direct bone marrow toxicity in dogs and monkeys. Markedly decreased absolute reticulocyte count is the best early evidence of direct bone marrow toxicity in rodents because they normally have relatively high absolute reticulocyte counts and relatively low absolute neutrophil counts. By the same token, recovery from bone marrow toxicity is most readily followed by increasing absolute neutrophil count for dogs and monkeys and absolute reticulocyte count for rodents. Negative effects on platelet count are often missed because the timing of blood sample collection tends to favor identification of changes in other cell lines, but a rebound increase in platelet count is sometimes observed during the recovery phase of studies with bone marrow toxins. Of the other white cell types, lymphocytes tend to be affected the least in terms of the magnitude of the reduction in absolute count, but they usually exhibit at least a modest decrease. Because hematopoietic tissue is so dynamic, the microscopic appearance of bone marrow is highly dependent on timing of necropsy in relation to the negative insult. Hypocellularity is the expected norm, but early in recovery, bone marrow may become hypercellular with a preponderance of early precursor cells that can give the impression of a maturation arrest or even leukemia. Timing is critical and one of the reasons that recovery of marrow function is best assessed by serial hematology collections and not the appearance of bone marrow sections or smears at a single time point. Toxicities severely affecting production of a single cell line, such as pure red cell aplasia, are rarely observed in nonclinical studies but would appear in peripheral blood as a single cell line cytopenia (e.g., nonregenerative anemia) and in histologic sections as depletion of a single cell line (e.g., absence of erythroid precursors only). At least some of these drug-induced toxicities in humans are idiosyncratic, immune-mediated conditions (Erslev 1995c) and would be difficult to predict or prove during nonclinical safety assessment.

6.4.3.4 Indirect Causes of Nonregenerative Conditions

Mildly decreased red cell mass with no regenerative response and no obvious cause is a relatively common finding in nonclinical studies. The difference in red cell mass from the respective control group is usually ≤10%, and a slightly lower MCV is sometimes present, especially in rodents. Although not always the case, affected animals frequently exhibit some evidence of poor health or malaise, such as poor grooming, decreased activity, reduced body weight or body weight gain, or reduced food consumption. Common concurrent clinical chemistry changes are mildly decreased serum total protein and albumin concentrations. These mild, nonspecific clinical pathology findings are most frequently identified in rat studies because of the relatively large number of animals tested, low interanimal variability, short circulating life span of rat red cells (approximately 45 to 65 days), and short circulating half-life of albumin compared with other species (Kaneko 1997). Although specific mechanisms are usually not identified, the overall constellation of findings suggests a generalized reduction of anabolic processes. Decreased physical activity and correspondingly decreased tissue oxygen demand may also contribute to reduced erythropoiesis.

Erythropoiesis and red cell survival are negatively affected by many other conditions, including chronic inflammatory diseases (Erslev 1995a; Feldman et al. 1981) and significant kidney (Caro and Erslev 1995), liver (Palek 1995), and endocrine dysfunction (e.g., hypothyroidism and hypo-adrenocorticism; Erslev 1995b). All these conditions can be associated with mildly to moderately reduced red cell mass without an appropriate regenerative response. These indirect, negative effects on red cell production and survival are relatively common in nonclinical studies as a result of toxic effects on other tissues or organ systems. The indirect effect on red cell mass, sometimes referred to as *anemia of chronic disease* (even though the animals are not anemic), is not as toxicologically important as the primary toxic effect.

On rare occasion, decreased red cell mass without an appropriate regenerative response is characterized by production of very small red cells (microcytosis; very low MCV) or very large red cells (macrocytosis; very high MCV). Relatively marked microcytosis usually indicates impaired hemoglobin synthesis (e.g., iron deficiency), while marked macrocytosis usually indicates impaired DNA synthesis (e.g., folate or B_{12} deficiency). In most cases, these outcomes are predictable on the basis of the pharmacologic activity of the test article, and the magnitudes of the effects on red cell size and mass are usually correlated with the duration of dosing.

Reduced red cell mass without an appropriate regenerative response is also a feature of cancer, especially hematopoietic cancers, owing to a variety of factors (Cazzola 2000). An occasional severely anemic animal as a result of naturally occurring leukemia is relatively common in carcinogenicity studies.

6.4.4 Physiological Leukocytosis

Physiological leukocytosis is caused by endogenous catecholamine release when animals become very excited or frightened (*fight or flight phenomenon*). Leukocytes acutely shift from the marginal pool (i.e., cells that adhere to endothelium or are sequestered in vascular tissue beds like the spleen) to the circulating pool as a result of increased heart rate, blood pressure, and muscular activity, and total WBC count may double. Cell types responsible for most of the increase vary among species because of differences in normal distribution. Neutrophils are the predominant increasing cell type in dogs, and lymphocytes predominate in rats. Physiological leukocytosis in monkeys can appear as relatively even increases in neutrophils and lymphocytes, but lymphocytes often predominate. Physiological leukocytosis occurs most frequently in animals not accustomed to handling or blood collection, is typically observed in only a few individuals, and is a key reason two baseline clinical pathology collections from large animals, especially monkeys, are beneficial for data interpretation. Reductions in leukocyte counts from a single baseline collection can easily be misinterpreted as a negative effect on myelopoiesis. Increases in red cell mass, due in part to splenic contraction, and serum glucose concentration, due to glycogenolysis, also occur in response to catecholamine release.

6.4.5 Stress-Induced Leukocyte Response

A stress-induced leukocyte pattern occurs when stressful conditions cause increased endogenous corticosteroid release and mimics that seen after exogenous corticosteroid administration. The pattern is characterized by increased absolute neutrophil count and decreased absolute lymphocyte and eosinophil counts. Immature neutrophils (e.g., bands) are absent, and increased absolute monocyte count may or may not be present. Animals in moribund condition often exhibit this pattern. It is unusual for an entire dose group to be affected, but it can occur in the presence of severe toxicity. Eosinophils are particularly sensitive to corticosteroids, and it is unusual for absolute lymphocyte count to decrease because of stress without a concurrent reduction in absolute eosinophil count.

6.4.6 Inflammation

Mildly to moderately increased absolute neutrophil count is a frequent response in all common laboratory animal species to toxicities or study-related procedures (e.g., chronic catheterization) with an inflammatory component. The magnitude of the neutrophil response to inflammation may appear smaller for rodents than for dogs and monkeys because their normal counts are so low, but when viewed as a multiple of concurrent controls, the response for rodents is comparable. Small concurrent increases in absolute monocyte count are common in response to inflammation. Concurrent increases in absolute lymphocyte count are less common but more apt to occur in rodents and in the presence of chronic inflammatory lesions. Immunogenic test articles that elicit a significant immune response may also be associated with increased absolute lymphocyte count. Platelet count is often mildly increased in association with increased absolute neutrophil count, similar to increases observed with notable erythroid regenerative responses. In addition to microscopic evidence of inflammation, other common correlative findings include increased fibrinogen, C-reactive protein (best for large animals), and globulin concentrations and decreased albumin concentration and albumin-to-globulin ratio. Large left shifts and degenerative left shifts are unusual findings in nonclinical studies and typically only occur for individual animals when a significant secondary bacterial infection is present (e.g., pneumonia associated with gavage accident or aspiration, septicemia associated with catheter-related infections, and peritonitis secondary to a perforating ulcerative lesion). On the other hand, left shifts and the appearance of toxic neutrophils are often observed upon administration of test articles that therapeutically stimulate granulopoiesis.

6.4.7 Miscellaneous Effects on Leukocytes

Although most leukocyte effects in nonclinical studies result from indirect mechanisms (e.g., in response to inflammation), more drugs are being developed that directly modify cell production and trafficking in an effort to minimize negative effects of chemotherapeutics (e.g., granulocyte colony-stimulating factor) or modulate the immune system to alleviate immune-mediated or allergic disorders. Effects of these drugs, such as increased absolute neutrophil count or decreased absolute lymphocyte or eosinophil count, are usually predictable and explained by pharmacologic activity.

Automated hematology analyzers have made detection of test article–related changes in the less numerous leukocyte types (i.e., monocytes, eosinophils, and basophils) much more common. Even though their numbers in peripheral blood are normally quite low, reductions in these cell types are often apparent with significant bone marrow toxicity. Small increases in these cell types are also more readily detected. Increased absolute monocyte count can occur in response to any condition involving significant tissue destruction, such as widespread inflammation, liver necrosis, or hemolytic anemia. Increased absolute eosinophil count can occur with test article–related hypersensitivity reactions. High absolute eosinophil count in response to parasitic infections unrelated to test article administration is an occasional finding in individual monkeys. Increased absolute basophil count is extremely rare, but basophils may also play a role in hypersensitivity reactions. *Large unstained cells* are a classification of cells enumerated only by ADVIA hematology analyzers manufactured by Siemens. The size and staining characteristics of these cells do not fit into one of the five major cell types, but they are generally thought to represent large lymphocytes or monocytes. Test article–related changes in absolute large unstained cell count are usually very small and most commonly observed in conjunction with changes in absolute lymphocyte count.

Drug-induced immune-mediated neutropenia (Bloom et al. 1988; Lorenz et al. 1999) is rare, typically idiosyncratic, and difficult to identify in nonclinical studies. As with immune-mediated hemolytic anemia, immune-mediated neutropenia is usually limited to one or two animals in a study and can occur at any dose level. Allowing recovery and then rechallenging the animal with the test article may be the simplest procedure leading to a tentative diagnosis. Detection of anti-neutrophil antibody is difficult.

A few animals will develop hematopoietic neoplasia, with or without leukemia, in most rodent carcinogenicity studies. Standard histopathology is superior to periodic or terminal hematologic evaluation for identification of hematopoietic neoplasia. Although some affected animals have markedly elevated total WBC count and circulating neoplastic cells (e.g., blasts), many animals do not. Lymphocytic leukemia is the most commonly observed leukemia in laboratory rats and is occasionally observed as an incidental finding in subchronic studies (Frith et al. 1993). Large granular lymphocyte leukemia (also called mononuclear cell leukemia) is a relatively common finding in older Fischer 344 rats (Stromberg 1985). Affected rats often develop an immune-mediated hemolytic anemia with increased total bilirubin and liver enzyme activities. In peripheral blood, neoplastic cells appear as large, immature lymphocytes, frequently containing prominent azurophilic granules.

With respect to determining toxicologic or biologic importance of various changes in leukocyte counts, small decreases in absolute lymphocyte count are most challenging because of their different subpopulations and the complicating factor of stress that is present in many situations. An important selective reduction of a specific lymphocyte subpopulation is possible with relatively little effect on total lymphocyte count (e.g., decreased CD^{4+} lymphocytes with human immunodeficiency virus). Consideration of all available data (e.g., clinical signs of illness, microscopic appearance of lymphoid tissues, and immunophenotyping results) is necessary to make the most informed interpretation.

6.4.8 PLATELETS

Relatively small test article–related increases or decreases in platelet count (e.g., ±20% from control or respective baseline) are often observed in nonclinical studies and generally result from indirect increases in platelet production or consumption, respectively. These small changes have little or no biologic significance regarding the likelihood of thromboembolism or inadequate hemostasis but can be markers for toxicologically important changes, such as a drug-induced vasculopathy. In the absence of concurrent vascular/endothelial damage or platelet dysfunction, clinical signs of decreased platelet count do not occur spontaneously unless the platelet count is extremely low (e.g., <20,000/μL; Boon 1993). Clinical signs include petechial and ecchymotic hemorrhages, epistaxis, melena, menorrhagia, and prolonged bleeding from venipuncture sites.

Reactive or *secondary thrombocytosis* are terms used to describe increased platelet count secondary to generalized bone marrow stimulation, as can occur in response to hemolysis, blood loss, and inflammation. Hematopoietic growth factors and cytokines (e.g., erythropoietin, interleukin-6, and interleukin-11) contribute to increased platelet production with these conditions (Beguin 1999; Williams 1995). Platelet count may transiently increase secondary to catecholamine-induced splenic contraction, much like red cell mass, and a rebound increase in platelet count often occurs during recovery from reversible bone marrow toxicity. Markedly increased platelet count (e.g., 3× to 4× control or respective baseline) is unlikely unless the test article specifically targets platelet production (e.g., thrombopoietin). The risk of thromboembolic sequelae with these test articles is clearly greater, but normal animals often tolerate extremely high counts without incident.

Decreased platelet count for individual animals, especially rodents, is a common spurious finding resulting from difficult sample collection owing to poor technique, poor condition of the animal, or a combination of both. Platelet clumps in these animals may be detected by an automated hematology analyzer, but blood smear examination confirms their presence. Occasionally, spuriously decreased platelet count may appear as a group effect because most or all animals in the group are more difficult to bleed than controls for a reason typically due to the test article (e.g., smaller size because of reduced growth rate or dehydration or low blood pressure because of poor health).

Mildly decreased platelet count due to increased platelet consumption is occasionally observed secondary to significant toxic injury to highly vascular tissues, such as the lung, liver, or gastrointestinal tract. Test articles that directly activate the clotting cascade, or directly target blood vessels/

endothelium, may result in greater platelet count reductions, and although rarely observed, disseminated intravascular coagulation with marked thrombocytopenia, prolonged clotting times, and decreased fibrinogen is a possible sequela. Immune-mediated thrombocytopenia, like other immune-mediated cytopenias, has been associated with many drugs (George et al. 1995) and is largely an idiosyncratic phenomenon unrelated to dose level and infrequently observed in nonclinical studies. Although detection of antiplatelet antibody may be possible using flow cytometry, rechallenging the affected animal after recovery is a relatively simple way to make a tentative diagnosis. Platelet count will decrease quickly after rechallenge with the test article. In all conditions that decrease platelet count owing to consumption, MPV may be increased as a reflection of increased platelet production in response to decreased circulating platelet mass. In addition, reticulated platelets (i.e., newly produced platelets with residual RNA that can be counted by flow cytometry in a manner similar to that for reticulocytes) will typically be increased in number.

Acute, profoundly decreased platelet count resulting from off-target platelet activation has recently been reported secondary to administration of therapeutic human monoclonal antibodies to cynomolgus monkeys (Everds et al. 2011a,b).

As previously described, decreased platelet count due to bone marrow toxicity typically occurs later than decreases for absolute reticulocyte and WBC counts because the circulating life span of platelets is approximately 5 to 10 days. MPV is typically not increased until platelet production increases during recovery.

Specialized tests of platelet function (Kurata and Horii 2004) are usually conducted in smaller investigational studies, most often when assessing test articles that specifically target platelet function (e.g., antithrombotic agents). Bleeding times (e.g., buccal mucosal bleeding time in dogs or anesthetized nonhuman primates) are *in vivo* tests of primary hemostasis that are relatively standardized but labor intensive. Platelet aggregation can be assessed by platelet aggregometers, but these are very low throughput instruments and not conducive to use in large nonclinical safety assessment studies. Platelet secretory functions are typically assessed via flow cytometric methods.

6.4.9 Bone Marrow Smear Evaluation

Preparation of bone marrow smears at necropsy is a common practice in most nonclinical studies, but bone marrow smear examination is rarely indicated. Routine hematology tests reflect bone marrow function, and if results from these tests are unaffected or only slightly affected, bone marrow smear examination has little or no benefit. In addition, bone marrow smear examination has no value if mechanisms for more pronounced hematology findings are clear from peripheral blood data and other findings. When indicated by one or more relatively pronounced peripheral blood cytopenias with *no apparent etiology* (e.g., the test article is not a cytotoxic chemotherapeutic), or by unusual peripheral blood cell morphologic abnormalities, bone marrow smear examination can assess the relative numbers, maturation, and appearance of precursor cells in order to help explain the peripheral blood changes (see Chapter 13, Hematopoietic System). Evaluation of histologic sections of the bone marrow is necessary to fully appreciate changes in cellularity.

Regardless of the type of examination performed, results of bone marrow smear examinations are always interpreted in conjunction with peripheral blood test results. The least informative or valuable type of bone marrow evaluation is determination of the M:E ratio. The most time-consuming and labor-intensive bone marrow evaluation is a manual bone marrow cell differential count. This thorough evaluation yields quantitative information but at a high cost. In large-animal studies with relatively few animals, differences must be fairly pronounced in order to have confidence that a difference between control and treated animals is real. Bone marrow differential counts by flow cytometry have the potential to increase the level of confidence in relatively small differences (Martin et al. 1992; Reagan et al. 2011). On the other hand, if differences are small, their toxicologic relevance may be moot. Cytologic bone marrow smear examination by an experienced veterinary pathologist is the most cost-effective and informative means of bone marrow evaluation.

The smear is examined microscopically, and findings are recorded in a manner similar to evaluating any histologic tissue section. Quality and suitability of the smear are first assessed, and then each cell line is assessed with respect to relative numbers, maturation, and morphology. Unusual findings for other cell types, such as plasma cells, macrophages, and mast cells, may also be recorded. A diagnosis or interpretation is determined on the basis of examination of the smear, concurrent peripheral blood results, and histologic findings. The primary goal is to assess the impact of the test article on the number and maturation of hematopoietic cell precursors (Bollinger 2004; Rebar 1993; Reagan et al. 2011).

6.4.10 COAGULATION

Concurrent with platelet aggregation and platelet plug formation at the site of vascular injury (primary hemostasis), insoluble fibrin is generated and deposited in a meshwork with platelets to form a stable clot (secondary hemostasis). Secondary hemostasis has traditionally been viewed as a cascade of plasma-based proteolytic reactions divided into the extrinsic pathway (begins with activation of factor VII by exposure to tissue thromboplastin in the vessel wall) and the intrinsic pathway (begins with activation of factor XII by exposure to subendothelial material, such as collagen, and uses factors XI, IX, and VIII) (Boon 1993; Jesty and Nemerson 1995). Under this paradigm, both pathways share the same terminal sequence, including activation of factor X, conversion of prothrombin to thrombin, and conversion of fibrinogen to fibrin. Although a new cell-based model of coagulation has emerged to better characterize the events of secondary hemostasis (Baker and Brassard 2011; Gale 2011), standard coagulation testing in nonclinical studies has not changed. The extrinsic and intrinsic pathways are routinely evaluated by PT and APTT, respectively (Kurata and Horii 2004). Fibrinogen is often measured concurrently using the same plasma sample and coagulation test instrument. Activated coagulation time is a simple test of the intrinsic pathway that does not require an automated analyzer (Byars et al. 1976; Schiffer et al. 1984). As with most tests, results vary among commonly tested laboratory animals. Of note, PT is relatively long for guinea pigs, and APTT for rabbits is highly dependent on the activator used in the reagent system. Ellagic acid functions well as an activator for rabbit APTT, but silica does not.

Coagulation times are occasionally spuriously prolonged and fibrinogen spuriously decreased because of difficult sample collection due to poor technique, poor condition of the animal, or a combination of both. Combined with low platelet count, these findings in an otherwise healthy animal indicate poor sample quality. Spuriously prolonged coagulation times also occur when the ratio of sodium citrate anticoagulant to plasma is too high, as happens when sample collection tubes are not filled with the proper volume of blood (Kurata et al. 1998). Hemoconcentration due to marked dehydration or test article–induced polycythemia will also affect the ratio of anticoagulant to plasma and prolong times (O'Brien et al. 1995). Mildly prolonged PT (e.g., 2 or 3 s) is observed in a small percentage of laboratory beagles because of inherited factor VII deficiency (Dodds 1997). These animals are clinically normal but would be inappropriate for use in studies of test articles known or suspected to affect clotting.

Although the speed of clot formation in coagulation assays differs between species, the range of results obtained from quality samples is generally small for a given species, and very small differences (e.g., <2 s) are frequently identified between large groups. While such differences may represent a real effect on the test result *in vitro*, they would have little or no effect on hemostasis *in vivo* and are only considered toxicologically relevant as a marker if correlated with other findings indicating a significant mechanistic origin (e.g., endothelial damage, liver toxicity, or thromboembolic lesions).

Because animals are repeatedly exposed to high concentrations of test article in nonclinical studies, any significant direct effect on clotting factor production, or inhibition of clotting factor activity, will likely result in a clinically obvious bleeding diathesis, as well as substantially prolonged PT or APTT (e.g., ≥1.5× control or baseline). Affected animals may exhibit prolonged bleeding from venipuncture sites or small wounds, such as torn nails, and mortality due to spontaneous hemorrhaging is possible. Vitamin K antagonists and poorly absorbed fat substitutes are examples of test articles associated with bleeding because fat-soluble vitamin K is required for production of several clotting factors. Theoretically, PT may be affected before APTT because factor VII has the shortest half-life of the vitamin K–dependent clotting factors.

As measures of liver function, PT and APTT are relatively insensitive, even though most clotting factors are produced by the liver. If coagulation times are prolonged as a result of liver injury, the liver effect is clearly adverse.

Coagulation assays can serve as pharmacodynamic markers for test articles that specifically target coagulation, such as anticoagulants to prevent/treat thromboembolism and clotting factors to treat inherited clotting factor deficiencies. With anticoagulants, it is often possible to demonstrate a gradation of effects dependent on dose; test results can therefore be used to determine a sublethal high dose. With clotting factors, accelerated clotting times and dose dependency are less easily demonstrated, and administration of activated clotting factors or test articles that specifically activate clotting have the potential to paradoxically prolong coagulation times as a result of excessive clotting factor consumption. In the latter case, correlative microscopic evidence of thrombi or emboli is likely.

A variety of more specialized coagulation tests are available (e.g., specific clotting factors, antithrombin III, D-dimer, and thromboelastograms) and used to address specific concerns, most frequently in investigational studies with test articles designed to affect some aspect of coagulation (Kurata and Horii 2004).

6.5 CLINICAL CHEMISTRY TESTS AND INTERPRETATION

Standard clinical chemistry tests assess liver integrity and function; kidney function; carbohydrate, lipid, and protein metabolism; and mineral and electrolyte balance.

6.5.1 TESTS OF LIVER INTEGRITY AND FUNCTION

Liver toxicity can affect many clinical pathology tests because of the varied metabolic, synthetic, and excretory functions of the liver and the enzymatic machinery needed to perform those functions (Sherwin and Sobenes 1996; Sturgill and Lambert 1997). The pattern of affected clinical pathology tests helps characterize the location, severity, and toxicologic relevance of test article–related liver effects (Boone et al. 2005; Carakostas et al. 1986). Although the search for more sensitive and specific translatable biomarkers of test article–induced liver toxicity has accelerated dramatically in recent years (Adler et al. 2010; Ozer et al. 2008; Ramaiah 2011), none of the potential candidates have yet been generally accepted to replace or supplement the following traditional tests.

6.5.1.1 Enzymes

Serum activities of liver enzymes are often referred to as liver function tests or *LFTs* by clinicians, but they provide little information about liver function and that term should be avoided. Some liver enzymes are used to assess hepatocellular integrity (e.g., ALT, AST, and GLDH) because their serum activities usually increase because of release from degenerating or necrotic hepatocytes. Other liver enzymes are used to assess hepatobiliary integrity and cholestasis (e.g., ALP and GGT) because their serum activities increase as a result of increased production (i.e., induction) by hepatobiliary cells in response to stimuli, such as increased biliary pressure or the presence of bile salts. Factors that determine the value of an enzyme to reflect liver effects include specificity to liver, intrahepatic location, intracellular location, the concentration gradient between hepatocyte and serum, serum half-life, *in vitro* stability, and economy of measurement (Boyd 1988).

ALT is the most common and generally most useful enzyme for detecting hepatocellular injury in nonclinical studies using mice, rats, dogs, and monkeys (Boone et al. 2005). Although the enzyme is present in many tissues, elevations of serum ALT activity usually indicate release of ALT from hepatocytes altered in some manner. ALT is less useful in a few laboratory animal species that have relatively low intrahepatocyte concentrations, most notably guinea pigs and minipigs (Clampitt and Hart 1978; Kramer and Hoffman 1997). ALT is primarily cytosolic and because intracellular concentration within hepatocytes is up to 10,000 times greater than that in plasma, ALT enters plasma easily if cell membrane is injured sufficiently. After an acute reversible hepatotoxic insult, serum ALT activity increases relatively quickly, peaking within 2 or 3 days, and decreases over the next few days. With repeated dosing, serum ALT activity will remain increased unless adaptive processes (e.g., drug metabolism) that reduce the insult occur (Davies 1992; O'Brien et al. 2000). When increased because of hepatocellular injury, the magnitude of increased serum ALT activity is dependent on the amount of affected tissue and does not necessarily indicate reversibility. As a general guideline, when serum ALT activity is increased because of hepatocellular injury, correlative microscopic evidence is usually present when serum ALT activity is >200 U/L for an individual or more than threefold control (or baseline for dogs and monkeys) for a group. More subtle increases are sometimes associated with single cell necrosis/apoptosis or centrilobular hypertrophy, but clearly correlative clinical pathology findings are often absent for these microscopic effects.

Unfortunately, increased serum ALT activity in nonclinical studies is not specific for test article–induced hepatocellular injury and may occur as a result of increased transport of the enzyme across an intact cell membrane (Solter 2005), increased hepatic intracellular concentration of the enzyme due to induction (Fuentealba et al. 2011; Hagopian et al. 2003), decreased clearance of the enzyme from circulation (Radi et al. 2011), severe damage to other tissue such as skeletal muscle (Swenson and Graves 1997; Watkins et al. 1989), subclinical infections such as enzootic hepatitis A in monkeys (Hall and Everds 2003; Slighter et al. 1988), and physical damage due to handling technique in mice (Swaim et al. 1985). In the absence of clear microscopic correlates for test article–related increases in serum ALT activity, all these are possibilities to consider. ALT isoenzymes (ALT1 and ALT2) are currently the focus of investigations to determine their potential to better characterize increases in serum ALT activity (Ramaiah 2011; Yang et al. 2009). In the rat, ALT1 is a cytoplasmic protein, and ALT2 is a mitochondrial protein. Both isoenzymes are found in multiple tissues, but ALT1 appears more widely distributed.

Serum GLDH and sorbitol dehydrogenase (SDH) activities are also used as markers for hepatocellular injury because, like ALT, they are considered relatively *liver specific* and sensitive (Boone et al. 2005; O'Brien et al. 2002; Travlos et al. 1996). GLDH is located in the mitochondrial matrix, and SDH is located in cytoplasm. In response to acute hepatotoxicity, serum GLDH activity increases may persist longer than those for ALT, while serum SDH activity increases tend to reverse quicker than those for ALT because of a shorter half-life. Although GLDH may have advantages over ALT with respect to certain models of hepatotoxicity (O'Brien et al. 2002), it is used infrequently in the United States, mostly owing to reagent/automated application availability.

As a marker for hepatocellular injury, serum AST activity is less sensitive and specific than serum ALT, GLDH, and SDH activities. Increases in serum AST activity are smaller in magnitude and tend to reverse quickly. AST activity is high in muscle, RBCs, and other tissues, and interanimal variability of serum activity is usually more prominent, especially in rodents that may be more difficult to bleed. As a marker of hepatocellular injury, LDH is similar to AST with regard to lack of specificity but appears even less sensitive because of greater interanimal variability. Although once commonly measured in nonclinical studies, the utility of LDH is questionable.

Decreased serum liver enzyme activities are occasionally observed but rarely associated with toxicologically important effects in the liver. Potential reasons for these decreased serum activities include reduced hepatocellular synthesis or release of the enzymes, inhibition of enzyme activity, and assay interference. The most widely recognized cause of decreased serum ALT and AST activities is a negative effect on plasma pyridoxal 5′-phosphate (vitamin B_6), a coenzyme cofactor for the aminotransferases (Cornish 1969; Dhami et al. 1979; Waner and Nyska 1991). If this cofactor is directly or indirectly affected, serum aminotransferase activities may appear to decrease unless the assay includes pyridoxal 5′-phosphate as one of the reagents. Decreased aminotransferase activities are sometimes observed in monkeys that develop chronic watery diarrhea because this water-soluble cofactor is lost.

Serum ALP activity increases as a result of induced synthesis and release from hepatocytes and biliary epithelial cells secondary to test article–related hepatobiliary effects involving cholestasis or biliary hyperplasia. In humans, at least four ALP isoenzymes have been identified: tissue non-specific (found in the liver, bone, and kidney), intestinal, placental, and germ cell. Most laboratory animals have only two ALP isoenzymes: tissue nonspecific and intestinal. Tissue-nonspecific ALP enzymes that originate from the liver, bone, and kidney are the product of the same gene and are, therefore, isoforms rather than isoenzymes. The isoforms are distinguished by differences in degree of posttranslational glycosylation and tissue of origin (Hoffmann et al. 1994; Hoffmann and Solter 1994; Kramer and Hoffmann 1997). The contribution of each isoenzyme/isoform to total serum ALP activity is dependent on tissue production and plasma half-life. Bone ALP originates from osteoblasts, and serum activity of this isoform is highest in young, growing animals and decreases with age. The liver isoform predominates in mature animals. Serum activity of the intestinal iso-enzyme increases substantially in rats after feeding (Waner and Nyska 1994). If rats are not fasted before sample collection and treated rats have a test article–related reduction in food consumption, there can be a difference in serum ALP activities between control and treated animals that is simply due to differences in food consumption. Intestinal ALP in other species and kidney ALP contribute little, if anything, to serum ALP activity because of short plasma half-lives and a cellular location that favors release into intestinal and renal tubular lumens, respectively. Dogs can produce a unique corticosteroid-induced ALP isoenzyme in response to exogenous or endogenous corticosteroid. This isoenzyme is absent from the serum of most dogs but can cause relatively mild to moderate increases in total serum ALP activity with long-term corticosteroid administration or chronic stress (Hoffmann and Solter 1994; Kidney and Jackson 1988; Solter et al. 1993).

Despite various ALP isoenzymes and isoforms, serum ALP activity remains beneficial as a marker for cholestasis, whether intrahepatic or extrahepatic, and hepatobiliary toxicity. It is espe-cially sensitive to cholestasis in dogs and increases before, or in the absence of, increases in other markers, such as serum GGT activity and total bilirubin concentration. Primary hepatocellular toxicities in dogs that cause cell swelling or inflammatory infiltrates frequently result in mildly increased serum ALP activity due to pressure obstruction of small bile ductules and ducts. Periportal injury results in higher serum ALP activities than centrilobular injury, and extrahepatic cholestasis (e.g., choleliths or bile duct cannulation complications) results in higher activities than intrahepatic cholestasis. Of the common laboratory animal species, serum ALP activity appears least beneficial as a marker of hepatobiliary toxicity in monkeys because of relatively marked, normal interanimal variability. A few drugs, such as anticonvulsants and corticosteroids, induce synthesis of liver ALP, with or without microscopic evidence of hepatobiliary disease.

Although infrequent, increased serum total ALP activity can be a marker for increased osteo-blast activity owing to test article effects on bone formation. Increases resulting from osteoblast activity are generally small (e.g., <3-fold control or baseline) but may be correlated with micro-scopic alterations in bone. More frequently, serum total ALP activity is decreased secondary to reduced osteoblast activity when test article administration significantly affects growth of young animals. Although a microscopic correlate in bone is usually absent when this occurs, body weight and body weight gain are almost always affected if the study duration is long enough.

Serum GGT activity is more specific for the hepatobiliary system than ALP and has been shown effective as a marker in certain models of biliary toxicity in the rat (Leonard et al. 1984). Although tissue concentrations of this membrane-localized enzyme are highest in the kidney and pancreas, increased serum activities typically occur only in conjunction with hepatobiliary lesions. Occasionally, serum GGT increases secondary to induction by test articles that also stimulate microsomal enzyme production (Goldberg 1980; Sherwin and Sobenes 1996). Serum GGT activity is unaffected by bone growth or toxicity. Because serum GGT activity in rodents and dogs is nor-mally very low and may not be measurable, small increases that appear relatively insignificant have greater importance. Monkeys normally have much higher serum GGT activities than rodents and dogs, and their serum GGT activities are less variable than serum ALP activities. For that reason, changes in serum GGT activity secondary to hepatobiliary lesions are easier to detect in monkeys than those for ALP. Of note, it is relatively common to observe simultaneous reductions in serum ALP and GGT activities in monkeys exhibiting general signs of poor health, such as reduced food consumption and body weight, fecal abnormalities, or lethargy.

6.5.1.2 Bilirubin

In contrast to serum liver enzyme activities, serum total bilirubin concentration can be a measure of liver function. In the absence of a significant hemolytic process, increased serum bilirubin concentration indicates general hepatic dysfunction due to hepatocellular injury; bile retention due to cholestasis; or altered bilirubin metabolism due to interference with the normal processes of bilirubin uptake, conjugation, secretion, and excretion. Secretion of conjugated bilirubin across the canalicular membrane is the rate-limiting step, and small amounts of conjugated or direct bilirubin normally escape into plasma. In contrast to unconjugated bilirubin, conjugated bilirubin is not bound to albumin, is freely filtered by the glomerulus, and can sometimes be detected in concentrated urine in the absence of toxicity or disease, especially in dogs.

Serum total bilirubin concentration in laboratory animals is relatively insensitive to test article–induced hepatocellular injury and cholestasis compared with serum ALT and ALP or GGT activities, respectively. Increases in total bilirubin concentration owing to these causes tend to occur only when effects are fairly pronounced and accompanied by microscopic evidence of hepatocellular degeneration/necrosis and bile stasis. Similar to increased serum ALP or GGT activities, periportal lesions are more likely to increase total bilirubin concentration.

Given all the information normally available in a nonclinical study, determination of direct/conjugated and indirect/unconjugated bilirubin is rarely necessary for understanding the origin of test article–induced increases in total bilirubin concentration. Hemolysis sufficient to overload a normal liver and cause increased serum indirect/unconjugated bilirubin concentration will produce other evidence of hemolysis (e.g., regenerative anemia, red cell morphology abnormalities, or hemosiderin accumulation in macrophages). Hepatic injury or cholestasis sufficient to increase direct/conjugated bilirubin concentration will also produce other correlative evidence, such as increased serum enzyme activities and microscopic changes. In addition, the standard test for direct and indirect bilirubin is too insensitive to accurately differentiate the two for the very small increases in total bilirubin concentration commonly observed (e.g., <0.5 mg/dL). However, bilirubin fractionation may be valuable when total bilirubin concentration is elevated in the absence of other findings. For example, test article–related inhibition of the bilirubin-conjugating enzyme, uridine diphosphate glucuronosyltransferase, may cause substantially increased indirect/unconjugated bilirubin (Boone et al. 2005; Zucker et al. 2001).

Drugs that induce microsomal enzyme production, like phenobarbital, sometimes result in decreased serum total bilirubin concentration as a result of accelerated bilirubin metabolism and excretion (Goldberg 1980; Robinson et al. 1971). Human patients receiving phenobarbital therapy have lower serum bilirubin levels than the general population (Jaynes 1984). Notably, however, induction of hepatic drug-metabolizing enzymes resulting in increased liver weight and centrilobular hepatocellular hypertrophy does not produce a consistent pattern of changes in clinical pathology test results (Ennulat et al. 2010). When changes do occur, especially increases in serum liver enzyme activities, they likely reflect concurrent hepatobiliary insult.

6.5.1.3 Other Liver-Related Analytes

Although serum total bile acid concentration can be a marker of liver toxicity and has proved useful in clinical veterinary medicine for identifying hepatobiliary disease (Center et al. 1985; Schlesinger and Rubin 1993), it has not proved effective at increasing identification of hepatotoxicity beyond the standard tests routinely performed in nonclinical studies, and it does not differentiate between different types of hepatic lesions. On the other hand, determination of fasted and postprandial total bile acid concentration may help quantify the magnitude of dysfunction in special circumstances.

The liver is at least partially responsible for synthesis of many clinical chemistry analytes, including glucose, cholesterol, urea, and a variety of proteins. Hepatocellular dysfunction can therefore be responsible for, or contribute to, decreased serum concentrations of glucose, cholesterol, urea nitrogen, and albumin and prolonged coagulation times owing to decreased synthesis of clotting factors. Because the liver has a large functional reserve, liver injury must be substantial before these effects occur solely as a result of liver dysfunction. Liver dysfunction can also be associated with increased serum concentrations of cholesterol and triglycerides owing to alterations in lipid metabolism.

Many new potential serum biomarkers of hepatotoxicity have been investigated, but at this time, no single test or group of tests has displayed the characteristics necessary to effectively improve early identification of drug-induced hepatobiliary injury in nonclinical studies (Adler et al. 2010; Ozer et al. 2008; Ramaiah 2011).

6.5.2 Tests of Kidney Function

Serum urea nitrogen (commonly referred to as blood urea nitrogen) and creatinine concentrations are standard tests to evaluate kidney function in nonclinical studies (Bovee 1986; Loeb 1998; Stonard 1990). Urea (and not urea nitrogen) is measured in many countries, but interpretation of results is the same. Although easy and inexpensive, serum urea nitrogen and creatinine concentrations are affected by nonrenal factors and relatively insensitive to minor kidney effects. Urinalysis and urine chemistry tests provide additional information concerning kidney integrity and function.

Serum urea nitrogen concentration is a product of the rate of urea production, glomerular filtration rate (GFR), and urine flow rate through the renal tubule (urea is reabsorbed passively with water in the proximal tubule). Causes of increased serum urea nitrogen concentration (i.e., azotemia) are categorized as prerenal, renal, or postrenal. Prerenal causes include those that increase urea synthesis (e.g., high protein diet or protein catabolic states, such as starvation, fever, tissue necrosis, and high gastrointestinal hemorrhage) and those that decrease renal blood flow (e.g., dehydration, shock, and cardiovascular disease). Increased urea synthesis typically results in minor increases in serum urea nitrogen concentration. The effect on serum urea nitrogen concentration caused by decreased renal blood flow is often relatively small, but if GFR is severely affected, the increase can mimic that observed with severe kidney toxicity. When increased serum urea nitrogen concentration is due to prerenal causes, renal concentrating ability is maintained. Urine volume will typically decrease, and urine concentration will increase, in response to dehydration, the most common cause of prerenal azotemia in nonclinical studies. Increased red cell mass and serum protein concentrations are additional evidence of dehydration, but these may appear unaffected if the growth and general health of the animals are compromised. Small increases in serum urea nitrogen concentration for dosed groups can occur because of minor changes in hydration status relative to the control group that are not evident as clinical dehydration.

Renal azotemia results from injury to kidney parenchyma. Kidneys have a large functional reserve capacity, and it is commonly stated that serum urea nitrogen concentration will not increase notably until approximately 75% of nephrons are nonfunctional. However, differences between control and treated animals for serum urea nitrogen concentration appear detectable before that degree of injury, at least on the basis of microscopic evidence of kidney injury. When increased serum urea nitrogen concentration is due to kidney toxicity, a correlative reduction in urine concentrating ability is often observed as increased urine volume and decreased urine specific gravity or osmolality. Correlative microscopic evidence of kidney injury is nearly always present (e.g., proximal tubular degeneration/regeneration, papillary necrosis, or increased severity of chronic progressive nephropathy). Additional clinical chemistry evidence of kidney dysfunction includes increased serum creatinine and inorganic phosphorus concentrations (owing to decreased GFR) and decreased serum sodium and chloride concentrations (owing to decreased reabsorption). Additional urinalysis evidence of kidney injury or dysfunction includes increased incidence and severity of urine protein, occult blood, glucose, RBCs, WBCs, or casts. Affected animals often exhibit clinical signs of poor health, such as decreased food consumption, body weight loss, or inactivity.

Postrenal azotemia occurs when GFR is reduced by obstructing urine flow. An obstructive nephropathy due to naturally occurring urinary calculi is an occasional incidental finding in older rats, but test articles that promote or form crystals/calculi can also cause obstructive nephropathy. When atypical urine crystals are present in urine sediment in conjunction with evidence of test article–related kidney dysfunction or injury, it is not unusual to observe intraluminal crystals, tubular degeneration/regeneration, and dilated tubules in kidney sections.

Serum creatinine concentration is not affected by diet or protein catabolism but is influenced by muscle mass and conditioning because it originates as a breakdown product of muscle phosphocreatine. Like urea nitrogen, creatinine is freely filtered through the glomerulus, but it is not reabsorbed by tubules. Changes in serum creatinine concentration tend to parallel those for serum urea nitrogen concentration that result from altered renal blood flow, kidney function, or urine outflow. The timing and magnitude of changes for serum creatinine concentration tend to lag behind those for serum urea nitrogen concentration. However, serum creatinine concentration is often a better reflection of GFR because fewer factors affect it. On rare occasion, increased serum creatinine concentration is observed in the absence of correlative effects on serum urea nitrogen concentration or kidney histopathology because of *noncreatinine chromogens* that interfere with the commonly used Jaffe method for measuring creatinine. Other analytical methods (e.g., enzymatic) are available to avoid the complication of interfering substances and may be necessary if the test article or metabolite is a noncreatinine chromogen. Although endogenous creatinine clearance is occasionally used as a noninvasive measure of GFR (Bovee 1986), results are generally more variable and less reliable than in a clinical setting for a single patient because completely emptying the bladder of every animal before and after the urine collection period is impractical in a typical nonclinical study.

Serum cystatin C concentration has drawn recent attention as a renal function biomarker that may be a better indicator of GFR than serum urea nitrogen or creatinine concentration because it is affected by fewer extrarenal influences (Ozer et al. 2010). Its increasing use clinically makes it an attractive candidate for potential use in nonclinical studies.

6.5.3 Proteins, Carbohydrates, and Lipids

6.5.3.1 Serum Proteins

Serum total protein concentration is approximately 0.3 to 0.5 g/dL lower than plasma total protein concentration because it does not include fibrinogen and other clotting factors consumed during clot formation. Albumin is the most abundant plasma protein, a labile storage reservoir of amino acids, and a transport protein for plasma constituents that lack specific transporter proteins, including many drugs that bind to it. Globulins are a heterogeneous population of proteins that include clotting factors, transport proteins (e.g., transferrin for iron and haptoglobin for hemoglobin), mediators of inflammation (e.g., complement), acute phase proteins, enzymes, and immunoglobulins. Globulins are loosely categorized by their electrophoretic migration pattern as α, β, and γ globulins; several different proteins are present in each region of the electrophoretic pattern (Kaneko 1997). Albumin and most globulin proteins are synthesized by the liver. Lymphocytes and plasma cells synthesize immunoglobulins. Serum total protein and albumin concentrations are measured directly; serum globulin concentration is simply the calculated difference between total protein and albumin.

A frequent cause for increased serum total protein concentration in nonclinical studies is dehydration of treated animals relative to control animals. The difference in hydration status may or may not be evident clinically. Albumin and globulin increase proportionately in simple dehydration, but other factors associated with the cause for dehydration often affect the ratio. The most frequent correlative findings are increased red cell mass and serum urea nitrogen concentration and clinical observations, such as vomiting, diarrhea, excessive salivation, and reduced water/food consumption. Water consumption in rodents, especially mice, is closely associated with food consumption, and abruptly reduced food consumption may result in insufficient water intake and increased serum protein concentrations. Conversely, decreased food consumption over a longer period resulting in decreased body weight gain is often associated with reduced serum albumin concentration that may be masked by dehydration.

Any test article–induced inflammatory condition that stimulates synthesis of acute phase proteins (e.g., C-reactive protein, haptoglobin, and α-2 macroglobulin) and immunoglobulin has the potential to increase serum total protein concentration because of increased globulin production. However, serum total protein concentration is often relatively unaffected secondary to inflammation because albumin is a negative acute phase protein, and reductions in serum albumin offset increased serum globulins. Albumin-to-globulin ratio is clearly decreased when this occurs. With respect to acute phase proteins and species differences, C-reactive protein works well as a marker for inflammation in dogs and monkeys, but not rats; α-2 macroglobulin is a major acute phase protein for rats (Watterson et al. 2009). Fibrinogen increases in response to inflammation in all three species, but the magnitude of the increase (i.e., fold change) is usually not as dramatic. Intravenous administration of therapeutic proteins, such as monoclonal antibodies, can increase serum total protein and globulin concentrations proportional to dose in the absence of a negative effect on albumin, provided blood samples are collected before the proteins are metabolized.

Decreased serum protein concentrations result from decreased synthesis or increased loss, but the exact mechanism for a decrease in a given study is often undetermined. For example, a small decrease in serum albumin concentration is a frequent finding in nonclinical studies with poorly tolerated test articles that also result in effects such as mildly decreased red cell mass, cholesterol concentration, and body weight or body weight gain. While reduced synthesis would appear to have caused the effect on serum albumin, a specific reason for reduced synthesis (e.g., reduced food consumption, maldigestion/malabsorption, or hepatic dysfunction) is often not apparent. Since plasma half-life of albumin is shorter for rodents than other laboratory animal species (Kaneko 1997), reductions in serum albumin levels may occur faster in rodents.

Concurrent losses of albumin and globulin occur with hemorrhage and some exudative lesions, such as might occur with severe dermal or intestinal toxicity, but acute phase protein synthesis often balances out any globulin loss resulting from an exudative inflammatory lesion. Because of its small size, albumin is the principal protein lost owing to a protein-losing glomerulopathy. Although relatively rare, administration of an immunogenic protein can result in an immune-complex glomerulonephritis with severely reduced serum albumin concentration. When observed, this condition typically affects only one or two animals in a given study, presumably because the necessary antigen-to-antibody ratio does not occur in every animal. Decreased serum globulin concentration in the absence of a concurrent or proportional decrease in serum albumin concentration may indicate decreased immunoglobulin synthesis. Microscopic evidence of a lymphoid tissue effect (e.g., reduced germinal centers) may or may not be present. Antibiotic administration to young animals has the potential to result in lower serum globulin concentration relative to controls because inhibition of normal bacterial flora reduces normal antigenic stimulation.

6.5.3.2 Serum Glucose

Serum glucose concentration reflects intestinal absorption, hepatic production (by gluconeogenesis and glycogenolysis), and tissue uptake and is affected by many hormones, including insulin, glucagon, glucagon-like peptide-1, glucocorticoids, growth hormone, and catecholamines. For individual animals, inadvertent failure to fast and catecholamine release secondary to fear or excitement are the most frequent reasons for increased serum glucose concentration. Marked hyperglycemia is occasionally observed in moribund animals, likely due to a combination of factors including catecholamine and glucocorticoid release. Marked hypoglycemia is also occasionally observed in moribund animals, sometimes the result of sepsis associated with a gavage accident or indwelling intravenous catheter contamination. Delays in sample processing result in spuriously low serum glucose concentrations because RBCs consume glucose for energy. This can create the appearance of a test article–related effect if samples are not collected and processed in a manner that eliminates time bias. Polycythemia caused by test articles that stimulate red cell production (e.g., erythropoietin) can create the appearance of a test article–related decrease in serum glucose concentration owing to more rapid glucose consumption in the blood sample. Relative to other laboratory animal species, serum glucose concentrations are highest for mice and lowest for monkeys. These species, especially mice, also have relatively broad reference intervals that may mask expected effects for test articles targeting glucose metabolism. Given the large number of test articles under investigation that specifically target diabetes, obesity, and metabolic syndrome, changes in serum glucose concentration are often expected, and control of preanalytical variables is critical.

The most common off-target, test article–related group effect on serum glucose concentration in nonclinical studies is a mild decrease (e.g., <15 mg/dL) in animals that fail to thrive and have lower body weight gains, with or without a concurrent reduction in food consumption. Similar to mild reductions in red cell mass and serum protein concentrations that are often observed concurrently, this minor effect on serum glucose concentration appears to reflect a negative effect on the overall health of the animals. Many clinical disease conditions that cause hyperglycemia (e.g., diabetes mellitus, hyperadrenocorticism, pancreatitis, and corticosteroid therapy) and hypoglycemia (e.g., hypoadrenocorticism, malabsorption syndromes, and insulinoma) are rarely observed in nonclinical studies. However, test article–related effects on serum glucose concentration are associated with alterations in the same *target tissues* (i.e., pancreas, adrenal and pituitary glands, liver, and intestinal tract).

6.5.3.3 Serum Lipids

Cholesterol and triglycerides are the two major serum lipids commonly measured in nonclinical studies. Serum cholesterol and triglyceride concentrations are affected by dietary intake, endogenous synthesis (primarily by the liver), and tissue uptake (Bruss 1997). Cholesterol and triglycerides circulate as components of chylomicrons and lipoprotein particles: high-density lipoprotein (HDL), low-density lipoprotein (LDL), and very-low-density lipoprotein (VLDL). Lipid metabolism is complex, and cholesterol transport differs considerably among species (Bauer 1996; Johnson 2005). LDL transports approximately two-thirds of circulating cholesterol in humans, while HDL transports the large majority of cholesterol for most laboratory animal species. Differences in lipid metabolism make translation of lipid effects from nonclinical to clinical studies problematic. In addition, species differences in lipoprotein composition complicate the accurate measurement of HDL, LDL, and VLDL cholesterol.

Small increases and decreases in serum cholesterol and triglyceride concentrations are common findings in nonclinical studies. Although the changes likely represent minor alterations in lipid metabolism, they would not be expected to adversely affect health. Specific mechanisms are usually undetermined, but concurrent alterations in food consumption and body weight or body weight gain are frequently present. Test article–related effects on the liver, gastrointestinal tract, and endocrine glands all have the potential to alter lipid metabolism.

Inadvertent failure to fast causes increased serum triglyceride concentration, but serum cholesterol concentration remains relatively stable. Significant anorexia, starvation, malabsorption/maldigestion, and diabetes cause increased serum triglyceride concentration as a result of fat mobilization for energy. Serum cholesterol concentrations in these conditions are less predictable. Markedly increased serum triglyceride concentration is a relatively common finding in moribund animals. Reduced thyroid function and liver injury, often with concurrent cholestasis, are two of the more frequent identifiable causes of increased serum cholesterol concentration in nonclinical studies. However, liver toxicity can also be associated with decreased serum cholesterol concentration. On rare occasion, increased serum cholesterol concentration is associated with a protein-losing glomerulopathy as a characteristic of nephrotic syndrome. Minor alterations in serum cholesterol concentration are identified most commonly in short-term rat studies because interanimal variability in young rats is small relative to other species and the number of animals tested is relatively large. In older rats (e.g., >1 year old), serum cholesterol and triglyceride concentrations are extremely variable owing to spontaneously occurring disease.

6.5.4 MINERALS AND ELECTROLYTES

6.5.4.1 Serum Calcium and Inorganic Phosphorus

Parathyroid hormone, calcitonin, and vitamin D act in concert to maintain plasma calcium and phosphorus concentrations via effects on intestinal calcium absorption, bone formation/reabsorption, and renal excretion/reabsorption (Rosol and Capen 1997). Serum calcium and inorganic phosphorus concentrations are potentially affected by alterations in multiple tissues (i.e., parathyroid and thyroid glands, kidney, bone, and intestine), but unless the test article specifically targets calcium/phosphorus metabolism (e.g., a drug for osteoporosis), changes in these analytes are most commonly affected by serum albumin concentration, food intake, and kidney function.

Approximately 40% of serum calcium is bound to albumin, and serum total calcium concentration usually parallels changes in serum albumin concentration, both increases and decreases. Because interanimal variability for serum calcium concentration is relatively small, surprisingly small differences between control and treated groups can be detected as a result of minor effects on albumin. These effects on serum total calcium concentration are typically not toxicologically or physiologically important because the biologically active ionized form of calcium is maintained at appropriate levels. Signs of hypocalcemia such as neurological or neuromuscular abnormalities are absent. Low food consumption and decreased GFR are the most common causes of decreased and increased serum inorganic phosphorus concentrations, respectively, in nonclinical studies. Increased serum inorganic phosphorus concentration resulting from decreased GFR typically parallels concurrent effects on serum urea nitrogen and creatinine concentrations.

6.5.4.2 Serum Sodium, Potassium, and Chloride

Reference intervals for serum electrolyte concentrations in clinical settings are relatively broad compared with the range of concentrations usually observed in controlled nonclinical studies, and very small but statistically significant differences between control and treated groups are a relatively frequent occurrence. Some of these small differences (e.g., 1 to 3 mmol/L for serum sodium or chloride concentration) are incidental, but others probably reflect subtle homeostatic effects associated with minor differences in food intake or fluid balance that are not indicative of significant toxicity. Effects on serum sodium and chloride concentrations usually parallel each other, and concurrent decreases are most commonly observed with gastrointestinal losses (i.e., vomiting or diarrhea) and renal losses (i.e., tubular dysfunction due to toxicity or a diuretic effect). Vomiting may decrease serum chloride concentration to a greater degree because of the loss of hydrochloric acid from the stomach. Slightly increased serum chloride concentration is observed on rare occasion as a result of secretory diarrhea and metabolic acidosis from loss of bicarbonate; decreased availability of bicarbonate causes increased renal tubular reabsorption of chloride.

Serum potassium concentration is relatively sensitive to dietary intake, and decreased concentrations are occasionally associated with substantially decreased food intake. However, similar to sodium and chloride, gastrointestinal and renal losses are the most common causes of decreased serum potassium concentration in nonclinical studies. Increased serum potassium concentration can occur in conditions causing acidosis (e.g., lactic acidosis associated with shock) because extracellular hydrogen ions are exchanged for intracellular potassium ions. The exchange of ions is the opposite with conditions causing metabolic alkalosis (e.g., persistent vomiting). Serum potassium concentration is higher than plasma potassium concentration because platelets release potassium into serum during clot formation *in vitro*. Substantial test article–related increases and decreases in platelet counts can therefore result in increased and decreased serum potassium concentrations, respectively, that do not reflect actual potassium concentrations in plasma (*in vivo*) and are toxicologically irrelevant. Species with high potassium concentrations within red cells (e.g., nonhuman primates) can have spuriously increased serum potassium concentrations owing to hemolysis associated with poor sample collection or handling technique. On rare occasion in nonclinical studies, severe test article–related necrosis of multiple tissues increases serum potassium concentration owing to release of intracellular potassium.

6.5.4.3 Miscellaneous Serum Chemistry Tests

Serum CK and aldolase activities are markers of striated muscle injury and used most commonly to assess skeletal muscle injury. Factors unrelated to test article administration, such as intramuscular ketamine injection in nonhuman primates, poor blood collection technique (especially cardiac puncture), and commingling injuries, affect these serum enzyme activities more frequently than test article–induced muscle toxicity. If skeletal muscle toxicity is a significant concern, sample collection should be avoided for at least 4 days after the use of ketamine in nonhuman primates, and an appropriate blood collection technique should be used to avoid muscle contamination of the sample.

Serum cardiac troponin (I or T) concentrations have become the tests of choice for assessment of myocardial injury in nonclinical studies (Berridge et al. 2009; Engle et al. 2009; O'Brien 2008; Reagan 2010; Schultze et al. 2009; Walker 2006), replacing tests such as CK-MB and LDH isoenzyme analyses. Cardiac troponin I is used most frequently because of assay availability, but it is essential to show that the assay used is appropriate for the species under study (Apple et al. 2008). There appears to be no advantage to measuring both I and T in a given study. While microscopic correlates (i.e., myocardial degeneration/necrosis) are commonly present with increases in serum cardiac troponin concentrations detected by early-generation assays (normal animals usually have levels below the detection limits of these assays), highly sensitive next-generation tests are able to detect smaller increases that may or may not be accompanied by microscopic correlates (Schultze et al. 2009, 2008). The toxicologic significance of such small increases is uncertain, but some may represent reversible injury.

Serum amylase and lipase activities are used clinically to diagnose acute pancreatic necrosis. These serum enzyme activities have limited value in nonclinical studies simply because test article–induced exocrine pancreas injury is rare and would likely cause marked clinical signs of illness and pronounced microscopic damage if it occurred in a repeat-dose study. In addition, these enzyme activities are insufficiently sensitive to serve as markers for test article–induced endocrine pancreas injury.

Thyroid hormones are perhaps the most commonly assessed hormones in nonclinical studies because of effects of microsomal enzyme inducers on thyroid hormone metabolism in rats. Accelerated metabolism of thyroxine (T_4) or triiodothyronine (T_3) by increased hepatic UDP-glucuronosyltransferase activity promotes increased release of thyroid-stimulating hormone (TSH) and proliferation of thyroid follicular cells (Klaassen and Hood 2001). Chronic stimulation of thyroid glands can ultimately result in follicular adenomas and carcinomas (Botts et al. 1991; McClain 1989). The most consistent hormone finding associated with microsomal enzyme induction that results in follicular cell proliferation in rats is increased serum TSH concentration. Effects on serum total and free T_3 and T_4 concentrations are more variable, but serum T_4 concentrations are more likely to be reduced than those of T_3.

Assessment of adrenal hormones in nonclinical studies is typically limited to test articles that have previously been shown to cause microscopic changes in the adrenal glands. Corticosterone is the principal glucocorticoid in mice, rats, and rabbits, and cortisol is the principal glucocorticoid in dogs and nonhuman primates (Rosol et al. 2001). Adrenocorticotropic hormone stimulation tests can be used to assess the functional status of adrenal glands with altered morphology but are typically limited to use in dogs for which more is known about the expected response (Hill et al. 2004).

Assessment of other hormones, including reproductive hormones, in laboratory animals is quite specialized and beyond the scope of this chapter (Capen 2010; Evans 2009; Woodman 1997).

6.6 URINALYSIS AND URINE CHEMISTRY TESTS AND INTERPRETATION

Standard urinalysis tests and commonly used urine chemistry tests primarily assess kidney function (in terms of concentrating ability and ability to reabsorb/retain analytes such as glucose and protein) and integrity. A few urine tests are markers for alterations in other tissues.

6.6.1 URINALYSIS

Although a standard component of most nonclinical studies in rats, dogs, and nonhuman primates, urinalysis has a relatively high cost/benefit ratio because sample collection and analysis are relatively labor intensive, sample quality is negatively affected by many factors, interanimal variability is often large, and significant kidney toxicity detected by light microscopy may fail to produce recognizable urinalysis effects. On the other hand, urinalysis results can provide information about urine function that other tests do not.

6.6.1.1 Physicochemical Properties of Urine

Physicochemical properties of urine include volume (for timed collections), color, clarity, specific gravity or osmolality, and reagent strip tests (i.e., pH, protein, glucose, ketones, bilirubin, urobilinogen, and blood). Tests for nitrite, indicating the presence of nitrite-producing bacteria, and leukocyte esterase are available on some reagent strips, but these are screening tests used clinically in human medicine to determine the need for sediment examination or bacterial culture and serve no purpose in nonclinical studies.

Timed urine volume (e.g., overnight or 16 h) and a measure of urine concentration (urine specific gravity or osmolality) are two of the most valuable urinalysis parameters because they can demonstrate the concentrating ability of the kidneys and help correctly interpret other findings. For example, animals with findings suggesting dehydration (e.g., increased red cell mass and serum protein and urea nitrogen concentrations) should not have increased urine volume or decreased urine specific gravity if the kidneys are functioning properly. Urine specific gravity is an approximation of urine solute concentration and most frequently measured by refractometry. Urine osmolality is a more accurate estimation of urine solute concentration, but the added expense is rarely justified. Reagent strip specific gravity measurements are inaccurate and should not be used in nonclinical studies. The potential for spurious results caused by problems with automatic watering systems should always be considered when evaluating urine volume and specific gravity data. Water contamination can result from faulty sipper tubes or animals that play with their water source, and inadvertent disruption of the water supply can cause dehydration.

When a test article impairs urine-concentrating ability, animals have increased urine volume and decreased urine specific gravity. Pharmacologic diuresis is not accompanied by increased serum urea nitrogen or creatinine concentrations unless the diuresis is so great that affected animals are unable to maintain their hydration status. Diuresis due to kidney toxicity is almost always accompanied by increased serum urea nitrogen and creatinine concentrations and correlative microscopic findings (e.g., tubular regeneration/degeneration or necrosis). On rare occasion, the timing of sample collection with respect to onset of toxicity and other factors (e.g., decreased food/protein consumption) may result in relatively unaffected serum measures of kidney dysfunction.

Urine concentration usually varies inversely with urine volume. However, recently developed test articles inhibiting renal tubular reabsorption of glucose as a means of treating diabetes mellitus present an exception. Treated animals have high urine specific gravity because of the presence of glucose and high urine volume as a result of osmotic diuresis.

6.6.1.2 Reagent Strip Tests

Reagent strip tests are only semiquantitative measures, and care must be taken to avoid overinterpretation of results. Animals with highly concentrated urine often appear to have a higher incidence of positive results, or greater amounts of an analyte, than animals with dilute urine simply because of urine concentration. A more quantitative measurement normalized for concentration may be desirable for proper interpretation of some test results (e.g., increased urine protein). Results from automated reagent strip readers using a gray-scale system can also be affected by urine color, and manual examination of reagent strips may be warranted if the test article or a metabolite causes an abnormal color.

Urine samples collected over a long period (e.g., overnight) often have spuriously high urine pH because of ammonia formation resulting from bacterial growth and loss of carbon dioxide from the sample. Collecting samples in a manner to prevent or slow bacterial growth (e.g., surrounding the collection container by wet ice) helps reduce this change. Test article–related effects on urine pH tend to be small and usually represent relatively subtle homeostatic changes and not renal tubular dysfunction. Urine pH is occasionally affected by the pH of the test article if it is administered in high enough quantities and the pH differs significantly from that of the vehicle control article.

A small amount of protein (e.g., trace or 1+) is normal in most animals, especially if the urine is concentrated. Higher protein concentrations may be abnormal, especially if the urine is dilute. Potential causes for increased urine protein include glomerular and tubular dysfunction and hemorrhage or inflammation anywhere along the urogenital tract. If the test article is responsible for increased urine protein, a microscopic correlate is usually apparent. Moderate to marked proteinuria is a common finding in older rats, especially males, owing to chronic progressive nephropathy. Increased urine protein is occasionally identified when a test article exacerbates chronic progressive nephropathy. Highly alkaline urine can spuriously increase urine protein measured by reagent strips.

Although glucose in glomerular filtrate is normally completely reabsorbed by renal tubules, reagent strip readers sometimes identify a small amount (e.g., trace) in urine from normal animals, especially if the urine is highly concentrated. Increased urine glucose due to test article administration usually occurs via one of three mechanisms: the test article causes markedly increased plasma glucose and the amount of glucose in glomerular filtrate exceeds the normal reabsorption capacity of renal tubules (typically a pharmacologic effect); the test article directly inhibits renal tubular glucose reabsorption (typically a pharmacologic effect); or the test article causes renal tubular injury and dysfunction. If increased urine glucose is caused by test article–related renal tubular injury, a microscopic correlate should be apparent.

Ketones are normally absent in the urine of most species, but fasted male rats and monkeys occasionally test positive. Anorectic animals and animals fasted for a prolonged period may have increased urine ketones as a result of incomplete oxidation of fatty acids during energy metabolism. Increased urine ketones owing to test article administration are often associated with decreased food consumption and body weight.

Bilirubin is normally absent in the urine of most laboratory animals, but reagent strip readers occasionally identify a small amount (e.g., trace or 1+), especially in concentrated urine or urine from male dogs. Increased urine bilirubin results from the same conditions that cause increased serum bilirubin and may precede an increase in serum.

A small amount of urobilinogen is normally present in urine. The test for urobilinogen has virtually no value in nonclinical studies because its theoretical purpose is to test for bile duct patency (indicated by the absence of urobilinogen). Although not necessary, urobilinogen is reported by most companies simply because it exists on standard reagent strips.

Although reagent strip tests for blood do not differentiate red cells from hemoglobin or myoglobin, correlative findings typically provide the information necessary to characterize test article–related increases in urine blood results. Hemoglobinuria and myoglobinuria would be associated with other evidence of significant intravascular hemolysis and muscle injury, respectively. Hematuria would be associated with other evidence of a bleeding diathesis or significant injury somewhere along the urogenital tract. Positive results for urine blood are occasionally present in normal animals. Blood from estrus is a common source in female dogs and monkeys, but the origin is often undetermined.

6.6.1.3 Microscopic Evaluation of Urine Sediment

Urine sediment is examined for the presence of cells (i.e., epithelial cells, WBCs, and RBCs), casts, crystals, bacteria, and other formed elements; results are only semiquantitative (e.g., 1+ to 3+). With few exceptions, significant test article–related effects on urine sediment (e.g., increased incidence of casts) are associated with microscopic findings that better characterize the nature and severity of the effect. Although urine sediment examination is a standard component of urinalysis in most nonclinical studies, the cost/benefit ratio is high. If nephrotoxicity is not considered a potential test article liability on the basis of early studies and drug class, eliminating urine sediment examination from the urinalysis presents little risk. However, if sediment detail is considered important (e.g., a unique crystal is suspected), then the method of urine sample collection is critical, and a standard timed collection (e.g., overnight) may be inappropriate. Cystocentesis at necropsy, free catch, or a limited time collection (e.g., 2 h) may be necessary to avoid deterioration of formed elements in the sample.

Small numbers of RBCs, WBCs, and epithelial cells are often present in urine sediment from normal animals. Test article–related increases in cell numbers are rare, but if one is detected on the basis of the number of treated animals affected and the number of cells present for affected animals, a microscopic correlate should be apparent and is necessary to determine the cause.

With exception of a few hyaline casts, urinary casts are rare in urine sediment from normal animals. Increased numbers of hyaline casts are occasionally observed in association with kidney lesions that result in excessive protein loss (e.g., a glomerulopathy). A test article–related increase in the incidence of cellular, granular, or waxy casts indicates significant renal tubular injury, and a microscopic correlate should be clearly evident. A few types of crystals are common in urine from normal animals. Triple phosphate, amorphous phosphate, and calcium carbonate are often observed in alkaline urine, and oxalate crystals are often observed in acid urine. Abnormal crystals associated with toxicity are rare, but ammonium biurate crystals, for example, might occur with severe liver toxicity. More importantly, crystals representing the test article or a metabolite may be identified. Test article–specific crystals are sometimes associated with the formation of calculi or obstructive nephropathy. Crystalluria may also play a role in rodent-specific mechanisms of bladder carcinogenesis (Cohen 2002; Cohen et al. 2002, 2007).

Unless the urine sample is collected by cystocentesis, bacteria are commonly observed in urine sediment of normal animals. Test article–related decreases in the number of bacteria are possible if the test article (or a metabolite) is excreted in urine and has properties that inhibit bacterial growth.

6.6.2 Urine Chemistry Tests

Several urine chemistry tests have been used or proposed to better identify early kidney injury (i.e., prior to changes in serum urea nitrogen or creatinine) and better determine the location of toxic injury within the nephron. At this time, none of these tests are practical or necessary as a standard screening procedure in nonclinical studies. However, many of these tests have merit if nephrotoxicity is an expected or suspected liability for a new test article based on early studies or known drug class effects. All urine chemistry tests should be normalized in some manner for effects of urine concentration and possible water contamination. This is commonly done by calculating the ratio of urine analyte concentration to urine creatinine concentration. Another means of normalizing for concentration is to calculate the total excretion of an analyte over a period (e.g., 16 or 24 h) by multiplying urine analyte concentration and urine volume.

Urine sodium, potassium, and chloride concentrations and timed total excretions (e.g., mmol/16 h) are of limited value but have frequently been measured because they were listed in nonclinical study guidelines for Japan's Ministry of Health, Labor, and Welfare. By themselves, urine electrolyte concentrations usually provide nothing more than information about urine concentration, similar to urine specific gravity. Timed total excretions have the potential to provide more information but can easily be misinterpreted. Increased total excretions can reflect a diuretic effect or renal tubular injury/dysfunction with decreased reabsorption. Decreased total excretions are most often a consequence of normal homeostatic mechanisms required to maintain fluid and electrolyte balance in response to effects such as decreased food/water intake or gastrointestinal losses (i.e., vomiting or diarrhea). Small effects are difficult to recognize because interanimal variability for urine electrolyte measurements is usually substantial. The time at which samples are collected can also influence interpretation. A short-acting test article causing diuresis that results in increased urine output and electrolyte excretion in the hours after dosing in the morning may have the opposite effect on those parameters overnight as animals compensate for earlier fluid and electrolyte losses.

Measurements of urine total protein, and more recently urine albumin, have commonly been used to assess glomerular and tubular integrity. These are typically reported as ratios to urine creatinine, but total excretions over time can also be calculated. Urinary protein loss from glomerular injury/dysfunction tends to be greater than that from tubular injury, but regardless of the source, microscopic correlates are usually present when test article–related increases in quantitative urine protein or albumin are present. Sodium dodecyl sulfate-polyacrylamide gel electrophoresis has been proposed as a means of differentiating the source of protein loss based on molecular weights of excreted proteins (Kolaja et al. 1992; Stonard et al. 1987). Glomerular injury is associated with loss of high-molecular-weight proteins, and tubular injury is associated with loss of low-molecular-weight proteins normally present in glomerular filtrate. β2-microglobulin is an example of a low-molecular-weight plasma protein that is freely filtered through glomeruli and almost completely reabsorbed by proximal tubular epithelium. β2-microglobulin has been proposed as a sensitive biomarker for tubular injury but may have stability issues that affect its value (Bonventre et al. 2010; Schardijn and van Eps 1987).

Urine activities of several enzymes have been evaluated as early markers of renal injury (Clemo 1998; Price 1982). Two of the most frequently measured enzymes are GGT and N-acetyl-p-glucosaminidase (NAG) because they are relatively stable and originate from different cell locations. GGT is a brush border enzyme located primarily in proximal tubular epithelial cells, and NAG is a lysosomal enzyme thought to be located in cells along most of the nephron. These and other urinary enzymes are best used to assess acute renal injury (e.g., within 1 or 2 days of insult) in studies of short duration. They are not indicators of renal function.

In recent years, technological advances and strong interest and cooperation among many different pharmaceutical industry stakeholders have resulted in identification of several urinary biomarkers with the potential to significantly improve early detection and localization of test article–induced renal injury (Bonventre et al. 2010). These urinary biomarkers include, but are not limited to, clusterin, cystatin C, α-glutathione-S-transferase (α-GST), kidney injury molecule-1 (KIM-1), neutrophil gelatinase–associated lipocalin (NGAL), osteopontin, renal papillary antigen-1 (RPA-1), and trefoil factor 3 (TFF3) (Chiusolo et al. 2010; Dieterle et al. 2010; Gautier et al. 2010; Harpur et al. 2011; Ozer et al. 2010; Price et al. 2010; Rouse et al. 2011; Tonomura et al. 2010; Vaidya et al. 2010; Yu et al. 2010). Although much is still to be learned about their utility in various forms of nephrotoxicity, it appears clear that a small, select panel of these or other biomarkers will ultimately become valuable tools for assessing test articles in the early stages of development that have a known or suspected renal liability. A few generalizations can be made at this time. Increased urine clusterin appears to correlate well with tubular injury, regardless of location along the nephron, and with tubular regeneration (Harpur et al. 2011; Rouse et al. 2011). Increased urine α-GST and KIM-1 appear to correlate well with proximal tubular injury (Chiusolo et al. 2010; Gautier et al. 2010; Harpur et al. 2011; Rouse et al. 2011; Tonomura et al. 2010; Vaidya et al. 2010). Increased urine

NGAL has been correlated with glomerular and tubular injury (Bonventre et al. 2010; Tonomura et al. 2010), and increased urine RPA-1 appears a good marker for distal tubule/collecting duct injury and regeneration (Harpur et al. 2011; Price et al. 2010; Rouse et al. 2011). Unlike the other urinary biomarkers, urine TFF3 decreases as a result of acute renal tubular injury (Yu et al. 2010).

REFERENCES

Adler, M., Hoffmann, D., Ellinger-Ziegelbauer, H., Hewitt, P. et al. 2010. Assessment of candidate biomarkers of drug-induced hepatobiliary injury in preclinical toxicity studies. *Toxicol Lett* 196:1–11.

Ameri, M. 2010. Laboratory diagnosis of malaria in nonhuman primates. *Vet Clin Pathol* 39:5–19.

Apple, F.S., Murakami, M.M., Ler, R., Walker, D., and M. York. 2008. Analytical characteristics of commercial cardiac troponin I and T immunoassays in serum from rats, dogs, and monkeys with induced acute myocardial injury. *Clin Chem* 54:1982–1989.

Baker, D.C. and J. Brassard. 2011. Review of continuing education course on hemostasis. *Toxicol Pathol* 39:281–288.

Bauer, J.E. 1996. Comparative lipid and lipoprotein metabolism. *Vet Clin Pathol* 25:49–56.

Beguin, Y. 1999. Erythropoietin and platelet production. *Haematologica* 84:541–547.

Bennett, J.S., Gossett, K.A., McCarthy, M.P., and E.D. Simpson. 1992. Effects of ketamine hydrochloride on serum biochemical and hematological variables in rhesus monkeys (*Macaca mulatto*). *Vet Clin Pathol* 21:15–18.

Berridge, B.R., Pettit, S., Walker, D.B., Jaffe, A.S. et al. 2009. A translational approach to detecting drug-induced cardiac injury with cardiac troponins: Consensus and recommendations from the Cardiac Troponins Biomarker Working Group of the Health and Environmental Sciences Institute. *Am Heart J* 158:21–29.

Bloom, J.C., Thiem, P.A., Sellers, T.S., Deldar, A. and H.B. Lewis. 1988. Cephalosporin-induced immune cytopenia in the dog: Demonstration of erythrocyte-, neutrophil-, and platelet-associated IgG following treatment with cefazedone. *Am J Hematol* 28:71–78.

Bollinger, A.P. 2004. Cytologic evaluation of bone marrow in rats: Indications, methods, and normal morphology. *Vet Clin Pathol* 33:58–67.

Bonventre, J.V., Vaidya, V.S., Schmouder, R., Feig, P., and F. Dieterle. 2010. Next-generation biomarkers for detecting kidney toxicity. *Nat Biotechnol* 28:436–440.

Boon, G.D. 1993. An overview of hemostasis. *Toxicol Pathol* 21:170–179.

Boone, L., Meyer, D., Cusick, P., Ennulat, D. et al. 2005. Selection and interpretation of clinical pathology indicators of hepatic injury in preclinical studies. *Vet Clin Pathol* 34:182–188.

Botts, S., Jokinen, M.P., Isaacs, K.R., Meuten, D.J., and N. Tanaka. 1991. Proliferative lesions of the thyroid and parathyroid glands. In: *Guides for Toxicologic Pathology*. STP/ARP/AFIP, Washington, DC, pp. 1–12.

Bovee, K.C. 1986. Renal function and laboratory evaluation. *Toxicol Pathol* 14:26–36.

Boyd, J.W. 1988. Serum enzymes in the diagnosis of diseases in man and animals. *J Comp Pathol* 98:381–404.

Bruss, M.L. 1997. Lipids and Ketones. In: *Clinical Biochemistry of Domestic Animals*, 5th ed. (J.J. Kaneko, J.W. Harvey, M.L. Bruss, eds) Academic Press, San Diego, pp. 83–115.

Byars, T.D., Ling, G.V., Ferris, N.A., and K.S. Keeton. 1976. Activated coagulation time (ACT) of whole blood in normal dogs. *Am J Vet Res* 37:1359–1361.

Capen, C.C. 2010. Toxic responses of the endocrine system. In: *Casarett and Doull's Essentials of Toxicology*, 2nd ed. (C.D. Klaasen, J.B. Watkins III, eds) McGraw-Hill, pp. 293–308.

Carakostas, M.C. and A.K. Banerjee. 1990. Interpreting rodent clinical laboratory data in safety assessment studies: Biological and analytical components of variation. *Fundam Appl Toxicol* 15:744–753.

Carakostas, M.C., Gossett, K.A., Church, G.E., and B.L. Cleghorn. 1986. Evaluating toxin-induced hepatic injury in rats by laboratory results and discriminant analysis. *Vet Pathol* 23:264–269.

Caro, J. and J.A. Erslev. 1995. Anemia of chronic renal failure. In: *Williams Hematology*, 5th ed. (E. Beutler, M.A. Lichtman, B.S. Coller, T.J. Kipps, eds) McGraw-Hill, New York, pp. 456–462.

Cazzola, M. 2000. Mechanisms of anaemia in patients with malignancy: Implications for the clinical use of recombinant human erythropoietin. *Med Oncol* 17:S11–16.

Center, S.A., Baldwin, B.H., Erb, H.N., and B.C. Tenant. 1985. Bile acid concentrations in the diagnosis of hepatobiliary disease in the dog. *J Am Vet Med Assoc* 187:935–940.

Chanter, D.O., Tuck, M.G., and D.W. Coombs. 1987. The chances of false negative results in conventional toxicology studies with rats. *Toxicology* 43:65–74.

Chiusolo, A., Defazio R., Zanetti, E., Mongillo, M. et al. 2010. Kidney injury molecule-1 expression in rat proximal tubule after treatment with segment-specific nephrotoxicants: A tool for early screening of potential kidney toxicity. *Toxicol Pathol* 38:338–445.

Clampitt, R.B. and R.J. Hart. 1978. The tissue activities of some diagnostic enzymes in ten mammalian species. *J Comp Pathol* 88:607–621.

Clemo, F.A.S. 1998. Urinary enzyme evaluation of nephrotoxicity in the dog. *Toxicol Pathol* 26:29–32.

Cohen, S.M. 2002. Comparative pathology of proliferative lesions of the urinary bladder. *Toxicol Pathol* 30:663–671.

Cohen, S.M., Johansson, S.L., Arnold, L.L., and T.A. Lawson. 2002. Urinary tract calculi and thresholds in carcinogenesis. *Food Chem Toxicol* 40:793–799.

Cohen, S.M., Ohnishi, T., Clark, N.M., He, J., and L.L. Arnold. 2007. Investigations of rodent urinary bladder carcinogens: Collection, processing, and evaluation of urine and bladders. *Toxicol Pathol* 35:337–347.

Cornish, H.H. 1969. The role of vitamin B_6 in the toxicity of hydrazines. *Ann NY Acad Sci* 166:136–145.

Dameron, G.W., Weingand, K.W., Duderstadt, J.M., Odioso, L.W. et al. 1992. Effect of bleeding site on clinical laboratory testing of rats: Orbital venous plexus versus posterior vena cava. *Lab Anim Sci* 42:299–301.

Davies, D.T. 1992. Enzymology in preclinical safety evaluation. *Toxicol Pathol* 20:501–505.

Dhami, M.S.I., Drangova, R., Farkas, R., Balazs, T., and G. Feuer. 1979. Decreases in aminotransferase activity of serum and various tissues in the rat after cefazolin treatment. *Clin Chem* 25:1263–1266.

Dieterle, F., Perentes, E., Cordier, A., Roth, D.R. et al. 2010. Urinary clusterin, cystatin C, β2-microglobulin and total protein as markers to detect drug-induced kidney injury. *Nat Biotechnol* 28:463–469.

Dodds, W.J. 1997. Hemostasis. In: *Clinical Biochemistry of Domestic Animals*, 5th ed. (J.J. Kaneko, J.W. Harvey, M.L. Bruss, eds) Academic Press, San Diego, pp. 241–283.

Donovan, J.C., Stokes, W.S., Montrey, R.D., and H. Rozmiarek. 1983. Hematologic characterization of naturally occurring malaria (*Plasmodium inui*) in cynomolgus monkeys (*Macaca fascicularis*). *Lab Anim Sci* 33:86–89.

Engle, S.K., Jordan, W.H., Pritt, M.L., Chiang, A.Y. et al. 2009. Qualification of cardiac troponin I concentration in mouse serum using isoproterenol and implementation in pharmacology studies to accelerate drug development. *Toxicol Pathol* 37:617–628.

Ennulat, D., Walker, D., Clemo, F., Magid-Slav, M. et al. 2010. Effects of hepatic drug-metabolizing enzyme induction on clinical pathology parameters in animals and man. *Toxicol Pathol* 38:810–828.

Erslev, A.J. 1995a. Anemia of chronic disease. In: *Williams Hematology*, 5th ed. (E. Beutler, M.A. Lichtman, B.S. Coller, T.J. Kipps, eds) McGraw-Hill, New York, pp. 518–524.

Erslev, A J. 1995b. Anemia of endocrine disorders. In: *Williams Hematology*, 5th ed. (E. Beutler, M.A. Lichtman, B.S. Coller, T.J. Kipps, eds) McGraw-Hill, New York, pp. 462–466.

Erslev, A.J. 1995c. Pure red cell aplasia. In: *Williams Hematology*, 5th ed. (E. Beutler, M.A. Lichtman, B.S. Coller, T.J. Kipps, eds) McGraw-Hill, New York, pp. 448–456.

Evans, G.O. 2009. Assessment of endocrine toxicity. In: *Animal Clinical Chemistry: A Practical Handbook for Toxicologists and Biomedical Researchers*, 2nd ed. (G.O. Evans, ed) Taylor & Francis, Boca Raton, pp. 201–242.

Everds, N., Santostefano, M.J., Vargas, H.M., Kirchner, J. et al. 2011a. Off-target platelet activation in macaques by a therapeutic monoclonal antibody. Society of Toxicologic Pathology Annual Symposium, Poster Abstracts, p. 10.

Everds, N., Sprugel, K., Bailey, K., Li, N. et al. 2011b. Thrombocytopenia and anemia caused by off-target species-specific activation of cynomolgus monocytes/macrophages by a human monoclonal therapeutic antibody. Society of Toxicologic Pathology Annual Symposium, Poster Abstracts, p. 11.

Feldman, B.F., Kaneko, J.J., and T.B. Farver. 1981. Anemia of inflammatory disease in the dog: Clinical characterization. *Am J Vet Res* 42:1109–1113.

Frith, C.H., Ward, J.M., and M. Chandra. 1993. The morphology, immunohistochemistry, and incidence of hematopoietic neoplasms in mice and rats. *Toxicol Pathol* 21:206–218.

Fuentealba, C., Bera, M., Jessen, B., Sace, F. et al. 2011. Evaluation of the effects of a VEGFR-2 inhibitor compound on alanine aminotransferase gene expression and enzymatic activity in the rat liver. *Comp Hepatol* 10:8.

Gale, A. 2011. Continuing education course #2: Current understanding of hemostasis. *Toxicol Pathol* 39:273–280.

Gautier, J.C., Riefke, B., Walter, J., Kurth, P. et al. 2010. Evaluation of novel biomarkers of nephrotoxicity in two strains of rat treated with Cisplatin. *Toxicol Pathol* 38:943–956.

George, J.N., El-Harake, M., and R.H. Aster. 1995. Thrombocytopenia due to enhanced platelet destruction by immunologic mechanisms. In: *Williams Hematology*, 5th ed. (E. Beutler, M.A. Lichtman, B.S. Coller, T.J. Kipps, eds) McGraw-Hill, New York, pp. 1315–1355.

Goldberg, D.M. 1980. The expanding role of microsomal enzyme induction, and its implications for clinical chemistry. *Clin Chem* 26:691–699.

Hagopian, K., Ramsey, J.J., and R. Weindruch. 2003. Caloric restriction increases gluconeogenic and transaminase enzyme activities in mouse liver. *Exp Gerontol* 38:267–278.

Hall, R.L. 1992. Clinical pathology for preclinical safety assessment: Current global guidelines. *Toxicol Pathol* 20:472–476.

Hall, R.L. 1997. Lies, damn lies, and reference intervals (or hysterical control values) for clinical pathology data. *Toxicol Pathol* 25:647–649.

Hall, R.L. and N.E. Everds. 2003. Factors affecting the interpretation of canine and nonhuman primate clinical pathology. *Toxicol Pathol* 31:6–10.

Harpur, E., Ennulat, D., Hoffman, D., Betton, G. et al. 2011. Biological qualification of biomarkers of chemical-induced renal toxicity in two strains of male rat. *Toxicol Sci* 122:235–252.

Hill, K., Scott-Moncrieff, J., and G. Moore. 2004. ACTH stimulation testing: A review and a study comparing synthetic and compounded ACTH products. *Vet Med* 99:134–147.

Hoffmann, W.E., Everds, N., Pignatello, M., and P.F. Solter. 1994. Automated and semiautomated analysis of rat alkaline phosphatase isoenzymes. *Toxicol Pathol* 22:633–638.

Hoffmann, W.E. and P.F. Solter. 1994. Alkaline phosphatase isoenzymes: Biochemistry and clinical evaluation in domestic and laboratory animals. *Curr Top Vet Res* 1:171–178.

Horowitz, G.L., Altaie, S., Boyd, J.C., Ceriotti, F. et al. Clinical and Laboratory Standards Institute (CLSI). 2008. *Defining, Establishing, and Verifying Reference Intervals in the Clinical Laboratory; Approved Guideline*, 3rd ed. CLSI document C28-A3.

Jaynes, P.K. 1984. Antiepileptic drug therapy: The laboratory effects on enzyme induction. *Lab Manage* March:40–46.

Jesty, J. and Y. Nemerson. 1995. The pathways of blood coagulation. In: *Williams Hematology*, 5th ed. (E. Beutler, M.A. Lichtman, B.S. Coller, T.J. Kipps, eds) McGraw-Hill, New York, pp. 1227–1238.

Johnson, M.C. 2005. Hyperlipidemia disorders in dogs. *Compend Contin Educ Pract Vet* 27:361–370.

Kaneko, J.J. 1997. Serum proteins and the dysproteinemias. In: *Clinical Biochemistry of Domestic Animals*, 5th ed. (J.J. Kaneko, J.W. Harvey, M.L. Bruss, eds) Academic Press, San Diego, pp. 117–138.

Khan, K.N.M., Komocsar, W.J., Das, I., Lazzaro, N.C. et al. 1996. Effect of bleeding site on clinical pathologic parameters in Sprague–Dawley rats: Retro-orbital venous plexus versus abdominal aorta. *Contemp Top* 35:63–66.

Kidney, B.A. and M.L. Jackson. 1988. Diagnostic value of alkaline phosphatase isoenzyme separation by affinity electrophoresis in the dog. *Can J Vet Res* 52:106–110.

Kimball, J.P., Eitzen, B.H., Lewandowski, A.D., Kirk, J.F.E. et al. 1995. Short-term carbon dioxide/oxygen anesthesia for laboratory rats and mice. *Clin Chem* 41:S163.

Klaassen, C.D. and A.M. Hood. 2001. Effects of microsomal enzyme inducers on thyroid follicular cell proliferation and thyroid hormone metabolism. *Toxicol Pathol* 29:34–40.

Kolaja, G.J., VanderMeer, D.A., Packwood, W.H., and P.S. Satch. 1992. The use of sodium dodecyl sulfate-polyacrylamide gel electrophoresis to detect renal damage in Sprague–Dawley rats treated with gentamicin sulfate. *Toxicol Pathol* 20:603–607.

Kramer, J.W. and W.E. Hoffmann. 1997. Clinical enzymology. In: *Clinical Biochemistry of Domestic Animals*, 5th ed. (J.J. Kaneko, J.W. Harvey, M.L. Bruss, eds) Academic Press, San Diego, pp. 303–325.

Kurata, M. and I. Horii. 2004. Blood coagulation tests in toxicological studies—review of methods and their significance for drug safety assessment. *J Toxicol Sci* 29:13–32.

Kurata, M., Noguchi, N., Kasuga, Y., Sugimoto, T. et al. 1998. Prolongation of PT and APTT under excessive anticoagulant in plasma from rats and dogs. *J Toxicol Sci* 23:149–153.

Leonard, T.B., Neptun, D.A., and J.A. Popp. 1984. Serum gamma glutamyl transferase as a specific indicator of bile duct lesions in the rat liver. *Am J Pathol* 116:262–269.

Loeb, W.F. 1998. The measurement of renal injury. *Toxicol Pathol* 26:26–28.

Lorenz, M., Evering, W.E., Provencher, A., Blue, J.T. et al. 1999. Atypical antipsychotic-induced neutropenia in dogs. *Toxicol Appl Pharmacol* 155:227–236.

Mansouri, A. and A.A. Luri. 1993. Concise review: Methemoglobinemia. *Am J Hematol* 42:7–12.

Martin, R.A., Brott, D.A., Zandee, J.C., and M.J. McKeel. 1992. Differential analysis of animal bone marrow by flow cytometry, *Cytometry* 13:638–643.

Matsuzawa, T., Nomura, M., and T. Unno. 1993. Clinical pathology reference ranges of laboratory animals. *J Vet Med Sci* 55:351–362.

Matsuzawa, T. and M. Sakazume. 1994. Effects of fasting on haematology and clinical chemistry values in the rat and dog. *Comp Haematol Int* 4:152–156.

Matsuzawa, T., Tabata, H., Sakazume, S., Yoshida, S. et al. 1994. A comparison of the effect of bleeding site on haematological and plasma chemistry values of F344 rats: The inferior vena cava, abdominal aorta, and orbital venous plexus. *Comp Haematol Int* 4:207–211.

McClain, R.M. 1989. The significance of hepatic microsomal enzyme induction and altered thyroid function in rats: Implications for thyroid gland neoplasia. *Toxicol Pathol* 17:294–306.

McGrath, J.P., Meador, V.P., Swain, R.R., and C.B. Jensen. 1993. Oxidative erythrocytic injury in preclinical toxicity testing. *Vet Pathol* 30:429.

Millis, D.L., Hawkins, E., Jager, M. and C.R. Boyle. 1995. Comparison of coagulation test results for blood samples obtained by means of direct venipuncture and through a jugular vein catheter in clinically normal dogs. *J Am Vet Med Assoc* 207:1311–1314.

Nemzek, J.A., Bolgos, G.L., Williams, B.A., and D.G. Remick. 2001. Differences in normal values for murine white blood cell counts and other hematological parameters based on sampling site. *Inflamm Res* 50: 523–527.

Neptun, D.A., Smith, C.N., and R.D. Irons. 1985. Effect of sampling site and collection methods on variations in baseline clinical pathology parameters in Fischer-344 rats. I. Clinical chemistry. *Fundam Appl Toxicol* 5:1180–1185.

O'Brien, P.J. 2008. Cardiac troponin is the most effective translational safety biomarker for myocardial injury in cardiotoxicity. *Toxicology* 245:206–218.

O'Brien, P.J., Slaughter, M.R., Polley, S.R., and K. Kramer. 2002. Advantages of glutamate dehydrogenase as a blood biomarker of acute hepatic injury in rats. *Lab Anim* 36:313–321.

O'Brien, P.J., Slaughter, M.R., Swain, A. et al. 2000. Repeated acetaminophen dosing in rats: Adaptation of hepatic antioxidant system. *Hum Exp Toxicol* 19:277–283.

O'Brien, S.R., Sellers, T.S., and D.J. Meyer. 1995. Artifactual prolongation of the activated partial thromboplastin time associated with hemoconcentration in dogs. *J Vet Intern Med* 9:169–170.

Ozer, J., Ratner, M., Shaw, M., Bailey, W., and S. Schomaker. 2008. The current state of serum biomarkers of hepatotoxicity. *Toxicology* 245:194–205.

Ozer, J.S., Dieterle, F., Troth, S., Perentes, E. et al. 2010. A panel of urinary biomarkers to monitor reversibility of renal injury and a serum marker with improved potential to assess renal function. *Nat Biotechnol* 28:486–494.

Packman, C.H. and J.P. Leddy. 1995. Drug-related immune hemolytic anemia. In: *Williams Hematology*, 5th ed. (E. Beutler, M.A. Lichtman, B.S. Coller, T.J. Kipps, eds) McGraw-Hill, New York, pp. 691–697.

Palek, J. 1995. Acanthocytosis, stomatocytosis, and related disorders. In: *Williams Hematology*, 5th ed. (E. Beutler, M.A. Lichtman, B.S. Coller, T.J. Kipps, eds) McGraw-Hill, New York, pp. 557–563.

Price, R.G. 1982. Urinary enzymes, nephrotoxicity, and renal disease. *Toxicology* 23:99–134.

Price, S.A., Davies, D., Rowlinson, R., Copley, C.G. et al. 2010. Characterization of renal papillary antigen 1 (RPA-1), a biomarker of renal papillary necrosis. *Toxicol Pathol* 38:346–358.

Radi, Z.A., Koza-Taylor, P.H., Bell, R.R., Obert, L.A. et al. 2011. Increased serum enzyme levels associated with Kupffer cell reduction with no signs of hepatic or skeletal muscle injury. *Am J Pathol* 179:240–247.

Ramaiah, S.K. 2011. Preclinical safety assessment: Current gaps, challenges, and approaches in identifying translatable biomarkers of drug-induced liver injury. *Clin Lab Med* 31:161–172.

Reagan, W.J. 2010. Troponin as a biomarker of cardiac toxicity: Past, present, and future. *Toxicol Pathol* 38:1134–1137.

Reagan, W.J., Irizarry-Rovira, A., Poitout-Belissent, F., Provencher Bolliger, A. et al. 2011. Best practices for evaluation of bone marrow in nonclinical toxicity studies. *Toxicol Pathol* 39:435–448.

Rebar, A.H. 1993. General responses of the bone marrow to injury. *Toxicol Pathol* 21:118–129.

Riley, J.H. 2005. Safety testing of immunomodulatory drugs in primates. Difficulties in differentiating test article effects from occult diseases—malaria. *Toxicol Pathol* 33:802.

Robinson, S.H., Yannoni, C., and S. Nagasawa. 1971. Bilirubin excretion in rats with normal and impaired bilirubin conjugation: Effect of phenobarbital. *J Clin Invest* 50:2606–2613.

Roncaglioni, M.C., de Gaetano, G., and M.B. Donati. 1982. Some aspects of hematological toxicity in animals. In: *Animals in Toxicological Research* (I. Bartosek, ed) Raven Press, New York, pp. 77–89.

Rosol, T.J. and C.C. Capen. 1997. Calcium-regulating hormones and diseases of abnormal mineral (calcium, phosphorus, magnesium) metabolism. In: *Clinical Biochemistry of Domestic Animals*, 5th ed. (J.J. Kaneko, J.W. Harvey, M.L. Bruss, eds) Academic Press, San Diego, pp. 619–702.

Rosol, T.J., Yarrington, J.T., Latendresse, J., and C.C. Capen. 2001. Adrenal gland: Structure, function, and mechanisms of toxicity. *Toxicol Pathol* 29:41–48.

Rouse, R.L., Zhang, J., Stewart, S.R., Rosenzweig, B.A. et al. 2011. Comparative profile of commercially available urinary biomarkers in preclinical drug-induced kidney injury and recovery in rats. *Kidney Int* 79:1186–1197.

Schardijn, G.H.C. and L.W.S. van Eps. 1987. β_2-Microglobulin: Its significance in the evaluation of renal function. *Kidney Int* 32:635–641.

Schiffer, S.P., Gillett, C.S., and D.H. Ringler. 1984. Activated coagulation time for rhesus monkeys (*Macaca mulatta*). *Lab Anim Sci* 34:191–193.

Schlesinger, D.P. and S.I. Rubin. 1993. Serum bile acids and the assessment of hepatic function in dogs and cats. *Can Vet J* 34:215–220.

Schnell, M.A., Hardy, C., Hawley, M., Propert, K.J., and J.M. Wilson. 2002. Effect of blood collection technique in mice on clinical pathology parameters. *Hum Gene Ther* 13:155–162.

Schultze, A.E., Carpenter, K.H., Wians, F.H., Agee, S.J. et al. 2009. Longitudinal studies of cardiac troponin-I concentrations in serum from male Sprague Dawley rats: Baseline reference ranges and effects of handling and placebo dosing on biological variability. *Toxicol Pathol* 37:754–760.

Schultze, A.E., Konrad, R.J., Credille, K.M., Lu, Q.A., and J. Todd. 2008. Ultrasensitive cross-species measurement of cardiac troponin-I using the Erenna immunoassay system. *Toxicol Pathol* 36:777–782.

Sherwin, J.E. and J.R. Sobenes. 1996. Liver function. In: *Clinical Chemistry: Theory, Analysis, Correlation*, 3rd ed. (L.A. Kaplan, A.J. Pesce, eds) Mosby, St. Louis, pp. 505–527.

Slighter, R.G., Kimball, J.P., Barbolt, T.A., Sherer, A.D., and H.P. Drobeck. 1988. Enzootic hepatitis A infection in cynomolgus monkeys (*Macaca fascicularis*). *Am J Primatol* 14:73–81.

Smith, C.N., Neptun, D.A., and R.D. Irons. 1986. Effect of sampling site and collection methods on variations in baseline clinical pathology parameters in Fischer-344 rats. II. Clinical hematology. *Fundam Appl Toxicol* 7:658–663.

Solter, P.F. 2005. Clinical pathology approaches to hepatic injury. *Toxicol Pathol* 33:9–16.

Solter, P.F., Hoffmann, W.E., Hungerford, L.L., Peterson, M.E., and J.L. Dorner. 1993. Assessment of corticosteroid-induced alkaline phosphatase isoenzyme as a screening test for hyperadrenocorticism in dogs. *J Am Vet Med Assoc* 203:534–538.

Stolk, J.M. and R.P. Smith. 1966. Species differences in methemoglobin reductase activity. *Biochem Pharmacol* 15:343–351.

Stonard, M.D. 1990. Assessment of renal function and damage in animal species. *J Appl Toxicol* 10:267–274.

Stonard, M.D., Gore, C.W., Oliver, G.J.A., and I.K. Smith. 1987. Urinary enzymes and protein patterns as indicators of injury to different regions of the kidney. *Fundam Appl Toxicol* 9:339–351.

Stringer, S.K. and B.E. Seligmann. 1996. Effects of two injectable anesthetic agents on coagulation assays in the rat. *Lab Anim Sci* 46:430–433.

Stromberg, P.C. 1985. Large granular lymphocyte leukemia in F344 rats. *Am J Pathol* 119:517–519.

Sturgill, M.G. and G.H. Lambert. 1997. Xenobiotic-induced hepatotoxicity: Mechanisms of liver injury and methods of monitoring liver function. *Clin Chem* 43:1512–1526.

Suber, R.L. and R.L. Kodell. 1985. The effect of three phlebotomy techniques on hematological and clinical chemical evaluation in Sprague–Dawley rats. *Vet Clin Pathol* 14:23–30.

Swaim, L.D., Taylor, H.W., and G.C. Jersey. 1985. The effect of handling techniques on serum ALT activity in mice. *J Appl Toxicol* 5:160–162.

Swenson, C.L. and T.K. Graves. 1997. Absence of liver specificity for canine alanine aminotransferase. *Vet Clin Pathol* 26:26–28.

Tonomura, Y., Tsuchiya, N., Torii, M., and T. Uehara. 2010. Evaluation of the usefulness of urinary biomarkers for nephrotoxicity in rats. *Toxicology* 273:53–59.

Travlos, G.S., Morris, R.W., Elwell, M.R., Duke, A. et al. 1996. Frequency and relationships of clinical chemistry and liver and kidney histopathology findings in 13-week toxicity studies in rats. *Toxicology* 107:17–29.

Upton, P.K. and D.J. Morgan. 1975. The effect of sampling technique on some blood parameters in the rat. *Lab Anim* 9:85–91.

Vaidya, V.S., Ozer, J.S., Dieterle, F., Collings, F.B. et al. 2010. Kidney injury molecule-1 outperforms traditional biomarkers of kidney injury in preclinical biomarker qualification studies. *Nat Biotechnol* 28:478–485.

Walker, D.B. 2006. Serum chemical biomarkers of cardiac injury for nonclinical safety testing. *Toxicol Pathol* 34:94–104.

Waner, T. and A. Nyska. 1991. The toxicological significance of decreased activities of blood alanine and aspartate aminotransferase. *Vet Res Commun* 15:73–78.

Waner, T. and A. Nyska. 1994. The influence of fasting on blood glucose, triglycerides, cholesterol, and alkaline phosphatase in rats. *Vet Clin Pathol* 23:78–80.

Waner, T., Nyska, A., and R. Chen. 1991. Population distribution profiles of the activities of blood alanine and aspartate aminotransferase in the normal F344 inbred rat by age and sex. *Lab Anim Sci* 25:263–271.

Wardrop, K.J. 2005. The Coombs' test in veterinary medicine: Past, present, future. *Vet Clin Pathol* 34:325–334.

Watkins, J.R., Gough, A.W., and E.J. McGuire. 1989. Drug-induced myopathy in beagle dogs. *Toxicol Pathol* 17:545–548.

Watterson, C., Lanevschi, A., Horner, J., and C. Louden. 2009. A comparative analysis of acute-phase proteins as inflammatory biomarkers in preclinical toxicology studies: Implications for preclinical and clinical translation. *Toxicol Pathol* 37:28–33.

Weil, C.S. and C.P. Carpenter. 1969. Abnormal values in control groups during repeated-dose toxicologic studies *Toxicol Appl Pharmacol* 14:335–339.

Weingand, K., Brown, G., Hall, R., Davies, D. et al. 1996. Harmonization of animal clinical pathology testing in toxicity and safety studies. *Fundam Appl Toxicol* 29:198–201.

Weiss, D.J. 1993. Leukocyte response to toxic injury. *Toxicol Pathol* 21:135–140.

Williams, W.J. 1995. Secondary thrombocytosis. In: Williams Hematology, 5th ed. (E. Beutler, M.A. Lichtman, B.S. Coller, T.J. Kipps, eds) McGraw-Hill, New York, pp. 1361–1363.

Woodman, D.D. 1997. *Laboratory Animal Endocrinology: Hormonal Action, Control Mechanisms, and Interactions with Drugs* (D.D. Woodman, ed) John Wiley and Sons Ltd, West Sussex, England.

Yang, R-Z., Park, S., Reagan, W.J., Goldstein, R. et al. 2009. Alanine aminotransferase isoenzymes: Molecular cloning and quantitative analysis of tissue expression in rats and serum elevation in liver toxicity. *Hepatology* 49:598–607.

Young, J.K., Hall, R.L., O'Brien, P., Strauss, V., and J.L. Vahle. 2011. Best practices for clinical pathology testing in carcinogenicity studies. *Toxicol Pathol* 39:429–434.

Yu, Y., Jin, H., Holder, D., Ozer, J.S. et al. 2010. Urinary biomarkers trefoil factor 3 and albumin enable early detection of kidney tubular injury. *Nat Biotechnol* 28:470–477.

Zucker, S.D., Qin, X., Rouster, S.D., Yu, F. et al. 2001. Mechanism of indinavir-induced hyperbilirubinemia. *Proc Natl Acad Sci* 98:12671–12676.

7 Toxicogenomics in Toxicologic Pathology

Mark J. Hoenerhoff and David E. Malarkey

CONTENTS

7.1 INTRODUCTION

7.1.1 -OMICS: THE BASICS

According to the latest calculations, there are about 20,000 genes in the mammalian genome (Carninci and Hayashizaki 2007; Claverie 2005) and, simply stated, up to 40% of them (~8000) may be actively transcribed (expressed as indicated by production of gene-specific messenger or mRNAs) at a baseline in normal tissues (Malarkey et al. 2005). This number is significantly lower than earlier estimates of 100,000 genes in the genome and reflects the complex efficiency of the genome to make multiple proteins from a single gene (Carninci and Hayashizaki 2007). Under environmental stressors or in disease states, there can be enhancement or suppression of baseline genes in addition to the expression of inactive genes. The study of the array of up- and downregulated genes under various conditions and disease states is the basis of the field called genomics. Genomics is also called transcriptomics because it refers to the process of transcription, that is, production of mRNA copies of coding DNA. Generally, but not always, the mRNA is spliced and translated into specific proteins. Proteomics refers to the study of translation and protein modification. Gene expression can be influenced by epigenetic events, or alterations in expression of genes without modification of the underlying genetic sequence, through such processes as methylation, microRNA, or histone deacetylation, whereby gene expression is suppressed or inhibited (Holliday

1994). Hypermethylation, for example, inhibits gene expression through methylation of CpG islands in DNA coding sequences. The large-scale investigation of global gene methylation is also called methylomics. MicroRNAs have more recently been identified to exert control of gene expression (Wang et al. 2009). The study of metabolites in body fluids is called metabolomics and the interaction of all the -omics is called interactomics. The various and increasing number of "-omics" fields are outside the scope of this chapter; instead, the focus of this chapter will be on the application of toxicogenomics.

Toxicogenomics is the functional application of genomics, or global gene expression changes within an organism or tissue, to toxicologic exposures (Boorman et al. 2002a,b; Morgan et al. 2004). This technology involves the collection and interpretation of genomic data in order to identify mechanism of action as well as prediction of potential toxicologic endpoints using microarray technology. This science is being applied for several uses in preclinical testing, including predicting toxicity, elucidating mechanisms of toxicity, and biomarker discovery (Decristofaro and Daniels 2008). Toxicogenomics may be viewed as a merger of toxicology and genomics and should be considered an interdisciplinary science requiring the input from multiple disciplines including toxicology, molecular biology, bioinformatics, and, importantly, pathology, among others, for proper study design, conduct, and interpretation of results (Boorman et al. 2002a,b; Irwin et al. 2004; Morgan et al. 2004). As an emerging, multidisciplinary science that affects the investigation of toxicologic responses, drug discovery, and therapeutics is performed, toxicologic pathologists will be called upon more and more to be a part of teams involved in the design, implementation, and interpretation of large data sets to answer important questions related to high-throughput differential gene expression analysis. Pathologists, in particular, are uniquely qualified to make significant contributions to the field of toxicogenomics, given their diverse training and background in systems biology (Boorman et al. 2002a). This systems biology training in multiple facets of science including biology, anatomy, disease processes, histology, and biochemistry makes the veterinary pathologist an integral part of any toxicogenomics team. The "whole animal" interpretation of large data sets brings biological relevance and meaning to large genomic data sets. As this technology advances, the role of the toxicologic pathologist will undoubtedly change as an important component of hypothesis generation, study design, sample acquisition, and interpretation of these very complex, large-scale genomic data sets. Therefore, a working understanding of this technology is becoming more critical in the toxicologic pathology arena in order to fully utilize the power of molecular biology in the context of toxicologic pathology. Furthermore, as toxicogenomics is often used to detect gene expression changes related to a "phenotypic anchor" (i.e., histological alterations), pathologists can help interpret the biological significance of gene expression changes as they relate to mechanisms and morphologic expression (alterations). This chapter focuses on the basic design, interpretation, and application of toxicogenomic studies as they relate to characterization of toxicity and carcinogenicity bioassays in toxicologic pathology.

7.1.2 -Omics Revolution

During the past 15 years, a tremendous amount of effort has been undertaken to develop high-throughput assays to evaluate large-scale gene expression changes in cells and tissues as a result of a disease state. In order to understand the mechanism of action of various perturbations in normal cellular function, a hypothesis-driven approach has traditionally been used to study a limited number of target genes at a time, on the basis of the general body of knowledge of those genes and their role in disease pathogenesis. The advent of microarray technology has allowed the assessment of the expression of literally thousands of genes at a time from a single sample of mRNA, revolutionizing the field of toxicology and significantly advancing the understanding of toxic mechanisms relevant to human health (Hamadeh et al. 2002a; Zidek et al. 2007).

To date, the "-omics" technologies have provided massive amounts of biological information and fewer-than-expected applications in predictive profiling in toxicologic pathology as well as human

---

TABLE 7.1

Functional Categories of Gene Responses to Rat Hepatotoxicants

Oxidative stress

DNA damage

Acute phase response

Cytoskeleton

DNA repair

Tissue repair/regeneration

Cell proliferation

Cell cycle

Apoptosis

Inflammation

Biotransformation/Drug metabolism

Metabolism (glucose, protein, carbohydrate, steroids)

Glutathione synthesis

Signal transduction

Energy loss (ATP)

Source: Adapted from Gerrish, K., Malarkey, D. E.: *Hepatotoxicity: From Genomics to In-Vitro and In-Vivo Models.* pp. 265–488. 2007. Copyright Wiley-VCH Verlag GmbH & Co. KGaA. Reproduced with permission.

---

medicine. The analysis and reporting of transcriptomic data have evolved over the last decade from an observational science, primarily reporting lists of differentially expressed genes in normal and abnormal conditions, to more in-depth, hypothesis-driven approaches utilizing advanced bioinformatics such as principal component analysis (PCA), biological networks, and pathway analyses. Over the past decade, investigators have incorporated transcriptomics research into a variety of studies, and genomics research is leading to new advances and applications that reveal biological insights, generate predictive gene profiles, and identify key genes and biomarkers of toxicity and carcinogenicity. Although predicting toxicity/disease outcomes is not yet reliable, but still promising, profiles of exposure and neoplastic growth are leading to new approaches to understand disease. Genomics research has contributed greatly to hepatology, with studies that report the ability to classify and identify hepatotoxicants (Gerrish and Malarkey 2007) (Table 7.1), carcinogens, and neoplasms; identify biological insights and pathways; discover new genes; assess similarities between species; validate animal models; and identify new biomarkers and therapeutic targets. Toxicogenomics can have a significant impact on drug discovery and development, including mechanisms of toxicity, discovery of novel drug targets, or diagnostic markers of efficacy or toxicity.

7.2 BASIC ARRAY TECHNOLOGIES

Several array platforms exist to evaluate large-scale changes in gene expression, and a more extensive technical description of various platforms is described elsewhere (Pandiri et al. 2011). The basic technology involves the concept that for every gene of interest, mRNA that is expressed represents a complementary copy of the DNA coding region of that gene, which, when transcribed into cDNA, binds to complementary sequences of DNA from the coding region of its respective gene (Boorman et al. 2002a). Microarray platforms are created by attaching DNA sequences (probes) of hundreds to thousands of genes to solid strata, such as plastic, nylon, or glass. Once samples are obtained, RNA purification must be performed. The output of any microarray study is influenced by the quality of the RNA sample being analyzed, and the reliability of the data is directly proportional to the quality of the RNA (Pandiri et al. 2011). Therefore, special care should be taken to properly

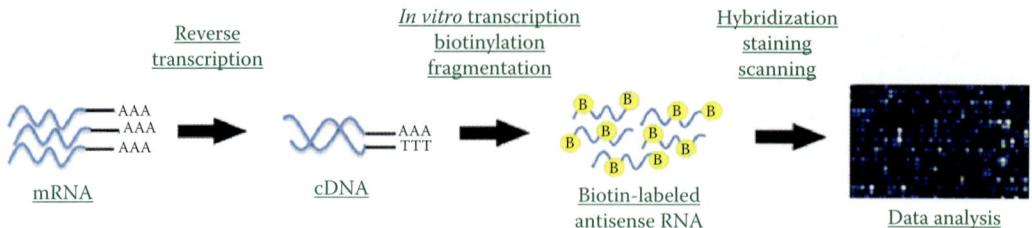

FIGURE 7.1 Test and control sample RNA is reverse transcribed to cDNA, biotinylated, fragmented, and hybridized to the microarray. The hybridized array is washed, labeled with streptavidin-phycoerythrin, and scanned. The ratio of fluorescent values of the test and control samples is calculated to determine the degree of differential gene expression. (From Pandiri, A. R. et al. *Fundamental Neuropathology for Pathologists and Toxicologists.* pp. 285–318. Copyright Wiley-VCH Verlag GmbH & Co. KGaA. Reproduced with permission.

and optimally collect the sample, ensure proper handling and storage, and achieve optimal RNA purification (Foley et al. 2006). After isolation, RNA samples from each group being investigated (treatment vs. control, for example) are reverse transcribed into cDNA, labeled with fluorescent markers, and allowed to competitively hybridize (bind) to the DNA sequences on the solid strata. After hybridization, the samples are scanned and the fluorescence signal is quantified with image analysis software. The resulting strength of fluorescent signal correlates with the relative expression of the transcript. While there are a number of platforms to evaluate gene expression changes, by far the most common involves the use of high-density synthetic oligonucleotide arrays (Figure 7.1). Regardless of the technique used, one must realize that the output of microarray platforms is not free from technical problems and may be influenced by sample selection, RNA purification and processing, data analysis, and issues with gene annotation or gene location on the array.

7.3 TOXICOLOGIC PATHOLOGIST'S ROLE IN TOXICOGENOMICS

The toxicologic pathologist plays a critical role in the study design, sample selection and acquisition, data analysis and interpretation, and validation of the toxicogenomics results. The pathologist has the appropriate background training in systems biology and various scientific disciplines that are important in the design of experiments utilizing animals and biologic materials. Since experimental animals are nonstatic biologic systems that are influenced by age, sex, diet, environment, and other factors, intricate knowledge of these variables is important in the design of a toxicogenomics study, since these factors will influence gene expression. Sample selection is of paramount importance, since the quality and appropriateness of the sample taken will directly influence the output of the gene expression analysis performed (i.e., the "garbage in, garbage out" theory). Also, when obtaining RNA from animal tissues, the pathologist plays a critical role in understanding the biology of the whole organism as it relates to changes in feeding patterns, diet, gender, circadian rhythm, and what the potential effects other stressors may have on gene expression (Boorman et al. 2002a; Irwin et al. 2004). These factors are critical in study design and sample acquisition, and the pathologist not only is uniquely qualified to understand the underlying components influencing systems biology but also has an understanding of the various different components of each tissue, as well as regional differences in gene expression within an organ (such as the liver).

Biologic and technical replicates are also of paramount importance when planning a toxicogenomics study in order to reduce error. Biologic replicates, representing the number of samples in each study group, are important in determining the inherent variability in gene expression between samples within each group (Boorman et al. 2002a). This is particularly important when comparing global gene expression changes in samples collected from animals exposed to different doses of a compound or when comparing gene changes associated with a particular lesion resulting from chemical exposure. There can be marked biologic variability between samples within a group, on the basis of heterogeneity of samples and mRNA expression; biological variations in individual mRNA expression is the largest source of error in microarray analysis (Hatfield et al. 2003). Given the degree of biological variability within groups and between animals, even within untreated control animals, and since changes in gene expression can be influenced by several factors other than chemical exposure, it is important to include a number of samples to provide as much statistical power as possible for analysis. This raises the question of whether individual samples should be pooled from a group of animals or if each animal should be evaluated separately. While pooling reduces cost in large-scale genomics studies, it may also be problematic if one of the animals shows a significantly different response, or a lack of a response, which could cause misinterpretation of the data if animals are pooled (Hamadeh et al. 2002a). When variability between samples is low, there is high confidence in the ability of statistical analysis to capture statistically significant, differentially expressed genes between groups while applying stringent analysis to minimize the false discovery rate. Technical replicates, on the other hand, are the number of measurements taken in each sample. A significant number of technical replicates are recommended to ensure proper handling and processing of samples to minimize internal variation within a study. For example, when subjecting samples to microarray analysis, ideally samples are assayed in triplicate, but at times duplicate samples are used for cost savings. This is done to minimize technical variation due to factors such as pipetting error in the case of sample handling and factors associated with evaporation or dissipation of samples in terms of processing error. In this way, measurements are averaged across samples, minimizing significant induced changes associated with artifact that would have otherwise significantly altered the output of gene expression analysis.

A statistically based approach to identification of significantly differentially regulated gene expression as a result of treatment or disease is of paramount importance in making sense of these very large data sets. All transcripts (~20,000) may be assessed at one time, with multiple probes per gene, such that the sheer volume of these data could not be realistically processed by the human brain alone. Therefore, it is necessary to apply a statistically based method of selection of significantly altered genes. Without a reliable method to obtain statistical significance of gene expression changes, it is impossible to determine whether or not the observed alterations in gene expression are actually real or only observed by chance. There are numerous statistical methods by which to analyze these data sets, and the output of the analysis will often depend on the type of statistical method used (Irwin et al. 2004). Thus, some differentially regulated genes of interest (target genes) identified after microarray analysis should be validated by other methods, including quantitative real-time polymerase chain reaction (QRT-PCR) analysis, immunohistochemistry, or in situ hybridization since mRNA data do not always correlate with protein production (Decristofaro and Daniels 2008; Guerreiro et al. 2003). In general, QRT-PCR results are used to verify the microarray findings. Furthermore, statistical analysis will only provide the first step in understanding the message behind the data; the most challenging and time-consuming aspect to global gene expression profiling in toxicogenomics is organizing the data into a biologically meaningful message. We will first discuss methods by which data are typically organized to provide a clearer understanding of the relevance of the gene changes observed. These methods typically involve PCA and hierarchical cluster analysis (HCA).

PCA is a means to compare global gene expression within and between each group being assayed in a spatial manner, in order to visualize significant differences in overall gene expression or to recognize overlap or congruence of gene expression changes on a global scale. It is a pattern recognition method representing a multivariate statistical method used to visualize high-density gene expression data up to three dimensions in order to easily comprehend global differences in gene expression between groups (Hamadeh et al. 2002b). PCA characterizes the variability in the data and may give clues to biologic meaning based on the interaction of samples within the analysis. For example, Figure 7.2a represents a PCA plot illustrating global gene expression in a recent National Toxicology Program (NTP) study, in which three groups of six biologic replicates were compared: (1) normal liver is represented by the red circles; (2) spontaneous hepatocellular carcinoma (HCC) is

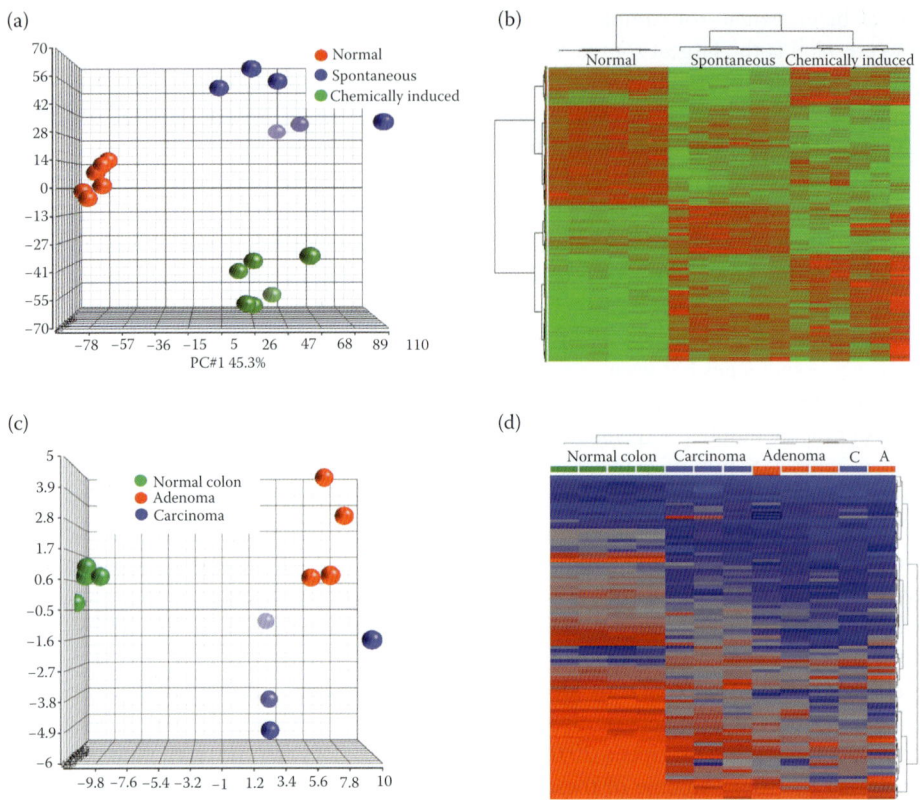

FIGURE 7.2 PCA (a and c) and HCA used in analysis of microarray data. (a) PCA plot illustrating significant differences in global gene expression between normal liver samples (red), spontaneously arising HCC (blue), and chemically induced HCC (green). (b) HCA heat map demonstrating differential gene expression in samples from a (green, downregulated; red, upregulated). These analyses provide important mechanistic information relevant to chemical exposures and cancer risk. (c) PCA plot demonstrating changes in global gene expression between normal colon (green), colonic adenoma (red), and colonic adenocarcinoma (blue). Significant differences in global gene expression between adenoma and carcinoma may be useful in confirming histologic diagnoses of these lesions in the continuum of colon cancer and may influence therapeutic success for patients with this disease. (d) HCA heat map shows that in one case, a carcinoma clusters with the adenoma signature, suggesting biological similarity of this neoplasm based on global gene expression (blue, downregulated; red, upregulated; C, carcinoma, A, adenoma).

represented by the blue circles; and (3) chemically induced HCC is represented by the green circles. From this plot, we can see that each sample clusters very closely with others from the same group. This indicates that there is very little biologic variability in the data within groups, illustrating that the overall global gene expression in each sample from its respective group is similar. This provides a means of internal validation to ensure that biologic replicates in each group are similar. In addition, there is appreciable separation of groups in space, with red circles (normal liver) a significant distance away from the blue (spontaneous HCC) and green (chemically induced HCC) samples. The significant separation between normal liver and HCC samples is to be expected, since there are naturally marked differences in gene expression between normal and tumor tissue; however, what is more significant is the clear separation between spontaneous and chemically induced HCC in this study, indicating that there are significant differences in overall global gene expression between these two tumor groups, in which the only predominant difference biologically is chemical treatment. Therefore, the marked differences in gene expression between these two HCC groups are based solely on chemical exposure.

Similar to PCA, HCA is another way to graphically depict global changes in gene expression between groups. This is an unbiased, unsupervised classification method for detecting similarities in patterns of gene expression across multiple profiles (Hamadeh et al. 2002a). Figure 7.2b represents a heat map depicting significant differences in global gene expression between normal liver, spontaneous HCC, and chemically induced HCC. In this output, upregulated genes are depicted in red, while downregulated genes are illustrated in green. The intensity of the red or green signal corresponds with the fluorescence signal data that are quantified with image analysis software after hybridization. Therefore, the resulting intensity of red or green color corresponds with the relative increase or decrease in gene expression, respectively. From Figure 7.2b, we can appreciate that there are obvious differences in overall gene expression that are associated with each group of samples being compared. These genes are further clustered based on similarities and differences in gene expression. From this clustering, one can gain information on the classification of groups of genes and their functional relevance to the disease or condition being studied. Analysis using both PCA and HCA is an effective way to visualize significant differences in global gene expression in a rapid and efficient manner. Furthermore, the illustration of significant changes in global gene expression between tumor samples (as shown in the above example) is of great significance, because it illustrates the utility that these studies have in the discovery of chemical effects on a global scale, even in tumor samples that may appear histologically identical, as in the case of HCC. Gene expression profiles and PCA have also been successfully applied to discriminate normal tissue from benign or malignant neoplasms, which not only supports published histopathologic diagnostic criteria but also provides key molecular pathways in cancer development and progression (Figure 7.2c and d). However, these analyses are merely first steps in evaluating such large data sets, and without a background in systems biology, an investigator is left with thousands of genes in these groups without any real appreciation of which changes are relevant and which are insignificant fluctuations ("background noise"). This is where the pathologist can make a further significant impact to any microarray study.

7.4 PATHWAY AND NETWORK ANALYSES

Once a set of statistically significant up- and downregulated genes is identified, the strategy of pathway and network analysis begins. The output of a global gene expression analysis typically results in lists of thousands of genes that are statistically significantly differentially expressed from a control (i.e., HCC vs. normal liver). These genes may then be uploaded into various software programs (Ingenuity Pathway Analysis [IPA], NextBio meta-analysis software, GeneGO, Gene Ontology Analysis, GeneSpring) and subjected to data processing in order to identify functionally and biologically relevant categories of gene expression. For example, when comparing gene expression between normal tissue and a neoplasm, data processing software can group genes in relevant pathways associated with the cell cycle, apoptosis, oncogenesis, or cellular growth and proliferation (Figure 7.3). Similarly, when comparing treatment groups to controls, pathway-based gene analysis can identify important pathways associated with toxicity or cellular damage. Through this pathway-based approach to gene expression analysis, significant information regarding biological processes relevant to mechanisms of action and tissue responses to injury or chemical exposure can be gained.

Pathway analyses and networks help group processes together to better understand mechanisms of toxicity. For example, the majority of hepatotoxicants studied have overwhelming responses in gene expression changes related to cell injury and degeneration, metabolism, DNA repair, and regeneration as the liver begins the healing process (Table 7.1). Our challenge is to find the key specific gene changes and molecular event(s) that play roles in chronic, debilitating diseases such as cancer. Network analysis can help investigators identify gene networks that may play a role in biologically relevant processes, including cancer.

Once a pathway-based approach has been used to evaluate gene expression and identify important alterations in networks responsible for mechanism of toxicity or carcinogenicity, it is often

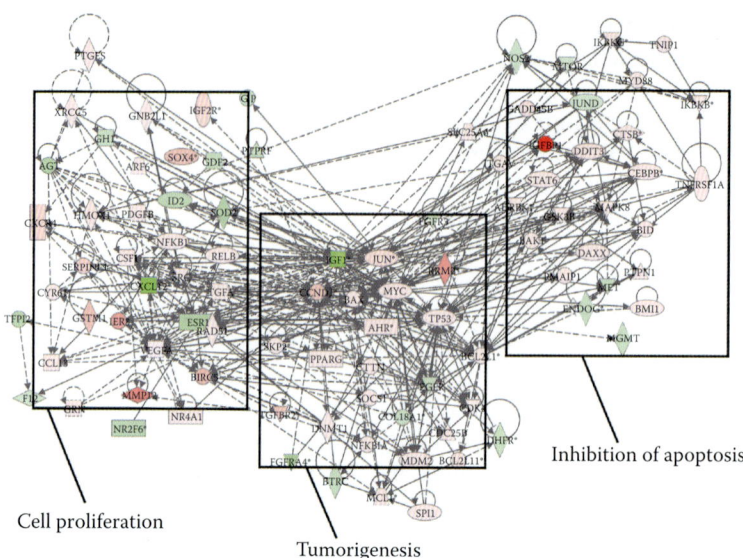

Cell proliferation

Tumorigenesis

Inhibition of apoptosis

FIGURE 7.3 IPA evaluation of gene networks associated with cell proliferation, tumorigenesis, and apoptosis inhibition in cancer. IPA may be used to visualize gene networks to understand alterations in biologic function resulting from aberrations in global gene expression (green, downregulated; red, upregulated).

necessary to further mine these large data sets in order to identify novel gene targets. For example, novel targets that are identified as highly up- or downregulated, and that may play an important role in the pathogenesis of a particular lesion, may not be represented in a pathway analysis–based approach. These targets need to be investigated individually and validated, and further study of each needs to be pursued to identify them as appropriate biomarkers of disease. Moreover, various targets of toxicity or carcinogenicity may be found to be highly dysregulated in a treatment group but poorly represented in a pathway-based approach depending on the curated literature and must therefore be evaluated on a gene-by-gene basis. Many targets are poorly characterized, and further investigation of their role in toxicity or carcinogenesis in the target organ, or other organs for that matter, should be done based on literature review and functional *in vitro* assays.

7.5 APPLICATIONS OF TOXICOGENOMICS

7.5.1 PHENOTYPIC ANCHORING

Toxicogenomics studies benefit greatly when combined with gross and histopathology. Pathology endpoints can provide a biologically relevant explanation for the gene changes seen in a microarray study. Integrating clinical or histopathology data with gene expression data in each analysis results in a better understanding of the significance of gene expression patterns in terms of biological relevance to a lesion or disease development (Bushel et al. 2007b). Linking array data to typical changes in tissue morphology as a result of toxicity or changes in clinical chemistry parameters, including liver (alanine aminotransferase [ALT], aspartate aminotransferase [AST], alkaline phosphatase [ALP]) or kidney (blood urea nitrogen [BUN], creatinine) is necessary to establish a cause-and-effect relationship between compound exposure and detrimental effects resulting from treatment. "Phenotypic anchoring" refers to the method of relating specific alterations in gene expression to adverse effects due to compound exposure (Paules 2003). Since the most common physiological processes involved in tissue injury and repair are similar between several different types of species (highly conserved), including degenerative processes (e.g., necrosis and apoptosis) and regenerative processes (e.g., DNA repair and hyperplasia), extrapolation between chemical effects in rodent models to humans are often made. However, one must take into account that chemical effects are influenced by dose and time of exposure, and chemical action in different species may be influenced by species/strain-specific gene expression or differences in metabolism (Paules 2003). By anchoring gene expression changes to a phenotypic alteration, this removes some variation owing to subjectivity of gene expression that may be due to nonchemical effects unrelated to toxicity. Anchoring gene expression changes to phenotype results in increased confidence in extrapolation between rodent models and humans and decreases in numbers of animals needed per study and increases mechanistic information regarding potential mechanisms of action of chemical effects or lesion development (Paules 2003). Phenotypic anchoring of gene expression data to histological alterations has linked biological data to specific gene regulation and raised the awareness of the cellular heterogeneity of samples and biological plausibility of genomics results. Histopathology of tissues provides a morphologic anchor by which gene expression changes may be corroborated and provides additional information for the interpretation of differential gene expression. Alternatively, data obtained through gene expression analysis that may indicate toxicity is validated through morphology; histopathologic evidence of tissue damage, necrosis, inflammation, or hyperplasia may be represented by certain changes in gene expression. Moreover, the pathologist is aware that there are subtypes of cell populations within each organ that have different functions. Therefore, depending on the aims of the study, or the question being asked, it may be crucial to collect a specific region of an organ for analysis. Pathologists have the knowledge and tools to identify subregions of various organs either grossly or through the use of microscopic technologies such as light microscopy and laser capture microdissection. For example, the differential gene expression within centrilobular areas of the liver after acetaminophen toxicity is significantly different (Irwin et al. 2004) than that in the periportal regions, and gene expression after exposure to a nephrotoxin targeting the renal cortex will be very different from that of a nontarget region such as the medulla. In this respect, the pathologist plays an important role in the selection of appropriate tissue samples that will dictate the success or failure of the entire project. Therefore, the pathologist can help put gene expression changes into context through an understanding of the whole animal, systems biology, and the interaction of multiorgan pathology and toxicities.

In conjunction with pathology endpoints, several investigators have established signatures of toxicity and predictive genomics related to exposure to various chemicals and compounds. These signatures provide a genomic link that may be used to predict toxicity in many studies or may be used to screen large numbers of compounds early on in the drug development process to streamline the production and development of numerous compounds. Much work has been done on the development and validation of prediction and mechanistic models, including signatures of renal, hepatic, and cardiac toxicity; early indicators of carcinogenicity; genotoxic versus nongenotoxic mechanisms; and other early biomarkers of disease.

7.5.2 Predictive versus Mechanistic Toxicogenomics

Generally, there are two principal methods of global gene expression analysis in toxicogenomics research, on the basis of the purpose of the study and the questions being asked: mechanistic and predictive (Ge and He 2009; Lord et al. 2006; Waters et al. 2010). Mechanistic toxicogenomics seeks to define biological pathways and molecular mechanisms through evaluation of alterations in genes comprising biologic pathways responsible for toxicity or carcinogenesis. Global gene expression data can be mined to determine which genes, out of thousands of altered transcripts in a data set, are relevant to a toxic exposure and can provide information regarding potential mechanism of action (Afshari et al. 1999). Toxicogenomics has had a very positive impact on the understanding of molecular mechanisms of toxicity and disease, and this is an arena in which the expertise and input of the toxicologic pathologist are especially impactful. This approach seeks to define and understand the underlying biological responses that result from exposure to a particular chemical, and how those responses influence lesion development in an adverse toxicologic outcome (Ge and

He 2009). For example, Yoon et al. (2003) utilized cDNA microarrays to investigate the mechanisms of benzene-induced bone marrow toxicity and leukemia development in mice. Comparing the p53 knockout mouse to wild-type C57BL/6 mouse in large-scale gene expression studies, they found that repeated genetic and epigenetic effects of benzene exposure resulted in DNA damage and dysfunction of p53, accompanied by dysregulation of the cell cycle, apoptosis, and DNA repair, ultimately culminating in leukemogenesis. This study is an example of a mechanistic toxicogenomics study, in which a focused question regarding the molecular mechanism of toxicity and carcinogenicity of a particular chemical is investigated. These studies often provide an important molecular link, such as alterations of conserved biologic pathways responsible for carcinogenesis between the rodent model and human disease, thus providing enhanced power in terms of extrapolation of toxicity or carcinogenicity findings in rodents to the human condition.

Predictive toxicogenomics, on the other hand, uses global molecular expression data resulting from genomic perturbation to predict a toxicologic outcome (Waters et al. 2010). The motivation behind predictive toxicogenomics lies in the fact that perturbations in global gene expression as a result of chemical exposure may provide an early warning of toxicity, prior to the development of clinical or histopathologic alterations (Ulrich and Friend 2002). Changes in gene expression resulting from toxicity can be noted using a database of validated gene expression changes anchored to known toxicologic and pathologic outcomes corresponding to a given toxicologic class; one seeks to identify compounds as potentially toxic or identify signatures or biomarkers to predict a toxicologic or carcinogenic outcome. Prediction of a toxicologic or carcinogenic outcome requires utilization of class prediction methods to develop a database of global gene expression changes based on compounds of a given toxicologic class that induce known toxicologic responses. Good examples are hepatotoxicity and nephrotoxicity wherein hepatocellular and renal tubular necrosis, respectively, are pathology endpoints (Ellinger-Ziegelbauer et al. 2008; Maggioli et al. 2006). These databases are then used to identify defined toxicologic gene signatures. Once these defined signatures are established and validated, candidate compounds with unknown toxicologic properties can be screened against these profiles for similarities in gene expression that might predict a toxicologic response. On the basis of this approach, compounds with unknown toxicity can be screened based on their genomic signatures early in the process, and those with a potential capacity to induce adverse toxicologic responses can be eliminated from a study sooner. This makes predictive toxicogenomics particularly attractive for preclinical drug development, in which companies may screen a number of compounds for gene expression signatures predictive of toxicity, thus providing additional information on potential adverse interactions in the research and discovery phase. Toxicogenomics data pertaining to potentially adverse outcomes are valuable in early pharmacology or safety studies to complement other assays when profiling for potential toxicity; however, one must keep in mind that it is important to consider toxicogenomics data in corporation with complementary toxicity assays rather than as a stand-alone measure of a toxicity risk, in order to avoid attrition of key lead molecules owing to a potential false-positive result. Outside the scope of drug development, numerous studies have been undertaken utilizing this approach in animal models in an attempt to predict carcinogenic (carcinogens vs. noncarcinogens, genotoxic vs. nongenotoxic carcinogens) or toxicologic (hepatotoxicity, nephrotoxicity, cardiotoxicity, etc.) responses in toxicology and carcinogenicity studies, providing a successful prediction of toxicity for uncharacterized compounds. Proper tissue sampling and careful study design are critical in the implementation of predictive and mechanistic toxicogenomics studies and may vary depending on the question being asked. For example, if predictive endpoints are desired, it is best to sample tissues for toxicogenomics early, prior to the onset of histopathologic findings, and at several time points. Depending on the chemical, dose, and duration of exposure, this may vary between hours and days. On the other hand, if sampling for mechanistic toxicogenomics endpoints, it is better to collect target organ tissue throughout the course of lesion development, so as to better understand how the lesion develops on the molecular scale, thus providing a better understanding of pathogenesis.

7.5.3 Prediction of Carcinogens Using Toxicogenomics

The 2-year rodent bioassay is the gold standard method used to evaluate compounds and chemicals for carcinogenic hazards relevant to humans. However, some view the bioassay as too time consuming, labor intensive, and costly, using hundreds of animals; therefore, there has been much interest recently in the predictive value of short-term bioassays (Thomas et al. 2007a,b; Tsujimura et al. 2006). Several studies utilizing global gene expression analysis and predictive toxicogenomics have attempted to predict the long-term carcinogenic effects of various chemicals based on short-term *in vivo* studies, in which a pathologic (tumor) response was defined. On the basis of gene expression signatures from early time points, investigators have shown significant predictive accuracy (ranging from 77.5% to 93.9%) in discriminating carcinogens from noncarcinogens when comparing carcinogenic endpoints in the chronic 2-year bioassay. For example, multiple 90-day studies were conducted in mice that were exposed to known lung or liver carcinogens (Thomas et al. 2007a,b), and through gene expression profiling, the investigators were able to identify multiple biomarkers at this early time point in each tissue that could discriminate between carcinogen and noncarcinogen (Thomas et al. 2007b). They further identified (within this data set) a six-gene classifier involving differentially expressed genes associated with endogenous and xenobiotic metabolism and growth factor signaling, commonly dysregulated pathways in neoplasia, that predicted the development of lung tumors by 2 years with 93.9% accuracy. Using 28-day exposures, Nakayama et al. (2006) identified differences in gene expression profiles related to the p53 DNA damage pathway between carcinogenic and noncarcinogenic isomers of various compounds, in order to develop an effective method of predicting hepatocarcinogenicity of compounds with similar chemical structure. Even earlier time points in exposure have been investigated as potentially useful in predicting tumor outcomes. Ellinger-Ziegelbauer et al. (2004) identified differentially expressed genes and pathways by 14 days of exposure associated with genotoxic compounds in the liver (Ellinger-Ziegelbauer et al. 2004), and a 5-day exposure of the nongenotoxic chemical, phenobarbital, was used by Kramer et al. (2004a) to establish biomarker genes that could distinguish carcinogens from noncarcinogens. Furthermore, Tsujimura et al. (2006) used an *in vitro* rat hepatoma cell model to accurately differentiate carcinogens from noncarcinogens, and hepatocarcinogens from noncarcinogens, with 88.9% accuracy, using a training set of known hepatocarcinogens, nonhepatic carcinogens, and noncarcinogens (Tsujimura et al. 2006). These studies demonstrated that liver and lung tumorigenesis could potentially be predicted by gene expression analysis using biomarkers from early and subchronic exposures, both *in vitro* and *in vivo*.

7.6 GENOTOXIC VERSUS NONGENOTOXIC

Carcinogens are generally divided into genotoxic and nongenotoxic compounds (Figure 7.4). Both classes induce tumors in rodents, most commonly in the lung, liver, mammary gland, stomach, vascular and hematopoietic systems, kidney, and urinary bladder (Gold et al. 1993; Waters et al. 2010). The classification of compounds as genotoxic or nongenotoxic in nature for cancer risk assessment

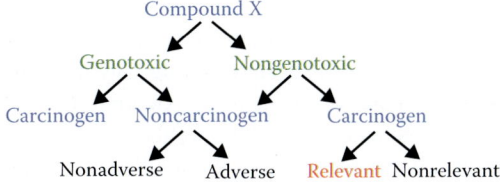

FIGURE 7.4 This algorithm demonstrates the potential strategy used to classify compounds using predictive gene expression profiles to identify genotoxic and nongenotoxic carcinogens as well as mechanistic relevance to humans to ultimately identify compounds relevant to human risk determination.

and drug development is very important, and means to predict the carcinogenic response to various genotoxic and nongenotoxic carcinogens is of great interest (Ellinger-Ziegelbauer et al. 2008, 2009). The link between genotoxicity and cancer is well known; genotoxic carcinogens directly alter DNA through point mutations, insertions, deletions, or changes in chromosome structure or number and form DNA adducts within the cells of target tissues, leading to initiation of neoplastic transformation (Butterworth 1990; Ellinger-Ziegelbauer et al. 2008, 2009; Waters et al. 2010). Nongenotoxic carcinogens are not DNA reactive, but rather act in an epigenetic fashion, or indirectly by inducing effects in target cells that either indirectly influence cellular transformation or promote initiated cells along the pathway of neoplastic transformation (Ellinger-Ziegelbauer et al. 2005, 2008). Nongenotoxic compounds act through various mechanisms to promote these carcinogenic pathways, including cell cycle dysregulation, increased mitogenesis, decreased apoptosis, or interference with intercellular signaling, endocrine, or immune function (Combes 2000; Ellinger-Ziegelbauer et al. 2008, 2009; Waters et al. 2010; Williams 2001). Furthermore, such compounds may result in genotoxicity as a secondary effect of toxicity by inducing cellular responses to toxicity such as marked regenerative cellular growth and proliferation or increased oxidative stress from excessive production of reactive oxygen and nitrogen species that damage DNA and other cellular constituents, which promote neoplastic transformation (Butterworth 1990; Cohen 1995; Cunningham 1996; Ellinger-Ziegelbauer et al. 2005, 2008; Klaunig et al. 1998; Waters et al. 2010; Williams 2001).

Genotoxic mechanisms of direct DNA damage are a hallmark of carcinogenesis. Prediction of carcinogenicity of compounds *in vitro*, using standard genotoxicity assays, is the current standard by which prediction of genotoxic mechanisms is measured. However, current assays that are used to detect genotoxicity are somewhat imprecise, have low specificity, and are generally insufficient to model the complex disease of cancer, and can often overpredict carcinogenesis, leading to false-positive results (Ellinger-Ziegelbauer et al. 2008, 2009; Kirkland et al. 2005, 2006; Ward 2007). In addition, over one-half of chemically induced tumors are caused by nongenotoxic compounds, which are difficult to predict in short-term assays (Nie et al. 2006). Furthermore, nongenotoxic compounds may induce a genotoxic response *in vitro* using current genotoxicity assays, owing to secondary mechanisms of DNA damage, as discussed previously. This makes interpretation of genotoxicity data for nongenotoxic compounds confusing and difficult in terms of human risk assessment. In fact, the ability to predict carcinogenicity in humans as a result of these assays has been questioned (Ellinger-Ziegelbauer et al. 2009; Kirkland et al. 2006; Waters et al. 2010). Additionally, since nongenotoxic mechanisms may be dictated or influenced by a dose response and be subject to a no-observable-adverse-affect level (NOAEL), both the assessment of mechanism and prediction of carcinogenesis based on dose response are important for nongenotoxic compounds relative to risk assessment.

The pathogenesis of cancer is complex and multifactorial, and its full complexity can only be examined using an *in vivo* rodent bioassay model that provides biologically relevant information, key events, and mechanism of action on target organ biology (Ellinger-Ziegelbauer et al. 2009; Holsapple et al. 2006). Utilizing predictive toxicogenomics at early time points, several investigators have examined differences in global gene expression between genotoxic and nongenotoxic compounds that are relevant to a carcinogenic endpoint in rodent models so as to establish early on key genomic events differentiating genotoxic from nongenotoxic mechanisms during the course of exposure (Waters et al. 2010). Genotoxic carcinogens have been shown to be associated with changes in gene expression indicative of a strong DNA damage response suggesting alteration in DNA structure, while induction of cell cycle genes and oxidative stress is consistent with nongenotoxic carcinogenesis (Ellinger-Ziegelbauer et al. 2005). Others have shown that nongenotoxic compounds are associated with prominent induction of metabolism genes, such as xenobiotic receptor agonists, peroxisome proliferator–activated receptors (PPARs), or hormonal responses (Fielden et al. 2007). For example, Ellinger-Ziegelbauer et al. (2005) studied the effects at 14 days on gene expression of a number of genotoxic and nongenotoxic compounds known to induce liver tumors in rats by 2 years, in order to define whether sets of dysregulated genes differentiated between genotoxic and nongenotoxic compounds and whether these gene sets represented relevant and logical biological pathways (Ellinger-Ziegelbauer et al. 2005). Genotoxic compounds elicited a gene expression signature involving induction of a p53 response, including upregulation of *Bax*, *p21*, *Btg2*, *Cccng1*, and *Mdm2*, suggestive of direct DNA damage and cell survival and proliferation pathways, while nongenotoxic compounds induced genes associated with cell cycle progression and a weaker p53 response, consistent with increased mitosis that was observed histologically. The latter was indicative of a strong oxidative stress response, which may often be responsible for secondary DNA damage and gene mutation, or enhancement of survival and proliferation of cells due to regenerative responses to lipid peroxidation or cellular damage and cytotoxicity (Ellinger-Ziegelbauer et al. 2005, 2008). In terms of predicting nongenotoxic carcinogens, Kramer et al. (2004a) identified several potential molecular markers of nongenotoxic carcinogenicity in rats that could differentiate carcinogens from noncarcinogens as early as 5 days of exposure using transcriptional profiling (sensitivity and specificity values of 86% and 81%, respectively) (Kramer et al. 2004a). Nie et al. (2006) identified a six-gene signature that was able to predict known nongenotoxic carcinogens at 24 h of exposure with an 88.5% accuracy predicted by cross-validation and 84% accuracy when samples were hybridized to commercially available oligo arrays (Nie et al. 2006). Fielden et al. (2007) established a predictive gene signature linked to preclinical anchors such as liver weight, hepatocellular hypertrophy and necrosis, serum ALT, and cytochrome p450 levels to predict hepatocarcinogenesis after 5 days of exposure to nongenotoxic compounds in rats. The addition of biologic and pathologic anchors allowed for increased accuracy in predicting nongenotoxic carcinogens, which elicited changes in gene expression consistent with proliferation due to regeneration, xenobiotic metabolism, peroxisome proliferation, and steroid hormone–mediated carcinogenesis (Fielden et al. 2007). In a follow-up study, the Carcinogenicity Working Group of the Predictive Safety Testing Consortium assessed the interlaboratory predictive accuracy of the Nie et al. (2006) and Fielden et al. (2007) data sets in a cross-laboratory meta-analysis validation study evaluating over 150 compounds and showed that while interlaboratory variation reduced predictive accuracy of the original data sets (Fielden et al., 63%–69%; Nie et al., 55%–64%), they were nonetheless deemed to be valuable in early assessment of drug development (Fielden et al. 2008).

Auerbach et al. (2010a) used a training set of known hepatocarcinogens and nonhepatocarcinogens in F344 rats treated for 2, 14, or 90 days to classify a series of alkenylbenzene flavoring agents using toxicogenomics and machine learning (Auerbach et al. 2010a) and showed that the model was able to accurately predict hepatocarcinogenic agents (safrole) from nonhepatocarcinogenic ones (anethole, eugenol, isoeugenol) that were previously evaluated in a carcinogenicity bioassay. Moreover, the model classified two previously unevaluated compounds as weak carcinogens, suggesting that these would be appropriate for further evaluation in a carcinogenicity bioassay (Auerbach et al. 2010a). These studies demonstrate that through the use of toxicogenomic methods, an understanding of the changes in gene expression associated with carcinogenesis of compounds with unknown mechanisms of action may be elucidated based on comparison to chemical classes that have a known mechanism (Fielden et al. 2007). Such predictive association of nongenotoxic compounds at early time points with an ultimate carcinogenic response in the 2-year bioassay would be extremely valuable for hazard identification and risk assessment (Ellinger-Ziegelbauer et al. 2009; Nie et al. 2006). Highly predictive short-term *in vivo* screening assays would provide more efficient means of identifying potential rodent carcinogens while at the same time providing mechanistic information that may be used to determine whether an exposure is relevant to human health (Fielden et al. 2007). However, much consideration must be given to whether or not firm conclusions can be made based on such early time points and the relationship of early gene changes and the ultimate carcinogenic properties of such a wide array of compounds, and how reliable early predictive toxicogenomics can be. For example, while toxicogenomics has potential value in determining dysregulation of gene expression related to early genotoxicity or nongenotoxic mechanisms, this only enables hypothesis generation in terms of whether or not a compound is ultimately carcinogenic. Thus, it is important to appreciate that not a single gene or a particular gene signature will necessarily be adequate for discrimination of genotoxic from nongenotoxic carcinogens, nor all carcinogens from noncarcinogens, and that a systems toxicology or biology paradigm is needed for adequate assessment of complex data sets and pathways related to target organ pathology and molecular mechanism (Ellinger-Ziegelbauer et al. 2009). The pathologist will ultimately play an integral role in connecting such changes in gene expression at such early time points with lesions associated with pre-neoplasia that will ultimately progress to neoplasia. Without this pathology anchor to validate these predictive toxicogenomic carcinogenicity profiles, these data may be viewed as subjective and too weak on which to base significant decisions regarding risk assessment. Validation of these signatures must include pathology assessment at 90-day and 2-year time points, coupled with gene expression validation by QRT-PCR and, ideally, protein evaluation by Western blotting or immunohistochemistry, to demonstrate that the gene changes demonstrated at early time points are part of a mechanism of the continuum of neoplastic transformation and that the alterations in gene expression result in biologically relevant protein signaling associated with tumorigenesis and a morphologic change ("profiling to the phenotype") (Waters et al. 2010).

7.7 TOXICOGENOMIC PROFILING OF HEPATOTOXICITY

The rodent liver transcriptome has been studied by numerous researchers worldwide for decades, and it has provided insight into the complex biological processes involved in liver injury, repair, and hepatocarcinogenesis. To date, hundreds of hepatotoxicants have been studied, and many are known to cause cancer in the rodent, and some are human carcinogens. Gene expression data could be used as an early indicator of liver toxicity because xenobiotic-mediated gene expression changes are often detectable before clinical chemistry, histopathology, clinical, or even ultrastructural changes are seen (Gerrish and Malarkey 2007). Liver injury also causes detectable changes in the transcriptome and microRNAs in blood (Bushel et al. 2007a; Lobenhofer et al. 2008).

The liver receives 25% of the total cardiac output, is the primary site of metabolism of drugs and xenobiotics, and is, therefore, one of the most common sites of toxicity; thus, it is one of the most common concerns of drug-related liability and withdrawals from the market (Huang et al. 2004; Zidek et al. 2007). The liver is a complex organ with multiple metabolic and physiologic functions, composed of various cell populations with differing roles in liver function. The liver is important in the efficient uptake of amino acids, carbohydrates, lipids, and vitamins for storage and metabolism, as well as release into the bloodstream. It plays a central role in biotransformation of xenobiotics and hydrophobic molecules to water-soluble forms, defense against foreign macromolecules, and regulation of blood volume (Malarkey et al. 2005).

While hepatocytes make up 75% of the cell population of the liver (and 80% of the volume), one must consider the various other cell populations within the liver to better interpret genomics data. The other cells include biliary epithelium, endothelial cells (sinusoidal, arteriolar, venular, lymphatic), Kupffer cells, hepatic stellate (Ito) fat-storing cells, resident lymphocytes (pit cells), progenitor cells (oval cells), neuroendocrine cell populations, hematopoietic cell clusters, blood cells, and various extracellular matrix constituents including mesenchymal cell populations (fibroblasts, smooth muscle cells, nerves, mesothelium) and extracellular matrix (5%–10% of the liver is collagen). In normal liver, approximately 40% of the entire genome (~8000 genes) is expressed (Malarkey et al. 2005), and the majority of RNA is derived from the hepatocytes, with smaller proportions contributed from the more minority cell populations such as biliary epithelium, oval cells, Kupffer cells, and mesenchymal components (Auerbach, unpublished data, Table 7.2). For example, it is estimated that hepatocytes contribute 75% of the total RNA in a whole liver specimen, while Kupffer cells, biliary epithelium, hepatic stellate cells, and sinusoidal endothelial cells each contribute approximately 5% of the total RNA in the liver. Not only is it critical to consider the various cell types in the liver when designing and performing a toxicogenomics study, but it is also imperative to understand that the complexities increase with disease as the number of genes being expressed can double (~16,000), and the proportion of contributing cells change (i.e., in cirrhosis). Further

TABLE 7.2
Top 20 Genes Expressed in Rat Liver

Rank	Gene Description
1	Albumin
2	Orosomucoid 1
3	Apolipoprotein A-II
4	Apolipoprotein C-III
5	Fibrinogen γ chain
6	Aldolase B, fructose-bisphosphate
7	Vitamin D binding protein
8	α-1-microglobulin
9	Cytochrome P450, family 2, subfamily E, polypeptide 1
10	Integral membrane protein 2B
11	CCR4-NOT transcription complex, subunit 2
12	Apolipoprotein A-I
13	Cytochrome P450, family 2, subfamily C, polypeptide 8
14	Fibrinogen β chain
15	Apolipoprotein B
16	Haptoglobin
17	Apolipoprotein H
18	Serpin peptidase inhibitor, clade C (antithrombin), member 1
19	Serpin peptidase inhibitor, clade A (α-1 antiproteinase, antitrypsin), member 1
20	Alcohol dehydrogenase 4 (class II), π polypeptide

Source: Auerbach, personal communication.

consideration should be given to variability related to lobe differences, fasting, time of day, and gender (Boorman et al. 2005a,b; Irwin et al. 2004; Morgan et al. 2005). Lobe differences in gene expression profiles may be related to blood flow, metabolic differences between regions within the hepatic lobule, and gene expression differences between the various cell types. For example, Irwin et al. (2004) showed significant differences in gene expression between the median and left liver lobes after treatment with acetaminophen in rats (Irwin et al. 2005). Other experimental variables such as age, strain, route of administration, vehicle, and stress should also be considered.

The various cell types in the liver are involved in different functions and, therefore, have different gene expression profiles under normal conditions as well as under conditions of toxicity. For example, the hepatocyte, containing large amounts of smooth endoplasmic reticulum and rough endoplasmic reticulum (15% of cell volume), numerous ribosomes, golgi, mitochondria (~1000 per cell), lysosomes, and glycogen, is the metabolic powerhouse of the liver and, thus, has a gene expression profile indicative of these cell-specific functions. Upregulation of genes encoding for various growth factors (*Tgfα, Fgf, Igf1*), metabolic enzymes (carboxykinases, glucokinases, glutamine synthetase, aminotransferases), and matrix enzymes and proteins (fibronectin, collagens, laminin, α1-antitrypsin) is also found in the normal liver. Biliary epithelium, involved in modification of canalicular bile and communication with other cell types during growth and response to injury, expresses genes associated with cellular growth and differentiation (*Egfr*), pancreatic peptide receptors (secretin receptor, somatostatin receptor), and cell communication and inflammation (MHC class I/II, cell matrix adhesion molecules, glutamyl transpeptidase, carcinoembryonic antigen [*Cea*], and epithelial membrane antigen [*Ema*]). Hepatic stellate cells, which play a major role in hepatocellular regeneration and hepatic fibrogenesis, express genes encoding for extracellular matrix proteins (fibronectin, others), cell proliferation and fibrogenesis genes (*Tgfβ, Hgf, Igf2*), and structural proteins (vimentin, desmin, smooth muscle actin), necessary for remodeling of the hepatic parenchyma in response to injury. The sinusoidal endothelial cell plays a role in filtration of fluid solutes and particles owing to its fenestrated structure and lack of a basal lamina. Moreover, it plays a significant role in endocytosis and various disease states such as atherosclerosis, cirrhosis, and tumor metastasis and, therefore, expresses various genes associated with vascular and cellular adhesion (*Icm1*, *F8ra*, *Icam1*), leukocyte cell surface markers (*Cd34*, *Cd4*, *Cd14*, *Cd16*), and immunomodulatory genes (*Il1*, *Il6*, *Nos1*). Finally, the Kupffer cell, which is considered the first line of defense in the liver, is a phagocytic resident cell within sinusoids (30% of sinusoidal cells) derived from circulating monocytes. These cells are mediators of inflammation and the major producers of cytokines; therefore, their gene expression signatures reflect their functions in antigen recognition and phagocytosis (*MhcII*) and inflammation (*Tnfα*, *Tgfβ*, *Il1*, *Il6*, *Il10*, *Infγ*). While the contributions to gene expression of the various cell populations in the liver are complex, the toxicologic pathologist, as a specialist in systems biology, plays an important role in understanding the interactions and response of each of these cell populations to toxicity and thus can relate transcriptomic responses to toxicity in the liver to biologically meaningful endpoints.

In addition to differences in gene expression between the constituent cell populations of the liver, there are lobular differences in gene expression. Specifically, vascular gradients exist within the lobule as blood travels from the portal veins, along the sinusoids, to the central vein within the hepatic lobule. For example, expression of glycogen-6-phosphatase is 8-fold increased in portal areas versus that in centrilobular areas, while expression of glucokinase is 3.4-fold increased in centrilobular zones as compared to periportal areas (Teutsch et al. 1999). The oxygen saturation in periportal areas is twice that in the centrilobular areas because of loss of oxygen tension as blood percolates from the hepatic artery to the central veins in the lobule. In periportal areas, there is increased expression of peroxisome proliferators, glutathione content, and bile acid uptake, and glycogen synthesis occurs first in this region. Glutamine synthetase is exclusively expressed in centrilobular areas, and other enzymes important in metabolism and biotransformation such as ethanol-inducible cyp2E1 and carboxylesterase are predominantly expressed here. Fenestrae of sinusoidal endothelial cells are of greater size and number as they progress toward the central veins, and Kupffer cells are larger with increased phagocytic ability in the periportal regions. Periportal hepatic stellate cells contain smaller volumes of lipid, whereas midzonal cells contain a large volume of lipid, and centrilobular hepatic stellate cells contain reduced amounts of vitamin A and desmin. Constituents of the extracellular matrix are also influenced by the architecture of the lobule, with laminin, collagen type IV, and heparan sulfate predominating in the space of Disse in periportal areas, while fibronectin, collagen type III, and dermatan sulfate are found in the centrilobular areas. Considering the variability in cell populations, as well as differences in gene expression within the hepatic lobule (centrilobular versus periportal) in response to various compounds, one method to minimize variability in sampling is the use of laser capture microdissection (LCM). With the ability to visualize the components of each section and isolate specific areas of the hepatic lobule, variation in toxicogenomics data resulting from differences in gene expression in various parts of the lobule, or in different cell populations, can be minimized. Furthermore, LCM can be used to answer specific questions that a whole tissue lyse cannot, such as gene expression in particular components of the lobule (hepatocytes, biliary epithelium, vascular components) owing to chemical exposure. This is of particular importance when studying modes of action of hepatotoxicity and biliary hyperplasia using mechanistic toxicogenomics methods.

Other experimental variables affecting gene expression in the liver include fasting, circadian rhythm, age, sex, strain, route of administration, vehicle, and stress. The state of fasting influences the physiologic state of the hepatocyte, including glycogen stores. As an animal is fasted, glycogen is metabolized to glucose for utilization, and thus, glycogen stores are depleted, as evidenced on hematoxylin and eosin–stained histologic specimens as a reduction of hepatocyte volume and loss of "moth-eaten" appearance of the hepatocyte cytoplasm. These histologic changes reflect alterations in gene expression, and unless all animals are fasted equally and sacrificed at the same time of day, the differences in hepatocyte appearance seen histologically will be evident in the gene expression profiles and could represent a significant confounding variable to proper interpretation of the toxicogenomic data (Boorman et al. 2005a). Increasing age also affects gene expression in the liver. With increasing age, there is a reduction in the overall number of hepatocytes but increased numbers that are hypertrophic and show polyploidy. Sex differences in the liver include significant contributions of gene expression due to estrogens in females and androgens in males, primarily related to the effects of growth hormone during puberty (Rogers et al. 2007). Given the potential significance of these changes in the analysis and interpretation of toxicogenomics data, animals on every toxicogenomics study should be age and sex matched. Route of administration and vehicle may alter gene expression results since route of administration affects toxicokinetics of the metabolism of compounds, and different vehicles may influence the metabolic status of the liver (e.g., methylcellulose versus corn oil). Stress from transport or chemical exposure may alter gene expression in the liver. Chida et al. (2006) documented that stress related to restraint leads to increases in ALT and that possible mechanisms for alterations in liver function due to stress include expansion of the natural killer cell population and inflammatory changes leading to hepatocellular damage and impairment of blood flow to regions of the brain responsible for proper hepatocellular function (Chida et al. 2006). Finally, strain differences account for a significant difference in the response of the liver to various compounds, which significantly influences gene expression. Bradford et al. (2011) showed considerable differences between 15 different mouse strains in the oxidation and conjugation of trichloroethylene (TCE), a well-known rodent carcinogen and probable human carcinogen (Bradford et al. 2011). They showed that treatment-specific effects of TCE on the liver transcriptome, particularly PPAR effects, are highly dependent on resistance and susceptibility differences in various strains of mice. The above data emphasize the fact that variability due to sampling, strain, sex, and age differences; vehicle; route of exposure; and circadian rhythm can all have a significant impact on the analysis and interpretation of toxicogenomics data, and all variables must be minimized to prevent misinterpretation of results.

There is much interest in early detection and prediction of hepatotoxicity of new compounds, and toxicogenomics approaches have been heavily used in the assessment of the toxic potential of compounds. In particular, prediction of compounds that elicit acute hepatotoxicity such as necrosis or steatosis is an important focus for predictive toxicogenomics studies (Ellinger-Ziegelbauer et al. 2008). Furthermore, in terms of elucidating molecular mechanisms of toxicity, mechanistic toxicogenomics is helpful when a common toxicologic phenotype such as hepatocellular hypertrophy, biliary hyperplasia, steatosis, or necrosis is produced by a variety of different compounds via several different mechanisms (Buck et al. 2008). Importantly, changes in gene expression resulting from hepatotoxin exposure can be more sensitive than traditional toxicologic assessments such as histopathology and clinical chemistry evaluations, which tend to be inadequate in terms of predictive ability as well as providing insight into the molecular mechanism of hepatotoxicity (Heinloth et al. 2004; Huang et al. 2004). Often, gene expression induced by a low or subclinical dose of a hepatotoxin may be reflective of subtle injury, which, at higher doses, would be evident histologically, making gene expression changes a more sensitive indicator of hepatotoxicity than the traditional endpoints (Heinloth et al. 2004; Ulrich and Friend 2002; Zidek et al. 2007). For example, Heinloth et al. (2004) showed that subclinical doses of acetaminophen elicited changes in gene expression in the liver that indicated adverse hepatocellular effects that were not detectable by histopathology or clinical chemistry (Heinloth et al. 2004). In fact, changes were only evident on transmission electron microscopy, consisting of occasional mitochondrial damage. Gene expression results indicated that the mechanism of action involved is cellular energy loss as a result of ATP depletion, oxidative stress, and DNA damage, and that the resulting signatures became more pronounced with increasing dose. In this way, predictive toxicogenomics allows detection of subtle changes of toxicity that may not be detectable using routine toxicologic endpoints. In another study, Foster et al. showed that a retrospective evaluation of 33 compounds from nonclinical toxicity studies led to the development of robust global gene expression changes that were predictive for toxicity and that transcriptional changes of toxicity observed before traditional study endpoints, including histopathology, occurred in 60% of cases (Foster et al. 2007). Importantly, it must be kept in mind that not all transcriptomic changes associated with toxicity are indeed indications of toxicity but may rather represent adaptive responses to exposures. It is also important to realize the limitations of toxicogenomics analyses in some responses to toxicity due to the differential response in some cases to exposures in target tissues. For example, significant histopathologic changes in a small subset of cells within an organ (single-cell hepatocellular necrosis, scattered single myofiber degeneration, Kupffer cell toxicity) may be difficult to interpret genomically and are better suited and more rapidly detected by histopathology (Foster et al. 2007). By incorporating phenotypic anchoring in toxicogenomic assessments, transcriptomic profiles indicative or suggestive of a toxic response can be confirmed by lesion development or alterations in clinical chemistry parameters for compounds of uncertain mechanism of action.

Because of this ability to detect early or subclinical changes representing adverse effects, toxicogenomics approaches have been used to fill the data gap between exposure and traditional toxicologic endpoints. Through predictive and mechanistic toxicogenomics approaches, researchers have utilized global gene expression profiling in rodent toxicity models to predict outcomes and elucidate mechanisms of hepatotoxicity (Zidek et al. 2007). As described for the prediction of carcinogens and noncarcinogens, as well as genotoxic and nongenotoxic hepatocarcinogens, toxicogenomic prognostication of hepatotoxicity relies on class prediction, based on training sets composed of gene expression profiles of known hepatotoxicants of differing mechanisms that are used to predict the hepatotoxic capacity of compounds with unknown toxicity (Maggioli et al. 2006; Schena et al. 1995; Zidek et al. 2007). Global gene expression profiling for the purpose of understanding hepatotoxicity and establishing a means to predict is of considerable importance. The utility of such an approach depends on whether hepatotoxicants can be distinguished based on their gene expression profiles in target organs that allows for classification of toxicity endpoints and mechanism of action (Hamadeh et al. 2002a). Since classification of compounds may be based on the similarity of the toxicologic endpoints they elicit, Hamadeh et al. (2002a) compared various peroxisome proliferators and phenobarbital using DNA microarrays to illustrate that compounds within the same chemical class, but of differing structure, induce similar gene expression profiles (peroxisome proliferators) but are still unique and discernable. Furthermore, they showed that chemicals from a different chemical class (phenobarbital) exhibit significantly different gene expression profiles in the liver, confirming that intraclass profiles are more similar to one another than those of a different class. This is particularly important when considering that compounds from different chemical classes may produce the same histopathologic endpoint; both peroxisome proliferators and phenobarbital induce centrilobular hepatocellular hypertrophy and are associated with tumor induction in rats and mice, although through differing mechanisms (Davies et al. 2008; Maronpot et al. 2010; Peters et al. 1997). Consistent with what is known about phenobarbital and PPAR mechanisms of hepatocellular hypertrophy and carcinogenesis, peroxisome proliferators induced gene expression changes associated with triglyceride metabolism, fatty acid uptake, and stimulation of the beta-oxidation pathway, while phenobarbital induced various cytochrome p450 genes (*Cyp2b2, 2c6, 3a9*) and several glutathione *S*-transferases. This study showed that it is possible to classify compounds on the basis of their gene expression profiles in rat liver and that these distinctions can be made despite similarities in toxicologic endpoints. Moreover, liver injury may be predicted using a more focused approach with smaller gene sets, rather than genome-wide analysis, to facilitate more rapid screening of chemicals for hepatotoxicity. For example, Zidek et al. (2007) developed a predictive screening system for acute hepatotoxicity through analysis of the gene expression profiles of well-known hepatotoxicants and nonhepatotoxicants in rats using focused gene microarrays of 550 genes after 6, 24, and 72 h of exposure (Zidek et al. 2007). Gene expression analysis accurately predicted hepatotoxicity in each of 64 compounds tested by 24 h, showing that gene expression analysis of a focused group of relatively few genes could discriminate between compounds that caused acute hepatotoxicity and those that did not. Furthermore, only 3 out of the 64 compounds tested (carbon tetrachloride, 1-naphthylisothiocyanate, and acetaminophen) showed evidence of histopathologic changes at 72 h.

Mechanistic toxicogenomics in the liver has facilitated the investigation of mechanisms of toxicity of various hepatotoxins, including carbon tetrachloride (Holden et al. 2000), arsenic (Lu et al. 2001), acetaminophen (Heinloth et al. 2004; Reilly et al. 2001), methapyriline (Hamadeh et al. 2002b), furan (Hamadeh et al. 2004), methotrexate and phenytoin (Huang et al. 2004), enzyme inducers (Bulera et al. 2001; Burczynski et al. 2000; Hamadeh et al. 2002a; Waring et al. 2001b), 2,3,7,8-tetrachlorodibenzo-*p*-dioxin [TCDD] and dioxin-like compounds (Boverhof et al. 2006; Kopec et al. 2008), benzene (Heijne et al. 2005), bromobenzene (Heijne et al. 2003, 2004), aromatic hydrocarbons, indomethacin, carbamazepine (Waring et al. 2001a,b), and oxidant stress/electrophilic reactive compounds (McMillian et al. 2004), among others. Furthermore, many investigators have shown a correlation between gene expression changes and histopathologic endpoints specific for a mechanism of action for a particular hepatotoxin. For example, in order to gain insight into the mechanisms of toxicity of methylpyrilene (MP), Hamadeh et al. (2002b) evaluated global gene expression in livers from rats exposed to MP for 1, 3, and 7 days and phenotypically anchored gene expression to resulting histopathologic lesions (Hamadeh et al. 2002b). Exposure of rats to MP resulted in hepatocellular necrosis, bile duct hyperplasia, periportal inflammatory cell infiltration, and microvesicular hepatocytic vacuolation in treated animals. Results of hierarchical clustering revealed that samples clustered, on the basis of the severity of histopathologic lesions and changes in gene expression, reflected alterations in genes associated with hepatocellular necrosis, biliary hyperplasia, altered fatty acid metabolism, and inflammation, increasing in severity with increasing dose. By phenotypically linking pathology endpoints with gene expression, the authors were able to associate the morphologic changes resulting from hepatotoxicity to specific changes in gene expression and identify low-dose effects that were undetectable by histopathology.

Huang et al. (2004) used gene expression profiling to define multiple toxicity endpoints correlating with histopathologic lesions using various hepatotoxicants (Huang et al. 2004). Using acetaminophen, methotrexate, methapyriline, furan, and phenytoin, each representing a hepatotoxicant that elicits a specific type of hepatic lesion, they showed that gene expression corresponded with a specific hepatic pathology, with dose- and time-related changes in gene expression being evident. Additionally, gene expression changes preceded morphologic alterations in tissue. PCA profiled a clear clustering of each compound, showing that gene expression differences correlated with specific hepatic histopathologic lesions, including centrilobular necrosis (acetaminophen), atrophy, steatosis and necrosis (methotrexate), periportal necrosis and biliary hyperplasia (methapyriline), cholangiofibrosis, biliary hyperplasia, HCC and cholangiocarcinoma (furan), and centrilobular hepatocellular hypertrophy (phenytoin). This study showed that toxicogenomics approaches allow differentiation of histopathologic endpoints based on gene expression, often before the onset of histopathologic lesions, and that these gene signatures can be used to help understand the mechanism of action of other hepatotoxins.

Similar mechanistic toxicogenomics studies by Waring et al. showed that gene expression analysis of rat hepatocytes *in vitro* (Waring et al. 2001a) and livers from rats *in vivo* (Waring et al. 2001b) exposed to 15 known hepatotoxins that induce specific histopathologic lesions (necrosis, hypertrophy, fibrosis, HCC) could be used to elucidate mechanisms of hepatotoxicity and correlate histopathologic and clinical chemistry endpoints. *In vitro*, they showed that each compound could result in a distinct gene expression profile and that similar profiles resulting from hepatotoxin exposure may reflect similar modes of action. Utilizing the same experimental design in rats exposed to the same 15 hepatotoxins *in vivo*, the investigators showed that the results of gene expression profiling of each compound correlated well with the observed histopathology and clinical chemistry endpoints (Waring et al. 2001b). Results of their *in vivo* study corroborated the findings of the *in vitro* study, in that chemicals clustered based on their gene expression in terms of molecular mechanism of hepatotoxicity. Compounds associated with induction of smooth endoplasmic reticulum and enzyme induction (aromatic hydrocarbons) and those causing midzonal and centrilobular (carbon tetrachloride) or periportal (allyl alcohol) necrosis and DNA damage (etoposide, monocrotaline) were evident by cluster analysis and correlated well with the histopathologic and clinical chemistry findings. These studies show that toxicogenomics methods can be used to elucidate mechanisms of hepatotoxicity and may provide a sensitive method for screening various compounds of unknown toxicity.

7.8 TOXICOGENOMIC PROFILING OF NEPHROTOXICITY

The kidney is one of the most common targets for toxicologic lesions, and drug-induced nephrotoxicity is one of the primary concerns in preclinical drug development and safety assessment (Jiang et al. 2007; Kondo et al. 2009; Wang et al. 2008). The kidney is the primary organ for filtration, metabolism, and excretion of drugs and chemicals, and because of its high blood flow (close to one-fourth the total cardiac output), rate of water, electrolyte, and nutrient exchange, and ability to concentrate compounds in urine resulting in exposure to high concentrations of chemicals, it is exposed to much higher concentrations of drugs and other chemicals than other organs (Khan and Alden 2001; Kondo et al. 2009; Thukral et al. 2005; Wang et al. 2008; Werner et al. 1995). Additionally, the kidney is able to dissociate protein-bound toxins that other organs otherwise do not come into contact with, alter the pH of the urinary solute, and, thus, contribute to the biotransformation of compounds to reactive forms. This organ is also directly involved in xenobiotic metabolism. Given the importance of the kidney in toxicologic exposures, better models of predicting human renal hazards are needed. There are numerous mechanisms of renal injury due to nephrotoxin exposure, whether a direct consequence of exposure to a compound or secondary to other injury. These compounds have been classified by Khan and Alden (2001) as follows: (1) compounds directly altering organelle function, (2) injury caused by reactive intermediates or oxidative stress, (3) compound causing alterations of substrates (cellular, interstitial, or luminal), (4) compounds that cause abnormalities in renal hemodynamics (increased or decreased glomerular filtration rate), and (5) compounds that elicit immune-mediated disease. Therefore, a good understanding of the molecular and biochemical effects of chemicals at all tissue levels and an understanding of tissue responses to various types of injury are important in defining a toxicologic risk, making the toxicologic pathologist critical as part of any toxicogenomics study interpreting gene expression changes resulting from nephrotoxin exposure.

Traditional biomarkers of kidney function such as BUN and creatinine are relatively insensitive in terms of identifying early nephrotoxicity since loss of three-fourths of the nephrons is necessary before significant elevations in these enzymes can be detected (Amin et al. 2004; Decristofaro and Daniels 2008; Price 1992; Wang et al. 2008). Additionally, alterations in BUN and creatinine give a general indication of nephrotoxicity, but they do not provide information on region of the kidney affected (Thukral et al. 2005). Therefore, a primary concern in safety assessment is early detection of kidney dysfunction as an indicator of nephrotoxicity before morphologic changes are evident to efficiently screen compounds of interest (Jiang et al. 2007; Kondo et al. 2009; Thukral et al. 2005). Changes in gene expression that correlate with nephron damage are much more sensitive, and detection of such changes are some of the earliest events that accompany kidney damage, even before histologic lesions are evident (Amin et al. 2004; Fielden et al. 2005; Kondo et al. 2009). To this end, microarray studies on prediction and diagnosis of renal tubular toxicity have been performed to identify early preclinical disease states and region-specific damage of the kidney (Fielden et al. 2005; Kondo et al. 2009; Thukral et al. 2005). Alterations in mRNA expression of specific targets associated with renal cellular damage are followed by general changes associated with either regeneration or repair of the nephron, or fibrosis and further kidney damage.

Toxicogenomics is becoming an attractive method for identifying compounds with possible toxic properties (Kondo et al. 2009), and several nephrotoxic agents have been studied using toxicogenomic methods. Most nephrotoxicants selectively injure the proximal tubule since this segment is the most sensitive component of the nephron and, thus, is most susceptible to injury (Jiang et al. 2007; Khan and Alden 2001; Thukral et al. 2005). For example, cisplatin is a chemotherapeutic agent that has nephrotoxic side effects. This drug injures the proximal tubule and glomerulus as a result of metabolism to toxic intermediates by proximal tubular epithelial cells, resulting in inhibition of DNA synthesis and induction of oxidative stress through glutathione depletion (Amin et al. 2004; Huang et al. 2001; Kramer et al. 2004b). Gentamycin is an aminoglycoside antibiotic that is nephrotoxic through a mechanism of inhibition of liposomal function in proximal tubular epithelial cells, resulting in phospholipidosis and tubular degeneration (Amin et al. 2004; Kramer et al. 2004b). Whereas cisplatin and gentamycin primarily injure the proximal tubule, puromycin (an animonucleoside antibiotic) selectively causes necrosis of glomerular podocytes (Amin et al. 2004) resulting in severe glomerular damage and protein loss with secondary tubular injury due to formation of protein casts in the proximal tubules (Kramer et al. 2004b). Given the differing mechanisms of action of these nephrotoxicants, much work has been done trying to predict nephrotoxicity and define molecular mechanisms using these compounds as models to study nephrotoxicity. Since the kidney is not a homogeneous organ, but rather performs specific and critical biologic functions depending on the segment of the nephron, damage to various segments of the nephron (proximal tubule, distal tubule, collecting ducts, loop of Henle, glomerulus) may be reflected in specific gene changes related to injury or toxicity to a specific segment (Amin et al. 2004). This provides important data on the mechanism of toxicity for various nephrotoxicants with unknown action.

Several groups have analyzed gene expression changes related to mechanism of toxicity for injury to various segments of the nephron *in vitro* and *in vivo* using the classic nephrotoxicants cisplatin, gentamycin, and puromycin (Amin et al. 2004; Huang et al. 2001; Thompson et al. 2004; Thukral et al. 2005; Wang et al. 2008) as well as other nephrotoxins (Kharasch et al. 2006; Luhe et al. 2003; Thukral et al. 2005). Microarray analysis of gene signatures in the kidneys of rats exposed to these drugs has defined novel changes associated with injury in specific portions of the nephron, reflecting site-specific mechanism of action. Using a panel of 48 genes associated with nephrotoxicity curated from the literature, Wang et al. (2008) identified a gene expression signature of acute tubular necrosis in rats exposed to the nephrotoxins gentamycin, bacitracin, vancomycin, or cisplatin (Wang et al. 2008). The alterations in gene expression were consistent with upregulation of the acute phase response, inflammatory, and tissue repair/regeneration/remodeling genes (Kim1, Spp1, Lnc2, Clu, and A2M) and downregulation of genes associated with apoptosis, necrosis, or energy transport (Egf, Rgn, Ngfg, G6pc, Oat, Slc21a1, Bmp4, and Calb1). From this signature, a select set of biomarkers for nephrotoxicity was identified: lipocalin 2 (Lcn2), kidney injury molecule 1 (Kim1), and osteopontin (Spp1). Similarly, Amin et al. (2004) performed microarray analysis of kidneys from rats exposed to cisplatin, gentamycin, and puromycin (Amin et al. 2004). They showed that PCA and hierarchical clustering could define signatures of gene expression and separate samples based on dose, time, and severity of toxicity in kidneys exposed to cisplatin, gentamycin, and puromycin. Using arrays, changes in gene expression due to cisplatin treatment reflected overrepresentation of biologic pathways, including cell cycle regulation, renal injury and regeneration, drug metabolism and detoxification, and creatinine synthesis and osmoregulation. These investigators identified alterations in several of the same genes as the Wang study, as well as other genes previously reported in other models of nephrotoxicity, including heme oxygenase-1, clusterin, thymosin beta-4, and other growth factors (Amin et al. 2004). In contrast, gentamycin induced a decrease in kallikrein, a protein produced in the distal nephron that controls water and sodium homeostasis and that has been implicated in renal injury. Puromycin treatment was associated with increases in several genes associated with glomerular injury or known biomarkers of glomerulopathy (serum amyloid p, cathepsins H and B, alcohol dehydrogenase, solute carrier 4, MIP1-alpha, interferon alpha-inducible protein, retinol binding protein).

Huang et al. (2001) demonstrated alterations in gene expression in kidneys of rats exposed to cisplatin consistent with a mechanism of apoptosis and disruption of intracellular calcium homeostasis, as well as upregulation of genes associated with tissue remodeling, cell proliferation, oxidative stress, and multidrug resistance (Huang et al. 2001). In order to develop a more rapid and less labor-intensive high-throughput assay, the authors used rat kidney epithelial cells and hepatocytes exposed to cisplatin to validate the gene expression changes observed *in vivo*. The results of microarray analysis of gene expression changes in cell lines revealed that the liver cells appeared more sensitive to cisplatin toxicity than kidney epithelial cells, which was the opposite effect than what was seen *in vivo*. Therefore, while cell lines are an efficient system to rapidly assess gene changes resulting from toxin exposure, they may not be the best system to examine an *in vivo* response, and extrapolation to *in vivo* data is unreliable and may not be a proper substitute for *in vivo* models (Huang et al. 2001). Pathologists play a significant role in assessment and relevance of *in vivo* changes as they relate to tissue morphology and toxic effects, such that relying strictly on gene expression changes in cell culture is not the best predictor of toxicity. Through correlation of pathology endpoints with gene expression patterns of nephrotoxicity, toxicogenomics methods may enhance our understanding of mechanisms of region-specific nephrotoxicity in risk assessment and drug development.

Since nephrotoxicity plays a critical role in the decision to pursue a drug for development, early detection of nephrotoxic compounds would greatly reduce labor and expense and increase the efficiency of drug development (Kondo et al. 2009). Therefore, in addition to the above mechanistic studies of nephrotoxicants, others have developed predictive studies to identify potential nephrotoxic compounds. Fielden et al. (2005) analyzed expression profiles from male rats exposed to 64 nephrotoxic or nonnephrotoxic treatments to develop a training data set to predict gene expression for tubular degeneration at early time points, weeks before histopathologic lesions were evident (Fielden et al. 2005). From this set of 64 compounds, 35-gene signatures accurately predicted structurally distinct nephrotoxic agents from the training set 76%, thus providing enhanced predictability, since clinical chemistry and histopathologic evaluations were unable to predict future lesion development. However, sensitivity of the predictive power of these toxicogenomic assays can be greatly improved when rooted in pathology endpoints. For example, Thukral et al. (2005) used toxicogenomics methods to identify biomarkers and evaluate mechanisms of nephrotoxicity linked to pathology endpoints of tubular degeneration, regeneration, and necrosis using various nephrotoxicants, including mercuric chloride, 2-bromoethylamine hydrobromide, hexachlorobutadiene, mitomycin, amphotericin, and puromycin (Thukral et al. 2005). They showed that gene expression profiles clustered based on the type and severity of renal pathology rather than by chemical type. Importantly, using these data as a training set, they were then able to predict the severity and type of pathology resulting from various nephrotoxin exposures on the basis of gene expression profiles, with 82% accuracy. These data show that changes in gene expression due to nephrotoxicity can be correlated with pathology endpoints to increase predictive power. Further, Jiang et al. (2007) showed that by correlating specific pathology endpoints such as proximal tubular damage to gene expression profiles in rats exposed to 10 different nephrotoxins, an improved sensitivity of 91% was achieved (Jiang et al. 2007). Kondo et al. (2009) performed global gene expression analysis on 33 nephrotoxicants in rats correlated with histopathologic findings. The results of this combined analysis was the development of a 92-gene signature that included both known biomarkers of nephrotoxicity, as well as novel targets reflecting activation of pathways associated with tissue remodeling, inflammation, cell proliferation and migration, and oxidative stress (Kondo et al. 2009). Most importantly, anchoring gene expression changes to histopathology endpoints of tubular injury resulted in improvement of prediction over that by either histopathology or gene expression analysis alone. However, while this 92-gene signature accurately identified nephrotoxins that would cause future tubular injury, some compounds that were considered negative by genomics analysis went on to cause histopathologic lesions of tubular damage. The occurrence of such false negatives in toxicogenomics studies is evidence of why genomics must always be rooted in pathology. Without a pathology outcome to anchor gene expression, predictive studies on nephrotoxicity, as with other endpoints, are problematic. While toxicogenomics is a powerful tool in the identification of potential nephrotoxicants, these studies show the importance of anchoring gene expression in pathology endpoints, in that correlations between well-known and novel biomarkers and functional groups of altered genes can be correlated with specific histopathologic lesions, thus providing important information both on the mechanism of action and on increasing the power of prediction in terms of toxicogenomics. When coupled with analysis of classic clinical and pathologic endpoints, renal gene expression profiling is a powerful tool to identify mechanisms of nephrotoxicity and potential bio-markers of kidney disease and may be useful in predicting nephrotoxicity of chemicals of unknown toxicity, including region-specific lesions within the nephron.

7.9 TOXICOGENOMIC PROFILING OF CARDIOTOXICITY

The heart is an important target for toxicity of natural toxins, industrial compounds, and almost every class of pharmaceutical (Buck et al. 2008; Decristofaro and Daniels 2008), including nonsteroidal anti-inflammatory drugs (Brophy 2007; Caporali and Montecucco 2005), chemotherapeutic agents (Albini et al. 2010; Broder et al. 2008; Keefe 2002; Krischer et al. 1997), antidiabetic, immunomodulatory, glucocorticoid, and antifungal agents (Slordal and Spigset 2006). It is also important to understand that there are significant strain differences in susceptibility between mice to cardiac pathology, which can be reflected in gene expression analysis (Auerbach et al. 2010b). Cardiotoxicity resulting from drug effects can be categorized according to (1) structural damage; (2) functional alterations, with or without morphologic change; and (3) altered tissue or cell homeostasis without observable changes in structure or function (Decristofaro and Daniels 2008; Wallace et al. 2004). Much of the -omics work done in cardiac studies has focused on biomarker development in terms of myocardial infarction, in which there is myofiber compromise due to ischemia, resulting in release of cellular proteins after myofiber damage, which are then detectable in serum, including creatinine kinase, lactate dehydrogenase, myoglobin, heart fatty acid–binding protein, and troponins T and I (Decristofaro and Daniels 2008; Mori et al. 2010). However, these cell damage markers are not necessarily increased in cases of drug-induced arrhythmias, valve disorders, or abnormalities in contractility, wherein there is no alteration of myofiber membrane permeability or cardiac cell injury (Decristofaro and Daniels 2008). Some changes in gene expression related to myocardial damage, including hypertrophy, include upregulation/re-expression of fetal oncogenes (myc, fos, jun) and fetal structural genes (β-myosin heavy chain, α-skeletal muscle actin), but these tend to occur along with histopathologic changes (Decristofaro and Daniels 2008; Mikaelian et al. 2008). There are relatively few ways the heart can respond to myocyte toxicity; usually, histologic findings of cardiotoxicity consist of myofiber degeneration, apoptosis, or necrosis, with variable replacement by interstitial fibrosis. Often, in safety studies of compounds, these morphologic changes are observed at a later stage in the study when lesions are well developed. Toxicogenomic analysis of compound-induced cardiotoxicity at early stages in the disease process would allow for a better understanding of mechanisms of cardiotoxicity. Furthermore, an understanding of early events in drug-induced cardiac lesions would allow identification of compounds with potential cardiac side effects earlier in the drug development process (Buck et al. 2008).

Although relatively fewer toxicogenomics studies have been performed on cardiotoxins compared to hepatotoxins and nephrotoxins, several investigators have utilized these applications for development of models of prediction or determination of molecular mechanisms of cardiotoxicity for various chemotherapeutics (doxorubicin) (Buck et al. 2008; Mori et al. 2010; Yi et al. 2006) and other pharmaceuticals (isoproterenol) (Mikaelian et al. 2008; Mori et al. 2010), environmental and occupational compounds (carbofuran, phthalates) (Mori et al. 2010; Singh and Li 2011), and other toxins (tobacco smoke) (Halappanavar et al. 2009). In terms of chemotherapeutics with cardiac toxicity side effects, doxorubicin has been extensively studied. Doxorubicin is an anthracycline antibiotic used as a chemotherapeutic agent for various cancers, including breast cancer, osteosarcoma, and lymphoma (Singal and Iliskovic 1998), but its use has been complicated by acute and chronic cardiotoxic side effects leading to cardiomyopathy and heart failure. Doxorubicin acts to destroy highly proliferative tumor cells through direct DNA damage and in the process contributes to a high degree of free-radical generation leading to detrimental effects on the cardiac myocyte, including cellular organelle damage, and subsequently cell death (Kalivendi et al. 2005; Yi et al. 2006). Exposure to doxorubicin in the rat, mouse, and rabbit recapitulates the cardiotoxic effects observed in humans treated with the drug, and as such, they have been used as models to study the mechanisms of doxorubicin-induced cardiotoxicity (Buck et al. 2008; Kalivendi et al. 2005; Robert 2007; Yi et al. 2006). While histopathologic and clinical chemistry evaluations are unremarkable after single treatments or early in the exposure period, several groups have used toxicogenomics applications to show marked changes in gene expression resulting from doxorubicin exposure that are consistent with the proposed mechanisms of toxicity (Buck et al. 2008; Mori et al. 2010; Yi et al. 2006). Using acute and chronic models of doxorubicin cardiotoxicity in mice, Yi et al. (2006) showed that while acute, single, large doses of the drug elicited changes in more transcripts than a low-dose chronic exposure, the chronic model better reflected the clinical disease caused by doxorubicin treatment in human patients: one of progressive myofiber degeneration and loss, resulting in replacement fibrosis, impairment of myocardial relaxation, and insufficient contractility, culminating in dilative cardiomyopathy (Yi et al. 2006). However, in both models, the significant changes in gene expression involved oxidative stress and metabolism, signal transduction, apoptotic mechanisms, and alteration of structural myofiber gene expression, illustrating that the same functional categories of genes were dysregulated in both models, providing early and late determinants of the molecular mechanism of cardiotoxicity leading to cardiomyopathy.

Using a rat model of doxorubicin-induced cardiotoxicity, Buck et al. (2008) showed that shortly after treatment with the drug, significant alterations in gene expression can be detected, primarily related to mitochondrial dysfunction and alterations in calcium regulation that occurred well before measureable decreases in ATP formation, showing that very early gene changes resulting from cardiotoxin exposure can be detected prior to physiologic and functional changes at the subcellular organelle level (Buck et al. 2008). This illustrates the utility of toxicogenomics applications for the identification of compounds with potential cardiac side effects early in the drug development process. In a follow-up study using doxorubicin as a positive control data set, the authors evaluated gene expression changes resulting from 3-day exposures in rats with various compounds in preclinical studies that produced cardiac toxicities by unknown mechanisms (Buck et al. 2008). Transcriptional profiles of these compounds were very similar to that of doxorubicin, suggesting similar mechanisms of toxicity.

Using single dosing of doxorubicin and two other prototypical cardiotoxins with differing mechanisms of toxicity, isoproterenol and carbofuran, Mori et al. (2010) evaluated the transcriptional response in the hearts of rats in conjunction with histopathology to detect potential genomic biomarkers of cardiotoxicity (Mori et al. 2010). Isoprotenerol is a catecholamine that induces acute tachycardia and myocardial infarction (Mikaelian et al. 2008; Mori et al. 2010), while carbofuran is an anticholinesterase pesticide (Gupta 1994). Using toxicogenomics to evaluate these different cardiotoxins, the authors identified gene signatures common between the three compounds that were functionally associated with cell proliferation, chemotaxis, regeneration, and morphogenesis, correlating with histopathologic findings of myofiber degeneration, edema, infiltration of inflammatory cells, and necrosis. Consistent with other studies, gene expression patterns correlated with the type of histopathologic lesion rather than the type of compound examined, suggesting that despite differing mechanisms of action, the morphologic endpoint of cardiotoxicity is consistent between compounds, illustrating the limited adaptive response of the heart to injury. Consistently upregulated genes throughout exposure included genes associated with cardiotoxicity, cardiac infarction, inflammation, dilative or hypertrophic cardiomyopathy, cardiac cytoskeletal proteins, myocarditis, and fibrosis (*Spp1, Fhl1, Timp1, Ccl7, Reg3b*), providing evidence that the upregulation of these common genes may be useful in predicting the cardiotoxicity of compounds with unknown cardiotropic effects (Mori et al. 2010).

Although isoproterenol has been used as a model of myocardial infarction for a number of years, the mechanisms leading to this cardiotoxicity are not well understood (Mikaelian et al. 2008). Several investigators have evaluated alterations of single or small numbers of genes to generate hypotheses regarding the mechanism(s) of myocardial necrosis as a toxic endpoint of exposure to this compound, which include increased myocardial oxygen demand due to tachycardia, electrolyte disturbances, coronary arterial vasoconstriction, and apoptotic mechanisms (Dhalla et al. 1992;

Mikaelian et al. 2008). Mikaelian et al. (2008) developed a model of acute myocardial necrosis to investigate the temporal global gene expression changes that occur after administration of isoproterenol and that correlated with histopathologic evidence of myocardial lesions (Mikaelian et al. 2008). Early in the disease process and occurring concurrently with histopathologic lesion development was upregulation of genes associated with cell death, myocardial damage, and re-expression of fetal genes, growth factors, and protooncogenes, followed by an adaptive response consisting of downregulation of fatty acid metabolism and upregulation of fetal genes, inflammation, and repair (Mikaelian et al. 2008). A very early signature of interleukin (IL)-6 activation was noted and is associated with myocardial ischemia and activation of the JAK/STAT and MAPK pathways, which are associated with myocardial necrosis. This IL-6 response corresponded to alterations in serum troponin levels and the histologic appearance of contraction bands and loss of cross-striations. Anchored to early clinical and histopathology endpoints, this study illustrated the temporal genomic changes related to the mechanism of isoproterenol-induced cardiotoxicity; an early IL-6-induced MAPK signaling response associated with myocardial necrosis and apoptosis, followed by an adaptive response of the myocardium to damage (Mikaelian et al. 2008). These studies stress the importance of early time points in transcriptional profiling in the determination of mechanism of toxicity of various compounds and the importance of anchorage of gene expression changes, particularly those occurring in a time-dependent or temporal manner, with clinical and histopathology findings to reveal biologically relevant mechanisms of toxicologic lesion development.

7.10 TOXICOGENOMIC DATABASES

Predictive toxicogenomics relies on the establishment of training sets of gene expression databases from compounds with known pharmacologic and toxicologic mechanisms of action. The establishment of such databases from a wide variety of chemicals through analysis by advanced bioinformatics methods enables a means by which compounds of unknown mechanism of action may be assayed for potential toxicity or carcinogenicity (Ge and He 2009). Those databases that provide information on histopathologic endpoints provide a more powerful means of prediction since gene expression can be related to lesion development and can provide the basis for mechanistic toxicogenomics as well, since different histopathologic lesions have been associated with distinct changes in gene expression and even specific gene signatures. Numerous toxicogenomics databases have been generated, many of which are available in the public domain. Such large-scale databases illustrating the effects on gene expression in multiple organs from different species at different time points and doses of various compounds provide the context to interpret mechanisms of toxicity and enhance prediction of toxicity or carcinogenicity endpoints.

The Chemical Effects in Biologic Systems database (http://www.niehs.nih.gov/research/resources/databases/cebs/index.cfm) is an integrated repository for toxicogenomics data designed and maintained by the National Institute of Environmental Health Sciences that is available publicly and includes microarray data, proteomics, and concurrent histopathologic lesions and clinical chemistry data in the context of biology in order to facilitate data integration across multiple studies (Waters et al. 2008). There are currently over 4000 microarray studies in this database, representing a significant wealth of information on toxicogenomics studies of interest to environmental scientists from academia, industry, and government laboratories. Submission of phenotypic anchoring data is required for this database, making it invaluable in terms of relating morphologic endpoints to gene expression induced by exposure to various compounds. Similarly, the Comparative Toxicogenomics Database is a cross-species reference database for establishing mechanisms of action and the effects of chemicals on susceptibility to disease (http://ctd.mdibl.org) (Mattingly et al. 2006). It provides curated information on compounds of toxicologic interest, gene expression data and proteomics, and general toxicology information in various animal species to facilitate integration of toxicogenomics data to better understand chemical–gene and chemical–protein interactions.

The Environment, Drugs, and Gene Expression Database (EDGE) was developed to address the problem of the use of multiple different microarray platforms, protocols, and informatics approaches when analyzing and generating toxicogenomics data and what the effect of the variables can be on the outcome of the interpretation of these findings between laboratories (Hayes et al. 2005; Vollrath et al. 2009). EDGE is a resource that enables scientists involved in toxicogenomics research to share data generated on a common platform, thus allowing the comparison of data sets. This database culminated in the generation of a training set of 117 genomic profiles linked to bioinformatics analysis software to serve as a resource for collaboration in the classification and prediction of hazardous compounds. DrugMatrix (http://ntp.niehs.nih.gov/drugmatrix/index.html), another resource for the sharing of toxicogenomics data, is a database containing microarray analysis of short-term (1-, 3-, and 5-day) studies of over 600 compounds, including industrial and environmental chemicals and pharmaceuticals. In order to facilitate the integration of toxicogenomics into toxicity assessment, NTP has acquired DrugMatrix and its associated assets (ToxFX and large rat tissue library). DrugMatrix is a huge relational database that relates traditional toxicity endpoints such as histopathology to gene expression patterns (derived from ~12,000 Codelink and 5,000 Affymetrix microarrays) from multiple rat tissues (Ganter et al. 2005). A user can upload normalized microarray data and score it against over 500 mode-of-action and pathology signatures, evaluate pathway perturbations, and perform hypergeometric analysis using a collection of toxicologically relevant ontologies, such as human toxicity. The interface allows users to perform extensive mining of the data and to formulate their own gene expression signatures.

ToxFX is an automated toxicogenomics analysis tool that employs the DrugMatrix data and signatures. Data are uploaded and a report is generated in minutes, containing an executive summary of the findings, analysis data, a list of toxicity mechanisms of action signatures present in the data, pathway analysis, and a list of differentially expressed genes. In addition to the analysis and data resources, the DrugMatrix acquisition came with a repository of well-curated frozen tissues that can be used to assess the value of future technologies in toxicity assessment.

There are a number of goals associated with NTP's acquisition of DrugMatrix: (1) make the database freely available to the toxicology community so that they can more effectively interpret toxicogenomics data; (2) make the underlying data freely available so that researchers can mine it and identify new ways of using it to characterize toxicity and disease processes; (3) help build the bridge between traditional toxicity metrics (histopathology) and molecular pathways, which can then be modeled *in vitro* and form the basis of *in vitro* toxicity assessment; and (4) provide a resource of fresh frozen tissues for evaluating new technologies in toxicity assessment.

7.11   SUMMARY AND CONCLUSIONS

As toxicogenomics studies become more and more prevalent in the study of toxicology, hazard identification, risk assessment, and drug development, toxicologic pathologists will be increasingly called upon to contribute their unique set of skills to the design, implementation, and analysis of large microarray experiments in an integrative systemic approach. As a discipline, toxicologic pathology must be a significant part of any toxicogenomics study, because without a phenotypic anchor, changes in gene expression are prone to misinterpretation. As toxicologic pathologists, we must understand that we possess a unique set of training and knowledge incorporating numerous disciplines including biology, anatomy, disease processes, histology, and biochemistry, among others, and this systems biology approach will be critical in the success of any toxicogenomics project. Those of us in a position to do so have a responsibility to ensure that studies are designed appropriately with pathology endpoints in mind, so that the data resulting from these high-throughput, large-scale genomic experiments are interpretable in terms of toxicologic pathology and successful in bringing about a better understanding of toxicologic responses, development of useful biomarkers of disease, and a more efficient means of detecting potentially harmful substances.

GLOSSARY

Bioset: a group of differentially expressed genes from a given set of samples in a microarray data set.

Canonical pathway: a classic or well-characterized biological pathway.

Dendrogram: a branching diagram representing a hierarchy of categories based on degree of similarity or number of shared characteristics.

Differential gene expression: differences in gene expression between biosets based on a response in gene regulation.

Genomics: study of alterations in gene expression, sequence, or structure of the entire genome.

Heat map: a graphical representation of data in which gene expression values are represented as colors in a two-dimensional table.

Hierarchical clustering: the process of organizing expression patterns into groups whose members share similar patterns of expression.

Methylomics: study of genome-wide alterations in methylation and histone codes.

Microarray: a collection of microscopic DNA spots attached to a solid surface used to measure the expression of large numbers of genes simultaneously.

Networks: an integrated collection of gene relationships as defined by biochemical, physical, or transcriptional interactions.

NOAEL: no-observable-adverse-effect level.

NOTEL: no-observable-transcriptomic-effect level.

Overrepresented genes: genes within a bioset that exhibit a high degree of variation in gene expression between study groups.

Pathway analysis: enrichment analysis to determine if genes from certain predefined signaling pathways are overrepresented in a transcriptome profile.

Phenotypic anchoring: the correlation of biologic endpoints including histopathology or clinical chemistry with specific alterations in gene expression due to compound exposure.

Principal component analysis (PCA): a method that reduces data dimensionality by performing a covariance analysis between factors in order to visualize significant differences in global gene expression.

Proteomics: large-scale study of alterations in the structure, function, or interaction of proteins within a biological sample.

Signature, molecular: a group of differentially expressed genes that correlate with, or predict, a biological outcome.

Toxicogenomics: the functional application of genomics to toxicologic exposures.

Training set: known and predictable global gene expression changes from exposures that are used to identify compounds with similar effects on gene expression in order to predict or classify toxicologic outcomes.

Transcriptomics: genome-wide study of changes in mRNA expression from coding DNA (also referred to as genomics).

REFERENCES

Afshari, C. A., Nuwaysir, E. F., and Barrett, J. C. (1999). Application of complementary DNA microarray technology to carcinogen identification, toxicology, and drug safety evaluation. *Cancer Res* **59**, 4759–60.

Albini, A., Pennesi, G., Donatelli, F., Cammarota, R., De Flora, S., and Noonan, D. M. (2010). Cardiotoxicity of anticancer drugs: the need for cardio-oncology and cardio-oncological prevention. *J Natl Cancer Inst* **102**, 14–25.

Amin, R. P., Vickers, A. E., Sistare, F., Thompson, K. L., Roman, R. J., Lawton, M., Kramer, J., Hamadeh, H. K., Collins, J., Grissom, S., Bennett, L., Tucker, C. J., Wild, S., Kind, C., Oreffo, V., Davis, J. W., 2nd, Curtiss, S., Naciff, J. M., Cunningham, M., Tennant, R., Stevens, J., Car, B., Bertram, T. A., and Afshari, C. A. (2004). Identification of putative gene based markers of renal toxicity. *Environ Health Perspect* **112**, 465–79.

Auerbach, S. S., Shah, R. R., Mav, D., Smith, C. S., Walker, N. J., Vallant, M. K., Boorman, G. A., and Irwin, R. D. (2010a). Predicting the hepatocarcinogenic potential of alkenylbenzene flavoring agents using toxicogenomics and machine learning. *Toxicol Appl Pharmacol* **243**, 300–14.

Auerbach, S. S., Thomas, R., Shah, R., Xu, H., Vallant, M. K., Nyska, A., and Dunnick, J. K. (2010b). Comparative phenotypic assessment of cardiac pathology, physiology, and gene expression in C3H/HeJ, C57BL/6J, and B6C3F1/J mice. *Toxicol Pathol* **38**, 923–42.

Boorman, G. A., Anderson, S. P., Casey, W. M., Brown, R. H., Crosby, L. M., Gottschalk, K., Easton, M., Ni, H., and Morgan, K. T. (2002a). Toxicogenomics, drug discovery, and the pathologist. *Toxicol Pathol* **30**, 15–27.

Boorman, G. A., Blackshear, P. E., Parker, J. S., Lobenhofer, E. K., Malarkey, D. E., Vallant, M. K., Gerken, D. K., and Irwin, R. D. (2005a). Hepatic gene expression changes throughout the day in the Fischer rat: implications for toxicogenomic experiments. *Toxicol Sci* **86**, 185–93.

Boorman, G. A., Haseman, J. K., Waters, M. D., Hardisty, J. F., and Sills, R. C. (2002b). Quality review procedures necessary for rodent pathology databases and toxicogenomic studies: the National Toxicology Program experience. *Toxicol Pathol* **30**, 88–92.

Boorman, G. A., Irwin, R. D., Vallant, M. K., Gerken, D. K., Lobenhofer, E. K., Hejtmancik, M. R., Hurban, P., Brys, A. M., Travlos, G. S., Parker, J. S., and Portier, C. J. (2005b). Variation in the hepatic gene expression in individual male Fischer rats. *Toxicol Pathol* **33**, 102–10.

Boverhof, D. R., Burgoon, L. D., Tashiro, C., Sharratt, B., Chittim, B., Harkema, J. R., Mendrick, D. L., and Zacharewski, T. R. (2006). Comparative toxicogenomic analysis of the hepatotoxic effects of TCDD in Sprague Dawley rats and C57BL/6 mice. *Toxicol Sci* **94**, 398–416.

Bradford, B. U., Lock, E. F., Kosyk, O., Kim, S., Uehara, T., Harbourt, D., DeSimone, M., Threadgill, D. W., Tryndyak, V., Pogribny, I. P., Bleyle, L., Koop, D. R., and Rusyn, I. (2011). Interstrain differences in the liver effects of trichloroethylene in a multistrain panel of inbred mice. *Toxicol Sci* **120**, 206–17.

Broder, H., Gottlieb, R. A., and Lepor, N. E. (2008). Chemotherapy and cardiotoxicity. *Rev Cardiovasc Med* **9**, 75–83.

Brophy, J. M. (2007). Cardiovascular effects of cyclooxygenase-2 inhibitors. *Curr Opin Gastroenterol* **23**, 617–24.

Buck, W. R., Waring, J. F., and Blomme, E. A. (2008). Use of traditional end points and gene dysregulation to understand mechanisms of toxicity: toxicogenomics in mechanistic toxicology. *Methods Mol Biol* **460**, 23–44.

Bulera, S. J., Eddy, S. M., Ferguson, E., Jatkoe, T. A., Reindel, J. F., Bleavins, M. R., and De La Iglesia, F. A. (2001). RNA expression in the early characterization of hepatotoxicants in Wistar rats by high-density DNA microarrays. *Hepatology* **33**, 1239–58.

Burczynski, M. E., McMillian, M., Ciervo, J., Li, L., Parker, J. B., Dunn, R. T., 2nd, Hicken, S., Farr, S., and Johnson, M. D. (2000). Toxicogenomics-based discrimination of toxic mechanism in HepG2 human hepatoma cells. *Toxicol Sci* **58**, 399–415.

Bushel, P. R., Heinloth, A. N., Li, J., Huang, L., Chou, J. W., Boorman, G. A., Malarkey, D. E., Houle, C. D., Ward, S. M., Wilson, R. E., Fannin, R. D., Russo, M. W., Watkins, P. B., Tennant, R. W., and Paules, R. S. (2007a). Blood gene expression signatures predict exposure levels. *Proc Natl Acad Sci U S A* **104**, 18211–6.

Bushel, P. R., Wolfinger, R. D., and Gibson, G. (2007b). Simultaneous clustering of gene expression data with clinical chemistry and pathological evaluations reveals phenotypic prototypes. *BMC Syst Biol* **1**, 15.

Butterworth, B. E. (1990). Consideration of both genotoxic and nongenotoxic mechanisms in predicting carcinogenic potential. *Mutat Res* **239**, 117–32.

Caporali, R., and Montecucco, C. (2005). Cardiovascular effects of coxibs. *Lupus* **14**, 785–8.

Carninci, P., and Hayashizaki, Y. (2007). Noncoding RNA transcription beyond annotated genes. *Curr Opin Genet Dev* **17**, 139–44.

Chida, Y., Sudo, N., and Kubo, C. (2006). Does stress exacerbate liver diseases? *J Gastroenterol Hepatol* **21**, 202–8.

Claverie, J. M. (2005). Fewer genes, more noncoding RNA. *Science* **309**, 1529–30.

Cohen, S. M. (1995). Role of cell proliferation in regenerative and neoplastic disease. *Toxicol Lett* **82–83**, 15–21.

Combes, R. D. (2000). The use of structure–activity relationships and markers of cell toxicity to detect nongenotoxic carcinogens. *Toxicol In Vitro* **14**, 387–99.

Cunningham, M. L. (1996). Role of increased DNA replication in the carcinogenic risk of nonmutagenic chemical carcinogens. *Mutat Res* **365**, 59–69.

Davies, R., Clothier, B., Robinson, S. W., Edwards, R. E., Greaves, P., Luo, J., Gant, T. W., Chernova, T., and Smith, A. G. (2008). Essential role of the AH receptor in the dysfunction of heme metabolism induced by 2,3,7,8-tetrachlorodibenzo-*p*-dioxin. *Chem Res Toxicol* **21**, 330–40.

Decristofaro, M. F., and Daniels, K. K. (2008). Toxicogenomics in biomarker discovery. *Methods Mol Biol* **460**, 185–94.

Dhalla, N. S., Yates, J. C., Naimark, B., Dhalla, K. S., Beamish, R. E., and Ostadal, B. (1992). Cardiotoxicity of catecholamines and related agents. In *Cardiovascular Toxicology* (D. Acosta, ed.), pp. 239–282. Raven Press, New York.

Ellinger-Ziegelbauer, H., Aubrecht, J., Kleinjans, J. C., and Ahr, H. J. (2009). Application of toxicogenomics to study mechanisms of genotoxicity and carcinogenicity. *Toxicol Lett* **186**, 36–44.

Ellinger-Ziegelbauer, H., Gmuender, H., Bandenburg, A., and Ahr, H. J. (2008). Prediction of a carcinogenic potential of rat hepatocarcinogens using toxicogenomics analysis of short-term in vivo studies. *Mutat Res* **637**, 23–39.

Ellinger-Ziegelbauer, H., Stuart, B., Wahle, B., Bomann, W., and Ahr, H. J. (2004). Characteristic expression profiles induced by genotoxic carcinogens in rat liver. *Toxicol Sci* **77**, 19–34.

Ellinger-Ziegelbauer, H., Stuart, B., Wahle, B., Bomann, W., and Ahr, H. J. (2005). Comparison of the expression profiles induced by genotoxic and nongenotoxic carcinogens in rat liver. *Mutat Res* **575**, 61–84.

Fielden, M. R., Brennan, R., and Gollub, J. (2007). A gene expression biomarker provides early prediction and mechanistic assessment of hepatic tumor induction by nongenotoxic chemicals. *Toxicol Sci* **99**, 90–100.

Fielden, M. R., Eynon, B. P., Natsoulis, G., Jarnagin, K., Banas, D., and Kolaja, K. L. (2005). A gene expression signature that predicts the future onset of drug-induced renal tubular toxicity. *Toxicol Pathol* **33**, 675–83.

Fielden, M. R., Nie, A., McMillian, M., Elangbam, C. S., Trela, B. A., Yang, Y., Dunn, R. T., 2nd, Dragan, Y., Fransson-Stehen, R., Bogdanffy, M., Adams, S. P., Foster, W. R., Chen, S. J., Rossi, P., Kasper, P., Jacobson-Kram, D., Tatsuoka, K. S., Wier, P. J., Gollub, J., Halbert, D. N., Roter, A., Young, J. K., Sina, J. F., Marlowe, J., Martus, H. J., Aubrecht, J., Olaharski, A. J., Roome, N., Nioi, P., Pardo, I., Snyder, R., Perry, R., Lord, P., Mattes, W., and Car, B. D. (2008). Interlaboratory evaluation of genomic signatures for predicting carcinogenicity in the rat. *Toxicol Sci* **103**, 28–34.

Foley, J. F., Collins, J. B., Umbach, D. M., Grissom, S., Boorman, G. A., and Heinloth, A. N. (2006). Optimal sampling of rat liver tissue for toxicogenomic studies. *Toxicol Pathol* **34**, 795–801.

Foster, W. R., Chen, S. J., He, A., Truong, A., Bhaskaran, V., Nelson, D. M., Dambach, D. M., Lehman-McKeeman, L. D., and Car, B. D. (2007). A retrospective analysis of toxicogenomics in the safety assessment of drug candidates. *Toxicol Pathol* **35**, 621–35.

Ganter, B., Tugendreich, S., Pearson, C. I., Ayanoglu, E., Baumhueter, S., Bostian, K. A., Brady, L., Browne, L. J., Calvin, J. T., Day, G. J., Breckenridge, N., Dunlea, S., Eynon, B. P., Furness, L. M., Ferng, J., Fielden, M. R., Fujimoto, S. Y., Gong, L., Hu, C., Idury, R., Judo, M. S., Kolaja, K. L., Lee, M. D., McSorley, C., Minor, J. M., Nair, R. V., Natsoulis, G., Nguyen, P., Nicholson, S. M., Pham, H., Roter, A. H., Sun, D., Tan, S., Thode, S., Tolley, A. M., Vladimirova, A., Yang, J., Zhou, Z., and Jarnagin, K. (2005). Development of a large-scale chemogenomics database to improve drug candidate selection and to understand mechanisms of chemical toxicity and action. *J Biotechnol* **119**, 219–44.

Ge, F., and He, Q. Y. (2009). Genomic and proteomic approaches for predicting toxicity and adverse drug reactions. *Expert Opin Drug Metab Toxicol* **5**, 29–37.

Gerrish, K., and Malarkey, D. E. (2007). Genomic profiling of liver injury. In *Hepatotoxicity: From Genomics to In-Vitro and In-Vivo Models*, pp. 465–488. Wiley and Sons, Hoboken.

Gold, L. S., Slone, T. H., Stern, B. R., and Bernstein, L. (1993). Comparison of target organs of carcinogenicity for mutagenic and non-mutagenic chemicals. *Mutat Res* **286**, 75–100.

Guerreiro, N., Staedtler, F., Grenet, O., Kehren, J., and Chibout, S. D. (2003). Toxicogenomics in drug development. *Toxicol Pathol* **31**, 471–9.

Gupta, R. C. (1994). Carbofuran toxicity. *J Toxicol Environ Health* **43**, 383–418.

Halappanavar, S., Stampfli, M. R., Berndt-Weis, L., Williams, A., Douglas, G. R., and Yauk, C. L. (2009). Toxicogenomic analysis of mainstream tobacco smoke-exposed mice reveals repression of plasminogen activator inhibitor-1 gene in heart. *Inhal Toxicol* **21**, 78–85.

Hamadeh, H. K., Bushel, P. R., Jayadev, S., Martin, K., DiSorbo, O., Sieber, S., Bennett, L., Tennant, R., Stoll, R., Barrett, J. C., Blanchard, K., Paules, R. S., and Afshari, C. A. (2002a). Gene expression analysis reveals chemical-specific profiles. *Toxicol Sci* **67**, 219–31.

Hamadeh, H. K., Jayadev, S., Gaillard, E. T., Huang, Q., Stoll, R., Blanchard, K., Chou, J., Tucker, C. J., Collins, J., Maronpot, R., Bushel, P., and Afshari, C. A. (2004). Integration of clinical and gene expression endpoints to explore furan-mediated hepatotoxicity. *Mutat Res* **549**, 169–83.

Hamadeh, H. K., Knight, B. L., Haugen, A. C., Sieber, S., Amin, R. P., Bushel, P. R., Stoll, R., Blanchard, K., Jayadev, S., Tennant, R. W., Cunningham, M. L., Afshari, C. A., and Paules, R. S. (2002b). Methapyrilene toxicity: anchorage of pathologic observations to gene expression alterations. *Toxicol Pathol* **30**, 470–82.

Hatfield, G. W., Hung, S. P., and Baldi, P. (2003). Differential analysis of DNA microarray gene expression data. *Mol Microbiol* **47**, 871–7.

Hayes, K. R., Vollrath, A. L., Zastrow, G. M., McMillan, B. J., Craven, M., Jovanovich, S., Rank, D. R., Penn, S., Walisser, J. A., Reddy, J. K., Thomas, R. S., and Bradfield, C. A. (2005). EDGE: a centralized resource for the comparison, analysis, and distribution of toxicogenomic information. *Mol Pharmacol* **67**, 1360–8.

Heijne, W. H., Jonker, D., Stierum, R. H., van Ommen, B., and Groten, J. P. (2005). Toxicogenomic analysis of gene expression changes in rat liver after a 28-day oral benzene exposure. *Mutat Res* **575**, 85–101.

Heijne, W. H., Slitt, A. L., van Bladeren, P. J., Groten, J. P., Klaassen, C. D., Stierum, R. H., and van Ommen, B. (2004). Bromobenzene-induced hepatotoxicity at the transcriptome level. *Toxicol Sci* **79**, 411–22.

Heijne, W. H., Stierum, R. H., Slijper, M., van Bladeren, P. J., and van Ommen, B. (2003). Toxicogenomics of bromobenzene hepatotoxicity: a combined transcriptomics and proteomics approach. *Biochem Pharmacol* **65**, 857–75.

Heinloth, A. N., Irwin, R. D., Boorman, G. A., Nettesheim, P., Fannin, R. D., Sieber, S. O., Snell, M. L., Tucker, C. J., Li, L., Travlos, G. S., Vansant, G., Blackshear, P. E., Tennant, R. W., Cunningham, M. L., and Paules, R. S. (2004). Gene expression profiling of rat livers reveals indicators of potential adverse effects. *Toxicol Sci* **80**, 193–202.

Holden, P. R., James, N. H., Brooks, A. N., Roberts, R. A., Kimber, I., and Pennie, W. D. (2000). Identification of a possible association between carbon tetrachloride-induced hepatotoxicity and interleukin-8 expression. *J Biochem Mol Toxicol* **14**, 283–90.

Holliday, R. (1994). Epigenetics: an overview. *Dev Genet* **15**, 453–7.

Holsapple, M. P., Pitot, H. C., Cohen, S. M., Boobis, A. R., Klaunig, J. E., Pastoor, T., Dellarco, V. L., and Dragan, Y. P. (2006). Mode of action in relevance of rodent liver tumors to human cancer risk. *Toxicol Sci* **89**, 51–6.

Huang, Q., Dunn, R. T., 2nd, Jayadev, S., DiSorbo, O., Pack, F. D., Farr, S. B., Stoll, R. E., and Blanchard, K. T. (2001). Assessment of cisplatin-induced nephrotoxicity by microarray technology. *Toxicol Sci* **63**, 196–207.

Huang, Q., Jin, X., Gaillard, E. T., Knight, B. L., Pack, F. D., Stoltz, J. H., Jayadev, S., and Blanchard, K. T. (2004). Gene expression profiling reveals multiple toxicity endpoints induced by hepatotoxicants. *Mutat Res* **549**, 147–67.

Irwin, R. D., Boorman, G. A., Cunningham, M. L., Heinloth, A. N., Malarkey, D. E., and Paules, R. S. (2004). Application of toxicogenomics to toxicology: basic concepts in the analysis of microarray data. *Toxicol Pathol* **32 Suppl 1**, 72–83.

Irwin, R. D., Parker, J. S., Lobenhofer, E. K., Burka, L. T., Blackshear, P. E., Vallant, M. K., Lebetkin, E. H., Gerken, D. F., and Boorman, G. A. (2005). Transcriptional profiling of the left and median liver lobes of male f344/n rats following exposure to acetaminophen. *Toxicol Pathol* **33**, 111–7.

Jiang, Y., Gerhold, D. L., Holder, D. J., Figueroa, D. J., Bailey, W. J., Guan, P., Skopek, T. R., Sistare, F. D., and Sina, J. F. (2007). Diagnosis of drug-induced renal tubular toxicity using global gene expression profiles. *J Transl Med* **5**, 47.

Kalivendi, S. V., Konorev, E. A., Cunningham, S., Vanamala, S. K., Kaji, E. H., Joseph, J., and Kalyanaraman, B. (2005). Doxorubicin activates nuclear factor of activated T-lymphocytes and Fas ligand transcription: role of mitochondrial reactive oxygen species and calcium. *Biochem J* **389**, 527–39.

Keefe, D. L. (2002). Trastuzumab-associated cardiotoxicity. *Cancer* **95**, 1592–600.

Khan, N. M. K., and Alden, C. L. (2001). Kidney. In *Handbook of Toxicologic Pathology* (W. M. Haschek, C. G. Rousseaux, and M. A. Wallig, eds.), Vol. 2, pp. 255–335. Academic Press, San Diego.

Kharasch, E. D., Schroeder, J. L., Bammler, T., Beyer, R., and Srinouanprachanh, S. (2006). Gene expression profiling of nephrotoxicity from the sevoflurane degradation product fluoromethyl-2,2-difluoro-1-(trifluoromethyl)vinyl ether ("compound A") in rats. *Toxicol Sci* **90**, 419–31.

Kirkland, D., Aardema, M., Henderson, L., and Muller, L. (2005). Evaluation of the ability of a battery of three in vitro genotoxicity tests to discriminate rodent carcinogens and non-carcinogens. I. Sensitivity, specificity and relative predictivity. *Mutat Res* **584**, 1–256.

Kirkland, D., Aardema, M., Muller, L., and Makoto, H. (2006). Evaluation of the ability of a battery of three in vitro genotoxicity tests to discriminate rodent carcinogens and non-carcinogens II. Further analysis of mammalian cell results, relative predictivity and tumour profiles. *Mutat Res* **608**, 29–42.

Klaunig, J. E., Xu, Y., Isenberg, J. S., Bachowski, S., Kolaja, K. L., Jiang, J., Stevenson, D. E., and Walborg, E. F., Jr. (1998). The role of oxidative stress in chemical carcinogenesis. *Environ Health Perspect* **106 Suppl 1**, 289–95.

Kondo, C., Minowa, Y., Uehara, T., Okuno, Y., Nakatsu, N., Ono, A., Maruyama, T., Kato, I., Yamate, J., Yamada, H., Ohno, Y., and Urushidani, T. (2009). Identification of genomic biomarkers for concurrent diagnosis of drug-induced renal tubular injury using a large-scale toxicogenomics database. *Toxicology* **265**, 15–26.

Kopec, A. K., Boverhof, D. R., Burgoon, L. D., Ibrahim-Aibo, D., Harkema, J. R., Tashiro, C., Chittim, B., and Zacharewski, T. R. (2008). Comparative toxicogenomic examination of the hepatic effects of PCB126 and TCDD in immature, ovariectomized C57BL/6 mice. *Toxicol Sci* **102**, 61–75.

Kramer, J. A., Curtiss, S. W., Kolaja, K. L., Alden, C. L., Blomme, E. A., Curtiss, W. C., Davila, J. C., Jackson, C. J., and Bunch, R. T. (2004a). Acute molecular markers of rodent hepatic carcinogenesis identified by transcription profiling. *Chem Res Toxicol* **17**, 463–70.

Kramer, J. A., Pettit, S. D., Amin, R. P., Bertram, T. A., Car, B., Cunningham, M., Curtiss, S. W., Davis, J. W., Kind, C., Lawton, M., Naciff, J. M., Oreffo, V., Roman, R. J., Sistare, F. D., Stevens, J., Thompson, K., Vickers, A. E., Wild, S., and Afshari, C. A. (2004b). Overview on the application of transcription profiling using selected nephrotoxicants for toxicology assessment. *Environ Health Perspect* **112**, 460–4.

Krischer, J. P., Epstein, S., Cuthbertson, D. D., Goorin, A. M., Epstein, M. L., and Lipshultz, S. E. (1997). Clinical cardiotoxicity following anthracycline treatment for childhood cancer: the Pediatric Oncology Group experience. *J Clin Oncol* **15**, 1544–52.

Lobenhofer, E. K., Auman, J. T., Blackshear, P. E., Boorman, G. A., Bushel, P. R., Cunningham, M. L., Fostel, J. M., Gerrish, K., Heinloth, A. N., Irwin, R. D., Malarkey, D. E., Merrick, B. A., Sieber, S. O., Tucker, C. J., Ward, S. M., Wilson, R. E., Hurban, P., Tennant, R. W., and Paules, R. S. (2008). Gene expression response in target organ and whole blood varies as a function of target organ injury phenotype. *Genome Biol* **9**, R100.

Lord, P. G., Nie, A., and McMillian, M. (2006). Application of genomics in preclinical drug safety evaluation. *Basic Clin Pharmacol Toxicol* **98**, 537–46.

Lu, T., Liu, J., LeCluyse, E. L., Zhou, Y. S., Cheng, M. L., and Waalkes, M. P. (2001). Application of cDNA microarray to the study of arsenic-induced liver diseases in the population of Guizhou, China. *Toxicol Sci* **59**, 185–92.

Luhe, A., Hildebrand, H., Bach, U., Dingermann, T., and Ahr, H. J. (2003). A new approach to studying ochratoxin A (OTA)-induced nephrotoxicity: expression profiling in vivo and in vitro employing cDNA microarrays. *Toxicol Sci* **73**, 315–28.

Maggioli, J., Hoover, A., and Weng, L. (2006). Toxicogenomic analysis methods for predictive toxicology. *J Pharmacol Toxicol Methods* **53**, 31–7.

Malarkey, D. E., Johnson, K., Ryan, L., Boorman, G., and Maronpot, R. R. (2005). New insights into functional aspects of liver morphology. *Toxicol Pathol* **33**, 27–34.

Maronpot, R. R., Yoshizawa, K., Nyska, A., Harada, T., Flake, G., Mueller, G., Singh, B., and Ward, J. M. (2010). Hepatic enzyme induction: histopathology. *Toxicol Pathol* **38**, 776–95.

Mattingly, C. J., Rosenstein, M. C., Davis, A. P., Colby, G. T., Forrest, J. N., Jr., and Boyer, J. L. (2006). The Comparative Toxicogenomics Database: a cross-species resource for building chemical–gene interaction networks. *Toxicol Sci* **92**, 587–95.

McMillian, M., Nie, A. Y., Parker, J. B., Leone, A., Bryant, S., Kemmerer, M., Herlich, J., Liu, Y., Yieh, L., Bittner, A., Liu, X., Wan, J., and Johnson, M. D. (2004). A gene expression signature for oxidant stress/ reactive metabolites in rat liver. *Biochem Pharmacol* **68**, 2249–61.

Mikaelian, I., Coluccio, D., Morgan, K. T., Johnson, T., Ryan, A. L., Rasmussen, E., Nicklaus, R., Kanwal, C., Hilton, H., Frank, K., Fritzky, L., and Wheeldon, E. B. (2008). Temporal gene expression profiling indicates early up-regulation of interleukin-6 in isoproterenol-induced myocardial necrosis in rat. *Toxicol Pathol* **36**, 256–64.

Morgan, K. T., Jayyosi, Z., Hower, M. A., Pino, M. V., Connolly, T. M., Kotlenga, K., Lin, J., Wang, M., Schmidts, H. L., Bonnefoi, M. S., Elston, T. C., and Boorman, G. A. (2005). The hepatic transcriptome as a window on whole-body physiology and pathophysiology. *Toxicol Pathol* **33**, 136–45.

Morgan, K. T., Pino, M., Crosby, L. M., Wang, M., Elston, T. C., Jayyosi, Z., Bonnefoi, M., and Boorman, G. (2004). Complementary roles for toxicologic pathology and mathematics in toxicogenomics, with special reference to data interpretation and oscillatory dynamics. *Toxicol Pathol* **32 Suppl 1**, 13–25.

Mori, Y., Kondo, C., Tonomura, Y., Torii, M., and Uehara, T. (2010). Identification of potential genomic biomarkers for early detection of chemically induced cardiotoxicity in rats. *Toxicology* **271**, 36–44.

Nakayama, K., Kawano, Y., Kawakami, Y., Moriwaki, N., Sekijima, M., Otsuka, M., Yakabe, Y., Miyaura, H., Saito, K., Sumida, K., and Shirai, T. (2006). Differences in gene expression profiles in the liver between carcinogenic and non-carcinogenic isomers of compounds given to rats in a 28-day repeat-dose toxicity study. *Toxicol Appl Pharmacol* **217**, 299–307.

Nie, A. Y., McMillian, M., Parker, J. B., Leone, A., Bryant, S., Yieh, L., Bittner, A., Nelson, J., Carmen, A., Wan, J., and Lord, P. G. (2006). Predictive toxicogenomics approaches reveal underlying molecular mechanisms of nongenotoxic carcinogenicity. *Mol Carcinog* **45**, 914–33.

Pandiri, A. R., Lahousse, S. A., and Sills, R. C. (2011). Molecular techniques in toxicological neuropathology. In *Fundamental Neuropathology for Pathologists and Toxicologists* (B. Bolon and M. T. Butt, eds.), pp. 285–318. Wiley, Hoboken.

Paules, R. (2003). Phenotypic anchoring: linking cause and effect. *Environ Health Perspect* **111**, A338–9.

Peters, J. M., Cattley, R. C., and Gonzalez, F. J. (1997). Role of PPAR alpha in the mechanism of action of the nongenotoxic carcinogen and peroxisome proliferator Wy-14,643. *Carcinogenesis* **18**, 2029–33.

Price, R. G. (1992). The role of NAG (*N*-acetyl-beta-D-glucosaminidase) in the diagnosis of kidney disease including the monitoring of nephrotoxicity. *Clin Nephrol* **38 Suppl 1**, S14–9.

Reilly, T. P., Bourdi, M., Brady, J. N., Pise-Masison, C. A., Radonovich, M. F., George, J. W., and Pohl, L. R. (2001). Expression profiling of acetaminophen liver toxicity in mice using microarray technology. *Biochem Biophys Res Commun* **282**, 321–8.

Robert, J. (2007). Preclinical assessment of anthracycline cardiotoxicity in laboratory animals: predictiveness and pitfalls. *Cell Biol Toxicol* **23**, 27–37.

Rogers, A. B., Theve, E. J., Feng, Y., Fry, R. C., Taghizadeh, K., Clapp, K. M., Boussahmain, C., Cormier, K. S., and Fox, J. G. (2007). Hepatocellular carcinoma associated with liver-gender disruption in male mice. *Cancer Res* **67**, 11536–46.

Schena, M., Shalon, D., Davis, R. W., and Brown, P. O. (1995). Quantitative monitoring of gene expression patterns with a complementary DNA microarray. *Science* **270**, 467–70.

Singal, P. K., and Iliskovic, N. (1998). Doxorubicin-induced cardiomyopathy. *N Engl J Med* **339**, 900–5.

Singh, S., and Li, S. S. (2011). Phthalates: toxicogenomics and inferred human diseases. *Genomics* **97**, 148–57.

Slordal, L., and Spigset, O. (2006). Heart failure induced by non-cardiac drugs. *Drug Saf* **29**, 567–86.

Teutsch, H. F., Schuerfeld, D., and Groezinger, E. (1999). Three-dimensional reconstruction of parenchymal units in the liver of the rat. *Hepatology* **29**, 494–505.

Thomas, R. S., O'Connell, T. M., Pluta, L., Wolfinger, R. D., Yang, L., and Page, T. J. (2007a). A comparison of transcriptomic and metabonomic technologies for identifying biomarkers predictive of two-year rodent cancer bioassays. *Toxicol Sci* **96**, 40–6.

Thomas, R. S., Pluta, L., Yang, L., and Halsey, T. A. (2007b). Application of genomic biomarkers to predict increased lung tumor incidence in 2-year rodent cancer bioassays. *Toxicol Sci* **97**, 55–64.

Thompson, K. L., Afshari, C. A., Amin, R. P., Bertram, T. A., Car, B., Cunningham, M., Kind, C., Kramer, J. A., Lawton, M., Mirsky, M., Naciff, J. M., Oreffo, V., Pine, P. S., and Sistare, F. D. (2004). Identification of platform-independent gene expression markers of cisplatin nephrotoxicity. *Environ Health Perspect* **112**, 488–94.

Thukral, S. K., Nordone, P. J., Hu, R., Sullivan, L., Galambos, E., Fitzpatrick, V. D., Healy, L., Bass, M. B., Cosenza, M. E., and Afshari, C. A. (2005). Prediction of nephrotoxicant action and identification of candidate toxicity-related biomarkers. *Toxicol Pathol* **33**, 343–55.

Tsujimura, K., Asamoto, M., Suzuki, S., Hokaiwado, N., Ogawa, K., and Shirai, T. (2006). Prediction of carcinogenic potential by a toxicogenomic approach using rat hepatoma cells. *Cancer Sci* **97**, 1002–10.

Ulrich, R., and Friend, S. H. (2002). Toxicogenomics and drug discovery: will new technologies help us produce better drugs? *Nat Rev Drug Discov* **1**, 84–8.

Vollrath, A. L., Smith, A. A., Craven, M., and Bradfield, C. A. (2009). EDGE(3): a web-based solution for management and analysis of Agilent two color microarray experiments. BMC Bioinformatics **10**, 280.

Wallace, K. B., Hausner, E., Herman, E., Holt, G. D., MacGregor, J. T., Metz, A. L., Murphy, E., Rosenblum, I. Y., Sistare, F. D., and York, M. J. (2004). Serum troponins as biomarkers of drug-induced cardiac toxicity. *Toxicol Pathol* **32**, 106–21.

Wang, E. J., Snyder, R. D., Fielden, M. R., Smith, R. J., and Gu, Y. Z. (2008). Validation of putative genomic biomarkers of nephrotoxicity in rats. *Toxicology* **246**, 91–100.

Wang, K., Zhang, S., Marzolf, B., Troisch, P., Brightman, A., Hu, Z., Hood, L. E., and Galas, D. J. (2009). Circulating microRNAs, potential biomarkers for drug-induced liver injury. *Proc Natl Acad Sci U S A* **106**, 4402–7.

Ward, J. A. (2007). The two-year rodent carcinogenesis bioassay—will it survive? *J Toxicol Pathol* **20**, 13–19.

Waring, J. F., Ciurlionis, R., Jolly, R. A., Heindel, M., and Ulrich, R. G. (2001a). Microarray analysis of hepatotoxins in vitro reveals a correlation between gene expression profiles and mechanisms of toxicity. *Toxicol Lett* **120**, 359–68.

Waring, J. F., Jolly, R. A., Ciurlionis, R., Lum, P. Y., Praestgaard, J. T., Morfitt, D. C., Buratto, B., Roberts, C., Schadt, E., and Ulrich, R. G. (2001b). Clustering of hepatotoxins based on mechanism of toxicity using gene expression profiles. *Toxicol Appl Pharmacol* **175**, 28–42.

Waters, M., Stasiewicz, S., Merrick, B. A., Tomer, K., Bushel, P., Paules, R., Stegman, N., Nehls, G., Yost, K. J., Johnson, C. H., Gustafson, S. F., Xirasagar, S., Xiao, N., Huang, C. C., Boyer, P., Chan, D. D., Pan, Q., Gong, H., Taylor, J., Choi, D., Rashid, A., Ahmed, A., Howle, R., Selkirk, J., Tennant, R., and Fostel, J. (2008). CEBS—Chemical Effects in Biological Systems: a public data repository integrating study design and toxicity data with microarray and proteomics data. *Nucleic Acids Res* **36**, D892–900.

Waters, M. D., Jackson, M., and Lea, I. (2010). Characterizing and predicting carcinogenicity and mode of action using conventional and toxicogenomics methods. *Mutat Res* **705**, 184–200.

Werner, M., Costa, M. J., Mitchell, L. G., and Nayar, R. (1995). Nephrotoxicity of xenobiotics. *Clin Chim Acta* **237**, 107–54.

Williams, G. M. (2001). Mechanisms of chemical carcinogenesis and application to human cancer risk assessment. *Toxicology* **166**, 3–10.

Yi, X., Bekeredjian, R., DeFilippis, N. J., Siddiquee, Z., Fernandez, E., and Shohet, R. V. (2006). Transcriptional analysis of doxorubicin-induced cardiotoxicity. *Am J Physiol Heart Circ Physiol* **290**, H1098–102.

Yoon, B. I., Li, G. X., Kitada, K., Kawasaki, Y., Igarashi, K., Kodama, Y., Inoue, T., Kobayashi, K., Kanno, J., Kim, D. Y., and Hirabayashi, Y. (2003). Mechanisms of benzene-induced hematotoxicity and leukemogenicity: cDNA microarray analyses using mouse bone marrow tissue. *Environ Health Perspect* **111**, 1411–20.

Zidek, N., Hellmann, J., Kramer, P. J., and Hewitt, P. G. (2007). Acute hepatotoxicity: a predictive model based on focused illumina microarrays. *Toxicol Sci* **99**, 289–302.

8 Spontaneous Lesions in Control Animals Used in Toxicity Studies

Robert C. Johnson, Robert H. Spaet, and Daniel L. Potenta

CONTENTS

8.1 INTRODUCTION

The development of a potential pharmaceutical requires establishing a risk profile that involves animal testing before human exposure. A pathologist is responsible for evaluating a representative list of tissues from study animals during the long, comprehensive toxicology screening process. During this review, the pathologist is often confronted with findings that are of uncertain relationship to the test substance. The comparison of findings in treated animal to those of the concurrent control group provides the initial (and most important) screen in order to make an assessment of a possible relationship to the test substance. There are those instances, however, wherein the concurrent control group will not contain sufficient numbers of animals to clearly make such an assessment. This is particularly true in toxicity studies with dogs and nonhuman primates wherein low numbers of animals are used, typically only 3/sex/group. Pathologists are often confronted with cases in which a finding in the high-dose group represents a tissue change that can represent an incidental finding, which might also be found in control group animals. In this example, as a result of biological variability, the incidence in the high-dose group might be elevated while the incidence in the control group is low or zero, implying a test substance relationship. A limited number of animals, again especially in dog and primate studies, make it difficult to dismiss a finding as unrelated to test substance unless there is a robust local historical control database that can be used to put the data into perspective. Lastly, for subtle changes, it is important to use reliable historical control data to make a proper assessment of potential compound-related effects (Dixon et al. 1995).

One major difficulty with historical control data is consistency. Different facilities quite naturally have different animal husbandry and laboratory animal management practices. Also, individual pathologists have varying thresholds for calling findings, as well as using analogous yet diverse descriptive terminology to describe what is seen. Factors such as food and ambient conditions in the animal room (e.g., water supply and light cycle) must be standardized in order to normalize influences on animal physiology and to minimize any changes that might occur as a result of peripheral, non-test article–related pressures. In addition to these factors, animal source/vendor (Engelhardt et al. 1993), body weight, age, sex, and tissue processing procedures and histopathology diagnostic criteria should also be standardized in a given facility to ensure the most uniform, reliable historical control database available.

The histopathological findings tabulated and discussed in this chapter were obtained from control animals in toxicity studies ranging from 4 to 52 weeks in duration:

1. Four-week studies: Wistar rats (300 animals/sex)
2. Twenty-six-week studies: Wistar rats (200 males, 201 females)
3. Thirteen-week studies: CD-1 mouse (100 animals/sex)
4. Four-week studies: beagle dogs (53 animals/sex)
5. Twenty-six-week and 39-week studies: beagle dogs (32 animals/sex)
6. Four-week studies: cynomolgus monkeys (64 males, 63 females)
7. Twenty-six-week and 52-week studies: cynomolgus monkeys (32 animals/sex)

For consistency, the data for each species and period were collected from one facility over a span of 4–6 years. The animals were bred for laboratory use and came from accredited suppliers. All animals were dosed with vehicle, typically by oral gavage (most studies) or intravenous routes. General trends that could be observed from the data provided are discussed.

8.2 RAT

The rat is the most commonly used species in toxicology testing. The tables below contain control data from the International Genetic Standard Wistar Hannover Rat; Crl:WI(Han), generated from 4-week (Table 8.1) and 26-week (Table 8.2) toxicology studies matching the duration of the most commonly used toxicity testing paradigms. The age of these animals at the start of dosing was typically 8–9 weeks. In general, the incidences of spontaneous findings were consistent with the published data (Stefanski et al. 1990; Tucker 1997).

The control data from the 4-week studies were generated from 300 rats/sex. The highest frequency of control incidental findings in both sexes occurred in the liver, followed by kidney and lung. The liver and lung findings were generally inflammatory in nature, characterized by mixed cell or mononuclear cell infiltrations (up to 40% in males and 60% in females); however, the incidence of extramedullary hematopoiesis (EMH) in the liver was also typically high, reaching 100% in both sexes in some studies. There was also a low incidence of alveolar foam cell accumulation in the lung (up to 10% in males and 30% in females). Kidney findings were frequently degenerative in nature, consisting of tubular epithelial basophilia (up to 40% in males and 20% in females), tubular hyaline droplets (up to 80% in males), and focal tubular mineralization (up to 60% in males and 80% in females). The incidence of pelvic dilation was up to 10% in males and 20% in females. In the lymphoid organs, lymph nodes had a high incidence of background findings, most typically lymphoid hyperplasia (up to 70% in males and 50% in females) and increased plasma cells (up to 50% in males and 20% in females) in addition to sinus histiocytosis (up to 40% in males and 50% in females) and erythrophagocytosis (up to 70% in males and 80% in females). The incidence of increased EMH (up to 60% in males and 90% in females) was generally high in the spleen. The number of findings in the gastrointestinal tract was modest and generally highest in the stomach, consisting of eosinophil accumulations (up to 90% in males and 60% in females), mixed cell inflammation (up to 80% in males and 10% in females), and epithelial vacuolation involving the limiting ridge (up to 80% in males and 40% in females). The stomach findings may have possibly been related to local trauma during the gavage procedure. There were generally few spontaneous findings in the primary and accessory sex organs, glandular tissues, bone marrow, and sensory organs. Notably, the incidence of cardiomyopathy was low in this 4-week data set.

While tubular basophilia in the kidney was higher in males than in females, females had a higher incidence of renal tubular mineralization. Both findings are consistent with the published data (McInnes 2011). The background incidence of inflammatory changes in the 4-week studies was generally higher in males than in females. Hematopoiesis in the spleen was higher in females, again consistent with the published control data (McInnes 2011). There was a moderately high incidence of background findings in the tongue due to bleeding from the sublingual vein and less so in the esophagus, most likely related to gavage. Hemorrhage in the thymus was a relatively common finding and is frequently associated with euthanasia in the absence of necrosis, inflammation, or hemosiderin accumulation (Dixon et al. 1995; Stefanski et al. 1990).

The spectrum of control animal findings in the 26-week rat studies (200 males, 201 females) was generally comparable to those in the 4-week studies; however, as might be anticipated, the incidence of degenerative findings was typically higher in the studies of longer duration (older animals). For example, the maximum incidence in a given study for renal tubular basophilia (up to 30% in males and 19% in females) and chronic progressive nephropathy (up to 25% in males and 15% in females) is highest for males, but higher for both sexes in the 26- versus 4-week studies. Mononuclear infiltrates (up to 55% in males and 20% in females) and tubular casts (up to 10% in males and 14% in females) in the kidney were also higher in the studies of longer duration. The highest number of findings occurred in the stomach of both sexes in the 26-week studies and consisted of epithelial hyperplasia (up to 25% in males and 20% in females), mixed cell inflammation (up to 20% in males and 5% in females), hemorrhage (up to 35% in males and 38% in females), and epithelial vacuolation involving the limiting ridge (up to 30% in males and 10% in females), the incidence of these lesions being generally higher in males. These gastric findings are typically attributed to mechanical trauma caused by the gavage procedure.

The incidence of cardiomyopathy was as high as 20% in males in the 26-week studies. In the liver, hepatocellular vacuolation (up to 15%) and clear cell focus (up to 30%) in the liver of male rats and basophilic cell focus (up to 15% in females) were observed in the 26-week studies. The incidence of mixed cell inflammation in the lung of male and female rats was about the same as that in the 4-week rat studies (up to 10% in males and 15% in females); however, the maximum incidence of alveolar foam cell accumulation/aggregates (up to 25% in males and 20% in females) was higher in the longer-term studies.

In the eye, retinal atrophy/degeneration (up to 15% in males and 5% in females) was observed in the 26-week studies. Mononuclear cell infiltration (up to 30%) and mixed cell inflammation (up to 10%) in the prostate gland, along with testicular tubular degeneration/atrophy (up to 10%), were observed in the 26-week studies. The incidence of hemorrhage (up to 45% in males and 54% in females) in the thymus is significantly elevated in the longer-term toxicity studies in both sexes while lymphoid depletion (up to 25%) is notably higher in male rats in the longer-term studies compared to male control incidences in the shorter-term studies (up to 10%).

TABLE 8.1

Spontaneous Lesions in Control Wistar Rats in Toxicity Studies of 4-Weeks Duration

Rat

4 weeks

		Males						Females					
Organ	Finding	Minimum	Minimum Range (%)	Maximum	Maximum Range (%)	Total Incidence	Total Incidence	Minimum	Minimum Range (%)	Maximum	Maximum Range (%)	Total Incidence	Total Incidence (%)
						300						300	
Adrenal	Accessory cortical tissue	0	0.0	5	50.0	6	2.0	0	0.0	4	40.0	9	3.0
Adrenal	Cortical hypertrophy, zona fasciculata	0	0.0	2	20.0	2	0.7	0	0.0	0	0.0	0	0.0
Adrenal	Cortical vacuolation, zona fasciculata	0	0.0	2	20.0	4	1.3	0	0.0	1	10.0	1	0.3
Adrenal	Cyst	0	0.0	1	10.0	1	0.3	0	0.0	0	0.0	0	0.0
Adrenal	Hematopoiesis	0	0.0	0	0.0	0	0.0	0	0.0	1	10.0	3	1.0
Adrenal	Infiltration, lymphoid cell	0	0.0	1	10.0	1	0.3	0	0.0	1	10.0	3	1.0
Adrenal	Necrosis/apoptosis, zona fasciculata	0	0.0	0	0.0	0	0.0	0	0.0	1	10.0	1	0.3
Bone marrow	Hypercellularity	0	0.0	2	20.0	2	0.7	0	0.0	2	20.0	2	0.7
Brain	Cyst	0	0.0	1	10.0	1	0.3	0	0.0	0	0.0	0	0.0
Brain	Hemorrhage	0	0.0	1	10.0	1	0.3	0	0.0	0	0.0	0	0.0
Brain	Inflammation, meningeal	0	0.0	0	0.0	0	0.0	0	0.0	1	10.0	1	0.3
Brain	Telangiectasia, focal	0	0.0	1	10.0	1	0.3	0	0.0	0	0.0	0	0.0
Cecum	Hyperplasia, mucosal	0	0.0	2	20.0	6	2.0	0	0.0	2	20.0	4	1.3
Cecum	Inflammation, mixed cell	0	0.0	3	30.0	12	4.0	0	0.0	5	50.0	10	3.3
Cervix	Inflammation, neutrophilic	0	0.0	0	0.0	0	0.0	0	0.0	1	10.0	1	0.3
Colon	Congestion	0	0.0	1	10.0	1	0.3	0	0.0	1	10.0	1	0.3
Colon	Hyperplasia, lymphoid	0	0.0	1	10.0	1	0.3	0	0.0	0	0.0	0	0.0
Colon	Hyperplasia, mucosal	0	0.0	2	20.0	2	0.7	0	0.0	1	10.0	1	0.3
Colon	Inflammation, mixed cell	0	0.0	1	10.0	2	0.7	0	0.0	1	10.0	1	0.3
Duodenum	Ectopic pancreas	0	0.0	1	10.0	1	0.3	0	0.0	0	0.0	0	0.0
Epididymides	Granuloma, spermatic	0	0.0	6	60.0	6	2.0	0	0.0	0	0.0	0	0.0
Epididymides	Infiltration, lymphoid cell	0	0.0	1	10.0	4	1.3	0	0.0	0	0.0	0	0.0
Epididymides	Oligospermia	0	0.0	1	10.0	1	0.3	0	0.0	0	0.0	0	0.0

Organ	Lesion	n	%	n	%	n	%	n	%	n	%	n	%
Esophagus	Infiltration, lymphoid cell	0	0.0	1	10.0	1	0.3	0	0.0	0	0.0	0	0.0
Esophagus	Inflammation, mixed cell	0	0.0	1	10.0	3	1.0	0	0.0	1	10.0	4	1.3
Esophagus	Degeneration/regeneration, muscle	0	0.0	2	20.0	4	1.3	0	0.0	2	20.0	6	2.0
Esophagus	Fibrosis	0	0.0	0	0.0	0	0.0	0	0.0	1	10.0	1	0.3
Esophagus	Granulation tissue	0	0.0	0	0.0	0	0.0	0	0.0	1	10.0	1	0.3
Esophagus	Hemorrhage	0	0.0	0	0.0	0	0.0	0	0.0	1	10.0	2	0.7
Eye	Rosette, retinal	0	0.0	1	10.0	3	1.0	0	0.0	0	0.0	0	0.0
Eye	Vacuolation, corneal	0	0.0	1	10.0	1	0.3	0	0.0	0	0.0	0	0.0
Femur	Fibrosis	0	0.0	1	10.0	2	0.7	0	0.0	1	10.0	1	0.3
Femur	Fracture	0	0.0	1	10.0	0	0.0	0	0.0	1	10.0	1	0.3
Femur	Increased trabeculae	0	0.0	2	20.0	0	0.0	0	0.0	2	20.0	3	1.0
Harderian gland	Atrophy	0	0.0	1	10.0	1	0.3	0	0.0	0	0.0	0	0.0
Harderian gland	Hemorrhage	0	0.0	1	10.0	0	0.0	0	0.0	1	10.0	1	0.3
Harderian gland	Infiltration, mononuclear cell	0	0.0	1	10.0	1	0.3	0	0.0	1	10.0	3	1.0
Harderian gland	Inflammation, mixed cell	0	0.0	1	10.0	1	0.3	0	0.0	1	10.0	2	0.7
Harderian gland	Inflammation, lymphocytic	0	0.0	3	30.0	10	3.3	0	0.0	1	10.0	6	2.0
Harderian gland	Mineralization	0	0.0	1	10.0	1	0.3	0	0.0	0	0.0	0	0.0
Harderian gland	Infiltration, lymphoid cell	0	0.0	0	0.0	0	0.0	0	0.0	1	10.0	1	0.3
Heart	Cardiomyopathy	0	0.0	1	10.0	1	0.3	0	0.0	0	0.0	0	0.0
Heart	Myxomatous change, valve	0	0.0	0	0.0	0	0.0	0	0.0	1	10.0	1	0.3
Heart	Fibrosis	0	0.0	0	0.0	0	0.0	0	0.0	1	10.0	2	0.7
Heart	Hemorrhage	0	0.0	0	0.0	0	0.0	0	0.0	1	10.0	1	0.3
Heart	Infiltration, mononuclear cell	0	0.0	1	10.0	3	1.0	0	0.0	1	10.0	3	1.0
Heart	Inflammation, mixed cell	0	0.0	1	10.0	5	1.7	0	0.0	1	10.0	1	0.3
Heart	Myocardial degeneration	0	0.0	1	10.0	1	0.3	0	0.0	0	0.0	0	0.0
Heart	Myxomatous change, valve	0	0.0	1	10.0	1	0.3	0	0.0	0	0.0	0	0.0
Ileum	Congestion	0	0.0	2	20.0	2	0.7	0	0.0	1	10.0	1	0.3
Jejunum	Congestion	0	0.0	1	10.0	1	0.3	0	0.0	0	0.0	0	0.0
Kidney	Basophilia, tubular	0	0.0	4	40.0	45	15.0	0	0.0	2	20.0	26	8.7
Kidney	Casts, tubular	0	0.0	1	10.0	6	2.0	0	0.0	1	10.0	4	1.3
Kidney	Cyst	0	0.0	2	20.0	6	2.0	0	0.0	1	10.0	3	1.0
Kidney	Dilation, pelvis	0	0.0	2	20.0	9	3.0	0	0.0	1	10.0	4	1.3
Kidney	Fibrosis	0	0.0	1	10.0	2	0.7	0	0.0	1	10.0	2	0.7
Kidney	Hyaline droplets, tubular	0	0.0	8	80.0	16	5.3	0	0.0	0	0.0	0	0.0

(continued)

TABLE 8.1 (Continued)
Spontaneous Lesions in Control Wistar Rats in Toxicity Studies of 4-Weeks Duration

Rat

Organ	Finding	Males (300)						Females (300)					
		Minimum	Minimum Range (%)	Maximum	Maximum Range (%)	Total Incidence	Total Incidence (%)	Minimum	Minimum Range (%)	Maximum	Maximum Range (%)	Total Incidence	Total Incidence (%)
Kidney	Dilation, pelvis	0	0.0	2	20.0	7	2.3	0	0.0	3	30.0	5	1.7
Kidney	Inflammation, lymphocytic	0	0.0	4	40.0	24	8.0	0	0.0	3	30.0	11	3.7
Kidney	Lipoma	0	0.0	1	10.0	1	0.3	0	0.0	0	0.0	0	0.0
Kidney	Tubular mineralization	0	0.0	6	60.0	8	2.7	0	0.0	8	80.0	77	25.7
Kidney	Pyelonephritis	0	0.0	0	0.0	0	0.0	0	0.0	1	10.0	1	0.3
Lacrimal gland	Atrophy	0	0.0	0	0.0	0	0.0	0	0.0	1	10.0	1	0.3
Lacrimal gland	Infiltration, lymphoid cell	0	0.0	2	20.0	8	2.7	0	0.0	0	0.0	0	0.0
Lacrimal gland	Inflammation, mixed cell	0	0.0	1	10.0	1	0.3	0	0.0	0	0.0	0	0.0
Lacrimal gland	Metaplasia	0	0.0	3	30.0	5	1.7	0	0.0	1	10.0	1	0.3
Lacrimal gland	Necrosis/vacuolation	0	0.0	1	10.0	1	0.3	0	0.0	0	0.0	0	0.0
Larynx	Edema	0	0.0	2	20.0	3	1.0	0	0.0	1	10.0	1	0.3
Larynx	Hemorrhage	0	0.0	1	10.0	1	0.3	0	0.0	0	0.0	0	0.0
Larynx	Hyperplasia, epithelial	0	0.0	1	10.0	1	0.3	0	0.0	0	0.0	0	0.0
Larynx	Infiltration, lymphoid cell	0	0.0	1	10.0	1	0.3	0	0.0	0	0.0	0	0.0
Larynx	Inflammation, mixed cell	0	0.0	1	10.0	2	0.7	0	0.0	1	10.0	1	0.3
Liver	Angiectasis	0	0.0	0	0.0	0	0.0	0	0.0	1	10.0	1	0.3
Liver	Apoptosis	0	0.0	1	10.0	1	0.3	0	0.0	0	0.0	0	0.0
Liver	Bile duct hyperplasia	0	0.0	0	0.0	0	0.0	0	0.0	1	10.0	1	0.3
Liver	Cyst	0	0.0	0	0.0	0	0.0	0	0.0	1	10.0	1	0.3
Liver	Degeneration, cystic	0	0.0	0	0.0	0	0.0	0	0.0	1	10.0	1	0.3
Liver	Deposition pigment	0	0.0	1	10.0	2	0.7	0	0.0	2	20.0	6	2.0
Liver	Fibrosis	0	0.0	3	30.0	3	1.0	0	0.0	1	10.0	3	1.0
Liver	Focus, clear	0	0.0	1	10.0	1	0.3	0	0.0	0	0.0	0	0.0
Liver	Glycogen increase, hepatocytes	0	0.0	2	20.0	2	0.7	0	0.0	0	0.0	0	0.0
Liver	Granuloma	0	0.0	0	0.0	0	0.0	0	0.0	1	10.0	1	0.3

Organ	Lesion												
Liver	Hematopoiesis	31.0	93	100.0	10	0.0	0	33.0	99	100.0	10	0.0	0
Liver	Hemorrhage	0.3	1	10.0	1	0.0	0	0.3	1	10.0	1	0.0	0
Liver	Infiltration, mixed cell	5.7	17	100.0	10	0.0	0	5.7	17	90.0	9	0.0	0
Liver	Inflammation, mixed cell	12.3	37	60.0	6	0.0	0	10.7	32	90.0	9	0.0	0
Liver	Inflammation, lymphoid cell	3.0	9	70.0	7	0.0	0	6.0	18	90.0	9	0.0	0
Liver	Mineralization	0.0	0	0.0	0	0.0	0	0.3	1	10.0	1	0.0	0
Liver	Mitosis increased	0.3	1	10.0	1	0.0	0	0.0	0	0.0	0	0.0	0
Liver	Infiltration, mononuclear cell	11.0	33	70.0	7	0.0	0	8.0	24	80.0	8	0.0	0
Liver	Necrosis, single cell, hepatocyte	8.0	24	70.0	7	0.0	0	8.0	24	70.0	7	0.0	0
Liver	Cytoplasmic vacuolation, hepatocyte	1.7	5	20.0	2	0.0	0	0.7	2	10.0	1	0.0	0
Lung	Alveolitis	1.0	3	20.0	2	0.0	0	0.3	1	10.0	1	0.0	0
Lung	Atelectasis	0.3	1	10.0	1	0.0	0	0.7	2	10.0	1	0.0	0
Lung	Epithelioma	0.3	1	10.0	1	0.0	0	0.0	0	0.0	0	0.0	0
Lung	Fibrosis	1.0	3	20.0	2	0.0	0	0.0	0	0.0	0	0.0	0
Lung	Alveolar foam cell aggregates	4.3	13	30.0	3	0.0	0	3.7	11	10.0	1	0.0	0
Lung	Hemorrhage	3.0	9	20.0	2	0.0	0	5.3	16	30.0	3	0.0	0
Lung	Inflammatory cell infiltration, perivascular	4.0	12	40.0	4	0.0	0	5.7	17	60.0	6	0.0	0
Lung	Inflammation, mixed cell	4.3	13	20.0	2	0.0	0	11.3	34	40.0	4	0.0	0
Lung	Inflammation, eosinophilic	0.3	1	10.0	1	0.0	0	1.7	5	40.0	4	0.0	0
Lung	Inflammation, lymphocytic	1.0	3	10.0	1	0.0	0	1.3	4	30.0	3	0.0	0
Lung	Inflammation, neutrophilic	0.3	1	10.0	1	0.0	0	0.3	1	10.0	1	0.0	0
Lung	Metaplasia, osseous	0.3	1	10.0	2	0.0	0	1.3	4	20.0	2	0.0	0
Lung	Mineralization	1.7	5	20.0	1	0.0	0	4.0	12	60.0	6	0.0	0
Lung	Pigmented macrophages	0.3	1	10.0	1	0.0	0	0.0	0	0.0	0	0.0	0
Mammary	Anomaly	0.0	0	0.0	0	0.0	0	0.3	1	10.0	1	0.0	0
Mammary	Fibrosis	0.3	1	10.0	1	0.0	0	0.0	0	0.0	0	0.0	0
Mammary	Galactocele	0.3	1	10.0	1	0.0	0	0.0	0	0.0	0	0.0	0
Mammary	Hyperplasia, lobular	0.3	1	10.0	1	0.0	0	0.0	0	0.0	0	0.0	0
Mandibular lymph node	Congestion	1.7	5	50.0	5	0.0	0	2.0	6	40.0	4	0.0	0
Mandibular lymph node	Dilation, sinusoid	0.0	0	0.0	0	0.0	0	0.7	2	20.0	2	0.0	0

(continued)

TABLE 8.1 (Continued)
Spontaneous Lesions in Control Wistar Rats in Toxicity Studies of 4-Weeks Duration

Rat

Organ	Finding	Males						4 weeks		Females					
		Minimum	Minimum Range (%)	Maximum	Maximum Range (%)	Total Incidence	Total Incidence (%)	Minimum		Minimum	Minimum Range (%)	Maximum	Maximum Range (%)	Total Incidence	Total Incidence (%)
						300								300	
Mandibular lymph node	Erythrophagocytosis	0	0.0	7	70.0	45	15.0	0		0	0.0	8	80.0	44	14.7
Mandibular lymph node	Sinus histiocytosis	0	0.0	4	40.0	8	2.7	0		0	0.0	4	40.0	9	3.0
Mandibular lymph node	Hyperplasia, plasma cell	0	0.0	5	50.0	14	4.7	0		0	0.0	2	20.0	10	3.3
Mandibular lymph node	Hyperplasia, lymphoid	0	0.0	7	70.0	11	3.7	0		0	0.0	5	50.0	9	3.0
Mesenteric lymph node	Congestion	0	0.0	0	0.0	0	0.0	0		0	0.0	1	10.0	1	0.3
Mesenteric lymph node	Cyst	0	0.0	0	0.0	0	0.0	0		0	0.0	1	10.0	1	0.3
Mesenteric lymph node	Depletion, lymphoid	0	0.0	1	10.0	1	0.3	0		0	0.0	0	0.0	0	0.0
Mesenteric lymph node	Dilation, sinusoid	0	0.0	2	20.0	2	0.7	0		0	0.0	0	0.0	0	0.0
Mesenteric lymph node	Erythrophagocytosis	0	0.0	2	20.0	6	2.0	0		0	0.0	4	40.0	6	2.0
Mesenteric lymph node	Sinus histiocytosis	0	0.0	1	10.0	5	1.7	0		0	0.0	3	30.0	11	3.7
Mesenteric lymph node	Hyperplasia, lymphoid	0	0.0	2	20.0	3	1.0	0		0	0.0	0	0.0	0	0.0
Mesenteric lymph node	Lymphangiectasia	0	0.0	1	10.0	1	0.3	0		0	0.0	0	0.0	0	0.0
Mesenteric lymph node	Macrophage aggregates	0	0.0	1	10.0	2	0.7	0		0	0.0	3	30.0	11	3.7
Muscle	Degeneration	0	0.0	1	10.0	1	0.3	0		0	0.0	1	10.0	3	1.0

Organ	Lesion												
Muscle	Infiltration, mononuclear cell	0	0.0	1	10.0	1	0.3	0	0.0	0	0.0	0	0.0
Muscle	Inflammation, mixed cell	0	0.0	1	10.0	1	0.3	0	0.0	0	0.0	0	0.0
Muscle	Mineralization	0	0.0	0	0.0	0	0.0	0	0.0	1	10.0	1	0.3
Nasal cavity	Inflammation, lymphocytic	0	0.0	1	10.0	1	0.3	0	0.0	0	0.0	0	0.0
Ovaries	Cyst	0	0.0	0	0.0	0	0.0	0	0.0	2	20.0	3	1.0
Ovaries	Degeneration, corpora lutea	0	0.0	0	0.0	0	0.0	0	0.0	6	60.0	6	2.0
Ovaries	Hemorrhage	0	0.0	0	0.0	0	0.0	0	0.0	2	20.0	6	2.0
Ovaries	Inflammation, mixed cell	0	0.0	0	0.0	0	0.0	0	0.0	1	10.0	1	0.3
Oviducts	Cyst	0	0.0	0	0.0	0	0.0	0	0.0	1	10.0	1	0.3
Oviducts	Inflammation, mixed cell	0	0.0	0	0.0	0	0.0	0	0.0	1	10.0	1	0.3
Pancreas	Adipose infiltration	0	0.0	1	10.0	1	0.3	0	0.0	0	0.0	0	0.0
Pancreas	Atrophy, acinar cell	0	0.0	1	10.0	3	1.0	0	0.0	2	10.0	2	0.7
Pancreas	Decrease, zymogen	0	0.0	0	0.0	0	0.0	0	0.0	4	40.0	9	3.0
Pancreas	Fibrosis	0	0.0	1	10.0	1	0.3	0	0.0	0	0.0	0	0.0
Pancreas	Hyperplasia, ductal	0	0.0	1	10.0	1	0.3	0	0.0	0	0.0	0	0.0
Pancreas	Hyperplasia, islet cell	0	0.0	1	10.0	1	0.3	0	0.0	0	0.0	0	0.0
Pancreas	Hypertrophy, acinar cell	0	0.0	0	0.0	0	0.0	0	0.0	1	10.0	1	0.3
Pancreas	Inflammation, mixed cell	0	0.0	1	10.0	3	1.0	0	0.0	0	0.0	0	0.0
Pancreas	Inflammation, lymphocytic	0	0.0	1	10.0	3	1.0	0	0.0	1	10.0	1	0.3
Pituitary	Cyst, pars distalis	0	0.0	2	20.0	5	1.7	0	0.0	2	20.0	6	2.0
Pituitary	Cyst, pars intermedia	0	0.0	1	10.0	2	0.7	0	0.0	1	10.0	2	0.7
Pituitary	Focus, basophilic, pars distalis	0	0.0	1	10.0	1	0.3	0	0.0	0	0.0	0	0.0
Prostate	Hemorrhage	0	0.0	1	10.0	1	0.3	0	0.0	0	0.0	0	0.0
Prostate	Hyperplasia, epithelial	0	0.0	1	10.0	1	0.3	0	0.0	0	0.0	0	0.0
Prostate	Infiltration, lymphoid cell	0	0.0	4	40.0	16	5.3	0	0.0	0	0.0	0	0.0
Prostate	Infiltration, mononuclear cell	0	0.0	2	20.0	2	0.7	0	0.0	0	0.0	0	0.0
Prostate	Inflammation, mixed cell	0	0.0	4	40.0	26	8.7	0	0.0	0	0.0	0	0.0
Prostate	Necrosis	0	0.0	1	10.0	1	0.3	0	0.0	0	0.0	0	0.0
Prostate	Vacuolation, epithelial	0	0.0	2	20.0	2	0.7	0	0.0	0	0.0	0	0.0
Rectum	Edema	0	0.0	0	0.0	0	0.0	0	0.0	1	10.0	1	0.3
Rectum	Erosion	0	0.0	0	0.0	0	0.0	0	0.0	1	10.0	1	0.3
Salivary gland	Atrophy, acinar	0	0.0	1	10.0	1	0.3	0	0.0	0	0.0	0	0.0
Salivary gland	Inflammation, lymphocytic	0	0.0	1	10.0	1	0.3	0	0.0	1	10.0	1	0.3
Salivary gland	Metaplasia, glandular	0	0.0	1	10.0	1	0.3	0	0.0	0	0.0	0	0.0

(continued)

TABLE 8.1 (Continued)
Spontaneous Lesions in Control Wistar Rats in Toxicity Studies of 4-Weeks Duration

Rat

Organ	Finding	Males (300)						Females (300)					
		Minimum	Minimum Range (%)	Maximum	Maximum Range (%)	Total Incidence	Total Incidence (%)	Minimum	Minimum Range (%)	Maximum	Maximum Range (%)	Total Incidence	Total Incidence (%)
Skin	Acanthosis	0	0.0	1	10.0	1	0.3	0	0.0	0	0.0	0	0.0
Skin	Cyst	0	0.0	0	0.0	0	0.0	0	0.0	1	10.0	1	0.3
Skin	Follicular atrophy	0	0.0	1	10.0	1	0.3	0	0.0	0	0.0	0	0.0
Skin	Hemorrhage	0	0.0	1	10.0	1	0.3	0	0.0	0	0.0	0	0.0
Skin	Hyperkeratosis	0	0.0	2	20.0	2	0.7	0	0.0	2	20.0	3	1.0
Skin	Inflammation, mixed cell	0	0.0	1	10.0	2	0.7	0	0.0	0	0.0	0	0.0
Skin	Serofibrinous debris (scab)	0	0.0	1	10.0	1	0.3	0	0.0	1	10.0	1	0.3
Spleen	Depletion, lymphoid	0	0.0	2	20.0	2	0.7	0	0.0	1	10.0	1	0.3
Spleen	Cyst	0	0.0	0	0.0	0	0.0	0	0.0	1	10.0	1	0.3
Spleen	Deposition pigment	0	0.0	0	0.0	0	0.0	0	0.0	1	10.0	1	0.3
Spleen	Hematopoiesis, increased	0	0.0	6	60.0	25	8.3	0	0.0	9	90.0	45	15.0
Spleen	Macrophage aggregates	0	0.0	1	10.0	1	0.3	0	0.0	1	10.0	1	0.3
Sternum	Chondromucinous degeneration	0	0.0	1	10.0	1	0.3	0	0.0	0	0.0	0	0.0
Stomach	Congestion	0	0.0	2	20.0	2	0.7	0	0.0	0	0.0	0	0.0
Stomach	Cyst	0	0.0	1	10.0	4	1.3	0	0.0	2	20.0	4	1.3
Stomach	Dilation, glandular	0	0.0	2	20.0	9	3.0	0	0.0	2	20.0	4	1.3
Stomach	Edema	0	0.0	1	10.0	1	0.3	0	0.0	0	0.0	0	0.0
Stomach	Globule leukocytes	0	0.0	4	40.0	4	1.3	0	0.0	2	20.0	2	0.7
Stomach	Hyperplasia, squamous cell, limiting ridge	0	0.0	1	10.0	2	0.7	0	0.0	0	0.0	0	0.0
Stomach	Hyperplasia, epithelial, non-glandular	0	0.0	0	0.0	0	0.0	0	0.0	1	10.0	1	0.3
Stomach	Hyperplasia, squamous cell, non-glandular	0	0.0	3	30.0	5	1.7	0	0.0	1	10.0	1	0.3
Stomach	Inflammation, mixed cell	0	0.0	8	80.0	22	7.3	0	0.0	1	10.0	4	1.3

Organ	Lesion	n	%	n	%	n	%	n	%	n	%	n	%
Stomach	Inflammation, neutrophilic	0	0.0	2	20.0	2	0.7	0	0.0	0	0.0	0	0.0
Stomach	Inflammation, lymphocytic	0	0.0	0	0.0	0	0.0	0	0.0	1	10.0	1	0.3
Stomach	Vacuolation, epithelial, limiting ridge	0	0.0	8	80.0	49	16.3	0	0.0	4	40.0	21	7.0
Stomach	Eosinophil accumulations	0	0.0	9	90.0	10	3.3	0	0.0	6	60.0	6	2.0
Testes	Atrophy, tubular	0	0.0	1	10.0	2	0.7	0	0.0	0	0.0	0	0.0
Testes	Degeneration, tubular	0	0.0	2	20.0	2	0.7	0	0.0	0	0.0	0	0.0
Thymus	Lymphocytolysis	0	0.0	2	20.0	3	1.0	0	0.0	0	0.0	0	0.0
Thymus	Congestion	0	0.0	1	10.0	1	0.3	0	0.0	0	0.0	0	0.0
Thymus	Cyst	0	0.0	0	0.0	0	0.0	0	0.0	1	10.0	2	0.7
Thymus	Depletion, lymphoid	0	0.0	1	10.0	1	0.3	0	0.0	1	10.0	1	0.3
Thymus	Edema	0	0.0	0	0.0	0	0.0	0	0.0	1	10.0	1	0.3
Thymus	Globule leukocytes	0	0.0	0	0.0	0	0.0	0	0.0	2	20.0	2	0.7
Thymus	Hemorrhage	0	0.0	3	30.0	21	7.0	0	0.0	5	50.0	21	7.0
Thymus	Inflammation, lymphocytic	0	0.0	1	10.0	1	0.3	0	0.0	0	0.0	0	0.0
Thymus	Inflammation, mixed cell	0	0.0	0	0.0	0	0.0	0	0.0	1	10.0	1	0.3
Thymus	Lymphocytolysis	0	0.0	5	50.0	5	1.7	0	0.0	2	20.0	5	1.7
Thymus	Macrophage aggregates	0	0.0	0	0.0	0	0.0	0	0.0	1	10.0	1	0.3
Thymus	Metaplasia, epithelial	0	0.0	1	10.0	1	0.3	0	0.0	0	0.0	0	0.0
Thyroid	Cyst, developmental	0	0.0	3	30.0	3	1.0	0	0.0	2	20.0	3	1.0
Thyroid	Cyst, follicular	0	0.0	2	20.0	3	1.0	0	0.0	0	0.0	0	0.0
Thyroid	Ectopic thymus	0	0.0	2	20.0	10	3.3	0	0.0	2	20.0	8	2.7
Thyroid	Hypertrophy, follicular	0	0.0	4	40.0	4	1.3	0	0.0	1	10.0	1	0.3
Tongue	Angiectasis	0	0.0	1	10.0	1	0.3	0	0.0	0	0.0	0	0.0
Tongue	Myofiber degeneration/regeneration	0	0.0	3	30.0	4	1.3	0	0.0	0	0.0	0	0.0
Tongue	Edema	0	0.0	1	10.0	1	0.3	0	0.0	0	0.0	0	0.0
Tongue	Fibrosis	0	0.0	3	30.0	4	1.3	0	0.0	4	40.0	8	2.7
Tongue	Hemorrhage	0	0.0	7	70.0	47	15.7	0	0.0	5	50.0	20	6.7
Tongue	Inflammation, neutrophilic	0	0.0	1	10.0	2	0.7	0	0.0	0	0.0	0	0.0
Tongue	Inflammation, mixed cell	0	0.0	3	30.0	28	9.3	0	0.0	5	50.0	17	5.7
Tongue	Myofiber degeneration/regeneration	0	0.0	4	40.0	12	4.0	0	0.0	4	40.0	13	4.3
Tongue	Thrombus	0	0.0	0	0.0	0	0.0	0	0.0	1	10.0	1	0.3
Tongue	Ulceration	0	0.0	1	10.0	3	1.0	0	0.0	0	0.0	0	0.0
Trachea	Congestion	0	0.0	2	20.0	2	0.7	0	0.0	0	0.0	0	0.0

(continued)

TABLE 8.1 (Continued)
Spontaneous Lesions in Control Wistar Rats in Toxicity Studies of 4-Weeks Duration

Rat

4 weeks

Organ	Finding	Males						Females					
		Minimum	Minimum Range (%)	Maximum	Maximum Range (%)	Total Incidence	Total Incidence (%)	Minimum	Minimum Range (%)	Maximum	Maximum Range (%)	Total Incidence	Total Incidence (%)
						300						300	
Tracheobronchial lymph node	Congestion	0	0.0	0	0.0	0	0.0	0	0.0	2	20.0	2	0.7
Tracheobronchial lymph node	Deposition pigment	0	0.0	3	30.0	5	1.7	0	0.0	3	30.0	5	1.7
Tracheobronchial lymph node	Erythrophagocytosis	0	0.0	5	50.0	14	4.7	0	0.0	6	60.0	25	8.3
Tracheobronchial lymph node	Sinus histiocytosis	0	0.0	2	20.0	6	2.0	0	0.0	5	50.0	6	2.0
Tracheobronchial lymph node	Hyperplasia, lymphoid	0	0.0	0	0.0	0	0.0	0	0.0	1	10.0	1	0.3
Urinary bladder	Hyperplasia, transitional cell	0	0.0	0	0.0	0	0.0	0	0.0	1	10.0	1	0.3
Urinary bladder	Infiltration, lymphoid cell	0	0.0	1	10.0	3	1.0	0	0.0	2	20.0	4	1.3
Urinary bladder	Inflammation, mixed cell	0	0.0	0	0.0	0	0.0	0	0.0	1	10.0	1	0.3
Urinary bladder	Plug, proteinaceous	0	0.0	1	10.0	1	0.3	0	0.0	0	0.0	0	0.0
Uterus	Dilation, luminal	0	0.0	0	0.0	0	0.0	0	0.0	3	30.0	8	2.7
Uterus	Dilation, glandular	0	0.0	0	0.0	0	0.0	0	0.0	2	20.0	6	2.0
Uterus	Infiltration, neutrophilic	0	0.0	0	0.0	0	0.0	0	0.0	1	10.0	2	0.7

TABLE 8.2

Spontaneous Lesions in Control Wistar Rats in Toxicity Studies of 26-Weeks Duration

Rat

Organ	Finding	Males						Females (26 weeks)					
		Minimum	Minimum Range (%)	Maximum	Maximum Range (%)	Total Incidence (200)	Total Incidence (%)	Minimum	Minimum Range (%)	Maximum	Maximum Range (%)	Total Incidence (201)	Total Incidence (%)
Adrenal	Angiectasis	0	0.0	0	0.0	0	0.0	0	0.0	1	5.0	1	0.5
Adrenal	Deposits, pigment	0	0.0	0	0.0	0	0.0	0	0.0	1	5.0	1	0.5
Adrenal	Hyperplasia, cortical, zona fasciculata	0	0.0	2	10.0	4	2.0	0	0.0	1	5.0	5	2.5
Adrenal	Congestion	0	0.0	1	5.0	1	0.5	0	0.0	2	10.0	4	2.0
Adrenal	Infiltration, mononuclear cell	0	0.0	0	0.0	0	0.0	0	0.0	4	20.0	4	2.0
Adrenal	Cortical hypertrophy, zona fasciculata	0	0.0	1	5.0	1	0.5	0	0.0	1	5.0	2	1.0
Adrenal	Hematopoiesis, extramedullary	0	0.0	0	0.0	0	0.0	0	0.0	1	4.8	1	0.5
Adrenal	Necrosis, cortex	0	0.0	0	0.0	0	0.0	0	0.0	1	5.0	1	0.5
Adrenal	Cortical vacuolation, zona fasciculata	0	0.0	2	10.0	3	1.5	0	0.0	0	0.0	0	0.0
Bone marrow	Hypocellularity	0	0.0	1	5.0	1	0.5	0	0.0	3	14.3	3	1.5
Bone marrow	Hypercellularity	0	0.0	1	5.0	2	1.0	0	0.0	1	4.8	1	0.5
Brain	Benign ependymoma	0	0.0	0	0.0	0	0.0	0	0.0	1	5.0	1	0.5
Brain	Glioma (b)	0	0.0	1	5.0	1	0.5	0	0.0	0	0.0	0	0.0
Brain	Malignant ependymoma	0	0.0	0	0.0	0	0.0	0	0.0	1	4.8	1	0.5
Brain	Malignant oligodendroglioma	0	0.0	0	0.0	0	0.0	0	0.0	1	5.0	1	0.5
Cecum	Hyperplasia, mucosal	0	0.0	0	0.0	0	0.0	0	0.0	1	5.0	1	0.5
Colon	Parasite	0	0.0	1	5.0	5	2.5	0	0.0	3	15.0	3	1.5
Duodenum	Inflammation, mixed cell	0	0.0	1	5.0	1	0.5	0	0.0	0	0.0	0	0.0
Epididymides	Cellular debris, intratubular	0	0.0	1	5.0	1	0.5	0	0.0	0	0.0	0	0.0
Epididymides	Granuloma, spermatic	0	0.0	1	5.0	1	0.5	0	0.0	0	0.0	0	0.0

(continued)

TABLE 8.2 (Continued)
Spontaneous Lesions in Control Wistar Rats in Toxicity Studies of 26-Weeks Duration

Rat

26 weeks

		Males						Females					
						Total Incidence 200						Total Incidence 201	
Organ	Finding	Minimum	Minimum Range (%)	Maximum	Maximum Range (%)	Total Incidence	Total Incidence (%)	Minimum	Minimum Range (%)	Maximum	Maximum Range (%)	Total Incidence	Total Incidence (%)
Epididymides	Oligospermia	0	0.0	1	5.0	2	1.0	0	0.0	0	0.0	0	0.0
Epididymides	Spermatocele	0	0.0	1	5.0	2	1.0	0	0.0	0	0.0	0	0.0
Eye	Degeneration/atrophy, retina	0	0.0	3	15.0	4	2.0	0	0.0	1	5.0	2	1.0
Eye	Inflammation, conjunctiva	0	0.0	1	5.0	1	0.5	0	0.0	0	0.0	0	0.0
Harderian gland	Atrophy	0	0.0	0	0.0	0	0.0	0	0.0	2	10.0	2	1.0
Harderian gland	Infiltration, mononuclear cell	0	0.0	3	15.0	3	1.5	0	0.0	3	15.0	3	1.5
Harderian gland	Inflammation, mixed cell	0	0.0	4	20.0	5	2.5	0	0.0	0	0.0	0	0.0
Harderian gland	Necrosis, single cell	0	0.0	1	5.0	1	0.5	0	0.0	2	10.0	2	1.0
Heart	Infiltration, mixed cell	0	0.0	3	15.0	3	1.5	0	0.0	1	5.0	1	0.5
Heart	Infiltration, mononuclear cell	0	0.0	2	10.0	4	2.0	0	0.0	0	0.0	0	0.0
Heart	Cardiomyopathy	0	0.0	4	20.0	6	3.0	0	0.0	2	9.5	2	1.0
Joint femorotibial	Hyperplasia, synovium	0	0.0	1	5.0	1	0.5	0	0.0	2	9.5	2	1.0
Kidney	Tubular basophilia	0	0.0	6	30.0	18	9.0	0	0.0	4	19.0	8	4.0
Kidney	Carcinoma, tubular cell	0	0.0	1	5.0	1	0.5	0	0.0	0	0.0	0	0.0
Kidney	Tubular casts, hyaline	0	0.0	2	10.0	3	1.5	0	0.0	3	14.3	3	1.5
Kidney	Chronic progressive nephropathy	0	0.0	5	25.0	5	2.5	0	0.0	3	15.0	3	1.5
Kidney	Congestion	0	0.0	0	0.0	0	0.0	0	0.0	1	5.0	1	0.5
Kidney	Cyst	0	0.0	1	5.0	2	1.0	0	0.0	2	10.0	2	1.0
Kidney	Dilation, pelvis	0	0.0	1	5.0	8	4.0	0	0.0	2	10.0	5	2.5
Kidney	Hyperplasia, transitional cell	0	0.0	0	0.0	0	0.0	0	0.0	2	10.0	2	1.0
Kidney	Infiltration, mononuclear cell	0	0.0	11	55.0	20	10.0	0	0.0	4	20.0	6	3.0
Kidney	Inflammation, mixed cell	0	0.0	1	5.0	2	1.0	0	0.0	0	0.0	0	0.0
Kidney	Pyelonephritis	0	0.0	1	5.0	1	0.5	0	0.0	1	5.0	2	1.0
Lacrimal gland	Metaplasia, Harderian gland	0	0.0	1	5.0	2	1.0	0	0.0	0	0.0	0	0.0
Lacrimal gland	Dilation	0	0.0	1	5.0	1	0.5	0	0.0	0	0.0	0	0.0

Organ	Lesion												
Lacrimal gland	Ectopic tissue	0	0.0	1	5.0	0.5	1	0	0.0	0	0.0	0	0.0
Lacrimal gland	Metaplasia, Harderian gland	0	0.0	1	5.0	0.5	1	0	0.0	0	0.0	0	0.0
Lacrimal gland	Inflammation, mixed cell	0	0.0	3	15.0	2.0	4	0	0.0	0	0.0	0	0.0
Larynx	Cyst	0	0.0	0	0.0	0.0	0	0	0.0	1	5.0	1	0.5
Larynx	Edema	0	0.0	1	5.0	0.5	1	0	0.0	0	0.0	0	0.0
Larynx	Granuloma	0	0.0	2	10.0	1.5	3	0	0.0	0	0.0	0	0.0
Larynx	Hemorrhage	0	0.0	1	5.0	0.5	1	0	0.0	0	0.0	0	0.0
Larynx	Inflammation, mixed cell	0	0.0	4	20.0	5.5	11	0	0.0	5	25.0	5	2.5
Liver	Atrophy, hepatocellular	0	0.0	0	0.0	0.0	0	0	0.0	3	15.0	4	2.0
Liver	Basophilic cell focus	0	0.0	1	5.0	0.5	1	0	0.0	3	15.0	7	3.5
Liver	Clear cell focus	0	0.0	6	30.0	3.0	6	0	0.0	1	5.0	2	1.0
Liver	Degeneration, cystic	0	0.0	0	0.0	0.0	0	0	0.0	1	5.0	1	0.5
Liver	Degeneration/necrosis, centrilobular	0	0.0	0	0.0	0.0	0	0	0.0	1	4.8	1	0.5
Liver	Deposition pigment	0	0.0	1	5.0	1.0	2	0	0.0	3	15.0	3	1.5
Liver	Dilation, sinusoidal	0	0.0	0	0.0	0.0	0	0	0.0	1	5.0	1	0.5
Liver	Fibrosis	0	0.0	1	5.0	0.5	1	0	0.0	1	5.0	1	0.5
Liver	Hematopoiesis	0	0.0	0	0.0	0.0	0	0	0.0	1	4.8	1	0.5
Liver	Infiltration, mixed cell	0	0.0	1	5.0	0.5	1	0	0.0	2	10.0	3	1.5
Liver	Inflammation, biliary	0	0.0	0	0.0	0.0	0	0	0.0	1	5.0	2	1.0
Liver	Inflammation, granulomatous	0	0.0	0	0.0	0.0	0	0	0.0	1	5.0	1	0.5
Liver	Infiltration, mononuclear cell	0	0.0	1	5.0	0.5	1	0	0.0	0	0.0	0	0.0
Liver	Necrosis	0	0.0	0	0.0	0.0	0	0	0.0	2	10.0	2	1.0
Liver	Reactive sinusoidal lining cells	0	0.0	0	0.0	0.0	0	0	0.0	2	10.0	2	1.0
Liver	Tension lipidosis	0	0.0	1	5.0	1.5	3	0	0.0	2	10.0	2	1.0
Liver	Vacuolation, hepatocellular	0	0.0	3	15.0	3.0	6	0	0.0	0	0.0	0	0.0
Lung	Congestion	0	0.0	1	5.0	1.0	2	0	0.0	0	0.0	0	0.0
Lung	Hemorrhage	0	0.0	2	10.0	2.0	4	0	0.0	1	5.0	1	0.5
Lung	Alveolar foam cell aggregates	0	0.0	4	20.0	2.0	4	0	0.0	2	9.5	2	1.0
Lung	Hyperplasia, bronchioloalveolar	0	0.0	1	5.0	0.5	1	0	0.0	0	0.0	0	0.0
Lung	Inflammation, mixed cell	0	0.0	3	15.0	2.0	4	0	0.0	2	10.0	2	1.0
Lung	Inflammation, pleura	0	0.0	0	0.0	0.0	0	0	0.0	1	4.8	1	0.5

(continued)

TABLE 8.2 (Continued)
Spontaneous Lesions in Control Wistar Rats in Toxicity Studies of 26-Weeks Duration

Rat		26 weeks											
		Males						Females					
		200						201					
Organ	Finding	Minimum	Minimum Range (%)	Maximum	Maximum Range (%)	Total Incidence	Total Incidence (%)	Minimum	Minimum Range (%)	Maximum	Maximum Range (%)	Total Incidence	Total Incidence (%)
Lung	Alveolar foam cell aggregates	0	0.0	5	25.0	12	6.0	0	0.0	4	20.0	13	6.5
Lymph node	Deposits, pigment	0	0.0	1	5.0	1	0.5	0	0.0	0	0.0	0	0.0
Lymph node	Erythrophagocytosis	0	0.0	5	25.0	20	10.0	0	0.0	4	20.0	20	10.0
Lymph node	Hemangioma	0	0.0	1	5.0	1	0.5	0	0.0	0	0.0	0	0.0
Lymph node	Hyperplasia, lymphoid	0	0.0	1	5.0	1	0.5	0	0.0	0	0.0	0	0.0
Lymph node	Sinus histiocytosis	0	0.0	1	5.0	1	0.5	0	0.0	1	5.0	1	0.5
Mammary	Increased vacuolation, acinar cell	0	0.0	0	0.0	0	0.0	0	0.0	2	9.5	2	1.0
Mandibular lymph node	Abscess	0	0.0	0	0.0	0	0.0	0	0.0	1	5.0	1	0.5
Mandibular lymph node	Lymphoid depletion	0	0.0	6	30.0	6	3.0	0	0.0	3	15.0	3	1.5
Mandibular lymph node	Erythrophagocytosis	0	0.0	6	30.0	21	10.5	0	0.0	6	30.0	21	10.4
Mandibular lymph node	Hyperplasia, lymphoid	0	0.0	1	5.0	1	0.5	0	0.0	2	10.0	4	2.0
Mandibular lymph node	Hyperplasia, plasma cell	0	0.0	1	5.0	1	0.5	0	0.0	2	10.0	6	3.0
Mesenteric lymph node	Erythrophagocytosis	0	0.0	7	35.0	16	8.0	0	0.0	2	10.0	9	4.5
Mesenteric lymph node	Granuloma	0	0.0	1	5.0	1	0.5	0	0.0	1	5.0	1	0.5
Mesenteric lymph node	Hyperplasia, lymphoid	0	0.0	2	10.0	2	1.0	0	0.0	2	10.0	3	1.5
Muscle	Degeneration, myofiber	0	0.0	0	0.0	0	0.0	0	0.0	1	4.8	1	0.5
Muscle	Hemorrhage	0	0.0	0	0.0	0	0.0	0	0.0	1	5.0	1	0.5

Organ	Lesion	n	%	n	%	n	%	n	%	n	%	n	%
Ovaries	Atrophy	0	0.0	0	0.0	0	0.0	0	0.0	1	5.0	1	0.5
Ovaries	Congestion	0	0.0	0	0.0	0	0.0	0	0.0	1	5.0	1	0.5
Ovaries	Cyst	0	0.0	0	0.0	0	0.0	0	0.0	2	10.0	7	3.5
Ovaries	Cystadenocarcinoma	0	0.0	0	0.0	0	0.0	0	0.0	1	4.8	1	0.5
Pancreas	Atrophy, acinar cell	0	0.0	1	5.0	3	1.5	0	0.0	1	5.0	1	0.5
Pancreas	Inflammation, mixed cell	0	0.0	3	15.0	3	1.5	0	0.0	1	5.0	2	1.0
Pituitary	Adenoma, pars distalis	0	0.0	1	5.0	1	0.5	0	0.0	1	5.0	2	1.0
Pituitary	Cyst, pars distalis	0	0.0	2	10.0	7	3.5	0	0.0	1	5.0	1	0.5
Pituitary	Hyperplasia, pars distalis	0	0.0	1	5.0	1	0.5	0	0.0	0	0.0	0	0.0
Pituitary	Vacuolation, pars distalis	0	0.0	3	15.0	3	1.5	0	0.0	0	0.0	0	0.0
Prostate	Infiltration, mononuclear cell	0	0.0	6	30.0	10	5.0	0	0.0	0	0.0	0	0.0
Prostate	Inflammation, mixed cell	0	0.0	2	10.0	4	2.0	0	0.0	0	0.0	0	0.0
Prostate	Vacuolation, epithelial	0	0.0	1	5.0	1	0.5	0	0.0	0	0.0	0	0.0
Rectum	Congestion	0	0.0	1	5.0	1	0.5	0	0.0	0	0.0	0	0.0
Rectum	Hyperplasia, lymphoid	0	0.0	3	15.0	3	1.5	0	0.0	0	0.0	0	0.0
Rectum	Parasite	0	0.0	2	10.0	2	1.0	0	0.0	0	0.0	0	0.0
Salivary gland	Atrophy, acinar	0	0.0	0	0.0	0	0.0	0	0.0	1	5.0	1	0.5
Salivary gland	Hemorrhage	0	0.0	0	0.0	0	0.0	0	0.0	1	5.0	1	0.5
Seminal vesicle	Dilation	0	0.0	1	5.0	1	0.5	0	0.0	0	0.0	0	0.0
Seminal vesicle	Infiltration, mononuclear cell	0	0.0	1	5.0	1	0.5	0	0.0	0	0.0	0	0.0
Seminal vesicle	Reduced colloid	0	0.0	1	5.0	1	0.5	0	0.0	0	0.0	0	0.0
Skin	Cyst	0	0.0	0	0.0	0	0.0	0	0.0	1	5.0	1	0.5
Skin	Erosion	0	0.0	1	5.0	1	0.5	0	0.0	0	0.0	0	0.0
Skin	Necrosis, muscle	0	0.0	1	5.0	1	0.5	0	0.0	0	0.0	0	0.0
Skin	Scab	0	0.0	1	5.0	1	0.5	0	0.0	0	0.0	0	0.0
Spleen	Depletion, lymphoid	0	0.0	1	5.0	1	0.5	0	0.0	3	15.0	5	2.5
Spleen	Deposition pigment	0	0.0	4	20.0	4	2.0	0	0.0	0	0.0	0	0.0
Spleen	Fibrosis, capsular	0	0.0	0	0.0	0	0.0	0	0.0	1	5.0	1	0.5
Spleen	Hematopoiesis, increased	0	0.0	0	0.0	0	0.0	0	0.0	3	14.3	4	2.0
Sternum	Fibrosis	0	0.0	0	0.0	0	0.0	0	0.0	1	5.0	1	0.5
Stomach	Congestion	0	0.0	2	10.0	2	1.0	0	0.0	0	0.0	0	0.0
Stomach	Hemorrhage, mucosa	0	0.0	7	35.0	13	6.5	0	0.0	8	38.1	9	4.5
Stomach	Cyst, squamous	0	0.0	0	0.0	0	0.0	0	0.0	1	5.0	3	1.5
Stomach	Erosion, mucosa	0	0.0	1	5.0	3	1.5	0	0.0	1	5.0	1	0.5

(continued)

TABLE 8.2 (Continued)
Spontaneous Lesions in Control Wistar Rats in Toxicity Studies of 26-Weeks Duration

Rat		Males						Females					
		26 weeks											
Organ	Finding	Minimum	Minimum Range (%)	Maximum	Maximum Range (%)	Total Incidence	Total Incidence (%)	Minimum	Minimum Range (%)	Maximum	Maximum Range (%)	Total Incidence	Total Incidence (%)
						200						201	
Stomach	Hyperplasia, epithelial, non-glandular	0	0.0	5	25.0	14	7.0	0	0.0	4	20.0	8	4.0
Stomach	Inflammation, mixed cell	0	0.0	4	20.0	4	2.0	0	0.0	1	4.8	1	0.5
Stomach	Necrosis, glandular	0	0.0	0	0.0	0	0.0	0	0.0	1	4.8	1	0.5
Stomach	Vacuolation, epithelial, non-glandular	0	0.0	6	30.0	6	3.0	0	0.0	2	9.5	2	1.0
Testes	Inflammation, mixed cell	0	0.0	1	5.0	1	0.5	0	0.0	0	0.0	0	0.0
Testes	Degeneration/atrophy, tubular epithelium	0	0.0	2	10.0	3	1.5	0	0.0	0	0.0	0	0.0
Testes	Hyperplasia, interstitial cell	0	0.0	1	5.0	1	0.5	0	0.0	0	0.0	0	0.0
Thymus	Cyst	0	0.0	0	0.0	0	0.0	0	0.0	1	5.0	1	0.5
Thymus	Depletion, lymphoid	0	0.0	5	25.0	7	3.5	0	0.0	1	4.8	1	0.5
Thymus	Hemorrhage	2	10.0	9	45.0	51	25.5	0	0.0	11	52.4	44	21.9
Thymus	Hyperplasia, epithelial	0	0.0	1	5.0	1	0.5	0	0.0	0	0.0	0	0.0
Thyroid	Hyperplasia, c-cell	0	0.0	1	5.0	2	1.0	0	0.0	0	0.0	0	0.0
Tracheobronchial lymph node	Erythrophagocytosis	0	0.0	0	0.0	0	0.0	0	0.0	2	10.0	3	1.5
Uterus	Cyst	0	0.0	0	0.0	0	0.0	0	0.0	1	5.0	1	0.5
Uterus	Decidual reaction	0	0.0	0	0.0	0	0.0	0	0.0	1	5.0	1	0.5
Uterus	Dilation, luminal	0	0.0	0	0.0	0	0.0	0	0.0	4	20.0	6	3.0
Uterus	Hemorrhage	0	0.0	0	0.0	0	0.0	0	0.0	1	5.0	1	0.5
Uterus	Polyp, endometrial stromal	0	0.0	0	0.0	0	0.0	0	0.0	1	5.0	2	1.0
Vagina	Abnormal mucification/keratinization	0	0.0	0	0.0	0	0.0	0	0.0	1	5.0	1	0.5

8.3   MOUSE

The mouse is a commonly used species for toxicology testing. Table 8.3 shows control data from the CD-1 mouse (Charles River Laboratories) generated from 200 control animals (100/sex) matching the duration of the most common studies that are used to select doses for the 104-week carcinogenicity studies in this species. Animals were approximately 8 weeks of age at the start of dosing.

The highest incidence of spontaneous findings, in descending order of frequency, occurred in the adrenal glands (females), the female reproductive tract, kidneys and lacrimal glands (males), and tracheobronchial lymph nodes and liver (both sexes). The most common findings in the adrenals were spindle cell hyperplasia (males up to 20% and females up to 80%) and cortical pigment in the zona reticularis, identified as lipofuscin/ceroid (males up to 20% and females up to 80%). In the female reproductive tract, the most common lesions were cysts: ovarian (up to 30%), ovarian bursal (up to 50%), and uterine (up to 50%). Common lesions in the kidney were tubular basophilia (up to 40% in both sexes) and hyaline tubular casts (up to 30% in males and 40% in females), while the most commonly observed lesion in the lacrimal gland consisted of mononuclear cell infiltration (up to 50% in males and 0% in females). In addition, an incidence of erythrophagocytosis of up to 70% in males and 80% in females occurred in the tracheobronchial lymph nodes. Mixed cell infiltration/inflammation and hepatocellular cytoplasmic vacuolation were also reported in the liver.

There are few published data on the incidences of spontaneous nonneoplastic lesions in mice. Some of the more common lesions observed in the CD-1 mouse have been described by Frith et al. (2007), but incidences are not given.

TABLE 8.3

Spontaneous Lesions in Control CD-1 Mice in Toxicity Studies of 13-Weeks Duration

Mouse

		Males						Females					
		13 weeks											
Organ	Finding	Minimum	Minimum Range (%)	Maximum	Maximum Range (%)	Total Incidence	Total Incidence (%)	Minimum	Minimum Range (%)	Maximum	Maximum Range (%)	Total Incidence	Total Incidence (%)
						100						100	
Adrenal	Ceroid/lipofuscin, zona reticulosa	0	0.0	2	20.0	2	2.0	0	0.0	8	80.0	14	14.0
Adrenal	Hyperplasia, spindle cell	0	0.0	2	20.0	2	2.0	0	0.0	8	80.0	23	23.0
Bone marrow	Hyperplasia, stromal	0	0.0	1	10.0	1	1.0	0	0.0	1	10.0	1	1.0
Cecum	Inflammation, mixed cell	0	0.0	0	0.0	0	0.0	0	0.0	1	10.0	1	1.0
Epididymides	Inflammation, mixed cell	0	0.0	1	10.0	1	1.0	0	0.0	0	0.0	0	0.0
Epididymides	Oligospermia	0	0.0	1	10.0	1	1.0	0	0.0	0	0.0	0	0.0
Esophagus	Infiltration, mixed cell	0	0.0	0	0.0	0	0.0	0	0.0	1	10.0	1	1.0
Esophagus	Inflammation, mixed cell	0	0.0	1	10.0	1	1.0	0	0.0	1	10.0	1	1.0
Eye	Mononuclear cellular infiltration	0	0.0	0	0.0	0	0.0	0	0.0	1	10.0	1	1.0
Eye	Rosette, retinal	0	0.0	1	10.0	1	1.0	0	0.0	1	10.0	1	1.0
Gallbladder	Colelithiasis	0	0.0	0	0.0	0	0.0	0	0.0	1	10.0	1	1.0
Harderian gland	Mononuclear cellular infiltration	0	0.0	0	0.0	0	0.0	0	0.0	1	10.0	1	1.0
Heart	Mononuclear cellular infiltration	0	0.0	1	10.0	1	1.0	0	0.0	0	0.0	0	0.0
Joint	Arteritis	0	0.0	0	0.0	0	0.0	0	0.0	1	10.0	1	1.0
Joint	Degeneration, cartilage	0	0.0	1	10.0	1	1.0	0	0.0	0	0.0	0	0.0
Joint	Hyperplasia, synovium	0	0.0	1	10.0	1	1.0	0	0.0	0	0.0	0	0.0
Joint	Infiltration, mixed cell	0	0.0	1	10.0	1	1.0	0	0.0	0	0.0	0	0.0
Kidney	Atrophy, tubular	0	0.0	0	0.0	0	0.0	0	0.0	1	10.0	2	2.0
Kidney	Cast, hyaline	0	0.0	3	30.0	5	5.0	0	0.0	4	40.0	9	9.0
Kidney	Cyst	0	0.0	2	20.0	3	3.0	0	0.0	2	20.0	3	3.0
Kidney	Dilatation, tubular	0	0.0	1	10.0	2	2.0	0	0.0	1	10.0	1	1.0
Kidney	Hyperplasia, tubular	0	0.0	1	10.0	1	1.0	0	0.0	0	0.0	0	0.0

Organ	Lesion												
Kidney	Mononuclear cellular infiltration	0	0.0	3	30.0	4	4.0	0	0.0	3	30.0	6	6.0
Kidney	Infiltration, mixed cell	0	0.0	5	50.0	5	5.0	0	0.0	4	40.0	4	4.0
Kidney	Inflammation, mixed cell	0	0.0	1	10.0	1	1.0	0	0.0	1	10.0	1	1.0
Kidney	Necrosis, tubular	0	0.0	1	10.0	1	1.0	0	0.0	0	0.0	0	0.0
Kidney	Nephropathy	0	0.0	0	0.0	0	0.0	0	0.0	1	10.0	1	1.0
Kidney	Tubular basophilia	0	0.0	4	40.0	15	15.0	0	0.0	4	40.0	15	15.0
Kidney	Vacuolation, tubular	0	0.0	1	10.0	2	2.0	0	0.0	0	0.0	0	0.0
Lacrimal gland	Atrophy	0	0.0	1	10.0	2	2.0	0	0.0	1	10.0	1	1.0
Lacrimal gland	Mononuclear cellular infiltration	0	0.0	5	50.0	14	14.0	0	0.0	0	0.0	0	0.0
Larynx	Cyst	0	0.0	0	0.0	0	0.0	0	0.0	1	10.0	1	1.0
Larynx	Degeneration, mucosal	0	0.0	0	0.0	0	0.0	0	0.0	3	30.0	4	4.0
Larynx	Infiltration, mixed cell	0	0.0	1	10.0	1	1.0	0	0.0	3	30.0	3	3.0
Larynx	Mononuclear cellular infiltration	0	0.0	1	10.0	1	1.0	0	0.0	0	0.0	0	0.0
Larynx	Inflammation, mixed cell	0	0.0	2	20.0	2	2.0	0	0.0	1	10.0	1	1.0
Liver	Clear cytoplasm, hepatocellular	0	0.0	8	80.0	8	8.0	0	0.0	9	90.0	9	9.0
Liver	Eosinophilic cytoplasm, hepatocellular	0	0.0	1	10.0	1	1.0	0	0.0	0	0.0	0	0.0
Liver	Infiltration, mixed cell	0	0.0	4	40.0	8	8.0	0	0.0	6	60.0	9	9.0
Liver	Mononuclear cellular infiltration	0	0.0	1	10.0	1	1.0	0	0.0	0	0.0	0	0.0
Liver	Inflammation, mixed cell	0	0.0	3	30.0	6	6.0	0	0.0	2	20.0	4	4.0
Liver	Necrosis, hepatocellular	0	0.0	2	20.0	4	4.0	0	0.0	1	10.0	2	2.0
Liver	Pigment deposit, hepatocytes	0	0.0	1	10.0	1	1.0	0	0.0	0	0.0	0	0.0
Liver	Tension lipidosis	0	0.0	1	10.0	1	1.0	0	0.0	0	0.0	0	0.0
Liver	Hepatocellular vacuolation, centrilobular	0	0.0	1	10.0	2	2.0	0	0.0	0	0.0	0	0.0
Liver	Hepatocellular vacuolation, periportal	0	0.0	1	10.0	1	1.0	0	0.0	0	0.0	0	0.0
Lung	Adenoma	0	0.0	1	10.0	1	1.0	0	0.0	0	0.0	0	0.0
Lung	Hemorrhage	0	0.0	0	0.0	0	0.0	0	0.0	3	30.0	5	5.0
Lung	Macrophage accumulation	0	0.0	1	10.0	2	2.0	0	0.0	0	0.0	0	0.0

(continued)

TABLE 8.3 (Continued)
Spontaneous Lesions in Control CD-1 Mice in Toxicity Studies of 13-Weeks Duration

Mouse

13 weeks

Organ	Finding	Males						Females					
		Minimum	Minimum Range (%)	Maximum	Maximum Range (%)	Total Incidence	Total Incidence (%)	Minimum	Minimum Range (%)	Maximum	Maximum Range (%)	Total Incidence	Total Incidence (%)
						100						100	
Lung	Mononuclear cellular infiltration	0	0.0	1	10.0	1	1.0	0	0.0	0	0.0	0	0.0
Lymph node mesenteric	Erythrophagocytosis	0	0.0	1	10.0	1	1.0	0	0.0	1	10.0	1	1.0
Lymph node mesenteric	Hyperplasia, lymphoid	0	0.0	0	0.0	0	0.0	0	0.0	1	10.0	1	1.0
Lymph node tracheobronchial	Erythrophagocytosis	0	0.0	7	70.0	11	11.0	0	0.0	8	80.0	9	9.0
Mandibular lymph node	Hematopoiesis	0	0.0	1	10.0	1	1.0	0	0.0	0	0.0	0	0.0
Mandibular lymph node	Sinus histiocytosis	0	0.0	1	10.0	1	1.0	0	0.0	4	40.0	5	5.0
Mandibular lymph node	Hyperplasia, lymphoid	0	0.0	1	10.0	1	1.0	0	0.0	1	10.0	1	1.0
Muscle	Degeneration, myofiber	0	0.0	1	10.0	1	1.0	0	0.0	0	0.0	0	0.0
Ovaries	Cyst	0	0.0	0	0.0	0	0.0	0	0.0	3	30.0	8	8.0
Ovaries	Cyst, bursa	0	0.0	0	0.0	0	0.0	0	0.0	5	50.0	16	16.0
Ovaries	Hemorrhage	0	0.0	0	0.0	0	0.0	0	0.0	1	10.0	1	1.0
Ovaries	Hyperplasia, stromal	0	0.0	0	0.0	0	0.0	0	0.0	1	10.0	1	1.0
Pancreas	Atrophy, acinar cell	0	0.0	0	0.0	0	0.0	0	0.0	1	10.0	1	1.0
Pancreas	Mononuclear cellular infiltration	0	0.0	1	10.0	1	1.0	0	0.0	1	10.0	1	1.0

Organ	Lesion	No.	%	No.	%	No.	%	No.	%	No.	%	No.	%
Parathyroid	Cyst	0	0.0	1	10.0	1	1.0	0	0.0	0	0.0	0	0.0
Prostate	Mononuclear cellular infiltration	0	0.0	2	20.0	4	4.0	0	0.0	0	0.0	0	0.0
Prostate	Inflammation, mixed cell	0	0.0	2	20.0	3	3.0	0	0.0	0	0.0	0	0.0
Salivary gland	Mononuclear cellular infiltration	0	0.0	1	10.0	1	1.0	0	0.0	0	0.0	0	0.0
Seminal vesicle	Mononuclear cellular infiltration	0	0.0	1	10.0	1	1.0	0	0.0	0	0.0	0	0.0
Skin	Inflammation, mixed cell	0	0.0	2	20.0	2	2.0	0	0.0	0	0.0	0	0.0
Skin	Ulceration	0	0.0	1	10.0	1	1.0	0	0.0	1	10.0	3	3.0
Spinal cord	Cyst	0	0.0	1	10.0	1	1.0	0	0.0	1	10.0	1	1.0
Spleen	Hematopoiesis increased	0	0.0	2	20.0	2	2.0	0	0.0	0	0.0	0	0.0
Spleen	Hyperplasia, lymphoid	0	0.0	2	20.0	3	3.0	0	0.0	1	10.0	1	1.0
Sternum	Hyperplasia, cartilage	0	0.0	1	10.0	1	1.0	0	0.0	0	0.0	0	0.0
Stomach	Cyst	0	0.0	1	10.0	1	1.0	0	0.0	1	10.0	1	1.0
Stomach	Erosion	0	0.0	1	10.0	1	1.0	0	0.0	1	10.0	1	1.0
Stomach	Mononuclear cellular infiltration	0	0.0	1	10.0	1	1.0	0	0.0	0	0.0	0	0.0
Testes	Degeneration, tubular	0	0.0	1	10.0	1	1.0	0	0.0	0	0.0	0	0.0
Testes	Dilatation, tubular	0	0.0	1	10.0	1	1.0	0	0.0	0	0.0	0	0.0
Testes	Mononuclear cellular infiltration	0	0.0	1	10.0	1	1.0	0	0.0	0	0.0	0	0.0
Testes	Single cell necrosis, germinal cells	0	0.0	1	10.0	1	1.0	0	0.0	0	0.0	0	0.0
Thymus	Atrophy, lymphoid	0	0.0	0	0.0	0	0.0	0	0.0	1	10.0	1	1.0
Thymus	Depletion, lymphoid	0	0.0	0	0.0	0	0.0	0	0.0	1	10.0	2	2.0
Thymus	Hemorrhage	0	0.0	1	10.0	4	4.0	0	0.0	2	20.0	5	5.0
Thymus	Hyperplasia, lymphoid	0	0.0	0	0.0	0	0.0	0	0.0	1	10.0	3	3.0
Thymus	Lymphocytolysis	0	0.0	0	0.0	0	0.0	0	0.0	1	10.0	2	2.0
Thyroid	Ectopic thymus	0	0.0	0	0.0	0	0.0	0	0.0	1	10.0	1	1.0
Tongue	Infiltration, mixed cell	0	0.0	1	10.0	1	1.0	0	0.0	0	0.0	0	0.0
Trachea	Infiltration, mixed cell	0	0.0	0	0.0	0	0.0	0	0.0	1	10.0	1	1.0
Urinary bladder	Perivasculitis	0	0.0	1	10.0	1	1.0	0	0.0	0	0.0	0	0.0
Uterus	Cyst	0	0.0	0	0.0	0	0.0	0	0.0	5	50.0	13	13.0

8.4 DOG

The purpose-bred beagle dog is the most commonly used large animal species in nonclinical safety studies. The historical control data in this review are taken from beagle dogs obtained from Marshall Farms (North Rose, New York) that served as controls in 4-week (Table 8.4) and 26- and 39-week (Table 8.5) studies, matching the study duration most often used when conducting toxicology evaluations in this species. The age of these animals at study start typically ranged from 9 to 12 months.

In the control data from the 4-week studies (53 animals/sex), the highest incidence of spontaneous findings was seen in the kidneys, lung, parathyroid gland, pituitary gland, mesenteric lymph nodes, prostate gland, and thymus. By far the most frequent observations in the kidneys consisted of focal, cortical tubular mineralization (mostly in the papilla) with an incidence of up to 80% in males and 100% in females and prostate gland wherein inflammatory foci were observed in up to 100% of the males, as was acinar gland dilation with an incidence of up to 100%. Other relatively common findings included focal/multifocal mixed cell inflammation in the lung (males, up to 67%; females, up to 100%), parathyroid gland cysts arising from the ultimobranchial duct (up to 67% in both sexes), and pituitary cysts derived from the craniopharyngeal conduit, primarily involving the pars distalis (up to 67% in males and females) and intermedia (up to 67% in males). Other findings included adrenal cortical vacuolation (zona glomerulosa or reticularis/fasciculata, up to 33% in males and 100% in females), thymic lymphoid depletion (males, up to 100%), salivary gland lymphoid cell infiltration (males, up to 100%), erythrophagocytosis in the mesenteric lymph nodes (up to 67% in both sexes), focal–multifocal mixed cell inflammation in the liver (up to 67% in males and 100% in females) as well as foci of extramedullary hematopoiesis (up to 67% in both sexes), renal tubular epithelial (brown) pigment deposition in males (up to 67%), alveolar foamy macrophages in the lung in males (up to 67%), testicular germinal epithelial (tubular) vacuolation (up to 33%), and focal glandular dilation in the duodenum of males (up to 33%).

In the control data from 26- and 39-week studies with a database containing 32 animals/sex, the highest incidence of spontaneous findings was observed in the mesenteric lymph nodes, lung, pituitary gland, and thymus. The percentage of incidence for a given finding was generally comparable between the sexes. The most frequent findings occurred in the mesenteric lymph nodes consisting of erythrophagocytosis (up to 100% in both sexes), followed by thymic lymphoid depletion (up to 100% in males and 75% in females), pituitary gland cysts, mostly involving the pars distalis (up to 75% in both sexes), and mixed cell inflammation in the lung (up to 25% in males and 50% in females). Other fairly common findings included thymic hemorrhage, focal fibrosis in the lung of females (mostly pleural/subcapsular), renal tubular basophilia and the presence of mononuclear cell infiltrates in males, and testicular germinal epithelial (tubular) degeneration and hypospermatogenesis and hepatocellular cytoplasmic (brown) pigment in males.

Where incidence comparisons can be made between the 4-week and 26-/39-week data, inflammatory foci in the lung and pituitary cysts were comparable while the incidence of thymic lymphoid depletion was increased in the studies of longer duration, most likely owing to physiological involution as related to aging. The incidence of erythrophagocytosis in the mesenteric lymph nodes was increased almost threefold and sixfold in males and females, respectively, in the chronic studies versus 4-week studies, respectively, suggesting a possible increased tendency for gastrointestinal microhemorrhage as a function of age. A relatively frequent finding in all studies consisted of inflammatory cell foci/infiltrates in various organs/tissues, notably liver, lung, prostate gland, and salivary glands. These are common sites for generally focal, minimal inflammation in beagle dogs used in toxicity studies (Chamanza et al. 2007; Maiti et al. 1977). Pituitary and parathyroid cysts are also often seen in control beagles (Capen 2007). Adrenal cortical vacuolation is another finding occasionally seen, mostly in females, as is thymic atrophy (depletion) with advancing age in both sexes (Morishima et al. 1990). Focal subpleural fibrosis (also called fibrosing alveolitis) has been described as a background lesion in the lungs of beagle dogs (Hahn and Dagle 2001) while vacuolation of the seminiferous tubular epithelium and hypospermatogenesis in the testes is not an uncommon spontaneous finding in laboratory beagles (Rehm 2000).

TABLE 8.4

Spontaneous Lesions in Control Beagle Dogs in Toxicity Studies of 4-Weeks Duration

Dog

| | | Males | | | | | | Females | | | | | |
| | | 4 weeks | | | | | | | | | | | |
Organ	Finding	Minimum	Minimum Range (%)	Maximum	Maximum Range (%)	Total Incidence	Total Incidence (%)	Minimum	Minimum Range (%)	Maximum	Maximum Range (%)	Total Incidence	Total Incidence (%)
						53						53	
Adrenal	Accessory cortical tissue	0	0.0	0	0.0	0	0.0	0	0.0	1	33.3	1	1.9
Adrenal	Vacuolation, cortex, zona fasciculata	0	0.0	1	33.3	3	5.7	0	0.0	3	100.0	7	13.2
Brain	Dilation, ventricle	0	0.0	1	33.3	1	1.9	0	0.0	0	0.0	0	0.0
Brain	Gliosis	0	0.0	0	0.0	0	0.0	0	0.0	1	33.3	1	1.9
Brain	Hemorrhage	0	0.0	1	33.3	1	1.9	0	0.0	0	0.0	0	0.0
Brain	Infiltration, lymphoid cell	0	0.0	1	33.3	1	1.9	0	0.0	0	0.0	0	0.0
Brain	Inflammation, lymphocytic	0	0.0	0	0.0	0	0.0	0	0.0	1	33.3	1	1.9
Cecum	Congestion	0	0.0	2	66.7	2	3.8	0	0.0	1	33.3	1	1.9
Cecum	Crypt plug	0	0.0	1	33.3	1	1.9	0	0.0	0	0.0	0	0.0
Cecum	Dilation, glandular	0	0.0	0	0.0	0	0.0	0	0.0	1	33.3	1	1.9
Cecum	Hemorrhage	0	0.0	1	33.3	2	3.8	0	0.0	1	33.3	1	1.9
Cecum	Infiltration, mixed cell	0	0.0	0	0.0	0	0.0	0	0.0	1	33.3	1	1.9
Cecum	Mineralization	0	0.0	1	33.3	1	1.9	0	0.0	0	0.0	0	0.0
Colon	Congestion	0	0.0	2	66.7	2	3.8	0	0.0	0	0.0	0	0.0
Colon	Infiltration, mixed cell	0	0.0	0	0.0	0	0.0	0	0.0	1	33.3	1	1.9
Duodenum	Congestion	0	0.0	2	66.7	3	5.7	0	0.0	1	33.3	1	1.9
Duodenum	Crypt plug	0	0.0	0	0.0	0	0.0	0	0.0	1	33.3	3	5.7
Duodenum	Dilation, glandular	0	0.0	1	33.3	4	7.5	0	0.0	2	66.7	3	5.7
Duodenum	Hemorrhage	0	0.0	1	33.3	1	1.9	0	0.0	0	0.0	0	0.0
Duodenum	Infiltration, lymphoid cell	0	0.0	0	0.0	0	0.0	0	0.0	1	33.3	1	1.9
Epididymides	Aspermia	0	0.0	2	66.7	3	5.7	0	0.0	0	0.0	0	0.0
Epididymides	Cellular debris	0	0.0	2	66.7	2	3.8	0	0.0	0	0.0	0	0.0
Epididymides	Vacuolation, epithelial	0	0.0	1	33.3	1	1.9	0	0.0	0	0.0	0	0.0
Esophagus	Inflammation, mixed cell	0	0.0	1	33.3	1	1.9	0	0.0	0	0.0	0	0.0
Gallbladder	Inflammation, lymphocytic	0	0.0	0	0.0	0	0.0	0	0.0	1	33.3	1	1.9

(continued)

TABLE 8.4 (Continued)
Spontaneous Lesions in Control Beagle Dogs in Toxicity Studies of 4-Weeks Duration

Dog — 4 weeks

Organ	Finding	Males						Females					
		Minimum	Minimum Range (%)	Maximum	Maximum Range (%)	Total Incidence	Total Incidence (%)	Minimum	Minimum Range (%)	Maximum	Maximum Range (%)	Total Incidence	Total Incidence (%)
						53						53	
Gallbladder	Vacuolation, epithelial	0	0.0	1	33.3	1	1.9	0	0.0	1	33.3	1	1.9
Heart	Myofiber degeneration	0	0.0	1	33.3	1	1.9	0	0.0	0	0.0	0	0.0
Heart	Infiltration, lymphoid cell	0	0.0	1	33.3	2	3.8	0	0.0	0	0.0	0	0.0
Heart	Medial hypertrophy, coronary artery	0	0.0	0	0.0	0	0.0	0	0.0	1	33.3	1	1.9
Ileum	Congestion	0	0.0	1	33.3	1	1.9	0	0.0	0	0.0	0	0.0
Ileum	Hemorrhage	0	0.0	1	33.3	1	1.9	0	0.0	0	0.0	0	0.0
Jejunum	Congestion	0	0.0	2	66.7	3	5.7	0	0.0	0	0.0	0	0.0
Jejunum	Dilation, glandular	0	0.0	1	33.3	1	1.9	0	0.0	0	0.0	0	0.0
Jejunum	Hemorrhage	0	0.0	1	33.3	1	1.9	0	0.0	0	0.0	0	0.0
Kidney	Basophilia, tubular	0	0.0	1	33.3	1	1.9	0	0.0	1	33.3	1	1.9
Kidney	Cast, hyaline	0	0.0	1	33.3	1	1.9	0	0.0	0	0.0	0	0.0
Kidney	Cyst	0	0.0	1	33.3	1	1.9	0	0.0	0	0.0	0	0.0
Kidney	Deposition pigment, tubular epithelium	0	0.0	4	80.0	4	7.5	0	0.0	0	0.0	0	0.0
Kidney	Dilation tubular	0	0.0	0	0.0	0	0.0	0	0.0	2	66.7	2	3.8
Kidney	Fibrosis	0	0.0	0	0.0	0	0.0	0	0.0	1	33.3	1	1.9
Kidney	Glomerular lipidosis	0	0.0	1	33.3	1	1.9	0	0.0	1	33.3	1	1.9
Kidney	Infiltration, lymphoid cell	0	0.0	1	33.3	1	1.9	0	0.0	1	33.3	1	1.9
Kidney	Inflammation, lymphocytic	0	0.0	1	33.3	2	3.8	0	0.0	2	33.3	2	3.8
Kidney	Inflammation, mixed cell	0	0.0	1	33.3	1	1.9	0	0.0	1	33.3	1	1.9
Kidney	Mineralization, tubular	0	0.0	4	80.0	25	47.2	0	0.0	5	100.0	26	49.1
Kidney	Vacuolation, tubular	0	0.0	0	0.0	0	0.0	0	0.0	1	33.3	1	1.9
Lacrimal gland	Infiltration, lymphoid cell	0	0.0	1	33.3	2	3.8	0	0.0	1	33.3	2	3.8
Larynx	Hyperplasia, lymphoid	0	0.0	2	66.7	2	3.8	0	0.0	1	33.3	4	7.5
Larynx	Infiltration, lymphoid cell	0	0.0	1	33.3	1	1.9	0	0.0	1	33.3	2	3.8
Liver	Atrophy, hepatocellular	0	0.0	1	33.3	1	1.9	0	0.0	0	0.0	0	0.0
Liver	Deposition, pigment	0	0.0	0	0.0	0	0.0	0	0.0	1	33.3	1	1.9

Organ	Lesion												
Liver	Fibrosis	0	0.0	1	33.3	1	1.9	0	0.0	1	33.3	1	1.9
Liver	Granuloma	0	0.0	1	33.3	1	1.9	0	0.0	0	0.0	0	0.0
Liver	Hematopoiesis	0	0.0	2	66.7	4	7.5	0	0.0	2	66.7	5	9.4
Liver	Infiltration, lymphoid cell	0	0.0	1	33.3	1	1.9	0	0.0	1	33.3	1	1.9
Liver	Infiltration, mixed cell	0	0.0	2	66.7	3	5.7	0	0.0	0	0.0	0	0.0
Liver	Infiltration, mononuclear cell	0	0.0	0	0.0	0	0.0	0	0.0	1	33.3	1	1.9
Liver	Inflammation, lymphocytic	0	0.0	1	33.3	1	1.9	0	0.0	0	0.0	0	0.0
Liver	Inflammation, mixed cell	0	0.0	3	100.0	6	11.3	0	0.0	3	100.0	5	9.4
Lung	Alveolitis	0	0.0	0	0.0	0	0.0	0	0.0	1	33.3	1	1.9
Lung	Congestion	0	0.0	1	33.3	1	1.9	0	0.0	1	33.3	2	3.8
Lung	Edema	0	0.0	0	0.0	0	0.0	0	0.0	1	33.3	1	1.9
Lung	Fibrosis	0	0.0	0	0.0	0	0.0	0	0.0	1	33.3	1	1.9
Lung	Granuloma	0	0.0	1	33.3	1	1.9	0	0.0	1	33.3	2	3.8
Lung	Infiltration, mixed cell	0	0.0	2	66.7	2	3.8	0	0.0	2	66.7	4	7.5
Lung	Infiltration, neutrophilic	0	0.0	0	0.0	0	0.0	0	0.0	1	33.3	1	1.9
Lung	Infiltration, perivascular lymphocytic	0	0.0	1	33.3	1	1.9	0	0.0	0	0.0	0	0.0
Lung	Inflammation, mixed cell	0	0.0	2	66.7	10	18.9	0	0.0	3	100.0	13	24.5
Lung	Inflammation, granulomatous	0	0.0	0	0.0	0	0.0	0	0.0	2	66.7	3	5.7
Lung	Inflammation, lymphocytic	0	0.0	1	33.3	2	3.8	0	0.0	0	0.0	0	0.0
Lung	Inflammation, perivascular/peribronchial	0	0.0	2	66.7	2	3.8	0	0.0	1	33.3	1	1.9
Lung	Inflammation, neutrophilic	0	0.0	0	0.0	0	0.0	0	0.0	1	33.3	1	1.9
Lung	Foamy macrophages, alveolar	0	0.0	2	66.7	4	7.5	0	0.0	2	66.7	2	3.8
Mammary	Hyperplasia, epithelial	0	0.0	0	0.0	0	0.0	0	0.0	1	33.3	1	1.9
Mammary	Increased secretory activity	0	0.0	0	0.0	0	0.0	0	0.0	2	66.7	2	3.8
Mammary	Functional hypertrophy	0	0.0	0	0.0	0	0.0	0	0.0	1	33.3	1	1.9
Mandibular lymph node	Sinus histiocytosis	0	0.0	1	33.3	1	1.9	0	0.0	0	0.0	0	0.0
Mandibular lymph node	Infiltration, mixed cell	0	0.0	1	33.3	2	3.8	0	0.0	0	0.0	0	0.0
Mandibular lymph node	Inflammation, mixed cell	0	0.0	1	33.3	1	1.9	0	0.0	0	0.0	0	0.0
Mesenteric lymph node	Congestion	0	0.0	0	0.0	0	0.0	0	0.0	1	33.3	1	1.9
Mesenteric lymph node	Erythrophagocytosis	0	0.0	2	66.7	8	15.1	0	0.0	2	66.7	5	9.4

(continued)

TABLE 8.4 (Continued)
Spontaneous Lesions in Control Beagle Dogs in Toxicity Studies of 4-Weeks Duration

Dog		Males (4 weeks)						Females					
Organ	Finding	Minimum	Minimum Range (%)	Maximum	Maximum Range (%)	Total Incidence	Total Incidence (%)	Minimum	Minimum Range (%)	Maximum	Maximum Range (%)	Total Incidence	Total Incidence (%)
						53						53	
Pancreas	Infiltration, lymphoid cell	0	0.0	1	33.3	1	1.9	0	0.0	0	0.0	0	0.0
Parathyroid	Cyst	0	0.0	2	66.7	8	15.1	0	0.0	2	66.7	10	18.9
Pituitary	Cyst, pars distalis	0	0.0	2	66.7	15	28.3	0	0.0	2	66.7	13	24.5
Pituitary	Cyst, pars intermedia	0	0.0	2	66.7	3	5.7	0	0.0	0	0.0	0	0.0
Pituitary	Dilation, Rathke's pouch	0	0.0	1	33.3	1	1.9	0	0.0	0	0.0	0	0.0
Prostate	Dilation, glandular	0	0.0	5	100.0	16	30.2	0	0.0	0	0.0	0	0.0
Prostate	Immature	0	0.0	2	66.7	2	3.8	0	0.0	0	0.0	0	0.0
Prostate	Infiltration, mixed cell	0	0.0	2	66.7	3	5.7	0	0.0	0	0.0	0	0.0
Prostate	Infiltration, lymphoid cell	0	0.0	2	66.7	5	9.4	0	0.0	0	0.0	0	0.0
Prostate	Inflammation, lymphocytic	0	0.0	1	33.3	1	1.9	0	0.0	0	0.0	0	0.0
Prostate	Inflammation, mixed cell	0	0.0	5	100.0	19	35.8	0	0.0	0	0.0	0	0.0
Prostate	Vacuolation, epithelial	0	0.0	2	66.7	2	3.8	0	0.0	0	0.0	0	0.0
Rectum	Dilation, glandular	0	0.0	1	33.3	1	1.9	0	0.0	0	0.0	0	0.0
Retropharyngeal lymph node	Deposition, pigment	0	0.0	0	0.0	0	0.0	0	0.0	1	33.3	1	1.9
Retropharyngeal lymph node	Erythrophagocytosis	0	0.0	0	0.0	0	0.0	0	0.0	1	33.3	1	1.9
Retropharyngeal lymph node	Hemorrhage	0	0.0	2	66.7	2	3.8	0	0.0	1	33.3	1	1.9
Retropharyngeal lymph node	Sinus histiocytosis	0	0.0	0	0.0	0	0.0	0	0.0	1	33.3	1	1.9
Retropharyngeal lymph node	Hyperplasia, lymphoid	0	0.0	2	66.7	2	3.8	0	0.0	0	0.0	0	0.0
Retropharyngeal lymph node	Lymphocytolysis	0	0.0	0	0.0	0	0.0	0	0.0	1	33.3	2	3.8
Salivary gland	Infiltration, lymphoid cell	0	0.0	3	100.0	6	11.3	0	0.0	3	100.0	4	7.5
Skin	Folliculitis	0	0.0	1	33.3	1	1.9	0	0.0	0	0.0	0	0.0

Organ	Lesion												
Skin	Infiltration, mixed cell	0	0.0	1	33.3	1	1.9	0	0.0	0	0.0	0	0.0
Skin	Inflammation, granulomatous	0	0.0	1	33.3	1	1.9	0	0.0	0	0.0	0	0.0
Skin	Inflammation, mixed cell	0	0.0	2	66.7	3	5.7	0	0.0	1	33.3	1	1.9
Skin	Ulceration	0	0.0	1	33.3	1	1.9	0	0.0	0	0.0	0	0.0
Spleen	Deposition, pigment	0	0.0	1	33.3	1	1.9	0	0.0	1	33.3	0	0.0
Spleen	Fibrosis	0	0.0	1	33.3	1	1.9	0	0.0	0	0.0	1	1.9
Spleen	Siderotic plaque	0	0.0	0	0.0	2	3.8	0	0.0	1	33.3	0	0.0
Stomach	Bacteria, luminal	0	0.0	1	33.3	0	0.0	0	0.0	0	0.0	1	1.9
Stomach	Congestion	0	0.0	0	0.0	1	1.9	0	0.0	0	0.0	0	0.0
Stomach	Dilation, glandular	0	0.0	1	33.3	0	0.0	0	0.0	1	33.3	3	5.7
Stomach	Hyperplasia, lymphoid	0	0.0	0	0.0	1	1.9	0	0.0	1	33.3	1	1.9
Stomach	Infiltration, mixed cell	0	0.0	1	33.3	0	0.0	0	0.0	1	33.3	1	1.9
Stomach	Inflammation, neutrophilic	0	0.0	1	33.3	1	1.9	0	0.0	0	0.0	0	0.0
Stomach	Inflammation, mixed cell	0	0.0	1	33.3	1	1.9	0	0.0	0	0.0	0	0.0
Testes	Atrophy, tubular	0	0.0	1	33.3	1	1.9	0	0.0	0	0.0	0	0.0
Testes	Degeneration, tubular	0	0.0	1	33.3	3	5.7	0	0.0	0	0.0	0	0.0
Testes	Depletion, germ cell	0	0.0	2	66.7	2	3.8	0	0.0	0	0.0	0	0.0
Testes	Giant cells	0	0.0	1	33.3	1	1.9	0	0.0	0	0.0	0	0.0
Testes	Hypospermatogenesis	0	0.0	2	66.7	1	1.9	0	0.0	0	0.0	0	0.0
Testes	Immature	0	0.0	2	66.7	2	3.8	0	0.0	0	0.0	0	0.0
Testes	Infiltration, mixed cell	0	0.0	2	66.7	1	1.9	0	0.0	0	0.0	0	0.0
Testes	Sperm stasis	0	0.0	3	100.0	3	5.7	0	0.0	0	0.0	0	0.0
Testes	Vacuolation, tubular	0	0.0	1	33.3	4	7.5	0	0.0	0	0.0	0	0.0
Thymus	Cyst	0	0.0	1	33.3	2	3.8	0	0.0	1	33.3	1	1.9
Thymus	Depletion, lymphoid	0	0.0	0	0.0	7	13.2	0	0.0	1	33.3	2	3.8
Thymus	Hematopoiesis	0	0.0	2	66.7	1	1.9	0	0.0	2	66.7	2	3.8
Thymus	Hemorrhage	0	0.0	1	33.3	1	1.9	0	0.0	1	33.3	1	1.9
Thymus	Hyperplasia, lymphoid	0	0.0	1	33.3	0	0.0	0	0.0	1	33.3	2	3.8
Thymus	Involution	0	0.0	1	33.3	2	3.8	0	0.0	1	33.3	2	3.8
Thymus	Lymphocytolysis	0	0.0	0	0.0	1	1.9	0	0.0	2	66.7	3	5.7
Thyroid	Cyst, follicular	0	0.0	1	33.3	1	1.9	0	0.0	1	33.3	1	1.9
Thyroid	Dilation, follicular	0	0.0	1	33.3	1	1.9	0	0.0	0	0.0	0	0.0
Thyroid	Infiltration, lymphoid cell	0	0.0	0	0.0	0	0.0	0	0.0	1	33.3	1	1.9
Thyroid	Inflammation, mixed cell	0	0.0	1	33.3	1	1.9	0	0.0	1	33.3	0	0.0

(continued)

TABLE 8.4 (Continued)

Spontaneous Lesions in Control Beagle Dogs in Toxicity Studies of 4-Weeks Duration

Dog		Males						Females					
		4 weeks											
Organ	Finding	Minimum	Minimum Range (%)	Maximum	Maximum Range (%)	Total Incidence	Total Incidence (%)	Minimum	Minimum Range (%)	Maximum	Maximum Range (%)	Total Incidence	Total Incidence (%)
						53						53	
Tracheobronchial lymph node	Thrombus, venule	0	0.0	1	33.3	1	1.9	0	0.0	0	0.0	0	0.0
Ureter	Inflammation, neutrophilic	0	0.0	1	33.3	1	1.9	0	0.0	0	0.0	0	0.0
Urinary bladder	Degeneration, mucosal	0	0.0	0	0.0	0	0.0	0	0.0	1	33.3	1	1.9
Urinary bladder	Edema	0	0.0	1	33.3	1	1.9	0	0.0	0	0.0	0	0.0
Urinary bladder	Erosion	0	0.0	1	33.3	1	1.9	0	0.0	0	0.0	0	0.0
Urinary bladder	Hemorrhage	0	0.0	1	33.3	3	5.7	0	0.0	1	33.3	2	3.8
Urinary bladder	Hyperplasia, transitional cell	0	0.0	1	33.3	1	1.9	0	0.0	1	33.3	1	1.9
Urinary bladder	Inflammation, mixed cell	0	0.0	1	33.3	1	1.9	0	0.0	1	33.3	1	1.9
Urinary bladder	Ulceration	0	0.0	0	0.0	0	0.0	0	0.0	1	33.3	1	1.9
Urinary bladder	Vacuolation, epithelial	0	0.0	0	0.0	0	0.0	0	0.0	1	33.3	1	1.9
Uterus	Infiltration, lymphoid cell	0	0.0	0	0.0	0	0.0	0	0.0	1	33.3	1	1.9
Vagina	Infiltration, mixed cell	0	0.0	0	0.0	0	0.0	0	0.0	1	33.3	1	1.9
Vagina	Infiltration, lymphoid cell	0	0.0	0	0.0	0	0.0	0	0.0	1	33.3	1	1.9

TABLE 8.5

Spontaneous Lesions in Control Beagle Dogs in Toxicity Studies of 26- and 39-Weeks Duration

Dog

Organ	Finding	Males (26 and 39 weeks)						Females (26 and 39 weeks)					
		Minimum	Minimum Range (%)	Maximum	Maximum Range (%)	Total Incidence	Total Incidence (%)	Minimum	Minimum Range (%)	Maximum	Maximum Range (%)	Total Incidence	Total Incidence (%)
						32						32	
Adrenal	Vacuolation, zona glomerulosa	0	0.0	0	0.0	0	0.0	0	0.0	1	25.0	1	3.1
Brain	Infiltration, mononuclear cell	0	0.0	0	0.0	0	0.0	0	0.0	1	25.0	1	3.1
Cecum	Hemorrhage	0	0.0	1	25.0	1	3.1	0	0.0	0	0.0	0	0.0
Colon	Hemorrhage	0	0.0	1	25.0	1	3.1	0	0.0	0	0.0	0	0.0
Duodenum	Hemorrhage	0	0.0	1	25.0	1	3.1	0	0.0	0	0.0	0	0.0
Epididymides	Cellular debris	0	0.0	1	25.0	1	3.1	0	0.0	0	0.0	0	0.0
Esophagus	Fibrosis	0	0.0	0	0.0	0	0.0	0	0.0	1	25.0	1	3.1
Esophagus	Infiltration, mononuclear cell	0	0.0	0	0.0	0	0.0	0	0.0	1	25.0	1	3.1
Gallbladder	Vacuolation, epithelial	0	0.0	0	0.0	0	0.0	0	0.0	1	25.0	1	3.1
Heart	Hemorrhage	0	0.0	1	25.0	1	3.1	0	0.0	0	0.0	0	0.0
Heart	Infiltration, mononuclear cell	0	0.0	1	25.0	1	3.1	0	0.0	0	0.0	0	0.0
Ileum	Depletion/necrosis, lymphoid	0	0.0	1	25.0	1	3.1	0	0.0	0	0.0	0	0.0
Kidney	Basophilia, tubular	0	0.0	1	25.0	4	12.5	0	0.0	1	25.0	1	3.1
Kidney	Cast, hyaline	0	0.0	0	0.0	0	0.0	0	0.0	2	50.0	2	6.3
Kidney	Dilation, pelvis	0	0.0	1	25.0	1	3.1	0	0.0	0	0.0	0	0.0
Kidney	Infiltration, mononuclear cell	0	0.0	2	50.0	3	9.4	0	0.0	1	25.0	1	3.1
Kidney	Inflammation, mixed cell	0	0.0	1	25.0	1	3.1	0	0.0	0	0.0	0	0.0
Kidney	Inflammation, neutrophilic	0	0.0	1	25.0	1	3.1	0	0.0	0	0.0	0	0.0
Kidney	Vacuolation, glomerular	0	0.0	1	25.0	1	3.1	0	0.0	0	0.0	0	0.0
Kidney	Vacuolation, tubular	0	0.0	0	0.0	0	0.0	0	0.0	1	25.0	2	6.3
Lacrimal gland	Infiltration, lymphoid cell	0	0.0	0	0.0	0	0.0	0	0.0	1	25.0	1	3.1
Liver	Deposition, pigment, hepatocyte	0	0.0	3	75.0	3	9.4	0	0.0	1	25.0	1	3.1
Liver	Fibrosis	0	0.0	1	25.0	1	3.1	0	0.0	0	0.0	0	0.0

(continued)

TABLE 8.5 (Continued)
Spontaneous Lesions in Control Beagle Dogs in Toxicity Studies of 26- and 39-Weeks Duration

Dog

26 and 39 weeks

Organ	Finding	Males						Females					
		Minimum	Minimum Range (%)	Maximum	Maximum Range (%)	Total Incidence	Total Incidence (%)	Minimum	Minimum Range (%)	Maximum	Maximum Range (%)	Total Incidence	Total Incidence (%)
						32						32	
Liver	Infiltration, mononuclear cell	0	0.0	1	25.0	1	3.1	0	0.0	0	0.0	0	0.0
Liver	Necrosis, hepatocellular	0	0.0	1	25.0	1	3.1	0	0.0	0	0.0	0	0.0
Lung	Fibrosis, pleura	0	0.0	1	25.0	1	3.1	0	0.0	2	50.0	5	15.6
Lung	Foreign material/body	0	0.0	1	25.0	1	3.1	0	0.0	0	0.0	0	0.0
Lung	Granuloma	0	0.0	2	50.0	2	6.3	0	0.0	1	25.0	1	3.1
Lung	Sinus histiocytosis	0	0.0	1	25.0	1	3.1	0	0.0	0	0.0	0	0.0
Lung	Infiltration, mixed cell	0	0.0	0	0.0	0	0.0	0	0.0	1	25.0	1	3.1
Lung	Inflammation, mixed cell	0	0.0	4	100.0	11	34.4	0	0.0	2	50.0	7	21.9
Lung	Accumulations, foam cell	0	0.0	0	0.0	0	0.0	0	0.0	2	50.0	2	6.3
Mandibular lymph node	Depletion, lymphoid	0	0.0	1	25.0	1	3.1	0	0.0	0	0.0	0	0.0
Mandibular lymph node	Deposits, pigment	0	0.0	1	25.0	1	3.1	0	0.0	0	0.0	0	0.0
Mandibular lymph node	Erythrophagocytosis	0	0.0	1	25.0	1	3.1	0	0.0	1	25.0	1	3.1
Mesenteric lymph node	Erythrophagocytosis	0	0.0	4	100.0	13	40.6	0	0.0	4	100.0	19	59.4
Parathyroid	Cyst	0	0.0	0	0.0	0	0.0	0	0.0	1	25.0	2	6.3
Pituitary	Cyst	0	0.0	3	75.0	11	34.4	0	0.0	3	75.0	8	25.0
Prostate	Dilation, glandular	0	0.0	1	25.0	1	3.1	0	0.0	0	0.0	0	0.0

Organ/Tissue	Lesion	n	%	n	%	n	%	n	%	n	%	n	%
Prostate	Infiltration, mononuclear cell	0	0.0	2	50.0	2	6.3	0	0.0	0	0.0	0	0.0
Rectum	Hemorrhage	0	0.0	1	25.0	1	3.1	0	0.0	0	0.0	0	0.0
Retropharyngeal lymph node	Depletion, lymphoid	0	0.0	0	0.0	0	0.0	0	0.0	1	25.0	1	3.1
Retropharyngeal lymph node	Erythrophagocytosis	0	0.0	1	25.0	3	9.4	0	0.0	2	50.0	4	12.5
Retropharyngeal lymph node	Hyperplasia, lymphoid	0	0.0	0	0.0	0	0.0	0	0.0	1	25.0	1	3.1
Skin	Granuloma	0	0.0	1	25.0	1	3.1	0	0.0	1	25.0	1	3.1
Skin	Infiltration, mononuclear cell	0	0.0	0	0.0	0	0.0	0	0.0	1	25.0	1	3.1
Skin	Inflammation, mixed cell	0	0.0	0	0.0	0	0.0	0	0.0	1	25.0	1	3.1
Spinal cord	Gliosis	0	0.0	0	0.0	0	0.0	0	0.0	1	25.0	1	3.1
Spleen	Depletion, lymphoid	0	0.0	0	0.0	0	0.0	0	0.0	1	25.0	1	3.1
Spleen	Deposition, pigment	0	0.0	1	25.0	1	3.1	0	0.0	1	25.0	1	3.1
Spleen	Fibrosis	0	0.0	0	0.0	0	0.0	0	0.0	1	25.0	2	6.3
Spleen	Siderotic plaque	0	0.0	0	0.0	0	0.0	0	0.0	1	25.0	2	6.3
Stomach	Hemorrhage	0	0.0	0	0.0	2	6.3	0	0.0	2	50.0	2	6.3
Testes	Degeneration, tubular	0	0.0	2	50.0	4	12.5	0	0.0	0	0.0	0	0.0
Testes	Hypospermatogenesis	0	0.0	2	50.0	3	9.4	0	0.0	0	0.0	0	0.0
Testes	Sperm stasis	0	0.0	1	25.0	1	3.1	0	0.0	0	0.0	0	0.0
Testes	Vacuolation, Sertoli cell	0	0.0	1	25.0	1	3.1	0	0.0	0	0.0	0	0.0
Thymus	Depletion, lymphoid	0	0.0	4	100.0	9	28.1	0	0.0	3	75.0	12	37.5
Thymus	Hemorrhage	0	0.0	3	75.0	5	15.6	0	0.0	2	50.0	4	12.5
Thyroid	Cyst	0	0.0	1	25.0	1	3.1	0	0.0	0	0.0	0	0.0
Thyroid	Infiltration, mononuclear cell	0	0.0	0	0.0	0	0.0	0	0.0	1	25.0	1	3.1
Trachea	Developmental malformation	0	0.0	0	0.0	0	0.0	0	0.0	1	25.0	1	3.1
Trachea	Inflammation, mixed cell	0	0.0	0	0.0	0	0.0	0	0.0	1	25.0	1	3.1
Tracheobronchial lymph node	Hyperplasia, lymphoid	0	0.0	1	25.0	1	3.1	0	0.0	0	0.0	0	0.0
Urinary bladder	Ectopic spleen	0	0.0	0	0.0	0	0.0	0	0.0	1	25.0	1	3.1

8.5 MONKEY

The historical control data reported in this section come from the most commonly used nonhuman primate in nonclinical safety studies: the cynomolgus monkey (*Macaca fascicularis*). The data are compiled from 4-week (Table 8.6) and 26- and 52-week (Table 8.7) toxicology studies matching the duration of those most commonly used in toxicity testing paradigms. Animals were approximately 2–4 years of age at the start of dosing.

In the control data from the 4-week studies with a database containing 64 males and 63 females, the most common incidental findings occurred in the kidney, lung, and gastrointestinal tract. These changes were typically inflammatory in nature and sometimes occurred at up to 100% incidence in individual studies and as high as approximately 40% incidence in animals across all studies and primarily involved the kidney. Mixed cell inflammation/infiltration in both the heart and kidney was present in all controls in several individual studies. Lymphoid and mononuclear cell infiltrates were also occasionally observed in the heart and kidney at an incidence of 100% in some studies. The incidence of these inflammatory cell foci in heart and kidney was roughly similar in both sexes. The lymphoid hyperplasia in the cecum and colon was most likely the result of gastrointestinal tract parasite migration (Chamanza et al. 2010).

In the chronic studies of 26- or 52-week duration, incidences of spontaneous lesions were compiled from 64 animals (32 male and 32 females). Similar to the data reported in the 4-week studies, the most common findings were inflammatory in nature for the gastrointestinal tract, particularly the cecum and colon. The incidence of mononuclear (inflammatory) cell infiltration in the kidney and heart was up to 25% and 50% across individual studies, respectively, and lower than what was seen in the 4-week studies. The incidence of interstitial inflammation as well as fibrosis in the lung was up to 25% in males and 50% in females. The incidence of mixed cell inflammation in the stomach was as high as 100% or 75% in individual studies for male and female monkeys, respectively. Pigment deposition and fibrosis were infrequently observed in the liver of control male and female monkeys. The incidence of thymic hemorrhage was as high as 50% in individual studies and averaged 9.4% for all animals, both males and females. There were no apparent sex differences for degenerative or inflammatory changes in control monkeys. Refer to Chamanza et al. (2010) for an excellent review of spontaneous findings in control cynomolgus monkeys.

TABLE 8.6
Spontaneous Lesions in Control Cynomolgous Monkeys in Toxicity Studies of 4-Weeks Duration

Monkey

		Males						Females					
		4 weeks											
Organ	Finding	Minimum	Minimum Range (%)	Maximum	Maximum Range (%)	Total Incidence	Total Incidence (%)	Minimum	Minimum Range (%)	Maximum	Maximum Range (%)	Total Incidence	Total Incidence (%)
						64						63	
Adrenal	Accessory cortical tissue	0	0.0	1	33.3	1	1.6	0	0.0	1	33.3	2	3.2
Adrenal	Anomaly	0	0.0	1	33.3	1	1.6	0	0.0	0	0.0	0	0.0
Adrenal	Cortical hypertrophy, zona fasciculata	0	0.0	0	0.0	0	0.0	0	0.0	1	33.3	2	3.2
Adrenal	Cortical vacuolation, zona fasciculata	0	0.0	1	33.3	1	1.6	0	0.0	1	33.3	1	1.6
Adrenal	Cyst	0	0.0	0	0.0	0	0.0	0	0.0	1	33.3	1	1.6
Adrenal	Hematopoiesis	0	0.0	0	0.0	0	0.0	0	0.0	1	33.3	1	1.6
Adrenal	Hemorrhage	0	0.0	1	33.3	1	1.6	0	0.0	0	0.0	0	0.0
Adrenal	Hyperplasia, zona fasciculata	0	0.0	0	0.0	0	0.0	0	0.0	1	33.3	2	3.2
Adrenal	Infiltration, lymphoid cell	0	0.0	1	33.3	1	1.6	0	0.0	1	33.3	1	1.6
Adrenal	Mineralization, zona fasciculata	0	0.0	1	33.3	2	3.1	0	0.0	2	66.7	4	6.3
Adrenal	Necrosis/apoptosis, zona fasciculata	0	0.0	0	0.0	0	0.0	0	0.0	1	33.3	1	1.6
Adrenal	Thrombus	0	0.0	0	0.0	0	0.0	0	0.0	1	33.3	1	1.6
Aorta	Inflammation, mixed cell	0	0.0	0	0.0	0	0.0	0	0.0	1	33.3	1	1.6
Bone marrow	Hemosiderosis	0	0.0	1	33.3	1	1.6	0	0.0	0	0.0	0	0.0
Bone marrow	Infiltration, lymphoid cell	0	0.0	1	33.3	1	1.6	0	0.0	0	0.0	0	0.0
Bone marrow	Lymphoid follicle	0	0.0	1	33.3	1	1.6	0	0.0	0	0.0	0	0.0
Brain	Cyst	0	0.0	1	33.3	1	1.6	0	0.0	0	0.0	0	0.0
Brain	Dilation, ventricular	0	0.0	1	33.3	1	1.6	0	0.0	0	0.0	0	0.0
Brain	Infiltration, lymphoid cell	0	0.0	1	33.3	1	1.6	0	0.0	0	0.0	0	0.0
Cecum	Congestion	0	0.0	1	33.3	1	1.6	0	0.0	0	0.0	0	0.0
Cecum	Edema	0	0.0	1	33.3	1	1.6	0	0.0	0	0.0	0	0.0
Cecum	Granuloma	0	0.0	0	0.0	0	0.0	0	0.0	1	33.3	2	3.2

(continued)

TABLE 8.6 (Continued)

Spontaneous Lesions in Control Cynomolgous Monkeys in Toxicity Studies of 4-Weeks Duration

Monkey

4 weeks

Organ	Finding	Males						Females					
		Minimum	Minimum Range (%)	Maximum	Maximum Range (%)	Total Incidence	Total Incidence (%)	Minimum	Minimum Range (%)	Maximum	Maximum Range (%)	Total Incidence	Total Incidence (%)
						64						63	
Cecum	Hemorrhage	0	0.0	1	33.3	1	1.6	0	0.0	1	33.3	1	1.6
Cecum	Hyperplasia, lymphoid	0	0.0	2	66.7	2	3.1	0	0.0	1	33.3	1	1.6
Cecum	Infiltration, lymphoid cell	0	0.0	0	0.0	0	0.0	0	0.0	1	33.3	1	1.6
Cecum	Inflammation, lymphocytic	0	0.0	1	33.3	1	1.6	0	0.0	0	0.0	0	0.0
Cecum	Inflammation, neutrophilic	0	0.0	1	33.3	1	1.6	0	0.0	1	33.3	1	1.6
Cecum	Parasite	0	0.0	2	66.7	2	3.1	0	0.0	0	0.0	0	0.0
Cervix	Inflammation, lymphocytic	0	0.0	0	0.0	0	0.0	0	0.0	3	100.0	3	4.8
Cervix	Inflammation, neutrophilic	0	0.0	0	0.0	0	0.0	0	0.0	1	33.3	2	3.2
Colon	Granuloma	0	0.0	0	0.0	0	0.0	0	0.0	1	33.3	1	1.6
Colon	Hyperplasia, lymphoid	0	0.0	2	66.7	2	3.1	0	0.0	1	33.3	2	3.2
Colon	Infiltration, mixed cell	0	0.0	1	33.3	1	1.6	0	0.0	0	0.0	0	0.0
Colon	Parasite	0	0.0	1	33.3	1	1.6	0	0.0	0	0.0	0	0.0
Duodenum	Atrophy, villous	0	0.0	1	33.3	1	1.6	0	0.0	0	0.0	0	0.0
Duodenum	Deposit, pigment	0	0.0	1	33.3	1	1.6	0	0.0	0	0.0	0	0.0
Duodenum	Diverticulum	0	0.0	1	33.3	1	1.6	0	0.0	0	0.0	0	0.0
Duodenum	Erosion	0	0.0	1	33.3	1	1.6	0	0.0	0	0.0	0	0.0
Duodenum	Hemosiderin deposits	0	0.0	1	33.3	1	1.6	0	0.0	0	0.0	0	0.0
Duodenum	Inflammation, lymphocytic	0	0.0	2	66.7	2	3.1	0	0.0	1	33.3	1	1.6
Duodenum	Inflammation, mixed cell	0	0.0	1	33.3	1	1.6	0	0.0	0	0.0	0	0.0
Duodenum	Necrosis, mucosal	0	0.0	2	66.7	2	3.1	0	0.0	0	0.0	0	0.0
Epididymides	Immaturity	0	0.0	4	100.0	39	60.9	0	0.0	0	0.0	0	0.0
Esophagus	Infiltration, lymphoid cell	0	0.0	1	33.3	3	4.7	0	0.0	1	33.3	1	1.6
Esophagus	Inflammation, lymphocytic	0	0.0	1	33.3	1	1.6	0	0.0	0	0.0	0	0.0
Esophagus	Necrosis, mucosal	0	0.0	1	33.3	1	1.6	0	0.0	0	0.0	0	0.0
Esophagus	Hyperplasia, epithelial	0	0.0	1	33.3	1	1.6	0	0.0	0	0.0	0	0.0
Eye	Corneal erosion	0	0.0	0	0.0	0	0.0	0	0.0	1	33.3	1	1.6

Eye	Degeneration, microcystoid	0	0.0	1	33.3	1	1.6	0	0.0	1	33.3	1	1.6
Eye	Gliosis	0	0.0	2	66.7	2	3.1	0	0.0	0	0.0	0	0.0
Eye	Infiltration, lymphoid cell	0	0.0	1	33.3	1	1.6	0	0.0	0	0.0	0	0.0
Femur	Fibrosis	0	0.0	2	66.7	4	6.3	0	0.0	1	33.3	1	1.6
Femur	Fracture	0	0.0	1	33.3	1	1.6	0	0.0	0	0.0	0	0.0
Femur	Necrosis	0	0.0	1	33.3	1	1.6	0	0.0	1	33.3	1	1.6
Gallbladder	Cystic dilation	0	0.0	1	33.3	1	1.6	0	0.0	0	0.0	0	0.0
Gallbladder	Infiltration, lymphoid cell	0	0.0	2	66.7	2	3.1	0	0.0	1	33.3	1	1.6
Gallbladder	Inflammation, lymphocytic	0	0.0	0	0.0	0	0.0	0	0.0	2	66.7	2	3.2
Heart	Degeneration/necrosis myocardium	0	0.0	0	0.0	0	0.0	0	0.0	1	33.3	1	1.6
Heart	Inflammation, mixed cell	0	0.0	1	33.3	1	1.6	0	0.0	2	66.7	4	6.3
Heart	Infiltration, lymphoid cell	0	0.0	3	100.0	14	21.9	0	0.0	3	100.0	18	28.6
Heart	Mononuclear cell infiltration	0	0.0	2	66.7	4	6.3	0	0.0	3	100.0	7	11.1
Heart	Inflammation, mixed cell	0	0.0	3	100.0	4	6.3	0	0.0	1	33.3	2	3.2
Ileum	Dilation, glandular	0	0.0	1	33.3	1	1.6	0	0.0	1	33.3	2	3.2
Ileum	Hemorrhage	0	0.0	1	33.3	1	1.6	0	0.0	0	0.0	0	0.0
Jejunum	Dilation, glandular	0	0.0	1	33.3	2	3.1	0	0.0	0	0.0	0	0.0
Jejunum	Inflammation, lymphocytic	0	0.0	1	33.3	1	1.6	0	0.0	0	0.0	0	0.0
Kidney	Basophilia, tubular	0	0.0	0	0.0	0	0.0	0	0.0	2	66.7	3	4.8
Kidney	Cast, hyaline	0	0.0	1	33.3	1	1.6	0	0.0	1	33.3	1	1.6
Kidney	Dilation, tubular	0	0.0	1	33.3	1	1.6	0	0.0	0	0.0	0	0.0
Kidney	Ectopic adrenal	0	0.0	0	0.0	0	0.0	0	0.0	1	33.3	1	1.6
Kidney	Fibrosis	0	0.0	1	33.3	1	1.6	0	0.0	1	33.3	2	3.2
Kidney	Glomerulosclerosis	0	0.0	1	33.3	1	1.6	0	0.0	0	0.0	0	0.0
Kidney	Infiltration, mixed cell	0	0.0	3	100.0	4	6.3	0	0.0	1	33.3	1	1.6
Kidney	Mononuclear cellular infiltration	0	0.0	2	66.7	19	29.7	0	0.0	3	100.0	25	39.7
Kidney	Inflammation, lymphocytic	0	0.0	2	66.7	3	4.7	0	0.0	2	66.7	5	7.9
Kidney	Inflammation, mixed cell	0	0.0	2	66.7	4	6.3	0	0.0	2	66.7	3	4.8
Kidney	Mineralization, tubular	0	0.0	1	33.3	2	3.1	0	0.0	0	0.0	0	0.0
Kidney	Infiltration, plasma cell	0	0.0	2	66.7	2	3.1	0	0.0	1	33.3	1	1.6
Lacrimal gland	Infiltration, lymphoid cell	0	0.0	3	100.0	22	34.4	0	0.0	3	100.0	20	31.7
Lacrimal gland	Inflammation, lymphocytic	0	0.0	1	33.3	1	1.6	0	0.0	0	0.0	0	0.0
Larynx	Degeneration, muscle	0	0.0	0	0.0	0	0.0	0	0.0	1	33.3	1	1.6
Larynx	Infiltration, lymphoid cell	0	0.0	2	66.7	3	4.7	0	0.0	1	33.3	3	4.8
Larynx	Inflammation, mixed cell	0	0.0	1	33.3	1	1.6	0	0.0	0	0.0	0	0.0

(continued)

TABLE 8.6 (Continued)
Spontaneous Lesions in Control Cynomolgous Monkeys in Toxicity Studies of 4-Weeks Duration

Monkey		Males 4 weeks (64)						Females (63)					
Organ	Finding	Minimum	Minimum Range (%)	Maximum	Maximum Range (%)	Total Incidence	Total Incidence (%)	Minimum	Minimum Range (%)	Maximum	Maximum Range (%)	Total Incidence	Total Incidence (%)
Liver	Fibrous adhesion	0	0.0	0	0.0	0	0.0	0	0.0	1	33.3	1	1.6
Liver	Atrophy, hepatocellular	0	0.0	1	33.3	1	1.6	0	0.0	0	0.0	0	0.0
Liver	Congestion	0	0.0	1	33.3	1	1.6	0	0.0	0	0.0	0	0.0
Liver	Deposition, pigment	0	0.0	2	66.7	3	4.7	0	0.0	0	0.0	0	0.0
Liver	Fibrosis	0	0.0	1	33.3	1	1.6	0	0.0	0	0.0	0	0.0
Liver	Hematopoiesis	0	0.0	2	66.7	2	3.1	0	0.0	2	66.7	2	3.2
Liver	Hyperplasia, Ito cell	0	0.0	0	0.0	0	0.0	0	0.0	1	33.3	1	1.6
Liver	Infiltration, mixed cell	0	0.0	3	100.0	5	7.8	0	0.0	2	66.7	6	9.5
Liver	Infiltration, lymphoid cell	0	0.0	3	100.0	4	6.3	0	0.0	3	100.0	7	11.1
Liver	Mononuclear cell infiltration	0	0.0	2	66.7	4	6.3	0	0.0	3	100.0	6	9.5
Liver	Inflammation, mixed cell	0	0.0	0	0.0	0	0.0	0	0.0	1	33.3	4	6.3
Liver	Necrosis, hepatocellular	0	0.0	1	33.3	1	1.6	0	0.0	0	0.0	0	0.0
Liver	Vacuolation, hepatocellular	0	0.0	1	33.3	1	1.6	0	0.0	1	33.3	1	1.6
Lung	Fibrous adhesion	0	0.0	0	0.0	0	0.0	0	0.0	1	33.3	2	3.2
Lung	Alveolitis	0	0.0	1	33.3	1	1.6	0	0.0	2	66.7	2	3.2
Lung	Bronchiolitis	0	0.0	1	33.3	1	1.6	0	0.0	0	0.0	0	0.0
Lung	Collagen increased	0	0.0	0	0.0	0	0.0	0	0.0	1	33.3	1	1.6
Lung	Congestion	0	0.0	0	0.0	0	0.0	0	0.0	2	66.7	2	3.2
Lung	Deposition, pigment	0	0.0	3	100.0	6	9.4	0	0.0	3	100.0	7	11.1
Lung	Edema	0	0.0	1	33.3	1	1.6	0	0.0	0	0.0	0	0.0
Lung	Fibrosis	0	0.0	0	0.0	0	0.0	0	0.0	1	33.3	2	3.2
Lung	Granuloma	0	0.0	0	0.0	0	0.0	0	0.0	1	33.3	1	1.6
Lung	Hemorrhage	0	0.0	1	33.3	2	3.1	0	0.0	1	33.3	2	3.2
Lung	Infiltration, lymphoid cell	0	0.0	2	66.7	2	3.1	0	0.0	1	33.3	4	6.3
Lung	Inflammation, mixed cell	0	0.0	3	100.0	7	10.9	0	0.0	3	100.0	10	15.9
Lung	Inflammation, lymphocytic	0	0.0	1	33.3	1	1.6	0	0.0	0	0.0	0	0.0

Organ	Lesion												
Lung	Macrophages, alveolar	0	0.0	1	33.3	2	3.1	0	0.0	0	0.0	0	0.0
Lung	Mineralization	0	0.0	0	0.0	0	0.0	0	0.0	1	33.3	1	1.6
Mammary gland	Fibrosis	0	0.0	0	0.0	0	0.0	0	0.0	1	33.3	1	1.6
Mandibular lymph node	Hyperplasia, lymphoid	0	0.0	2	66.7	3	4.7	0	0.0	2	66.7	4	6.3
Mesenteric lymph node	Deposition, pigment	0	0.0	1	33.3	1	1.6	0	0.0	2	66.7	3	4.8
Mesenteric lymph node	Dilation, sinusoid	0	0.0	0	0.0	0	0.0	0	0.0	2	66.7	2	3.2
Mesenteric lymph node	Sinus histiocytosis	0	0.0	0	0.0	0	0.0	0	0.0	2	66.7	3	4.8
Mesenteric lymph node	Hyperplasia lymphoid	0	0.0	2	66.7	5	7.8	0	0.0	1	33.3	3	4.8
Mesenteric lymph node	Sinus histiocytosis	0	0.0	1	33.3	1	1.6	0	0.0	1	33.3	1	1.6
Mesenteric lymph node	Macrophage aggregate(s)	0	0.0	1	33.3	1	1.6	0	0.0	0	0.0	0	0.0
Muscle	Degeneration	0	0.0	1	33.3	1	1.6	0	0.0	0	0.0	0	0.0
Muscle	Deposition, pigment	0	0.0	1	33.3	1	1.6	0	0.0	0	0.0	0	0.0
Muscle	Infiltration, lymphoid cell	0	0.0	0	0.0	0	0.0	0	0.0	1	33.3	1	1.6
Muscle	Mononuclear cell infiltration	0	0.0	1	33.3	1	1.6	0	0.0	0	0.0	0	0.0
Muscle	Inflammation, lymphocytic	0	0.0	0	0.0	0	0.0	0	0.0	1	33.3	1	1.6
Muscle	Inflammation, mixed cell	0	0.0	2	66.7	3	4.7	0	0.0	0	0.0	0	0.0
Muscle	Protozoal cyst	0	0.0	0	0.0	0	0.0	0	0.0	1	33.3	1	1.6
Ovaries	Cyst, corpus luteum	0	0.0	0	0.0	0	0.0	0	0.0	1	33.3	2	3.2
Ovaries	Dilation, bursa	0	0.0	0	0.0	0	0.0	0	0.0	1	33.3	1	1.6
Ovaries	Hemorrhage	0	0.0	0	0.0	0	0.0	0	0.0	1	33.3	1	1.6
Ovaries	Immature	0	0.0	0	0.0	0	0.0	0	0.0	1	33.3	2	3.2
Ovaries	Mineralization	0	0.0	0	0.0	0	0.0	0	0.0	2	66.7	6	9.5
Oviducts	Hyperplasia, epithelial	0	0.0	0	0.0	0	0.0	0	0.0	1	33.3	1	1.6
Pancreas	Decreased, zymogen	0	0.0	1	33.3	1	1.6	0	0.0	0	0.0	0	0.0
Pancreas	Ectopic spleen	0	0.0	1	33.3	1	1.6	0	0.0	1	33.3	1	1.6
Pancreas	Fibrosis	0	0.0	1	33.3	2	3.1	0	0.0	0	0.0	0	0.0
Pancreas	Hyperplasia, ductal	0	0.0	0	0.0	0	0.0	0	0.0	1	33.3	1	1.6
Pancreas	Infiltration, lymphoid cell	0	0.0	1	33.3	2	3.1	0	0.0	1	33.3	2	3.2
Pancreas	Inflammation, lymphocytic	0	0.0	0	0.0	0	0.0	0	0.0	1	33.3	2	3.2

(continued)

TABLE 8.6 (Continued)
Spontaneous Lesions in Control Cynomolgous Monkeys in Toxicity Studies of 4-Weeks Duration

Monkey		Males						Females					
		4 weeks											
Organ	Finding	Minimum	Minimum Range (%)	Maximum	Maximum Range (%)	Total Incidence	Total Incidence (%)	Minimum	Minimum Range (%)	Maximum	Maximum Range (%)	Total Incidence	Total Incidence (%)
						64						63	
Pancreas	Inflammation, mixed cell	0	0.0	1	33.3	1	1.6	0	0.0	0	0.0	0	0.0
Parathyroid	Cyst	0	0.0	1	33.3	1	1.6	0	0.0	0	0.0	0	0.0
Parathyroid	Ectopic thymus	0	0.0	0	0.0	0	0.0	0	0.0	1	33.3	1	1.6
Pituitary	Cyst	0	0.0	1	33.3	1	1.6	0	0.0	1	33.3	4	6.3
Pituitary	Infiltration, lymphoid cell	0	0.0	1	33.3	1	1.6	0	0.0	1	33.3	1	1.6
Prostate	Immature	0	0.0	4	100.0	39	60.9	0	0.0	0	0.0	0	0.0
Prostate	Infiltration, mixed cell	0	0.0	1	33.3	1	1.6	0	0.0	0	0.0	0	0.0
Prostate	Infiltration, lymphoid cell	0	0.0	1	33.3	3	4.7	0	0.0	0	0.0	0	0.0
Prostate	Inflammation, lymphocytic	0	0.0	1	33.3	1	1.6	0	0.0	0	0.0	0	0.0
Rectum	Hyperplasia, lymphoid	0	0.0	2	66.7	2	3.1	0	0.0	1	33.3	1	1.6
Rectum	Inflammation, lymphocytic	0	0.0	1	33.3	1	1.6	0	0.0	0	0.0	0	0.0
Retropharyngeal lymph node	Depletion, lymphoid	0	0.0	1	33.3	1	1.6	0	0.0	1	33.3	2	3.2
Retropharyngeal lymph node	Hyperplasia, lymphoid	0	0.0	1	33.3	1	1.6	0	0.0	0	0.0	0	0.0
Salivary gland	Dilation, duct	0	0.0	1	33.3	1	1.6	0	0.0	0	0.0	0	0.0
Salivary gland	Infiltration, lymphoid cell	0	0.0	3	100.0	25	39.1	0	0.0	3	100.0	14	22.2
Salivary gland	Mononuclear cell infiltration	0	0.0	1	33.3	1	1.6	0	0.0	1	33.3	1	1.6
Salivary gland	Inflammation, mixed cell	0	0.0	0	0.0	0	0.0	0	0.0	2	66.7	2	3.2
Salivary gland	Inflammation, lymphocytic	0	0.0	1	33.3	1	1.6	0	0.0	2	66.7	3	4.8
Salivary gland	Mineralization	0	0.0	1	33.3	1	1.6	0	0.0	0	0.0	0	0.0
Sciatic nerve	Infiltration, lymphoid cell	0	0.0	1	33.3	1	1.6	0	0.0	0	0.0	0	0.0
Seminal vesicles	Immature	0	0.0	4	100.0	43	67.2	0	0.0	0	0.0	0	0.0
Skin	Acanthosis	0	0.0	0	0.0	0	0.0	0	0.0	0	0.0	0	0.0
Skin	Hyperkeratosis	0	0.0	1	33.3	1	1.6	0	0.0	1	33.3	2	3.2
Skin	Hyperplasia, squamous cell	0	0.0	1	33.3	1	1.6	0	0.0	0	0.0	0	0.0

Organ	Lesion												
Skin	Infiltration, lymphoid cell	0	0.0	0	0.0	0	0.0	0	0.0	1	33.3	2	3.2
Skin	Inflammation, neutrophilic	0	0.0	0	0.0	0	0.0	0	0.0	1	33.3	2	3.2
Skin	Inflammation, mixed cell	0	0.0	0	0.0	0	0.0	0	0.0	1	33.3	2	3.2
Skin	Serofibrinous debris (scab)	0	0.0	1	33.3	2	3.1	0	0.0	1	33.3	1	1.6
Skin	Ulceration	0	0.0	1	33.3	1	1.6	0	0.0	1	33.3	3	4.8
Spleen	Depletion, lymphoid	0	0.0	0	0.0	0	0.0	0	0.0	1	33.3	1	1.6
Spleen	Deposition, pigment	0	0.0	2	66.7	2	3.1	0	0.0	0	0.0	0	0.0
Spleen	Ectopic spleen	0	0.0	0	0.0	0	0.0	0	0.0	1	33.3	1	1.6
Spleen	Fibrosis	0	0.0	1	33.3	1	1.6	0	0.0	0	0.0	0	0.0
Spleen	Hyaline change, lymphoid follicle	0	0.0	1	33.3	2	3.1	0	0.0	1	33.3	3	4.8
Spleen	Hyperplasia, lymphoid	0	0.0	2	66.7	7	10.9	0	0.0	2	66.7	5	7.9
Sternum	Infiltration, lymphoid cell	0	0.0	1	33.3	1	1.6	0	0.0	1	33.3	1	1.6
Stomach	Cyst	0	0.0	0	0.0	0	0.0	0	0.0	2	66.7	2	3.2
Stomach	Erosion	0	0.0	1	33.3	1	1.6	0	0.0	0	0.0	0	0.0
Stomach	Hemorrhage	0	0.0	1	33.3	2	3.1	0	0.0	0	0.0	0	0.0
Stomach	Hyperplasia, lymphoid	0	0.0	1	33.3	1	1.6	0	0.0	2	66.7	4	6.3
Stomach	Hyperplasia, epithelial	0	0.0	1	33.3	2	3.1	0	0.0	1	33.3	3	4.8
Stomach	Infiltration, mixed cell	0	0.0	1	33.3	1	1.6	0	0.0	0	0.0	0	0.0
Stomach	Infiltration, lymphoid cell	0	0.0	3	100.0	6	9.4	0	0.0	2	66.7	4	6.3
Stomach	Inflammation, mixed cell	0	0.0	3	100.0	8	12.5	0	0.0	3	100.0	6	9.5
Stomach	Inflammation, lymphocytic	0	0.0	1	33.3	1	1.6	0	0.0	1	33.3	1	1.6
Stomach	Necrosis, single cell	0	0.0	2	66.7	2	3.1	0	0.0	1	33.3	1	1.6
Stomach	Parietal cell decrease	0	0.0	1	33.3	1	1.6	0	0.0	1	33.3	1	1.6
Testes	Fibrosis	0	0.0	1	33.3	1	1.6	0	0.0	0	0.0	0	0.0
Testes	Immature	0	0.0	4	100.0	44	68.8	0	0.0	0	0.0	0	0.0
Thymus	Cyst	0	0.0	1	33.3	2	3.1	0	0.0	1	33.3	2	3.2
Thymus	Depletion, lymphoid	0	0.0	2	66.7	3	4.7	0	0.0	1	33.3	4	6.3
Thyroid	Cyst	0	0.0	1	33.3	4	6.3	0	0.0	1	33.3	3	4.8
Thyroid	Cyst, follicular	0	0.0	2	66.7	2	3.1	0	0.0	1	33.3	1	1.6
Thyroid	Dilation, follicular	0	0.0	2	66.7	2	3.1	0	0.0	0	0.0	0	0.0
Thyroid	Ectopic thymus	0	0.0	1	33.3	4	6.3	0	0.0	2	66.7	18	28.6
Thyroid	Hypertrophy, follicular cell	0	0.0	0	0.0	0	0.0	0	0.0	1	33.3	1	1.6
Thyroid	Infiltration, mixed cell	0	0.0	1	33.3	3	4.7	0	0.0	0	0.0	0	0.0
Thyroid	Inflammation, mixed cell	0	0.0	1	33.3	1	1.6	0	0.0	0	0.0	0	0.0

(continued)

TABLE 8.6 (Continued)
Spontaneous Lesions in Control Cynomolgous Monkeys in Toxicity Studies of 4-Weeks Duration

Monkey		Males						Females					
		4 weeks											
		64						63					
Organ	Finding	Minimum	Minimum Range (%)	Maximum	Maximum Range (%)	Total Incidence	Total Incidence (%)	Minimum	Minimum Range (%)	Maximum	Maximum Range (%)	Total Incidence	Total Incidence (%)
Tongue	Myofiber degeneration/regeneration	0	0.0	1	33.3	2	3.1	0	0.0	1	33.3	1	1.6
Tongue	Infiltration, lymphoid cell	0	0.0	1	33.3	4	6.3	0	0.0	2	66.7	3	4.8
Tongue	Inflammation, neutrophilic	0	0.0	0	0.0	0	0.0	0	0.0	1	33.3	1	1.6
Tongue	Inflammation, mixed cell	0	0.0	2	66.7	6	9.4	0	0.0	1	33.3	2	3.2
Trachea	Infiltration, lymphoid cell	0	0.0	1	33.3	1	1.6	0	0.0	0	0.0	0	0.0
Trachea	Inflammation, mixed cell	0	0.0	1	33.3	1	1.6	0	0.0	1	33.3	1	1.6
Trachea	Inflammation, lymphocytic	0	0.0	1	33.3	1	1.6	0	0.0	0	0.0	0	0.0
Tracheobronchial lymph node	Depletion, lymphoid	0	0.0	1	33.3	1	1.6	0	0.0	0	0.0	0	0.0
Tracheobronchial lymph node	Deposition, pigment	0	0.0	1	33.3	2	3.1	0	0.0	1	33.3	3	4.8
Tracheobronchial lymph node	Hyperplasia, lymphoid	0	0.0	1	33.3	1	1.6	0	0.0	0	0.0	0	0.0
Urinary bladder	Eosinophilic droplets, transepithelial	0	0.0	1	33.3	1	1.6	0	0.0	0	0.0	0	0.0
Urinary bladder	Hyperplasia, lymphoid	0	0.0	1	33.3	1	1.6	0	0.0	0	0.0	0	0.0
Urinary bladder	Infiltration, mixed cell	0	0.0	0	0.0	0	0.0	0	0.0	1	33.3	1	1.6
Urinary bladder	Infiltration, lymphoid cell	0	0.0	1	33.3	3	4.7	0	0.0	1	33.3	2	3.2
Urinary bladder	Inflammation, mixed cell	0	0.0	1	33.3	1	1.6	0	0.0	0	0.0	0	0.0
Urinary bladder	Inflammation, lymphocytic	0	0.0	0	0.0	0	0.0	0	0.0	1	33.3	2	3.2
Urinary bladder	Syncytia, epithelium	0	0.0	1	33.3	1	1.6	0	0.0	0	0.0	0	0.0
Urinary bladder	Vacuolation, epithelial	0	0.0	0	0.0	0	0.0	0	0.0	1	33.3	1	1.6
Uterus	Immature	0	0.0	0	0.0	0	0.0	0	0.0	1	33.3	1	1.6
Uterus	Infiltration, lymphoid cell	0	0.0	0	0.0	0	0.0	0	0.0	1	33.3	2	3.2
Vagina	Infiltration, mixed cell	0	0.0	0	0.0	0	0.0	0	0.0	1	33.3	1	1.6
Vagina	Infiltration, lymphoid cell	0	0.0	0	0.0	0	0.0	0	0.0	1	33.3	1	1.6
Vagina	Inflammation, lymphocytic	0	0.0	0	0.0	0	0.0	0	0.0	3	100.0	4	6.3

TABLE 8.7

Spontaneous Lesions in Control Cynomolgous Monkeys in Toxicity Studies of 26- and 52-Weeks Duration

Monkey		Males — 26 and 52 weeks						Females					
Organ	Finding	Minimum	Minimum Range (%)	Maximum	Maximum Range (%)	Total Incidence	Total Incidence (%)	Minimum	Minimum Range (%)	Maximum	Maximum Range (%)	Total Incidence	Total Incidence (%)
						32						32	
Adrenal	Cortical hypertrophy, zona fasciculata	0	0.0	0	0.0	0	0.0	0	0.0	1	25.0	1	3.1
Adrenal	Ectopic liver	0	0.0	1	25.0	1	3.1	0	0.0	0	0.0	0	0.0
Brain	Mononuclear cell infiltration	0	0.0	1	25.0	1	3.1	0	0.0	1	25.0	2	6.3
Cecum	Infiltration, mixed cell	0	0.0	0	0.0	0	0.0	0	0.0	1	25.0	1	3.1
Cecum	Inflammation, mixed cell	0	0.0	2	50.0	2	6.3	0	0.0	1	25.0	1	3.1
Cecum	Inflammation, granulomatous	0	0.0	1	25.0	1	3.1	0	0.0	0	0.0	0	0.0
Cecum	Parasite	0	0.0	1	25.0	1	3.1	0	0.0	0	0.0	0	0.0
Colon	Inflammation, granulomatous	0	0.0	1	25.0	2	6.3	0	0.0	2	50.0	3	9.4
Colon	Hemorrhage	0	0.0	1	25.0	2	6.3	0	0.0	1	25.0	1	3.1
Colon	Inflammation, mixed cell	0	0.0	2	50.0	2	6.3	0	0.0	0	0.0	0	0.0
Duodenum	Hemorrhage	0	0.0	1	25.0	2	6.3	0	0.0	0	0.0	0	0.0
Epididymides	Oligo/aspermia	0	0.0	4	100.0	20	62.5	0	0.0	0	0.0	0	0.0
Eye	Atrophy, retina	0	0.0	1	25.0	1	3.1	0	0.0	1	25.0	1	3.1
Eye	Dysplasia, retina	0	0.0	1	25.0	1	3.1	0	0.0	0	0.0	0	0.0
Heart	Inflammation, mixed cell	0	0.0	0	0.0	0	0.0	0	0.0	1	25.0	1	3.1
Heart	Mononuclear cell infiltration	0	0.0	2	50.0	3	9.4	0	0.0	2	50.0	3	9.4
Ileum	Hyperplasia, lymphoid (gut-associated lymphoid tissue)	0	0.0	0	0.0	0	0.0	0	0.0	1	25.0	1	3.1
Jejunum	Hyperplasia, lymphoid	0	0.0	0	0.0	0	0.0	0	0.0	1	25.0	1	3.1
Kidney	Mononuclear cell infiltration	0	0.0	1	25.0	1	3.1	0	0.0	1	25.0	3	9.4
Lacrimal gland	Mononuclear cell infiltration	0	0.0	0	0.0	0	0.0	0	0.0	1	25.0	1	3.1
Liver	Deposition, pigment	0	0.0	0	0.0	0	0.0	0	0.0	1	25.0	1	3.1
Liver	Fibrosis	0	0.0	1	25.0	1	3.1	0	0.0	1	25.0	1	3.1

(continued)

TABLE 8.7 (Continued)

Spontaneous Lesions in Control Cynomolgous Monkeys in Toxicity Studies of 26- and 52-Weeks Duration

Monkey		Males (26 and 52 weeks)						Females					
Organ	Finding	Minimum	Minimum Range (%)	Maximum	Maximum Range (%)	Total Incidence	Total Incidence (%)	Minimum	Minimum Range (%)	Maximum	Maximum Range (%)	Total Incidence	Total Incidence (%)
						32						32	
Liver	Hemorrhage	0	0.0	1	25.0	1	3.1	0	0.0	0	0.0	0	0.0
Liver	Hypertrophy, hepatocellular	0	0.0	1	25.0	1	3.1	0	0.0	1	25.0	1	3.1
Liver	Inflammation, mixed cell	0	0.0	1	25.0	1	3.1	0	0.0	0	0.0	0	0.0
Lung	Deposition, pigment	0	0.0	1	25.0	1	3.1	0	0.0	0	0.0	0	0.0
Lung	Fibrosis	0	0.0	1	25.0	1	3.1	0	0.0	2	50.0	6	18.8
Lung	Granuloma	0	0.0	0	0.0	0	0.0	0	0.0	1	25.0	1	3.1
Lung	Hemorrhage	0	0.0	0	0.0	0	0.0	0	0.0	1	25.0	1	3.1
Lung	Mononuclear cell infiltration	0	0.0	0	0.0	0	0.0	0	0.0	1	25.0	1	3.1
Lung	Inflammation, mixed cell	0	0.0	0	0.0	0	0.0	0	0.0	1	25.0	1	3.1
Lung	Inflammation, interstitial	0	0.0	1	25.0	1	3.1	0	0.0	2	50.0	2	6.3
Lung	Inflammation, pleura	0	0.0	0	0.0	0	0.0	0	0.0	1	25.0	1	3.1
Lung	Mineralization	0	0.0	0	0.0	0	0.0	0	0.0	1	25.0	1	3.1
Lymph node	Erythrophagocytosis	0	0.0	1	25.0	1	3.1	0	0.0	1	25.0	1	3.1
Mammary	Cyst	0	0.0	1	25.0	1	3.1	0	0.0	0	0.0	0	0.0
Mandibular lymph node	Hematopoiesis	0	0.0	0	0.0	0	0.0	0	0.0	1	25.0	1	3.1
Mesenteric lymph node	Hyperplasia, lymphoid	0	0.0	0	0.0	0	0.0	0	0.0	1	25.0	1	3.1
Muscle	Myofiber degeneration	0	0.0	4	100.0	5	15.6	0	0.0	4	100.0	5	15.6
Ovaries	Cyst	0	0.0	0	0.0	0	0.0	0	0.0	1	25.0	2	6.3
Ovaries	Hemorrhage	0	0.0	0	0.0	0	0.0	0	0.0	1	25.0	1	3.1
Ovaries	Mineralization	0	0.0	0	0.0	0	0.0	0	0.0	1	25.0	1	3.1

Organ	Lesion												
Pituitary	Cyst	0	0.0	1	25.0	1	3.1	0	0.0	1	25.0	1	3.1
Prostate	Immature	0	0.0	4	100.0	15	46.9	0	0.0	0	0.0	0	0.0
Retropharyngeal lymph node	Erythrophagocytosis	0	0.0	0	0.0	0	0.0	0	0.0	1	25.0	2	6.3
Retropharyngeal lymph node	Hyperplasia, lymphoid	0	0.0	1	25.0	1	3.1	0	0.0	1	25.0	1	3.1
Salivary gland	Cyst	0	0.0	0	0.0	0	0.0	0	0.0	1	25.0	1	3.1
Sciatic nerve	Hemorrhage	0	0.0	1	25.0	2	6.3	0	0.0	0	0.0	0	0.0
Sciatic nerve	Mononuclear cell infiltration	0	0.0	1	25.0	1	3.1	0	0.0	1	25.0	1	3.1
Seminal vesicles	Immature	0	0.0	4	100.0	16	50.0	0	0.0	0	0.0	0	0.0
Skin biopsy	Inflammation, dermis	0	0.0	1	25.0	1	3.1	0	0.0	0	0.0	0	0.0
Skin biopsy	Hemorrhage	0	0.0	3	75.0	3	9.4	0	0.0	4	100.0	4	12.5
Spinal cord	Hemorrhage	0	0.0	0	0.0	0	0.0	0	0.0	1	25.0	1	3.1
Spleen	Fibrosis	0	0.0	1	25.0	3	9.4	0	0.0	2	50.0	2	6.3
Spleen	Hyperplasia, lymphoid	0	0.0	2	50.0	3	9.4	0	0.0	1	25.0	1	3.1
Stomach	Dilation, glandular	0	0.0	0	0.0	0	0.0	0	0.0	1	25.0	1	3.1
Stomach	Erosion, glandular mucosa	0	0.0	1	25.0	1	3.1	0	0.0	0	0.0	0	0.0
Stomach	Hemorrhage	0	0.0	1	25.0	1	3.1	0	0.0	1	25.0	1	3.1
Stomach	Inflammation, mixed cell	0	0.0	4	100.0	6	18.8	0	0.0	3	75.0	4	12.5
Testes	Dilation, tubular	0	0.0	1	25.0	1	3.1	0	0.0	0	0.0	0	0.0
Testes	Hypo/aspermatogenesis	0	0.0	4	100.0	16	50.0	0	0.0	0	0.0	0	0.0
Testes	Mononuclear cell infiltration	0	0.0	2	50.0	2	6.3	0	0.0	0	0.0	0	0.0
Thymus	Depletion, lymphoid	0	0.0	2	50.0	2	6.3	0	0.0	2	50.0	2	6.3
Thymus	Hemorrhage	0	0.0	2	50.0	3	9.4	0	0.0	2	50.0	3	9.4
Thyroid	Inflammation, mixed cell	0	0.0	0	0.0	0	0.0	0	0.0	1	25.0	1	3.1
Tongue	Hyperplasia, epithelial	0	0.0	0	0.0	0	0.0	0	0.0	1	25.0	1	3.1
Tongue	Inflammation, mixed cell	0	0.0	0	0.0	0	0.0	0	0.0	1	25.0	1	3.1
Tracheobronchial lymph node	Erythrophagocytosis	0	0.0	0	0.0	0	0.0	0	0.0	1	25.0	1	3.1

8.6 SUMMARY

During the toxicology review process, the pathologist is often confronted with findings that are of uncertain relationship to the test article. A comparison of findings in treated animals versus the concurrent controls provides the initial and most important screen to make an assessment of a possible relationship to the test substance. In some instances, the concurrent control group does not contain sufficient numbers of animals to make a valid assessment. In addition, it is important to have a reliable historical control database to ensure proper evaluation of subtle compound-related changes. One major difficulty with historical control data is consistency, which is critical if it is to be used properly. The incidence of spontaneous lesions in commonly used species and strains varies considerably. In the Wistar rat, the highest frequency of incidental findings occurred in the liver (inflammatory), followed by kidney (degenerative) and lung (alveolar foam cell accumulation). In mouse, the highest incidence of spontaneous findings occurred in the adrenal glands (spindle cell hyperplasia and cortical pigment in the zona reticularis), the female reproductive tract (ovarian and uterine cysts), kidneys (tubular basophilia and hyaline tubular casts), lacrimal glands (mononuclear cell infiltration), tracheobronchial lymph nodes (erythrophagocytosis), and liver (mixed cell inflammation/infiltration and hepatocellular cytoplasmic vacuolation). In dog, the highest incidences of spontaneous findings were observed in the kidneys (focal, tubular mineralization, mostly in the papilla), lung (focal mixed cell inflammation), parathyroid gland (ultimobranchial duct cysts), pituitary gland (cysts), mesenteric lymph nodes (erythrophagocytosis), prostate gland (inflammatory foci), and thymus (lymphoid depletion). Finally, in the cynomolgus monkey, the most common spontaneous findings were observed in the kidney (inflammatory), lung (interstitial inflammation, fibrosis), and gastrointestinal tract (lymphoid hyperplasia in the cecum and colon).

REFERENCES

Capen, C.C. 2007. Endocrine glands. In: Grant Maxie, M. (Ed.), *Jubb, Kennedy and Palmer's Pathology of Domestic Animals.* Vol. 2, 5th ed. Saunders, Philadelphia, p. 360.

Chamanza, R., Marxfeld, H., Blanco, A., Garcia, B., Kubiliene, J. and Bradley, A. 2007. STP Annual Symposium, Puerto Rico: Incidences and Range of Spontaneous Lesions in Control Laboratory Beagle Dogs Used in Toxicity Studies. Charles River Laboratories Preclinical Services, Edinburgh.

Chamanza, R., Marxfeld, H.A., Blanco, A.I., Naylor, S.W., and Bradley, A.E. 2010. Incidences and range of spontaneous findings in control cynomolgus monkeys (*Macaca fascicularis*) used in toxicity studies. *Toxicol Pathol* 38(4): 642–57. Epub May 6, 2010.

Dixon, D., Heider, K., and Elwell, M. 1995. Incidence of non-neoplastic lesions in historical control male and female Fischer-344 rats from 90-day toxicity studies. *Toxicol Pathol* 23(3): 338–48.

Engelhardt, J.A., Gries, C.L., and Long, G.G. 1993. Incidence of spontaneous neoplastic and non-neoplastic lesions in Charles River CD-1 mice varies with breeding origin. *Toxicol Pathol* 21(6): 538–41.

Frith, C.H., Goodman, D.G., and Boysen, G.G. 2007. Mouse, pathology. In: Gad, S.C. (Ed.), *Animal Models in Toxicology,* 2nd ed. CRC Press (Taylor and Francis Group), Boca Raton, FL.

Hahn, F.F. and Dagle, G.E. 2001. Non-neoplastic pulmonary lesions. In: Mohr, U., Carlton, W.W., Dungworth, D.L. et al. (Eds.), *Pathobiology of the Aging Dog.* International Life Sciences Institute, Iowa State University Press, Ames.

Maita, K., Masuda, H., Suzuki, Y. 1977. Spontaneous lesions detected in Beagles used in toxicity studies. *Jikken Dobutsu* 26: 161–167.

McInnes, E.F. 2011. Background lesions in laboratory animals: A color atlas. Saunders/Elsevier, Philadelphia.

Morishima, H., Nonoyama, T., Sasaki, S., and Miyajima, H. 1990. Spontaneous lesions in beagle dogs used in toxicity studies. *Jikken Dobutsu* 39: 239–48.

Rehm, S. 2000. Spontaneous testicular lesions in purpose-bred beagle dogs. *Toxicol Pathol* 28(6): 782–87.

Stefanski, A.S., Elwell, M.R., and Stromberg, P.C. 1990. Spleen, lymph nodes and thymus. In: Boorman, G.A., Eustis, S.L., Elwell, M.R., Montgomery, C.A. Jr., and MacKenzie, W.F. (Eds.), *Pathology of the Fischer Rat.* San Diego, CA: Academic Press, pp. 369–93.

Tucker, M.J. 1997. *Diseases of the Wistar Rat.* 18th Ed., Taylor and Francis, Bristol, PA.

Section II

Organ Systems

9 Gastrointestinal Tract

Judit E. Markovits, Graham R. Betton,
Donald N. McMartin, and Oliver C. Turner

CONTENTS

9.1 INTRODUCTION

Components of the gastrointestinal (GI) tract serve as the first interface of a host organism with xenobiotics by oral dosing. The tract may be affected by this initial exposure but may also be impacted by systemic exposure via the vasculature or due to enterohepatic circulation. Additionally, the GI tract is important in maintaining the general health of the organism if for no other reason than its role in providing nutrients for the host; furthermore, the intestine has significant metabolic activities on its own (similar to liver), and its luminal contents contain modifying factors for xenobiotics (such as bacteria and bile salts) as well as dietary components, including fiber. Its gross structure varies by species, primarily influenced by diet and its biochemical features such as enzyme activity; cell products including mucus contents may be altered by environmental factors including bacteria and diet along with genetic influences. Perhaps due to the vulnerability to many of these external influences, much of the GI tract has a rapid turnover rate. The high metabolic activity makes many of its cells (especially the surface epithelium) and the GI tract as a whole sensitive to hypoxia, which is reflected in functional/morphological changes in the living organism and presents a challenge to pathologists because of rapid autolysis. This chapter provides information on the integrated assessment of this complex organ system in the most commonly used toxicologic species, from rodents (mice and rats) to large animals (dogs and nonhuman primates). Detailed evaluation by the toxicologic pathologist requires familiarity with the anatomic and physiologic differences along with molecular events and conventional morphological characteristics of various tissues, including their pathological responses.

9.2 EMBRYOLOGY

The general stages of development are the same for all mammalian species, the only difference being the timing of the actual events. The upper digestive tract (mouth, pharynx, salivary glands, esophagus, stomach, and proximal duodenum) develops by infolding of the foregut, whereas the rest of the small intestine and the proximal portion of the large intestine originate from the midgut. The hindgut gives rise to the distal large intestine including the rectum and anal canal. Much of the epithelial lining of the digestive tract has an endodermal origin, except the epithelium of the stomadeum (mouth and salivary glands) and the proctodeum corresponding to the caudal portion of the antral canal. Additionally, the supportive tissues and muscle of the digestive tract are formed from the splanchnic mesoderm. In general, embryonal development involves sequential modifications of structures by closing/fusion of segments such as separation of the embryonal pharynx by a septum that is lost in the fully developed animal. Other modifications include elongation, rotation (stomach 90° and intestines 360°), and temporal atresia (occlusion because of epithelial proliferation of esophagus and intestine that resolves by the vacuolation of cells and lumen formation at later stages) (Fletcher and Weber 2011). Based on this brief description of events, it is easy to understand that embryonic development of the digestive tract is patterned along multiple axes: a left–right axis that develops earlier than the anterior–posterior axis. The molecular events driving the morphogenetic signaling pathways are well preserved phylogenetically and involve the hedgehog signaling pathway that was reviewed in detail by van den Brink (2007). Hedgehog signaling is also important in the development and differentiation of regionally differing cell populations lining the digestive tract. Many of these processes are complex and involve regional differentiation of mucosal components in the stomach (nonglandular region and fundus and antrum with several cell types) and villus formation in the small intestine. Mice null for either the Sonic or the Indian hedgehog (Shh or Ihh) indicate that hedgehog signaling is important for the development of the circular layer of muscle and appropriate migration of neurons and innervations of the gut (Parkin and Ingham 2007). In addition to hedgehog signaling, the canonical Wnt (after wingless + integration) pathway is important in GI organogenesis. The apparent default mode is under the influence of Wnt signaling and produces intestinal differentiation. Stomach-specific epithelium develops when stomach mesenchyme regionally produces Barx1, which stimulates sFRPs that, in turn, locally inhibit Wnt signaling and allow the development of stomach-specific epithelium (Kim et al. 2005). It has been suggested that intestinal metaplasia following chronic injury of gastric mucosa represents a reversal of normal development. Toxicologic pathologists seldom deal with developmental abnormalities because most of the studies requiring their involvement are conducted in young adult animals that were deemed to be healthy by clinical evaluation. The most common anomaly of the digestive system found incidentally in adult animals in toxicity studies is the Meckel's diverticulum, an appendix-like remnant of the yolk stalk whose mucosa is similar to normal ileum and appears on the antimesenteric border of the intestine. Other congenital changes rarely observed include telescoping of the intestine into the thorax via a diaphragmatic hernia and mirror translocation of the viscera.

9.3 FUNCTIONAL ANATOMY

9.3.1 ORAL CAVITY

Much of the oral cavity is evaluated in toxicologic studies only grossly as part of the general examination of the body when the lips, palate, pharynx and buccal mucosa (including cheek pouch in macaques), and tongue are inspected. In most toxicologic studies in a pharmaceutical setting, the tongue is the only one of these tissues that is evaluated routinely histologically. Additionally, the palate is included in the tissue section in studies where the nasal cavity is examined microscopically. In rodents, the function of the oral cavity is limited to accepting, processing, and transporting food, whereas the oral cavity also contributes to vocalization and/or heat control in large animals. The hard palate contains several ridges in rodents and dogs, whereas macaques have palatine rugae that are not as prominent as those of other species of interest. The incisive papilla (covered by keratinized squamous epithelium) is a cartilaginous projection of the hard palate between the incisors and the first palatal ridge. The oral mucosa has a similar microscopic appearance to skin but typically has a higher epithelial proliferation rate. In the rat, the oral mucosal cell turnover rate varies between 3.2 and 5.8 days (Brown and Hardisty 1990). Of some curiosity is the presence of sebaceous glands (in the absence of hair) in the oral mucosa of most species (referred to as Fordyce's granules in humans) with predictive distribution and increasing numbers/incidence with age. In rats, most often, these glands are located in the gingiva between the first and third upper molars (Imaoka et al. 2003).

9.3.2 TONGUE

The tongue is important in mastication and taste as well as grooming and vocalization; furthermore, in dogs, it may serve as an additional cooling surface if needed. It is composed of three layers: (1) the muscularis, (2) the lamina propria, and (3) the epithelium. The center of the tongue is composed of striated muscle organized into bundles; it is well vascularized and contains a large population of mast cells. The lamina propria is composed of a collagen-rich loose connective tissue that connects the muscle to the mucosa. It contains lingual salivary glands (serous and mucinous at the base of the tongue), lymphatics, and nerves serving the taste buds. The tongue is covered by stratified squamous epithelium. The taste buds are composed of epithelial cells that are specialized gustatory sensory cells and are organized into filiform, conical, fungiform, foliate, and circumvallate papillae (Boughter et al. 1997; Abayomi et al. 2009).

9.3.3 SALIVARY GLANDS

Rodents have mixed mandibular salivary glands, serous parotid glands, and mucous sublingual glands. The sublingual glands are located adjacent to the mandibular salivary glands, whereas minor salivary glands are also present within the tongue. The parotid gland covers a large area extending from the mandibular glands to the ear and clavicle in mice. In dogs, the parotid and zygomatic glands empty into the dorsal vestibule, whereas the mandibular and sublingual glands open rostral to the frenulum of the tongue. The salivary glands of large animals are not characterized in as much detail as those of rodents. In dogs, the parotid is a mixed-type salivary gland whose secretion contains both acidic and neutral mucus in contrast to the mostly neutral secretum of rodents. In primates, parotids are serous or mixed, the mandibular glands are mixed, and the sublingual ones are mostly mucous.

The salivary glands of mice and rats are characterized in great detail. Microscopically, the mandibular gland is composed of the acini, intercalated ducts, convoluted (granular) ducts, intralobular (striated) ducts, interlobular ducts, and a single excretory duct emptying into the oral cavity. The convoluted (granular) glands are unique to the mandibular gland, produce polypeptides, and exhibit sexual dimorphism (the granules are larger in males; Figure 9.1a and b) (Barka 1980). In males, these ducts are tall columnar and contain prominent granules, whereas in females, the ducts are lined by shorter columnar cells with fewer cytoplasmic granules than males (Botts et al. 1999). This sexual dimorphism is not evident at the time of birth and develops later with sexual maturity, about 7 weeks of age in rats (Neuenschwander and Elwell 1990). Histologically, the acini in the murine parotid are composed of small basophilic cells resembling cells in the exocrine pancreas.

The intercalated glands of rodents contain large granules that contain epidermal growth factor (EGF). The salivary glands of mice have been found to have complex endocrine functions by demonstration of polypeptides in both saliva and blood, including erythropoietin, renin, gastrin, and nerve growth factors. Perhaps the best characterized is the range of effects of the EGF in

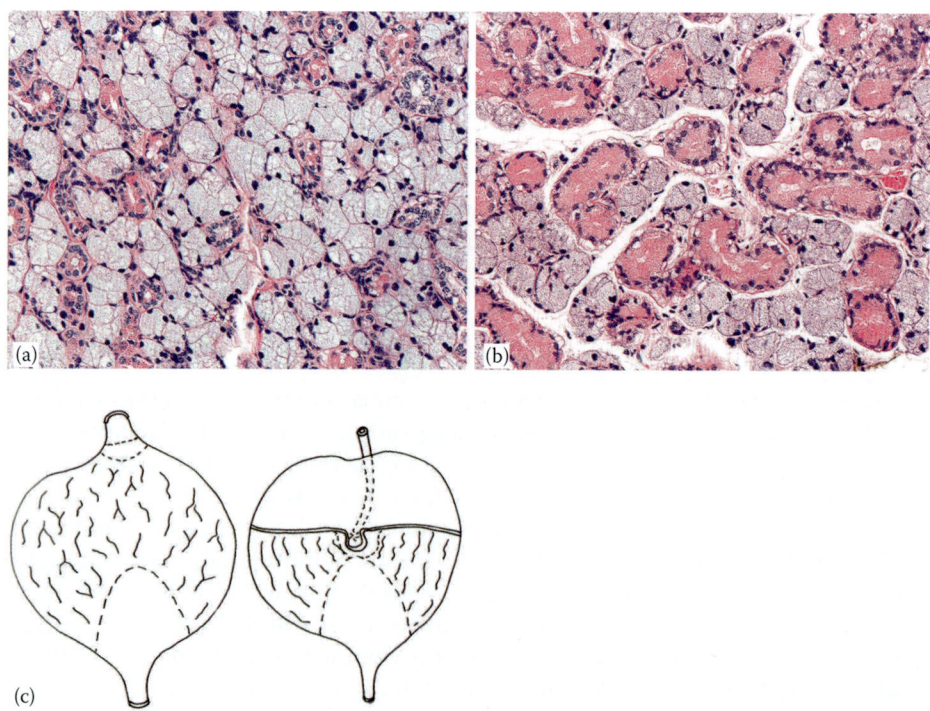

FIGURE 9.1   (a) Female mouse, submandibular salivary gland, HE stain. The convoluted ducts have low columnar epithelial cells with inconspicuous granules. (b) Male mouse, submandibular salivary gland, HE stain. In contrast to the female, the convoluted ducts in males have tall low columnar epithelial cells that contain prominent eosinophilic cytoplasmic granules. (c) Diagram of stomach in dog, primate (left), and rodent (right).

mice, functioning as a secretagogue and trophic factor in mucosal healing in the digestive tract through reproductive effects and having a potential role in mammary gland tumor development. It is assumed that other species also have EGF activity in salivary glands with similar effects (Lantini et al. 2006). The life spans of various cells of rat salivary glands were estimated to vary from 41 days (parotid acini) to 95 days (secretory tubules of the submandibular salivary gland) (Neuenschwander and Elwell 1990).

The functions of the salivary gland include lubrication of food by saliva to aid in swallowing, control of pH in the oral cavity, and initiation of digestion by amylase production. The secretory activity is under sympathetic and parasympathetic control. The multiple nervous controls for the salivary gland include the salivary nuclei of the medulla oblongata, the appetite center of the hypothalamus, and reflex pathways of the upper digestive tract.

Saliva is primarily composed of water and also contains amylase, mucin, electrolytes, immunoglobulins, and other components.

9.3.4 ESOPHAGUS

Starting with the esophagus, the GI tract is mainly structured as a tube with some surface/structural modifications. The general architecture is similar in all regions and includes the mucosa surrounding the lumen, submucosa, and muscularis. The first segment of the tubular digestive tract is the esophagus, which is essentially a conduit between the oral cavity and the stomach. Its mucosa is similar to that of the oral cavity and is composed of stratified squamous epithelium arranged in longitudinal folds. The poorly vascularized esophagus has delayed wound healing. In different regions of the submucosa, serous glands are present (especially in dogs). Noteworthy is the muscular layer of the esophagus because its composition determines whether luminal contents can move only in one direction or both directions. Species with only smooth muscle in the muscularis, such as mice and rats, are not able to vomit. In contrast, dogs have only striated muscle, whereas primates have a mixture of smooth and striated muscle in the muscularis of the esophagus, and these species are able to vomit. Emesis is initiated either by mucosal information or by direct central nervous stimuli. In the context of toxicity testing in dogs, occasionally a change of large animal species from dogs to nonhuman primates is needed because nonhuman primates are generally less sensitive to emetic stimuli than dogs who are prone to emesis due to mucosal stimuli that may cause limited bioavailability.

9.3.5 STOMACH

The nonglandular (fore-) stomach in rodents is covered by squamous epithelium and differs from that in dogs, nonhuman primates, and humans, where the squamous epithelium of the esophagus terminates at the cardiac sphincter (Figure 9.1c). This relates to the diet of rodents and other herbivores having lower nutritional content, thus requiring a larger food intake. To allow safe feeding during the hours of darkness, the nonglandular stomach serves as a reservoir permitting continual digestion.

Where the nonglandular stomach joins the glandular stomach of the rodent, there is a thickened and elevated limiting ridge (Figure 9.2a), which is curved around the entry of the esophagus at the cardia. There is a short region of mucus-secreting cardiac glands before the glandular stomach becomes the acid-secreting thicker oxyntic mucosa of the fundus and body. Oxyntic glands in this region contain a mixture of cell types (Figure 9.2b). In the deeper parts of the gland are the zymogen granule containing chief cells, mitochondrial rich parietal cells with an acid secretory canalicular system, and neuroendocrine cells with secretory vacuoles containing amines and peptide hormone granules (Figure 9.2c). The antral mucosa at the lower end leading to the pylorus is thinner, smoother, and comprised simpler glands (Figure 9.2d). In nonrodents, the esophageal entry is direct into the cardiac region, fundus, body, and antrum. These regions can be identified macroscopically at necropsy once the stomach is opened out by incising along the greater curvature (Vidal et al. 2008).

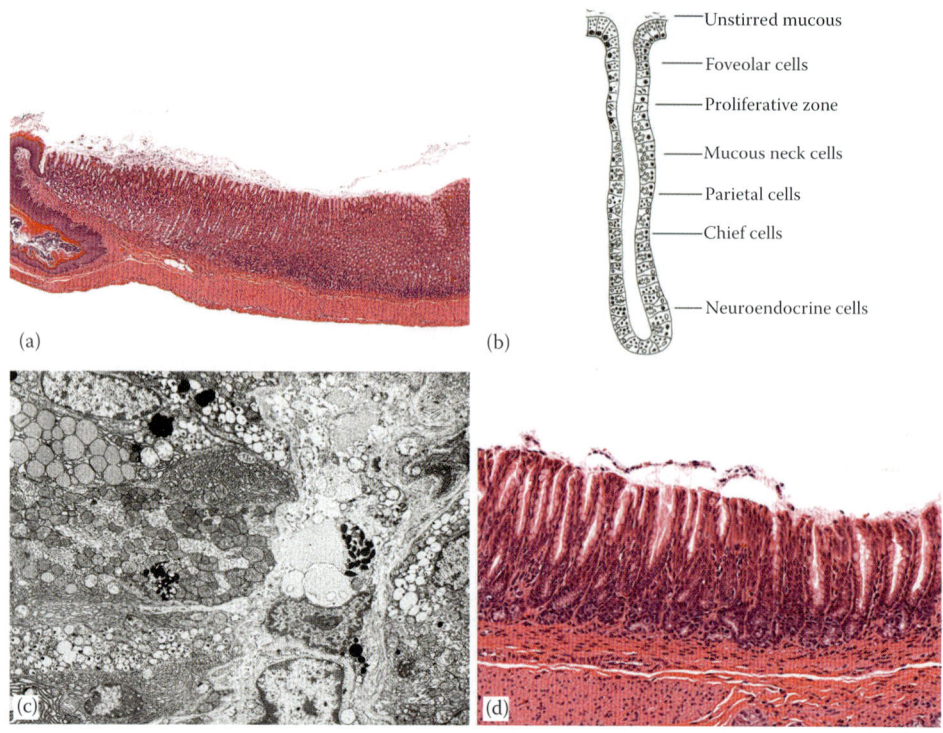

FIGURE 9.2 (a) Rat, stomach, HE stain. The nonglandular stomach and limiting ridge are present on the left, cardiac glands on the center, and oxyntic glands on the right. The oxyntic mucosa thickness is approximately 720 μm. (b) Diagram of oxyntic gland showing distribution of main cell types. (c) Rat, oxyntic gland, transmission electron microscopy. Chief cells with large zymogen granules, parietal cells rich in mitochondria with canalicular system, and ECL neuroendocrine cells with open neurosecretory vesicles with small dense cores. (d) Rat, antral mucosa, HE stain. This region of the stomach is composed of simple glands with basal mucin. Note that the antrum is thinner than the fundus and has an approximate thickness of 225 μm.

Histologically, the cardiac glands around the cardiac sphincter at the entry point of the esophagus are a narrow band of short, mainly mucus-secreting glands. The fundus and body are covered by oxyntic mucosa, which functions to secrete gastric juice containing pepsin, acid, and various growth factors. In primates, parietal cells are present only in the body. In the body of the stomach, the oxyntic glands contain a proliferative compartment, which is relatively superficial, with mucus-secreting foveolar cells forming the gastric pits above with a 6-day turnover and oxyntic glands below. The proliferative compartment contains progenitor cells in the isthmus of normal glands, which express the marker doublecortin and calcium/calmodulin protein kinase-like-1 (DCAMKL1), which under pathological conditions becomes less localized (Kikuchi et al. 2010). Gastric oxyntic glands have a life span of about 100 days, and cell types can be identified using immunohistochemical markers such as H^+/K^+ ATPase for parietal cells; *Mist1* and pepsinogen II for chief cells; trefoil factor 2 (TFF2) and Muc6 for mucous neck cells; and chromogranin A, neuron-specific enolase (NSE), synaptophysin (Gould et al. 1987; Hanby et al. 1999), and anti-protein gene product (PGP9.5; UCHL1) for neuroendocrine cells. The pyloric antrum is lined by simpler antral glands with mucous cells at the base, leading into the pyloric sphincter at the entry to the duodenum, where Brunner's glands are present, with bicarbonate secretions to raise the pH.

The gastric content varies with time of day and feeding patterns. In toxicology studies, the pH can also change with buffers or with the pharmacological mode of action of antisecretory drugs reducing proton pump secretion of hydrochloric acid from the tubulo-canalicular system of parietal cells. The low pKa of some xenobiotics means that they exist in non-ionized form in the stomach, and this can lead to direct uptake by the mucosa. Excipients in formulations may influence local uptake, affect gastric emptying time, or cause other changes, for example, osmotic effect of poly-ethylene glycols (PEGs). Local irritancy may be modified according to timing of dosing and fed-versus-fasted administration. Diets with abrasive high-fiber composition, helminth parasites, and long gavage needles can traumatize the gastric mucosa.

Gastric physiology is complex, with individual cell types in the oxyntic glands of the fundic mucosa being regulated by autonomic nerves, peptide hormones, amines, and local paracrine and autocrine signals (Håkanson et al. 1994). Mucus, spasmolytic polypeptide/TFF2, and bicarbonate are secreted by surface foveolar cells, mucous neck cells, plus cardiac and antral glands. Mucus and bicarbonate are critical for cytoprotection of the mucosa from acid attack by gastric juice.

Pepsinogens, intrinsic factor (in rodents; Shao et al. 2000), and leptin are secreted by chief cells. Hydrochloric acid, intrinsic factor (in man), and sonic hedgehog ligand are secreted by parietal cells. Neuroendocrine (enteroendocrine) cells secrete gastrin, somatostatin, ghrelin (Woods and D'Alessio 2008), and other peptide hormones from secretory vesicles with peptide cores and amines (histamine, serotonin/5HT; Håkanson et al. 1986) of the amine precursor uptake and decarboxylase (APUD) neuroendocrine system of the GI tract.

Parietal cells are specialized cells for acid secretion and are located in oxyntic (fundic and body) mucosa. They derive from the progenitor cells as pre-parietal cells before migrating down the gland to form mature parietal cells (Karam 2010). They have receptors for histamine, ACTH, acetylcho-line, and gastrin (CCK2 receptor), which raise cAMP to activate the proton pump H^+/K^+ ATPase. Vesicles form into a canalicular system when stimulated to secrete H^+ ions into the oxyntic gland and into the stomach lumen. With acid secretion by parietal cells, there is a balancing rise in pH of the venous outflow from the oxyntic mucosa called the "alkaline tide." Deep antral gland cells all immunostain for trefoil factor 2 (TFF2) and mucin MUC6 and are strongly stained with Alcian blue.

9.3.6 SMALL AND LARGE INTESTINES

The diet and feeding behavior (composition, frequency, need for storage, and availability of water) of any given species along with body size has the greatest impact on the gross anatomic character-istics of the intestines. Most of the species we are discussing in this chapter are characterized as omnivorous by Stevens (1980), on the basis of their diet composition being some type of a mixture of plant and animal material. Hence, rodents with a substantial proportion of plant-based fiber-rich diet have a relatively long large intestine and a cecum with large capacity and complex wall due to sacculation and longitudinal bands of teniae. In contrast, dogs whose diet is high in animal protein have a relatively simple and small cecum. Macaques, with respect to the complexity of the large intestine, fall between these two extremes. It is useful for a pathologist to understand the general function of each segment of the gut and to be able to identify them. In this regard, the reader is directed to an excellent paper by Kararli (1995) that compares gut function and length of several laboratory species. Briefly, the duodenum is the first segment of the small intestine whose proximal portion contains the specialized submucosal Brunner's glands. Brunner's glands are located only in the most proximal portion of the duodenum adjacent to the gastric pylorus in rats and produce mucin and bicarbonate-containing secretum in order to increase the luminal pH of the duodenum from the acidic pH of the stomach. In rats, however, bicarbonate production by Brunner's glands is not prominent (Ainsworth et al. 1995). The proximal duodenum also contains papillae with species-specific distribution where bile ducts and pancreatic ducts empty. In dogs, as in humans, the com-mon bile duct enters the duodenum at the duodenal papilla. In these species, the pancreatic duct unites with the bile duct at the sphincter of Oddi. In contrast, in rats, the pancreatic duct directly flows into the common bile duct (Kararli 1995). The distal portion of the duodenum is easy to rec-ognize grossly *in situ* in the animal as the ligament of Treitz serves as the landmark, connecting the small intestine at the duodeno-jejunal junction to the diaphragm. The longest segment of the small intestine, the jejunum in the species of interest, is being supported by the mesentery, as is the third shortest segment, the ileum, which measures approximately 3 cm in rats. A little-recognized noteworthy species difference is that in humans, the length of the jejunum and that of the ileum are quite similar, as both measure approximately 300 cm, whereas in mice, the jejunum is approximately ten times longer than the ileum (Kararli 1995). The small intestine is the major site of absorption for nutrients and xenobiotics, whereas the primary role of the colon is the absorption of water and ions, including Na^+. Solubility, dissolution, and absorption of drugs depend on whether they are ionizable, a pH-dependent process. Intestinal luminal contents have an increasing pH from oral to caudal regions. Bile fluids containing bile acids are important for solubilizing drugs, and it is also a major route of excretion for drugs. Bile secretion depends on circadian rhythm and digestion under secretin and CCK regulation and also on whether the animal has a gallbladder or not.

The microscopic structure of the intestine is in keeping with the general morphology of the GI tract, as it is composed of mucosa, muscularis mucosa, submucosa, muscularis, and serosa. The muscularis is composed of two layers of smooth muscle and contains the nervous tissue between its layers. The interstitial cells of Cajal are located within the muscularis and are the pacemakers of the intestine by propagating electrical events and modulating neurotransmitters. In the small intestine, the mucosa is composed of villi and crypts along the full length, with subtle differences in the crypt-to-villus ratio and cell components. In the adult mouse, villi are interspersed with varying numbers of crypts. In the duodenum, the crypt-to-villus ratio is 14:1 compared to 6:1 in the jejunum and ileum, respectively. The length of villi shortens in the distal segments of the small intestine. Each duodenal villus in the mouse contains approximately 7800 cells, whereas in the ileum, each villus contains about 2100 cells.

The large-intestinal mucosa contains straight intestinal tubules/crypts with occasional branching at the base. The surface epithelium contains enterocytes, whereas much of the crypts are taken up by mucus-producing goblet cells. The colonic mucosa contains mucosal folds that are especially prominent in rodents.

The adult small intestine is organized into crypts containing the proliferative regions interspersed with Paneth cells (their location and cytoplasmic granules first described by Joseph Paneth in the nineteenth century) and villi composed of the differentiated cells of secretory and enterocyte lineages (Figure 9.3a). In fetal and suckling mice, the intervillous epithelium has a similar function as that of the crypt in adults. In species with Paneth cells (rodents and primates among those species toxicologic pathologists work with most frequently), the deeper regions (positions 1–3) of the crypt are taken up by Paneth cells, and stem cells are present higher in the crypts (at position +4) as well as individually between Paneth cells. Using a cell sorting method of mouse jejunal cells with CD24, the resulting cell fractions included the lysozyme-rich Paneth cells and cells that also contained the leucine-rich repeat-containing G protein–coupled receptor 5 (Lgr5) (von Furstenberg et al. 2011). In the colon, CD24+ cells are also present adjacent to Lgr5 cells, indicating that those cells are related to Paneth cells (this will need to be confirmed by other investigators) (Sato et al. 2011). In culture systems, Paneth cells express several factors that are important for the maintenance of the culture and improve organoid formation when co-cultured with stem cells, including EGF, TGFα, Wnt3, and the Notch ligand Dll4. Exogenous Wnt may be substituted for the Paneth cells *in vitro*, whereas *in vivo*, removal of Paneth cells results in concomitant loss of Lgr5 cells. When in an experimental system, a small molecule of Wnt secretion inhibitor (porcupine inhibitor) was added, organoids were lost, and proliferation stopped. Under normal conditions *in vivo*, the Wnt signaling pathway is the dominant pathway in control of the crypt–villus axis through secreted signaling proteins. A key component of the pathway is the cytoplasmic β catenin that is regulated by the destruction complex. The destruction complex is composed of the tumor suppressor adenomatous polyposis coli (APC) and axin bind β catenin if Wnt receptors are not engaged. In case APC function is lost, cytoplasmic and nuclear β catenin accumulates. Nuclear β catenin binds with Tcf proteins to activate Wnt target genes, ultimately impacting cell cycle. In summary, the Wnt signaling pathway is considered to be a key factor in intestinal tumorigenesis. In addition to Wnt signaling, the bone morphogenic protein

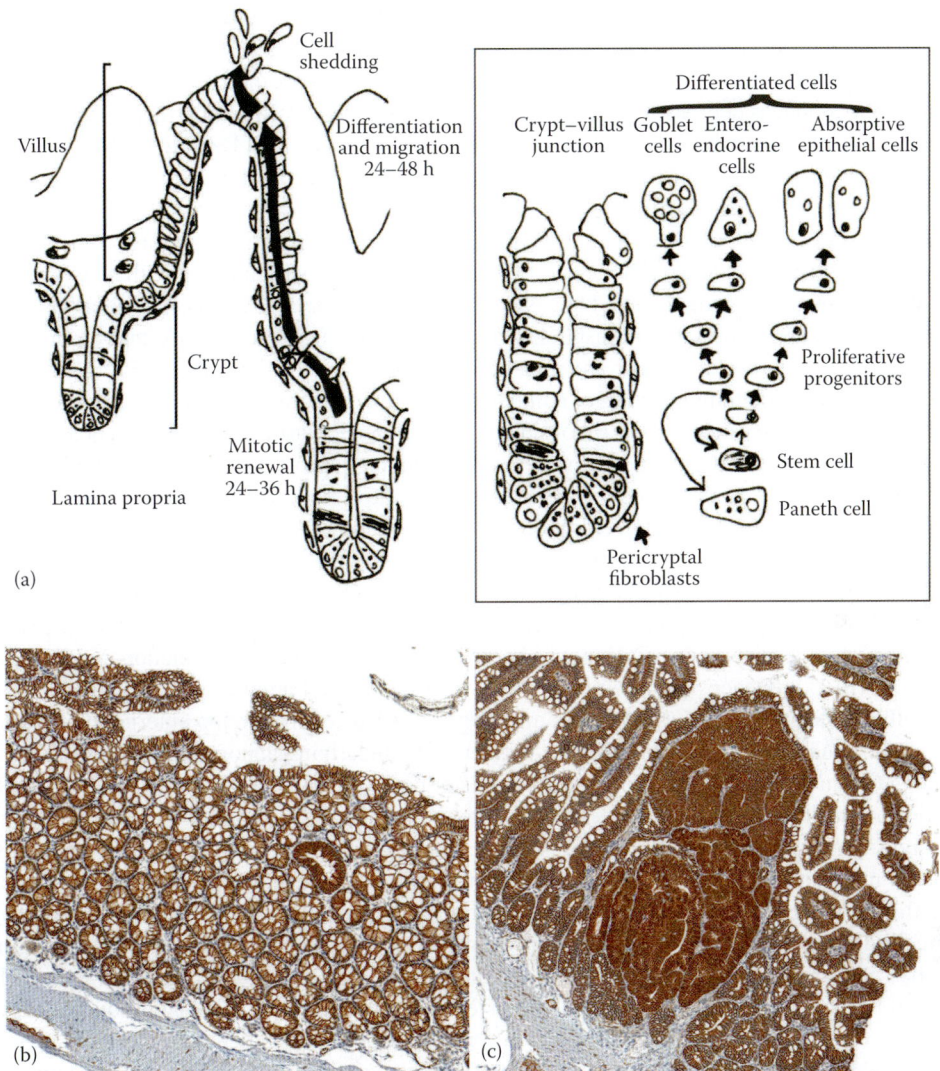

FIGURE 9.3 (a) Diagram of intestinal proliferation and self-renewal. The small intestine is organized into crypts and villi lined in adults by clonal epithelial cells. Stem cells give rise to transit-amplifying cells that after three to four cycles of self-renewal (taking 24–36 h in mice) give rise (in 24–48 h) to differentiated goblet, enteroendocrine, and absorptive epithelial cells (inset). Cells move upward along the villi and are eventually shed by apoptosis. Myo-epithelial fibroblasts (i.e., pericryptal fibroblasts) are closely apposed to crypt basal lamina and are important for establishment of the crypt niche. (After Radtke F., Clevers H., *Science* 307, 1904–1909, 2005.) (b) Apc^Min/+ mouse, colon, IHC for β catenin. ACF is easily recognized by dense immunoreactivity due to cytoplasmic translocation of β catenin (compare neighboring normal crypts with membranous immunoreactivity). (Courtesy of Dr. C. Ibebunjo and Dr. M. McLaughlin, NIBRI, Cambridge, MA.) (c) Apc^Min/+ mouse, small intestine, IHC for β catenin. An adenoma is characterized by compression and cytoplasmic and nuclear translocation of β catenin immunoreactivity from the membranous immunoreactivity in surrounding normal regions. (Courtesy of Dr. C. Ibebunjo and Dr. M. McLaughlin, NIBRI, Cambridge, MA.)

(BMP) pathway plays a role in maintenance of normal intestinal structure; BMPs are expressed in the stroma of villi (Radtke and Clevers 2005). The stem cells self-renew and give rise to transit-amplifying cells that undergo three to four cycles of division to give rise to the differentiated cells (goblet cells, enteroendocrine cells, and absorptive cells) (Radtke and Clevers 2005). Cells that migrate upward in the villus are eventually shed by apoptosis up to 1400 cells per villi within a

24-h period. In the large intestine, intercryptal tables are formed by cells originating from colonic crypts. The cell turnover in the large intestine is increased approximately to 8 days from 2–3 days in the small intestine (Johnson 2006). Both proliferation and apoptosis increase with age in the small intestine, but apoptosis decreases with age in the colon, although proliferation increases; this apparent change may have a role in intestinal carcinogenesis (Majumdar and Basson 2006).

Hyperproliferation due to disturbance of the orderly proliferation and differentiation may be visualized as individual crypts or clusters of crypts that are larger than normal, often with a slit-like opening (Figure 9.3b and c) (Fenoglio-Preiser and Noffsinger 1999). In a clinical setting, aberrant crypt foci (ACFs) may be visualized at the time of endoscopy or as in nonclinical samples, with *en face* preparations that are stained with methylene blue as darkly stained clusters of crypts. These crypts contain abnormal mucus and microsatellite instability (repeats of short DNA sequences) and often have ras mutations. Based on morphological and genetic evidence as well as because of the circumstances under which lesions are found in a larger number (after carcinogen treatment of animals or in patients with high risk of colon cancer), ACF is considered to be a preneoplastic lesion (Alrawi et al. 2006).

Paneth cells as part of the innate immune system function to protect stem cells in small-intestinal crypts provide defense against ingested pathogens and control both the number and composition of commensal bacteria (Bevins 2004). Additionally, based on mouse studies, the interaction of Paneth cells and bacteria is needed for appropriate angiogenesis in villi for the development of adult-type villi that become well vascularized during weaning. Paneth cells carry out these important functions in host defense by the secretion of lysozyme, zinc, and antimicrobial molecules (defensins). The unfolding protein response gene and autophagy have key roles in Paneth cell function. X-Box binding protein 1 (XBP1) influences antimicrobial activity and Paneth cell number and decreases responses to proinflammatory stimuli. Furthermore, mice with XBP1 deletion develop enteritis (Garrett et al. 2010). Several human diseases have been identified with underlying abnormal Paneth cell function, including Crohn's disease, necrotizing enterocolitis of newborns, and cystic fibrosis (Bevins 2004).

Intestinal stromal cells impact regeneration, wound repair, and communication between epithelium and immune cells (primarily macrophages) (Stappenbeck and Miyoshi 2009). Intestinal subepithelial myofibroblasts form a network of fenestrated cells as they merge with vascular pericytes while they are also closely apposed to the epithelial cell layer (Vidrich et al. 2006). Mesenchymal stem cell–derived cells have a key function coordinating macrophage-driven events to eliminate microbes and the epithelial repair. Wound repair is quite similar across different organs with an epithelial lining (such as lung and gut) and involves the epithelial stem cells that produce differentiated cells away from the wound bed and less differentiated cells associated with it. The exact nature of either stem cell type (mesenchymal and epithelial) is poorly understood during tissue repair. As alluded to earlier, Lgr5 epithelial stem cells are sensitive to injury. Hence, it is believed that long-lived "label-retaining" cells (characterized by their ability to retain BrDU labeling for a long time) may be the source to repopulate the injured epithelium (Cordero and Sampson 2011).

9.3.7 Intestinal Absorption and Secretion

Nutrients and drugs are taken up by a number of mechanisms including passive, active, and pinocytotic uptake, and these processes are influenced by the lipid composition of enterocyte membranes, among other factors. Most nutrients are absorbed through the apically located brush border of the small-intestinal epithelium. The brush border contains several biotransforming and metabolizing enzymes and is being supported by cytoskeletal elements of microvilli, referred to as the terminal web. Dietary components such as carbohydrates are absorbed by specific translocators using cAMP as a messenger (Stumpel et al. 2000). A unique transport mechanism was identified for the transfer of minute amounts of protein or peptides from the intestinal lumen into the blood via surface invaginations of the intestinal epithelium and subsequent cytoplasmic vesicle formation of the endosomal structures. Within minutes, the process is completed by the release of peptides through the basolateral membrane into the interstitial space to reach circulation (Ziv and Bendayan 2000).

Xenobiotic absorption in the GI tract is influenced by the mucosal unstirred water layer, luminal pH, and the relative length of different gut regions as well as intestinal flora. Dogs are often considered to be good for modeling drug absorption, although they have some differences from humans. Dogs may have a delayed gastric emptying, a shorter small-intestinal transit time, and a greater individual variation in luminal pH than humans do (Dressman 1986). Many pathways of the intestinal transport are energy-dependent processes using several ATPases.

The intestinal lumen contains a larger number of bacteria than the number of cells in the host body, without triggering an inflammatory reaction. Other luminal contents include components of the adaptive and innate immune systems (e.g., secretory IgA, lysozyme, and antibacterial peptides). Recent advances in the evaluation of mucus in the colon provided greater understanding of the production and structure of the colonic mucus blanket and its interaction with luminal bacteria (Figure 9.4a). The turnover of goblet cells and mucin is a complex mechanism. Goblet differentiation from

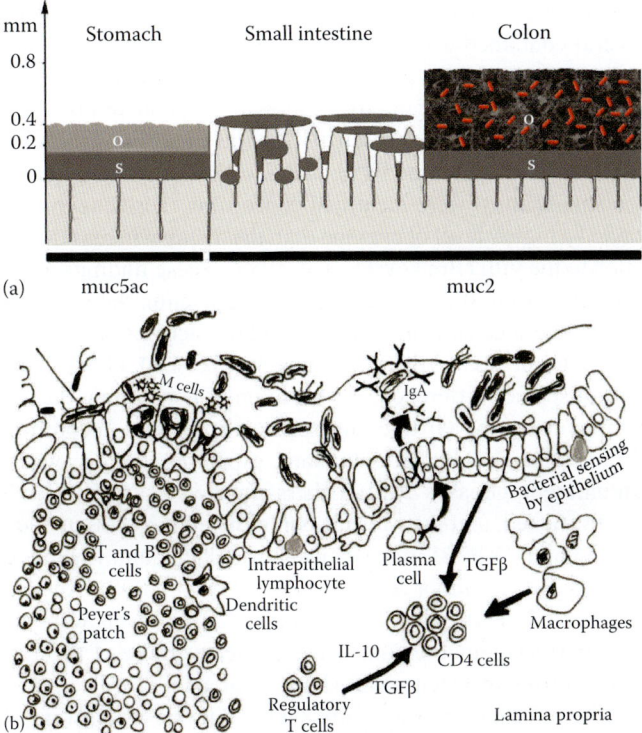

FIGURE 9.4 (a) Diagram of gastrointestinal mucus production. The approximate thickness of mucus layers is indicated for the rat. The primary mucin type in the stomach is Muc5ac, and in the small and large intestines, it is Muc2. The structures of the mucus blankets of the stomach and colon both have two diffuse layers: a stratified inner layer (s) firmly attached to the epithelium and an outer layer (o) that is loose and, in the colon, contains commensal bacteria (red rods). The mucin layer in the small intestine is not continuous and is a single layer produced at the top of crypts and moves up the villi, some of which may be exposed. (After Johansson M. E. V. et al., *PNAS* 108, 4659–4665, 2011.) (b) Diagram of Peyer's patch. The Peyer's patch is covered by epithelium containing antigen-presenting M cells that introduce antigens to dendritic cells (DCs) in the underlying subepithelial dome that contains naive T and B cells. Enteric antigens may also be sampled from the lumen by DC in lamina propria. Activated T cells or antigen-containing DCs may migrate to regional mesenteric lymph nodes via lymphatics to interact with naive T cells. CD8+ T lymphocytes are intraepithelial, whereas CD4 T cells, macrophages, and IgA-producing plasma cells are in the lamina propria. Regulatory T lymphocytes interacting with immunosuppressive cytokines may protect against tissue damage by T cells. (After MacDonald T. T., Monteleone G., *Science* 307, 1920–1925, 2005.)

stem cells is under the influence of wnt signaling; as goblet cells mature and move upward in the crypt, they acquire the ability to produce Muc2. Upon release of mucus from goblet cells (usually at the opening of the crypt), the mucus expands up to 1000 folds when exposed to water. This newly released mucus forms the inner mucus layer that is impervious to bacteria. The outer layer of the mucus is less dense, may be broken down by bacteria, and provides the environment for commensal bacteria. The loose outer mucus layer is eventually removed from the body via the feces (Johansson et al. 2011). The above is further confirmed by Muc2$^{-/-}$ knockout (KO) mice that have bacteria attached to exposed epithelium and have inflammation in the GI tract.

9.3.8 Biotransformation

The liver is recognized as the primary site for first-pass metabolism of compounds delivered orally (because of its cytochrome P450 enzyme content) and for control of the systemic drug levels. However, similar enzyme activity to that of the liver is also recognized in tissues that serve as portals of entry for drug delivery, the respiratory and GI tract, for example (Ding and Kaminsky 2003). The intestines in general contained about 10% of the P450 enzyme levels of the liver in rats in a study investigating enzyme induction by phenobarbital (Bonkovsky et al. 1985). The intestinal P450 was found to be inducible just as that of the liver following phenobarbital dosing and dietary components such as broccoli (Kaminsky and Fasco 1992). The small intestine was studied in greatest detail as to the distribution of cytochrome P450, and two axes (one along the length of the gut and another along the intestinal villus) were identified concerning these enzyme levels. The proximal small intestine contained a higher level of enzyme than the distal, whereas the P450 levels increased from mid villous region to the villi (Bonkovsky et al. 1985). These findings indicated that soon after the entry of oral xenobiotics from the stomach into the duodenum, they may undergo metabolism. Furthermore, as a protective mechanism, cells have higher activity to produce potentially active metabolites as they move to the tip of villi where they may be shed. Other than the general aspects outlined above, details of species differences among animals concerning the CYP subfamilies represented in different regions of the GI tract are still controversial. According to one source, the mouse and dog small intestine, just as that of humans, expresses CYP3A, whereas in rats, CYP2C appears to be more prominent (Greaves 2012). Others reported a surprising individual variation in the cohort of rats they evaluated, and their results contradicted those discussed above. Han–Wistar rats had abundant CYP3A and CYP2B1 in the duodenum and jejunum, whereas CYP2D1, CYP2C6, and CYP2C11 were expressed in minor levels (Mitschke et al. 2008). An interesting age-related regional difference was noted in rats when liver and gut CYP3A levels were compared. Following weaning, hepatic enzyme levels remained unchanged, whereas those of the gut increased, perhaps as a protective mechanism from ingested toxins (Johnson et al. 2000). The intestinal mucosa is also rich in peroxisome. Little information is available on CYP levels in extra-intestinal regions of the GI tract, even in humans. Esophageal enzyme activity in humans was compared from the United States and regions of China with a high incidence of esophageal cancer because of an interest in metabolic activation of carcinogens in tobacco smoke. Microsomal preparations had a higher level of bioactivation from samples originating from high-risk regions of China (Ding and Kaminsky 2003). In general, no significant P450 activity was reported in human stomach, but there is some suggestion that areas of intestinal metaplasia in the pyloric antrum have primarily CYP1A activity. Most investigators report that both humans and animals have low levels of cytochrome P450 in the colon compared to the small intestine—an interesting observation especially from a human epidemiological perspective in light of the high prevalence of cancer, at least in the human colon (Ding and Kaminsky 2003).

Glutathione-related activities are also varied along the previously identified axes in the gut. Enzyme activities were higher orally than aborally, and they also had a differential expression along the villi. Glutathione content was lower in the tips of villi than deeper in the crypts, whereas the related enzymes, γ glutamyl transpeptidase and glutathione S transferase, were higher toward the tip of villi than in the crypts (Ogasawara et al. 1985).

9.3.9 ENTEROHEPATIC CIRCULATION

Bile formation is important for intestinal lipid digestion and absorption and excretion of lipid soluble xenobiotics. Enterohepatic circulation allows the recycling of bile acids (and metabolized or non-metabolized compounds) and involves a number of transport proteins through different epithelia, including hepatocytes, cholangiocytes, ileal enterocytes, and renal proximal tubular cells (Dawson et al. 2006). The rate of enterohepatic circulation is linked to diet intake and to either contraction of gall bladder in species with a gall bladder or the propelling of bile from the proximal small intestine, where bile is stored in species without a gall bladder. The terminal ileum is the primary site of bile acid reabsorption involving active transport through the ileal brush border membranes. Glucuronide metabolites can be deconjugated by the gut microflora and resorbed. Bile acids regulate gene transcription for components of lipid metabolism either by up- or downregulating different components. Bile acid reabsorption is downregulated in different inflammatory diseases, including *Eimaeria magna* infection in rabbits and inflammatory bowel disease (IBD) in humans. If bile acid production cannot keep up with bile acid reabsorption, it may cause malabsorption of fat-soluble vitamins and water-insoluble fatty acids. Exogenous corticosteroids (used for a long time for treatment of IBD) upregulate bile acid reabsorption by directly acting on transporter gene expression. Xenobiotics may interact with intestinal contents during enterohepatic circulation. Decreased bile acid reabsorption is claimed to be at least part of the reason for the positive effects of increased dietary fibers on health. Indomethacin toxicity is a classic example of the impact enterohepatic circulation may have on the manifestation of species-specific toxicity. In dogs, most of the indomethacin is excreted as a conjugate and is not reabsorbed. In contrast, nonhuman primates excrete much of the dose as the parent compound that is readily reabsorbed. This species difference plays an important role in the ulcerogenic effect of indomethacin in dogs (Rozman 1988).

9.3.10 BACTERIA

Microbiologists from Louis Pasteur to Ilya Mechnikov recognized the diversity and significance of intestinal microbiota to health and disease. Its function includes energy production (may be favorable for the host by salvaging otherwise indigestible dietary components), chemical transformations, and self-renewal (replication). Microbiota contributes to glucose uptake by the host epithelium, elevating serum glucose and insulin, and to lipogenesis. Studies in mice and human populations indicated that certain intestinal microbiota may enhance energy harvest (referred to as "obesity-associated gut microbiome") (Turnbaugh et al. 2006). The human gut exhibited a limited microbial diversity; only 8 of the 55 known bacterial divisions were represented (compared to soil, which contained 20 of 55 divisions) (Backed et al. 2005). An interesting finding was that in the human intestine, bacterial populations were remarkably stable in any given individual, implying that mechanisms either promoted or suppressed certain subpopulations. It should be noted, however, that a change in the diet of mice (from predominantly plant based to a western type) caused a shift in the microbiota composition within a day and changed the represented metabolic pathways (Turnbaugh et al. 2009).

Another aspect of intestinal microflora that needs further probing is the apparent spatial organization of microbiota within the gut (Nava et al. 2011). Morphologically distinct populations representing microbiologically distinct organisms were present close to the transverse folds in the colon and were distinct from those of the digesta. Such differential distribution may indicate a specific role in physiological or barrier functions.

Compounds that alter bacterial composition may cause malabsorption by changing the intestinal brush border enzymes. In contrast to mammalian metabolic pathways that are oxidative, intestinal bacterial pathways are anaerobic and include reduction and hydrolysis. Bacterial β glucuronidase in the intestine may produce toxic and carcinogenic aglycones (Tamura et al. 1996). Another example is the production of methylazoxymethanol from cycasin by Streptobacillus glycosidase.

9.3.11 LYMPHOID TISSUE

The lymphoid system, including functional anatomy, is discussed in detail in Chapter 14; hence, only a brief overview of the GI immune system is presented here. Regionally diverse components form the lymphoid tissue of the digestive tract, whose function is defense against environmental pathogens (especially in the microorganism-rich gut) and tolerance to dietary components. In most species, but not in rodents, the oropharynx is encircled by the tonsil (Casteleyn et al. 2011). In rats, nasal-associated lymphoid tissue (NALT) is located at the ventral nasal meatus and can be found at level III of the nasal turbinates (Elmore 2006). A less organized cluster of lymphoid tissue is found at the gastric cardia adjacent to the esophageal sphincter, which is referred to as mucosa-associated lymphoid tissue (MALT), along with the similar lymphoid aggregate at the pyloric antrum. Similarly to MALT, lymphoid nodules are associated with minor salivary glands, referred to as duct-associated lymphoid tissue (DALT) (Nair and Schroeder 1986). Newborn animals seem to have no or minimal DALT at birth, but just as MALT, DALT develops as animals mature and are exposed to environmental factors and bacteria. Secretory ducts of minor salivary glands are associated with follicles or lymphoid nodules, whereas plasma cells are interacinar. In mature animals, DALT is part of the integrated immune system of the GI tract, contributing to the secretory immunoglobulin mediated immunity of the oral cavity. The intestine contains the gut-associated lymphoid tissue (GALT), which is organized into Peyer's patches in the antimesenteric aspect of the small intestine and lymphoid nodules in the cecum and colon. Components of GALT are not easily recognized grossly in large animals but often appear as light gray serosal nodules in mice. Additionally, upon careful inspection of the intestinal mucosa, oval structures aligned along the long axis of the gut may be recognized on mucosal surfaces, especially in dogs. Caudal segments of the small intestine contain a larger number of Peyer's patches than the proximal ones, but Peyer's patches are present in all segments of the small intestine. Peyer's patches are formed in the lamina propria extending into the submucosa by multiple domes that somewhat protrude into the gut lumen and are covered by follicle-associated epithelium, which contain M cells that serve as antigen-presenting cells (Figure 9.4b). Luminal contents are also sampled by antigen-presenting dendritic cells as their cell processes extend between epithelial cells. Additional components of the lymphoid system include intraepithelial lymphocytes that are mostly CD8 and CD4 cells in the lamina propria. The lamina propria also contains macrophages, plasma cells, mast cells, eosinophils, and regulatory and other T lymphocytes. Furthermore, the intestinal defense mechanism contains pro-inflammatory components composed of cell membrane–associated toll-like receptors (TLRs) and cytosolic nucleotide-binding oligomerization domain molecules (Nod). Different TLRs and Nods recognize different components of bacteria and viruses and in some way are also able to distinguish pathogens from commensal organisms. In an interesting symbiosis, normal intestinal flora assures cytoprotection by inducing certain types of heat shock proteins to be produced by epithelial cells (MacDonald and Monteleone 2005). This anti-inflammatory function is confirmed by mice that are deficient in TLR signaling, do not express Hsp25 and Hsp72 in their colonic epithelium, and have greater sensitivity to dextran sulfate–induced colitis than wild-type mice, suggesting that normal flora may be protective against nonspecific damage through intact TLR signaling of the host. Much of the dome of the Peyer's patch is taken up by B lymphocytes organized into follicles, whereas interfollicular regions are populated by T cells. Once B and T cells are activated in the Peyer's patch, they migrate to the blood. Immune cells enter the lamina propria via a homing function that is achieved by high endothelial cell-lined postcapillary venules (HEVs). A unique feature of gut immunity is that circulating lymphocytes that were primed in the gut may populate other mucosal sites such as the respiratory or genital tract. Hence, there is a unified mucosal immune system wherever the host may be exposed to environmental stimulus. The colonic GALT is organized similarly, except it contains lymphoglandular structures that are formed by invaginations of the surface epithelium. Both the MALT and the GALT predominantly provide humoral immunity of the IgA isotype with or without a secretory component.

Related to immunity is the control of inflammation in the gut by regulatory T cells that can suppress immune responses. These T cells regulate through IL10 and transforming growth factor 1B signaling. In a recent review by Erdman and Poutahidis (2010), a mouse model was presented to illustrate how disruption of immune homeostasis leads to a pro-inflammatory process with elevated IL6 and a Th-17 host response. There is evidence in mice and humans that weakened IL10 and T regulatory cell functions result in an increased risk of inflammation and associated cancers (Erdman and Poutahidis 2010).

9.3.12   ENTERIC NERVOUS SYSTEM

The nervous system of the GI tract is a highly organized complex system albeit widely dispersed in the body. Hirschprung, a Danish pediatrician, published the first case of megacolon about 100 years ago and recognized at least part of the general architecture of the enteric nervous system. The enteric nervous system from the esophagus to the rectum is composed of the myenteric (Auerbach), inner and outer submucosal (Meissner and Schabadasch), and mucosal plexuses (sub/periglandular, vascular, and villous subepithelial), which we know to be interconnected and ganglionated. Intestinal sensory receptors continuously monitor luminal components for a wide range of characteristics, including texture, temperature, fluidity, volume, and chemical composition (Cooke 1986; Hansen 2003a). Neurons of the submucosal ganglia seem to project toward the mucosa and coordinate and control absorptive and secretory functions, along with blood flow and control of muscularis mucosa. In contrast, myenteric neurons are involved in the generation of motility. More than 30 neurotransmitters have been identified from small molecules (5-hydroxytryptophen [5HT]) to peptides (substance P) and gases (NO). Functionally, the neurons are divided into sensory neurons, orally and aborally directed interneurons, short and long excitatory muscle motor neurons, inhibitory muscle neurons, and secretomotor neurons. Secretomotor neurons stimulate epithelial secretion of Cl$^-$ by a cAMP or Ca-dependent mechanism, depending on their neurotransmitters (vasoactive intestinal peptide [VIP] or acetylcholine). While the basic organization of the system is similar across species and age of individuals, both species-specific and age-related differences are present. An additional layer of complexity is provided by the interaction of the nervous system with enteroendocrine cells, which provide information via mediators about luminal contents. With the exception of gastrin-producing G, somatostatin-containing D, and enterochromaffin cells, little is known about the neuronal control of enteroendocrine cells. The enteroendocrine cell of the GI tract represents the largest endocrine organ in the body, but because the cell types of this diffuse neuroendocrine system are widely dispersed along the GI tract, showing 15 specific cell types, most with a single peptide hormone product and located along the GI tract (Solcia et al. 1998), they pass unnoticed unless immunostained or form tumors. For example, gastrin-secreting G cells are located in the gastric antral mucosa and regulate the pH of gastric juice by stimulating acid secretion in the oxyntic mucosa of the stomach. Adjacent somatostatin-secreting D cells downregulate gastrin secretion in a paracrine manner. In addition, autonomic innervation modulates gastrin secretion via acetylcholinergic signals. Other cell types of the diffuse neuroendocrine system of the GI tract are involved in pancreatic and biliary secretion, glucose homeostasis, and satiety signals. Enterochromaffin cells contain several neuroactive substances, including 5HT, which may be released following a number of mucosal stimuli and contribute to sensory, peristaltic, and secretory reflexes. In the contemporary view of GI disease, 5HT has a central role in irritable bowel disease, response to cholera, and *Clostridium difficile* and *Escherichia coli* toxins, among others; the reader is referred to references provided for greater detail (Goyal and Hirano 1996; Hansen 2003b). The interaction of nerves and mast cells regulates blood flow and mucosal function and is important in the local inflammatory response (either by a direct effect or through interactions with nerves). Because the enteric nervous system is involved in many processes of the GI tract, targeting mediators may impact diseases of motility (diarrhea, constipation), inflammation, and non-occlusive ischemia (Hansen 2003c). In the organization of the enteric nervous system, in addition to local influences, reflexes involve distant regions. In terms of motility, such interactions are relatively well understood: paralytic ileus involves the stretching of one region, resulting in decreased motility in a distant region of the GI. The basal smooth muscle activity of the intestine is maintained by the interstitial cells of Cajal. Enteric nerves may alter smooth muscle membrane polarization such that the contractions of muscle cells become more or less frequent. Although the enteric nervous system for the most part is independent of the central nervous system (CNS), there is two-way trafficking to further modulate gut function via the vagal fibers (Hansen 2003b).

The vomiting reflex occurs in many species, dogs being the most important in toxicologic pathology. Emesis may occur due to a local irritant effect or a central reflex. Chemotherapy-related emesis has been studied in detail and will be discussed here briefly. It is believed that 5HT originating from enterochromaffin cells is the most important mediator of the emesis reflex. 5HT interacts with vagal terminals in the intestinal wall, resulting in the stimulus of the dorsal vagal complex in the brainstem. Receptors for some of the neurotransmitters that may be important in the emesis reflex are located in the dorsal vagal complex. The neurotransmitters identified to be important include substance P, 5HT, and dopamine. A second mechanism may involve regions around the fourth ventricle, where opioids and dopamine may bind. Finally, the amygdala is considered to have a role in the stimulation of emesis reflex. In the last two decades, selective antagonists of the key neurotransmitters were developed to prevent chemotherapy-related nausea and vomiting (Hesketh 2008).

9.4 NONPROLIFERATIVE AND PROLIFERATIVE MORPHOLOGICAL RESPONSES

International regulatory guidelines (Reni trimming guide) require the examination of the luminal GI tract (esophagus, stomach, and the three segments each of small and large intestines represented); most health authorities, but not the US Food and Drug Administration (FDA), require the microscopic examination of the tongue. Additionally, the FDA requires only the examination of only one of the salivary glands (typically the submandibular one), whereas the European Medicines Agency (EMA) also requires the examination of parotid and sublingual salivary glands. Other than the tongue, the oral mucosa is seldom examined routinely unless lesions are recognized at necropsy. An exception is the palate, which is included in sections of the nasal cavity and apparently routinely examined by National Toxicology Program (NTP) and in all inhalation studies by others. The cheek pouches of macaques are not routinely examined but should at least be evaluated grossly since they are often the site of opportunistic infections such as candidiasis.

9.4.1 ORAL CAVITY AND TONGUE

Regardless of the location within the oral cavity, inflammatory and/or necrotizing changes may be the most common ones in toxicity studies. Such lesions may occur spontaneously in small and large animals, including mechanical injuries or rarely in conjunction with intestinal shigellosis in macaques (Lowenstein 2003). Sunitinib, a broad-spectrum tyrosine kinase inhibitor, was reported to cause gingival necrosis and erosion in nonhuman primates, but not in rats, along with esophageal and lingual epithelial atrophy (Patyna et al. 2008). Pigmentary changes in dogs (including lips and palate), suggestive of abnormal melanosome formation or melanization, were described after dosing of dogs with an inhibitor of platelet aggregation (Walsh and Gough 1989). Increased pigmentation of skin and oral mucosa is reported more frequently in human patients (since most toxicity studies are conducted in albino rats) but also has been described in pigmented rats following subacute treatment with antimalarial agents (Savage et al. 1986). Gingival hyperplasia has been described in rats and dogs (and human patients) associated with calcium channel blockers and phenytoin (Figure 9.5a)

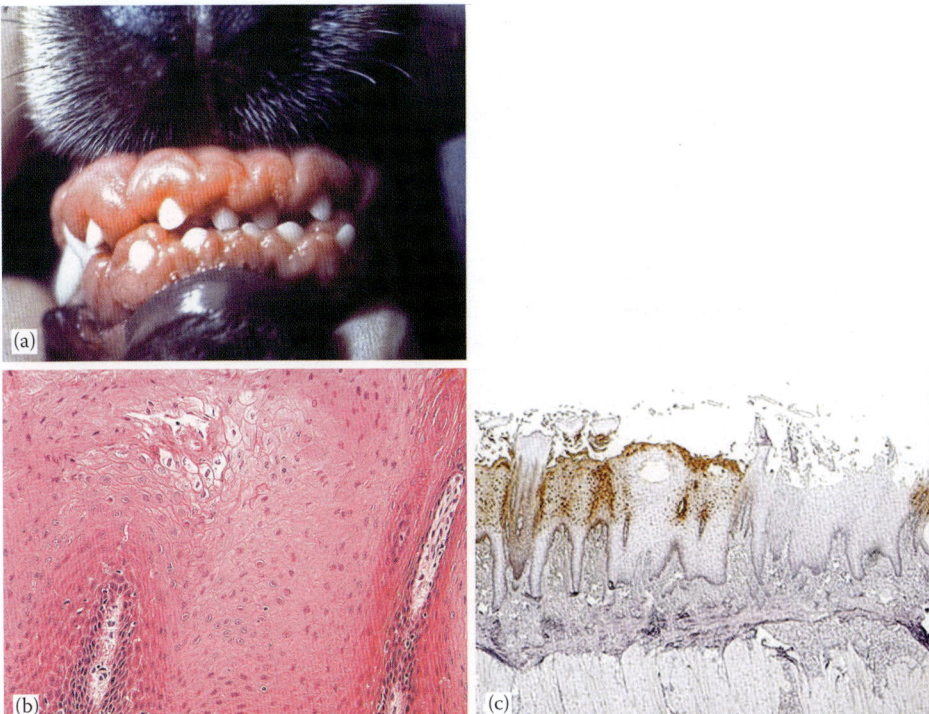

FIGURE 9.5   (a) Dog, gingiva, gross. The coalescing nodular gingival hyperplasia effaces the teeth. (b) Macaque, tongue, HE stain. Leukoplakia-like lesion in an immunosuppressed cynomolgus monkey is characterized by ballooning degeneration and intranuclear inclusions of the epithelium. (c) Macaque, tongue, IHC for sVCA of EBV that cross-reacts with monkey lymphocryptovirus. Same samples as those in (b). Immunoreactivity in the epithelium indicates areas of viral infection.

(Nyska et al. 1990). These lesions in humans and in animals are composed of epithelial proliferations forming rete pegs and being supported by proliferative fibrovascular stroma. Fibroepithelial gingival proliferation was also described in several species, including humans, following cyclosporin A treatment (Cetinkaya et al. 2006).

Orderly proliferation of oral mucosal epithelium being supported with thin fibrovascular stalks occurs in dogs infected with canine oral papilloma virus. Generalized cutaneous involvement as an extension of the oral involvement may occur in immunosuppressed animals (Sundberg et al. 1998).

In addition to changes described above for the oral mucosa in general, a spectrum of changes occurs specifically in the tongue. Mineralization of the tongue muscle occurs in mouse strains that have a high incidence of myocardial mineralization such as the DBA strain. Another local manifestation of generalized disease occurs in amyloidosis involving the tongue vasculature. The tongue is a common site of candidiasis of immunocompromised nonhuman primates. A finding less commonly seen following administration of immunosuppressive agents is the activation of a lymphocryptoviral (LCV) lytic infection, resulting in changes similar to those seen in models of simian acquired immunodeficiency syndrome (SAIDS) and human patients with hairy cell leukoplakia (Baskin et al. 1995; Kutok et al. 2004; Kutok and Wang 2006). The lesion is often not appreciated grossly and identified only microscopically. The tongue epithelium is thickened and hyperkeratotic, and in keeping with a viral infection, cells undergo ballooning degeneration and contain intranuclear inclusions (Figure 9.5b and c). Ultrastructurally, viral factories are recognized within epithelial cells, and enveloped viral particles are intercellular. The tongue squamous epithelium, among other tissues of the GI tract, and other organs underwent hyperplasia following dosing of rodents and

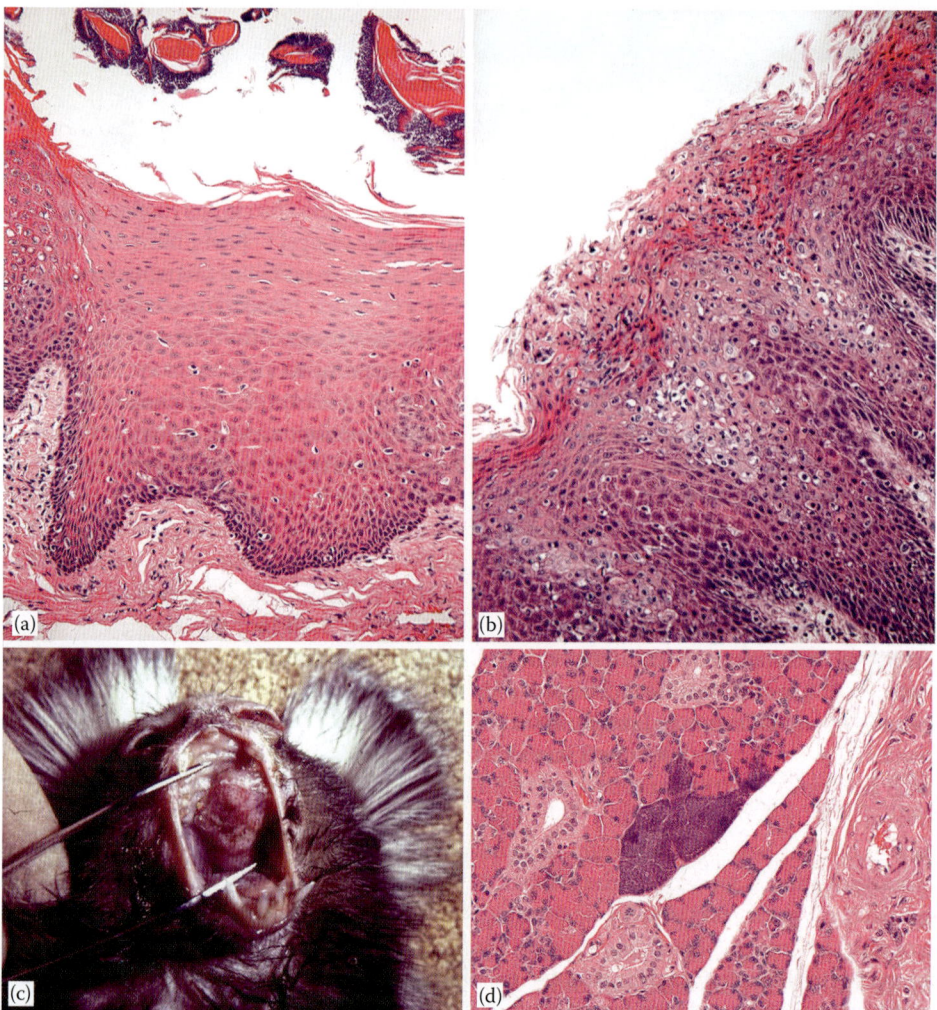

FIGURE 9.6 (a) Macaque, tongue, HE stain. In the control animal, orderly maturation of the keratinized stratified epithelium is present. (b) Macaque, tongue, HE stain. Multifocal epithelial degeneration and necrosis are present following dosing with a xenobiotic for 2 weeks. (c) Marmoset, palate, gross. A space-occupying, mottled mass is present asymmetrically. It was diagnosed histologically as a squamous cell carcinoma. (d) Rat, parotid salivary gland, HE stain. A basophilic hypertrophic focus is composed of larger-than-normal deeply basophilic cells whose apical cytoplasm is finely vacuolated.

monkeys with EGF (Reindel et al. 1996). Inflammation and myositis were noted in a ventral subepithelial distribution in the tongue following dosing with a ricin A-chain immunotoxin. The specific distribution was considered to be due to either local macrophages or mannose receptor disposition (Westwood et al. 1996). Disruption of normal epithelial keratinization and single cell necrosis was produced by a xenobiotic in the tongue and esophagus of nonhuman primates (Figure 9.6a and b).

9.4.1.1 Proliferative Changes of Oral Cavity and Tongue

9.4.1.1.1 Hyperplasia, Squamous Cell

Squamous cell hyperplasia is composed of focal or multifocal well-differentiated squamous cells with appropriate orderly maturation with or without keratinization. The lesion is well circumscribed, and finger-like projections are supported by a nonbranching fibrovascular stroma.

9.4.1.1.2 Papilloma, Squamous

Squamous papillomas are well-circumscribed single or multiple finger-like projections supported by branching fibrovascular stroma containing nests of epithelial cells due to invaginations, but no real invasion. The epithelium is less differentiated and may be traumatized and infiltrated by inflammatory cells.

9.4.1.1.3 Carcinoma, Squamous

The pleomorphic epithelial cells form irregular cords, nests, or clusters and invade the underlying stroma (Figure 9.6c). Dyskeratosis and keratin pearls may be present.

9.4.1.1.4 Sarcoma

A spontaneous angiosarcoma with lung metastasis was reported in the tongue of a young Wistar rat. The irregularly shaped vascular spaces were lined by pleomorphic endothelial cells that were positive for FVIIIRA and vimentin (Pace et al. 2010).

9.4.2 SALIVARY GLANDS

Congenital lesions of the salivary glands are rare, but an ectopic parotid gland within the sublingual salivary gland has been recognized by the presence of small mucinous acini (Neuenschwander and Elwell 1990). Although rodents used for toxicological testing are bred and maintained in a highly controlled environment and undergo rigorous health screening in order to qualify as specific pathogen free (SPF), occasionally vendors report the occurrence of classical infectious diseases that may endanger colonies in institutional vivaria. One of these infections that may affect salivary glands is the highly contagious infection with the sialodacryoadenitis virus, a corona virus rendering animals unsuitable for toxicity studies. In acute infections, salivary (especially parotid), lacrimal, and Harderian glands are edematous, necrotic, and infiltrated with neutrophils (Jones et al. 1997; Percy et al. 1989). In a study of disease progression, early changes were recognized primarily in the parotid and submandibular salivary glands, whereas in subchronic disease, Harderian glands and exorbital salivary glands were more frequently affected (Percy et al. 1989). In an enzootic outbreak, it was noted that spontaneously hypertensive rats had a more severe involvement and a lower serological response to the virus than seen in Sprague–Dawley rats (Carthew and Slinger 1981). Bacterial infections, including abscess formation, are common incidental findings in chronic mouse studies. Sialolithiasis can occur sporadically both in rodents and large animals and is typically found incidentally. Salivary mucocele may develop secondary to obstruction by calculi. Bacterial infection and/or desquamated epithelial cells form the nidus for the stone formation. The distended ducts may be surrounded by fibrosis and atrophic acini. Certain mouse strains with a tendency for autoimmune disease, such as NZB or BDF1 mice, may develop a spontaneous age-related sialoadenitis resembling Sjogren's syndrome (Hayashi et al. 1988). Salivary glands are infiltrated with lymphocytes effacing the glandular architecture. Affected animals had circulating antibodies against salivary gland ducts, while the majority of infiltrating cells are T lymphocytes. Among toxicologic changes of the salivary glands, atrophy is relatively often encountered due to marked reduction of food consumption. In contrast, theophylline, a phosphodiesterase (PDE) inhibitor used for asthma and emphysema, caused an increase in the basophilic basal portion of acinar cells and enlargement of nuclei. These morphological changes were associated with changes in gene expression of secretory proteins, PDE3A, and cyclic AMP. It was assumed that PDE inhibition resulted in an increase in cyclic AMP, which in turn regulated the expression of secretory protein genes (Greaves 2012). Systemic exposure to isoproterenol, a β adrenergic agonist, also caused glandular enlargement, increased DNA, and protein synthesis (Ten Hagen et al. 2002). In contrast, β adrenergic antagonists resulted in atrophy characterized by decreased secretory granules, decreased cellular height, and acinar vacuolation (Gopinath et al. 1987). The effect of ionizing radiation was investigated on all three types of salivary glands. The parotid was the most sensitive and had low regenerative capacity following even mild damage (Denny et al. 1997). In the mouse, castration of males caused loss of duct granulation in the submandibular salivary gland, whereas the administration of testosterone to females resulted in duct morphology similar to those of males (Gopinath et al. 1987).

Basophilic hypertrophic foci of salivary glands in mice and rats are composed of enlarged acinar cells that are typically intensely basophilic and contain a decreased amount of cytoplasmic granules (Figure 9.6d) (Chiu and Chen 1986). The incidence of this spontaneous lesion increases with aging.

9.4.2.1 Proliferative Changes of Salivary Glands

Spontaneous proliferative changes (other than basophilic foci) are very rare in rodents. Salivary gland neoplasms were induced by the infection of neonatal mice with polyoma virus. The most common morphology was a mixed type of tumor containing both mesenchymal and epithelial cells. Additionally, poorly differentiated epithelial and scirrhous forms were described (Botts et al. 1999).

9.4.2.1.1 Hyperplasia

Multifocal hyperplasia of the intercalated ducts was associated with a novel steroid treatment of Wistar rats (de Rijk et al. 2003). Microcystic ducts were surrounded by numerous myoepithelial cells. The epithelial cells were positive for progesterone receptors and negative for estrogen receptors. Some features of these hyperplastic changes (including major cell type, morphology, and progesterone receptor positivity) were compared to the adenoid cystic–type salivary gland tumor in humans.

9.4.2.1.2 Adenoma

Adenomas may be recognized grossly due to color changes. Microscopically, adenomas are well demarcated with or without compression and capsule; they are generally composed of cells that are either larger or smaller than normal, that are arranged in an acinar or papillary pattern, and that contain secretory granules. The nuclei are hyperchromatic and basally located; mitotic figures are rare. Differential diagnosis includes regenerative hyperplasia characterized by chronic inflammation/fibroplasia, cytoplasmic basophilia, and acinar and ductal proliferation.

9.4.2.1.3 Adenocarcinoma

Adenocarcinoma (Figure 9.7a) may be apparent grossly either due to differences in color from the normal glandular tissue or due to causing enlargement or nodularity of the gland. In rats, spontaneous tumors of the salivary glands are rare and have been reported mostly to be epithelial in origin with morphology of adenocarcinoma, papillary cystadenocarcinoma, or pleomorphic adenoma. Recently, a poorly differentiated carcinoma was reported with vimentin immunoreactivity that was negative for smooth muscle–specific actin, and most cells were also positive for keratin. Neoplastic cells ultrastructurally contained desmosome-like structures suggestive of an acinar or ductal origin (Nishikawa et al. 2010).

Adenocarcinomas originate from ductal and acinar epithelium and have a varying growth pattern, which may range from whorls and spindle pattern to solid, papillary, or mixed morphologies. The neoplastic cells are large, polyhedral epithelial cells with high nuclear-to-cytoplasmic ratio or are smaller than normal, exhibiting cellular atypia and numerous mitotic figures. They may be locally invasive or may have distant metastasis.

9.4.2.1.4 Squamous Cell Carcinoma

The origin of squamous cell carcinomas involving the salivary glands is debated: they may be in Zymbal's gland instead. Zymbal's glands are sebaceous glands of the rodent's auditory canal and are located near salivary glands. Also, Zymbal's gland tumors are more common than salivary gland tumors. Hence, care must be taken when squamous cell carcinomas are diagnosed as primary salivary gland tumors. The composition of squamous cell tumors is the same as those found elsewhere. Microscopically, the morphology varies from well-differentiated squamous epithelium to anaplastic spindle cells.

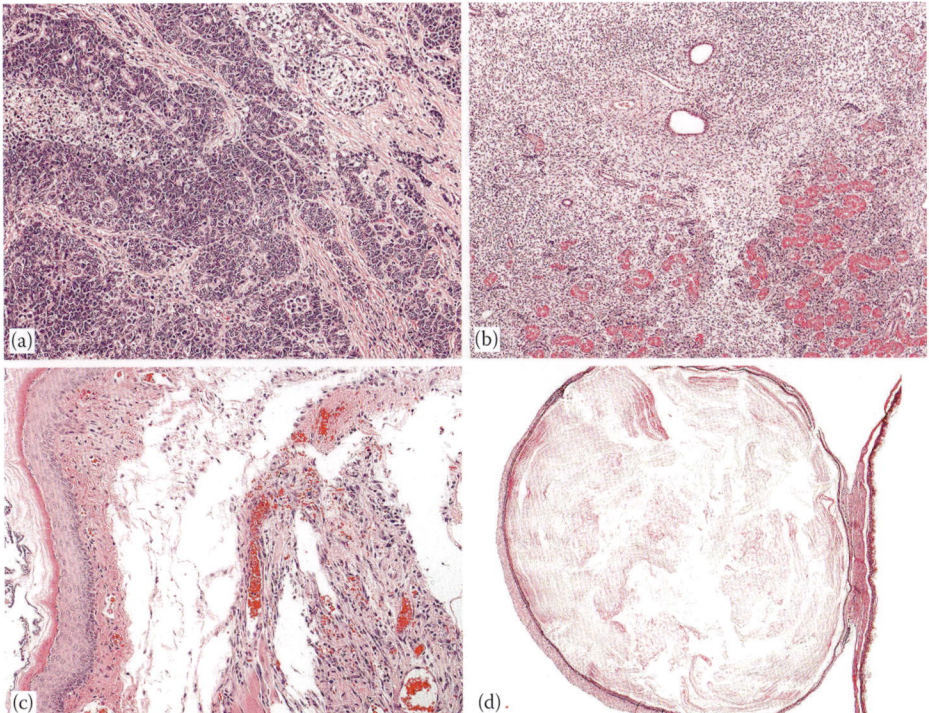

FIGURE 9.7 (a) Rat salivary gland, HE stain. Adenocarcinoma. Irregularly shaped lobules composed of poorly differentiated cells are separated with a fibrovascular stroma. (b) Rat salivary gland, HE stain. Schwannoma. Normal tissue has been replaced and effaced by a dense network of swirling, pale spindloid cells with two cystic spaces in the center. (c) Rat, esophagus, HE stain. Transmural myodegeneration, inflammation, and hemorrhage, secondary to gavage trauma. (d) Mouse, nonglandular stomach, HE stain. Cyst filled with keratin just below the mucosa.

9.4.2.1.5 Myoepithelioma

Originating from myoepithelial cells of the salivary glands, the unencapsulated myoepithelioma extends into neighboring tissues and is composed of spindle cells without acinar or ductal morphology. The pleomorphic cells resemble spindle or epithelial cells and may have multiple necrotic foci. The neoplasm may be locally invasive or may have distant metastases in the lung. In contrast to polyoma-induced tumors, there is no evidence of mononuclear cellular infiltrates. Myoepitheliomas stain positively by immunohistochemical methods for actin and cytokeratin.

9.4.2.1.6 Tumor, Mixed, Benign

Mixed benign tumors originate from glandular epithelium and myoepithelial mesenchymal components of salivary glands and lack pleomorphism.

9.4.2.1.7 Tumor, Mixed Malignant

These neoplasms originate from glandular epithelial and myoepithelial cells exhibiting cellular pleomorphism with features of both sarcoma and carcinoma.

9.4.2.1.8 Mesenchymal Tumors, Benign and Malignant

Although mesenchymal tumors are rare both in mice and rats (Figure 9.7b), they were more common than epithelial tumors in the NTP database for B6C3F1 mice. These mesenchymal tumors included hemangioma and hemangiosarcoma, fibrosarcoma, leiomyoma, and malignant schwannoma (Botts et al. 1999).

9.4.3 ESOPHAGUS

Esophageal mucosal changes and/or muscular injury due to gavage errors have been decreasing in frequency in recent years with the introduction of soft gavage needles and increased awareness of correct animal handling. When present, muscle degeneration/regeneration may be focal or may extend along much of the circumference of the cross-sectional esophageal area examined. Epithelial damage may be erosion when the mucosal deficit is superficial or may be ulcer/perforation when the deficit extends into the lamina propria or muscularis (Figure 9.7c). These lesions are typically associated with a mixed cellular infiltrate containing a varying number of neutrophils. Undetected esophageal mucosal damage may present at the end of a study with stricture, obstruction of the lumen due to fibroplasias, and scar formation. Although not associated with morphological changes in the esophagus, but rather in the nasal cavity and lung, toxicologic pathologists should be aware of gavage-related reflux in rats (Damsch et al. 2011). Important factors in the pathogenesis of reflux included viscous and/or irritant test article, increased volume/contents of stomach, increased gastric acid secretion, and delayed gastric emptying for a variety of reasons.

Disturbance of esophageal motility indicated by megaloesophagus may be due to congenital defects of innervation or may be secondary to acquired neuropathy because of acrylamide or organophosphate toxicity (Betton 1998). The esophagus may also be a site of candidiasis in immunosuppressed animals. Zinc and vitamin A are important for the maintenance for appropriate thickness of layers of the esophageal squamous epithelium. Both zinc and vitamin A deficiencies cause hyperkeratosis, and zinc deficiency also causes esophageal epithelial thickening. If zinc levels are marginal, rats become more sensitive to esophageal carcinogens, and this effect is further increased by alcohol (Brown and Hardisty 1990).

9.4.3.1 Proliferative Changes of Esophagus

Recently, epithelial hyperplasia and hyperkeratosis were described in the esophagus and other tissues composed of squamous epithelial cells of rodents and dogs after being treated with RAF inhibitors independent of their scaffolds since different chemotypes produced these changes (Carnahan et al. 2010; John-Baptiste et al. 2010; Wisler et al. 2011). Molecular investigations indicated that a single dose of B-RAF inhibitors could alter the homeostasis of the MAPK pathway in nonmutant B-RAF cells, resulting in cell proliferation.

Neoplastic changes of the esophagus are not common in toxicity studies in a pharmaceutical setting. Rats may develop epithelial proliferations ranging from hyperplasia and hyperkeratosis through papilloma to carcinoma after exposure to nitrosoaniline or nitrosourea compounds. In a comparative study with the rat esophageal carcinogen N-nitrosomethylbenzylamine (NBZA) probing the role of microsomal metabolism from several tissues, it was found that NBZA had to be metabolized by microsomal activation in order to produce toxicity. Although both rat hepatocytes and esophageal epithelium could metabolize NBZA, only the esophagus was damaged when rats were dosed, suggesting that additional factors were needed for lesion development (Mehta et al. 1984).

9.4.3.1.1 Hyperplasia, Squamous

The stratified squamous epithelium may be thickened focally or diffusely. Papillomatous projections may overlie the convoluted lamina propria, but there is no single fibrovascular core. The growth pattern is either exophytic or endophytic; when endophytic, the muscularis may be replaced in a keratoacanthomatous pattern. Epithelial cells may exhibit parakeratosis or hyperkeratosis.

9.4.3.1.2 Papilloma, Squamous

Most commonly squamous cell papillomas are pedunculated masses with branched stalks (exophytic) or less frequently appear as endophytic growths. The fibrovascular supportive stroma is covered by well-differentiated epithelial cells that may have acanthosis with normal maturation. Mitotic figures are rare, and an inflammatory reaction may be present. Papillomas can be differentiated from hyperplasia by the more complex branching morphology.

9.4.3.1.3 Carcinoma, Squamous

This lesion may have an exophytic or endophytic growth pattern, and in case a carcinoma arises within a papilloma, the stalk is invaded. Most of the carcinomas are composed of relatively well-differentiated large cells; however, anaplastic carcinomas may have areas of basal cell morphology. Mitotic figures are common, and local invasion may occur.

9.4.4 STOMACH

The nonglandular and glandular stomach will be treated as if they were two organs because of their different structures and often differing pathogenesis of lesions.

9.4.4.1 Nonglandular Stomach

Keratin cysts are common findings below the mucosa of the nonglandular stomach (Figure 9.7d). Erosion is defined as a partial necrosis or loss of the stratified squamous epithelium, usually associated with irritant suspensions or solutions administered orally. It may also be accompanied by intra-epithelial vesicle formation, although this can also be observed in the thicker epithelium covering the limiting ridge. Full-thickness necrosis and loss of epithelium (through the muscularis mucosa) lead to focal or multifocal ulceration. Macroscopically, the regenerative hyperplasia of the surrounding epithelium leads to a volcano-shaped macroscopic appearance (Figure 9.8a).

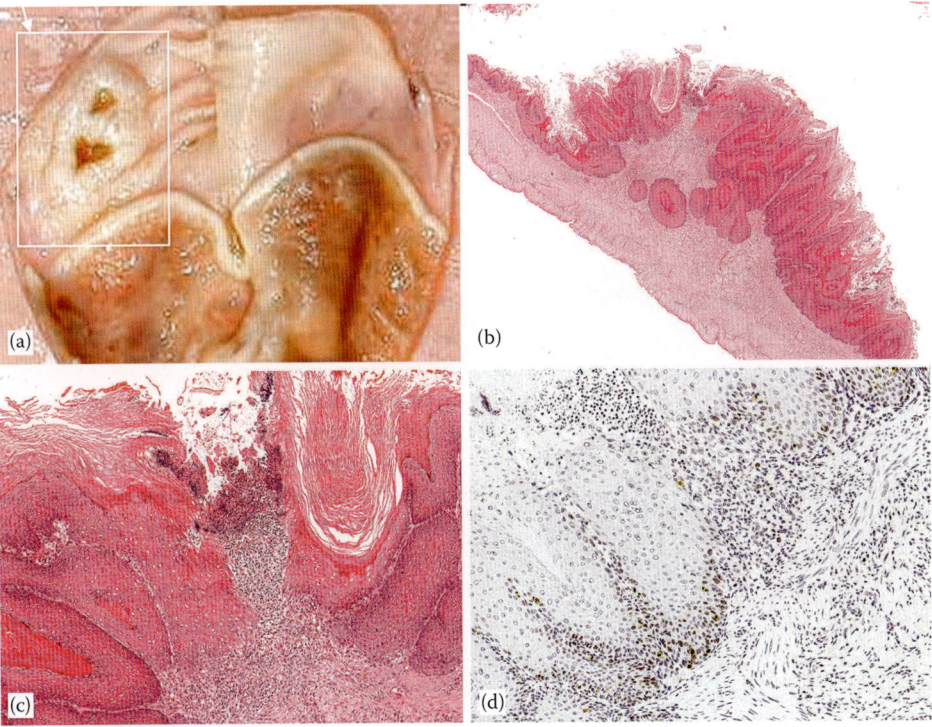

FIGURE 9.8 (a) Rat, nonglandular stomach, gross. Ulcers in nonglandular stomach are surrounded by thickened reactive hyperplastic epithelium. (b) Rat, nonglandular stomach, HE stain. Histological appearance of area marked with rectangle in (a). The ulcer is surrounded by reactive hyperplasia, hyperkeratosis, convoluted germinal epithelium with penetration into submucosa, and central inflammatory cell infiltration. (c) Rat, nonglandular stomach, HE stain. Higher-power view of (b) illustrating mitoses in germinal layer and disruption of muscularis mucosa. (d) Rat, nonglandular stomach IHC for Ki67. Same lesion as in (a) through (c). Immunoreactivity is present in many cells in area of reactive hyperplasia adjacent to ulcer.

Inflammation may be acute, chronic, or granulomatous. The lamina propria of the gastric mucosa and the submucosa of control animals contain a low degree of inflammatory cell infiltration. In rodents, this is mainly along the limiting ridge. With irritants or ulcerogenic compounds, damage to the simple stratified squamous epithelium of the nonglandular stomach typically induces an inflammatory reaction with edema, hyperemia, and inflammatory cell infiltration. Traumatic injury by long dosing needles may also occur. Anti-inflammatory agents may suppress inflammatory responses.

Hyperkeratosis and parakeratosis with increased thickness of keratinized squamous epithelial cell layers can be seen in response to irritants, either directly or as a reactive hyperplasia around ulcers (Figure 9.8b). The basal germinal epithelium is typically folded in appearance and may penetrate the muscularis mucosa but is still well polarized to differentiate through to keratinized squames (Figure 9.8c). The germinal layer shows increased cell proliferation and Ki67 staining (Figure 9.8d). Squames can also accumulate on the surface when food consumption is reduced because of general toxicity or unpalatability of formulated diet. Some compounds induce foci or plaques of hyperplastic squamous epithelium where squamous epithelial cells do not mature fully and retain nuclei to form parakeratosis (Figure 9.9a and b) (Betton and Salmon 1984). With some statins, HMGCoa accumulates within hyperplastic keratinocytes (Singer et al. 1991).

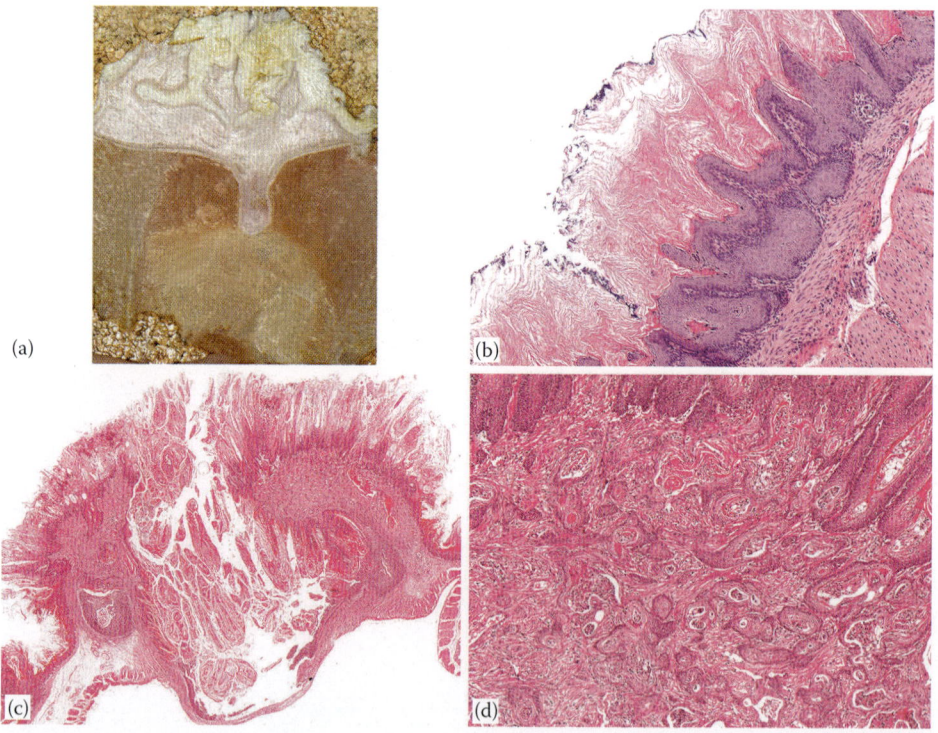

FIGURE 9.9   (a) Rat, nonglandular stomach, gross. Contrast gross appearance of squamous epithelial hyperplasia with well-demarcated plaques of hyperkeratotic epithelium with that of Figure 9.8a containing crater-like regions of ulcer. (b) Rat, nonglandular stomach, HE stain. Squamous epithelial hyperplasia and parakeratosis from case in (a). (c) Rat, nonglandular stomach, HE stain. Squamous cell carcinoma arising in area of squamous cell hyperplasia. Invasion through muscularis mucosa is disorganized, and cells are not keratinized and have lost polarity. (d) Rat, nonglandular stomach, HE stain. Squamous cell carcinoma from (c). Multiple nests and "pearls" of malignant keratinized epithelium replace normal submucosa.

In parakeratosis, there is retention of nuclei as seen with zinc deficiency or in association with squamous epithelial hyperplasia (Figure 9.9b).

9.4.4.1.1 Proliferative Changes of Nonglandular Stomach

9.4.4.1.1.1 Hyperplasia—Simple, Diffuse, Focal
The hyperplasia at the border of the nonglandular (fore) stomach and glandular stomach (limiting ridge) is normal. Hyperkeratosis or parakeratosis alone should be distinguished from hyperplasia. Acanthosis is a synonym for hyperplasia of the squamous cell epithelium of the skin and should not be used in this organ. Focal hyperplasia may result from gavage procedures. Areas of hyperplasia of the germinal layer are often convoluted and may "invade" the muscularis mucosa, but this is reversible (Betton and Salmon 1984; Masui et al. 1987). Unlike reactive hyperplasia, no erosion, ulceration, or inflammation is present.

9.4.4.1.1.2 Reactive Hyperplasia
This is usually present around the margin of pinpoint foci of erosion and ulceration. The center of the lesion shows necrosis and acute inflammatory cell infiltration (except after NSAID administration with anti-inflammatory action). Edema and/or congestion of lamina propria and intra-epithelial vesicle formation may be present. If hyperplasia is observed without an ulcer in the section but inflammatory responses are present, additional sectioning will usually reveal the cause as being due to irritants causing erosion or ulceration.

9.4.4.1.1.3 Papilloma—Exophytic, Endophytic
Benign tumors are usually exophytic squamous papillomas with a single or branched connective tissue stalk or multiple papillae and may arise within the area of epithelial hyperplasia (Fukushima and Ito 1985). The epithelium may be hyperkeratotic or parakeratotic but is well differentiated. There should be no invasion of the stalk or muscularis mucosa, although some displacement of the muscularis may occur. In the endophytic subtype, downgrowth resembling an acanthoma displaces the muscularis mucosa.

9.4.4.1.1.4 Squamous Cell Carcinoma
Squamous cell carcinomas display epithelial nests (with or without keratinized cysts) or cords showing true invasion of the submucosa, often arising in the base of papillomas (Figure 9.9c and d). The poorly differentiated type is arranged as solid sheets or as strands infiltrating the submucosa or adjacent tissue. Keratinization may be difficult to detect. Tumors may metastasize to the abdominal cavity, regional lymph nodes, or the lung.

This neoplasm is a relatively frequent finding in carcinogenicity studies with irritants, promoters, and genotoxins (Brown and Hardisty 1990; Frantz et al. 1991; Fukushima and Ito 1985; Greaves 2012; Maekawa 1994; Stinson and Kovatch 1990; Takahashi and Hasegawa 1990; Chandra et al. 2010). Examples of genotoxins targeting the nonglandular stomach are polycyclic aromatic hydrocarbons (BP, MCA, DMBA), N-nitroso compounds (DEN, MNNG, MNU, 4-NQA), urethane, and dibenzocarbazole. Metabolic activation of genotoxins to generate proximate carcinogens in the squamous epithelium can be via cytochrome P450 activity. Nonglandular stomach and esophageal P450 isozymes differ, explaining the targeting of the site of carcinogenesis within the nitrosamine family. Also, gastric carcinogens such as MNNG target the nonglandular stomach more when administered by gavage and the glandular stomach more when delivered in drinking water, and carcinogenicity can be modified by coadministration of salt, bile acids, aspirin, and butylated hydroxyanisole (BHA) (Newberne et al. 1986). Chemically depleting sulfhydryl groups in the nonglandular stomach can progress through ulceration, from hyperplasia to neoplasia (Frederick et al. 1990).

Brca1-mutated mice show increased sensitivity to genotoxic carcinogenesis of the nonglandular stomach with increased oxidative stress and loss of *p53* (Cao et al. 2007).

Nongenotoxins acting as nonglandular stomach carcinogens include citrus oils, limonene, aristolochic acid, BHA antioxidant, ascorbic acid, and lipophilic statins. Because there is no direct counterpart of the nonglandular stomach in the human, changes there induced by nongenotoxins generally considered not to be a risk for man.

9.4.4.2 Glandular Stomach

The glandular stomach commences at the esophageal cardia located on the lesser curvature. In rodents, this is situated in a distinct notch on the limiting ridge at the margins of the nonglandular stomach. Examination of the gastric mucosa after opening along the greater curvature is strongly recommended as mucosal lesions may be pinpoint in size and not reliably detected after sectioning.

Inflammation can be acute, chronic, or granulomatous. The lamina propria of the gastric mucosa and the submucosa of control animals contain a moderate degree of inflammatory cell infiltration. In rodents, this can have a significant eosinophil content. In dogs and nonhuman primates, inflammatory infiltrates are primarily composed of mononuclear cells. In the cardiac and antral regions, these may be slight to moderate in severity, and lymphoid follicles with active germinal centers may be present, indicative of enzootic bacterial infection, for example, *Helicobacter* spp. (Figure 9.10a and b). Unlike *Helicobacter pylori,* the human pathogen in man, a number of *Helicobacter* spp including, *Helicobacter felis, H. bizzozeroni* and *H. salomonsis* are not considered pathogenic and may colonize clinically normal dogs (Baele et al. 2004; Jalava et al. 1998; Van den Bulck et al. 2005), unlike *H. pylori*, the main human pathogen. Dogs experimentally infected with *H. pylori* show gastritis, erosions, and lymphoid follicle formation (Rossi et al. 1999). The microbiological status of treated versus control dogs can be assessed using special stains on tissue, polymerase chain reaction (PCR), or *Helicobacter* [13C] urea breath tests (Cornetta et al. 1998). *H. pylori* induces gastritis, intestinal metaplasia, and ulcer formation in Mongolian gerbils (Ikeno et al.

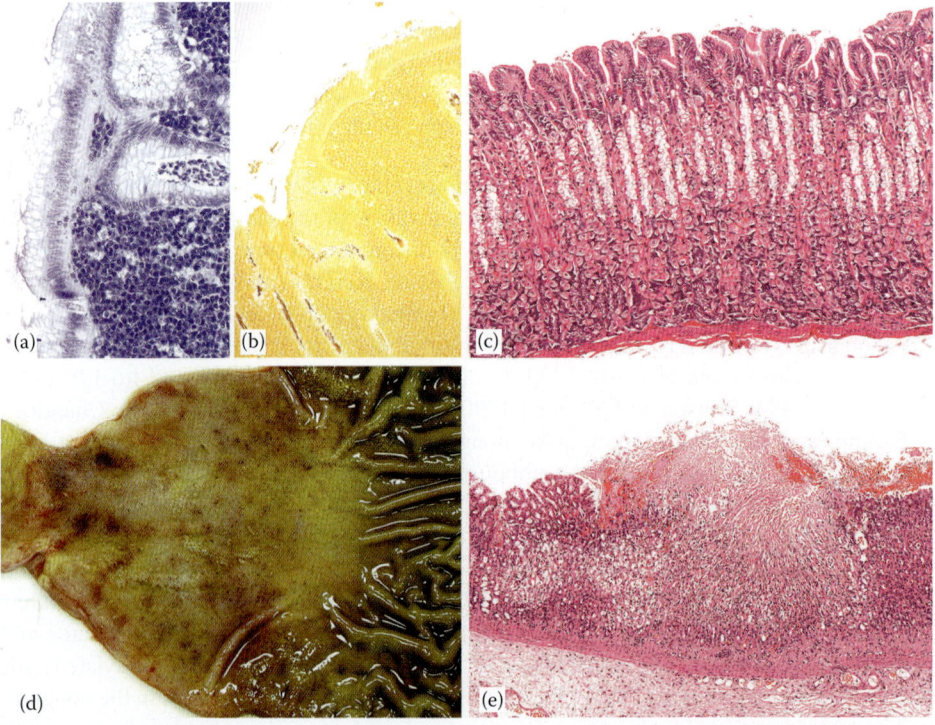

FIGURE 9.10 (a) Macaque, stomach, Giemsa stain. *H. pylori* infection demonstrated as delicate S-shaped bacteria admixed with inflammatory cells in gland. The lamina propria is expanded by a mononuclear cellular infiltrate. (b) Macaque, stomach, Steiner's stain. Same stomach as in (a). Silver stain demonstrates a large number of bacteria in gastric glands. (c) Rat, stomach, HE stain. Mucous neck cell hypertrophy/hyperplasia is present after prostaglandin E agonist administration for 7 days. Foveolar cell region is also expanded. (d) Dog, stomach, gross. The antrum and pylorus show multiple punctate red-brown erosions. (e) Rat, stomach, HE stain. The fundic mucosal erosion has a central area of necrosis, hemorrhage, and inflammation with viable cells in base and at margins.

1999). Experimental infection of pigs with *H. pylori* produces a lymphocytic gastritis (Poutahidis et al. 2001) similar to the human disease. The inflammation and cell death caused by *Helicobacter* are believed to be caused by oxygen free radical formation leading to adenocarcinoma in a subset of humans (Konturek et al. 2006).

Mucous neck cell hypertrophy represents an adaptive response to increase mucosal cytoprotection, which depends on the secretion of an unstirred mucous layer by foveolar cells and on mucus secretion by mucous neck cells in the oxyntic glands (Hanby et al. 1999). Expansion of the mucous neck cell region is seen after administration of a variety of irritants, exposure to prostaglandins (Figure 9.10c), and interferon gamma (Kang et al. 2005).

Erosion and ulceration of the gastric mucosa can result from chemical, pH, mechanical, hypoxia, hypovolemia, or vasoconstriction challenges. The unstirred layer of the gastric mucus provides a pH gradient between the acidic lumen and bicarbonate secreting surface cells. In oral toxicology studies, direct exposure, especially to gavage formulations, activates uptake into acidic compartments for compounds with low pKas. This direct exposure as well as systemic plasma exposure can lead to gastric mucosal erosion or ulceration. Macroscopically, erosions are more common in the antral mucosa and pylorus, commencing as brown pinhead foci (Figure 9.10d). Histologically, erosions show focal necrosis and an inflammatory cell infiltrate, usually centered above an arteriole (Figure 9.10e). Cytoprotection requires prostaglandins and mucosal blood flow, and NSAIDs block prostacyclin production required to maintain local perfusion. Inhibitors of the cyclooxygenase (COX-1) enzyme prevent eicosanoid synthesis, reducing production of prostaglandins, prostacyclins, and thromboxanes. 5-Lipoxygenase inhibitors and pranlukast, a leukotriene antagonist, can negate NSAID-induced ulceration (Nakamori et al. 2010). The hypergastrinemia seen after antisecretory drug treatment upregulated COX-2, and prostaglandin E_2 conferred cytoprotection against ethanol-induced gastric injury (Tsuji et al. 2002). Trefoil factor family 2 (TFF2) produced by mucous neck cells is also cytoprotective against NSAID-induced ulceration in mice (Farrell et al. 2002).

Hypovolemia and shock can exacerbate erosion and ulceration. Gastric mucus is produced by foveolar and surface cells of fundic pits (Class II mucins), cardiac glands (mixed mucins), and mucous neck cells of fundus and antral glands (Class III mucins).

Erosion affects less than full thickness of mucosa, commencing as necrosis or fluid accumulation. Hemorrhage from exposed capillaries of the lamina propria can result in red cell lysis, and hemoglobin changed to acid hematin conferring brown specks on the mucosal surface (Figure 9.10d).

Ulceration penetrates the mucosal basement membrane, exposes submucosal connective tissue, and typically attracts an inflammatory cell infiltration. Because full-thickness destruction of the mucosal epithelial population has taken place, repair must begin from the margins. Arterial bleeding or perforation of the wall causes additional complications as the ulcer erodes through the submucosa, muscularis externa, and serosal surface, progressing to peritonitis. Peptic ulcers are typically located in the antrum or proximal duodenum and can be stress related or, in humans, due to gastrinomas in Zollinger–Ellison syndrome, causing hypersecretion of gastric acid.

Rats show marked reactive hyperplasia with basophilic "dysplastic" glands, yet progression to adenocarcinoma is rare. Hyperplastic antral glands often penetrate the muscularis mucosa; this process is not a criterion for malignancy. Chronic "adenomatous" submucosal cysts show foveolar differentiation and have been described as *gastritis cystica profunda* when ulcers undergoing repair recruit progenitor cells into the regenerating glands, and glands trapped below the muscularis mucosa differentiate into cystic or foveolar glandular structures (Figure 9.11a).

EGF (saliva, Brunner's glands), sonic hedgehog (parietal cells), and gastrin (antral G cells) are potent trophic factors involved in the growth and repair of the gastric mucosa.

Amyloidosis is the deposition of amyloid in a wide range of organs and is a feature of aging mice of a number of strains such as C57Bl. The amyloid has been shown to comprise Type A AApoAII fibrils (Korenaga et al. 2004) (Figure 9.11b).

Arteritis as a result of vascular injury can present in many organs, depending on species and inducing agent. Lesions in gastric vessels, usually in small- to medium-sized arteries, can be

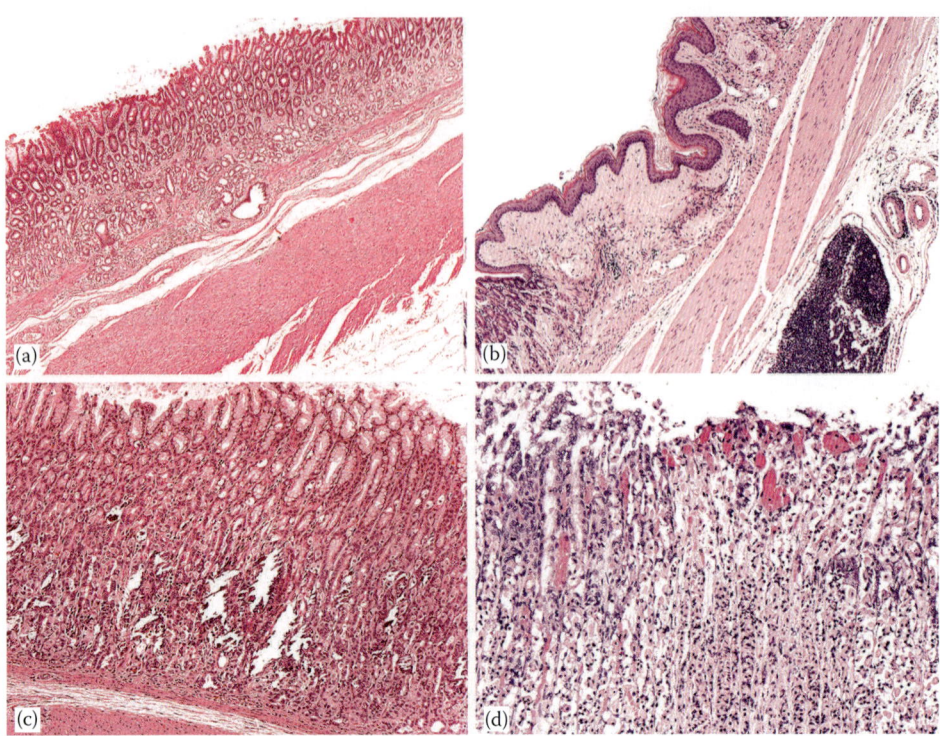

FIGURE 9.11   (a) Rat, stomach, HE stain. Regenerative hyperplasia of antral glandular epithelium post-ulceration. Glandular structures have protruded through muscularis mucosa and are forming a cystic foveolar lined diverticulum ("gastritis cystica profunda"). (b) Mouse, stomach, HE stain. Amyloidosis in the nonglandular region causes focal expansion of the lamina propria. (c) Rat, stomach, HE stain. Metastatic calcification of fundic mucosa post-MEK inhibitor related to calcium phosphate deposition. Von Kossa was positive. (d) Rat, stomach, HE stain. Uremic gastropathy characterized by mineralization, congestion, and necrosis.

observed in rodents and nonrodents and range from acute necrotizing lesions in canine necrotizing vasculitis (Beagle pain syndrome) to rat mesenteric arteritis.

Mineralization can be present in both the mucosa and muscle layers of the stomach. Metastatic mineralization of many organs takes place when calcium phosphate homeostasis is disrupted, causing calcium hydrogen phosphate deposition in tissues such as the gastric mucosa (Figure 9.11c and d) and uremic gastropathy also affecting the muscularis externa and other sites. This is commonly observed in aging male rats as part of the chronic progressing nephropathy syndrome where failure to excrete phosphate results in saturation of $calcium^3 \times phosphate^2$ in the blood, exceeding solubility limits and causing precipitation in blood vessels and tissues. It is also seen after short-term treatment with gadolinium (III) (Rees et al. 1997), inhibitors of the FGFR/MEK/ERK pathway (Brown et al. 2005), or a range of nephrotoxin administrations. In the case of MEK inhibitors, inhibition of FGF23 signaling in the kidney upregulated 1,25 dihydroxy vitamin D synthesis to increase serum phosphate (Diaz et al. 2012).

Parietal cell vacuolation is seen after high-dose administration of antisecretory compounds. Omeprazole is acid-activated to covalently bind to H^+/K^+ ATPase proton pump to suppress gastric acid output to treat peptic ulcer disease and gastro-esophageal reflux disease (GERD). At high toxicological doses, proton pump inhibitors (PPIs) can cause selective parietal cell vacuolation and single cell necrosis. The parietal cell protonophore DMP-777 depletes parietal cells (Nomura et al. 2005; Nozaki et al. 2008).

Eosinophilic chief cells occur as glandular nests in oxyntic glands, are seen in rats more than in mice, and are associated with mucosal hyperplasia and neuroendocrine cell hyperplasia after antisecretory drug treatment (Figure 9.12a). The nature of these eosinophilic cells is the subject of debate, with claims that the eosinophilic granules contain pepsinogen and are chief cells (Frantz et al. 1991), whereas others describe these as a pancreatic metaplasia (Buettner et al. 2004). It is believed to be a metaplasia. In humans, an eosinophilic variant of fundic adenocarcinoma has been reported by Ueyama et al. (2010), but this has not been reported in rodents.

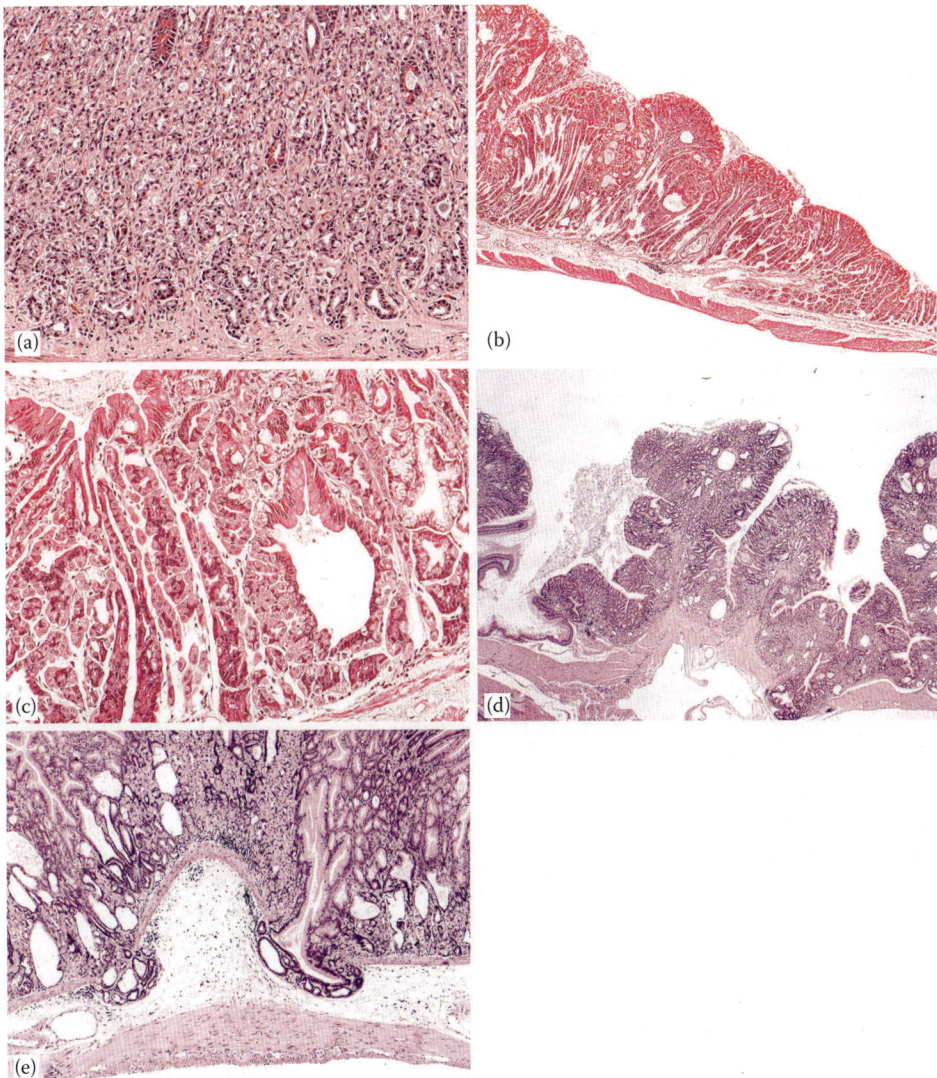

FIGURE 9.12 (a) Rat, stomach, HE stain. Eosinophilic chief cells (top-center) in a 2-year H_2RA-treated rat. Pale neuroendocrine cell hyperplasia is also present. (b) Mouse, stomach, HE stain. There is fundic mucosal hypertrophy following dosing for 2 years with H_2RA. Although oxyntic glands are convoluted and sometimes cystic, differentiation paths are retained. (c) Mouse, stomach, HE stain. Fundic mucosal hypertrophy in a 2-year H_2RA-treated CD1 mouse, higher power of (b). Glands are less well organized, and some mucous neck cell–chief cell intermediate stages are present. (d) Mouse, stomach, HE stain. Spontaneous hypertrophy/ hyperplasia in a CD1 mouse from a carcinogenicity study. The mucosal surface is multinodular, and glands are dilated. (e) Mouse, stomach, HE stain. Spontaneous hypertrophy/hyperplasia in a CD1 mouse from a carcinogenicity study. There is loss of specialized cells in several of the glands that also microherniated into the submucosa. A minimal mononuclear cellular infiltrate is present.

Metaplasia can be of intestinal type, with goblet cells and lysozyme present (rare in animals), or pseudo-pyloric metaplasia of the fundic mucosal, with loss of parietal and chief cells and replacement by pale basal cells containing fine mucus with lesser amounts of lysozyme (Rubio and Befrits 2009). Areas of pseudopyloric metaplasia in nonhuman primates are often colonized with *H. pylori*–like bacteria. This spasmolytic polypeptide/TFF2-expressing pseudopyloric metaplasia (SPEM) involves chief cell–mucous cell transdifferentiation (Nozaki et al. 2008; Goldenring and Nomura 2006). TFF2 KO mice infected with *H. pylori* showed increased antral dysplasia and intra-epithelial neoplasia compared with wild-type mice (Fox et al. 2007). Parietal cell metaplasia progressing to neuroendocrine gastric cancer has been reported in 44-week-old Atp4b-SV40 TAg mice. Hyperplasia progressing to neoplasia is characterized by increased expression of NE markers and loss of a parietal cell marker (Syder et al. 2004).

Gastric mucosal atrophy consists of a reduced mucosal thickness and loss of secretory output (Faller and Kirchner 2005). In chronic atrophic gastritis of man, this can be caused by antiparietal cell antibodies and results in reduced gastric acid secretion with consequent hypergastrinemia (Borch et al. 1986a,b). Intrinsic factor is secreted by parietal cells in man, and in atrophy, the deficit leads to pernicious anemia through B_{12} deficiency. Cytotoxic and cytostatic anticancer agents cause necrosis or apoptosis of gastric glandular epithelial populations, which can progress to mucosal atrophy (Ramiro-Ibáñez et al. 2005). High doses of PPIs causing parietal cell vacuolation and death can cause gastric mucosal atrophy in toxicology studies. Depletion of parietal cells with the compound DMP-777 causes a mucosal atrophy followed by metaplasia (Goldenring and Nomura 2006). Achlorhydria predisposes to bacterial overgrowth, and nitrosation of dietary components in the presence of nitrite has been linked to gastric carcinogenesis in man. Gastric mucosal atrophy is also associated with "wasting" syndrome of marmosets.

9.4.4.2.1 Proliferative Changes of Glandular Stomach

9.4.4.2.1.1 Fundic Mucosal Hyperplasia The oxyntic (fundic) mucosa has deep glands with long cell life span (100+ days) and gastric pits above proliferative zone (life span approximately 6 days). Hypertrophy and hyperplasia can be observed with gastrin, EGF, RegIII beta and gamma (Franic et al. 2004), growth hormone (in pregnancy), and prostaglandin E analogues. Fundic mucosal hypertrophy resembling Menetrier's disease of man is observed post PPI treatment in dogs and mice (Figure 9.12b and c). Depletion of parietal cells with the ionophore DMP-777 leads to gastric mucosal hyperplasia and to spasmolytic polypeptide/TFF2-positive metaplasia through transdifferentiation of chief cells (Nozaki et al. 2008). In histamine-deficient HDC KO mice, maturation of mucous neck cells to chief cells was increased (Nozaki et al. 2009). Mouse fundic mucosal hypertrophy/hyperplasia is a common spontaneous lesion related to strain (especially NMRI, CD-1; Figure 9.12d and e). Control incidences also vary according to diet and housing. The incidence is exacerbated by antisecretory agents, together with neuroendocrine tumors. Increased parietal cells and delayed mucous neck cell to chief cell maturation were observed following lansoprazole treatment (Matsuzaki et al. 2010). It is also seen in TGFalpha transgenic mice (Takagi et al. 1992) and following induction of an autoimmune gastritis by thymectomy in mice.

9.4.4.2.1.2 Neuroendocrine Cells Hyperplasia Neuroendocrine cells (formerly cells of the APUD system) were all thought to originate from the neural crest. However, pancreatic–gastroenteral endocrine cells are able to proliferate from progenitor cells in the proliferative zone of the gastric glands and in intestinal crypts. The enterochromaffin-like (ECL) cell is the main cell type in the rat fundic mucosa, mainly in the basal third. It may be increased focally at the base of the mucosa. Hyperplasia of neuroendocrine cells can be induced by antisecretory drugs (PPIs, histamine H_2 receptor antagonists [H_2RAs]), which raise the serum gastrin level due to an acid-inhibiting effect. Potent long-acting H_2RAs loxtidine (Poynter et al. 1985), SKF93479 (Betton et al. 1988), BL-6341

(Hirth et al. 1988), and ICI162846 (Streett et al. 1988) caused a new type of tumor in the fundic mucosa of rats and (some) mice (Nilsson et al. 1993; Poynter et al. 1986). The new class of anti-secretory PPIs (Shin and Sachs 2008) such as omeprazole (Ekman et al. 1985) and lansoprazole (Tanabe et al. 2003) caused the same type of hyperplasia and tumor. Also, the *Mastomys natalensis* rat has hypergastrinemia, causing fundic mucosal hyperplasia and neuroendocrine hyperplasia and neoplasia (Chiba et al. 1998; Kidd et al. 2007). H^+/K^+ ATPase proton pump KO mice show severe hyperplasia and metaplasia (Judd et al. 2005). These tumors were argyrophilic, NSE and chromogranin A positive by immunohistochemistry (IHC) and therefore of neuroendocrine origin and were positive for histidine decarboxylase (HDC), a marker of histamine-producing ECL cells (Håkanson et al. 1986, 1994). The drug ciprofibrate also produced ECL cell hyperplasia and neoplasia in rats and was subsequently shown to have antisecretory properties (Spencer et al. 1989). Gastric neuro-endocrine tumors in mice unrelated to treatment were reported by Thoolen et al. (2002). The relationship of ECL cell neuroendocrine hyperplasia and neoplasia to the antisecretory mode of action causing hypergastrinemia (Chen et al. 1998) and proliferation has been generally accepted and confirmed in H_2RA and histamine KO mice (Chen et al. 2006; Ogawa et al. 2003). Hypergastrinemia after pharmacological doses of antisecretory agents falls below the degree of hypergastrinemia required to induce neuroendocrine neoplasia in humans (Borch et al 1986a; Håkanson and Sundler 1990; Creutzfeld and Lamberts 1991; IARC 1999). Neuroendocrine "carcinoid" tumor induction is accepted as a nongenotoxic gastrin-mediated class effect of long-acting antisecretory drugs. Potassium-competitive acid blockers are potent antisecretory agents (Simon et al. 2007; Kirchhoff et al. 2006), and KO mouse models show mucosal hyperplasia and metaplasia (Kuwamura et al. 2008; Lee et al. 2000; Roepke et al. 2006, 2010).

9.4.4.2.1.3   Neuroendocrine Tumor: Benign/Malignant (Synonym: Gastric Carcinoid)   Neuro-endocrine ECL cells are situated in the basal part of the oxyntic glands and undergo diffuse then focal hyperplasia following prolonged marked hypergastrinemia. Clusters of cells fill the base of glands (up to 3 glands' diameter). Larger lesions are classified as benign tumors, and when there is invasion into the submucosa (more than isolated cells in lymphatics) taking place, tumors are classified as malignant (Figure 9.13a and b). Benign neuroendocrine tumor cells are clear or pale staining, becoming more eosinophilic as tumors develop. Nuclei are uniform and oval and show few mitoses. Malignant neuroendocrine tumors become more eosinophilic or basophilic with solid or glandular structures and sometimes mitotic figures (Figure 9.13c). The overlying glands may become necrotic and ulcerated. Local invasion progresses to lymphatic and hematogenous metastasis to regional lymph nodes, the liver (Figure 9.13d), or, rarely, the lung.

9.4.4.2.1.4   Adenoma: Exophytic, Endophytic   The earliest dysplastic lesions seen are altered single basophilic glands with hyperchromatic nuclei (Figure 9.14a) and usually arise in the antral mucosa. Benign exocrine tumors show atypical architecture composed of exocrine branching or tubular crypts present, usually forming a polypoid tumor with a stromal stalk (Figure 9.14b), or a sessile structure may be present. Most adenomas have a well-organized glandular pattern, but additionally, areas of cystic tubular arrangement with distorted branching glands may be present. Tumor cells form a single layer of columnar cells, which are mostly hyperchromatic and show distinct cell boundaries. Exocrine adenomas are seen in the pylorus of mice following glucocorticoid and gonadorelin administration. If there is either a diffuse thickening of the mucosa or a focal proliferation of some gastric glands within otherwise normal mucosal architecture, the lesion is considered hyperplastic.

The differentiation between regenerative hyperplasia and adenoma may be difficult, and criteria for carcinoma *in situ* taken from human pathology (Watanabe et al. 1990) are not always appropriate. Regenerating glands following erosion or ulceration form undifferentiated glandular structures, which sometimes penetrate the muscularis mucosa to form *diverticula*, which can become cystic with foveolar cytology.

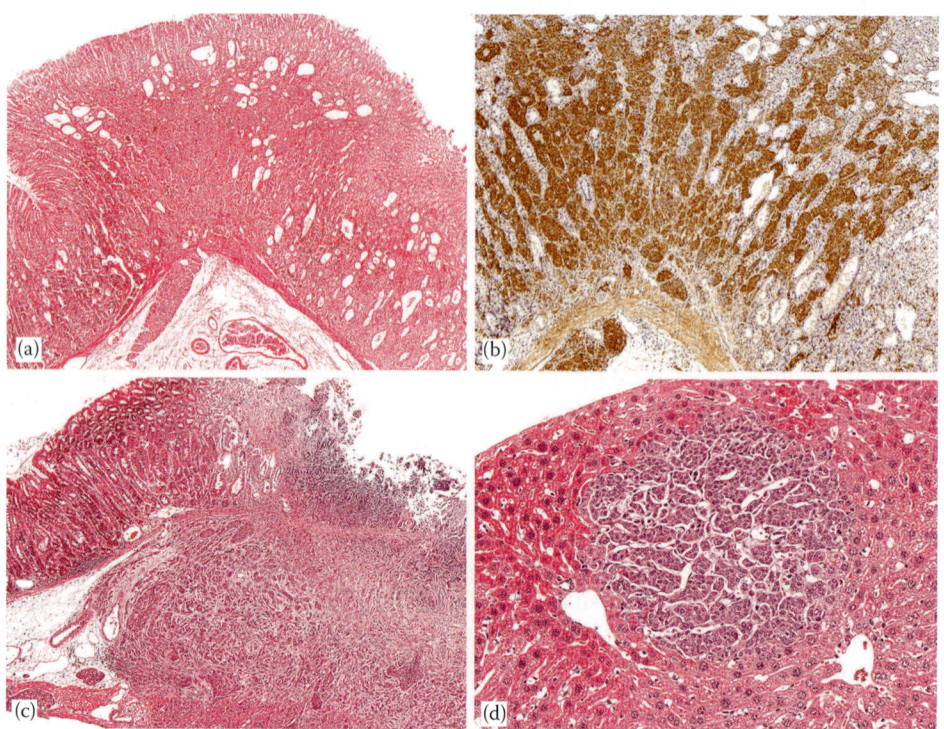

FIGURE 9.13   (a) Rat, stomach, HE stain. Fundic malignant neuroendocrine tumor in a 2-year H₂RA-treated Wistar rat exhibiting multiple gland bases filled with tumor cells, which have invaded submucosa as a solid cord. (b) Rat, stomach, IHC for NSE. Immunoreactivity demonstrated in a fundic malignant neuroendocrine tumor in a 2-year H₂RA-treated Wistar rat stomach showing infiltrative growth up and across oxyntic glands and into submucosa. Adjacent oxyntic mucosa shows diffuse and (right) focal neuroendocrine cell hyperplasia. (c) Mouse, stomach, HE stain. Fundic malignant neuroendocrine tumor in a 2-year H₂RA-treated CD1 mouse stomach. Tumor has destroyed overlying glands and has invaded submucosa as small nests of proliferating cells. (d) Mouse, liver, HE stain. Metastasis of case in (c). Neuroendocrine cells show some nested and glandular patterns and are basophilic.

9.4.4.2.1.5 Adenocarcinoma   Malignancy is based on invasion of muscularis mucosa (Figure 9.14c) or budding into lamina propria. Tumors may be tubular endophytic, nodular, cystic, or solid, composed of either cuboidal cells with varying polarity and round or oval sometimes vesicular nuclei and basophilic cytoplasm or columnar cells with atypia, and sometimes may produce abundant mucus (*signet ring type*). Induced adenocarcinomas usually occur in the antrum and are seen with genotoxins such as MNNG, DEN, irradiation, dietary nitroso compounds, and opioids. Promoters include salt, helminths, bile salts, and pyloric reflux with fundic–duodenal anastomosis (Bilroth A surgical model). Aroclor 1254 caused intestinal metaplasia with true goblet cell formation followed by adenocarcinoma in F344 rats (Morgan et al. 1981).

Although *H. pylori* gastritis can progress to gastric cancer in humans (Wee et al. 1992; Polk and Peek 2010), there is no evidence of *Helicobacter* spp.–related carcinogenesis in laboratory animals apart from the Mongolian gerbil (Pritchard and Przemek 2004), although *H. pylori* caused preneoplastic changes in B6219 mice (Rogers et al. 2005) and potentiated ENNG genotoxic gastric carcinogenesis in the rhesus monkey (Liu et al. 2009). *H. felis* infection of mice produced metaplastic and dysplastic lesions (Takaishi et al. 2009).

9.4.4.2.1.6 GI Stromal Tumor—Benign/Malignant   In humans, nearly all GI stromal tumors (GIST) are classified on the basis of c-*kit* gene CD117 expression, and these soft tissue tumors are

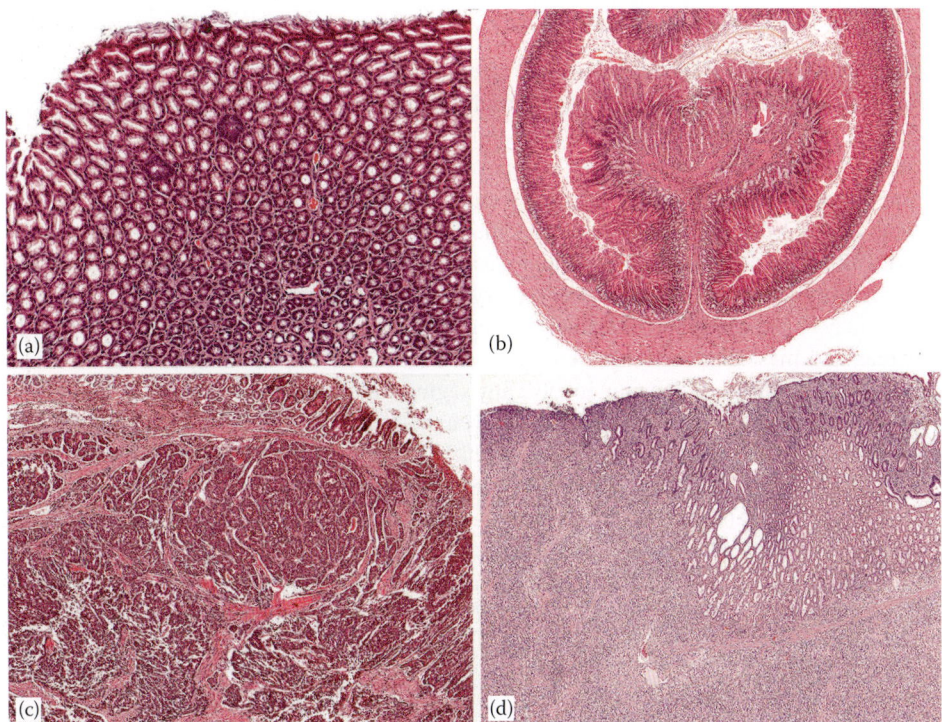

FIGURE 9.14 (a) Rat, stomach, HE stain. Transverse section through old rat antrum showing dysplastic glands. (b) Mouse, stomach, HE stain. Antral adenoma after gonadorelin treatment. Polypoid tumor retains antral gland organization. The borderline invasion of stalk was not enough for a diagnosis of malignant tumor. (c) Rat, stomach, HE stain. Antral adenocarcinoma with well-differentiated glandular structures in submucosal invasive nodule. (d) Rat, stomach, HE stain. Antral leiomyosarcoma. Bundles and whorls of elongated cells with cigar-shaped nuclei replace large areas of normal tissue.

believed to derive from the interstitial cells of Cajal, which have both smooth muscle and autonomic neuronal features. These cells are pacemakers for contractility of the GI tract. *C-kit* K461E knock-in mice develop hyperplasia of Cajal cells, GI distention, and GIST neoplasia (Rubin et al. 2005).

9.4.4.2.1.7 Leiomyoma   Leiomyoma is a benign smooth muscle cell tumor, composed of well-circumscribed bundles and whorls of spindle-shaped smooth muscle cells with abundant eosinophilic cytoplasm. Cytoplasm is positive for smooth muscle–specific actin and desmin immunoreactivity. Few mitoses and little pleomorphism are present. Fibrous connective tissue and vascular components are variable.

9.4.4.2.1.8 Leiomyosarcoma   Leiomyosarcoma is composed of smooth muscle cells derived from mesenchymal stem cells and characterized by the presence of interwoven bundles of eosinophilic spindle cells with cigar-shaped blunt-ended nuclei (Figure 9.14d). Undifferentiated cells may be polygonal. Frequent mitoses with pleomorphic hyperchromatic nuclei are present. Immunohistochemical characteristics of leiomyosarcoma are the same as those of leiomyoma.

9.4.4.2.1.9 Sarcoma, NOS (Synonym: Sarcoma Undifferentiated)   This is a malignant tumor derived from mesenchymal stem cells comprising poorly differentiated round or spindle cells exhibiting pleomorphism and anaplasia.

9.4.5 SMALL AND LARGE INTESTINES

Rare spontaneous lesions of the intestines in different rat strains include the presence of ectopic exocrine pancreas (Figure 9.15a) and, in aging animals, focal mineralization of the mucosa in any intestinal segment or osseous metaplasia in the submucosa or lamina propria usually associated with inflammation. Epithelial inclusion cysts, composed of squamous epithelium, have been described in the muscularis of the colon and rectum of rodents (Elwell and McConnell 1990; Shackelford and Elwell 1999). Aging rodents have a thickened lamina propria supporting the villi causing an increased width of intestinal villi. A spontaneous mutant mouse strain is being used as a model of intestinal malformations of the enteric nervous system (Nishijima et al. 1990). Spontaneous vascular changes may be present in the intestine of aging animals as part of polyarteritis nodosa, although the pancreas and mesentery are more common sites. Another important spontaneous disease of aging mice is amyloidosis, which may involve any segment of the GI tract, including the small intestine, and when extensive, it may cause death. The characteristic pale eosinophilic material replaces and distorts the normal structures of the intestinal lamina propria. Osseous metaplasia associated with ulceration was reported in Fischer rats (Elwell and McConnell 1990).

As with other segments of the GI tract, inflammatory changes and mucosal necrosis/deficits (erosion in case the muscularis mucosa remains intact and ulcer when it is perforated) are common changes in all species either due to infections or exposure to xenobiotics. Small-intestinal ulcerations associated with nonselective NSAIDs (nsNSAIDs) such as diclofenac in a rat model were

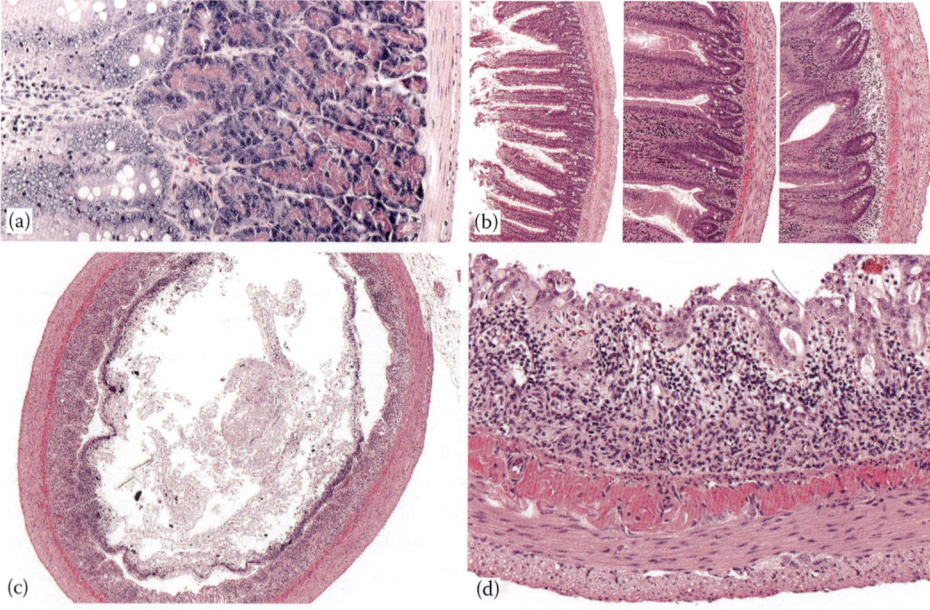

FIGURE 9.15 (a) Rat, small intestine, HE stain. Ectopic pancreatic tissue expands to the muscularis. (From Bertram T.A. et al., *Guides for Toxicologic Pathology* GI-1, 1996. With permission.) (b) Rat, small intestine, HE stain. Dose-related changes are present following treatment with a Wnt inhibitor. Note the number of goblet cells and slender villi in left panel (control). Animals receiving low (middle panel) and intermediate dose (right panel) have an expanded lamina propria and decreased specialized cells. (c) Rat, small intestine, HE stain. Mucosal collapse with loss of villi following high-dose treatment with a Wnt inhibitor. (d) Rat, small intestine, HE stain. Higher power of (c) showing the loss of villous architecture and crypt epithelium in mucosal collapse. Due to loss of crypt epithelium, including stem cells and Paneth cells, this mucosa cannot regenerate.

not due to changes in intestinal prostaglandins but, rather, were due to enterohepatic circulation, increased enteric gram-negative bacteria, bile, and impaired enteric barrier (Reuter et al. 1997; Seitz and Boelsterli 1998). Additional contributing factors were suggested such as TLR-4-dependent mechanisms based on KO mouse studies. There is a species-specific difference in sensitivity to GI changes associated with nsNSAIDs, and COX-2 selective NSAIDs have an improved GI safety profile compared with those of nonselective ones (Radi 2009).

Inflammatory changes may be due to infections but may also be produced by test articles that affect the immune system and host resistance. Infectious agents and parasites are not often encountered in the pharmaceutical industry because of improved husbandry conditions and extensive preventative care in cases of large animals, including primates.

Motility disorders may be observed as intussusception when a segment of the intestine telescopes into another. Such changes are seen associated with euthanasia in rodents and dogs when they are not characterized by segmental mucosal or serosal changes (redness, fibrin precipitation, or necrosis) and can be corrected with ease at necropsy. Centrally acting α adrenergic agonists in rats were associated with intussusception probably due to increased peristalsis, and, although were considered to be test article related, no morphological changes occurred (Gopinath et al. 1987). Pseudo-obstruction may be seen as a complication of anesthesia (due to neurogenic disturbance) and is also encountered in breeder mice (Feinstein et al. 2008). Mortality in these animals was due to necrosis and inflammation of segments of the distended small intestine.

Cecal enlargement was reported in rats following poor digestion of dietary starches and sugar alcohols. Animals had grossly distended abdomen and osmotic changes in cecal luminal contents, and the mucosal hyperplasia and hypertrophy were accompanied by increased ^{3}H-thymidine incorporation (Newberne et al. 1988).

Because of the high proliferation rate of the small intestine, insults that impact cell proliferation will result in architectural changes from villous blunting and fusion to mucosal collapse (loss of all epithelial cells), depending on the severity of the insult. Radiomimetic agents, ionizing radiation, antimitotics, and compounds targeting the wnt pathway may have such effects (Figure 9.15b through d). In the case of radiation injury, free radicals are formed by the interaction of radiation and cell components; subsequently, apoptosis is produced by breaks in single- and double-stranded DNA. Additionally, following radiation, endothelial damage occurs allowing for vascular leakage and cellular infiltrates (Wang and Hauer-Jensen 2003). A distinguishing feature of radiation injury from toxic insult is the presence of thickened submucosal vasculature (Greaves 2012). An unusual metaplastic change was produced by a local irritant in the ileum when apical enterocytes were replaced by goblet cells (Figure 9.16a through d).

In addition to increased apoptosis of the surface and/or crypt epithelium, decreased apoptosis of surface epithelium may occur due to a number of etiologies, including infectious agents and xenobiotics. In these cases, the surface epithelium has an abnormally uneven, lace-like morphology (Figure 9.17a through c).

Infections or infestations may occur in nonhuman primates, especially in studies with immunosuppressive agents, although the ciliate protozoa, *Balantidium* spp., may be seen in the large-intestinal lumen in immunocompetent nonhuman primates or dogs. Invasive balantidiasis (associated with mucosal damage and the presence of organisms extending into the submucosa) or flask-shaped ulcers due to *Entamoeba histolytica* may occur in immunosuppressed nonhuman primates. In the small intestine, the most commonly encountered infestation is cryptosporidiosis resulting in villus blunting. The organism is recognized as 1–4 µm round structures. *Giardia* appearing as racquet-shaped delicate organism adjacent to the epithelium of the proximal small intestine may be present in immunosuppressed nonhuman primates or mice and are easily overlooked because they may appear as mucus droplets in crypts. Viral inclusions and associated mucosal changes are not common in the gut of nonhuman primates dosed with immunosuppressive xenobiotics and include adenoviral and cytomegaloviral infections. Activation of an LCV in macaques may result in lymphoproliferative changes that involve segments of the intestinal tract and are typically

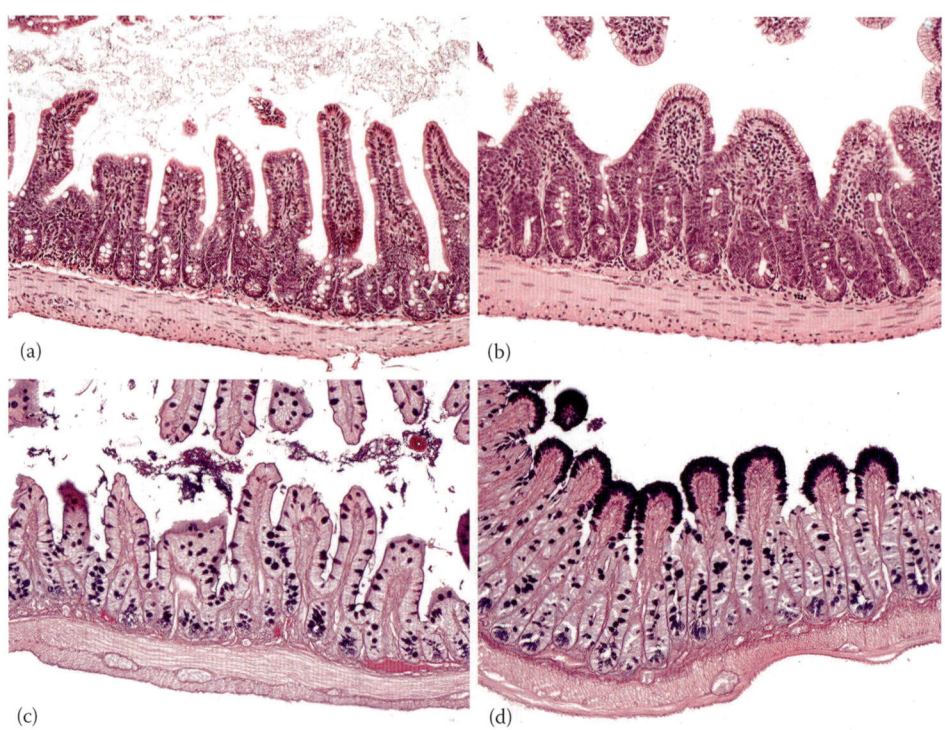

FIGURE 9.16 (a) Rat, small intestine, HE stain. Control small intestine with slender, long villi and goblet cell. (b) Rat, small intestine, HE stain. Villous blunting, fusion with increased basophilia following treatment with a xenobiotic. Note the tall columnar cells forming a "crown" along the tip of villi. (c) Rat, small intestine, PAS/AB stain. Control small intestine has mucus-positive cells within crypts and along villi, but not on tip of villi. (d) Rat, small intestine, PAS/AB stain. Strong mucus staining is present in metaplastic cells forming tip of villi.

composed of B lymphocytes (Figure 9.18a through d). Other organisms in nonhuman primates encountered include *Spironucleus*, a delicate flagellate organism in the large intestine. Nodular worms (*Oesophagostomum* sp.) were seen most frequently spontaneously in nonhuman primates (the nodules being composed of a granulomatous reaction associated with the intralesion parasite), whereas whip worms (*Trichuris* sp.) are encountered less frequently and mostly in immunosuppressed animals. Nematodes are seldom seen in rodents due to modern animal husbandry, but occasionally, pinworms (*Syphacia muris* or *Aspicularis tetraptera*) may be encountered in rats (Elwell and McConnell et al. 1990). Bacterial infections that are commonly seen in outdoor-housed macaques (campylobacteriosis and shigellosis) are uncommon in animals on toxicity studies. In addition to nonhuman primates, *Campylobacter jejuni* may be encountered as an etiology of acute enteric inflammation in dogs. Yersiniosis is another bacterial infection that occurs primarily in outdoor-housed macaques in wet, colder months, but this etiology, as others, may also be seen indoors in a quarantine setting. Yersiniosis is characterized by large flower petal-like bacterial colonies surrounded by neutrophils. During testing of antibiotics, the toxicologic pathologist may encounter pseudomembranous colitis characterized by a necrotizing colitis containing small mucosal deficits being covered by a "volcanic eruption" of exudates composed of neutrophils and fibrin (Lowenstein 2003). New World monkeys (especially callitrichids) are not commonly used as toxicologic species, but the practicing toxicologic pathologist needs to be aware of the widespread chronic colitis present in many colonies that may be part of the marmoset wasting disease (Lowenstein

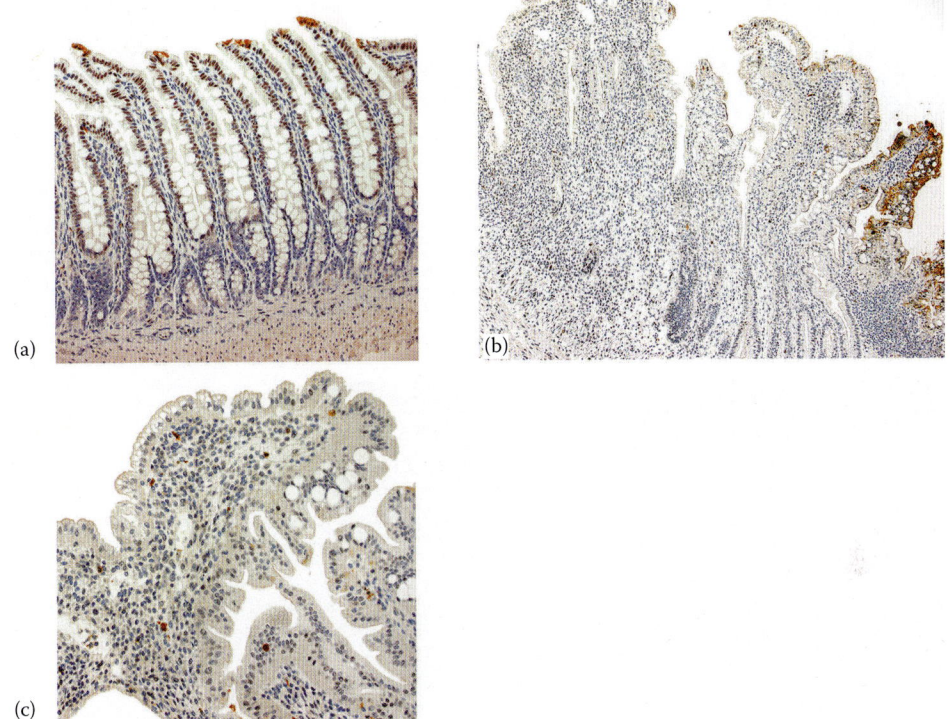

FIGURE 9.17 (a) Rat, small intestine, IHC for activated caspase-3. In control small intestine, caspase-3 immunoreactivity corresponds to these cells undergoing apoptosis as they are being shed. (b) Rat, small intestine, IHC for activated caspase-3. Note the lack of caspase-3 apoptosis in the center of the field in the tip of villi after dosing with a Wnt inhibitor. (c) Rat, small intestine, IHC for activated caspase-3. Higher magnification of (b) illustrating the lace-like appearance of villous epithelium that lacks caspase-3 immunoreactivity. Such lace-like surface alterations are common in animals with intestinal changes, especially monkeys, perhaps corresponding to delayed apoptosis in those cases as well.

2003; Chalmers et al. 1983). The lesion varies in morphology from a primarily mononuclear infiltrate to mucosal deficits along with neutrophilic infiltrate and crypt abscesses.

Recently, a series of p38MAPK inhibitors was studied in acute and 7-day repeat-dose studies in both rats and dogs. In these studies, GI changes were present in dogs but not rats. The changes included necrosis in GALT and mucosal epithelium along with hemorrhage in the colon and cecum. The hemorrhage was noted grossly and was considered to be due to ischemia and reperfusion of the large-intestinal mucosa. Although there was evidence of peripheral neutrophilia, and splenic follicles were infiltrated by neutrophils, inflammatory changes in the large intestine were not prominent in this cohort of animals. The preliminary conclusion of these studies was that at least in dogs, the p38MAPK signaling pathway is important in maturation of B cell subpopulations and their survival after activation through cellular caspases (Morris et al. 2010).

Indomethacin in rats caused mucosal deficits adjacent to Peyer's patches, suggesting that an exuberant immune response to intestinal antigens produced the lesion following local depression of prostaglandin synthetase (Greaves 2012).

Intestinal damage is often produced by anticancer drugs including those that act on the microtubule cytoskeleton (e.g., taxol) or are mitotic kinesin inhibitors. These compounds cause mitotic arrest, the formation of large abnormal ring mitotic figures, karyomegaly, pseudostratification of the epithelium, and epithelial apoptosis (Greaves 2012). Methotrexate, the much-studied antifolate cytotoxic drug, causes inhibition of proliferation and apoptosis of crypt epithelium, resulting in

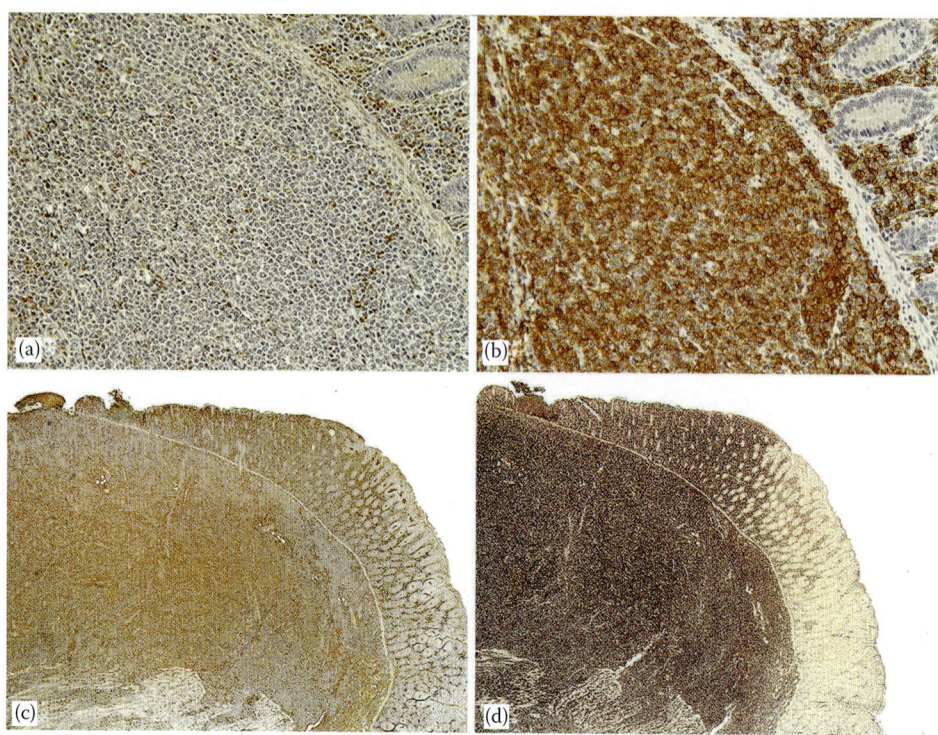

FIGURE 9.18   (a) Macaque, large intestine, IHC for CD3. Lymphoproliferative changes in an immunosup-pressed animal. Lymphocytes present in the mucosa and submucosa are not T cells as indicated by the lack of immunoreactivity to CD3. (b) Macaque, large intestine, IHC for CD20. Lymphoproliferative changes in an immunosuppressed animal. Lymphocytes present in the mucosa and submucosa are B cells as indicated by the immunoreactivity to CD20. (c) Macaque, large intestine, IHC for EBNA-2. The majority of lymphocytes present in the mucosa and submucosa are positive for EBNA-2, an antibody for EBV, confirming a viral etiol-ogy. (d) Macaque, large intestine, *in situ* hybridization for EBER-1. The majority of lymphocytes present in the mucosa and submucosa are positive for EBER-1, confirming an LCV-related lesion.

villus atrophy, crypt loss, and attenuation of epithelium. Some of the terminally differentiated cells (goblet and Paneth cells) and cells associated with the Peyer's patch appeared to be spared. When non-Peyer's patch epithelium was compared to that of the Peyer's patch, the former had diminished proliferation and enterocyte-specific gene expression, suggesting that retention of the ability to pro-liferate was needed for unperturbed enterocyte function (Renes et al. 2002).

Vacuolation of Brunner's glands has been described at all doses in dogs treated with a β adren-ergic receptor blocker (Atenolol 2011) (Figure 9.19a).

In a study with several γ-secretase inhibitors in rats, crypt epithelial apoptosis in the small and large intestines was followed by goblet cell metaplasia. Gene expression profiling indicated a mech-anism for lesion development involving the Rath1-dependent Notch pathway alteration (Milano et al. 2004).

Anti-obesity drugs may cause lipid accumulation within intestinal epithelium and lipid phagocy-tosis by macrophages in the tips of villi. Lipid could be demonstrated either by the oil red O method in frozen sections or by osmium tetroxide. Other drugs associated with lipid accumulation in rats included an ester of erythromycin and inhibitors of protein synthesis, puromycin, and ethionine (Greaves 2012). Among accumulation enteropathies, phospholipidosis has been described more fre-quently following exposure to cationic amphiphilic drugs than lipid accumulation (Halliwell 1997). Many drugs on the market cause phospholipidosis without adverse effects, often in a species-specific

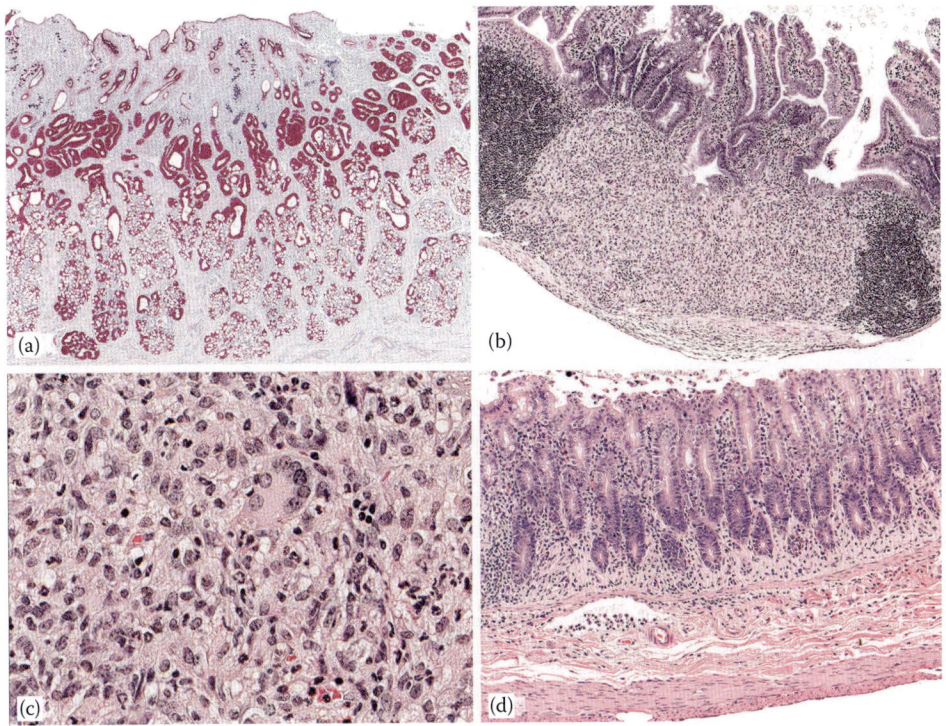

FIGURE 9.19 (a) Dog, duodenum, PAS stain. Decreased PAS staining is present in vacuolated epithelial cells of Brunner's glands. (b) Mouse, small intestine, HE stain. Accumulation enteropathy following dosing with nanoparticles. (c) Mouse, small intestine, HE stain. Higher magnification of (b) showing foamy macrophages and multinucleated giant cell. (d) Rat, cecum, HE stain. Cecal hyperplasia in a control rat; note the lack of goblet cells and increased basophilia in intestinal tubules.

distribution in a number of tissues depending on drug distribution and metabolism. Phospholipidosis in the intestine is mainly characterized by the accumulation of foamy macrophages that contain lysosomal myelin figures ultrastructurally. Intestinal phospholipidosis is significant if the villus architecture is distorted such that there is either an interference with normal intestinal function, especially absorption, or increased permeability because of epithelial damage. Similar accumulation enteropathy was seen following exposure to nanoparticles (Figure 9.19b and c).

9.4.5.1 Proliferative Changes of Small and Large Intestines

The most common spontaneous GI change in rats is a diffuse hyperplasia of cecal mucosa with or without mixed cellular infiltrate (Figure 9.19d). Mucosal and glandular hyperplasia occurs in aging CD1 mice in the ampulla of Vater accompanied by eosinophilic degeneration with or without crystalline structures (Shackelford and Elwell 1999). An inotropic phosphodiesterase inhibitor caused diffuse, reversible hyperplasia of all segments of the small and large intestines. In addition to the lengthening of the intestinal tubules (that contained appropriate goblet cell populations based on PAS/AB staining), the muscularis mucosa was also thickened (Westwood et al. 1991). In contrast, atrophy of intestinal mucosa characterized by small epithelial cells lining slender, somewhat collapsed-appearing intestinal villi or, more frequently, short intestinal tubules in the large intestine may be associated with chronic inflammation or poor general body condition. Test article–related hyperplasia may be associated with increased lengthening of intestinal tubules accompanied by increased or decreased goblet cell populations. Hyperplasia of GALT may occur with antigenic stimulus.

Citrobacter rodentium, the etiologic agent of murine transmissible colonic hyperplasia, is associated with a cellular infiltrate of CD4 cells and a Th1 cytokine response (TNF α, IL 12, and γ-interferon), similar to that of murine models of IBD (Higgins et al. 1999).

Sunitinib, a potent tyrosine kinase inhibitor, caused hyperplasia or decrease of goblet cell populations with or without a cellular infiltrate of the small intestine of rats and nonhuman primates (Patyna et al. 2008). Cellular hyperplasia of the intestine in addition to that of the stomach, salivary gland, and urinary system was due to treatment with recombinant human EGF in rats and nonhuman primates (Breider et al. 1996; Reindel et al. 1996). In all tissues and both species, the proliferative response was composed of somewhat undifferentiated cells.

A unique partially reversible lesion, referred to as adenosis of duodenal Brunner's glands, was produced by a vascular endothelial growth factor (VEGF) receptor inhibitor in chronic studies (Figure 9.20a through c) (Ettlin et al. 2010). In short-term studies, degeneration and inflammatory changes occurred with other VEGF inhibitors, suggesting that these changes may precede the proliferative changes observed in the 26-week study (Inomata et al. 2011).

As discussed earlier, the intestine has a high proliferation rate that, under normal conditions, is in balance, maintaining the villus-to-crypt ratio and mucosal thickness in all segments of the gut. This delicate balance, however, may be disrupted by many factors either to cause decreased mucosal thickness (intestinal blunting and shortening in the small intestine) or increased mucosal thickness and lengthening of intestinal tubules. Factors that decrease mucosal thickness include reduced food intake, hypophysectomy, thyroidectomy, and bypass surgery. Other factors that cause decreased proliferation in mice include stimulation of α1 or β receptors at least in part because of

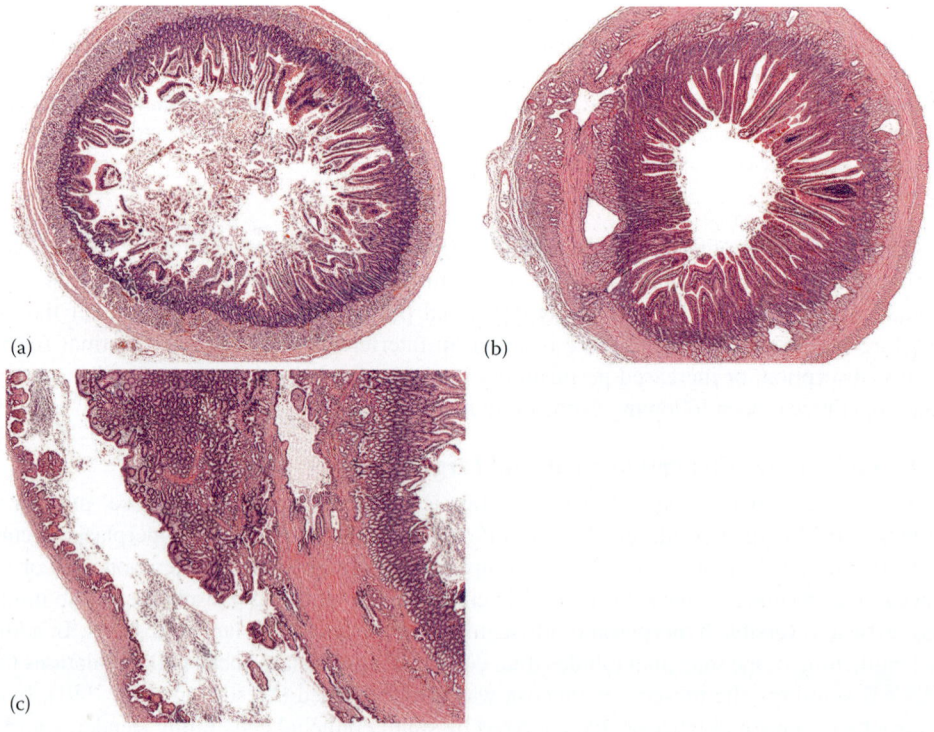

(a)

(b)

(c)

FIGURE 9.20   (a) Rat, duodenum, HE stain. Brunner's glands of a control rat are uniformly spaced around the circumference of the proximal duodenum within the submucosa. (b) Rat, duodenum, HE stain. Following chronic dosing with a VEGF inhibitor, Brunner's gland hyperplasia with extension into muscularis and serosa is present. (c) Rat, duodenum, HE stain. Higher magnification of (b). Note the markedly dilated proliferative Brunner's glands.

decreased blood flow (Greaves 2012). Additionally, anticancer and antiviral drugs decrease proliferation in the intestine, causing shortened intestinal villi. Other compounds may have antimitotic and direct toxic effects on the surface epithelium, resulting in villus atrophy and loss of enzyme activity of the surface epithelium. Several factors increase intestinal proliferation, including several hormones (e.g., gastrin, glucagon, thyroxin, corticosteroids, and GLP-2), neurotransmitters, and partial intestinal resection. Hyperplasia of the gut may be accompanied by a normal, decreased, or increased goblet cell population. Furthermore, a change in the composition of mucus in goblet cells may be compensatory to irritant effects as seen following partial intestinal resection (Greaves 2012). Atypical hyperplasia in the colon (produced by carcinogens such as azoxymethane) is characterized by increased numbers of goblet cells containing abnormal mucus (indicated by changes in sialo- and sulfomucin contents) or a decreased goblet cell population containing decreased amounts of mucin, and crypt branching or increased tortuosity. Crypts in the areas of atypical hyperplasia exhibit increased basophilia, with pseudostratification of enlarged and vesicular nuclei.

9.4.5.1.1 Hyperplasia and Reactive Hyperplasia

The lesion is characterized by the lack of compression, although cells may penetrate the muscularis mucosa into the submucosa, but the basement membrane remains intact. There is no prominent cell type. In the large intestine, reactive hyperplasia is often composed of cells producing a decreased amount of mucus exhibiting increased basophilia and may be associated with an inflammatory infiltrate. Nuclei may be vesicular and elongated with prominent nucleoli. Less frequently, an increased goblet cell population is present. Diffuse hyperplasia may occur in lactating rodents in response to increased metabolic demands of lactation and increased food intake.

9.4.5.1.2 Atypical Hyperplasia

In areas of atypical hyperplasia, the villous or intestinal tubular structure is maintained, but cells may be crowded and pseudostratified. Cellular atypia and loss of polarity may be present. In the large intestine, whole crypts or parts of crypts may be enlarged and have a dilated lumen. These crypts are lined by cells with different degrees of dysplasia and decreased goblet cell differentiation. The lesion typically is not associated with inflammation.

9.4.5.1.3 Avillous Hyperplasia

Avillous hyperplasia may be associated with inflammation and characterized by crypts interspersed between hyperplastic Brunner's glands. This is a common lesion in aged male DBA mice and in both sexes of C57BL. Because of the presence of inflammation and concurrent hyperplasia of several cell types, this lesion is considered to be a reactive hyperplasia (Betton et al. 2001).

Spontaneous intestinal neoplasias are not common. In the small intestine, epithelial and mesenchymal tumors occur with similar incidence, whereas most tumors are of epithelial origin in the large intestine. In the NTP program, several compounds, including N-nitroso compounds and dimethylhydrazine, among others, caused epithelial neoplasias that could typically be identified grossly (Elwell and McConnell 1990). The earliest lesions involved only one or two crypts that were lined by closely packed hyperchromatic dysplastic epithelial cells that contained frequent mitotic figures. Test article–related intestinal tumorigenesis is unusual in pharmaceutical testing. An interesting presentation was a life span study in rats with Sporanox (itraconazole), an antifungal agent formulated in a cyclodextrin vehicle. Colonic hyperplasia and a minimally increased incidence of colonic adenocarcinoma in rats were considered to be due to an adaptive response to the vehicle and hence did not indicate liability to patients receiving intravenous dosing of the drug (Greaves 2012).

9.4.5.1.4 Adenoma

Adenomas (Figure 9.21a) are distinguished from focal atypical hyperplasia based on the presence of compression. Adenoma may develop as a polypoid growth supported by a stalk or sessile, endophytic growth of the mucosa. The intestinal epithelium may exhibit some stratification or, if in a

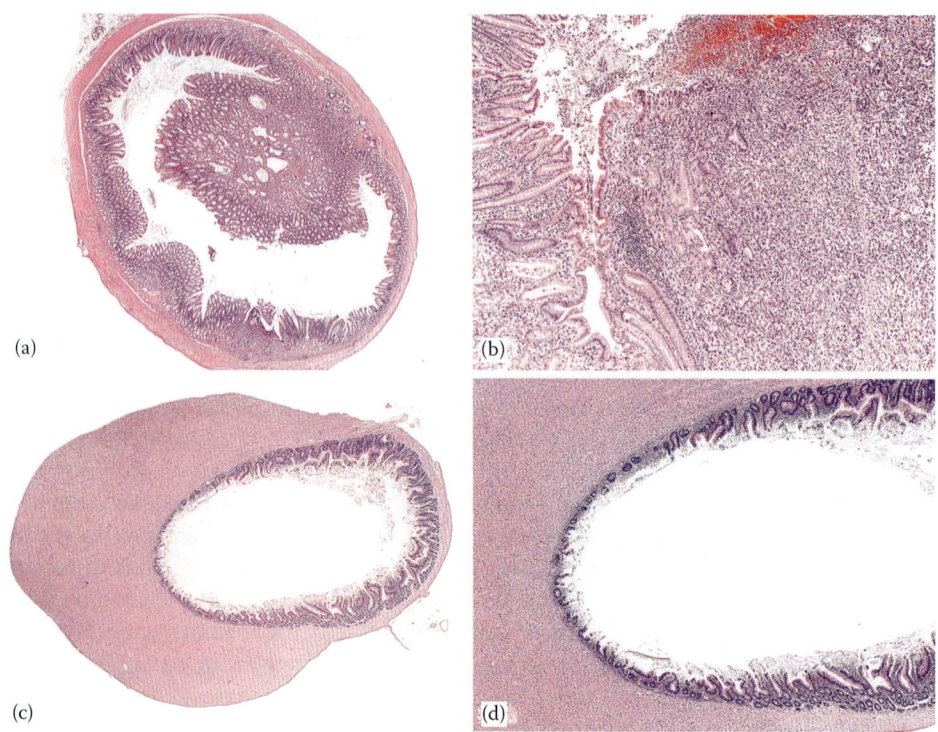

FIGURE 9.21 (a) Rat, colon, HE stain. Adenoma composed of an exophytic mass lined by mucosal epithelium extends into the lumen. (b) Rat cecum HE stain. Adenocarcinoma composed of poorly differentiated invasive epithelial cells that have replaced and effaced the normal architecture. Focal erosion and hemorrhage are present. (c) Rat, jejunum, HE stain. Leiomyoma is causing an asymmetric nodular thickening of the gut wall. (d) Rat, jejunum, HE stain. Higher magnification of (c). Well-differentiated smooth muscle cells replaced the normal muscularis.

monolayer, will exhibit some nuclear atypia. Crypts may be microherniated by penetrating muscularis mucosa, but the basement membrane remains intact. Small-intestinal adenomas may contain goblet cells and Paneth cells. Depending on the method of evaluation and strain of mice, the incidence in the proximal small intestine may be up to 50%, whereas in other segments, it may be as low as 5% (Betton et al. 2001).

9.4.5.1.5 Adenocarcinoma

Malignant epithelial tumors are either endophytic or nodular and are composed of cells arranged in varying morphologic patterns from solid to cystic. Cells are pleomorphic, and their polarity may be lost; mitotic figures are common, and cells invade the lamina propria by penetrating the basement membrane or may invade the submucosa. Large-intestinal adenocarcinomas (Figure 9.21b) may arise within adenomas or may originate from dysplastic areas of "flat" mucosa. Adenocarcinomas must be distinguished from areas of atypical epithelium herniating into the submucosa in areas of scirrhous reaction. Large-intestinal sessile tumors metastasize more readily than those that are pedunculated. Furthermore, at least in rats, adenocarcinomas of the small intestine metastasize more frequently than those of the large intestine.

9.4.5.1.6 Mucinous Adenocarcinoma

A special morphology refers to signet ring appearance as intracellular mucus accumulates in a characteristic pattern, while other tumors may have extracellular accumulation of mucus in the form of mucus lakes. These tumors are typically sessile and locally invasive. Mucinous adenocarcinomas may be associated with lymphoid nodules in both the small and large intestines of rats. Osseous metaplasia may occur.

9.4.5.1.7   Mesenchymal Benign and Malignant Tumors

The cellular origin of mesenchymal tumors is difficult to identify without immunohistochemistry. The majority of the tumors are considered to be of smooth muscle origin (Figure 9.21c and d). Schwannomas in rats tend to be malignant, often originating in the mesentery and invading multiple tissues. In contrast, most GI mesenchymal tumors in humans are considered to be of interstitial cells of Cajal origin based on immunoreactivity to CD117. Other sporadic mesenchymal tumors include hemangioma and hemangiosarcoma, fibroma and fibrosarcoma, and manifestations of systemic tumors (lymphoma, histiocytic sarcoma, and mast cell tumors).

9.5   METHODS OF EVALUATION

The fixative for the evaluation of the GI tract should be selected based on the focus of the evaluation. For most purposes, formalin-fixed tissue will suffice; however, should the mucus layers be of primary interest, Carnoy's fixative is recommended as it is not a cross-linking fixative and does not contain water, being composed of chloroform, dry methanol, and glacial acetic acid. Carnoy's fixative or methacarn will ensure that the *in vivo* thickness of the mucus layer is maintained as well as the spatial organization of the luminal contents (Johansson et al. 2011; Nava et al. 2011). The best methods for detailed histological evaluation of the stomach were described earlier. Because of the length of the intestine, specialized evaluation of the rodent small intestine is best carried out by rolling up its full length around a supporting axis of a slender rod or even a toothpick for small rodents following the gentle flushing of the luminal contents (Figure 9.22a and b). Similar preparations may be made of rodent large intestine as well as segments of the gut of large animals. Such preparations allow the evaluation of the full length of the intestine as well as the Peyer's patches. In large animals, once the full length of the gut is opened, segments of the intestine may be pinned to a corkboard to ensure flat fixation and subsequent sampling with ideal perpendicular orientation of the mucosa. Careful macroscopic inspection of both mucosal and serosal surfaces with a separate sample for brown hematin deposits indicative of pinhead erosions, inclusion of Peyer's patch samples, are recommended. Histologically, histochemical or immunohistochemical stains may facilitate the detailed evaluation of GI morphology. Mucous epithelial cells can be characterized by PAS-AB and HID-AB stains in order to distinguish neutral and acid mucus substances including sialo and sulfated mucus (Figure 9.22c and d). A less frequently used method takes advantage of the characteristics of lectins to bind to specific sugar moieties of mucus. Using the binding pattern of several lectins, mucins may be evaluated in segments of the GI tract in health and disease (Kuhlmann et al. 1983; Kitajima et al. 1990). GI mucus may also be characterized by its staining in the so-called paradoxical concanavalin A staining by a modification of the concanavalin A-horseradish peroxidase method using a variety of oxidative methods with or without reduction. The mucin of the GI tract falls into four categories by this method: Class I, Class II, and stable and labile Class III mucins. Class I mucin was present in the absorptive epithelial cells of normal rat colon, whereas Class II mucin was present in the surface mucus layer. Additionally, labile Class III mucin and Class II mucin were present in the normal goblet cells of rat colon. Stable Class III mucins were described in the different regions of the stomach of rats (Katsuyama and Spicer 1978; Uchida et al. 2001).

Lesion components can be further characterized by immunohistochemical methods demonstrating specific mucus and by flow cytometry of inflammatory components as used in the investigation of the impact of antibody treatment on *Citrobacter*-associated colitis (Wlodarska et al. 2011).

Immunohistochemical methods can be further used to identify different cellular components such as lysozyme for Paneth cells, specific products for the subtypes of enteroendocrine cells, or NSE or chromogranin A as a general marker. As in other tissues, proliferation may be assessed by

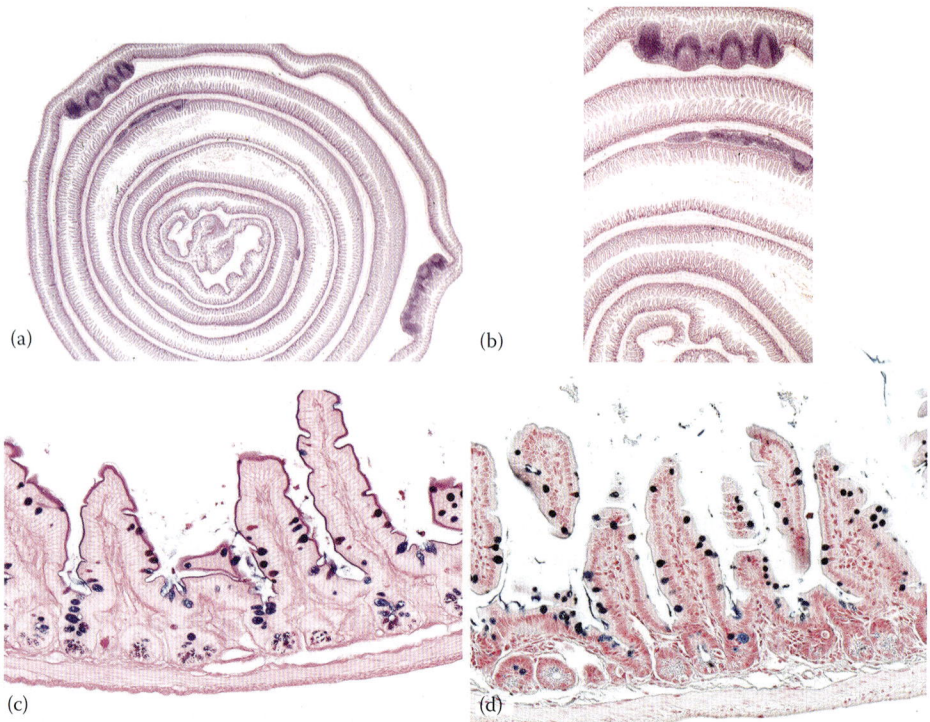

FIGURE 9.22 (a) Mouse, small intestine, HE stain. Swiss role method allows the microscopic examination of the full length of the intestine. Peyer's patches can be identified with ease, and all of them can be evaluated. (b) Mouse, small intestine, HE stain. Higher magnification of (a). Notice the well-preserved villous architecture that can be evaluated in detail. (c) Mouse, small intestine, periodic acid Schiff and alcian blue stain pH 2.5 (PAS/AB). In this stain, neutral mucosubstances stain red, acid mucin stains blue, whereas purple granules are those that contain a mixture of neutral and acid mucin. (d) Mouse, small intestine, high iron diamine, and alcian blue stain pH 2.5 (HID/AB). This stain distinguishes acid mucosubstances if they are nonsulfated (blue) sialo mucosins or sulfated (black) sulfomucin. Bluish gray color indicates that a mixture of sialo and sulfomucins is present.

immunohistochemical staining for BrDU (following timed pretreatment of animals) or Ki67 (without pretreatment) and subsequent image analysis.

In vitro evaluation of cells may be used in order to characterize the absorption, metabolism, and toxicity of xenobiotics. The cell cultures may be based on primary cells, cell lines from normal tissues, or normal cell lines transfected with regulatory genes (Sambruy et al. 2001). The utility of the *in vitro* systems includes screening permeability properties of drugs and drug candidates, identifying transport mechanisms, and evaluating cellular sites of metabolism.

9.5.1 Assessment of Structural Integrity and Biomarkers

GI diseases are often associated with clinical signs of vomiting, diarrhea or constipation, and changes in some routine clinical pathology parameters, especially in levels of monovalent electrolytes and proteins (although panhypoproteinemia is not specific to enteric disease) (Stockham and Scott 2008a,b). Antisecretory drugs typically elevate gastrin levels in the blood. Intestinal malabsorption may involve several nutrients, including fats, proteins, and sugars, and may result in decreased levels of serum folate or cobalamin. Additional ancillary tests include absorption, and intestinal tolerance tests may indicate malassimilation, without being specific for maldigestion or malabsorption (Bounous 2003). The tests evaluate lipid, carbohydrate, or protein assimilation.

These indicators, however, do not allow the recognition of early events or follow progression of diseases. Finally, a fecal occult blood test is easily performed on laboratory animals and is a sensitive indication of GI blood loss. From a clinical perspective, early detection of disease progression, especially cancer or adverse events following treatment of cancer, is of interest. One effort focused on monitoring and detection of progression of mucositis using noninvasive methods of sucrose breath tests in animal models and patients (Butler 2008). The evaluation of mitochondrial DNA in patients with preneoplastic lesions as well as chemotherapy-related toxicity in rats has been published. Mitochondrial DNA damage was considered to be important in the evaluation of pathogenesis of GI toxicity of chemotherapeutic agents and nonsteroidal anti-inflammatory drugs and may be also used as a biomarker for early cancer diagnosis (Sui et al. 2006; Yanez et al. 2003). Additional efforts to date were not successful for identification of miRNA in digestive tract cancers of patients (Albulescu et al. 2011).

The intestinal changes produced by γ secretases due to disruption of notch signaling were described earlier. Adipsin was found to be a fecal marker in animals treated with a novel γ secretase presumably because of perturbation of cell differentiation in the small intestine due to Notch/hes-1 signaling disruption (Searfoss et al. 2003).

New promising biomarkers of GI toxicity were identified in rats treated with a PAK-4 inhibitor. Preliminary findings indicated the utility of plasma citrulline and fecal miRNA194, at least in the model used (John-Baptiste et al. 2012). Additional method validation will be needed to confirm if these analytes could be accepted as biomarkers of GI damage.

ACFs have been suggested as a morphological biomarker for malignancy based on experimental evidence in a variety of models. Morphological categories of nondysplastic, hyperplastic, and dysplatic ACFs were correlated with molecular markers and possible progression to adenocarcinoma. The authors acknowledge that ACF is not well characterized in humans, and the tracking of its progression in a clinical setting is limited (Wargovich et al. 2010).

9.5.2 ASSESSMENT OF PROLIFERATION OF MUCOSAL CELLS

During the practice of toxicologic pathology, assessment of proliferation of the GI tract is called for from time to time. Most commonly (as in other tissues), immunohistochemical methods are used to demonstrate Ki67 or immunoreactivity to exogenously administered BrDU, and the evaluation involves image analysis of decorated and undecorated nuclei in order to determine a labeling index to indicate proliferation (Hormi and Lehy 1996). Less frequently used methods involve the separation of the epithelial components of the intestine that then can be evaluated for their DNA content by flow cytometry (Walsh 1994).

9.5.3 TOXICOGENOMICS AND METABONOMICS

Nuclear magnetic resonance (NMR)-based metabonomics was used on fecal samples from patients with Crohn's disease, and several metabolites were identified to either positively or negatively correlate with the disease. Serum metabolites from obese patients were also evaluated by NMR after gastric bypass surgery in order to characterize the metabolic adaptation process. It is too early to tell if any of the novel methods outlined above will be rewarding and gain broader acceptance (Mutch et al. 2009; Jansson et al. 2009).

9.6 ANIMAL MODELS

9.6.1 SJOGREN'S SYNDROME

Sjogren's syndrome is an important autoimmune disease of humans (either as a primary disease or associated with other autoimmune diseases such as lupus), causing dry mouth and other clinical signs due to lymphocytic infiltrates in salivary glands. The syndrome also includes changes in the lacrimal glands, resulting in keratoconjunctivitis sicca, which is not discussed further here. Sjogren's syndrome is poorly understood as most patients present with advanced disease, making it difficult to identify a pathogenesis. The wide range of mouse models used to study the disease further indicates that the syndrome is poorly understood, and each model may represent different aspects of the syndrome. The mouse models can be divided into primary and secondary, and in both categories, spontaneous, immunization-induced, KO, and transgenic models were developed (Lavoie et al. 2011). The salivary glands in these models contain necrotic ducts and lymphocytic infiltrates and capture different aspects of the syndrome.

9.6.2 Gastritis

Models of *Helicobacter*-associated gastritis are of great interest because of the relatively high incidence of infection (especially in developing countries) and its association with peptic ulcer disease and cancer in humans. Since its identification in 1982, a number of animal models have been used in order to study the pathogenesis and in search of treatment modalities. These models included the use of gnotobiotic piglets and macaques and the utilization of related organisms in different species, including *H. mustelae* in ferrets and mice. More recently, however, mouse models have emerged as preferred systems because of the possibility of developing a more reproducible model using a small animal species (Marchetti et al. 1995). To that end, a reproducible quantification of the histological changes with relevance to disease biology was developed because the Updated Sydney System for the evaluation of human gastric biopsies was not considered to be relevant in animal models (due to differences in type of samples and features of lesions between the clinical and preclinical settings). In the new scoring system for mice, neutrophils, gastritis, and metaplasia were scored based on the percentage of microscopic fields exhibiting the change (Eaton et al. 2007). When scores were compared from different experiments and different pathologists, the results correlated well.

9.6.3 Mucositis

Mucositis (meaning damage to the GI epithelium, including that of tongue) is a common and painful toxicity associated with radiotherapy and chemotherapy and targeted anti-EGFR therapies in humans. The clinical presentation is complex as it involves direct damage due to the offending agents and secondary bacterial or fungal infections. Models for oral mucositis focus on the initial insult and include the radiation-induced mouse model, where changes in the ventral tongue are assessed following acute irradiation of the head, and the hamster buccal mucosa model, which involves the combination of dosing with 5-fluorouracil and superficial irradiation. Intestinal damage is modeled following irradiation of mice. These models have been used to study the pathogenesis of lesion development and to preclinically test treatment modalities. Oral mucositis is characterized by the attenuation of epithelium with secondary inflammatory changes in the lamina propria and muscle of the tongue. In the small intestine, apoptosis and crypt loss are present. Keratinocyte growth factor (KGF), IL11, and transforming growth factor β were efficacious in these models by sparing most of the epithelium of the tongue and maintaining the proliferative region of the small-intestinal crypt (Bowen et al. 2011; Booth and Potten 2001; Chen et al. 2011).

9.6.4 Inflammatory Bowel Disease

IBD is a multifactorial disease in humans with a spectrum of clinical and morphological manifestations from the inflammatory, granulomatous Crohn's disease to ulcerative colitis characterized by mucosal deficits, inflammation, and epithelial changes. Because the human disease is multifactorial, stemming from environmental to genetic and immune mechanisms, which all contribute to the manifestation of disease, no ideal animal model has been identified. An overview by Blumberg et al.

(1999) is provided on inflammatory models, some of which are spontaneous (cotton top tamarin); others require the administration of exogenous material as enema (acetic acid), oral (carrageenan, dextran sulfate sodium [DSS]), subcutaneous (cyclosporine A), or intracolonic administration (peptidoglycan polysaccharide). Additional models are either transgenic or KO targeting specific genes of cytokine function (IL10$^{-/-}$), T cell function (HLA-B27 transgenic rat), or IEC barrier function (trefoil factor$^{-/-}$) (Figure 9.23a and b) (Blumberg et al. 1999; Hammer et al. 1990). A final category of induced models involves cell transfer into immunodeficient animals (CDεTg26 into SCID mice). One of the most commonly used animal models using DSS recapitulates certain features of IBD. Dextran is a complex polymer of glucose with varying molecular weight of 5000 to over 1 million Da. DSS is a highly water-soluble polyanionic derivative of dextran containing close to 20% sulfate. The model in mice is induced by providing varying concentrations of DSS in drinking water to animals for 4 to 14 days, often in a cycling manner. The morphological changes depend on the mouse strain and experimental protocol used and include crypt loss, erosion/ulcer, inflammatory infiltrate, and hyperplastic/dysplastic epithelial changes (Figure 9.23c) (Solomon et al. 2010). The reader is referred to a scoring scheme of mouse IBD presented by Mahler et al. (1998) for details of systematic evaluation of the lesions that consider loss of crypts, erosion/ulcer, hyperplastic and dysplastic changes, and the extent and composition of inflammatory reaction. A recent study of temporal genome-wide expression profiling in a mouse model of DSS-induced colitis revealed similarities to ulcerative colitis in immune responses, tissue remodeling, and angiogenesis (Fang et al.

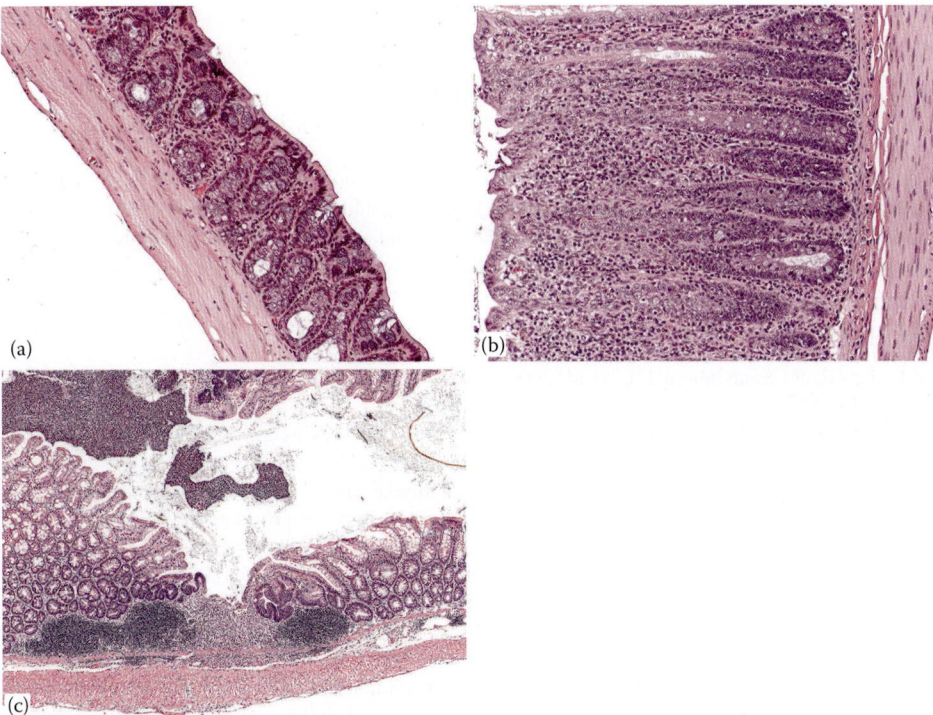

FIGURE 9.23 (a) Rat, colon, HE stain. The sample originated from a control Fischer 344 rat. Note mucosal thickness and numerous goblet cells. In this control animal, the lamina propria contains very few cells. (Courtesy of Dr. M. Harbison, Roche Pharmaceuticals, Nutley, NJ.) (b) Rat, colon, HE stain. Colon of HLA-B27 transgenic rat at same magnification as that in (a). The mucosa is markedly thickened due to epithelial hyperplasia and cellular infiltrate in the lamina propria. (Courtesy of Dr. M. Harbison, Roche Pharmaceuticals, Nutley, NJ.) (c) Mouse, colon, HE stain. In this model of DSS colitis, crypt loss, erosion, cellular infiltrate, crypt hyperplasia, and branching are present.

2011). Furthermore, multicyclic administration of DSS was associated with β catenin translocation, an early event in human colorectal carcinogenesis (Cooper et al. 2000).

9.6.5 MODELS OF COLORECTAL NEOPLASIA

DSS may be coadministered with carcinogens such as azoxymethane (AOM) to mice or rats in order to produce a higher incidence of adenocarcinomas. The model has been used to study pathogenesis, inflammatory mediators, and inflammation-associated carcinogenesis. The pathogenesis of carcinogenesis in ulcerative colitis models is not clear but may indicate (as human epidemiologic studies do as well) that underlying inflammation may have a key role. Both in the human disease and in models of inflammation, the two key genes contributing to the inflammatory process were COX-2 and nuclear factor K (NF-κB). In the aforementioned combination model of AOM/DSS, tumor necrosis factor alpha (TNF α) was found to be elevated, which regulated the trafficking of inflammatory cells, which were the source for expression of COX-2. Inflammatory models also implicated NF-κB regulating pro-inflammatory cytokines, including IL-6. Increased IL-6 levels were also demonstrated in the AOM/DSS model (Kraus and Arber 2009).

As discussed earlier, APC^{min} mice heterozygous for the multiple neoplasia allele primarily develop small-intestinal polyps. However, upon infection with *C. rodentium*, a fourfold increase of neoplasia occurred in the distal colon, where this bacterium-induced hyperplasia occurred (Newman et al. 2001).

REFERENCES

Abayomi T. A., Ofusori D. A., Ayoka O. A. et al. 2009. A comparative histological study of the tongue of rat (*Rattus norvegicus*), bat (*Eidolon helvum*) and pangolin (*Manis tricuspis*). *Int J Morphol* 27(4):1111–9.
Ainsworth M. A., Koss M. A., Hogan D. L., Isenberg J. I. 1995. Higher proximal duodenal mucosal bicarbonate secretion is independent of Brunner's glands in rats and rabbits. *Gastroenterology* 109:1160–6.
Albulescu R., Neagu M., Albulescu L. et al. 2011. Tissular and soluble miRNAs for diagnostic and therapy improvement in digestive tract cancers. *Expert Rev Mol Diagn* 11:101–20.
Alrawi S. J., Schiff M., Carroll R. E. et al. 2006. Aberrant crypt foci. *Anticancer Res* 26:107–20.
Atenolol. 2011. http://www.astrazeneca.ca/documents/ProductPortfolio/TENORMIN_PM_en.pdf (accessed April 2012).
Backed F., Ley R. E., Sonnenburg J. L. et al. 2005. Host-bacterial mutualism in the human intestine. *Science* 307:1915–20.
Baele M., Van den Bulck K., Decostere A. et al. 2004. Multiplex PCR assay for differentiation of *Helicobacter felis*, *H. bizzozeronii*, and *H. salomonis*. *J Clin Microbiol* 42:1115–22.
Barka T. 1980. Biologically active polypeptides in submandibular glands. *J Histochem Cytochem* 28:836–59.
Baskin G. B., Roberts E. D., Kuebler D. et al. 1995. Squamous epithelial proliferative lesions associated with rhesus Epstein–Barr virus in simian immunodeficiency virus-infected monkeys. *JID* 172:535–9.
Bertram TA, Markovits JE, Juliana MM. 1996. Non-proliferative lesions of the alimentary canal in rats. In *Guides for Toxicologic Pathology*. STP/ARP/AFIP, Washington, DC GI-1.
Betton G. 1998. The digestive system I: The gastrointestinal tract and exocrine pancreas. In *Target Organ Pathology. A Basic Text* (Eds J. Turton and J. Hooson). Taylor and Francis, London, pp. 29–60.
Betton G. R., Salmon G. K. 1984. Pathology of the forestomach in rats treated for 1 year with a new histamine H2-receptor antagonist, SK&F 93479 trihydrochloride. *Scand J Gastroenterol Suppl* 101:103–8.
Betton G. R., Dormer C. S., Wells T. et al. 1988. Gastric ECL-cell hyperplasia and carcinoids in rodents following chronic administration of H2-antagonists SK&F 93479 and oxmetidine and omeprazole. *Toxicol Pathol* 16:288–98.
Betton G. R., Whiteley L. O., Anver M. R. et al. 2001. Gastrointestinal tract. In *International Classification of Rodent Tumors the Mouse* (Ed U. Mohr). Springer Verlag, Berlin, Germany, pp. 23–58.
Bevins C. L. 2004. The Paneth cell and the innate immune response. *Curr Opin Gastroenterol* 20:572–80.
Blumberg R. S., Saubermann L. J., Strober W. 1999. Animal models of mucosal inflammation and their relation to human inflammatory bowel disease. *Curr Opin Immunol* 11:648–56.

Bonkovsky H. L., Hauri H. P., Marti U. et al. 1985. Cytochrome P450 of small intestinal epithelial cells. Immunohistochemical characterization of the increase in cytochrome P450 caused by phenobarbital. *Gastroenterology* 88:458–67.

Booth D., Potten C. S. 2001. Protection against mucosal injury by growth factors and cytokines. *J Natl Canc Inst Monogr* 29:16–20.

Borch K., Renvall H., Liedberg G. et al. 1986a. Relations between circulating gastrin and endocrine cell proliferation in the atrophic gastric fundic mucosa. *Scand J Gastroenterol* 21:357–63.

Borch K., Renvall H., Liedberg G. 1986b. Endocrine cell proliferation and carcinoid development: a review of new aspects of hypergastrinaemic atrophic gastritis. *Digestion* 35 (Suppl 1):106–15.

Botts S., Jokinen M., Gaillard E. T. et al. 1999. Salivary, Harderian and lacrimal gland. In *Pathology of the Mouse* (Eds R. R. Maronpot, G. A. Borman, and B. W. Gaul). Cache River Press, Saint Louis, MO, pp. 48–79.

Boughter J. D., Pumplin D. W., Yu C. et al. 1997. Differential expression of a-gustducin in taste bud populations in the rat and hamster. *J Neurosci* 17:2852–8.

Bounous D. I. 2003. Digestive system. In *Duncan and Prasse's Veterinary Laboratory Medicine Clinical Pathology*, 4th edition (Eds K. S. Latimer, E. A. Mahaffey, and K. W. Prasse). Iowa State Press, Ames, IA, pp. 215–30.

Bowen J. M., Gibson R. J., Keefe D. M. 2011. Animal models of mucositis: implications. *J Support Oncol* 9:161–8.

Breider M. A., Bleavins M. R., Reindel J. F. et al. 1996. Cellular hyperplasia in rats following continuous intravenous infusion of recombinant human epidermal growth factor. *Vet Pathol* 33:184–93.

Brown A. P., Courtney C. L., King L. M. et al. 2005. Cartilage dysplasia and tissue mineralization in the rat following administration of a FGF receptor tyrosine kinase inhibitor. *Toxicol Pathol* 33:449–55.

Brown H. R., Hardisty J. F. 1990. Oral cavity, esophagus and stomach. In *Pathology of the Fischer Rat. Reference and Atlas.* (Eds G. A. Boorman, S. L. Eustis, M. R. Elwell, C. A. Montgomery, Jr., and W. F. MacKenzie), Academic Press, San Diego, pp. 9–30.

Buettner M., Dimmler A., Magener A. et al. 2004. Gastric PDX-1 expression in pancreatic metaplasia and endocrine cell hyperplasia in atrophic corpus gastritis. *Mod Pathol* 17: 56–61.

Butler R. N. 2008. Measuring tools for gastrointestinal toxicity. *Curr Opin Supp Pall Care* 2:35–9.

Cao L., Xu X., Cao L. L. et al. 2007. Absence of full-length Brca1 sensitizes mice to oxidative stress and carcinogen-induced tumorigenesis in the esophagus and forestomach. *Carcinogenesis* 28:1401–7.

Carnahan J., Beltran P. J., Babij C. et al. 2010. Selective and potent RAF inhibitors paradoxically stimulate normal cell proliferation and tumor growth. *Mol Cancer Ther* 9:2399–410.

Carthew P. and Slinger R. P. 1981. Diagnosis of sialodacryoadenitis virus infection of rats in a virulent enzootic outbreak. *Lab Anim* 15:339–42.

Casteleyn C., Breugelmans S., Simoens P. et al. 2011. The tonsils revisited: review of the anatomical localization and histological characteristics of the tonsils of domestic and laboratory animals. *Clin Dev Immunol* doi:10.1155/2011/472460.

Cetinkaya B. O., Acikgoz G., Aydin O. et al. 2006. The relationship between proliferating cell nuclear antigen expression and histomorphometric alterations in cyclosporine A-induced gingival overgrowth in rats. *Toxicol Pathol* 34:180–6.

Chalmers D. T., Murgatroyed L. B., Wadsworth P. F. 1983. A survey of the pathology of marmosets (*Callithrix jacchus*) derived from a marmoset breeding unit. *Lab Anim* 17:270–9.

Chandra S. A., Nolan M. W., Malarkey D. E. 2010. Chemical carcinogenesis of the gastrointestinal tract in rodents: an overview with emphasis on NTP carcinogenesis bioassays. *Toxicol Pathol* 38:188–97.

Chen D., Zhao C. M., Andersson K. et al. 1998. ECL cell morphology. *Yale J Biol Med* 71:217–31.

Chen D., Aihara T., Zhao C. M. et al. 2006. Differentiation of the gastric mucosa. I. Role of histamine in control of function and integrity of oxyntic mucosa: understanding gastric physiology through disruption of targeted genes. *Am J Physiol Gastrointest Liver Physiol* 291:G539–44.

Chen P., Lingen M., Sonis S. T. et al. 2011. Role of AMP-18 in oral mucositis. *Oral Oncol* 47:831–9.

Chiba T., Kinoshita Y., Sawada M. et al. 1998. The role of endogenous gastrin in the development of enterochromaffin-like cell carcinoid tumors in Mastomys natalensis: a study with the specific gastrin receptor antagonist AG-041R. *Yale J Biol Med* 71:247–55.

Chiu T., Chen H. C. 1986. Spontaneous basophilic hypertrophic foci of the parotid glands of rats and mice. *Vet Pathol* 23:606–9.

Clayson D. B., Iverson F., Nera E. A. et al. 1990. The significance of induced forestomach tumors. *Ann Rev Pharmacol Toxicol* 30: 441–463.

Cooke H. J. 1986. Neurobiology of the intestinal mucosa. *Gastroenterology* 90:1057–81.

Cooper H. S., Murthy S., Kido K. et al. 2000. Dysplasia and cancer in the dextran sulfate sodium mouse colitis model. Relevance to colitis-associated neoplasia in human: a study of histopathology, b catenin and p53 expression and the role of inflammation. *Carcinogenesis* 21:757–68.

Cordero J. B., Sampson O. J. 2011. Wnt signaling and its role in stem cell-driven intestinal regeneration and hyperplasia. *Acta Physiol* doi:10.1111/j1748-1716.2011.02288x.

Cornetta A.M., Simpson K.W., Strauss-Ayali D. et al. Use of a [13C]urea breath test for detection of gastric infection with *Helicobacter* spp in dogs. *Am J Vet Res* 59:1364–9.

Creutzfeldt W., Lamberts R. 1991. Is hypergastrinaemia dangerous to man? *Scand J Gastroenterol Suppl* 180:179–91.

Damsch S., Eichenbaum G., Tonelli A. et al. 2011. Gavage-related reflux in rats: identification, pathogenesis, and toxicological implications (review). *Toxicol Pathol* 39:348–59.

Dawson P. A., Shneider B. L., Hofman A. F. 2006. Bile formation and the enterohepatic circulation. In *Physiology of the Gastrointestinal Tract*, 4th edition (Ed L. R. Johnson), Academic Press, Waltham, MA, pp. 1438–62.

Denny P. C., Ball W. D., Redman R. S. 1997. Salivary glands: a paradigm for diversity of gland development. *Crit Rev Oral Biol Med* 8:51–75.

de Rijk E. P. C. T., Ravesloot W. T. M., Hafmans T. G. M. et al. 2003. Multifocal ductal cell hyperplasia in the submandibular salivary glands of Wistar rats chronically treated with a novel steroid compound. *Toxicol Pathol* 31:1–9.

Diaz D., Allamnent K., Tarant J. M. et al. 2012. Phosphorous dysregulation induced by MEK small molecule inhibitors in rats involves blockade of FGF-23 signaling in kidney. *Toxicol Sci* 125:187–95.

Ding X., Kaminsky L. S. 2003. Human extrahepatic cytochromes P450: function in xenobiotic metabolism and tissue-selective chemical toxicity in the respiratory and gastrointestinal tracts. *Annu Rev Pharmacol Toxicol* 43:149–73.

Dressman J. B. 1986. Comparison of canine and human gastrointestinal physiology. *Pharm Res* 3:123–31.

Eaton K. A., Danon S. J., Krakowka S. et al. 2007. A reproducible scoring system for quantification of histologic lesions of inflammatory disease in mouse gastric epithelium. *Comp Med* 57:57–65.

Ekman L., Hansson E., Havu N. et al. 1985. Toxicological studies on omeprazole. *Scand J Gastroenterol* 108 (Suppl.):53–69.

Elmore S. A. 2006. Enhanced histopathology of mucosa-associated lymphoid tissue. *Toxicol Pathol* 34:687–96.

Elwell M. R., McConnell E. E. 1990. Small and large intestine. In *Pathology of the Fischer Rat. Reference and Atlas.* (Eds G. A. Boorman, S. L. Eustis, M. R. Elwell, C. A. Montgomery, Jr, and W. F. MacKenzie), Academic Press, San Diego, pp. 43–61.

Erdman S. E., Poutahidis T. 2010. Roles of inflammation and regulatory T cells in colon cancer. *Toxicol Pathol* 38:76–87.

Ettlin R. A., Kuroda J., Plassmann S. et al. 2010. Successful drug development despite adverse preclinical findings. Part 2: Examples. *J Toxicol Pathol* 23:213–34.

Faller G., Kirchner T. 2005. Immunological and morphogenic basis of gastric mucosa atrophy and metaplasia. *Virchows Arch* 446:1–9.

Fang K., Bruce M., Pattillo C. B. et al. 2011. Temporal genomewide expression profiling of DSS colitis reveals novel inflammatory and angiogenesis genes similar to ulcerative colitis. *Physiol Genomics* 43:43–56.

Farrell J. J., Taupin D., Koh T. J. et al. 2002. TFF2/SP-deficient mice show decreased gastric proliferation, increased acid secretion, and increased susceptibility to NSAID injury. *J Clin Invest* 109:193–204.

Feinstein R. E., Morris W. E., Waldemarson A. H. et al. 2008. Fatal acute intestinal pseudoobstruction in mice. *JAAALAS* 47:58–63.

Fenoglio-Preiser C. M., Noffsinger A. 1999. Aberrant crypt foci: a review. *Toxicol Pathol* 27:632–42.

Fletcher T. F., Weber A. F. 2011. Veterinary developmental anatomy. Veterinary embryology class notes (CVM 6100). Available at http://vanat.cvm.umn.edu/vanatpdf/EmbryoLectNotes.pdf (accessed May 2012).

Fox J.G., Rogers A.B., Whary M.T. et al. 2007. Accelerated progression of gastritis to dysplasia in the pyloric antrum of TFF2–/–C57BL6 × Sv129 *Helicobacter pylori*-infected mice. *Am J Pathol* 171:1520–8.

Franic T. V., Judd L. M., Nguyen N. V. et al. 2004. Growth factors associated with gastric mucosal hypertrophy in autoimmune gastritis. *Am J Physiol Gastrointest Liver Physiol* 287:G910–8.

Frantz J. D., Betton G., Cartwright M. E. et al. 1991. Proliferative lesions of the non-glandular and glandular stomach in rats. In *GI-3 Guides for Toxicol Pathology*, STP/ARP/AFIP, Washington, DC.

Frederick C. B., Hazelton G. A., Frank J. D. 1990. The histopathological and biochemical response of the stomach of male rats following two weeks of oral dosing with ethyl acrylate. *Toxicol Pathol* 18:247–56.

Fukushima S., Ito N. 1985. Papilloma, forestomach, rat. In *Monographs on Pathology of Laboratory Animals. Digestive System.* (Eds T. C. Jones, U. Mohr, and R. D. Hunt), Springer Verlag, Berlin, pp. 289–92.

Garrett W. S., Gordon J. I., Glimcher L. H. 2010. Homeostasis and inflammation in the intestine. *Cell* 140:859–70.

Goldenring J. R., Nomura S. 2006. Differentiation of the gastric mucosa III. Animal models of oxyntic atrophy and metaplasia. *Am J Physiol Gastrointest Liver Physiol* 291:G999–1004.

Gopinath C., Prentice D. E., Lewis D. J. 1987. The alimentary system and pancreas. In *Atlas of Experimental Toxicological Pathology*. Current Histopathology Series, vol. 13, G. Austin Gresham (series consultant editor), MTP Press Limited, Lancaster, UK, pp. 61–76.

Gould V. E., Wiedenmann B., Lee I. et al. 1987. Synaptophysin expression in neuroendocrine neoplasms as determined by immunocytochemistry. *Am J Pathol* 126:243–57.

Goyal R. K., Hirano I. 1996. The enteric nervous system. *NEJM* 334:1106–15.

Greaves P. 2012. Digestive system. In *Histology of Preclinical Toxicity Studies*, 4th edition, Elsevier, London, pp. 325–431.

Håkanson R., Sundler F. 1990. Proposed mechanism of induction of gastric carcinoids: the gastrin hypothesis. *Eur J Clin Invest* 20 (Suppl. 1):S65–71.

Håkanson R., Böttcher G., Ekblad E. et al. 1986. Histamine in endocrine cells in the stomach: a survey of several species using a panel of histamine antibodies. *Histochemistry* 86:5–17.

Håkanson R., Chen D., Sundler F. 1994. The ECL cells. In *Physiology of the Gastrointestinal Tract*, 3rd edition (Ed L. R. Johnson), Raven Press, New York, pp. 1171–84.

Halliwell W. H. 1997. Cationic amphiphilic drug-induced phospholipidosis. *Toxicol Pathol* 25:53–60.

Hammer R. E., Maika S. D., Richardson J. A. et al. 1990. Spontaneous inflammatory disease in transgenic rats expressing HLS-B27 and human B$_2$m: an animal model of HLA-B27-associated human disorders. *Cell* 63:1099–112.

Hanby A. M., Poulsom R., Playford R. J. et al. 1999. The mucous neck cell in the human gastric corpus: a distinctive, functional cell lineage. *J Pathol* 187(3):331–7.

Hansen M. B. 2003a. The enteric nervous system I: organization and classification. *Pharmacol Toxicol* 92:105–13.

Hansen M. B. 2003b. The enteric nervous system II: gastrointestinal functions. *Pharmacol Toxicol* 92:249–57.

Hansen M. B. 2003c. The enteric nervous system III: a targeting for pharmacological treatment. *Pharmacol Toxicol* 93:1–13.

Hayashi Y., Kurashima C., Utsuyama M. et al. 1988. Spontaneous development of autoimmune sialadenitis in aging BDF1 mice. *Am J Pathol* 132:173–9.

Hesketh P. J. 2008. Chemotherapy-induced nausea and vomiting. *N Engl J Med* 358:2482–94.

Higgins L. M., Frankel G., Douce G. et al. 1999. *Citrobacter rodentium* infection in mice elicits a mucosal Th1 cytokine response and lesions similar to those in murine inflammatory bowel disease. *Infect Immun* 67:3031–9.

Hirth R. S., Evans L. D., Buroker R. A. et al. 1988. Gastric enterochromaffin-like cell hyperplasia and neoplasia in the rat: an indirect effect of the histamine H2-receptor antagonist BL-6341. *Toxicol Pathol* 16:273–87.

Hormi K., Lehy T. 1996. Transforming growth factor a *in vivo* stimulates epithelial cell proliferation in digestive tissues of suckling rats. *Gut* 39:532–8.

IARC. 1999. Predictive value of rodent forestomach and gastric neuroendocrine tumors in evaluating carcinogenic risks to humans. In *Views and Expert Opinions of an IARC Working Group*, IARC Technical Publication No. 39 Lyon, 29 November–1 December 1999.

Ikeno T., Ota H., Sugiyama A. et al. Helicobacter pylori-induced chronic active gastritis, intestinal metaplasia, and gastric ulcer in Mongolian gerbils. *Am J Pathol* 154:951–60.

Imaoka M., Satoh H., Kai K. et al. 2003. Spontaneous ectopic sebaceous glands (Fordyce's granules) in the oral mucosa of Sprague Dawley rats. *J Toxicol Pathol* 16:253–7.

Inomata A., Nakano K., Hosokawa S. et al. 2011. Bruner's gland lesions in rats induced by vascular endothelial growth factor receptor-2 inhibitor. Pg 217 Cutting Edge Pathology, ESTP Uppsala 2011. Available at http://www.esvp.eu/site/index.php?option=com_content&view=section&layout=blog&id=8&Itemid=32 (accessed April 2012).

Jalava K., On S.L., Vandamme P.A. et al. 1998. Isolation and identification of *Helicobacter* spp. from canine and feline gastric mucosa. *Microbiol* 64:3998–4006.

Jansson J., Willing B., Lucio M. et al. 2009. Metabolomics reveals metabolic biomarkers of Crohn's disease. *PLoS One* 4:26386–95.

Johansson M. E. V., Larsson J. M. H., Hansson G. C. 2011. The two mucus layers of colon are organized by the MUC2 mucin, whereas the outer layer is a legislator of host-microbial interactions. *PNAS* 108:4659–65.

John-Baptiste A., Lettiere D., Giovanelli M. et al. 2010. Paradoxical induction of epithelial hyperplasia by a selective Raf inhibitor. American Association for Cancer Research 101st Annual Meeting, Washington,

DC. Available at http://www.abstractsonline.com/Plan/ViewAbstract.aspx?sKey=21e1dba3-e367-4f22-b284-4492fe1f1aa7&cKey=84ae9abc-8d2b-40d8-aa40-7d5a4af44ce7&mKey=%7b0591FA3B-AFEF-49D2-8E65-55F41EE8117E%7d (accessed May 2012).

John-Baptiste A., Huang W., Kindt E. et al. 2012. Evaluation of potential gastrointestinal biomarkers in a PAK4 inhibitor-treated preclinical toxicity model to address unmonitorable gastrointestinal toxicity. *Toxicol Pathol* 40:482–90.

Johnson L. R. 2006. Apoptosis in the gastrointestinal tract. In *Physiology of the Gastrointestinal Tract*. 4th edition (Ed L. R. Johnson), Academic Press, Waltham, MA, pp. 345–74.

Johnson T. N., Tanner M. S., Tucker G. T. 2000. A comparison of the ontogeny of enterocytic and hepatic cytochrome P450 3A in the rat. *Biochem Pharmacol* 60:1601–10.

Jones T. C., Hunt R. D., King N. W. 1997. *Veterinary Pathology*, 6th edition, Lippincott Williams and Wilkins, Baltimore, MD, p. 354.

Judd L. M., Andringa A., Rubio C. A. et al. 2005. Gastric achlorhydria in H/K-ATPase-deficient (Atp4a(–/–)) mice causes severe hyperplasia, mucocystic metaplasia and upregulation of growth factors. *J Gastroenterol Hepatol* 20:1266–78.

Kaminsky L. S., Fasco M. 1992. Small intestinal cytochrome P450. *Critical Review Toxicol* 21:407–22.

Kaneko M., Morimura K., Nishikawa T. et al. 2002. Different genetic alterations in rat forestomach tumors induced by genotoxic and non-genotoxic carcinogens. *Carcinogenesis* 23:1729–35.

Kang W., Rathinavelu S., Samuelson L. C. et al. 2005. Interferon gamma induction of gastric mucous neck cell hypertrophy. *Lab Invest* 85:702–15.

Karam S. M. 2010. A focus on parietal cells as a renewing cell population. *World J Gastroenterol* 16:538–46.

Kararli T. T. 1995. Comparison of the gastrointestinal anatomy, physiology and biochemistry of humans and commonly used laboratory animals. *Biopharm Drug Disposition* 16:351–80.

Katsuyama T., Spicer S. 1978. Histochemical differentiation of complex carbohydrates with variants of the concanavalin A-horseradish peroxidase method. *J Histochem Cytochem* 26:233–50.

Kidd M., Modlin I. M., Eick G. N. et al. 2007. Role of CCN2/CTGF in the proliferation of Mastomys enterochromaffin-like cells and gastric carcinoid development. *Am J Physiol Gastrointest Liver Physiol* 292:G191–200.

Kikuchi M., Nagata H., Watanabe N. et al. 2010. Altered expression of a putative progenitor cell marker DCAMKL1 in the rat gastric mucosa in regeneration, metaplasia and dysplasia. *BMC Gastroenterology* 10:65. doi:10.1186/1471-230X-10-65.

Kim B. M., Buchner G., Miletich I. et al. 2005. The stomach mesenchymal transcription factor Barx1 specifies gastric epithelial identity through inhibition of transient Wnt signaling. *Dev Cell* 8:611–22.

Kirchhoff P., Andersson K., Socrates T. et al. 2006. Characteristics of the K+-competitive H+,K+-ATPase inhibitor AZD0865 in isolated rat gastric glands. *Am J Physiol Gastrointest Liver Physiol* 291:G838–43.

Kitajima M., Mogi M., Kiuchi T. et al. 1990. Alteration of gastric mucosal glycoprotein (lectin-binding pattern) in gastric mucosa in stress. *J Clin Gastroenterol* 12: S1–S7.

Konturek P. C., Konturek S. J., Brzozowski T. 2006. Gastric cancer and *Helicobacter pylori* infection. *J Physiol Pharmacol* 57 (Suppl 3):51–65.

Korenaga T., Fu X., Xing Y. et al. 2004. Tissue distribution, biochemical properties, and transmission of mouse type A AApoAII amyloid fibrils. *Am J Pathol* 164:1597–606.

Kraus S., Arber N. 2009. Inflammation and colorectal cancer. *Curr Opin Pharmacol* 9:1–6. doi:10.1016/j.coph.2009.06.006.

Kuhlmann W. D., Peschke P., Wurster K. 1983. Lectin–peroxidase conjugates in histopathology of gastrointestinal mucosa. *Virchows Arch (Pathol Anat)* 398:319–28.

Kutok J. L., Wang F. 2006. Spectrum of Epstein–Barr virus-associated disease. *Annu Rev Pathol Mech Dis* 1:375–404.

Kutok J. L., Klumpp S., Simon M. et al. 2004. Molecular evidence for rhesus lymphocryptovirus infection of epithelial cells in immunosuppressed rhesus macaques. *Virology* 78:3455–61.

Kuwamura M., Okajima R., Yamate J. et al. 2008. Pancreatic metaplasia in the gastro-achlorhydria in WTC-dfk rat, a potassium channel Kcnq1 mutant. *Vet Pathol* 45:586–91.

Lantini M. S., Cossu M., Isola M. et al. 2006. Subcellular localization of epidermal growth factor receptor in human submandibular gland. *J Anat* 208:595–9.

Lavoie T. N., Lee B. H., Nguyen C. Q. 2011. Current concepts: mouse models of Sjögren's syndrome. *J Biomed Biotechnol*. doi.org/10.1155/2011/549107.

Lee M. P., Ravenel J. D., Hu R. J. et al. 2000. Targeted disruption of the Kvlqt1 gene causes deafness and gastric hyperplasia in mice. *J Clin Invest* 106:1447–55.

Liu H., Merrell D. S., Semino-Mora C. et al. 2009. Diet synergistically affects helicobacter pylori-induced gastric carcinogenesis in nonhuman primates. *Gastroenterology* 137:1367–79.

Lowenstein L. J. 2003. A primer of primate pathology: lesions and non-lesions. *Toxicol Pathol* 31 (Suppl):92–102.

MacDonald T. T., Monteleone G. 2005. Immunity, inflammation, and allergy in the gut. *Science* 307:1920–5.

Maekawa A. 1994. Changes in the esophagus and stomach. In *Pathobiology of the Aging Rat*. Vol 2 (Eds U. Mohr, C. C. Capen, and D. L. Dungworth), ILSI Press, Washington, DC, pp. 323–31.

Mahler M., Bristol I. J., Leiter E. H. et al. 1998 Differential susceptibility in inbred mouse stains to dextrane sulfate sodium-induced colitis. *Am J Physiol Gastrointest Liver Physiol* 274:G544–G51.

Majumdar A. P. N., Basson M. D. 2006. Effect of aging on the gastrointestinal tract. In *Physiology of the Gastrointestinal Tract*, 4th edition (Ed L. R. Johnson), Academic Press, Waltham, MA, pp. 406–34.

Marchetti M., Arico B., Burroni D. et al. 1995. Development of a mouse model of *Helicobacter pylori* infection that mimics human disease. *Science* 267:1655–8.

Masui T., Asamoto M., Hirose M. et al. 1987. Regression of simple hyperplasia and papillomas and persistence of basal cell hyperplasia in the forestomach of F344 rats treated with butylated hydroxyanisole. *Cancer Res* 47:5171–74.

Matsuzaki J., Suzuki H., Minegishi Y. et al. 2010. Acid suppression by proton pump inhibitors enhances aquaporin-4 and KCNQ1 expression in gastric fundic parietal cells in mouse. *Dig Dis Sci* 55:3339–48.

Mehta R., Labuc G. E., Archer M. C. 1984. Organ specificity in the microsomal activation and toxicity of N-nitrosomethylbenzylamine in various species. *Cancer Res* 44:4017–22.

Milano J., McKay J., Dagenais C. et al. 2004 Modulation of notch processing by gamma-secretase inhibitors causes intestinal goblet cell metaplasia and induction of genes known to specify gut secretory lineage differentiation. *Toxicol Sci* 82:341–58.

Mitschke D., Reichel A., Fricker G. et al. 2008. Characterization of cytochrome P450 protein expression along the entire length of the intestine of male and female rats. *Drug Metabol Dispos* 36:1039–45.

Morgan R. W., Ward J. M., Hartman P. E. 1981. Aroclor 1254-induced intestinal metaplasia and adenocarcinoma in the glandular stomach of F344 rats. *Cancer Res* 41: 5052–59.

Morris D. L., O'Neil S. P., Devraj R. V. et al. 2010. Acute lymphoid and gastrointestinal toxicity induced by selective p38a map kinase and MAP kinase activated protein kinase-2 (MK2) inhibitors in the dog. *Toxicol Pathol* 38:606–18.

Mutch D. M., Fuhrman J. C., Rein D. et al. 2009. Metabolite profiling identifies candidate markers reflecting the clinical adaptations associated with Roux-en-Y gastric bypass surgery. *PLoS One* 4:e7905–16.

Nair P. N. R., Schroeder H. E. 1986. Duct-associated lymphoid tissue (DALT) of minor salivary glands and mucosal immunity. *Immunology* 57:171–80.

Nakamori Y., Komatsu Y., Kotani T. et al. 2010. Pathogenic importance of cysteinyl leukotrienes in development of gastric lesions induced by ischemia/reperfusion in mice. *J Pharmacol Exp Ther* 333:91–8.

Nava G. M., Friedrichsen H. J., Stappenbeck T. S. 2011. Spatial organization of intestinal microbiota in the mouse ascending colon. *ISME J* 5:627–38.

Neuenschwander S. B., Elwell M. R. 1990. Salivary glands. In *Pathology of the Fischer Rat. Reference and Atlas* (Eds G. A. Boorman, S. L. Eustis, M. R. Elwell, C. A. Montgomery, Jr, and W. F. MacKenzie), Academic Press, San Diego, pp. 31–42.

Newberne P. M., Charnley G., Adams K. et al. 1986. Gastric and oesophageal carcinogenesis: models for the identification of risk and protective factors. *Food Chem Toxicol* 24:1111–9.

Newberne P., Conner M. W., Estes P. 1988. The influence of food additives and related materials on lower bowel structure and function. *Toxicol Pathol* 16:184–97.

Newman J. V., Kosaka T., Sheppard B. J. et al. 2001. Bacterial infection promotes colon tumorigenesis in APC[min/+] mice. *J Inf Dis* 184:227–30.

Nilsson O., Wängberg B., Johansson L. et al. 1993. Rapid induction of enterochromaffin like cell tumors by histamine2-receptor blockade. *Am J Pathol* 142:1173–85.

Nishijima E., Meijers J. H., Tibboel D. et al. 1990. Formation and malformation of the enteric nervous system in mice: an organ culture study. *J Ped Surg* 25:627–31.

Nishikawa S., Sano F., Takagi K. et al. 2010. Spontaneous poorly differentiated carcinoma with cells positive for vimentin in a salivary gland of a young rat. *Toxicol Pathol* 38:315–8.

Nomura S., Yamaguchi H., Ogawa M. et al. 2005. Alterations in gastric mucosal lineages induced by acute oxyntic atrophy in wild-type and gastrin-deficient mice. *Am J Physiol Gastrointest Liver Physiol* 288:G362–75.

Nozaki K., Ogawa M., Williams J. A. et al. 2008. A molecular signature of gastric metaplasia arising in response to acute parietal cell loss. *Gastroenterology* 134:511–22.

Nozaki K., Weis V., Wang T. C. et al. 2009. Altered gastric chief cell lineage differentiation in histamine-deficient mice. *Am J Physiol Gastrointest Liver Physiol* 296:G1211–20.

Nyska A., Waner T., Zlotogorski A. et al. 1990. Animal model of human disease. Oxodipine-induced gingival hyperplasia in beagle dogs. *Am J Pathol* 137:737–9.

Ogasawara T., Hoensh H., Ohnhaus E. E. 1985. Distribution of glutathione and its related enzymes in the small intestinal mucosa of rats. *Arch Toxicol Suppl* 8:110–3.

Ogawa T., Maeda K., Tonai S. et al. 2003. Utilization of knockout mice to examine the potential role of gastric histamine H2-receptors in Menetrier's disease. *J Pharmacol Sci* 91:61–70.

Pace V., Wieczorek G., Pace M. et al. 2010. Spontaneous metastatic angiosarcoma of the tongue in a Wistar rat: morphological and immunohistochemical characterization. *Toxicol Pathol* 38:472–5.

Parkin C. A., Ingham P. W. 2007. The adventures of sonic hedgehog in development and repair. I hedgehog signaling in gastrointestinal development and disease. *Am J Physiol Gastrointest Liver Physiol* 294:G363–7.

Patyna S., Arrigoni C., Terron A. et al. 2008. Nonclinical safety evaluation of Sunitinib: a potent inhibitor of VEGF, PDGF, KIT, FLT3 and RET receptors. *Toxicol Pathol* 36:905–16.

Percy D. H., Wojcinski Z. W., Schunk M. K. 1989. Lacrimal glands in Wistar rats infected with sialodacryoadenitis virus. *Vet Pathol* 26:238–45.

Polk D. B., Peek R. M. 2010. *Helicobacter pylori*: gastric cancer and beyond. *Nat Rev Cancer* 10:403–14.

Poutahidis T., Tsangaris T., Kanakoudis G. et al. Helicobacter pylori-induced gastritis in experimentally infected conventional piglets. *Vet Pathol* 38:667–78.

Poynter D., Pick C. R., Harcourt R. A. et al. 1985. Association of long lasting unsurmountable histamine H2 blockade and gastric carcinoid tumors in the rat. *Gut* 26:1284–95.

Poynter D., Selway S. A., Papworth S. A. et al. 1986. Changes in the gastric mucosa of the mouse associated with long lasting unsurmountable histamine H2 blockade. *Gut* 27:1338–46.

Pritchard D. M., Przemeck S. M. 2004. Review article: how useful are the rodent animal models of gastric adenocarcinoma? *Aliment Pharmacol Ther* 19:841–59.

Proctor D. M., Gatto N. M., Hong S. J. et al. 2007. Mode-of-action framework for evaluating the relevance of rodent forestomach tumors in cancer risk assessment. *Toxicol Sci* 98:313–26.

Radi Z. 2009. Pathophysiology of cyclooxygenase inhibition in animal models. *Toxicol Pathol* 37:34–46.

Radtke F., Clevers H. 2005. Self-renewal and cancer of the gut: two sides of a coin. *Science* 307:1904–9.

Ramiro-Ibáñez F., Trajkovic D., Jessen B. 2005. Gastric and pancreatic lesions in rats treated with a pan-CDK inhibitor. *Toxicol Pathol* 33:784–91.

Rees J., Spencer A., Wilson S. et al. 1997. Time course of stomach mineralization, plasma, and urinary changes after a single intravenous administration of gadolinium(III) chloride in the male rat. *Toxicol Pathol* 25:582–9.

Reindel J. F., Pilcher G. D., Gough A. W. et al. 1996. Recombinant human epidermal growth factor 1-48-induced structural changes in the digestive tract of cynomolgus monkeys (*Macaca fascicularis*). *Toxicol Pathol* 24:669–80.

Renes I. B., Verburg M., Bulsing N. P. et al. 2002. Protection of the Peyer's patch-associated crypt and villus epithelium against methotrexate-induced damage is based on its distinct regulation of proliferation. *J Pathol* 198:60–8.

Reuter B. K., Davies N. M., Wallace J. L. 1997. Nonsteroidal anti-inflammatory drug enteropathy in rats: role of permeability, bacteria, and enterohepatic circulation. *Gastroenterology* 112:109–17.

Reni: Revised guides for organ sampling and trimming in rats and mice. Available at http://reni.item.fraunhofer.de/reni/trimming/index.php (accessed January 2012).

Roepke T. K., Anantharam A., Kirchhoff P. et al. 2006. The KCNE2 potassium channel ancillary subunit is essential for gastric acid secretion. *J Biol Chem* 281:23740–7.

Roepke T. K., Purtell K., King E. C. et al. 2010. Targeted deletion of Kcne2 causes gastritis cystica profunda and gastric neoplasia. *PLoS One* 5:e11451.

Rogers A. B., Taylor N. S., Whary M. T. et al. 2005. *Helicobacter pylori* but not high salt induces gastric intraepithelial neoplasia in B6129 mice. *Cancer Res* 65:10709–15.

Rozman K. 1988. Disposition of xenobiotics: species differences. *Toxicol Pathol* 16:123–9.

Rubin B. P., Antonescu C. R., Scott-Browne J. P. et al. 2005. A knock-in mouse model of gastrointestinal stromal tumor harboring kit K641E. *Cancer Res* 65:6631–9.

Rubio C.A, Befrits R. 2009. Increased lysozyme expression in gastric biopsies with intestinal metaplasia and pseudopyloric metaplasia. *Clin Exp Med* 2:248–53.

Sambruy Y., Ferruzza S., Ranaldi G. et al. 2001. Intestinal cell culture models. *Cell Biol Toxicol* 17:301–17.

Sato T., van Es J. H., Snippert H. J. et al. 2011. Paneth cells constitute the niche for Lgr5 stem cells in intestinal crypts. *Nature* 469:415–9.

Savage N. W., Barber M. T., Adkins K. F. 1986. Pigmentary changes in the rat oral mucosa following antimalarial therapy. *J Oral Pathol* 15:468–71.

Searfoss G. H., Jordan W H., Calligaro D. O. et al. 2003. Adipsin, a biomarker of gastrointestinal toxicity mediated by a functional g secretase inhibitor. *J Biol Chem* 278:46107–16.

Seitz S., Boelsterli U. A. 1998. Diclofenac acyl glucuronide, a major biliary metabolite, is directly involved in small intestinal injury of rats. *Gastroenterology* 115:1476–82.

Shackelford C. C., Elwell M. R. 1999. Small and large intestine, and mesentery. In *Pathology of the mouse* (Ed R. Maronpot), Cache River Press, Saint Louis, MO, pp. 81–118.

Shao J., Sartor R. B., Dial E. et al. 2000. Expression of intrinsic factor in rat and murine gastric mucosal cell lineages is modified by inflammation. *Am J Pathol* 157:1197–205.

Shin J. M., Sachs G. 2008. Pharmacology of proton pump inhibitors. *Curr Gastroenterol Rep* 10:528–34.

Simon W. A., Herrmann M., Klein T. et al. 2007. Soraprazan: setting new standards in inhibition of gastric acid secretion. *J Pharmacol Exp Ther* 321(3):866–74.

Singer I. I., Kawka D. W., Scott S. et al. 1991. Inhibitors of 3-hydroxy-3-methylglutaryl coenzyme A reductase induce reductase accumulation and altered lamellar bodies in rat forestomach keratinocytes. *Arterioscler Thromb* 11:1156–65.

Solcia E., Capella C., Fiocca R. et al. 1998. Disorders of the endocrine system. In *Pathology of the Gastrointestinal Tract* (Eds S. C. Ming and H. Goldman), Williams and Wilkins, Philadelphia, pp. 295–322.

Solomon L., Mansor S., Mallon P. et al. 2010. The dextran sulphate sodium (DSS) model of colitis: an overview. *Comp Clin Pathol* 19:235–9.

Spencer A. J., Barbolt T. A., Henry D. C. et al. 1989. Gastric morphological changes including carcinoid tumors in animals treated with a potent hypolipidemic agent, ciprofibrate. *Toxicol Pathol* 17:7–15.

Stappenbeck T. S., Miyoshi H. 2009. The role of stromal cells in tissue regeneration and wound repair. *Science* 324:1666–9.

Stevens C. E. 1980. The gastrointestinal tract of mammals: major variations. In *Comparative Physiology: Primitive Mammals* (Eds K. Schmidt-Nielsen, L. Bolis, and C. R. Taylor), University Press, New York, pp. 52–62.

Stinson S. F., Kovatch R. M. 1990. Tumors of the upper digestive tract (oral cavity, esophagus, forestomach). In *Atlas of Tumor Pathology of the Fischer Rat* (Eds S. F. Stinson, H. M. Schuller, and G. K. Reznik), CRC Press, Boca Raton, pp. 69–93.

Stockham S. L., Scott M. A. 2008a. Exocrine pancreas and intestine. In *Fundamentals of Veterinary Clinical Pathology*, 2nd edition, Blackwell Publishing, Ames, IA, pp. 739–62.

Stockham S. L., Scott M. A. 2008b. Monovalent electrolytes and osmolality. In *Fundamentals of Veterinary Clinical Pathology*, 2nd edition, Blackwell Publishing, Ames, IA, pp. 497–557.

Streett C. S., Robertson J. L., Crissman J. W. 1988. Morphologic stomach findings in rats and mice treated with the H2 receptor antagonists, ICI 125.211 and ICI 162.846. *Toxicol Pathol* 16:299–304.

Stumpel F., Scholtka B., Jungermann K. 2000. Stimulation by portal insulin of intestinal glucose absorption via hepatoenteral nerves and prostaglandin e2 in the isolated, jointly perfused small intestine and liver of the rat. *Ann NY Acad Sci* 915:111–6.

Sui G., Zhou S., Wang J. et al. 2006. Mitochondrial DNA mutations in preneoplastic lesions of the gastrointestinal tract: a biomarker for early detection of cancer. *Mol Cancer* 5:73–81.

Sundberg J. P., Schlegel R., Jenson A. B. 1998. Mucosotropic papillomavirus infections. *Lab Anim Sci* 48:240–2.

Syder A. J., Karam S. M., Mills J. C. et al. 2004. A transgenic mouse model of metastatic carcinoma involving transdifferentiation of a gastric epithelial lineage progenitor to a neuroendocrine phenotype. *Proc Natl Acad Sci U S A* 101:4471–6.

Takagi H., Jhappan C., Sharp R. et al. 1992. Hypertrophic gastropathy resembling Ménétrier's disease in transgenic mice overexpressing transforming growth factor alpha in the stomach. *J Clin Invest* 90:1161–7.

Takahashi M., Hasegawa R. 1990. Tumors of the stomach. In *Pathology of Tumors in Laboratory Animals. Vol I. Tumors of the Rat*, 2nd edition (Eds V. S. Turusov and U. Mohr), IARC Scientific Publications No. 99, Lyon, pp. 129–57.

Takaishi S., Tu S., Dubeykovskaya Z. A. et al. 2009. Gastrin is an essential cofactor for helicobacter-associated gastric corpus carcinogenesis in C57BL/6 mice. *Am J Pathol* 175:365–75.

Tamura M., Hirayam K., Itoh K. 1996. Comparison of colonic bacterial enzymes in gnotobiotic mice monoassociated with different intestinal bacteria. *Microbiol Ecol Health Dis* 9:287–94.

Tanabe T., Murata I., Karasuyama M. 2003. Immunoelectron microscopic study for histamine in the gastric enterochromaffin-like cells of rats treated with the proton pump inhibitor lansoprazole. *Histochem Cell Biol* 120:401–8.

Ten Hagen K. G., Balys M. M., Tabak L. A. et al. 2002. Analysis of isoproterenol-induced changes in parotid gland gene expression. *Physiol Genomics* 8:107–14.

Thoolen B., Koster H., van Kolfschoten A. et al. 2002. Gastric neuroendocrine tumors in a 2-year oncogenicity study with CD-1 mice. *Toxicol Pathol* 30(3):322–7.

Tsuji S., Sun W. H., Tsujii M. et al. 2002. Lansoprazole induces mucosal protection through gastrin receptor-dependent up-regulation of cyclooxygenase-2 in rats. *J Pharmacol Exp Ther* 303:1301–8.

Turnbaugh P. J., Ley R. E., Mahowald M. A. et al. 2006. An obesity-associated gt microbiome with increased capacity for energy harvest. *Nature* 444:1027–31.

Turnbaugh P. J., Ridaura V. K., Faith J. J. et al. 2009. The effect of diet on the human gut microbiome: a meta-genomic analysis in humanized gnotobiotic mice. *Sci Transl Med* 1:1–10.

Uchida K., Kado S., Ando M. et al. 2001. A mucinous histochemical study on malignancy of aberrant crypt foci (ACF) in rat colon. *J Vet Med Sci* 63:145–9.

Ueyama H., Yao T., Nakashima Y. et al. 2010. Gastric adenocarcinoma of fundic gland type (chief cell predominant type): proposal for a new entity of gastric adenocarcinoma. *Am J Surg Pathol* 34:609–19.

van den Brink G. 2007. Hedgehog signaling in development and homeostasis of the gastrointestinal tract. *Physiol Rev* 87:1343–75.

Van den Bulck K., Decostere A., Baele M. et al. 2005. Identification of non-*Helicobacter pylori* spiral organisms in gastric samples from humans, dogs, and cats. *J Clin Microbiol* 43:2256–60.

Vidal J. D., Mirabile R. C., Thomas H. C. 2008. Evaluation of the cynomolgus monkey stomach: recommendations for standard sampling procedures in nonclinical safety studies. *Toxicol Pathol* 36:250–5.

Vidrich A., Buzan J. M., De La Rue S. A. et al. 2006. Physiology of the gastrointestinal stem cells. In *Physiology of the Gastrointestinal Tract*, 4th edition (Ed L. R. Johnson), Academic Press, Waltham, MA, pp. 307–44.

von Furstenberg R. J., Gulati A. S., Bassi A. et al. 2011. Sorting mouse jejuna cells with CD24 yields a population with characteristics of intestinal stem cells. *Am J Physiol Gastrointest Liver Physiol* 300:G409–17.

Walsh C. 1994. Methods in gastrointestinal toxicology. In *Principles and Methods in Toxicology*, 3rd edition (Ed A. W. Hayes), Raven Press, New York, pp. 895–916.

Walsh K. M., Gough A. W. 1989. Hypopigmentation in dogs treated with an inhibitor of platelet aggregation. *Toxicol Pathol* 17:549–53.

Wang J., Hauer-Jensen M. 2003. Radiation toxicity and proteinase-activated receptors. *Drug Dev Res* 60:1–8.

Wargovich M. J., Brown V. R., Morris J. 2010. Aberrant crypt foci: the case for inclusion as a biomarker for colon cancer. *Cancers* 2:1705–16.

Watanabe H., Jass J. R., Sobin L. H. 1990. Histological typing of oesophageal and gastric tumors. In *WHO, International Histological Classification of Tumors*, 2nd edition, Springer Verlag, Berlin, pp. 19–39.

Wee A., Kang J. Y., Teh M. 1992. *Helicobacter pylori* and gastric cancer: correlation with gastritis, intestinal metaplasia, and tumor histology. *Gut* 33:1029–32.

Westwood F. R., Iswaran T. J., Greaves P. 1991. Long-term effects of an inotropic phosphodiesterase inhibitor (ICI153,110) on the rat salivary gland, Harderian gland, and intestinal mucosa. *Toxicol Pathol* 19:214–23.

Westwood F. R., Jones D. V., Aldridge A. 1996. The synovial membrane, liver and tongue: target organs for a Ricin A-chain immunotoxin (ZD0490). *Toxicol Pathol* 24:477–83.

Wisler J. A., Afshari C., Fielden M. et al. 2011. RAF inhibition causes extensive multiple tissue hyperplasia and urinary bladder neoplasia in the rat. *Toxicol Pathol* 39:809–22.

Wlodarska M., Willing B., Keeney K. M. et al. 2011. Antibiotic treatment alters the colonic mucus layer and predisposes the host to exacerbated *Citrobacter rodentium*-induced colitis. *Inf Immun* 79: 1536–45.

Woods S. C., D'Alessio D. A. 2008. Central control of body weight and appetite. *J Clin Endocrinol Metab* 93(11 Suppl 1):S37–50.

Yanez J. A., Teng X. W., Roupe K. A. et al. 2003. Chemotherapy induced gastrointestinal toxicity in rats: involvement of mitochondrial DNA, gastrointestinal permeability and cyclooxygenase-2. *J Pharm Pharmaceut Sci* 6:308–14.

Ziv E., Bendayan M. 2000. Intestinal absorption of peptides through the enterocytes. *Microsc Res Tech* 49:346–52.

10 Liver, Gallbladder, and Exocrine Pancreas

Russell C. Cattley, James A. Popp, and Steven L. Vonderfecht

CONTENTS

10.1 LIVER

10.1.1 Introduction

The liver is an important target organ for toxicity. It is especially susceptible to toxic agents absorbed from the gastrointestinal (GI) tract as well as substances that must be metabolically activated to produce cellular injury. In addition, the liver is susceptible to carcinogenesis, notably in rodents, which are typically used in long-term studies to assess carcinogenic activity for predicting risk to humans. Most importantly, hepatotoxicity in humans has been a major reason for product development failures and withdrawal or significant limitation in use of marketed products (Chen et al. 2011). Since the liver performs critical functions to support the life of the organism, significant injury to the liver, ultimately leading to liver failure in humans, often results in death unless its function can be restored by transplantation (Soltys et al. 2010).

The liver is a multilobed organ located in the cranial abdomen (Si-Tayeb et al. 2010). It has two blood supplies, including an arterial supply via the hepatic artery and a venous supply via the portal vein. Following passage through the microcirculation, blood exits the liver via the hepatic veins, which enter the caudal vena cava. The liver excretes bile, which, in many species, flows from the liver to the gallbladder via the common hepatic duct and is conducted from the gallbladder to the duodenum via the common bile duct. In some species, notably rats, there is no gallbladder, and bile is directly secreted from the liver into the duodenum.

The liver parenchyma has a generally similar gross and microscopic appearance among various mammalian species. The liver consists of lobes, which vary in number and shape between species but have consistent anatomic features across species. In toxicology studies, sample collection of the liver should be consistently conducted for histopathology and for other endpoints since differences in response may be noted between different lobes and even within a single lobe of the liver. This includes the protocol-defined lobes as well as the position and orientation for histopathology. Consistency of this sampling in small animals such as rats and mice will often enable identification of individual lobes from sections based upon the two-dimensional appearance of the sections.

In the embryo, the liver arises from foregut endoderm (Si-Tayeb et al. 2010). Formation is believed to be the response to fibroblast growth factor (FGF)-1 and FGF-2 produced by the mesoderm of the developing heart. A liver bud from the anterior foregut endoderm is the first morphological structure observed in hepatic organogenesis. A variety of developmental pathways regulate the further growth and differentiation of the hepatic parenchyma, as well as its vascularization. The fetal liver is transiently colonized by hematopoietic progenitors and is the source of fetal blood cells. Neonatal mammals have remnants of hematopoietic tissue that are not retained during postnatal maturation. However, in instances of extreme demand or inadequate bone marrow response, livers of adult animals may contain foci of hematopoietic tissue.

The parenchymal cell of the liver, the hepatocyte, is responsible for the key metabolic and exocrine functions of the liver and is most often the target cell of hepatotoxicity. Hepatocytes are structurally arranged in cords that are lined by a specialized sinusoidal endothelium that is fenestrated and lacks basement membrane (Braet and Wisse 2002). This facilitates free exchange of blood solutes with the sub-endothelial membrane of the hepatocytes. Hepatocytes are connected to each other by gap junctions and tight junctions, the latter forming bile canaliculi, which are lined by the plasma membrane at the excretory pole of adjacent hepatocytes. The canaliculi form the channels for bile flow from the hepatocytes through the canals of Herring, into the portal bile ducts that ultimately merge and conduct the bile out of the liver.

The blood supply to the hepatocytes via the sinusoids reflects a mixture of two sources: the major one (75%) being the portal vein wherein the flow is composed of blood exiting from the splanchnic beds (spleen, pancreas, stomach, small and large intestines) and the minor one (25%) from the hepatic artery derived from abdominal aortic supply. Blood flow arrives via small branches of the portal vein and hepatic artery that travel together along the portal areas of the liver parenchyma. These portal areas, which also contain the smallest bile ducts and a meager stromal component, define the periphery of adjacent hepatic structures known as lobules. The lobule is considered to be a microanatomic unit describing the organization of the hepatic tissue. At the center of each lobule is the small central vein, through which blood collects into larger veins and, ultimately, the caudal vena cava. Within this microarchitecture of the lobule, the blood flows from portal areas into the sinusoids and out through the central vein. The direction of blood flow across sinusoids accounts for metabolic differences between periportal and pericentral hepatocytes, influencing susceptibility to drug-induced injury (Jungermann and Kietzmann 1996).

Residing along the intravascular surface of the hepatic sinusoids are the Kupffer cells, which are phagocytic cells that share common lineage and many characteristics with monocytes derived from the bone marrow (Klein et al. 2007). These cells are activated by opsonized and particulate materials in the circulation, produce cytokines, and locally, by phagocytosis, can perpetuate injury and/or resolve necrotic tissue.

Among other nonparenchymal cells, the stellate cells (sometimes called *Ito cells*) reside in the peri-sinusoidal space (so-called space of Disse) between the endothelial-lined sinusoids and the cords of hepatocytes (Senoo 2004). The stellate cells store vitamin A and other lipid substances and may participate in local repair of injured tissue by differentiating into myofibroblasts. Another less common cell type residing along the sinusoidal endothelial surface was originally termed the *pit cell* but actually represents both natural killer (NK) and natural killer-T (NK-T) cells (Gao et al. 2009). In fetal liver, the space also contains hematopoietic tissue, but in adult animals, the bone marrow is the primary site of hematopoiesis, and the liver contains only readily detectable hematopoietic cells during conditions of extreme demand.

10.1.2 HEPATOCELLULAR DEGENERATION, NECROSIS, AND REGENERATION

Hepatocellular injury caused by drugs and chemical agents may lead to cellular degeneration and death, which typically can be recognized by light microscopy and, in many cases, by altered clinical pathology parameters. An important role of the toxicological pathologist is to recognize and describe the pattern of injury, in addition to identifying no-effect levels and reversibility. The injury is commonly recognized as occurring in a lobular pattern, in which the mechanism of toxicity accounts for localization of injury and its histological manifestation to central, periportal, or midzonal regions of the lobule (Thoolen et al. 2010). Less commonly, injury may affect random areas that are focal and smaller than the lobule or may affect the entirety of some or many lobules in various regions of the liver.

Hepatocytes may undergo sublethal injury, characterized by cellular enlargement and pallor due to fluid accumulation. By transmission electron microscopy (TEM), fluid accumulates within the endoplasmic reticulum (ER) and/or mitochondria (Figure 10.1a). This change is recognized as hepatocellular degeneration and may be reversible or may progress to irreversible injury (though degeneration is not an obligatory step toward irreversible injury). Theoretically, irreversible injury may involve two distinct (but in many instances simultaneous and overlapping) types of processes, leading to necrosis (Malhi et al. 2006). The first type is oncotic necrosis, which reflects the inability

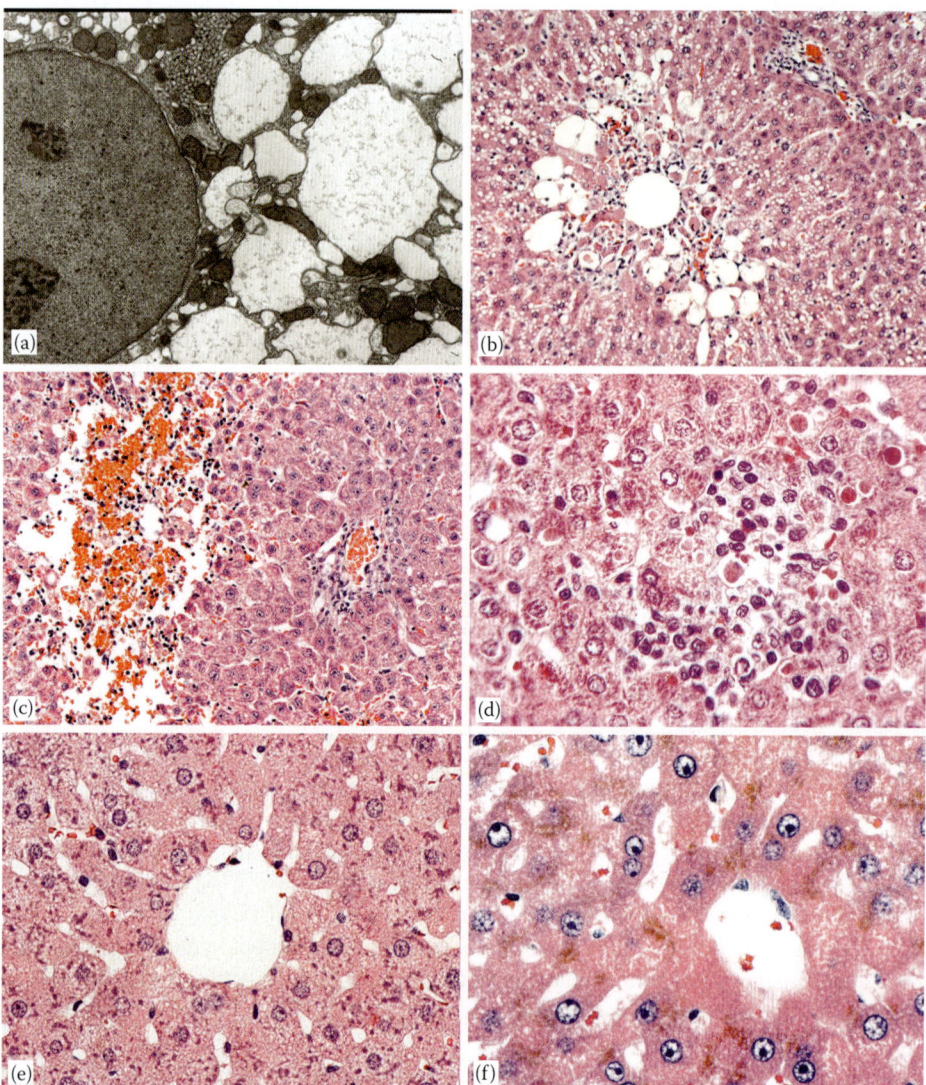

FIGURE 10.1 (a) Hepatocellular fluid accumulation within ER, electron micrograph. This change often leads to a decrease in cytoplasmic staining intensity by light microscopy, referred to as hydropic degeneration. (b) Ballooning degeneration of hepatocytes adjacent to zonal (central lobular) necrosis. (c) Zonal (central lobular) hemorrhage associated with hepatocellular necrosis. This finding indicates injury and necrosis of sinusoidal endothelial cells. (d) Focal necrosis of hepatoctyes. There is necrosis and loss of hepatocytes as well as accumulation of mononuclear inflammatory cells. (e) Hepatocellular hypertrophy, central lobular. The appearance of homogeneously eosinophilic cytoplasm is suggestive of classic P450 inducers such as phenobarbital. (f) Hepatocellular hypertrophy, central lobular. The appearance of granular intensely eosinophilic cytoplasm is suggestive of peroxisome proliferators such as gemfibrozil. The pericanalicular brown pigment is lipofuscin.

of the cell to adapt and maintain homeostasis, leading to ion shifts, calcium influx, and failure to maintain the cell membrane. The other form is apoptotic necrosis, which reflects the activation of specific signal transduction pathways that lead to enzymatic destruction of nuclear constituents but maintenance of the cell membrane and organelles, at least in the initial phase.

Practically speaking, it is difficult to consistently distinguish oncotic from apoptotic necrosis by light microscopy or by any other means. The processes are overlapping in that both may occur in the same population of injured hepatocytes and probably because oncotic necrosis may supervene in hepatocytes about to undergo apoptosis. In addition, the light microscopic criteria for distinguishing oncotic from apoptotic necrosis are time-dependent, so that an assessment that does not allow sampling times to approximate critical events may be too limited (Bursch et al. 1986).

By light microscopy, oncotic necrosis generally appears as coagulative necrosis in individual and groups of hepatocytes, with retention of cell outlines, increased cytoplasm eosinophilia, and nuclear changes such as pyknosis, karyorrhexis, and karyolysis. Inflammatory cells and activated Kupffer cells are often present but may be quite limited and partly dependent on the time point evaluated relative to the toxic insult. In contrast, apoptosis is more often limited to single or very few cells, perhaps reflecting the extremely short duration of time (hours) during which affected hepatocytes may be recognized microscopically, a feature that has been established through time course studies. The cells are typically round and may be fragmented into multiple round "apoptotic bodies." These affected hepatocytes often have distinct borders reflecting their ultimate locations inside phagocytic vacuoles within adjacent hepatocytes. Inflammatory cell infiltrate and Kupffer cell activation are not typical features of apoptosis (Levin 1999; Levin et al. 1999).

The distinction between oncotic and apoptotic forms of hepatocellular necrosis has been described by TEM. In oncotic necrosis, the cell organelles undergo swelling and breakage, and the cell membrane integrity is lost. The nucleus also undergoes dissolution. In apoptotic necrosis, the cell organelles remain intact, and the cell membrane forms blebs but remains intact. The nucleus in apoptotic hepatocytes will have peripheral aggregation of chromatin but often remains intact until late in the process when it becomes fragmented. Apoptotic bodies within the cytoplasm of adjacent hepatocytes and Kupffer cells may also be observed by TEM (Dini et al. 2002).

Various light microscopic methods have been used to characterize apoptosis, but these methods are not entirely specific. Apoptotic cells have been identified by immunohistochemical detection of activated caspase 3, an important step in the apoptotic signal transduction pathway. Alternatively, the detection of endonuclease-mediated nuclear DNA fragmentation by the TUNEL (terminal deoxynucleotidyl transferase dUTP nick end labeling) method has been used to identify cells undergoing apoptosis. Both activated caspase 3 and TUNEL have, on occasion, been observed to label cells undergoing oncotic necrosis, so that lack of specificity makes reliability uncertain.

There are several common mechanisms of hepatocellular necrosis (Grattagliano et al. 2009). Some drugs and chemicals may deplete critical proteins by reacting with sulfhydryl groups, typically upon overwhelming the cellular concentration of glutathione (Han et al. 2006). Others interfere with mitochondrial energy metabolism, so that adenosine triphosphate is depleted and homeostatic ion and fluid balance cannot be maintained (Scatena et al. 2007; Jaeschke et al. 2002). Still others may target the cytoskeleton (Wickstrom et al. 1995) or block maintenance of protein synthesis either by blocking transcription or translation (Herzog et al. 1975; Yu et al. 1988). The underlying mechanism of acute hepatocellular injury is seldom recognized by the nature of the light or electron microscopic findings but may, in some instances, be elucidated by specialized biochemical or molecular biological investigations.

The loss of hepatocytes through necrosis decreases the functional mass of the liver, and, with few exceptions, this leads to a regenerative response by hepatocytes. The regenerative response occurs in surviving hepatocytes, which undergo proliferation due to a complex interplay between endocrine and paracrine growth factors and activation of signal transduction (Michalopoulos 2010; Michalopoulos and DeFrances 1997). Although hepatocytes in the normal adult liver are often considered to be quiescent, it is their relatively long life span (several months) that results in very low demand for renewal. However, a decreased number of hepatocytes due to drug-induced injury will result in regenerative proliferation of hepatocytes that restores the functional mass. This increased proliferation is striking if there is acute and substantial injury or loss. Regenerative proliferation is not limited to drug-induced injury, as viral injury and surgical hepatectomy will also elicit a considerable hepatoproliferative response if hepatocyte loss is substantial.

The normally low frequency of proliferating hepatocytes in the adult liver enables regeneration to be readily monitored by a variety of approaches. One approach to monitoring hepatocellular proliferation is by conventional histology. By light microscopy, hepatocellular regeneration may be detected as increased mitotic figures or by nuclear changes such as nucleolar enlargement and, usually, increase in cytoplasmic basophilia. Hepatocellular regeneration may also be detected histologically as an increased frequency of certain markers using techniques that directly or indirectly label proliferating cells. Among direct methods, immunohistochemical detection of proliferation markers such as Ki67, phospho-histone H3, or proliferating cell nuclear antigen (PCNA) has been utilized (Nolte et al. 2005). Hepatocellular proliferation may also be monitored indirectly by analysis of replicative DNA synthesis in nuclei following premortem labeling with tritiated thymidine (detected autoradiographically) or the thymidine analog, bromodeoxyuridine (detected immunohistochemically) (Eldridge et al. 1990). An advantage of the indirect labeling method is that the duration of labeling can be extended to integrate the frequency of S-phase over time. This increases the sensitivity and reduces the variability in response that may occur among groups of animals. Furthermore, the use of both direct and indirect labeling methods for proliferating cells is amenable to automated image analysis to increase the number of cells evaluated.

10.1.2.1 Morphological Patterns of Hepatocellular Necrosis

Centrilobular necrosis is the most common pattern of liver necrosis. It is typically oncotic or coagulative necrosis and involves hepatocytes adjacent to the central vein in many lobules (Hinson et al. 2010; Thoolen et al. 2010). This pattern of necrosis following treatment with chemicals or drugs has been established for some time (Graham 1915). The central lobular areas of necrosis not only can affect a single row of hepatocytes around the central vein but also can extend to involve up to one-half the width of the lobule. In some instances, the non-necrotic hepatocytes immediately peripheral to the necrotic area are enlarged and pale, reflecting fluid accumulation (sometimes referred to as "balloon cells"; Figure 10.1b) or the presence of lipid-containing vacuoles (Popp et al. 1978). Upon gross examination, the capsular and cut surfaces of the liver with significant central lobular necrosis may be characterized by a prominently visible lobular architecture but not distinguishable from other lobular patterns of necrosis.

Resolution of centrilobular necrosis is initiated by phagocytic elimination of dead hepatocytes by activated Kupffer cells and infiltrating leukocytes. In most, but not all, cases, regeneration occurs by mitotic cell division of surviving hepatocytes with restoration of the normal architecture of cords of hepatocytes with intervening sinusoids. In some instances where the sinusoidal endothelium is damaged or there is persistent or repeated episodic hepatocellular injury with inadequate regeneration, repair may involve activation of stellate cells that are able to differentiate into myofibroblasts with production of collagen, resulting in a scar. There are potential species (and in humans, interindividual) differences in the likelihood of repair by fibrosis. Although not entirely refractory, rodents are generally less likely to exhibit repair by collagenous scarring compared to dogs and macaques. With any animal species, fibrosis is viewed as a significant concern for safety assessment because it is most typically associated with significant parenchymal injury and considered irreversible.

Central lobular necrosis is a common pattern observed with drugs and chemicals that are not injurious as parent compounds but require metabolic activation resulting in hepatocellular injury caused by a toxic metabolite. Hepatocytes are heterogeneous with respect to xenobiotic metabolism, and those CYP enzymes most often responsible for metabolic activation are expressed at the highest levels in central lobular hepatocytes (Buhler et al. 1992). As a result, these hepatocytes achieve the highest rates of formation of reactive metabolites and are thereby most susceptible to injury (Sinclair et al. 2000).

In rare instances, reactive metabolites may be released by hepatocytes and cause injury to adjacent sinusoidal endothelium (Jin et al. 2003). When this occurs, centrilobular hepatocellular necrosis may be associated with hemorrhage (Figure 10.1c). Damage to the sinusoidal architecture increases the likelihood that repair will involve some degree of scar formation.

Periportal necrosis, while less common than centrilobular necrosis, is occasionally encountered in the evaluation of drugs (Graichen et al. 1985). It is typically an oncotic or coagulative necrosis and involves hepatocytes adjacent to the portal areas in many lobules. The periportal areas of necrosis can affect only those hepatocytes immediately adjacent to the portal areas but can also involve up to one-half the width of the lobule. Normally, hepatocytes form the so-called limiting plate where cords of hepatocytes converge at the margin of the portal area. Disruption of the limiting plate is a feature of periportal necrosis. Upon gross examination, the capsular and cut surfaces of the liver with significant periportal lobular necrosis may be characterized by a prominently visible lobular architecture but not distinguishable from other lobular patterns of necrosis.

Resolution of periportal necrosis involves phagocytic elimination of dead hepatocytes by activated Kupffer cells and infiltrating leukocytes. In most cases, regeneration occurs by mitotic cell division of surviving hepatocytes with restoration of the normal architecture of cords of hepatocytes with intervening sinusoids. In some instances, proliferation of bile duct epithelial cells in the adjacent portal areas may also be observed. In addition, proliferation of oval cells, believed to derive from cells lining the connection between the canaliculi and the bile ducts (canal of Hering), may accompany periportal necrosis (see discussion on oval cells below). If regeneration is limited or injury is prolonged, deposition of collagenous scar may occur in the periportal areas. The development of collagenous scar may result from stellate cells but may also involve fibroblasts derived from portal connective tissue.

The appearance of periportal necrosis raises several possible mechanisms of pathogenesis. One potential mechanism is suggested by the concentration gradient across the lobule, whereby toxic substances that are rapidly removed by hepatocytes reach the highest possible concentration nearest the region where portal and arterial blood enters the lobule. Another potential mechanism for the increased sensitivity of periportal hepatocytes may be the higher oxygen tension in this region of the lobule. This factor has been established for the sensitivity of hepatocytes to some compounds that depend upon high oxygen tension for metabolism to a reactive metabolite (Belinsky et al. 1986). A third reason may be the participation of Kupffer cells in hepatocellular injury, as Kupffer cells in the periportal region are slightly more numerous and may have a lower threshold for activation (Bykov et al. 2003). Despite the experimental evidence supporting these potential mechanisms, the actual mechanism for any particular instance of periportal necrosis cannot be discerned from the morphological features of the lesion.

Midzonal necrosis is a rarely observed pattern of liver injury. It is characterized by oncotic necrosis that appears coagulative by light microscopy and is specifically seen as bands of affected hepatocytes that are located midway between the periportal and central lobular hepatocytes. Resolution and repair of midzonal necrosis is similar to that for other lobular patterns of necrosis, to the extent that it involves phagocytic removal of necrotic hepatocytes and regeneration by adjacent viable hepatocytes. Although plausible, however, the possibility of repair by collagenous scarring has not been described. Upon gross examination, the capsular and cut surfaces of the liver with significant midzonal necrosis may be normal or have only a slight accentuation of the lobular appearance.

The mechanistic basis of midzonal hepatocellular injury is unknown. It has been observed with selected toxic substances (Mackie et al. 2009), and the midzonal necrosis observed with one of these toxic substances in one species often fails to produce a similar pattern of necrosis in studies conducted in another species. There is recent evidence that midzonal necrosis might arise due to ischemia following changes in hepatic sinusoidal circulation associated with lipopolysaccharide-mediated increases in induced nitric oxide synthase (iNOS) (Rose et al. 2006).

Diffuse necrosis (synonymous with panlobular necrosis or massive necrosis) is a consequence of hepatocellular injury involving the entirety of some or many lobules in various regions of the liver. It appears as coagulative necrosis of entire lobules and typically affects some or many adjacent lobules in one or more regions of the liver. Diffuse necrosis does not affect the entire liver. Upon gross examination, the capsular surface in affected areas may often appear collapsed.

Resolution of diffuse necrosis involves the removal of dead hepatocytes by phagocytic cells. However, the extensive nature of the lesions and the distance of penetration into the necrotic parenchyma by neutrophils and monocytes probably allow the presence of necrosis to persist for longer periods of time than that observed in other patterns of injury. Often the neutrophils and macrophages may appear more numerous at the periphery of areas of necrosis. Regeneration of hepatocytes may contribute to repair, but the lack of surviving hepatocytes in some lobules makes this prospect slow or unlikely to occur. Areas of connective tissue accumulation may occur, but it is often difficult to ascertain the degree to which this results from active collagen production and/or collapse of preexisting matrix.

The presence of massive necrosis should alert the pathologist to ensure that a random versus selective distribution to one area or lobe should be documented and may be important in the consideration of mechanism. Several mechanisms have been suggested. One hypothesis is that extremely high doses of the toxic agent may favor its appearance and that incomplete mixing of portal blood in the relatively short portal vein can lead to preferential streaming of the toxic agent to achieve high concentrations in certain areas of the liver (Daniel et al. 2004).

Another theory for the pathogenesis of massive necrosis invokes the occurrence of pressure-induced ischemia, secondary to rapidly developing and marked adaptive hepatomegaly that may result from hepatocellular hypertrophy and/or hyperplasia (see below) (Maronpot et al. 2010). When diffuse necrosis occurs with hepatomegaly, the lesion is often noted in areas immediately subjacent to the capsule. This subcapsular pattern is reminiscent of necrosis observed in rats with tightly applied bandaging of the abdominal torso, where the pathogenesis is assumed to involve compression of the capsule of the liver (Parker and Gibson 1995). However, a review of a series of studies in rats (Amacher et al. 1998) suggested that the association of subcapsular necrosis with drug-induced hepatomegaly was inconsistent at best, leaving open the possibility that other drug effects could be as (or more) important in the pathogenesis.

Focal necrosis is an occasionally observed pattern of hepatocellular injury consisting of oncotic or apoptotic necrosis that affects individual or small discrete clusters of hepatocytes that are distributed randomly with respect to lobular location (Spencer et al. 1997). The necrotic hepatocytes are sometimes associated with mononuclear cells and/or neutrophils, and this is probably dependent on the time from the initial necrogenic insult (Figure 10.1d). The lesion appears to readily resolve by phagocytosis and regeneration and fibrosis, and generally does not recur. Focal necrosis is typically not detected upon gross examination. In toxicology studies, this pattern of necrosis may occur in association with test article treatment or may occur spontaneously. Careful comparison of the frequency and severity of this lesion among treatment and control groups (and in some instances, historical control groups) is necessary to determine its association with the test article. Due to the random location and variable frequency of this lesion, slight increases in incidence among treated animals are often not interpreted as treatment effects, unless the severity in affected animals is clearly increased.

Definitive mechanisms of focal necrosis as a response to toxic injury of hepatocytes have not been identified. The pattern resembles the response to infectious agents, and a role for immune response and cytokine-mediated hepatocellular injury has been theorized (Car et al. 1999; Shibayama et al. 1994). This raises the possibility that some instances of focal necrosis might be mediated by activation of Kupffer cells or NK cells.

10.1.2.2 Clinical Chemistry Biomarkers of Hepatocellular Injury

Beyond the application of light microscopy, clinical chemistry is also used to detect and monitor the severity and course of hepatocellular degeneration and necrosis. Several enzymes, notably alanine aminotransferase (ALT) and aspartate aminotransferase (AST), circulate in the blood, and their activities in sera or plasma are typically monitored. ALT and AST are sometimes monitored before and during the in-life phase of a toxicology study but, most frequently, at termination of the in-life and recovery phases. In medical parlance, ALT and AST are sometimes called "liver function tests (LFTs)," but this is a misnomer as elevated test results reflect injury, not function. Other enzyme activities have been similarly evaluated for monitoring liver injury, with some success, but none have been as commonly applied as ALT and AST. Elevations of circulating enzyme activities are most often attributable to increased release of enzyme from cells undergoing degeneration or oncotic necrosis.

Increased ALT is most commonly derived from injured hepatocytes, while increased AST may be derived from injured hepatocytes but also from injured skeletal and cardiac muscle. ALT is located in the cytosol, while AST is present in the cytosol and the mitochondria. It has been estimated that approximately 80% of hepatic AST is mitochondrial in rats, while 30%–40% of hepatic AST is mitochondrial in dogs (Solter 2005).

Hepatocellular degeneration (reversible injury) typically results in more subtle increases in ALT and cytosolic AST and has been attributed to widespread release of cytoplasmic blebs from the apical surface of the injured hepatocytes (Lemasters et al. 1983). These increases, attributable to reversible injury without histological evidence of necrosis, sometimes create an erroneous assumption that a disparity exists between the elevation of circulating enzyme and injury, since blebbing is not detected histologically. In contrast, substantial increases in ALT and AST (both cytosolic and mitochondrial) are associated with oncotic necrosis, when loss of membrane integrity leads to rapid and robust release of cytoplasmic proteins into the circulation. Increased ALT and AST are not usually attributable to apoptotic necrosis, as apoptotic cells and cell fragments are ingested and thus contained within neighboring viable hepatocytes, before the cell membrane becomes permeable.

The magnitude of increase in circulating ALT and AST associated with liver degeneration and necrosis depends on the rate of release into the circulation, so that the simultaneous release of enzyme from many cells is expected to cause greater increases than protracted release of enzyme from fewer cells. The levels of ALT and AST represent a steady state that depends on the rate of release and removal into and from the circulation, respectively. Steady-state levels may vary slightly between animals on study. In some studies with low group sizes, typically in dogs and nonhuman primates (large animals), comparing ALT and AST values to one or two pretest values will aid in accurately detecting treatment-related increases. Slight variation between repeated measurements in the same animal may be observed, but consistently increased values over pretreatment baselines may indicate that a subtle treatment effect is present if absolute values exceed concurrent controls. However, pretest values are seldom available in rodents, in part due to concern about the effects of prior sampling (always a larger fraction of blood volume is sampled in smaller animals) on results of subsequent collections.

Increases in ALT and AST are sometimes associated with compounds that are so-called "enzyme inducers." As will be discussed later in this chapter, these agents cause variable and often selective increases in hepatocellular enzymes that enable phase 1 (typically monooxygenation) and phase 2 (typically conjugation) drug metabolism. Hepatomegaly (due to hypertrophy and hyperplasia) and increased organellar content (often of smooth ER) of hepatocytes are sometimes associated with this response. A recent review notes this association but also cautions against an assumption of a causal relationship. As summarized, the available data collectively indicated that in the absence of hepatocellular injury, induction of drug metabolizing enzymes is not expected to be associated with consistent or substantive changes in ALT or AST (Ennulat et al. 2010). Rather, increases in ALT and AST were considered to reflect hepatobiliary insult rather than enzyme induction.

Among the various morphological patterns of oncotic necrosis, some are more likely to be associated with detectable elevations in ALT and AST. The lobular patterns of hepatocellular necrosis, namely, centrilobular, periportal, and midzonal patterns, are more likely to cause increased ALT and AST. ALT and AST elevations may be variably associated with focal necrosis. This variability is thought to reflect a lack of sensitivity in instances where the focal necrosis involves only a small fraction of the hepatocellular mass. In addition, focal lesions may lack synchrony that would enhance sensitivity. Diffuse necrosis often affects a significant portion of the liver, which should translate into elevations in ALT and AST. However, it has been suggested that any impairment of sinusoidal circulation in areas of multiple, adjacent, necrotic lobules might slow the entry of leaked proteins into the circulation and thus limit detection in the peripheral circulation.

Plasma proteins are removed from the circulation by the resident mononuclear phagocytes in tissues, especially in the liver and spleen (Kamimoto et al. 1985). There is evidence that the clearance of enzymes from the circulation may occur at different rates. In humans, the half-lives of ALT and mitochondrial AST (47 and 87 h, respectively) vary (Giannini et al. 2005), though the relative variability in other species has not been compared; thus, it is possible that the rate of rise and recovery among these enzyme markers may vary and that mononuclear phagocytes may assume other functions that compete with these clearance processes. Moreover, in certain instances, elevations in circulating ALT and AST have been associated with drugs that impair the function of mononuclear phagocytes in the absence of evidence of hepatocellular injury (Radi et al. 2011). In such cases, enzyme elevations are explained by prolonged retention in the circulation rather than an increased rate of release by injured hepatocytes into the circulation.

As may be inferred from the preceding discussion, ALT and AST enzyme levels are useful in the analysis of liver injury by potential therapeutic agents. These enzymes are often of interest in preclinical safety assessment because of their widespread utilization in clinical research, particularly in clinical trials of new drug candidates. Although there are subtle differences in the approaches to interpretation of these enzyme activities between preclinical and clinical studies, the specificity and sensitivity of these enzymes are generally accepted in both applications. It is important to understand the processes that cause and modify their release and subsequent clearance from the circulation to ensure that appropriate inferences are drawn from study datasets. (See Chapter 7 for additional discussion on ALT and AST.)

10.1.2.3 Differential Diagnosis

It is important to distinguish hepatocellular necrosis that is caused by the toxicity of a drug from that caused by other mechanisms. Among the patterns of necrosis, the zonal patterns (centrilobular, periportal, and midzonal) are practically never observed as spontaneous lesions, so that these findings are easily attributed to the test article. These forms of zonal necrosis and degeneration usually arise as direct effects of the toxic agent or toxic metabolite(s) of the administered agent, with one rare exception being centrilobular necrosis, which, in some instances, may be simulated by ischemic change secondary to circulatory shock. This is especially true for hypovolemic shock, as has been observed in association with hemorrhage secondary to intended but exaggerated pharmacologic activity of anticoagulant drugs in nonclinical toxicology studies. The presence of other findings in circulatory shock should prevent any confusion regarding this cause of centrilobular necrosis.

Diffuse necrosis is practically never observed as a spontaneous lesion. The threshold for considering this lesion as treatment-related is low. Though it may reflect a compound's toxicity, it is important to distinguish diffuse necrosis caused directly by toxins from infarction, which may or may not be attributed to the test article.

Focal necrosis is often observed as a background lesion. In untreated control animals, it may be associated with bacterial infections and endotoxemia. It also may occur for reasons that are not apparent (Spencer et al. 1997). Thus, it is very important to compare the incidence and severity of focal necrosis in treated and control groups and judge whether a treatment effect actually exists. In studies where the finding of focal necrosis is considered to be treatment related, it may be necessary to evaluate possible secondary effects. Focal necrosis may sometimes occur as the result of a test article that compromises intestinal integrity or significantly alters intestinal microflora. If secondary mechanisms cannot be identified, then it should be assumed that focal necrosis may have been caused by the test article.

10.1.2.4 Significance in Safety Assessment

In safety assessment, treatment-related hepatocellular necrosis is a significant issue that must be addressed for a compound to be considered a viable product candidate. First of all, evaluation of the dose response based on internal parameters of dose such as peak concentration or area under curve is an important exercise to see if the desired pharmacology can be achieved at doses significantly lower than the threshold for hepatocellular injury. Alternatively, in the case of grievous unmet need (such as cancer), the dose-response evaluation is crucial for selection of a reasonable starting dose in the clinic. It is also important to evaluate metabolite profiles for susceptible animal species and determine if the predicted metabolite profile for humans is similar and, if not, whether a reactive metabolite is responsible for hepatocellular injury. These investigations may suggest that the susceptible animal species is not appropriate for predicting risk in humans and that another species may be more appropriate.

Additional considerations are important in establishing the context in which hepatocellular necrosis may be observed. First of all, there should be evidence that noninvasive monitoring, usually through clinical chemistry parameters, will be effective in the clinical setting. Second, the transient or sustained nature of hepatocellular injury upon repeated dosing should be evaluated, as transient injury may not require as large a margin of safety as sustained injury. Finally, the reversibility of the effect should be established, although this consideration is probably more useful when the duration of systemic exposure after a single dose is short, as with small molecule drug candidates. However, for drug candidates with a long exposure after a single dose, such as proteins and monoclonal antibodies, establishing reversibility is difficult and less meaningful for clinical extrapolation.

10.1.3 CELLULAR ADAPTATIONS AND ACCUMULATIONS

Cellular adaptations and accumulations are frequently noted in the histological evaluation of the liver in toxicity studies but not upon gross examination. While the histological appearance of these changes may be subtle and require careful observation to detect, they can have important implications for determining the effects of an experimental agent. The type, character, and extent of the cellular alteration may provide a clue for further exploration of other less subtle hepatic effects or effects occurring in other organs. It is stressed that cellular changes should be used as a starting point for understanding the effects of drugs on the liver. Identification and diagnosis of a cellular change should never be considered as the final answer regarding the effect on the liver. While cellular adaptations and accumulations most frequently affect the hepatocyte, these changes may also be noted in other cell types, most notably the Kupffer cells.

10.1.3.1 Alterations in Hepatocyte Size and Number

In the normal liver, the size of hepatocytes is generally similar across the various lobular locations, though the central lobular hepatocytes may appear to be somewhat larger than the periportal hepatocytes, an observation supported by stereological analysis of rat liver (Schmucker et al. 1978). This difference in size is histologically quite subtle.

Hypertrophy of hepatocytes is a frequent response following drug administration in toxicity studies and is generally associated with increased liver size, grossly and/or by liver weight (Amacher et al. 1998). While hepatocellular hypertrophy is most frequently noted in rodents compared to other species, hypertrophy can also be observed in dogs and monkeys. When noted in rodents, a centrilobular distribution of the hypertrophic hepatocytes is the norm, though a periportal distribution can occasionally be noted. Hypertrophy is most frequently characterized by increased cytoplasm with little to no effect on the nuclear size, though nuclear size may be increased and in some cases associated with nuclear inclusions or increased ploidy. The histological characteristics of an enlarged cytoplasm are variable, ranging from vacuolation, the presence of cytoplasmic inclusions, and/or alterations of tinctorial properties, most frequently enhanced eosinophilia. If cytoplasmic vacuolation is not the cause of hepatocellular hypertrophy, the increased ER as a consequence of induction of P450-related enzymes is frequently the reason. Indeed, the histological appearance of hypertrophic hepatocytes is frequently interpreted as an indication that the drug is a "P450 inducer" in the species being evaluated. However, the toxicological pathologist should be careful not to over-commit based on the histological appearance. For example, drugs that cause peroxisome proliferation also cause hypertrophic hepatocytes with an eosinophilic cytoplasm. Peroxisome proliferation is characterized by a bright red, finely granular cytoplasm (Figure 10.1f) versus the homogeneously eosinophilic cytoplasm (Figure 10.1e) that generally characterizes the P450 inducers (Cattley and Popp 2002). The cytoplasmic features of peroxisome inducers are not always specific, as rare agents that cause mitochondrial proliferation result in a similar histological appearance (Reznik-Schuller and Lijinsky 1981). While the histological distinction between classic P450 inducers and peroxisome proliferating agents is possible in extreme cases, additional techniques should also be used to provide further direction for investigation. Biochemical parameters will provide confirmatory evidence and, often being more sensitive than histopathology, provide data to establish a no observed effect level for induction. Based on the experience of many toxicological pathologists who have compared histopathology to biochemical results, hypertrophy of hepatocytes can be appreciated only when enzyme induction is greater than 20%, as determined in in vivo enzyme induction studies. Similarly, pathologists are unlikely to observe hepatocellular hypertrophy when liver weight increases are less than 20% (Amacher et al. 1998).

While hepatocellular hypertrophy is often associated with ultrastructural and biochemical evidence of enzyme induction, the reverse is not commonly true. Some drugs may induce xenobiotic metabolizing enzymes (phase I [P450 monooxygenases] and/or phase II [conjugating enzymes]) without histological evidence of hypertrophy or ultrastructural (organellar) alterations. In particular, many drugs may induce CYP3A through activation of the pregnane-X-receptor (PXR) without causing significant hypertrophy or ultrastructural alterations (Maronpot et al. 2010). Another example is omeprazole, an atypical AhR-type inducer that increases CYP1A1 but does not cause hepatomegaly or hepatocellular hypertrophy (Kashfi et al. 1995).

Atrophy of hepatocytes is rarely observed in the histological evaluation of drug candidates. When present, there is generally no lobular distribution and no alteration in nuclear size. The mechanism of hepatocyte atrophy has been rarely investigated in drug evaluation studies. However, atrophy would be expected in cases where an agent causes inhibition of protein synthesis to a degree that was still compatible with cell viability and may also be observed in instances of chronic passive congestion (Yu et al. 1994) or prolonged starvation (Belloni et al. 1988).

Hyperplasia of hepatocytes is characterized by cell proliferation that causes or contributes to increased liver mass (hepatomegaly). Hyperplasia of hepatocytes may be difficult to assess by standard histological evaluation, in part due to the insensitivity of using light microscopic evaluation of routinely stained sections to detect mitotic figures. However, more sensitive methods (e.g., markers that directly or indirectly label proliferating cells, see below) often improve the ability to detect hepatocyte proliferation. Regardless of the method, the sampling interval for detection of proliferating hepatocytes is critical, as the hyperplasia that many drugs cause is transient. In such cases, proliferating hepatocytes may not be detected once the increase in liver weight has stabilized, even if drug treatment continues (Jones and Clarke 1993; Furukawa et al. 2000; Peraino et al. 1971).

In rodents, direct and indirect methods to label proliferating hepatocytes are often applied to evaluate hyperplasia. These methods are the same as used to evaluate regeneration (discussed above). Among direct methods, immunohistochemical detection of proliferation markers such as Ki67, phospho-histone H3, or PCNA has been utilized. Hepatocellular proliferation may also be monitored indirectly by analysis of replicative DNA synthesis in nuclei following premortem labeling with tritiated thymidine (autoradiographically detected) or the thymidine analog, bromodeoxyuridine (immunohistochemically detected). An advantage of the indirect labeling method is that the duration of labeling can be extended to integrate the frequency of S-phase over time.

Since both regeneration and hyperplasia involve hepatocellular proliferation, it is necessary to distinguish these fundamentally distinct processes. In general, evaluation of liver weight is the best approach to addressing this distinction. If liver weights are not increased (either decreased or unchanged), hepatocellular proliferation is likely related to regeneration. If liver weights are increased, hepatocellular proliferation is likely related to hyperplasia. However, the direct documentation of an increase in hepatocyte number (hyperplasia) requires stereological evaluation. One method for stereological evaluation, the physical dissector method, involves generation of sections taken randomly but at systematic intervals and a robust analysis using advanced digital imaging integrated with appropriately designed software (Boyce et al. 2010). In current practice, this is not typically performed because liver samples are not optimally collected and retained from routine toxicology studies, necessitating a second study and more extensive histology lab support.

Liver enlargement associated with enzyme induction often occurs from a combination of hepatocellular hypertrophy and hyperplasia. The relative contribution of these two processes is not easily determined without intensive stereological procedures to determine cell size and number estimations. As mentioned earlier, this stereological analysis requires detailed tissue sampling protocols.

The induction of hepatocellular enzymes, hypertrophy, hyperplasia, and hepatomegaly are generally considered to be reversible and adaptive in nature when noted in the absence of indicators of toxicity (Amacher et al. 1998; Crampton et al. 1977; Williams and Iatropoulos 2002). The mechanism of these changes has been actively investigated and characterized in recent literature, and in most cases, the mechanism involves activation of usually one of several receptors by the drug or its metabolite (di Masi et al. 2009; Hu et al. 2007; Moore et al. 2006; Plant and Aouabdi 2009). Most are members of the steroid-thyroid hormone receptor family, such as CAR, PXR, and PPAR-alpha. Another important nuclear receptor, the Ah receptor, is a member of the basic Helix–Loop–Helix (bHLH) receptors. The receptors function as transcription factors that regulate genes responsible for drug-induced changes such as enzyme induction, hypertrophy, organellar increases, and hyperplasia. Unless the drug or its active metabolite persists within the hepatocyte cytoplasm, cessation of treatment reverses the activation of transcription, resulting in a return to the pretreatment morphological and biochemical status.

The reversal of hepatocellular hypertrophy, enzyme levels, and organellar changes appears to depend on the normally short (hours to days) half-life of the respective cellular constituents, and achievement of steady state occurs within a few days or less. However, hepatocytes normally have a life span of several months or longer, so that prompt reversal of hyperplasia depends on activation of apoptotic cell death and elimination. The induction of apoptosis appears to be rapidly activated upon elimination of the drug, and it is a more or less synchronous response. Given the synchronous nature of induction of apoptosis, and the relatively short span of the morphologically observed stages, its appearance can be undetected unless detailed time course studies are conducted. In a time course study, the apoptosis observed during the regression of hyperplasia caused by cyproterone acetate preferentially occurred in hepatocytes that did not replicate during hyperplasia (Bursch et al. 1985). However, it is not known whether this observation applies to the regression of hyperplasia caused by other drugs.

The toxicological significance of drug-induced adaptive effects such as hepatomegaly, hypertrophy, hyperplasia, and enzyme induction for clinical safety assessment of a drug candidate should be carefully considered (Maronpot et al. 2010). If toxicology studies reveal other liver endpoints that suggest toxicity, these additional findings should be the basis for defining hepatotoxicity and used for determining safe human doses. If the adaptive changes are unaccompanied by other liver effects, then species and dose extrapolation must be considered. If adaptive changes are limited to rats and mice and not observed in large animal species (dog or nonhuman primate (NHP)), it is generally accepted that rodent-specific adaptive effects are not limiting with respect to entry into human trials. If adaptive changes are found in both small and large animal test species, then the dose response is evaluated to determine if humans should be dosed only at subthreshold levels to lessen the possibility that similar adaptive changes might occur in them. If the dose response indicates plausibility of similar adaptive changes in humans, clinical trials are plausible; concern may exist, though typically not based on expectations that adaptive effects would be adverse. Rather, the primary concern would be based on the risk of future drug–drug interactions, as the ultimate patient populations are often dependent upon one or several therapeutic agents that may be metabolized via the same phase I and/or phase II enzymes as the drug candidate. In this scenario, the adverse effects of the drug candidate are attributed to diminished effectiveness or enhanced toxicity of concurrent medications. It should be remembered that the ultimate assessment of drug–drug interactions is not the primary responsibility of the toxicologic pathologist and that additional information and assessment should come from experts in drug metabolism and clinical pharmacology.

Another practical consideration regarding the safety assessment of hepatic adaptive effects arises from the possibility of inducing increased incidences of hepatocellular neoplasms in carcinogenicity (1.5- to 2-year) studies that are required for the final marketing approval of drugs for chronic treatment (Maronpot et al. 2010). The association between liver adaptive effects and liver tumor formation is not without exception but is common enough to suggest a reasonable potential of hepatocarcinogenicity with any potential therapeutic agent that demonstrates a liver adaptive response. While it is still possible to gain approval for drugs that cause hepatocellular neoplasia in rodents, the process may require additional effort and cost to the sponsor. In addition, the drug candidate may face hurdles in regulatory approval and marketing disadvantage compared to competitors that lack this liability, even if its significance for human safety is considered to be negligible. To provide data that will assist in determining human risk, pathology and biochemical assessment of liver enzyme induction, as well as assessment of hepatocyte replication, should be used in setting doses in the carcinogenicity study (Rhomberg et al. 2007).

10.1.3.2 Cytoplasmic Accumulations and Inclusions (Nonpigment)

Lipid accumulation is by far the most frequent hepatocellular cytoplasmic accumulation noted in toxicology studies. The appearance is similar in all species and can vary from very fine cytoplasmic vacuolation to large vacuoles that exceed the size of the nucleus (Figure 10.2a). While it has been common practice to subclassify hepatic lipidosis based on the size of the vacuoles, this effort has limited value in the context of drug development. More importantly, the diagnosis and histological descriptions of hepatic lipidosis should give an indication of the degree of lipid accumulation since massive accumulation implies more serious consequences than minimal lipidosis. As pointed out in all standard pathology texts, the vacuoles represent the spaces left when the cytoplasmic lipid is removed during tissue processing. Therefore, special stains have limited value since the material to be defined by the stain has been largely removed. However, special stains of frozen sections of fixed but unprocessed tissues can clearly identify intracytoplasmic lipid. The interpretation of the significance of hepatic lipidosis must be made in the context of other information available in the study. Minimal to moderate lipidosis frequently occurs in higher dose groups that have other toxic manifestations or where the animals refused food or at least manifested reduced food intake. In these cases, the resulting moderate lipidosis simply represents a secondary physiological effect where the metabolism had shifted to the use of stored lipid as a primary energy source. In contrast, moderate to severe lipidosis, in the absence of other significant toxicities and of reduced food intake, likely indicates a primary drug effect that should be seriously investigated. In summary, it is important that hepatic lipidosis be neither overinterpreted when it is simply a consequence of altered physiology nor underinterpreted in regard to biological significance when the effect may represent a primary toxic response.

Phospholipid accumulation occurs in a well-characterized syndrome referred to as phospholipidosis, in which the accumulation can be found in a wide array of cell types in multiple organs (Halliwell 1997; Nonoyama and Fukuda 2008). While the liver is rarely, if ever, the primary site of phospholipid accumulation, it can certainly be affected. The Kupffer cells are most frequently affected, though concurrent accumulation may occur in hepatocytes. However, unusual cellular distributions of phospholipids have been noted, including instances where the condition is restricted to the bile duct epithelium in the liver, though cells in other organs were also affected. Phospholipidosis is histologically characterized by a finely vacuolated cytoplasm where the vacuoles represent removal of the phospholipid during tissue processing. While both phospholipidosis and lipidosis of the liver may be characterized by finely vacuolated cytoplasm, the cell distribution of the lesion is an important tip as to which accumulation is being represented. The definitive diagnosis of phospholipidosis is based on either phospholipid analysis or TEM, which is still considered the final diagnostic criterion of the lesion (Reasor et al. 2006). In the electron micrograph, phospholipid accumulation

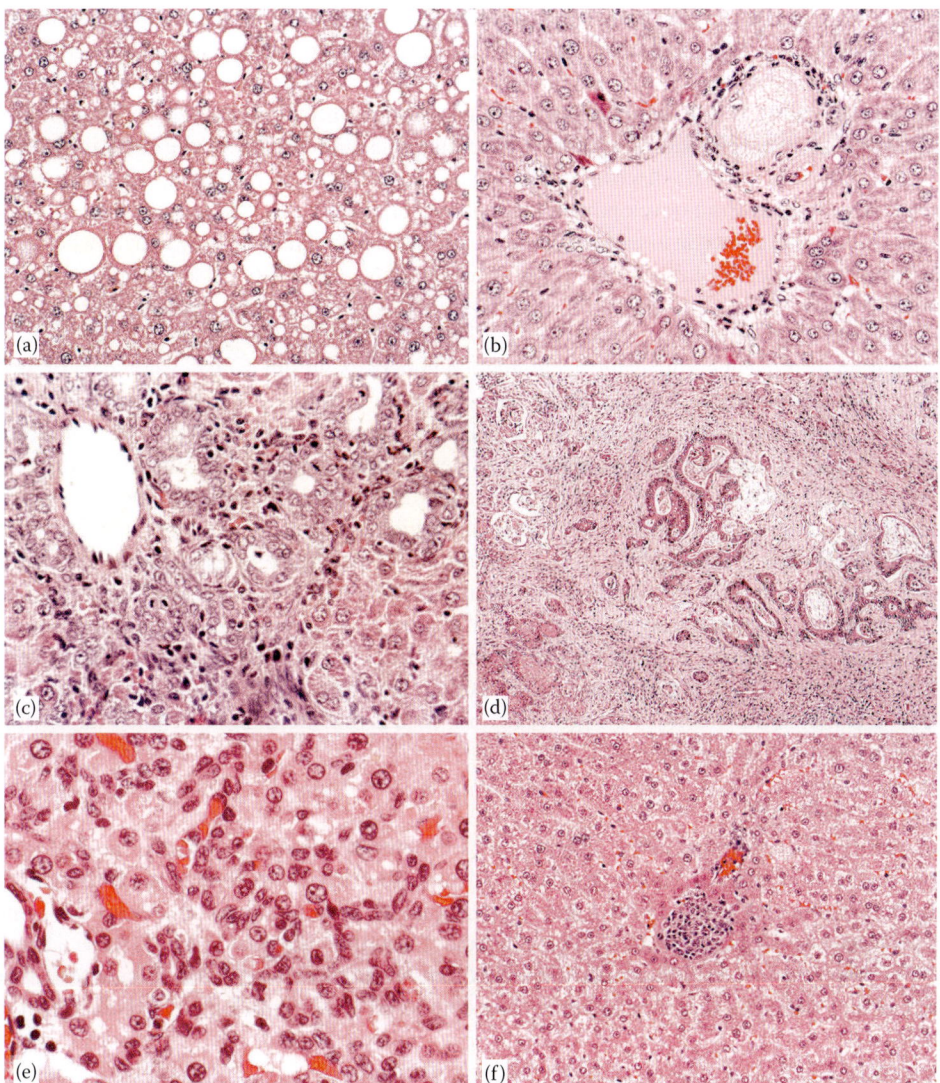

FIGURE 10.2 (a) Hepatocellular vacuolation (lipidosis). The vacuoles may vary in size and appear empty due to the extraction of lipid during processing of tissue for histology. (b) Bile duct necrosis. There is kary-olysis and loss of cytoplasmic detail of biliary epithelium, accompanied by infiltration of neutrophils. (c) Bile duct proliferation. There are several bile ducts, one with a mitotic figure, within the portal region. (d) Cholangiofibrosis. There are numerous bile ducts, some with irregular branching and variable epithelial height, and marked fibrous connective tissue formation. (e) Oval cell proliferation (ductular reaction). The oval cells have oval basophilic nuclei and scant, often imperceptible cytoplasm. The oval cells are present between rows of hepatocytes. (f) Focal inflammatory cell infiltrate. This lesion may occur spontaneously but also may be caused or exacerbated by infectious agents or hepatotoxins.

is characterized by rather equal-sized, membrane-bound structures (lysosomes) that have internal lamellated structures (membrane whorls) that are electron dense. Phospholipid accumulation results from interference of the normal processing of phospholipids that are primarily derived from nor-mal turnover of cellular membranes (Halliwell 1997). Due to drug interference with one or several steps in phospholipid catabolism within lysosomes, the remnant material remains in the lysosomes and progressively accumulates over time as an undigested residue. Due to the mechanism of phos-pholipid accumulation, phospholipidosis is infrequently observed in short-term toxicity studies but appears as a new and unexpected finding in longer-term studies (e.g., 3- to 12-month studies). The implication for human risk assessment has been debated for many years, though phospholipidosis has certainly been observed in humans receiving drugs that cause phospholipidosis in animals (Chatman et al. 2009). While there are questions concerning animal predictivity of phospholipidosis in humans, screening based on chemical characteristics and biochemical effects in short-term tests is now part of many drug discovery programs. Drug candidates that result in phospholipidosis are frequently dropped from development; thus, phospholipidosis is not as frequently seen today as in the past but may occur as an unexpected finding missed by screening or may appear when screening has not occurred in drug discovery.

10.1.3.3 Glycogen

Glycogen is an infrequent cytoplasmic accumulation in hepatocytes in drug development programs. However, this accumulation is occasionally observed with molecules that cause alteration of glucose or glycogen metabolism. Feeding versus fasting prior to termination of study animals can dramatically impact the glycogen content of the liver. In nonfasted animals, the liver may contain glycogen up to 3% by weight, while fasting will result in essentially complete removal of glycogen from the hepatocyte; both conditions are easily discernible by light microscopy. In the absence of standardized overnight fasting, there may be a substantial difference in glycogen level in animals terminated early in the day versus those terminated late in the day. While overnight fasting is a standard procedure for most drug development GLP studies, it may not be standard for animals in drug discovery protocols. When glycogen is present, hepatocytic cytoplasm is finely vacuolated and may be indistinguishable from minimal lipid accumulation. Special stains are required to confirm glycogen accumulation, which is best performed on tissues that are unfixed or fixed for short periods of time to avoid glycogen removal.

10.1.3.4 Cytokeratin

Accumulation of cytokeratin in the cytoplasm of hepatocytes is rarely noted in animal studies. Mallory bodies composed of cytokeratin have been described in mice receiving the antifungal agent griseofulvin (Denk et al. 1975, 1979). Light microscopically, accumulations of keratins can be noted as small, bright, eosinophilic structures usually adjacent to the nucleus. On TEM, these accumulations are composed of fine, rod-shaped filaments that are randomly oriented. Characterization of Mallory bodies indicates that they are primarily composed of keratins 8 and 18 (Nakamichi et al. 2002).

10.1.3.5 Drug or Drug Metabolite

Accumulations of drug or drug metabolite may be found within hepatocytic cytoplasm and can have a variable appearance by both light and electron microscopy. Such accumulations may appear as irregular microscopic structures and can be accentuated by standard stains or, alternatively, may demonstrate an inherent color, most frequently a dark brown. These accumulations may be noted by TEM where the structure may again be variable depending on the crystal or aggregate that is being viewed. The histological appearance of the structure is unlikely to be helpful in identifying the accumulated material, with identification best left to chemical analysis.

10.1.3.6 Cytoplasmic Pigments

Lipofuscin is primarily observed in hepatocytes but may also be found concurrently in Kupffer cells. This pigment is generally found to a minimal degree in control animals in standard toxicology studies, even in chronic studies, in part due to the relatively young age of the animals. Lipofuscin may be noted, but still to a minimal degree, in control rodents in carcinogenicity studies, where the animals approach living an entire life span. With such a low background of lipofuscin, a compound-related increase is relatively easy to detect and should be given more serious attention. An increase in lipofuscin may be the first, and perhaps only, suggestion that there is a compound-related enhancement of oxidative injury, and its appearance may represent more serious injury, which requires biochemical follow-up. Lipofuscin in Kupffer cells may occur either alone or in conjunction with accumulation of other pigments, most notably hemosiderin.

Hemosiderin is generally noted in Kupffer cells when associated with enhanced red cell removal. While this pigment is generally dark brown, it is important to use special stains to distinguish from other brown pigments such as lipofuscin and possible drug or metabolite accumulation. In rodents, hemosiderin accumulation may be associated with extramedullary hematopoiesis.

Bile accumulation can occur in hepatocytes, Kupffer cells, and/or bile canaliculi, though the location may be different in the various species used in toxicology studies. In dogs and nonhuman primates, bile may accumulate at any or all of these locations. In some instances, canalicular accumulation predominates, particularly in nonrodent species, while canalicular accumulation rarely, if ever, occurs in the rodent. Interpretation of bile accumulation is dependent on other data, primarily the evaluation of direct and indirect bilirubin during clinical chemistry assessments. Bile is generally a light yellow color but may have a green tinge. As noted for other pigments, special stains should be used to distinguish the various pigments, though the simultaneous accumulation of more than one pigment is not uncommon.

10.1.4   Nuclear Alterations

Nuclear alteration of hepatocytes is relatively uncommon in the evaluation of molecules for drug development. In some instances, the nuclei may be enlarged and somewhat hyperchromatic due to increased DNA content associated with increased ploidy. In evaluation of nuclear size and staining characteristics, the toxicological pathologist must carefully compare treated subjects to controls, particularly in rodents, since ploidy states above 2X are normal in both rats and mice and generally increase with age. Increased ploidy with enlarged hyperchromatic nuclei is more common in control mice compared with control rats. However, various xenobiotic agents will increase the ploidy in rodents (Miller et al. 1996), though the implication of this alteration is not clear. Assessment of hepatocyte proliferation, as determined by a number of techniques previously mentioned, is a measure of DNA synthesis, which is assumed to lead to cell proliferation. However, in some cases, the increased DNA synthesis may result, at least partially, in increased ploidy rather than an increase in cell number.

Large nucleoli may occasionally be seen in hepatocytes following administration of a compound and simply reflects increased processing of RNA and increased activity. Increased nucleolar size is frequently an indirect indication, but not a sensitive indicator, of increased cell proliferation. In addition, while the active proliferative phase may have already passed, the enlarged nucleoli often remain for some period after.

Nuclear inclusions are rarely found in the evaluation of drug candidates. Apparent nuclear inclusions can be observed in control mice and, rarely, in rats, secondary to cytoplasmic invagination into the nucleus. The invaginated cytoplasm is characterized by an eosinophilic appearance similar to the cytoplasm and may appear to be totally circumscribed by nuclear material in the plane of the section being examined. Similar-appearing structures may appear more frequently in treated versus control livers, but the implication of this is unknown.

10.1.4.1   Multinucleated Hepatocytes

Multinucleated hepatocytes are not frequently seen in rodents in toxicology studies but have raised concern when observed, and literature on the topic is sparse. Numbers of nuclei can range from 3 to 15 or even 20 within a single hepatocyte. These nuclei appear normal, based on size and staining characteristics. A cluster of nuclei is typically surrounded by a thin zone of normal-staining cytoplasm. Multinucleated hepatocytes have been identified in various toxicological studies (Cattley et al. 1994), including those from the National Toxicology Program. Multinucleated hepatocytes have been described in detail in rats receiving the antimycobacterial agent rifabutin (Scampini et al. 1993). They are not always associated with other morphologic alterations in the liver, including toxicity or hepatocellular hypertrophy. Based on the rifabutin study, multinucleated hepatocytes appear to have a normal life span, indicating that their formation is not simply a step in cell injury leading to cell loss. Multinucleated hepatocytes typically first appear after at least several weeks of compound administration and have not been observed as an acute response. Based on the available information, multinucleated hepatocytes should be considered an adaptive response and not an indication of hepatotoxicity. Moreover, their presence in subchronic studies is not an indication of potential carcinogenicity.

10.1.5 BILIARY CHANGES, NON-NEOPLASTIC

Injury to the biliary epithelium represents an unusual form of hepatic toxicity that is only rarely described in the scientific literature related to drug development. It has been studied and reported for the model toxicant alpha-napthyisothiocyanate (Leonard et al. 1984) and the chemotherapeutic agent ET-743 (trabectidin) (Donald et al. 2002). The effects following treatment with these agents are bile duct degeneration and bile duct necrosis. By light microscopy, degeneration of biliary epithelial cells appears as cell swelling, and necrosis appears as coagulative change with sloughing of cells into the duct lumens (Figure 10.2b). The resolution of bile duct necrosis may be regeneration, but if injury is severe or sustained, there may be peribiliary fibrosis. Ultrastructural examination is not typically performed but may detect apoptotic biliary epithelial cells early in the course of injury, in addition to degeneration and necrosis. By clinical pathology, injury to the biliary epithelial cells may be recognized in plasma or serum samples by modest elevations in alkaline phosphatase and AST activity and dramatic elevations in conjugated bilirubin in all species. In rodents, increased activity of gamma glutamyl-transpeptidase (GGT) is an additional marker of biliary epithelial injury (Leonard et al. 1984). Due to species differences in GGT levels in rodent versus nonrodent species, elevations of circulating enzyme require differing interpretations for different species. The rat hepatocyte has 1/30 of the GGT levels compared with hepatocytes in other species so that virtually all the GGT is contained in bile duct epithelium. This is in contrast to other species in which GGT is normally found in high concentrations in both the hepatocyte and bile duct epithelium. Therefore, elevation of circulating GGT in the rat is a greater indication of bile duct injury compared to its elevation in other species.

It is suspected that the mechanism of bile duct injury involves exposure of the biliary epithelium to reactive metabolites that either are excreted into the bile or may form in the bile via breakdown of conjugated metabolite(s) that are excreted in the bile. It is uncertain whether this event is rare or whether it is recognized and underreported in the course of screening for new drug candidates, as deselection is routinely decided.

In safety assessment studies, biliary epithelial degeneration and necrosis are not recognized as a background lesion. As a result, the threshold is low for attributing the lesion to the test article. In humans, injury to the biliary epithelium occurs with certain infections and autoimmune diseases, and in these conditions, the injury is accompanied by significant morbidity and mortality. Despite the potential reversibility and ability to monitor biliary epithelial injury by clinical chemistry parameters, it remains a serious obstacle to clinical development.

Following either acute or chronic insults, bile duct epithelium readily responds by cellular proliferation to replace the damaged cells. However, this response may overcompensate, resulting in various types of biliary epithelial responses.

Biliary hyperplasia can occur as a lesion independent of other evidence of hepatic toxicity but is more frequently found in conjunction with other chronic hepatic effects such as continuing hepatocyte loss and/or fibrosis. When present, biliary hyperplasia can take several forms. In a mild form and when independent of other hepatic effects, the portal tracts have an increase in normal-appearing bile ducts (Figure 10.2c). With greater proliferation, usually related to sustained injury to the biliary epithelium, the proliferating ducts may at first compress adjacent periportal hepatocytes and may even extend between them, causing pressure atrophy. Mitotic figures may be present but are frequently not obvious. The absence of mitotic figures cannot be used as an indication that the proliferative response has subsided. An inflammatory response generally does not accompany mild bile duct hyperplasia. With greater injury, for example, when related to bile leakage and/or sustained biliary necrosis, the proliferating ducts may become surrounded by variable numbers of mixed inflammatory cells and collagen, depending on the severity and duration of injury. Bile duct proliferation may not be accompanied by an increase in circulating bilirubin unless there is significant ongoing injury resulting in leakage of bilirubin. The longer-term consequences of bile duct injury are extremely variable. When biliary hyperplasia occurs following acute injury to the epithelium, the proliferated ducts will generally regress over several weeks, with no residual evidence of the hyperplasia. However, when biliary hyperplasia is accompanied by inflammation and collagen deposition, regression of the proliferated ducts may be accompanied by mild portal fibrosis, though without obvious long-term consequences based on morphology and clinical chemistry parameters. When hyperplasia occurs over an extended period of time and is accompanied by inflammation and fibroplasia, periportal fibrosis will most likely result. Despite these potential long-term consequences of bile duct proliferation, it is generally difficult for the pathologist to be certain of the outcome simply based on examination of the lesion at a single time point in a toxicology study.

Cholangiofibrosis is a special form of biliary hyperplasia that is observed primarily, if not exclusively, in rats and has been well characterized in part due to the unusual morphologic characteristics (Elmore and Sirica 1991). In the most florid yet simple form, the lesion is characterized by significant bile duct proliferation that extends beyond the immediate portal area and is associated with extensive collagen deposition (Figure 10.2d). Inflammation is frequently present but not a dominant characteristic of the lesion. The lesion is focal and adjacent to portal areas during early development and does not involve all or even a majority of the portal areas. The lesions may be variable in size from a few bile ducts to a lesion that in unusual instances may approach the size of a lobule. While this description of cholangiofibrosis covers the classical lesion, it represents only a single phase in the pathogenesis and eventual regression of the lesion. Sequential studies have shown that cholangiofibrosis generally originates as a simple form of biliary hyperplasia (as described above) or oval cell proliferation (as described below). Fibrosis develops secondarily, though it is frequently an early companion bile duct proliferation. The proliferated ducts become irregular in shape and lined by cuboidal to columnar to single-layered, flattened biliary epithelium. Unexpected cell types, such as intestinal epithelial cells (as defined by brush borders on TEM) and goblet cells, are found in variable numbers. In some areas, cysts will form and may contain periodic acid Schiff (PAS)–positive staining material with some necrotic debris. The classic lesion may remain for varying periods of time but generally regresses over weeks to months if the inciting agent is removed. During regression, cysts become more prominent with greater accumulations of PAS-positive material. The epithelium lining the cysts and channels (formerly lined by biliary epithelium) is mainly flattened epithelium with little to no resemblance to the original biliary epithelium. Cysts may lose this epithelial lining and become surrounded by dense connective tissue. Over time, these cysts may become reduced in size with little or no lining epithelium, leaving a smaller, residual mass of dense connective tissue. Cholangiofibrosis is unique to rodents and without a human counterpart. Therefore, its relevance for human risk assessment is uncertain.

Oval cell proliferation is a form of bile duct proliferation that was first described in the rodent using experimental models of hepatotoxicity and carcinogenesis. While the term is widely accepted and utilized in rodent studies, this lesion is infrequently observed in studies evaluating potential pharmaceuticals. In contrast to use of the term *oval cell proliferation* in rodents, the term is infrequently used in other species. Some forms of ductular reaction in humans resemble this lesion, with some important differences (Bird 2008; Desmet 2011; Gouw et al. 2011). Ductular reactions have been infrequently described in dogs (Yoshioka et al. 2004; Ilzer et al. 2010); therefore, it is uncertain whether there is a canine counterpart to oval cell proliferation in rodents. The oval cell is considered to be a hepatic progenitor cell or intrahepatic stem cell (Bird et al. 2008). The oval cell is named for the oval appearance of the nucleus within scanty cytoplasm with indistinct borders. Therefore, histologically, the lesion is characterized by numerous small, closely spaced nuclei seemingly without cytoplasm. Oval cell proliferation begins in the portal area and rapidly extends into the hepatic lobule (Figure 10.2e). At first, oval cells will insinuate between normal-appearing hepatocytes, while greater numbers will replace the atrophic periportal hepatocytes. In the most florid forms of oval cell proliferation, oval cells may extend half the distance between the portal and central lobular areas. Initial oval cell proliferation is generally not accompanied by inflammation or collagen deposition. The lesion may be observed grossly only when the oval cell proliferation is most pronounced. Oval cells represent proliferation of the cells in the small biliary passages (canals of Hering) that connect the peripheral lobular canaliculi to the small bile ducts of the portal area. The oval cell proliferation can take several courses. Removal of the inciting agent usually results in regression of the oval cells with no residual evidence of the lesion once regression is complete. With retention of the proliferated oval cells when the inciting agent is not removed, more obvious forms of bile ducts may appear within the field of oval cells, although this is not a progression of all or even a majority of oval cells. Oval cell hyperplasia can, in some cases, progress to cholangiofibrosis.

The importance of oval cell proliferation has been studied and debated for decades. Today, the oval cell is considered to be a pluripotent cell or stem cell with the ability to differentiate into either bile duct epithelium or hepatocytes (Bird et al. 2008). This concept is supported by characterization of the cell, which has both biliary and hepatocytic markers. Oval cell proliferation has been linked to hepatocarcinogenesis, with the oval cell a reputed cell of origin of hepatocellular tumors. However, these studies frequently utilized agents that cause DNA alterations. This and the fact that hepatocellular tumors occur in the absence of oval cell proliferation (in many cases including essentially all cases of hepatocarcinogenesis associated with nongenotoxic agents) demonstrate that oval cell proliferation is not a prerequisite for hepatic tumor formation in rodents. In addition, it is well known that oval cell proliferation caused by short period of treatment with a known hepatocarcinogen will not result in carcinogenesis if treatment is stopped. Based on the accumulated knowledge to date, chronic oval cell proliferation should be considered a potential indicator of risk of hepatocarcinogenesis in rodents, though the relevance to humans is not clear.

10.1.6 INTERSTITIAL AND VASCULAR CHANGES, NON-NEOPLASTIC

10.1.6.1 Hepatic Inflammatory Cells, Kupffer Cells, and Hematopoietic Cells

The appearance of inflammatory cells accumulating within the vascular and interstitial areas of the liver may be a primary response or secondary to necrosis of hepatic parenchyma. When secondary to necrosis, the inflammatory cell infiltrate may be documented as part of the description or pathology narrative, rather than a diagnosis. However, an inflammatory cell infiltrate may occur as a primary lesion, in response to either a test article or to infectious agents or autoimmunity (Sneed et al. 1997; Thoolen et al. 2010). If considered to be a primary response, the inflammatory cell infiltration should be a primary diagnosis.

In the generation of histopathology data for safety assessment studies, the infiltration of inflammatory cells in the hepatic parenchyma is termed "inflammatory cell infiltration" and not "inflammation" or "hepatitis." This practice is preferred for two reasons. One reason is that, in safety assessment studies, inflammatory cell infiltration in the liver is seldom accompanied by other morphological indicators of inflammation such as congestion and edema (if acute) or fibrovascular tissue formation, macrophage epithelioid differentiation, or lymphocytic aggregates (if chronic). A second reason is that the term "hepatitis" has connotations in humans that indicate specific causes of liver disease such as viral or autoimmune hepatitis. These connotations may lead to misunderstanding that can otherwise be avoided. As a result, unless there are sufficient additional features to support the use of the term "hepatitis," the infiltration of inflammatory cells in the liver is given a descriptive diagnosis.

Inflammatory cell infiltration of the liver is typically subdivided based upon the types of inflammatory cell infiltrates. If the response is predominantly one type of inflammatory cell, then that cell type is added as a modifier. If two or more cell types are involved, then the term "mixed inflammatory cell" is added as a modifier, and the types of cells should be characterized in the narrative description.

Inflammatory cell infiltration is usually characterized by light microscopy (Figure 10.2f). Gross findings are likely only when severity is moderate or marked, and these will appear as white-tan discoloration on capsular and cut surfaces of the liver, with either a lobular or diffuse pattern. In rare instances, TEM may be used to detect or confirm the presence of infectious agents, but not for the morphological diagnosis. Clinical pathology parameters are seldom significantly or specifically altered, except in cases where there is extensive secondary hepatocellular injury.

Neutrophilic and eosinophilic inflammatory cell infiltrations are two types of inflammatory cell infiltration that may be diagnosed based on identification of the predominant cell type. These types of inflammatory cell infiltration are rarely considered to be a primary response of the liver to the test article but may be secondary to hepatocellular necrosis or infectious disease. The lesion may be either lobular or random (focal but not specific to any area within the lobule) in distribution and is characterized by accumulation of neutrophils (or eosinophils) filling and expanding the hepatic parenchyma, sometimes adjacent to hepatocellular atrophy, degeneration, or necrosis.

Mononuclear inflammatory cell infiltration may be diagnosed based upon identification of mononuclear round cells as the predominant cell type. The cells are either lymphocytes or monocytes/macrophages (macrophages may be derived from circulating monocytes in addition to the resident macrophages or Kupffer cells), and often, both are involved. The differentiation of monocytes and lymphocytes in tissue lesions by light microscopy is often difficult, and immunohistochemical markers are usually required. This determination is occasionally needed to develop a hypothesis regarding mechanism, when the finding is treatment related. However, in practice, this is rarely done. There are several different complex mechanisms of immune-mediated liver injury (Adams et al. 2010), meaning that the characterization of types of inflammatory cells may provide only part of the mechanistic characterization. Furthermore, even though mononuclear inflammatory cell infiltration often includes lymphocytes and monocytes/macrophages, attempts to determine ratios of cell types from a single or few sections often do not provide useful information.

Mononuclear inflammatory cell infiltration is only occasionally considered to be a primary response of the liver to the test article but may be secondary to hepatocellular necrosis or infectious disease. The lesion may be either lobular or random in distribution and is characterized by foci of mononuclear cells occasionally adjacent to a focus of hepatocellular necrosis. In some cases, monocytes/macrophages may differentiate to form epithelioid cells and multinucleate giant cells. When this is a common feature, it may be addressed in the narrative, but some prefer to diagnose the lesion as focal granulomatous inflammation.

Mixed inflammatory cell infiltrate is used to designate the accumulation of mononuclear cells along with neutrophils and/or eosinophils. The lesion may be either lobular or random in distribution and is characterized by inflammatory cells occasionally adjacent to a small focus of hepatocellular necrosis.

Considerable judgment may be required to determine if inflammatory cell infiltration is related to treatment with a test article. Both incidence and severity must be considered in comparing treatment groups to controls. Occasional foci of inflammatory cell infiltrate often may occur as a background lesion of unknown pathogenesis in most animal species. A variety of infectious agents (see Table 10.1) produce inflammatory cell infiltration and often other features of hepatic inflammation. Several of these infectious agents should also be considered as potential contributors to either inflammatory cell infiltrates or inflammation in the liver, especially if the pharmacology of the test article is to suppress or activate the immune system.

In rare instances, inflammatory cell infiltration plus additional features of inflammation may be observed despite the apparent absence of an infectious agent. These cases may be appropriately

TABLE 10.1

Infectious Agents That May Produce Inflammatory Cell Infiltration or Inflammation in Liver, by Species

Species	Infectious Agent
Mouse	Helicobacter, norovirus, MHV
Rat	*Corynebacterium kutscheri*, parvovirus
Dog	Canine adenovirus Type 1, canine herpesvirus
Macaque	Cytomegalovirus, Shigella
Several species	Salmonella, Tyzzer's disease

diagnosed as hepatic inflammation or hepatitis, although there is a tendency to instead use descriptive terms, unless the number of descriptive terms becomes excessive. Although drug-induced hypersensitivity may be suspected, attempts to provide objective evidence of hypersensitivity are rarely obtained. Furthermore, although certain drugs may cause immune-mediated hepatitis in humans, these drugs do not seem to produce similar effects in nonclinical animal studies.

When inflammatory cell infiltration or inflammation is attributable to the test article, it represents a potentially significant safety concern in clinical trials. Theoretically, the findings could involve a pathogenesis that is specific for some animal species but would not be predicted to occur in humans; however, in practice, the pathogenesis is often difficult to establish. As a result, the confidence in a proposed species-specific mechanism is often weak.

Opportunities to use a proposed mechanism of inflammatory cell infiltration or inflammation to contextualize the potential risks in the clinical setting should be rationally approached. If the pathogenesis of inflammatory cell infiltrate or inflammation is related to immune modulation and secondary infection, it may be possible to establish a safety margin between the intended pharmacological and the immunomodulatory doses and thus determine a safe starting dose in the clinic. This would be further supported by the application of biomarkers that could be used to monitor the specific effects of the drug on the immune system. In the unlikely event that the pathogenesis of inflammatory cell infiltrate or inflammation is related to hypersensitivity, a margin approach would not be considered appropriate. However, if a species-specific small molecule metabolite was responsible for the hypersensitivity, there might be an opportunity to proceed. For protein therapeutic agents, hypersensitivity could be related to the foreignness of an engineered human protein in a nonhuman species, and a clinical approach might proceed if human immune response to the drug could be monitored.

Kupffer cell hypertrophy and hyperplasia is a lesion that is distinct from mononuclear cell infiltration that represents the activation of Kupffer cells. The Kupffer cells may be increased in number or size, or both, but retain their normal distribution along the sinusoidal surface. The lesion is often diffuse in distribution. By light microscopy, increased numbers of Kupffer cells may be observed, but it is the enlargement of Kupffer cell cytoplasm and nucleus that is more apparent. Kupffer cells are readily identifiable because of the presence of ingested material (cells, cell debris, or particulate material) within an expanded cytoplasm, owing to their specialized phagocytic capacity. Kupffer cells are distinct from the endothelial cells that line the sinusoids that may also undergo hypertrophy and karyomegaly. Differentiation of Kupffer cells from endothelial sinusoidal lining cells can be done using immunohistochemical markers or by TEM. Kupffer cells are recognized by immunostaining for markers such as F4/80 (mouse), ED1 and ED2 (aka CD68 and CD163, respectively) (rat), and CD68 (dog and NHP), while endothelial cells are usually recognized by expression of CD31 in many species (Baluk and McDonald 2008; Fan et al. 2009; Kinoshita et al. 2010; Lapis et al. 1995). By TEM, Kupffer cells contain many primary and secondary lysosomes, as well as phagocytic vacuoles.

Kupffer cell hypertrophy and hyperplasia are seldom a spontaneous finding. They are often associated with test articles (or their carriers) wherein their physicochemical characteristics result in clearance from circulation by the Kupffer cells and perhaps other tissue macrophages in the spleen. In some cases, uptake by Kupffer cells is accompanied by uptake into sinusoidal endothelial cells. The materials associated with this mechanism include nonionic detergents (Warren et al. 2011), pegylated and other types of nanoparticles (Fawaz et al. 1993; Xiao et al. 2011), and antisense oligonucleotides (Butler et al. 1997; Henry et al. 1997a,b). The significance of the finding in such cases is seldom related to any real or theoretical adverse effects. It is significant, however, if the efficiency of the uptake of the experimental therapeutic agent is high enough to preclude delivery to the intended target cells or tissues.

Extramedullary hematopoietic cell proliferation (EMH) may be observed in the liver as a spontaneous or treatment-related lesion in toxicology studies (Thoolen et al. 2010). By light microscopy, this lesion appears as aggregates of hematopoietic cells that are subendothelial and randomly distributed along the hepatic sinusoids or in portal or centrilobular areas. The hematopoietic cells may include immature erythroid and myeloid cell aggregates. Megakaryocytes are inconsistently present. The mechanism is considered unlikely to involve a direct effect on the hematopoietic cells, unless the test article is a hematopoietic growth factor. More typically, it represents an adaptive response to increased turnover of erythrocytes or neutrophils. Evidence of such increased turnover is typically accompanied by clinical pathology findings such as altered erythrocytic morphology and increased counts of immature forms in the circulation. The lesion is occasionally mistaken for mononuclear or mixed inflammatory cell infiltration. While seldom done, this may be resolved by demonstrating immunohistochemical markers of erythroid lineage (TER119) (Hintze et al. 2009) or myeloid lineage (BM1, also known as myeloperoxidase) (O'Malley et al. 2005; Swirski et al. 2010).

10.1.7 ENDOTHELIAL CELL RESPONSE

Endothelial cell injury is an unusual form of liver injury. As a primary event, it is variably observed by light microscopy as necrosis and/or loss of endothelial cells, sinusoidal congestion, and perisinusoidal hemorrhage in the early stages, accompanied by central lobular necrosis and fibrosis in later stages. It has been described in humans in two scenarios: high-dose cytoablative chemotherapy with bone marrow transplantation and ingestion of herbal remedies containing pyrrolizidine alkaloids (Rubbia-Brandt 2010). It has been produced in the rat by the pyrrolizidine alkaloid monocrotaline (DeLeve et al. 1999), and a similar form of injury has been described in dogs treated with an imidazopyridine proton pump inhibitor (Berg et al. 2008). Time course studies in rats suggest that the initial injury is to the sinusoidal endothelium wherein loss or contraction of these cells permits blood cells to enter the space of Disse, thereby obstructing sinusoidal blood flow.

Endothelial cell injury is also observed as a secondary event with certain agents that cause centrilobular hepatocellular necrosis (Anderson et al. 1986; Butler and Hard 1971; Oyaizu et al. 1997). This has been observed in rats following treatment with agents that are activated to a stable reactive metabolite that is produced in central lobular hepatocytes where it induces hepatocellular injury. The low molecular weight of the metabolite may promote diffusion and subsequent contact with the endothelium. The endothelial cell injury is presumed to be a bystander event. This mechanism is supported by time course studies that demonstrate hepatocellular necrosis preceding endothelial cell necrosis.

Endothelial cell injury is considered a rarity in toxicology studies. However, given its association with the development of sinusoidal obstruction syndrome (formerly known as veno-occlusive disease) in humans (Rubbia-Brandt 2010), its appearance in a safety assessment study would represent a serious concern for clinical investigators.

Angiectasis is a distinct lesion of uncertain pathogenesis that is characterized by formation of blood-filled spaces within the hepatic parenchyma (Figure 10.3a). It is often, but not always, regarded as synonymous with the term "peliosis." By light microscopy, its appearance varies between two forms. The first is described as "cystic" or "phlebectatic," in which the blood-containing spaces are lined by normal-appearing endothelial cells and are separated by cords of hepatocytes. The second is described as "cavernous" or "parenchymal," in which the blood-containing spaces mostly lack endothelial lining cells and contact the intervening (if present) and adjacent cords of hepatocytes. Most theories concerning the pathogenesis of angiectasis (Thoolen et al. 2010) consider damage and disruption of sinusoidal endothelial cells as the primary event, though it is apparently accompanied by focal atrophy and/or loss of hepatocytes.

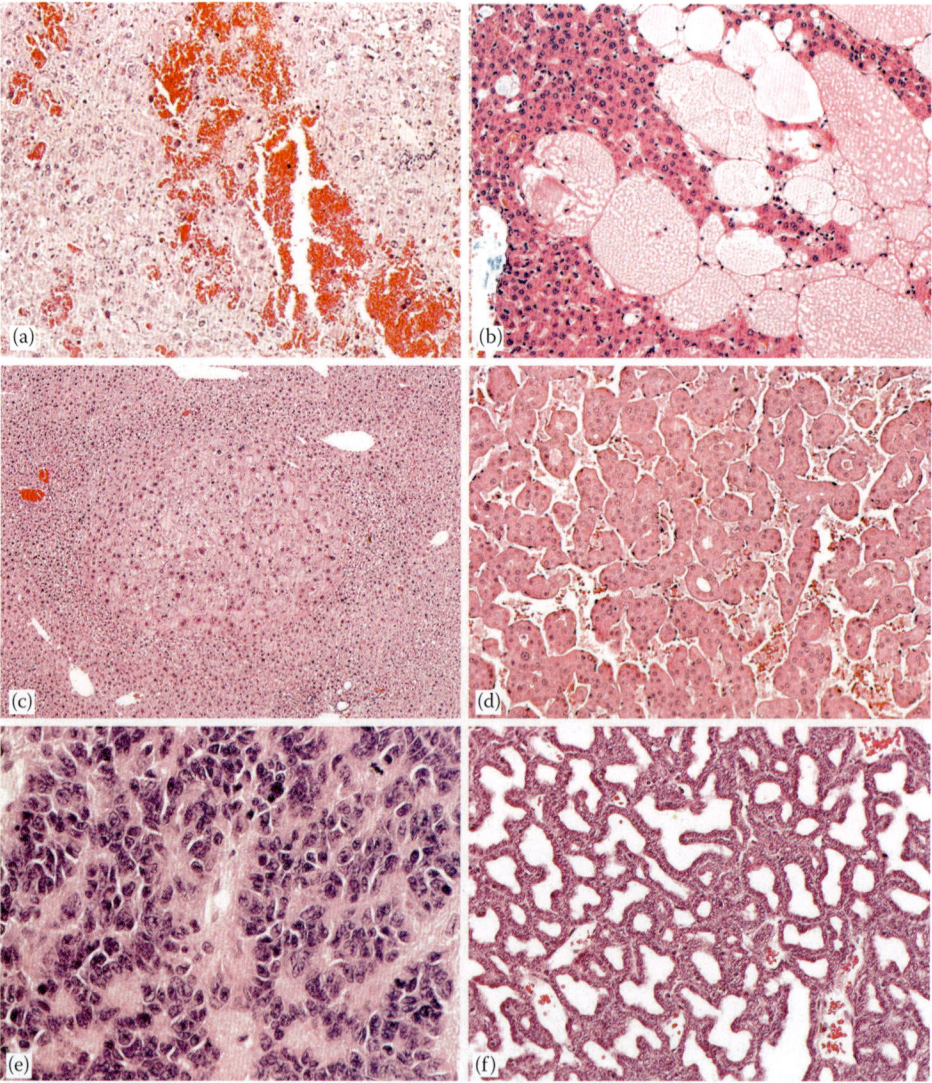

FIGURE 10.3 (a) Angiectasis (peliosis). Sinusoids are irregularly dilated and contain erythrocytes. (b) Spongiosis. The lesion contains several irregularly sized cystic spaces that contain reticulated eosinophilic material. (c) Focus of hepatocellular alteration, eosinophilic. The focus is composed of enlarged hepatocytes with increased cytoplasmic eosinophilia. (d) Hepatocellular carcinoma. This lesion contains variably sized trabeculae of neoplastic hepatocytes. The trabecular pattern is the most commonly observed pattern in rodents. (e) Hepatoblastoma. The neoplastic cells are characterized by darkly stained nuclei and scant cytoplasm and may form rosettes. (f) Cholangioma (bile duct adenoma). Neoplastic epithelial cells are arranged in well-defined ductal structures.

Angiectasis has been associated with a variety of natural and environmental toxins, but among drugs, it appears that only anabolic and contraceptive steroids have been reported to cause this change in humans (Tsokosa and Erbersdobler 2005). Angiectasis has also been associated with long-term administration of tezapam in mice (Robison et al. 1984) and repeat dosing of CKD-602 (camptothecin analog) in rats (Kim et al. 2004). It has also been described as an aging lesion in animals. Functionally, it does not appear to be associated with progressive liver disease and, as such, may represent an end-stage lesion. As a result, the significance of angiectasis for safety assessment is uncertain.

10.1.8 Stellate Cell Response

An unusual lesion involving stellate cells has been termed cystic degeneration or spongiosis hepatis (Thoolen et al. 2010). This lesion is characterized by the formation of multiple, sometimes coalescing, cystic structures separated by fine septa but lacking endothelium (Figure 10.3b). The cystic spaces contain finely reticulated eosinophilic material that is PAS-positive and may contain a few erythrocytes and leukocytes in some areas. Immunohistochemically, the lesions stain for desmin and vimentin but not for alpha smooth muscle actin (Stroebel et al. 1995). An increase in replicative DNA synthesis among nuclei in the lesion has been demonstrated (Karbe and Kerlin 2002; Stroebel et al. 1995). The lesion causes no significant compression of the adjacent hepatic parenchyma.

Cystic degeneration/spongiosis hepatis occurs as a spontaneous lesion in aging rats or, rarely, in mice (Karbe and Kerlin 2002). Its incidence in chronic studies may be increased by the administration of chemicals that often, but not always, cause hepatocellular neoplasia. Some divergent views have been expressed in the literature concerning whether cystic degeneration/spongiosis hepatis may represent a pre-neoplastic or neoplastic lesion of stellate cells (Bannasch 2003; Kerlin and Karbe 2004).

The occurrence of cystic degeneration/spongiosis hepatis in studies of drugs or drug candidates has not been published. As a result, there is no apparent precedent for addressing its impact upon drug safety. However, this lesion has not been described in studies of typical nonrodent species (dogs, NHP). Moreover, this lesion has not been reported in humans. As a result, it seems unlikely that development of a drug candidate would be obstructed, assuming demonstrable medical need, by the appearance or an increased incidence of cystic degeneration/spongiosis hepatis in a chronic rodent study.

10.1.9 Hepatic Proliferative Lesions

Proliferative lesions in the liver can involve multiple cell types including the hepatocyte, bile duct epithelium, vascular endothelium, and, rarely, Kupffer and stellate cells, though there is a vast difference in both spontaneous and treatment-related incidence of proliferative lesions of these diverse cell types. In toxicology studies, proliferative lesions of the liver are an issue in the 2-year carcinogenicity studies in rats and mice or in the 6-month carcinogenicity studies using alternative mouse models. However, early hyperplastic lesions can be found in the chronic toxicity study of rodents that may suggest development of tumors on longer administration. While hyperplastic lesions (as discussed earlier in the chapter) may be found in nonrodent species used in toxicity studies, a neoplasm in the liver of a dog or nonhuman primate in a chronic toxicity study is an extremely rare event.

Since neoplastic lesions are important endpoints in toxicity studies that can have serious implications on drug approvability or utilization, the toxicologic pathologist evaluating tissues in a carcinogenicity study must be familiar with background lesions in older rodents and the morphological criteria of neoplasms that are not observed in shorter-term studies. The morphologic criteria for the various diagnoses of hepatocellular neoplastic lesions have become standardized over the years through discussion at numerous workshops and extensive consultation of toxicologic pathologists.

These criteria have been summarized in several publications of different groups, each primarily based in different parts of the world. Most recently, the criteria for histological diagnoses in rodents have been summarized by a single international group (Thoolen et al. 2010). Such standardization has enhanced the rigor of interpretation but, more importantly, provides a better basis for comparison of liver effects across studies when similar diagnostic approaches have been used. While there is very consistent agreement of diagnostic criteria for the most common proliferative liver lesions, there are still variations in terminology and criteria for diagnosis for the less common ones.

10.1.9.1 Hepatocytes

Proliferative lesions of the hepatocyte are by far the most frequent spontaneous and drug-induced proliferative lesions in rodents. The incidence of spontaneous proliferative lesions will be variable across the strains of rodents used and will also be variable based on the laboratory where the studies are performed. These points are important when selecting historical control data to assist in the interpretation of hepatocellular tumors.

Proliferative lesions of hepatocytes include a range of non-neoplastic lesions to malignant neoplasms. While diffuse and zonal hyperplasia have been addressed earlier under hyperplasia, the important non-neoplastic proliferative lesion formation is the "focus of cellular alteration" most frequently found in rats, less frequently in mice, and rarely in dogs and NHPs. [Foci of cellular alteration have been described in the human liver (Su and Bannasch 2003).] In rodents, these foci are noticeable primarily due to altered tinctorial properties of the cytoplasm (Figure 10.3c) that distinguishes the lesion from the surrounding parenchyma (Popp and Goldsworthy 1989). While there have been multiple types of foci described in the diagnostic and experimental carcinogenesis literature, there are only a few that are commonly found in the evaluation of the liver in drug development, for example, basophilic, eosinophilic, and clear cell foci. As the name implies, basophilic foci have basophilic cytoplasm compared to the more eosinophilic cytoplasm of the surrounding hepatocytes. The cytoplasm is sparse, but the nuclei are similar in size and staining compared to normal-appearing hepatocytes. In contrast, eosinophilic foci have cytoplasm that stains slightly more eosinophilic than the surrounding normal hepatocytes, though this staining difference may be subtle, making these foci less apparent at low magnifications than basophilic foci. The amount of cytoplasm is somewhat greater in eosinophilic foci than normal hepatocytes, while the nuclei appear comparable. Both focus types retain normal lobular architecture, though there may be evidence of compression along the circumference of the lesion in eosinophilic versus basophilic foci. Eosinophilic and basophilic foci appear as spontaneous lesions in multiple strains of rats beginning at about 1 year of age (Popp et al. 1985; Harada et al. 1989). The incidence of animals with foci and the number of spontaneous foci per liver increase with increasing age, making the lesion very common in control as well as treated animals at the end of a typical 2-year carcinogenicity study. The number and size of foci tend to increase when rats are treated with genotoxic or nongenotoxic hepatocarcinogens, and progression from foci to tumors does occur but is infrequently observed. Foci of cellular alteration are proliferative lesions as demonstrated by an increased number of cells synthesizing DNA compared to normal hepatocytes (Marsman and Popp 1994). Animals treated with nongenotoxic hepatocarcinogens also demonstrate a greater proliferation rate in focal hepatocytes than is found in focal hepatocytes of nontreated animals. Although some types of foci in the rat are generally believed to be precursors to hepatic tumors, the frequency of progression from focus to tumor is extraordinarily low. Stereological analysis in time sequence studies with several different experimental nongenotoxic carcinogens in rats indicates that only one in several thousand foci will progress to neoplasia, though this number may be somewhat different for different compounds. While hepatocellular tumors are generally believed to develop from foci of cellular alteration, it is important to note that the presence of drug-enhanced numbers of foci does not necessarily indicate that the molecule will be a hepatocarcinogen when evaluated over a 2-year time period (Wood et al. 1991). Since tumor development occurs in multiple steps, some compounds that may readily cause foci to form lack the ability to make them progress to tumors. There is frequent discussion as to whether basophilic or eosinophilic foci have the greater potential to develop into hepatocellular tumors. While basophilic foci are often considered to be of greater concern, there are examples of drugs that almost exclusively induce eosinophilic foci that do progress to hepatocellular tumors. Increases in clear cell foci may occur in treated animals, though these foci tend to be a mixture of clear cells and eosinophilic cells and are less common with continued administration of the drug. Vacuolated foci generally represent focal lipidosis, which should not be considered as a precursor to tumor formation.

There are substantial differences in foci formation in various species. Foci of cellular alteration are most numerous in the rat compared with the mouse for both spontaneous and compound-induced foci. Mice have a very low incidence of spontaneous foci, and these are very few in number within a single liver. Likewise, foci of cellular alteration tend to be much less frequently observed in mice administered with hepatocarcinogens. Foci of cellular alteration are also rare in dogs, non-human primates, and humans, though they have been described.

Hepatocellular adenomas occur spontaneously in a relatively low incidence that is somewhat dependent on strain and can also vary between laboratories. These lesions are characterized by a loss of lobular pattern and demonstrate obvious compression along the edge of the lesion but lack the highly disorganized characteristics and cellular atypia commonly observed in the hepatocellular carcinoma. The tinctorial properties of the cytoplasm are variable. While adenomas are frequently composed of more basophilic-appearing hepatocytes, this is not always the case. The tinctorial properties of adenomas that are related to test article administration, particularly the smaller ones, tend to be similar to the tinctorial properties of the most common type of focus of cellular alteration associated with administration of that particular compound.

Spontaneous hepatocellular carcinomas are less frequent than spontaneous adenomas in both rats and mice. An increased incidence of this neoplasm in treated animals is an important indication of a carcinogenic response in rodents but should also be evaluated in the context of latency period and rate of metastasis. Decreased latency and increased rates of metastasis are important indicators of the biological activity of the material being administered. Hepatocellular carcinomas manifest the classical criteria of malignancy, including local invasion and cellular atypia. Variation of cellular size and staining may be the first indication of a malignant lesion when examined at low power. While increased mitotic figures may be noted, many hepatocellular carcinomas tend to have few mitotic figures. Hepatocellular carcinomas cause compression of adjacent parenchyma, and the lobular architecture is replaced by a variety of abnormal tissue patterns (Figure 10.3d). Historically, these patterns have led to many different subclassifications of hepatocellular carcinomas having entered the literature, for example, trabecular (cords > 3 cells in width), acinar, and solid. While this is an interesting exercise and may have value in experimental carcinogenesis, the subclassification of hepatocellular carcinomas does not serve a useful purpose in drug development, while the metastatic rate is much more important.

Hepatocellular tumors, especially benign tumors, must be distinguished from localized hepatocellular hyperplasia/foci of cellular alteration. While the histological distinction between adenomas and localized hepatocellular hyperplasia is difficult and subtle, this distinction should be considered based on the histological distinctions described (Thoolen et al. 2010). Localized hepatocellular hyperplasia is most frequently found in livers with previous or ongoing substantial hepatocellular injury.

Hepatodiaphragmatic nodules represent congenital anomalies and are not neoplasms, though they can be confused with neoplasms by an inexperienced pathologist. These lesions are located at the hilus of the liver on the diaphragmatic surface and are generally noted grossly. When carefully dissected, the nodule appears to extend through the diaphragm, although there is a thin fibrous component of the diaphragm that separates the lesion from the thoracic cavity. Histologically, the nodule is composed of relatively normal-appearing hepatic architecture, including identifiable lobular structures with central veins and portal triads. Hepatodiaphragmatic nodules are found in rats but not mice and are relatively common in Fischer 344 rats compared with rats of other strains (Rittinghausen et al. 1998; Eustis et al. 1990).

While a drug-related increase in incidence of any neoplasm in a rodent carcinogenicity study raises concern for potential human risk, this occurs more often with rodent hepatocytic tumors. Multiple factors must be considered in assessing risk. First, the compound's genotoxic potential must be considered, though most molecules being developed for human therapy that require carcinogenicity studies are negative, or they would have been previously removed from clinical development. Nevertheless, a positive and unexpected liver tumor finding indicates that the genotoxicity data should be reevaluated, including consideration of the potential effects of metabolites and impurities. The results of this reevaluation may suggest a need for additional genotoxicity studies to be certain that the molecule is clearly negative. Once negative genotoxicity has been established, based on the data and best scientific judgment, assessment of the relevance of the carcinogenic response for human subjects or patients may proceed. If an increased tumor incidence occurred with an apparent dose response leading to the identification of a noncarcinogenic dose, efforts should focus on what nontumor effects may be associated with the tumor response and not present in the livers from nontumor doses. While there are many possibilities, a specific example would be to consider that low-grade toxicity may be occurring as demonstrated by chronic enhancement of hepatocyte proliferation at the carcinogenic dose but not at the noncarcinogenic dose. If chronic toxicity is related to the development of tumors, this information should be used in assessing human risk. It is very common that the highest dose levels selected for carcinogenicity studies lead to exposures that are several multiples higher than would occur in humans. These highest exposure levels may produce a rodent hepatocarcinogenic response that is secondary to chronic toxicity. A reasonable safety margin between the highest exposure that does not produce tumors in the rodent and intended human exposure greatly reduces the concern for human carcinogenic potential, when the mode of action resulting in carcinogenicity does not occur at human exposures.

10.1.9.2 Hepatoblastoma

Hepatoblastomas are uncommon tumors in mice, whether in treated or control groups, and have not been reported in the liver of rats. While this tumor continues to be very rare in Swiss Webster mice, there have been increasing incidences in B6C3F1 mice in the National Toxicology Program (NTP), though the tumor still remains relatively rare in this mouse strain (Turusov et al. 2002). Although the lesion has been well described in both mice and humans, its rarity in mice had resulted in limited information on its biology until the increased incidence in the NTP has allowed limited assessment of the origin and biological potential, at least in the B6C3F1 mouse. It is unclear whether this information is also applicable to the Swiss Webster mouse. (The Swiss Webster strain is closely related to the CD-1 strain that is most commonly used in pharmaceutical development at this time.) Hepatoblastomas have been observed in B6C3F1 mice in three NTP studies evaluating pharmaceuticals (primidone, oxazepam, and methylphenidate) (Turusov et al. 2002). It is interesting that in the oxazepam studies where the drug was evaluated in both B6C3F1 and Swiss Webster strains of mice, hepatoblastomas were noted only in the B6C3F1 strain. Grossly, hepatoblastomas are most frequently observed as single lesions. Microscopically, hepatoblastomas are very cellular and characterized by dark, basophilic staining, resulting from the intense staining of the nuclei, surrounded by scant, slightly basophilic cytoplasm (Figure 10.3e). The cells may form sheets or, in some cases, small rosettes around vascular spaces, which may be cystic. Mitotic figures may be numerous. Squamous and osteoid differentiation may be observed. In the NTP series of tumors, most hepatoblastomas appeared to develop within a hepatocellular adenoma or carcinoma rather than de novo. Metastases may occur to the lung, lymph node, mesentery, and kidney, where the morphology of the primary tumor is maintained. Since the rate of metastases is low, hepatoblastomas are considered a low-grade malignancy. Hepatoblastomas are also found in humans, though almost exclusively in children. In contrast, these neoplasms are found in aged mice, similar to the age when other hepatocellular tumors occur in mice. Based on current knowledge, the mouse hepatoblastoma should be considered in conjunction with other hepatocellular tumors for the purpose of human risk assessment.

10.1.9.3 Bile Duct Epithelium

Bile duct tumors and related proliferative lesions (other than simple bile duct hyperplasia) are rare spontaneous lesions in rats and mice (Thoolen et al. 2010) and are also uncommon as a response to drug administration in comparison to the much more frequent appearance of spontaneous and drug-induced hepatocellular tumors.

Cholangiomas are well-circumscribed lesions composed of relatively well-formed acini that are lined by cuboidal basophilic epithelial cells (Figure 10.3f). In some instances, the spaces may become cystic with papillary projections. This lesion must be distinguished from cystic bile duct hyperplasia, as well as cholangiocarcinoma and early forms of cholangiofibrosis, which contain significant fibrous connective tissue.

Cholangiocarcinomas may have a glandular structure similar to cholangiomas but may also be solid or appear in cystic forms. The cells are typically more basophilic and are more irregular in size, shape, and organization compared to the cholangioma. Local invasion into lymphatics and blood vessels is expected. Metastasis is common. While cholangiocarcinomas must be differentiated from cholangiomas, this distinction is not difficult based on classical criteria. However, the distinction between cholangiocarcinoma and cholangiofibrosis (discussed above) may be diagnostically challenging. While the cholangiocarcinoma may contain significant fibrosis, the degree of fibrosis is generally much less compared to cholangiofibrosis. In addition, cholangiofibrosis is characterized by mucin-filled cysts, regressing ducts, and ducts lined by intestinal or goblet-type cells that are not typical for cholangiocarcinoma.

Since bile duct tumors are rarely found in carcinogenicity testing of pharmaceuticals, there is little precedent in addressing human risk based on these tumor types. Obviously, genotoxicity of the potential therapeutic agent and/or bile-excreted metabolites should be given serious consideration as there are a few examples of nongenotoxic bile duct carcinogens.

Combined carcinomas with both hepatocellular and cholangiocellular differentiation have been described as rare spontaneous lesions in B6C3F1 mice (Bach et al. 2010). These lesions are diagnosed as hepatocholangiocellular carcinomas (or hepatocholangiocarcinomas). Histologically, these neoplasms are characterized by proliferative hepatocellular and biliary epithelial components in addition to a poorly differentiated, often sarcomatous component. These neoplasms have a high propensity to metastasize. Hepatocholangiocellular carcinomas have not been reported to occur in other mouse strains.

10.1.9.4 Endothelial Tumors

Hemangiomas and hemangiosarcomas spontaneously occur in rats and mice, though they are more common in mice. Since these are vascular tumors that can occur in many different organs, the liver is rarely the only, or even the predominant, site of such neoplasms. While these tumors can be induced by a number of chemicals and pesticides, there has been increased interest in the induction of these tumors by pharmaceuticals in the last decade. Tumors of endothelial origin are associated with drugs of several different chemical structures and therapeutic indications (Cohen et al. 2009). There has been a heightened interest in these tumors as they appear to be increased in animals given PPAR gamma agonists, though these tumors generally originate in adipose tissue and do not primarily involve the liver. Pharmaceutical-induced tumors of endothelial origin occur primarily in mice and rarely in rats.

Hemangiomas consist of blood-filled spaces lined by a single layer of endothelial cells. They tend to be discrete lesions causing compression of the surrounding tissue but are rarely encapsulated. In some tumors, the spaces are cystic and filled with blood. Mitotic figures are rare. Hemangiomas rarely, if ever, demonstrate progression to hemangiosarcomas, which appear to arise independently of hemangiomas.

Hemangiosarcomas are composed of proliferating endothelial cells that may form vascular spaces but may also form solid sheets of neoplastic cells, at least in some areas of the neoplasm, making identification of the parent cell difficult. However, most, if not all, hemangiosarcomas will have areas that are clearly composed of vascular spaces (Figure 10.4a), though they may be difficult to distinguish. The individual cells will demonstrate atypia, including variation of nuclear size and staining intensity. Mitotic figures are usually present. The tumor has indistinct borders as a result of local invasion, and metastasis is fairly common.

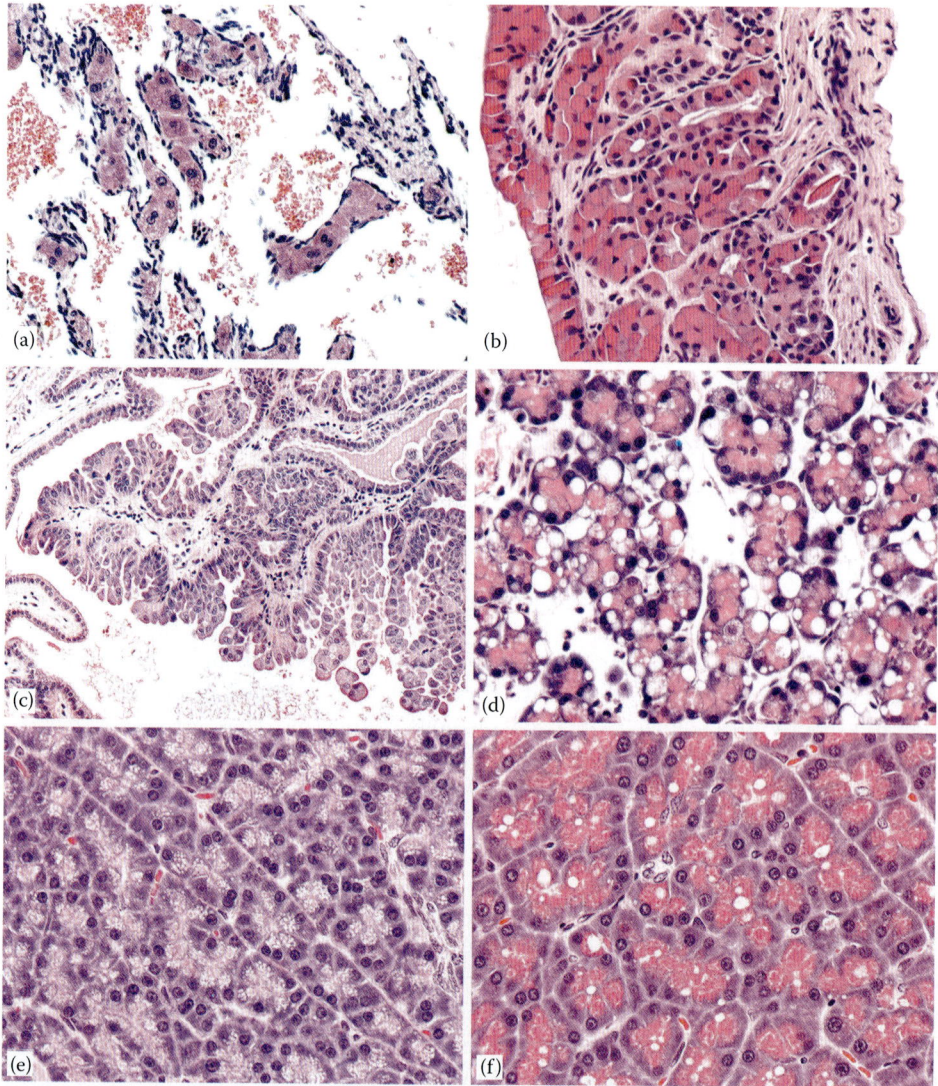

FIGURE 10.4 (a) Hemangiosarcoma. Neoplastic endothelial cells are plump and line vascular spaces between remnants of hepatocellular parenchyma. (b) Epithelial alteration, gallbladder epithelium. The epithelial cells contain prominent hyaline cytoplasm, and there is hyperplasia and inflammatory cell infiltration of the gallbladder mucosa. (c) Gallbladder adenoma. The neoplastic mucosal epithelium lines a fibrovascular stroma that forms a mass within the gallbladder lumen. (d) Pancreatic vacuolation, degenerative. This form of vacuolation is considered to result from autophagy in response to acinar cell injury, leading to the appearance of variably sized vacuoles that occasionally contain inclusions. (e) Pancreatic vacuolation, storage form. This form of vacuolation is considered to result from accumulation of material within lysosomes, leading to the appearance of small, uniformly sized vacuoles. (f) Pancreatic vacuolation, artifactual. These vacuoles appear in patchy distribution, may contain amorphous eosinophilic material, and often vary in size and shape. Ultrastructurally, these vacuoles are not associated with cellular organelles.

The lack of obvious precursor lesions and the late appearance of these tumors have hindered studies on the biology of tumor induction that would assist human risk assessment. Important information relative to the mechanism of endothelial tumor induction has been obtained in the case of the PPAR-gamma agonists (Cohen et al. 2009). Multiple mechanisms of endothelial tumor induction are likely so that the pathogenesis with a given molecule may not be applicable to human risk assessment with another molecule.

10.1.9.5 Stellate Cell Tumors (Ito Cell Tumors)

Stellate cell tumors are very rare as spontaneous and drug-induced neoplasms; therefore, the biology and human risk assessment consequences are unknown. The tumor may occur at a single site or may be multicentric. At the edge of the lesion, the tumor cells appear to dissect between hepatocytes. The individual cells may be finely vacuolated. While the tumor is rare, it should be distinguished from tumors of Kupffer cell origin.

10.1.9.6 Kupffer Cell Tumors

Kupffer cell tumors are very rare as spontaneous or drug-induced neoplasms. They may be single or multicentric and form small clusters between adjacent hepatocytes. A neoplasm termed "histiocytic sarcoma," which is found in rats, has been considered to be of Kupffer cell origin, though this point has not been well documented (Thoolen et al. 2010).

10.1.9.7 Histiocytic Sarcoma

Histiocytic sarcomas generally appear as multicentric nodules in the liver, but the lesion is also frequently found in other organs of the same animal and is rarely restricted to the liver. Many nodules will have a central necrotic zone surrounded by palisading cells. Neoplastic cells have nuclei of variable size and shape but are typically oval. The cell cytoplasm is modest in extent with indistinct borders, and multinucleated giant cells can be observed.

10.2 GALLBLADDER

The gallbladder is a hollow organ that receives bile from the liver, stores and concentrates bile, and excretes it into the duodenum. It is thin-walled and lined by a mucosa that is surrounded by a muscular tunic and serosa. In addition to its serosal and vascular attachments, it is secured to the biliary tree by the duct that joins with the common bile duct. The gallbladder is stimulated to secrete its contents by increasing blood levels of cholecystokinin, a peptide hormone released by endocrine cells of the small intestine. Among animal species typically found in safety assessment studies, rats lack gallbladders, but mice, dogs, and NHPs do have gallbladders. Given in part that many safety assessment programs rely heavily upon the rat in toxicology studies, the gallbladder is only rarely a toxicologically significant target organ.

Cystic mucinous hyperplasia is a lesion of the gallbladder in dogs that is characterized by formation of intraluminal projections of the mucosa with abundant accumulation of mucin within the lumen and within cystic structures formed by the mucosa (Kovatch et al. 1965). Grossly, this appears as a thick, white material continuous with the wall of the gallbladder, and that fills and replaces, or dramatically reduces, the bile containing luminal space. By light microscopy, the relative amounts of epithelial proliferation, cyst formation, and PAS-positive mucin accumulation may vary. The mucosal epithelium is cuboidal to columnar, and squamous metaplasia is rarely noted. Electron microscopy does not add any additional information, and clinical pathology does not provide any reliable parameters for monitoring this condition.

In the evaluation of safety assessment studies in dogs, it is first important to determine whether cystic mucinous hyperplasia represents a spontaneous background finding or may be related to the test article. While the cause in spontaneous cases is unknown, as is the mechanism of drug-induced lesions, mucin secretion has been shown to be modulated by specific bile salts in dog gallbladder epithelium (Klinkspoor et al. 1995). However, the lesion has been associated with administration of steroids with progestational activity (Geil and Lamar 1977; Mawdesley-Thomas and Noel 1967). The lesion is generally accepted as being irrelevant to the prediction of human risk in clinical studies or approved usage of drugs. This is, at least in part, because the widespread use of progestins in humans has not been associated with a risk of gallbladder disease.

A potential confounder of cystic mucinous hyperplasia is the occurrence of gallbladder mucocoeles in dogs (Worley et al. 2004). This condition has been described as a spontaneous cause of morbidity and an indication for cholecystectomy in clinical veterinary medicine. Mucocoele is characterized by accumulation of a green-black, bile-laden, semisolid to immobile mucoid mass within the fundus of the gallbladder and in some cases may lead to compromised integrity of the gallbladder and sequelae (e.g., secondary peritonitis). The light microscopic features of gallbladders with mucocoele have variably included mucosal epithelial necrosis, inflammation, and/or cystic hyperplasia. The pathogenesis is unknown, but a possible association with hyperadrenalcorticism has been identified. Mucocoeles have not been reported as spontaneous or test article–related findings in safety studies.

Cholecystitis (inflammation of the gallbladder) is occasionally observed in safety assessment studies (Glaze et al. 2005). By light microscopy, cholecystitis is variably characterized by congestion, hemorrhage, and edema of the lamina propria and serosa, mucosal ulceration, and inflammatory cell infiltration. The inflammatory cells may be neutrophilic in the early stages, but macrophages and lymphocytes may be more frequently observed in the later stages. Regenerative proliferation of mucosal epithelium and fibrovascular tissue formation represent the repair phase, and these features may be present either following exudation and mucosal ulceration or while they are still occurring. Clinical pathology provides reliable parameters for monitoring inflammatory processes, but none are specific for the gallbladder. Elevations in circulating bilirubin levels and activities of AST and amylase may be inconsistently observed in cholecystitis and are not specific for the lesion. In dogs, it is possible to monitor wall thickness by CT or by ultrasonography, and wall thickness may be increased due to inflammation. Such imaging techniques for gallbladder are not well established for toxicology studies.

In toxicology studies involving dogs, cholecystitis is infrequent as a spontaneous lesion; therefore, its presence in treated animals is often considered as attributable to the test article. In dogs, cholecystitis has been reported following treatment with cholesterol-lowering agents that inhibit HMG-CoA reductase (Gerson et al. 1991; Hartman et al. 1996). However, the use of these drugs in humans has not been associated with gallbladder disease. In humans, cholecystitis is a common disease that is almost always secondary to the formation of gallstones. Gallstones are a fairly common occurrence in humans (in contrast to most animal species, including mice, dogs, and NHP), and the etiology includes many factors such as heredity, ethnicity, age, and sex, as well as drugs including clofibrate, oral contraceptives, and octreotide (Davidson et al. 2007; Redfern and Fortuner 1995). Taken together, these data indicate that cholecystitis in the dog is not predictive of human risk, and with an appropriate noninvasive monitoring strategy, clinical studies may proceed.

In toxicology studies of mice and NHP, cholecystitis may be more commonly found as a background lesion. In mice, it appears as a spontaneous lesion of unknown pathogenesis, typically in aged mice (Lewis 1984). In macaques, cholecystitis has been associated with infection by *Enterocytozoon bieneusi* (Wachtman and Mansfield 2008). This microsporidian parasite has also been associated with cholecystitis in immunosuppressed human patients, so that a secondary effect of immunosuppression could be considered a contributing factor of an apparent test article association of this lesion in the macaques. With respect to safety assessment, it is not possible to generalize regarding the implications of cholecystitis in mice or NHPs regarding risk to humans. If related to a test article, cholecystitis in these species may represent an impediment to human clinical studies unless a safety margin is established, a plausible mechanism is elucidated, and an appropriate noninvasive monitoring strategy can be pursued.

In some instances, cholecystitis must be differentiated from *vasculitis*, at least in dogs and, to a limited extent, in macaques. A variety of drugs have been associated with vasculitis (see discussion in Chapter 17). Although not strictly limited to the gallbladder, the segmental nature of vasculitis probably leads to an underestimation of its distribution. In addition, the wall of the gallbladder is not thick, and evidence of edema and hemorrhage, which may occur as a consequence of vasculitis, is readily detected at gross examination. It is also possible, but not known, that the blood vessels of the gallbladder may be at greater risk for certain mechanisms of vasculitis. Despite the overlap in the gross appearance, it is usually possible to distinguish vasculitis of the gallbladder from cholecystitis by light microscopic detection of vessel lesions, which are usually also present elsewhere.

Epithelial alteration has been described in the gallbladder of mice and dogs. Given the diverse nature of the changes, it is often useful to describe the appearance of epithelial alteration in the comment to the diagnosis and/or in the report narrative.

In mice, epithelial alteration has various synonyms (hyalinosis, crystals, cytoplasmic inclusions) that reflect its light microscopic appearance of a uniform and prominent hyaline eosinophilic cytoplasm of the mucosal epithelial cells (Figure 10.4b) (Thoolen et al. 2010; Ward et al. 2001). Its appearance usually results from the accumulation of YM1 (also called Chi313), a chitinase-like protein that may be confirmed by immunohistochemistry. In the gallbladder and other tissues (notably lung, kidney, and stomach), this protein has often (but not exclusively) been reported in association with inflammation and proliferative lesions. Its appearance in the gallbladder and other tissues has been reported as a treatment effect in chronic studies. The presence of this epithelial alteration in mice does not cause morbidity or mortality. Its association with penicillin as a test article in mice (National Toxicology Program 1988) suggests that, by itself, it should not present serious concerns for human safety.

A different form of epithelial alteration has been described as epithelial vacuolation and macrophage infiltration in dogs (Molon-Noblot et al. 1996). By light microscopy, this lesion appears as vacuoles that are demonstrated to contain neutral lipid using histochemical stains such as Sudan black or oil red O. By TEM, the lesion was characterized by accumulation of lipid droplets and a loss of the mucosal epithelial cell microvilli, with increased numbers of macrophages containing cytoplasmic myelin figures. The pathogenesis of this lesion and its significance for safety assessment are unknown.

Epithelial proliferative lesions of the gallbladder are rare in mice, dogs, and NHPs. As a result, it is not possible to generalize about the light microscopic or ancillary findings in species commonly used for safety assessment. In mice, hyperplasias and papillomas (adenomas) have been described as exceedingly rare spontaneous findings (Lewis 1984). The gallbladder adenoma typically appears as a solitary mass of well-differentiated epithelial cells that line a predominantly papillary fibrovascular stroma, arising from the wall of the gallbladder (Figure 10.4c). Gallbladder adenomas in mice have been reported as test article–related findings in safety assessment studies of a PPAR-alpha/gamma agonist (though the reported incidence was low, the rarity of the lesion as a spontaneous finding suggested a test article–related effect) (Waites et al. 2007). In dogs, proliferative lesions of the gallbladder are similarly rare as spontaneous or test article–related findings. A gallbladder carcinoma and an extrahepatic bile duct carcinoma were reported as spontaneous lesions in companion dogs (Patnaik et al. 1981). It has been reported that experimental carcinogens can cause gallbladder tumors in dogs, but there are no reports implicating drugs or drug candidates. In NHPs, gallbladder carcinoma is a rare spontaneous lesion that has not been reported in association with drug administration but was associated with aflatoxin treatment (Sieber et al. 1979).

10.3 EXOCRINE PANCREAS

10.3.1 Introduction

The pancreas is an unpaired, secretory digestive organ composed of an exocrine portion in the form of acini and ducts, an endocrine portion largely in the form of the islets of Langerhans, and sparse loose connective tissue comprising the interstitium (Klimstra 1997). In comparison with the liver, the exocrine pancreas makes an insignificant contribution to drug metabolism and detoxification and is seldom identified as a target organ of xenobiotic toxicity (Longnecker and Wilson 2002).

However, when it is identified as a target, a heightened sense of concern is warranted because of the potentially serious clinical implications related to acinar cell injury (pancreatic inflammation/ autodigestion) and acinar/ductal cell proliferation (pancreatic cancer).

10.3.2 Embryology

The pancreas develops from the endoderm of the foregut near the transition to the midgut in a region known as the hepatopancreatic ring. This region gives rise to the liver, pancreas, and a series of mucinous glands. The pancreas in humans originates from two diverticula of the foregut producing ventral and dorsal pancreatic primordia. In most other mammals, one dorsal and two ventral pancreatic diverticula are formed; however, the left ventral diverticulum remains small and eventually disappears. Changes in topography resulting from differential growth of the duodenal wall eventually bring the dorsal and ventral primordia into contact. The dorsal primordium forms part of the head, the body, and the tail of the pancreas, and the ventral primordium contributes to the head of the pancreas. Since the dorsal and ventral primordia arise from separate evaginations of the foregut, these connections to the intestine will serve as the draining ducts. In humans, the duct systems of dorsal and ventral pancreas become connected, and the ventral duct becomes the main duct, which empties with the common bile duct into the duodenum. The former connection of the dorsal pancreas to the duodenum is generally lost; however, in other mammals, persistence of both ducts is regularly seen (Böck et al. 1997; Foster 2009).

The endodermal sprouts, destined to give rise to the pancreas, proliferate and develop as solid cords of cells that push into the surrounding mesenchyme and become enveloped by condensed mesodermal cells. These endodermal sprouts produce both the exocrine and endocrine pancreas. The cellular cords gradually acquire lumina that extend from the openings of the main ducts to the periphery of the developing gland. These cells demonstrate polarity with apical microvilli and are joined by terminal bars. The cells at the termination of this extensive network of branched cords develop into acinar cells, and this differentiation is reflected by the accumulation of rough ER, Golgi areas, and secretory granules (Böck et al. 1997; Klimstra 1997).

10.3.3 Gross Anatomy

The pancreas is a faintly lobulated, pale, yellow to tan-pink organ that extends from the duodenum to the hilum of the spleen. The gross anatomy of the pancreas varies substantially between humans and domestic or laboratory animals; therefore, the terminology used from humans is not adequate for animals. The head of the pancreas in humans is adjacent to the superior duodenal flexure, extending to the left as the body of the pancreas and eventually elongating toward the spleen as the tail of the pancreas. In many domestic animals, including dogs, the body or middle part of the pancreas is adjacent to the duodenum, and left and right lobes extend from it to the respective sides. Small laboratory rodents have duodenal, gastric, and splenic lobes of the pancreas, and each lobe has a main excretory duct that joins the common bile duct before reaching the duodenum. Additionally, accessory or aberrant lobes of pancreas are common in mice and rats, and each of these lobes has its own excretory duct (Böck et al. 1997; Longnecker and Wilson 2002; Sisson and Grossman 1953).

10.3.4 Microscopic Anatomy

Microscopically, the pancreas is arranged in multiple lobules separated by loose connective tissue septa that often contain adipocytes. Each lobule is highly cellular, containing both exocrine and endocrine pancreas. The exocrine pancreas is composed of two epithelial cell types, acinar and ductal, with the acinar epithelium making up the major portion of the pancreas. By routine light microscopy, the acinar cells are triangular to polygonal with basally located, round nuclei that generally have distinct central nucleoli and are arranged around a central lumen to form a glandular acinus. The basal cytoplasm is basophilic due to the high content of ribonucleoproteins owing to the abundant rough ER in the acinar cells. A clear zone of cytoplasm, just above the nucleus, is often observed and corresponds with the Golgi zone. The apical cytoplasm is granular and eosinophilic, reflecting the accumulation of numerous zymogen granules containing the secretory products of the exocrine pancreas. The accumulation of zymogen granules is variable depending upon the secretory state of the pancreas. Immunohistochemical stains of acinar cells show that the cells contain trypsin, chymotrypsin, carboxypeptidases A and B, lipase, amylase, elastase, DNase, and RNase. Each of these enzymes is present in the zymogen granules in a proenzyme form (Bendayan and Ito 1979; Böck et al. 1997; Kraehenbuhl et al. 1977; Longnecker and Wilson 2002), and detailed immunocytochemical analysis has shown that all exocrine cells in the gland and all zymogen granules and Golgi in each cell are qualitatively alike with regard to their content of secretory proteins (Kraehenbuhl et al. 1977). Each acinar cell is adjoined to adjacent acinar cells by zonula occludens– and zonula adherens–type junctions near the acinar lumen. Each acinus is surrounded by a continuous basement membrane, and no myoepithelial or basal cells have been recognized (Klimstra 1997). Although the acinar cells from different areas of the pancreas are morphologically and functionally similar, the size of nuclei and quantity of zymogen granules are often increased in acinar cells surrounding the islets. It has been suggested that this "halo effect" is due to the connections between the vessels of the islets and capillaries of the adjacent acinar cells and the resulting exposure of these peri-islet acini to high levels of insulin or other hormones from the islets (Henderson et al. 1981).

The ductal system is composed of five components consisting of centroacinar cells (located in the middle of the exocrine acini), followed in order by the intercalated, intralobular, interlobular, and main ducts. The centroacinar cells are small, flat to cuboidal cells that border the acinar lumina along with the acinar cells, to which they are joined by tight junctions. The lining of the acinus is incompletely bordered by centroacinar cells, and the lumen formed by the acinar and centroacinar cells drains into the intercalated ducts. The intercalated ducts are low cuboidal and resemble the centroacinar cells. Neither of these cell types contains zymogen, neurosecretory, or mucin granules (Klimstra 1997).

The intercalated ducts fuse imperceptibly to form the intralobular ducts. Neither of these ducts has a significant collagen matrix around them; however, once the ducts leave the lobules, they acquire a variably thick rim of collagen and are termed interlobular ducts. The epithelium of intralobular and interlobular ducts progresses from cuboidal to low columnar and contains sulfomucins. As the interlobular ducts approach the main pancreatic ducts, they develop an increasingly thick collagenous wall. The epithelium becomes columnar, and epithelial mucins are more abundant. Each main pancreatic duct receives numerous tributaries of interlobular ducts (Klimstra 1997).

Acinar and ductal cells of the exocrine pancreas can undergo mitosis, and mitotic figures are occasionally seen in acinar and, less often, in duct epithelium of control animals. Ki67 expression and BrdU incorporation in acinar cells expressing amylase suggest that acinar cells can enter the cell cycle in a differentiated state (Strobel et al. 2007a). Cell lineage tracing studies have demonstrated that both of these epithelial cell components are important in establishing the exocrine cell mass during normal physiological processes and following acinar cell injury. It appears that centroacinar/terminal duct cells are important progenitors of acinar cells during physiologic organ maintenance (Furuyama et al. 2011), while surviving acinar cells are important in regeneration of the acinar cell mass after injury or partial pancreatectomy (Desai et al. 2007; Hess et al. 2011; Jensen et al. 2005; Strobel et al. 2007a).

Although the exocrine pancreas contains the expected vascular, neural, and connective tissue support structures, these features will not be discussed further. However, an additional cell type, the pancreatic stellate cell, deserves additional mention since it has attracted attention as an important element in the reparative response to exocrine pancreatic injury. Pancreatic stellate cells are myofibroblast-like cells that are present in the periacinar space of the exocrine pancreas and have long cytoplasmic processes that encircle the base of the acinus. The cells are also found in the periductal and perivascular regions of the pancreas (Omary et al. 2007). They are similar to hepatic stellate cells and, in the quiescent state, are characterized by the presence of the intermediate filament proteins, desmin and glial fibrillary acidic protein (GFAP), and intracellular fat droplets. These features together distinguish pancreatic stellate cells from normal fibroblasts (Apte et al. 1998; Bachem et al. 1998). Pancreatic stellate cells are activated by a variety of factors such as cytokines, growth factors, and angiotensin II and, when activated, lose their fat droplets and express α-smooth muscle actin (-SMA) and extracellular matrix proteins such as collagen types I and III and fibronectin. Given the expression of such a diversity of proteins and the ability to respond to a variety of "inflammatory" mediators, it is not surprising that pancreatic stellate cells are thought to have a key role in the fibrosis that accompanies chronic pancreatitis and pancreatic adenocarcinoma (Omary et al. 2007).

10.3.5 Immunohistochemical Markers

A variety of immunohistochemical markers can be used to differentiate the epithelial components of the exocrine pancreas, although some species differences are noted. In the rat, cytokeratins 19 and 20 were detected only in cells of the ductal system, from centroacinar cells to the main ducts. Antibodies to cytokeratin 7 labeled epithelial cells of the islets and of the main, interlobular, and intralobular ducts, but not the centroacinar or terminal duct cells. All three of these cytokeratins were expressed in proliferating ducts during tissue regeneration following partial pancreatectomy (Bouwens et al. 1995).

Protein markers of acinar epithelium include any of the digestive enzymes or their proenzyme forms including amylase, carboxypeptidase, chymotrypsin, elastase, lipase, and trypsin (Bendayan and Ito 1979; Hansen et al. 1981). Amylase appears to be used more often than the other markers as an experimental tool for demonstrating acinar cell differentiation (Desai et al. 2007; Furuyama et al. 2011; Hess et al. 2011). MIST1 has been used similarly as a marker of differentiated acinar epithelium (Hess et al. 2011). Trypsinogen-activation peptide (TAP), an amino-terminal peptide released from trypsinogen when trypsin is formed, can be used as a marker to demonstrate intracellular activation of trypsinogen (Hofbauer et al. 1998; Seyama et al. 2003) Antibodies to cytokeratins 8 and 18 label acinar epithelium; however, these antibodies also label islet and duct epithelium (Schüssler et al. 1992).

10.3.6 Physiology of Secretion

Secretion of pancreatic juice is primarily under hormonal control. Cholecystokinin (CCK) secreted from the upper small intestine acts on the acinar cells of the pancreas via their CCKA receptor (CCKAR) to cause release of zymogen granules rich in pancreatic proenzymes and augments the action of secretin on pancreatic ducts to cause secretion of bicarbonate-rich fluid. Acetylcholine may also act on acinar cells to cause the release of zymogen granules, and this effect appears to be mediated through vagal nerve stimulation. The enzymes of the pancreas are secreted as inactive proenzymes into the duodenum where the intestinal brush border enzyme, enteropeptidase (enterokinase), converts trypsinogen to its active form. Trypsin can also activate trypsinogen; therefore, once trypsin is formed, there is an autocatalytic chain reaction. Trypsin subsequently converts other secreted pancreatic enzymes, such as proelastase, procarboxypeptidases, and chymotrypsinogens, to their active forms (Ganong 1991; Longnecker and Wilson 2002). Given the autocatalytic capacity of trypsin and its ability to activate other proenzymes in zymogen granules, it is not surprising that intra-acinar activation of trypsinogen to trypsin is central to the pathogenesis of acute pancreatitis (Chan and Leung 2007; Dawra et al. 2011).

10.3.7 Pathology of Exocrine Pancreas

Vacuolation of acinar epithelium has been described following treatment with numerous agents including arginine, (Tani et al. 1990), supraphysiologic stimulation with cerulein, a CCK receptor agonist, cyclosporine A (Hirano et al. 1992), choline-deficient, ethionine-supplemented diet (Mareninova et al. 2009), palmitoylpentachlorophenol (PPCP) (Ansari et al. 1987), puromycin (Longnecker et al. 1975), and 2,3,7,8-tetrachlorodibenzo-*p*-dioxin (TCDD) (Nyska et al. 2004; Yoshizawa et al. 2005). In these instances, it is generally accompanied by other changes in the exocrine pancreas such as apoptosis or necrosis of acinar cells and/or edema, hemorrhage, or inflammation. The vacuoles in affected acinar epithelium examined by light microscopy are solitary to numerous, variable in size, and often empty, but may contain eosinophilic or basophilic inclusions (Longnecker and Wilson 2002) (Figure 10.4d). They are a long-noted, but poorly understood, morphologic feature generally accompanied by other evidence of acinar cell injury or inflammation and are formed by autophagy (Grasso et al. 2011; Hashimoto et al. 2008; Mareninova et al. 2009; Ropolo et al. 2007) and/or endocytosis of post-exocytic structures.

Autophagy associated with acute pancreatitis is one of the earliest descriptions of this process in human tissues (Vaccaro 2008), and the formation of autophagic vacuoles has been extensively studied in rodent models of acute pancreatitis. The role of autophagy in acute pancreatitis has been debated for decades. Some work suggests that excess (Hashimoto et al. 2008), impaired, or incomplete (Fortunato et al. 2009; Mareninova et al. 2009) autophagy has an important role in trypsinogen activation and subsequent acinar cell injury. Others believe that a form of autophagy ("zymophagy") involves a recently identified autophagy-related transmembrane protein, vacuole membrane protein 1 (VMP1) (Dusetti et al. 2002; Ropolo et al. 2007), to control intracellular zymogen activation. This process serves to protect the acinar cell from irreversible injury (Grasso et al. 2011) or eliminates the cell by apoptosis (Dusetti et al. 2002) and thereby prevents acinar cell necrosis and extracellular release of activated trypsin causing more extensive pancreatic injury. The electron microscopic appearance of autophagic vacuoles in pancreatitis induced by cerulein is that of a double membrane-bound vesicle containing zymogen granules. Other organelles and cellular material may (Hashimoto et al. 2008; Mareninova et al. 2009) or may not (Grasso et al. 2011) be present. Other vacuoles, also noted in the acinar epithelium, are filled with homogeneous or partially condensed protein content and have been interpreted as autolysosomes (Hashimoto et al. 2008) or endocytic vacuoles (Sherwood et al. 2007). Activated trypsinogen has been demonstrated in vacuoles that appear within the acinar epithelium soon after cerulein exposure (Grasso et al. 2011; Hofbauer et al. 1998; Raraty et al. 2000; Sherwood et al. 2007). It appears that subsequent to this activation, trypsin can move from this compartment into the cytosol (Hofbauer et al. 1998), initiating the intracellular digestion that leads to irreversible acinar cell injury and acute pancreatitis.

Other forms of vacuolation are also noted in the acinar epithelium. Vacuoles that are found in nearly every acinar cell and are small, round, uniform in size, and not accompanied by other changes in the exocrine pancreas should raise the suspicion of a lysosomal storage disorder (Figure 10.4e). By TEM, these vacuoles are shown to be tightly clustered in the Golgi to apical zones. Such disorders include those produced by cationic amphiphilic drugs causing accumulation of membrane phospholipids (phospholipidosis) (Fedorko 1968) and by toxins, such as the plant toxin swainsonine, which causes a specific type of glycogen storage disorder (mannosidosis) (Stegelmeier et al. 2008). Immunohistochemical staining for lysosome-associated membrane protein-2 (LAMP-2) will demonstrate that the observed vacuoles are lysosomes, and histochemical stains for lipids (Sudan Black, Oil-Red-O, Nile Red) or glycoconjugates (PAS) may help to characterize the material within the vacuoles (Obert et al. 2007). However, the histochemical stains for lipids are not particularly sensitive and require the use of material that has not been embedded in paraffin. Examination of affected exocrine cells by TEM is ultimately needed to confirm these disorders. The presence of characteristic lysosomal lamellar bodies is considered a morphologic hallmark and is diagnostic of phospholipidosis (Reasor 1989). If the vacuolated cells contain numerous lysosomes filled with any other type of material, the diagnosis of phospholipidosis can be eliminated, and biochemical analyses are likely necessary to identify the source of the vacuolation. Although the epithelium of pancreatic ducts is rarely, if ever, described as a target for drug-induced lysosomal storage disorders, the fact that this epithelium can be affected in inherited lysosomal storage diseases (Knowles et al.

1993; Schott et al. 2001) indicates that this site should be carefully examined when a drug-induced lysosomal disorder is suspected.

The possibility that the vacuoles in exocrine epithelium represent the presence of intracellular fat should also be considered, though it is unclear how commonly this is observed. Some suggest that this change does take place (Longnecker and Wilson 2002), while others imply that it does not (Omary et al. 2007). Intracellular fat vacuoles are described in ultrastructural studies of pancreatic acinar cells from rats subjected to starvation (Kitagawa and Ono 1986; López et al. 1996) or a zinc-deficient diet (Koo and Turk 1977). The presence of fat in intracellular vacuoles could be demonstrated by histochemical staining as noted above. Alternatively, the presence of fat in the vacuoles can be demonstrated by immunohistochemical staining for adipophilin, a protein that encircles intracellular fat droplets (Obert et al. 2007). This immunohistochemical procedure can be used on routine, formalin-fixed, paraffin-embedded tissues.

If the vacuolation of the acinar epithelium is generally patchy and occurs in the absence of other indications of acinar cell injury, the possibility that the vacuoles are a postmortem artifact should be seriously considered. Vacuoles in this case are irregular in size and shape and either are empty or sometimes contain a small amount of eosinophilic material (Figure 10.4f). Examination of the vacuoles by TEM shows that they are irregular in shape, are generally not membrane bound, and are either empty or contain a small amount of finely granular or membranous material (Tapp 1970). Although adjacent organelles may protrude into the vacuoles, organelles are not found within the vacuoles and appear.

10.3.7.1 Decreased Zymogen Granules

Decreased amount of zymogen granules is occasionally noted in toxicity studies and is often ascribed to decreased food consumption. Ultrastructural examination of pancreatic exocrine cells from rats subjected to starvation supports this notion (Kitagawa and Ono 1986). Decreased zymogen granules in the absence of other significant changes in exocrine pancreas have been reported in rats given a zinc-deficient diet (Koo and Turk 1977) and as a test article–related change in rats and monkeys given sunitinib, a potent inhibitor of several receptor tyrosine kinases (VEGF, PDGF, KIT, FLT3, and RET receptors) (Patyna et al. 2008). Similar alterations in exocrine pancreas did not occur in animals given a monoclonal antibody to VEGF receptor (Ryan et al. 1999), suggesting that the change caused by administration of sunitinib was not likely related to inhibition of VEGF signaling (Patyna et al. 2008).

10.3.7.2 Increased Zymogen Granules

As noted above, the quantity of zymogen granules in acini surrounding the islets is often increased in control animals, and it has been suggested that this "halo effect" is due to the connections between the vessels of the islets and capillaries of the adjacent acinar cells and the resulting exposure of these peri-islet acini to high levels of insulin or other hormones from the islets (Henderson et al. 1981). Additionally, an irregular pattern of acini containing increased zymogen granules, without the peri-islet orientation, is sometimes observed in control animals. This is particularly common in mice, so caution is warranted when considering increased zymogen granules as a drug-related effect in this species.

Inhibition of pancreatic exocrine secretion by reduction of CCK stimulus would be expected to cause accumulation of zymogen granules in the acinar epithelium. Decreased CCK signaling caused either by blockade of the CCK receptor, as seen in male Wistar rats given the CCK antagonist L-364,718 (Rodriguez et al. 1997), or by deficiency of CCK-producing cells in the intestine, as seen in BETA2/NeuroD-deficient mice (Naya et al. 1997), causes increased zymogen granules in pancreatic acini.

Exocytosis of zymogen granules from acinar epithelium is a highly regulated process, and disruption of this process at any point in the pathway could lead to increased zymogen granules in the affected epithelium. This has been demonstrated in pancreatic acini from mice genetically deficient in various components of the exocytic pathway, including interferon regulatory factor-2 (Mashima et al. 2011), Noc2 (Matsumoto et al. 2004), or Slp1 (Saegusa et al. 2008).

Administration of soybean trypsin inhibitor to male rats causes increased numbers of acinar cells and increased zymogen granule mass per acinar cell accompanied by ultrastructural changes indicative of increased zymogen granule production (Sato and Herman 1990). These observations suggest that increased production of zymogen granules, without a concomitant increase in secretion, could also cause increased zymogen granules in pancreatic acini.

10.3.7.3 Apoptosis, Necrosis, and Regeneration of Acinar Epithelium

Many agents can cause cytotoxic effects in the exocrine pancreas (Longnecker and Wilson 2002). The morphologic features of apoptotic and oncotic necrosis of acinar epithelium are similar to those already described for hepatocytes. Apoptosis of scattered acinar cells is a common finding in sections of pancreas from control animals, and the number of apoptotic bodies can vary widely from animal to animal and even within different areas of the pancreas from the same animal. Therefore, due consideration should be given before attributing to a test compound finding of increased acinar cell apoptosis if observed in the absence of other changes in the pancreas. Reports of chemicals that cause increased apoptosis without other changes in the pancreas are rare. Apoptosis of acinar cells is a notable feature in the pancreas of mice and rats given a single intravenous injection of the naturally occurring plant toxin, nitrile 1-cyano-2-hydroxy-3-butene (CHB), though decreased zymogen granules, paleness, and fine vacuolation were also prominent features. In some instances, edema and a light inflammatory cell infiltrate were noted (Wallig et al. 1988). Apoptosis of pancreatic acinar cells has been described in mice fed with a soya diet for several weeks, followed by a return to normal diet. Presumably, the trypsin-inhibiting properties of the soya diet interfere with the breakdown of trypsin-sensitive CCK-releasing peptide in the intestine and a subsequent rise in CCK leading to a trophic stimulus on the exocrine pancreas. Once this stimulus is removed by placing the mice on a normal diet, the pancreas undergoes a reduction in exocrine parenchymal cell number, attributable to increased apoptosis (Saluja et al. 1996). Apoptosis is a major component induced by conditional knockout in acinar epithelium of the Xbp1 gene, which is important for the unfolded protein response (UPR) to ER stress (Hess et al. 2011). Acinar cells from these animals also have substantial reduction in zymogen granules and cytoplasmic area associated with a greatly reduced cytoplasmic footprint. The changes in pancreas were thought to be mediated through the ER stress pathway. On the other hand, ablation of another distinct signaling arm of the UPR, protein kinase RNA-like ER kinase (PERK), in acinar epithelium causes loss of acinar cells by oncotic necrosis (oncosis) and is associated with an inflammatory cell infiltrate; however, ER stress is not considered to be the cause of acinar cell injury in this model (Iida et al. 2007).

Acinar cells in pancreatitis undergo attrition through apoptosis and oncotic necrosis. In several models of experimental pancreatitis, it has been shown that severe pancreatitis is associated with marked necrosis and little apoptosis, while mild pancreatitis is associated with little necrosis and marked apoptosis (Gukovskaya and Pandol 2004; Gukovskaya et al. 1996; Kaiser et al. 1995). Additionally, experimental manipulations to induce apoptosis have been demonstrated to reduce the severity of pancreatitis (Bhatia et al. 1998; Saluja et al. 1996), while inhibiting apoptosis worsens the severity of pancreatitis (Kaiser et al. 1996). These observations have led to discussion of therapeutic strategies to either decrease the severity of both types of cell death or to induce apoptosis as a means to decrease the severity of pancreatitis and improve clinical outcome (Gukovskaya and Pandol 2004).

Regardless of whether acinar cells are lost by apoptosis or necrosis, or by partial pancreatectomy, the pancreas demonstrates a remarkable regenerative capacity. Models of acute pancreatitis induced by injection of cerulein (Reid and Walker 1999) or arginine (Delaney et al. 1993; Tani et al. 1990) show interstitial edema and neutrophil infiltration within the first 12 h, followed by apoptosis or necrosis of acinar epithelium that peaks in severity within 72 h. Despite the severity of acinar cell injury, the lobular architecture of the pancreas returns to near-normal appearance within 7 (Desai et al. 2007; Jensen et al. 2005; Reid and Walker 1999) to 14 (Tani et al. 1990) days. Cell replacement is largely due to proliferation of surviving acinar cells (Desai et al. 2007; Jensen et al. 2005; Strobel et al. 2007a) that appear to repress the terminal acinar epithelial gene program and induce genes normally associated with pancreatic progenitor cells (Jensen et al. 2005). Similarly, surviving acinar cells appear to be the source for regeneration of new cells following extensive loss of acinar epithelium in models such as partial pancreatectomy (Desai et al. 2007) and induction of apoptosis by conditional knockout in acinar epithelium of the Xbp1 gene (Hess et al. 2011). The proliferating acinar cells do not appear to contribute to regeneration of β cells of the pancreatic islets (Desai et al. 2007) and only rarely give rise to structures having features of the terminal pancreatic ducts (Strobel et al. 2007a). In contrast, during physiologic maintenance of the pancreas, it has been shown that almost all of the exocrine duct and centroacinar and acinar cells, but none of the endocrine cells, are supplied from exocrine-specific progenitors that express the protein Sox9 and are located in the pancreatic duct structure (duct or centroacinar cells) (Furuyama et al. 2011). Taken together, these observations suggest that the source of cells responsible for acinar cell regeneration may differ when considering physiological maintenance versus response to injury and could vary depending upon the specific type of injury as has been shown for the liver (Furuyama et al. 2011).

10.3.7.4 Tubular Complexes and Metaplastic Ductal Lesions

In diseases of the pancreas such as pancreatitis and pancreatic cancer, lesions described as tubular complexes (TCs) are commonly observed (in humans and experimental animals). The TCs are defined as cylindrical tubes, often with wide lumens, lined by a monolayer of flattened, duct-like cells. Studies of TCs formed after injection of cerulein (Reid and Walker 1999) or cyanohydroxy-butene (CHB) (Kelly et al. 1999), or by intrapancreatic implantation of dimethylbenzanthracene (DMBA) (Bockman et al. 1978, 2003), indicate that TCs arise by loss of zymogen granules and/or apoptosis of acinar epithelium, accompanied by persistence of ductal cells expressing cytokeratins and the anti-apoptotic protein bcl-2.

It has been suggested that TCs are part of a group of lesions collectively described as metaplastic ductal lesions (MDLs) (Strobel et al. 2007a,b). The MDL can be subdivided based on morphologic features into TC and mucinous metaplastic lesions (MMLs), with the TC further subdivided into types 1 and 2. The tubules of the type 1 lesions are lined by a few large, flat cells that have staining characteristics similar to acinar cells and lack markers of duct cells. Tubules of the type 2 lesions are lined by many small cells and arranged in groups with branching and anastomoses and are stained for markers of duct cells. The epithelial cells of MML are not flat but vary in height depending on the amount of mucin present. The mucin is stained by PAS and Alcian blue stains. The MML may be of pure ductal phenotype or have a mixture of ductal and acinar morphology. The significance of the various forms of MDL has been controversial. The TCs are observed in pancreatitis and pancreatic cancer in humans and in animal models of pancreatic injury and chemical carcinogenesis. However, in recent years, the altered expression of mucins in pancreatic cancer has shifted the focus from the TC to MML as direct precursors of cancer (Konieczny and Leach 2007; Strobel et al. 2007a).

The distinct cellular origins of the various forms of MDL have been extensively studied in mice using genetic markers to trace cell lineage in pancreatitis induced by either a single, acute series of injections with cerulein or repeated injections of cerulein over periods of several weeks (Strobel et al. 2007a,b). These studies have shown that type 1 TCs are derived from acinar cells and that any cytokeratin positive duct-like cells in the lesions are not derived from acinar cells but likely represent persistent adjacent cells of the terminal ductal compartment. The type 2 lesions are composed of non-acinar cells, presumably of centroacinar and/or terminal duct origin, since the flattened cells are stained for cytokeratins and Hes1. Thus, these lesions represent duct cells that persist and proliferate after selective loss of acinar cells. The vast majority of MMLs are not of acinar origin. This is true whether the MMLs are of mixed or ductal morphology, suggesting that these two morphologies represent one type of lesion that appears as mixed or ductal, depending on the plane of section.

However, a small percentage (~5%) of mixed MML and a similar percentage of MML with purely ductal morphology express markers suggesting true acinar-to-ductal transdifferentiation. Though the MMLs observed in this model of repeated pancreatic injury are the only MDL with some morphologic similarities to mouse pancreatic intraepithelial neoplasia (mPanIN; considered a murine cancer precursor) (Hruban et al. 2006), progression of MML to lesions with higher atypia or to invasive neoplasia was not observed.

A low incidence of lesions morphologically consistent with TCs have been described in human islet amyloid polypeptide (HIP) transgenic mice (Matveyenko et al. 2009) and Sprague–Dawley (Nachnani et al. 2010) rats treated with GLP-1 mimetics. These lesions were attributed to the test compounds; however, this conclusion should be approached with some caution. Foci of TCs are occasionally observed as background lesions in sections of pancreas from control or vehicle-treated animals. TCs have been observed following surgical manipulation of the pancreas (Bockman et al. 1978, 2003), so it is possible that the TCs seen as a spontaneous change result from abdominal trauma. The spontaneous TC could reflect obstruction of the duct draining this specific region of the exocrine pancreas, resulting in atrophy of the associated acinar tissue (Sarles et al. 1993). The incidence of TC as a background lesion should be well documented in the specific age, sex, and strain of laboratory animal being used in experimental studies before attributing a low incidence of TC to a test compound.

10.3.7.5 Chronic Pancreatitis

Chronic pancreatitis, defined as a progressive inflammatory disease with a prominent component of fibrosis, as occurs in humans, is apparently uncommon as a drug-induced change in toxicology studies. Chronic pancreatitis in humans is often associated with chronic alcohol abuse; however, long-term ethanol feeding alone does not induce a similar effect in animals (Braganza et al. 2011; Otsuki et al. 2010). Repetitive intraperitoneal injection of arginine (Delaney et al. 1993), intraductal infusion of zein–oleic acid–linoleic acid (Kataoka et al. 1998), or copper deficiency in rats (Rao et al. 1989) cause persistent damage to the pancreas, but these treatments result in replacement of exocrine tissue by adipose tissue rather than the fibrosis typical of chronic pancreatitis in humans. A surgical model that produced persistent hypertension in pancreatic ducts of rats resulted in significant interlobular and intralobular fibrosis and clinical signs of pancreatic insufficiency (Yamamoto et al. 2006). This indicates that pancreatic ductal hypertension could play an important role in the pathogenesis of chronic pancreatitis. Similarly, it was suggested that duct obstruction is important in the development of the chronic lesions that persist after acute pancreatic injury induced by intraductal infusion with sodium taurodeoxycholate (Sarles et al. 1993).

10.3.7.6 Hepatocyte Metaplasia (Pancreatic Hepatocytes)

Given that the liver and pancreas have a common embryologic origin, a structure composed of functioning units (hepatic plates and pancreatic acini) connected to a ductal tree, and appear to be physiologically supplied from Sox9-expressing progenitor epithelial cells in this ductal tree (Furuyama et al. 2011), it might be expected that under certain conditions, liver cells could be found in pancreas or vice versa. A number of experimental manipulations in rats, including prolonged feeding of copper- or methyl-group-deficient diets, followed by return to normal diet (Hoover and Poirier 1986; Rao et al. 1989, 1993; Rao and Reddy 1995), repeated injections of $CdCl_2$ (Konishi et al. 1990), and chronic administration of ciprofibrate (a PPARα agonist) (Reddy et al. 1984), cause the development of pancreatic hepatocytes. These are also seen in the regenerating pancreas of hamsters given a single injection of the pancreatic carcinogen N-nitrosobis(2-oxypropyl)amine (NBOP) (Rao et al. 1983; Scarpelli and Rao 1981), in hamsters injected intraperitoneally with TCDD (Rao et al. 1988), and in the islets of transgenic mice in which keratinocyte growth factor is ectopically expressed (Krakowski et al. 1999). In the diet deficiency models in rats and the NBOP model in hamsters, pancreatic hepatocytes are seen under conditions that first cause massive destruction of acinar epithelium followed by a return to conditions that support or promote proliferation. The pancreatic hepatocytes are often located adjacent to islets and have morphologic, antigenic, and functional characteristics identical to or nearly identical to those of hepatocytes in the liver (Hoover and Poirier 1986; Rao et al. 1982, 1983; Reddy et al. 1984; Scarpelli and Rao 1981). Electron microscopic examination of hepatocytes in pancreas from ciprofibrate-treated rats showed occasional cells having features of liver cells (uricase-positive, nucleoid-containing peroxisomes) and acinar or endocrine pancreatic epithelium (zymogen and/or β-cell granules) (Reddy et al. 1984); however, these intermediate or transitional cells were not observed in the copper deficiency model in rats (Rao et al. 1989). The origin of the pancreatic hepatocytes in the latter model appears to be ductal epithelial cells or other cells of uncertain origin, referred to as interstitial cells.

10.3.7.7 Biomarkers

The devastating nature of pancreatic neoplasia in humans has led to a great deal of research to identify early biomarkers of pancreatic neoplasia, as well as biomarkers of neoplastic progression. Relatively less attention has been given to biomarkers of injury to the exocrine pancreas, and much of this has been focused on identifying biomarkers of acute pancreatitis in humans. Serum amylase and lipase have historically been the most widely used tests to support the diagnosis of acute pancreatic injury; however, they have significant limitations. Both are good diagnostic indicators once clinical signs are present, though amylase is not specific to the pancreas, and neither is particularly sensitive or has the ability to separate mild cases of pancreatitis from those that are severe and life threatening (Walgren et al. 2007b). The ideal biomarker would appear early in the course of the disease, accurately stage and predict severity, and be easy and inexpensive to measure (Dambrauskas et al. 2010). A variety of other analytes have been investigated in serum and urine as biomarkers of acute pancreatitis. C-reactive protein, a nonspecific acute phase protein, has utility in predicting severity of pancreatitis in the clinical setting; however, it is hampered since differentiation between mild and severe disease occurs, at best, 3 to 4 days after disease onset (Büchler et al. 1998). Many other markers have been evaluated, including trypsinogen-1, trypsinogen-2, trypsin-1-α_1-antitrypsin, and trypsin-2-α_1-antitrypsin complexes (Hedstrom et al. 2001; Lempinen et al. 2003), procarboxypeptidase B and its activation peptide (Appelros et al. 1998; Müller et al. 2002), trypsinogen activation peptide (Lempinen et al. 2003), IL-6 (Dambrauskas et al. 2010), and neutrophil gelatinase-associated lipocalin (Chakraborty et al. 2010).

Because of the infrequency of xenobiotic-induced exocrine injury, even less attention has been given to biomarkers of pancreatic injury in laboratory animals. Recently, proteomics techniques were used to identify two novel peptides that show promise as safety markers of pancreatic toxicity (Walgren et al. 2007a,b). These peptides, referred to as RA1609 and RT2864, were initially investigated as alternative biomarkers to address the deficiencies of serum amylase and lipase as markers of acute pancreatic injury in rats (Walgren et al. 2007b). Peptide RA1609 is a fragment of rat albumin and decreases with acute pancreatic injury, while RT2864 is a portion of rat trypsin III and increases with acute pancreatic injury. A subsequent study showed that the same peptide markers were altered in mice with acute pancreatic injury and suggested that corresponding peptides were also altered in humans with acute pancreatitis (Walgren et al. 2007a). Another novel approach is the measurement of organ-specific microRNA (miRNA) biomarkers in the circulation. In this regard, levels of a pancreas-specific miRNA, designated miR-216a, were elevated in the sera of rats with arginine-induced pancreatitis but not in sera from rats with acute peritonitis and sepsis. Amylase and lipase levels were elevated in both conditions (Kong et al. 2010). Further investigative work will be needed to confirm the usefulness of these markers in a drug development setting.

10.3.7.8 Pancreatic Proliferative Lesions

The exocrine pancreas is susceptible to spontaneous and xenobiotic-induced proliferative lesions, both neoplastic and non-neoplastic. Spontaneous proliferative lesions are rarely observed in young adult dogs and NHPs in toxicology studies, and xenobiotic-induced proliferative lesions are not described in these species. In mice and rats, spontaneous and xenobiotic-induced proliferative lesions of exocrine pancreas may occur, though not as commonly as in the liver.

Foci of cellular alteration and *focal hyperplasia* have been described among the non-neoplastic proliferative lesions of the rat pancreas (Eustis et al. 1990). In the mouse pancreas, only focal hyperplasia has been described among the non-neoplastic proliferative lesions described in the current literature on nomenclature (Boorman and Sills 1999; Deschl et al. 2001).

Foci of cellular alteration are focal lesions composed of acinar cells that have altered staining characteristics but cause little or no compression of adjacent pancreatic parenchyma. The subclassification of these foci, and the relative significance of the subtypes, varies among various reported studies. These foci are often described as basophilic foci owing to decreased cytoplasmic content of eosinophilic zymogen granules and contain an abundance of rough ER by TEM. However, some studies have reported the occurrence of eosinophilic foci. While they may occur spontaneously, both types of foci have been associated with treatments that increase the incidence of exocrine neoplasia. Basophilic foci do not have elevated indices of cell proliferation such as mitotic figures or S-phase nuclei, suggesting that these lesions are not part of the pathogenesis of neoplasia. In contrast, eosinophilic foci have been reported to have increased mitotic activity and may be part of the pathogenesis of neoplasia under certain circumstances.

Focal hyperplasia is a focal lesion composed of acinar cells with altered staining characteristics, variable mitotic activity, and compression of the adjacent pancreatic parenchyma. Focal hyperplasia is associated with treatments that increase the incidence of exocrine neoplasia and is considered to be part of the continuum of lesions that include adenomas and carcinomas of the exocrine epithelium. Moreover, the distinction between focal hyperplasia and adenoma is subtle. Some classifications depend upon the arbitrary feature of size, with larger lesions more likely to be diagnosed as adenomas.

The significance of pancreatic exocrine neoplasia in long-term carcinogenicity studies in rodents requires some perspective. While these lesions may occur spontaneously, the historical incidence in controls is exceedingly rare, so that in most studies, the control incidence is 0%, and an incidence of 2 or more (~5%) in a group of 50 treated animals in a 2-year study (compared to 0% among controls) warrants consideration of a treatment-related effect, even if not statistically significant.

Pancreatic acinar adenomas are benign proliferative lesions composed of acinar cells arranged in branching tubules. While part of a morphological continuum with focal hyperplasia, adenomas are larger and usually grossly apparent as nodular or multinodular, well-demarcated masses. Mitotic figures and slight atypia may be present, but evidence of local invasion is absent. In contrast to adenomas, *pancreatic acinar carcinomas* are malignant proliferative lesions that are usually grossly apparent as poorly demarcated masses. Carcinomas are composed of acinar cells arranged in glands, trabeculae, and sheets. The neoplastic cells are often pleomorphic and atypical. Loss of demarcation and invasion of adjacent parenchyma are present. Fibrosis may be present but often is not.

The induction of pancreatic acinar neoplasia has been reported with a number of genotoxic and nongenotoxic substances in rodents. A variety of experimental models of pancreatic carcinogenesis in rats have been reported in the literature, but these more often than not involve genotoxic, non-pharmaceutical chemicals, including N-nitroso compounds.

The nongenotoxic substances that cause proliferative lesions of the exocrine pancreas include drugs that are activators of PPAR-alpha, such as fibrates, that cause acinar lesions in rats, particularly in males. Similar responses are not observed in mice. It has been postulated that PPAR-alpha activators cause acinar hyperplasia and adenoma by decreasing flow or altering composition of bile in a manner that results in cholestasis and increased cholecystokinin (CCK) secretion by duodenal endocrine cells. CCK stimulates proliferation of pancreatic acinar cells, and there is evidence that, if sustained, this is sufficient to cause acinar hyperplasias and adenomas in rats (Biegel et al. 2001; Klaunig et al. 2003). This evidence is based in part on the similar role of increased CCK stimulation in rats that developed acinar proliferative lesions following prolonged (1) feeding with raw soy flour diets that contain a naturally occurring trypsin inhibitor or (2) daily corn oil gavage.

Besides PPAR-alpha activators, pancreatic acinar adenomas and carcinomas were also reported following chronic treatment with the nongenotoxic neuroactive drug gabapentin (Sigler et al. 1995). This response was observed in male rats but not in similar studies of gabapentin in female rats or in mice of either sex. Gabapentin causes proliferation of pancreatic acinar cells, though this does not involve CCK. Although the mechanism of gabapentin acinar cell proliferation is unknown, the proliferative response is thought to cause acinar lesions following prolonged administration (Dethloff et al. 2000).

The implications of pancreatic neoplasia for safety assessment are somewhat context dependent. Assuming that a drug candidate in development is not genotoxic, any increase in incidence of pancreatic exocrine neoplasia would have to be evaluated to elucidate a possible mechanism. If the increased incidence of neoplasms was limited to rats, and if the drug candidate caused acinar cell proliferation in the same sex and strain of rats (through CCK or independent of CCK), there may be sufficient rationale for establishing a threshold for carcinogenesis that could be extrapolated to patients.

In humans, pancreatic cancer is a significant cause of morbidity and mortality, and it is most often not detected until it has reached a stage where treatment is often not successful. Interestingly, pancreatic cancer in humans is considered to nearly always arise from the pancreatic ducts. In contrast, pancreatic neoplasia in rats is considered to nearly always arise from the pancreatic acini. The significance of this difference for safety assessment has not been established.

REFERENCES

Adams, D.H., Ju, C., Ramaiah, S.K., Uetrecht, J.P., Jaeschke, H., 2010. Mechanism of immune-mediated liver injury. *Toxicological Sciences* 115, 307–321.

Amacher, D.E., Schomaker, S.J., Burkhardt, J.E., 1998. The relationship among microsomal enzyme induction, liver weight and histological change in rat toxicology studies. *Food and Chemical Toxicology* 36, 831–839.

Anderson, L.M., Harrington, G.W., Pylypiw, H.M., Jr., Hagiwara, A., Magee, P.N., 1986. Tissue levels and biological effects of N-nitrosodimethylamine in mice during chronic low or high dose exposure with or without ethanol. *Drug Metabolism and Disposition: The Biological Fate of Chemicals* 14, 733–739.

Ansari, G.A.S., Kaphalia, B.S., Boor, P.J., 1987. Selective pancreatic toxicity of palmitoylpentachorophenol. *Toxicology* 46, 57–63.

Appelros, S., Thim, L., Borgström, A., 1998. Activation peptide of carboxypeptidase B in serum and urine in acute pancreatitis. *Gut* 42, 97–102.

Apte, M.V., Haber, P.S., Applegate, T.L. et al., 1998. Periacinar stellate shaped cells in rat pancreas: identification, isolation, and culture. *Gut* 43, 128–133.

Bach, U., Hailey, J.R., Hill, G.D. et al., 2010. Proceedings of the 2009 National Toxicology Program Satellite Symposium. *Toxicologic Pathology* 38, 9–16.

Bachem, M.G., Schneider, E., Groß, H. et al., 1998. Identification, culture, and characterization of pancreatic stellate cells in rats and humans. *Gastroenterology* 115, 421–432.

Baluk, P., McDonald, D.M., 2008. Markers for microscopic imaging of lymphangiogenesis and angiogenesis. *Annals of the New York Academy of Sciences* 1131, 1–12.

Bannasch, P., 2003. Comments on R. Karbe and R. L. Kerlin (2002). Cystic degeneration/spongiosis hepatis (Toxicol Pathol 30 (2), 216-227). *Toxicologic Pathology* 31, 566–570.

Belinsky, S.A., Badr, M.Z., Kauffman, F.C., Thurman, R.G., 1986. Mechanism of hepatotoxicity in periportal regions of the liver lobule due to allyl alcohol: studies on thiols and energy status. *Journal of Pharmacology and Experimental Therapeutics* 238, 1132–1137.

Belloni, A.S., Rebuffat P., Gottardo G. et al., 1988. A morphometric study of the effects of short-term starvation on rat hepatocytes. *Journal of Submicroscopic Cytology and Pathology* 20, 751–757.

Bendayan, M., Ito, S., 1979. Immunohistochemical localization of exocrine enzymes in normal rat pancreas. *Journal of Histochemistry and Cytochemistry* 27, 1029–1034.

Berg, A.L., Bottcher, G., Andersson, K. et al., 2008. Early stellate cell activation and veno-occlusive-disease (VOD)-like hepatotoxicity in dogs treated with AR-H047108, an imidazopyridine proton pump inhibitor. *Toxicologic Pathology* 36, 727–737.

Bhatia, M., Wallig, M.A., Hofbauer, B. et al., 1998. Induction of apoptosis in pancreatic acinar cells reduces the severity of acute pancreatitis. *Biochemical and Biophysical Research Communications* 246, 476–483.

Biegel, L.B., Hurtt, M.E., Frame, S.R., O'Connor, J.C., Cook, J.C., 2001. Mechanisms of extrahepatic tumor induction by peroxisome proliferators in male CD rats. *Toxicological Sciences* 60, 44–55.

Bird, T.G., Lorenzini, S., Forbes, S.J., 2008. Activation of stem cells in hepatic disease. *Cell Tissue Research* 331, 283–300.

Böck, P., Abdel-Moneim, M., Egerbacher, M., 1997. Development of pancreas. *Microscopy Research and Technique* 37, 374–383.

Bockman, D.E., Black, O., Jr., Mills, L.R., Webster, P.D., 1978. Origin of tubular complexes developing during induction of pancreatic carcinoma by 7, 12-dimethylbenz(a)anthracene. *American Journal of Pathology* 90, 645–658.

Bockman, D.E., Guo, J., Buchler, P., Muller, M.W., Bergmann, F., Friess, H., 2003. Origin and development of the precursor lesions in experimental pancreatic cancer in rats. *Laboratory Investigation* 83, 853–859.

Boorman, G.A., Sills, R.C., 1999. Exocrine and endocrine pancreas. In: *Pathology of the Mouse*, Maronpot, R., Boorman, G., Gaul, B. (editors), Cache River Press, Vienna, IL, pp. 185–205.

Bouwens, L., Braet, F., Heimberg, H., 1995. Identification of rat pancreatic duct cells by their expression of cytokeratins 7, 19, and 20 in vivo and after isolation and culture. *Journal of Histochemistry and Cytochemistry* 43, 245–253.

Boyce, R.W., Dorph-Petersen, K.A., Lyck, L., Gundersen, H.J., 2010. Design-based stereology: introduction to basic concepts and practical approaches for estimation of cell number. *Toxicologic Pathology* 38, 1011–1025.

Braet, F., Wisse, E., 2002. Structural and functional aspects of liver sinusoidal endothelial cell fenestrae: a review. *Comparative Hepatology* 1, 1.

Braganza, J.M., Lee, S.H., McCloy, R.F., McMahon, M.J., 2011. Chronic pancreatitis. *The Lancet* 377, 1184–1197.

Büchler, M.W., Uhl, W., Andrén-Sandberg, Å., 1998. CAPAP in acute pancreatitis: just another marker or real progress? *Gut* 42, 8–9.

Buhler, R., Lindros, K.O., Nordling, A., Johansson, I., Ingelman-Sundberg, M., 1992. Zonation of cytochrome P450 isozyme expression and induction in rat liver. *European Journal of Biochemistry* 204, 407–412.

Bursch, W., Taper, H.S., Lauer, B., Schulte-Hermann, R., 1985. Quantitative histological and histochemical studies on the occurrence and stages of controlled cell death (apoptosis) during regression of rat liver hyperplasia. *Virchows Archiv. B, Cell Pathology Including Molecular Pathology* 50, 153–166.

Bursch, W., Dusterberg, B., Schulte-Hermann, R., 1986. Growth, regression and cell death in rat liver as related to tissue levels of the hepatomitogen cyproterone acetate. *Archives of Toxicology* 59, 221–227.

Butler, M., Stecker, K., Bennett, C.F., 1997. Cellular distribution of phosphorothioate oligodeoxynucleotides in normal rodent tissues. *Laboratory Investigation* 77, 379–388.

Butler, W.H., Hard, G.C., 1971. Hepatotoxicity of dimethylnitrosamine in the rat with special reference to veno-occlusive disease. *Experimental and Molecular Pathology* 15, 209–219.

Bykov, I., Ylipaasto, P., Eerola, L., Lindros, K.O., 2003. Phagocytosis and LPS-stimulated production of cytokines and prostaglandin E2 is different in Kupffer cells isolated from the periportal or perivenous liver region. *Scandinavian Journal of Gastroenterology* 38, 1256–1261.

Car, B.D., Eng, V.M., Lipman, J.M., Anderson, T.D., 1999. The toxicology of interleukin-12: a review. *Toxicologic Pathology* 27, 58–63.

Cattley, R.C., Popp, J.A., 2002. Liver. In: *Handbook of Toxicologic Pathology*, Haschek, W., Rousseaux, C., Walling, M. (editors), Academic Press, San Diego, CA, pp. 187–225.

Cattley, R.C., Everitt, J., Gross, E.A., Moss, O.R., Hamm, T.E. Jr., Popp, J.A., 1994. Carcinogenicity and toxicity of inhaled nitrobenzene in B6C3F1 Mice and F344 and CD rats. *Fundamental and Applied Toxicology* 22, 328–340.

Chakraborty, S., Kaur, S., Muddana, V. et al., 2010. Elevated serum neutrophil gelatinase-associated lipocalin is an early predictor of severity and outcome in acute pancreatitis. *American Journal of Gastroenterology* 105, 2050–2059.

Chan, Y.C., Leung, P.S., 2007. Acute pancreatitis. Animal models and recent advances in basic research. *Pancreas* 34, 1–14.

Chatman, L.A., Morton, D., Johnson, T.O., Anway, S.D., 2009. A strategy for risk management of drug-induced phospholipidosis. *Toxicologic Pathology* 37, 997–1005.

Chen, M., Vijay, V., Shi, Q., Liu, Z., Fang, H., Tong, W., 2011. FDA-approved drug labeling for the study of drug-induced liver injury. *Drug Discovery Today* 16, 697–703.

Cohen, S. M., Storer, R.D., Criswell, K.A. et al., 2009. Hemangiosarcoma in rodents: mode-of-action evaluation and human relevance. *Toxicological Sciences* 111, 4–18.

Crampton, R.F., Gray, T.J.B., Grasso, P., Parke, D.V., 1977. Long-term studies on chemically induced liver enlargement in the rat, 1. Sustained induction of microsomal enzymes with absence of liver damage on feeding phenobarbitone and butylated hydroxytoluene. *Toxicology* 7, 289–306.

Dambrauskas, Z., Gulbinas, A., Pundzius, J., Barauskas, G., 2010. Value of the different prognostic systems and biological markers for predicting severity and progression of acute pancreatitis. *Scandinavian Journal of Gastroenterology* 45, 959–970.

Daniel, G.B., DeNovo, R.C., Sharp, D.S., Tobias, K., Berry, C., 2004. Portal streamlining as a cause of non-uniform hepatic distribution of sodium pertechnetate during per-rectal portal scintigraphy in the dog. *Veterinary Radiology and Ultrasound* 45, 78–84.

Davidson, M.H., Armani, A., McKenney, J.M., Jacobson, T.A., 2007. Safety considerations with fibrate therapy. *American Journal of Cardiology* 99, 3C–18C.

Dawra, R., Sah, R.P., Dudeja, V. et al., 2011. Intra-acinar trypsinogen activation mediates early stages of pancreatic injury but not inflammation in mice with acute pancreatitis. *Gastroenterology* 141, 2210–2217.

Delaney, C.P., McGeeney, K.F., Dervan, P., Fitzpatrick, J.M., 1993. Pancreatic atrophy: a new model using serial intra-peritoneal injections of L-arginine. *Scandinavian Journal of Gastroenterology* 28, 1086–1090.

DeLeve, L.D., McCuskey, R.S., Wang, X. et al., 1999. Characterization of a reproducible rat model of hepatic veno-occlusive disease. Hepatology 29, 1779–1791.

Denk, H., Gschnait, F., Wolff, K., 1975. Hepatocellular hyaline (Mallory bodies) in long term griseofulvin-treated mice, a new experimental model for the study of hyaline formation. *Laboratory Investigation* 32, 773–776.

Denk H., Franke W.W., Eckerstorfer R., Schmid, E., Kerjaschki, D., 1979. Formation and involution of Mallory bodies ("alcoholic hyaline") in murine and human liver revealed by immunofluorescence microscopy with antibodies to prekeratin. *Proceedings of the National Academy of Sciences* 76, 4112–4116.

Desai, B.M., Oliver-Krasinski, J., De Leon, D.D. et al., 2007. Preexisting pancreatic acinar cells contribute to acinar cell, but not islet β cell, regeneration. *The Journal of Clinical Investigation* 117, 971–977.

Deschl, U., Cattley, R.C., Harada, T. et al., 2001. Liver, gallbladder, and exocrine pancreas. In: *International Classification of Rodent Tumors—The Mouse*. Mohr, U. (editor), Springer, Berlin, pp. 59–86.

Desmet, V.J., 2011. Ductular plates in hepatic ductular reactions. Hypothesis and implications. I. Types of ductular reactions reconsidered. *Virchows Archives* 458, 251–259.

Dethloff, L., Barr, B., Bestervelt, L. et al., 2000. Gabapentin-induced mitogenic activity in rat pancreatic acinar cells. *Toxicological Sciences* 55, 52–59.

di Masi, A., De Marinis, E., Ascenzi, P., Marino, M., 2009. Nuclear receptors CAR and PXR: Molecular, functional, and biomedical aspects. *Molecular Aspects of Medicine* 30, 297–343.

Dini, L., Pagliara, P., Carla, E.C., 2002. Phagocytosis of apoptotic cells by liver: a morphological study. *Microscopy Research and Technique* 57, 530–540.

Donald, S., Verschoyle, R.D., Edwards, R. et al., 2002. Hepatobiliary damage and changes in hepatic gene expression caused by the antitumor drug ecteinascidin-743 (ET-743) in the female rat. *Cancer Research* 62, 4256–4262.

Dusetti, N.J., Jiang, Y., Vaccaro, M.I. et al., 2002. Cloning and expression of the rat vacuole membrane protein 1 (VMP1), a new gene activated in pancreas with acute pancreatitis, which promotes vacuole formation. *Biochemical and Biophysical Research Communications* 290, 641–649.

Eldridge, S.R., Tilbury, L.F., Goldsworthy, T.L., Butterworth, B.E., 1990. Measurement of chemically induced cell proliferation in rodent liver and kidney: a comparison of 5-bromo-2'-deoxyuridine and [3H]thymidine administered by injection or osmotic pump. *Carcinogenesis* 11, 2245–2251.

Elmore, L.W., Sirica, A.E., 1991. Phenotypic characteristics of metaplastic intestinal glands and ductular hepatocytes in cholangiofibrotic lesions rapidly induced in the caudate liver lobe of rats treated with furan. *Cancer Research* 51, 5752–5759.

Ennulat, D., Walker, D., Clemo, F. et al., 2010. Effects of hepatic drug-metabolizing enzyme induction on clinical pathology parameters in animals and man. *Toxicologic Pathology* 38, 810–828.

Eustis, S.L., Boorman, G.A., Harada, T., Popp, J.A., 1990. Liver. In: *Pathology of the Fisher Rat*, Boorman, G., Eustis, S., Elwell, M., Montgomery Jr., C., MacKenzie W. (editors), Academic Press, San Diego, CA, pp. 95–108.

Fan, Y., Yamada, T., Shimizu, T. et al., 2009. Ferritin expression in rat hepatocytes and Kupffer cells after lead nitrate treatment. *Toxicologic Pathology* 37, 209–217.

Fawaz, F., Bonini, F., Guyot, M., Lagueny, A.M., Fessi, H., Devissaguet, J.P., 1993. Influence of poly(DL-lactide) nanocapsules on the biliary clearance and enterohepatic circulation of indomethacin in the rabbit. *Pharmaceutical Research* 10, 750–756.

Fedorko, M.E., 1968. Effect of chloroquine on morphology of leukocytes and pancreatic exocrine cells from the rat. *Laboratory Investigation* 18, 27–37.

Fortunato, F., Bürgers, H., Bergmann, F. et al., 2009. Impaired autolysosome formation correlates with lamp-2 depletion: role of apoptosis, autophagy, and necrosis in pancreatitis. *Gastroenterology* 137, 350–360.

Foster, J.R. 2009. Toxicology of the exocrine pancreas. In: *General, Applied and Systems Toxicology*, John Wiley & Sons, Ltd., Hoboken, NJ, pp. 1413–1455.

Furukawa, S., Usuda, K., Fujieda, Y. et al., 2000. Apoptosis and cell proliferation in rat hepatocytes induced by barbiturates. *Journal of Veterinary Medical Science* 62, 23–28.

Furuyama, K., Kawaguchi, Y., Akiyama, H. et al., 2011. Continuous cell supply from a Sox9-expressing progenitor zone in adult liver, exocrine pancreas and intestine. *Nature Genetics* 43, 34–41.

Ganong, W.F. 1991. Regulation of gastrointestinal function, In: *Review of Medical Physiology*. Appleton & Lange, Norwalk, CT, pp. 448–477.

Gao, B., Radaeva, S., Park, O., 2009. Liver natural killer and natural killer T cells: immunobiology and emerging roles in liver diseases. *Journal of Leukocyte Biology* 86, 513–528.

Geil, R.G., Lamar, J.K., 1977. FDA studies of estrogen, progestogens, and estrogen/progestogen combinations in the dog and monkey. *Journal of Toxicology and Environmental Health* 3, 179–193.

Gerson, R.J., Allen, H.L., Lankas, G.R., MacDonald, J.S., Alberts, A.W., Bokelman, D.L., 1991. The toxicity of a fluorinated-biphenyl HMG-CoA reductase inhibitor in beagle dogs. *Fundamental and Applied Toxicology* 16, 320–329.

Giannini, E.G., Testa, R., Savarino, V., 2005. Liver enzyme alteration: a guide for clinicians. *CMAJ* 172, 367–379.

Glaze, E.R., Lambert, A.L., Smith, A.C. et al., 2005. Preclinical toxicity of a geldanamycin analog, 17-(dimethylaminoethylamino)-17-demethoxygeldanamycin (17-DMAG), in rats and dogs: potential clinical relevance. *Cancer Chemotherapy and Pharmacology* 56, 637–647.

Gouw, S.H., Clouston, A.D., Theise N.D., 2011. Ductular reactions in human liver: diversity at the interface. *Hepatology* 54, 1853–1863.

Graham, E.A., 1915. The resistance of pups to late chloroform poisoning in its relation to liver glycogen. *Journal of Experimental Medicine* 21, 185–191.

Graichen, M.E., Neptun, D.A., Dent, J.G., Popp, J.A., Leonard, T.B., 1985. Effects of methapyrilene on rat hepatic xenobiotic metabolising enzymes and liver morphology. *Fundamental and Applied Toxicology* 5, 165–174.

Grasso, D., Ropolo, A., Lo Ré, A. et al., 2011. Zymophagy, a novel selective autophagy pathway mediated by VMP1-USP9x-p62, prevents pancreatic cell death. *Journal of Biological Chemistry* 286, 8308–8324.

Grattagliano, I., Bonfrate, L., Diogo, C.V., Wang, H.H., Wang, D.Q., Portincasa, P., 2009. Biochemical mechanisms in drug-induced liver injury: certainties and doubts. World Journal of Gastroenterology 15, 4865–4876.

Gukovskaya, A.S., Pandol, S.J., 2004. Cell death pathways in pancreatitis and pancreatic cancer. *Pancreatology* 4, 567–586.

Gukovskaya, A.S., Perkins, P., Zaninovic, V. et al., 1996. Mechanisms of cell death after pancreatic duct obstruction in the opossum and the rat. *Gastroenterology* 110, 875–884.

Halliwell, W.H., 1997. Cationic amphophilic drug-induced phospholipidosis. *Toxicologic Pathology* 25, 53–60.

Han, D., Hanawa, N., Saberi, B., Kaplowitz, N., 2006. Mechanisms of liver injury. III. Role of glutathione redox status in liver injury. American Journal of Physiology—Gastrointestinal and Liver Physiology 291, G1–G7.

Hansen, L.J., Mangkornkanok/Mark, M., Reddy, J.K., 1981. Immunohistochemical localization of pancreatic exocrine enzymes in normal and neoplastic pancreatic acinar epithelium of rat. *Journal of Histochemistry and Cytochemistry* 29, 309–313.

Harada, T., Maronpot, R.R., Morris, R.W., Stitzel, K.A., Boorman, G.A., 1989. Morphological and stereological characterization of hepatic foci of cellular alteration in control Fischer 344 rats. *Toxicologic Pathology* 17, 579–593.

Hartman, H.A., Myers, L.A., Evans, M., Robison, R.L., Engstrom, R.G., Tse, F.L., 1996. The safety evaluation of fluvastatin, an HMG-CoA reductase inhibitor, in beagle dogs and rhesus monkeys. *Fundamental and Applied Toxicology* 29, 48–62.

Hashimoto, D., Ohmuraya, M., Hirota, M.I. et al., 2008. Involvement of autophagy in trypsinogen activation within the pancreatic acinar cells. *The Journal of Cell Biology* 181, 1065–1072.

Hedstrom, J., Kemppainen, E., Andersen, J., Jokela, H., Puolakkainen, P., Stenman, U.-H., 2001. A comparison of serum trypsinogen-2 and trypsin-2-[alpha]1-antitrypsin complex with lipase and amylase in the diagnosis and assessment of severity in the early phase of acute pancreatitis. *American Journal of Gastroenterology* 96, 424–430.

Henderson, J.R., Daniel, P.M., Fraser, P.A., 1981. The pancreas as a single organ: the influence of the endocrine upon the exocrine part of the gland. *Gut* 22, 158–167.

Henry, S.P., Grillone, L.R., Orr, J.L., Bruner, R.H., Kornbrust, D.J., 1997a. Comparison of the toxicity profiles of ISIS 1082 and ISIS 2105, phosphorothioate oligonucleotides, following subacute intradermal administration in Sprague–Dawley rats. *Toxicology* 116, 77–88.

Henry, S.P., Zuckerman, J.E., Rojko, J. et al., 1997b. Toxicological properties of several novel oligonucleotide analogs in mice. *Anti-Cancer Drug Design* 12, 1–14.

Herzog, J., Serroni, A., Briesmeister, B.A., Farber, J.L., 1975. N-hydroxy-2-acetylaminofluorene inhibition of rat live RNA polymerases. *Cancer Research* 35, 2138–2144.

Hess, D.A., Humphrey, S.E., Ishibashi, J. et al., 2011. Extensive pancreas regeneration following acinar-specific disruption of Xbp1 in mice. *Gastroenterology* 141, 1463–1472.

Hinson, J.A., Roberts, D.W., James, L.P., 2010. Mechanisms of acetaminophen-induced liver necrosis. Handbook of Experimental Pharmacology, 369–405.

Hintze, C., Strobele, C., Ruster, B. et al., 2009. Erythrocytic precursor cells show potent shear stress resistant adhesion and home to hematopoietic tissue in vivo. *Transfusion* 49, 2122–2130.

Hirano, T., Manabe, T., Ando, K., Tobe, T., 1992. Acute cytotoxic effect of cyclosporin A on pancreatic acinar cells in rats: protective effect of the synthetic protease inhibitor E3123. *Scandinavian Journal of Gastroenterology* 27, 103–107.

Hofbauer, B., Saluja, A.K., Lerch, M.M. et al., 1998. Intra-acinar cell activation of trypsinogen during caerulein-induced pancreatitis in rats. *American Journal of Physiology—Gastrointestinal and Liver Physiology* 275, G352–G362.

Hoover, K.L., Poirier, L.A., 1986. Hepatocyte-like cells within the pancreas of rats fed methyl-deficient diets. *The Journal of Nutrition* 116, 1569–1575.

Hruban, R.H., Adsay, N.V., Albores-Saavedra, J. et al., 2006. Pathology of genetically engineered mouse models of pancreatic exocrine cancer: consensus report and recommendations. *Cancer Research* 66, 95–106.

Hu, W., Sorrentino, C., Denison, M.S., Kolaja, K., Fielden, M.R., 2007. Induction of cyp1a1 is a nonspecific biomarker of aryl hydrocarbon receptor activation: results of large scale screening of pharmaceuticals and toxicants in vivo and in vitro. *Molecular Pharmacology* 71, 1475–1486.

Iida, K., Li, Y., McGrath, B., Frank, A., Cavener, D., 2007. PERK eIF2 alpha kinase is required to regulate the viability of the exocrine pancreas in mice. *BMC Cell Biology* 8, 38.

Ilzer J., Schotanus B.A., Vander Borght, S. et al., 2010. Characterization of the hepatic progenitor cell compartment in normal liver and in hepatitis, an immunohistochemical comparison between dog and man. *Veterinary Journal* 184, 308–314.

Jaeschke, H., Gores, G.J., Cederbaum, A.I., Hinson, J.A., Pessayre, D., Lemasters, J.J., 2002. Mechanisms of hepatotoxicity. *Toxicological Sciences* 65, 166–176.

Jensen, J.N., Cameron, E., Garay, M.V.R., Starkey, T.W., Gianani, R., Jensen, J., 2005. Recapitulation of elements of embryonic development in adult mouse pancreatic regeneration. *Gastroenterology* 128, 728–741.

Jin, Y.L., Enzan, H., Kuroda, N. et al., 2003. Tissue remodeling following submassive hemorrhagic necrosis in rat livers induced by an intraperitoneal injection of dimethylnitrosamine. *Virchows Archives* 442, 39–47.

Jones, H.B., Clarke, N.A., 1993. Assessment of the influence of subacute phenobarbitone administration on multi-tissue cell proliferation in the rat using bromodeoxyuridine immunocytochemistry. *Archives of Toxicology* 67, 622–628.

Jungermann, K., Kietzmann, T., 1996. Zonation of parenchymal and nonparenchymal metabolism in liver. *Annual Review of Nutrition* 16, 179–203.

Kaiser, A.M., Saluja, A.K., Sengupta, A., Saluja, M., Steer, M.L., 1995. Relationship between severity, necrosis, and apoptosis in five models of experimental acute pancreatitis. *American Journal of Physiology—Cell Physiology* 269, C1295–C1304.

Kaiser, A.M., Saluja, A.K., Lu, L., Yamanaka, K., Yamaguchi, Y., Steer, M.L., 1996. Effects of cycloheximide on pancreatic endonuclease activity, apoptosis, and severity of acute pancreatitis. *American Journal of Physiology—Cell Physiology* 271, C982–C993.

Kamimoto, Y., Horiuchi, S., Tanase, S., Morino, Y., 1985. Plasma clearance of intravenously injected aspartate aminotransferase isozymes: evidence for preferential uptake by sinusoidal liver cells. *Hepatology* 5, 367–375.

Karbe, E., Kerlin, R.L., 2002. Cystic degeneration/spongiosis hepatis in rats. *Toxicologic Pathology* 30, 216–227.

Kashfi, K., McDougall, C.J., Dannenberg, A.J., 1995. Comparative effects of omeprazole on xenobiotic metabolizing enzymes in the rat and human. *Clinical Pharmacology and Therapeutics* 58, 625–630.

Kataoka, K., Sasaki, T., Yorizumi, H., Sakagami, J., Kashima, K., 1998. Pathophysiologic studies of experimental chronic pancreatitis in rats induced by injection of zein-oleic acid-linoleic acid solution into the pancreatic duct. *Pancreas* 16, 289–299.

Kelly, L., Reid, L., Walker, N.I., 1999. Massive acinar cell apoptosis with secondary necrosis, origin of ducts in atrophic lobules and failure to regenerate in cyanohydroxybutene pancreatopathy in rats. *International Journal of Experimental Pathology* 80, 217–226.

Kerlin, R.L., Karbe, E., 2004. Response to comments on E. Karbe and R.L. Kerlin (2002). Cystic degeneration/spongiosis hepatis (Toxicol Pathol 30 (2), 216-227). *Toxicologic Pathology* 32, 271.

Kim, J.C., Shin, D.H., Kim, S.H. et al., 2004. Subacute toxicity evaluation of a new camptothecin anticancer agent CKD-602 administered by intravenous injection to rats. *Regulatory Toxicology and Pharmacology* 40, 356–369.

Kinoshita, M., Uchida, T., Sato, A. et al., 2010. Characterization of two F4/80-positive Kupffer cell subsets by their function and phenotype in mice. *Journal of Hepatology* 53, 903–910.

Kitagawa, T., Ono, K., 1986. Ultrastructure of pancreatic exocrine cells of the rat during starvation. *Histology and Histopathology* 1, 49–57.

Klaunig, J.E., Babich, M.A., Baetcke, K.P. et al., 2003. PPARalpha agonist-induced rodent tumors: modes of action and human relevance. *Critical Reviews in Toxicology* 33, 655–780.

Klein, I., Cornejo, J.C., Polakos, N.K. et al., 2007. Kupffer cell heterogeneity: functional properties of bone marrow derived and sessile hepatic macrophages. *Blood* 110, 4077–4085.

Klimstra, D.S., 1997. Pancreas. In: *Histology for Pathologists*, Sternberg, S.S. (editor), Lippincott-Raven, Philadelphia, PA, pp. 613–647.

Klinkspoor J.H., Ruver R., Savard C.E. et al., 1995. Model bile and bile salts accelerate mucin secretion by cultured dog gallbladder epithelium. *Gastroenterology* 109, 264–274

Knowles, K., Alroy, J., Castagnaro, M., Raghavan, S.S., Jakowski, R.M., Freden, G.O., 1993. Adult onset lysosomal storage disease in a Schipperke dog: clinical, morphological and biochemical studies. *Acta Neuropathologica* 86, 306–312.

Kong, X.-Y., Du, Y.-Q., Li, L. et al., 2010. Plasma miR-216a as a potential marker of pancreatic injury in a rat model of acute pancreatitis. *World Journal of Gastroenterology* 16, 4599–4604.

Konieczny, S.F., Leach, S.D., 2007. Metaplastic metamorphoses in the mammalian pancreas. *Gastroenterology* 133, 2056–2059.

Konishi, N., Ward, J.M., Waalkes, M.P., 1990. Pancreatic hepatocytes in Fischer and Wistar rats induced by repeated injections of cadmium chloride. *Toxicology and Applied Pharmacology* 104, 149–156.

Koo, S.I., Turk, D.E., 1977. Effect of zinc deficiency on the ultrastructure of the pancreatic acinar cell and intestinal epithelium in the rat. *The Journal of Nutrition* 107, 896–908.

Kovatch, R.M., Hildebrandt, P.K., Marcus, L.C., 1965. Cystic mucinous hypertrophy of the mucosa of the gall bladder in the dog. *Pathologia Veterinaria* 2, 574–584.

Kraehenbuhl, J.P., Racine, L., Jamieson, J.D., 1977. Immunocytochemical localization of secretory proteins in bovine pancreatic exocrine cells. *The Journal of Cell Biology* 72, 406–423.

Krakowski, M.L., Kritzik, M.R., Jones, E.M. et al., 1999. Pancreatic expression of keratinocyte growth factor leads to differentiation of islet hepatocytes and proliferation of duct cells. *American Journal of Pathology* 154, 683–691.

Lapis, K., Zalatnai, A., Timar, F., Thorgeirsson, U.P., 1995. Quantitative evaluation of lysozyme- and CD68-positive Kupffer cells in diethylnitrosamine-induced hepatocellular carcinomas in monkeys. *Carcinogenesis* 16, 3083–3085.

Lemasters, J.J., Stemkowski, C.J., Ji, S., Thurman, R.G., 1983. Cell surface changes and enzyme release during hypoxia and reoxygenation in the isolated, perfused rat liver. *Journal of Cell Biology* 97, 778–786.

Lempinen, M., Stenman, U.-H., Puolakkainen, P., Hietaranta, A., Haapiainen, R., Kemppainen, E., 2003. Sequential changes in pancreatic markers in acute pancreatitis. *Scandinavian Journal of Gastroenterology* 38, 666–675.

Leonard, T.B., Neptun, D.A., Popp, J.A., 1984. Serum gamma glutamyl transferase as a specific indicator of bile duct lesions in the rat liver. *American Journal of Pathology* 116, 262–269.

Levin, S., 1999. Commentary: implementation of the STP recommendations on the nomenclature of cell death. Society of Toxicologic Pathologists. *Toxicologic Pathology* 27, 491.

Levin, S., Bucci, T.J., Cohen, S.M. et al., 1999. The nomenclature of cell death: recommendations of an ad hoc Committee of the Society of Toxicologic Pathologists. *Toxicologic Pathology* 27, 484–490.

Lewis, D.J., 1984. Spontaneous lesions of the mouse biliary tract. *Journal of Comparative Pathology* 94, 263–271.

Longnecker, D.S., Crawford, B.G., Nadler, D.J., 1975. Recovery of pancreas from mild puromycin-induced injury. A histologic and ultrastructural study in rats. *Archives of Pathology* 99, 5–10.

Longnecker, D.S., Wilson, G., 2002. Pancreas. In: *Handbook of Toxicologic Pathology*, Haschek, W.M., Rousseaux, C.G., Wallig, M.A. (editors), Academic Press, London, pp. 227–254.

López, J.M., Bombi, J.A., Valderrama, R. et al., 1996. Effects of prolonged ethanol intake and malnutrition on rat pancreas. *Gut* 38, 285–292.

Mackie, J.T., Atshaves, B.P., Payne, H.R., McIntosh, A.L., Schroeder, F., Kier, A.B., 2009. Phytol-induced hepatotoxicity in mice. *Toxicologic Pathology* 37, 201–208.

Malhi, H., Gores, G.J., Lemasters, J.J., 2006. Apoptosis and necrosis in the liver: a tale of two deaths? *Hepatology* 43, S31–S44.

Mareninova, O.A., Hermann, K., French, S.W. et al., 2009. Impaired autophagic flux mediates acinar cell vacuole formation and trypsinogen activation in rodent models of acute pancreatitis. *The Journal of Clinical Investigation* 119, 3340–3355.

Maronpot, R.R., Yoshizawa, K., Nyska, A. et al., 2010. Hepatic enzyme induction: histopathology. *Toxicologic Pathology* 38, 776–795.

Marsman, D.S., Popp, J.A., 1994. Biological potential of basophilic hepatocellular foci and hepatic adenoma induced by the peroxisome proliferator, Wy-14,643. *Carcinogenesis* 15, 111–117.

Mashima H., Sato T., Horie, Y. et al., 2011. Interferon regulatory factor-2 regulates exocytosis mechanisms mediated by SNAREs in pancreatic acinar cells. *Gastroenterology* 141, 1102–1113.

Matsumoto M., Miki T., Shibasaki T. et al., 2004. Noc2 is essential in normal regulation of exocytosis in endocrine and exocrine cells. *Proceedings of the National Academy of Sciences* 101, 8313–8318.

Matveyenko, A.V., Dry, S., Cox, H.I. et al., 2009. Beneficial endocrine but adverse exocrine effects of sitagliptin in the human islet amyloid polypeptide transgenic rat model of type 2 diabetes: interactions with metformin. *Diabetes* 58, 1604–1615.

Mawdesley-Thomas, L.E., Noel, P.R., 1967. Cystic hyperplasia of the gall bladder in the beagle, associated with the administration of progestational compounds. *Veterinary Record* 80, 658–659.

McConnell, E.E., Solleveld, H.A., Swenberg, J.A., 1986. Guidelines for combining neoplasms for evaluation of rodent carcinogenesis studies. *Journal of the National Cancer Institute* 76, 283–289.

Michalopoulos, G.K., 2010. Liver regeneration after partial hepatectomy: critical analysis of mechanistic dilemmas. *American Journal of Pathology* 176, 2–13.

Michalopoulos, G.K., DeFrances, M.C., 1997. Liver regeneration. *Science* 276, 60–66.

Miller, R.T., Shah, R.S., Cattley, R.C., Popp, J.A., 1996. The peroxisome proliferators WY-14,643 and methylclofenapate induce hepatocyte ploidy alterations and ploidy-specific DNA synthesis in F344 rats. *Toxicology and Applied Pharmacology* 138, 317–323.

Molon-Noblot, S., Gillet, J.P., Durand-Cavagna, G., Huber, A.C., Patrick, D.H., Duprat, P., 1996. Lipidosis induced in the dog gallbladder by a direct 5-lipoxygenase inhibitor. *Toxicologic Pathology* 24, 231–237.

Moore, J.T., Collins, J.L., Pearce, K.H., 2006. The nuclear receptor superfamily and drug discovery. *ChemMedChem* 1, 504–523.

Müller, C.A., Appelros, S., Uhl, W., Büchler, M.W., Borgström, A., 2002. Serum levels of procarboxypeptidase B and its activation peptide in patients with acute pancreatitis and non-pancreatic diseases. *Gut* 51, 229–235.

Nachnani, J.S., Bulchandani, D.G., Nookala, A. et al., 2010. Biochemical and histological effects of exendin-4 (exenatide) on the rat pancreas. *Diabetologia* 53, 153–159.

Nakamichi, I., Hatakeyama, S., Nayayama, K.I., 2002. Formation of Mallory body-like inclusions and cell death induced by deregulated expression of keratin 18. *Molecular Biology of the Cell* 13:3441–3451.

National Toxicology Program, 1988. NTP toxicology and carcinogenesis studies of penicillin VK (CAS No. 132-98-9) in F344/N rats and B6C3F1 mice (gavage studies). National Toxicology Program Technical Report Series 336, 1–170.

Naya, F.J., Huang, H.-P., Qiu, Y. et al., 1997. Diabetes, defective pancreatic morphogenesis, and abnormal enteroendocrine differentiation in BETA2/NeuroD-deficient mice. *Genes and Development* 11, 2323–2334.

Nolte, T., Kaufmann, W., Schorsch, F., Soames, T., Weber, E., 2005. Standardized assessment of cell proliferation: the approach of the RITA-CEPA working group. *Experimental and Toxicologic Pathology* 57, 91–103.

Nonoyama, T., Fukuda, R., 2008. Drug-induced phospholipidosis—pathological aspects and its prediction. *Journal of Toxicology and Pathology* 21, 9–24.

Nyska, A., Jokinen, M.P., Brix, A.E. et al., 2004. Exocrine pancreatic pathology in female Harlan Sprague–Dawley rats after chronic treatment with 2,3,7,8-tetrachlorodibenzo-*p*-dioxin and dioxin-like compounds. *Environmental Health Perspectives* 112, 903–909.

Obert, L.A., Sobocinski, G.P., Bobrowski, W.F. et al., 2007. An immunohistochemical approach to differentiate hepatic lipidosis from hepatic phospholipidosis in rats. *Toxicologic Pathology* 35, 728–734.

O'Malley, D.P., Kim, Y.S., Perkins, S.L., Baldridge, L., Juliar, B.E., Orazi, A., 2005. Morphologic and immuno-histochemical evaluation of splenic hematopoietic proliferations in neoplastic and benign disorders. *Modern Pathology* 18, 1550–1561.

Omary, M.B., Lugea, A., Lowe, A.W., Pandol, S.J., 2007. The pancreatic stellate cell: a star on the rise in pancreatic diseases. *The Journal of Clinical Investigation* 117, 50–59.

Otsuki, M., Yamamoto, M., Yamaguchi, T., 2010. Animal models of chronic pancreatitis. In: *Gastroenterology Research and Practice*, Hindawi Publishing Corporation, New York.

Oyaizu, T., Shikata, N., Senzaki, H., Matsuzawa, A., Tsubura, A., 1997. Studies on the mechanism of dimethylnitrosamine-induced acute liver injury in mice. *Experimental and Toxicologic Pathology* 49, 375–380.

Parker, G.A., Gibson, W.B., 1995. Liver lesions in rats associated with wrapping of the torso. *Toxicologic Pathology* 23, 507–512.

Patnaik, A.K., Hurvitz, A.I., Lieberman, P.H., Johnson, G.F., 1981. Canine bile duct carcinoma. *Veterinary Pathology* 18, 439–444.

Patyna, S., Arrigoni, C., Terron, A. et al., 2008. Nonclinical safety evaluation of sunitinib: A potent inhibitor of VEGF, PDGF, KIT, FLT3, and RET receptors. *Toxicologic Pathology* 36, 905–916.

Peraino, C., Fry, R.J., Staffeldt, E., 1971. Reduction and enhancement by phenobarbital of hepatocarcinogenesis induced in the rat by 2-acetylaminofluorene. *Cancer Research* 31, 1506–1512.

Plant, N., Aouabdi, S., 2009. Nuclear receptors: the controlling force in drug metabolism of the liver? *Xenobiotica* 39, 597–605.

Popp, J.A., Goldsworthy, T.L., 1989. Defining foci of cellular alteration in short-term and medium term rat liver tumor models. *Toxicologic Pathology* 17, 561–568.

Popp, J.A., Shinozuka, H., Farber, E., 1978. The protective effects of diethyldithiocarbamate and cyclohexi-mide on the multiple hepatic lesions induced by carbon tetrachloride in the rat. *Toxicology and Applied Pharmacology* 45, 549–564.

Popp, J.A., Scortichini, B.H. Garvey, L.K., 1985. Quantitative evaluation of hepatic foci of cellular alteration occurring spontaneously in Fischer-344 rats. *Fundamental and Applied Toxicology* 5, 314–319.

Radi, Z.A., Koza-Taylor, P.H., Bell R.R. et al., 2011. Increased serum enzyme levels associated with Kupffer cell reduction with no signs of hepatic or skeletal muscle injury. *American Journal of Pathology* 179, 240–247.

Rao, M.S., Reddy, J.K., 1995. Hepatic transdifferentiation in the pancreas. *Seminars in Cell Biology* 6, 151–156.

Rao, M.S., Reddy, M.K., Reddy, J.K., Scarpelli, D.G., 1982. Response of chemically induced hepatocytelike cells in hamster pancreas to methyl clofenapate, a peroxisome proliferator. *The Journal of Cell Biology* 95, 50–56.

Rao, M.S., Subbarao, V., Luetteke, N., Scarpelli, D.G., 1983. Further characterization of carcinogen-induced hepatocytelike cells in hamster pancreas. *American Journal of Pathology* 110, 89–94.

Rao, M.S., Subbarao, V., Scarpelli, D.G., 1988. Development of hepatocytes in the pancreas of hamsters treated with 2,3,7,8-tetrachlorodibenzo-p-dioxin. *Journal of Environmental Health* 25, 201–205.

Rao, M.S., Dwivedi, R.S., Yeldandi, A.V. et al., 1989. Role of periductal and ductular epithelial cells of the adult rat pancreas in pancreatic hepatocyte lineage. A change in differentiation commitment. *American Journal of Pathology* 134, 1069–1086.

Rao, S.M., Yeldandi, A.V., Subbarao, V., Reddy, J.K., 1993. Role of apoptosis in copper deficiency-induced pancreatic involution in the rat. *American Journal of Pathology* 142, 1952–1957.

Raraty, M., Ward, J., Erdemli, G. et al., 2000. Calcium-dependent enzyme activation and vacuole formation in the apical granular region of pancreatic acinar cells. *Proceedings of the National Academy of Sciences* 97, 13126–13131.

Reasor, M.J., 1989. A review of the biology and toxicologic implications of the induction of lysosomal lamellar bodies by drugs. *Toxicology and Applied Pharmacology* 97, 47–56.

Reasor, M.J., Hastings, K.L., Ulrich, R.G., 2006. Drug-induced phospholipidosis, issues and future direction. *Expert Opinions on Drug Safety* 5, 567–583.

Reddy, J.K., Rao, M.S., Qureshi, S.A., Reddy, M.K., Scarpelli, D.G., Lalwani, N.D., 1984. Induction and origin of hepatocytes in rat pancreas. *The Journal of Cell Biology* 98, 2082–2090.

Redfern, J.S., Fortuner, W.J., 2nd, 1995. Octreotide-associated biliary tract dysfunction and gallstone formation: pathophysiology and management. *American Journal of Gastroenterology* 90, 1042–1052.

Reid, L.E., Walker, N.I., 1999. Acinar cell apoptosis and the origin of tubular complexes in caerulein-induced pancreatitis. *International Journal of Experimental Pathology* 80, 205–215.

Reznik-Schuller, H.M., Lijinsky, W., 1981. Morphology of early changes in liver carcinogenesis induced by methapyrilene. *Archives of Toxicology* 49, 79–83.

Rhomberg, L.R., Baetchke, K., Blancato, J. et al., 2007. Issues in the design and interpretation of chronic toxicity and carcinogenicity studies in rodents, approaches to dose selection. *Critical Reviews in Toxicology* 37, 729–837.

Rittinghausen, S., Ernst, H., Ashswede-Sannecke, F., 1998. Incomplete herniation of liver lobes through the diaphragm in Han:WIST rats. *Zeitschrift für Versuchstierkunde* 31, 151–154.

Robison, R.L., Van Ryzin, R.J., Stoll, R.E., Jensen, R.D., Bagdon, R.E., 1984. Chronic toxicity/carcinogenesis study of temazepam in mice and rats. *Fundamental and Applied Toxicology* 4, 394–405.

Rodriguez, A.I., Manso, M.A., Garcia-Montero, A.C., Orfao, A., de Dois, I., 1997. Long-term blockade of cholecystokinin (CCK): effects of L-364,718 (a CCK receptor antagonist) on pancreatic enzyme storage and secretion. *Pancreas* 15, 314–322.

Ropolo, A., Grasso, D., Pardo, R. et al., 2007. The pancreatitis-induced vacuole membrane protein 1 triggers autophagy in mammalian cells. *Journal of Biological Chemistry* 282, 37124–37133.

Rose, R., Banerjee, A., Ramaiah, S.K., 2006. Calpain inhibition attenuates iNOS production and midzonal hepatic necrosis in a repeat dose model of endotoxemia in rats. *Toxicologic Pathology* 34, 785–794.

Rubbia-Brandt, L., 2010. Sinusoidal obstruction syndrome. *Clinics in Liver Disease* 14, 651–668.

Ryan, A.M., Eppler, D.B., Hagler, K.E. et al., 1999. Preclinical safety evaluation of rhuMAbVEGF, an antiangiogenic humanized monoclonal antibody. *Toxicologic Pathology* 27, 78–86.

Saegusa, C., Kanno, E., Itohara, S., Fukuda, M., 2008. Expression of Rab27B-binding protein Slp1 in pancreatic acinar cells and its involvement in amylase secretion. *Archives of Biochemistry and Biophysics* 475, 87–92.

Saluja, A., Hofbauer, B., Yamaguchi, Y., Yamanaka, K., Steer, M., 1996. Induction of apoptosis reduces the severity of caerulein-induced pancreatitis in mice. *Biochemical and Biophysical Research Communications* 220, 875–878.

Sarles, H., Camarena-Trabous, J., Gomez-Santana, C., Choux, R., Iovanna, J., 1993. Acute pancreatitis is not a cause of chronic pancreatitis in the absence of residual duct strictures. *Pancreas* 8, 354–357.

Sato T., Herman L., 1990. Morphometry and elemental analysis of rat exocrine pancreas following administration of trypsin inhibitor. *Acta Anatomica (Basel)* 137, 65–76.

Scampini, G., Nava, A., Newman, A.J. et al., 1993. Multinucleated hepatocytes induced by rifabutin in rats. *Toxicologic Pathology* 21, 369–376.

Scarpelli, D.G., Rao, M.S., 1981. Differentiation of regenerating pancreatic cells into hepatocyte-like cells. *Proceedings of the National Academy of Sciences* 78, 2577–2581.

Scatena, R., Bottoni, P., Botta, G., Martorana, G.E., Giardina, B., 2007. The role of mitochondria in pharmacotoxicology: a reevaluation of an old, new emerging topic. *American Journal of Physiology Cell Physiology* 293, C12–C21.

Schmucker, D.L., Mooney, J.S., Jones, A.L., 1978. Stereological analysis of hepatic fine structure in the Fischer 344 rat. Influence of sublobular location and animal age. *Journal of Cell Biology* 78, 319–337.

Schott, I., Hartmann, D., Gieselmann, V., Lüllmann-Rauch, R., 2001. Sulfatide storage in visceral organs of arylsulfatase A-deficient mice. *Virchows Archives* 439, 90–96.

Schüssler, M.H., Skoudy, A., Ramaekers, F., Real, F.X., 1992. Intermediate filaments as differentiation markers of normal pancreas and pancreas cancer. *American Journal of Pathology* 140, 559–568.

Senoo, H., 2004. Structure and function of hepatic stellate cells. *Medical Electron Microscopy* 37, 3–15.

Seyama, Y., Otani, T., Matsukura, A., Makuuchi, M., 2003. The pH modulator chloroquine blocks trypsinogen activation peptide generation in cerulein-induced pancreatitis. *Pancreas* 26, 15–17.

Sherwood, M.W., Prior, I.A., Voronina, S.G. et al., 2007. Activation of trypsinogen in large endocytic vacuoles of pancreatic acinar cells. *Proceedings of the National Academy of Sciences* 104, 5674–5679.

Shibayama, Y., Asaka, S., Nakata, K., 1994. Role of activated macrophages in augmentation of endotoxin hepatotoxicity. *Experimental and Toxicologic Pathology* 45, 497–502.

Sieber, S.M., Correa, P., Dalgard, D.W., Adamson, R.H., 1979. Induction of osteogenic sarcomas and tumors of the hepatobiliary system in nonhuman primates with aflatoxin B1. *Cancer Research* 39, 4545–4554.

Sigler, R.E., Gough, A.W., de la Iglesia, F.A., 1995. Pancreatic acinar cell neoplasia in male Wistar rats following 2 years of gabapentin exposure. *Toxicology* 98, 73–82.

Sinclair, J.F., Szakacs, J.G., Wood, S.G. et al., 2000. Acetaminophen hepatotoxicity precipitated by short-term treatment of rats with ethanol and isopentanol: protection by triacetyloleandomycin. *Biochemical Pharmacology* 59, 445–454.

Sisson, S., Grossman, J.D. 1953. The digestive system, In: *The Anatomy of the Domestic Animals*. W. B. Saunders Company, Philadelphia, pp. 387–516.

Si-Tayeb, K., Lemaigre, F.P., Duncan, S.A., 2010. Organogenesis and development of the liver. *Developmental Cell* 18, 175–189.

Sneed, R.A., Grimes, S.D., Schultze, A.E., Brown, A.P., Ganey, P.E., 1997. Bacterial endotoxin enhances the hepatotoxicity of allyl alcohol. *Toxicology and Applied Pharmacology* 144, 77–87.

Solter, P.F., 2005. Clinical pathology approaches to hepatic injury. *Toxicologic Pathology* 33, 9–16.

Soltys, K.A., Soto-Gutierrez, A., Nagaya, M. et al., 2010. Barriers to the successful treatment of liver disease by hepatocyte transplantation. *Journal of Hepatology* 53, 769–774.

Spencer, A.J., Everett, R, Popp, J.A., 1997. Multifocal inflammation, liver, rat. In: *Digestive System, Monographs on Pathology of Laboratory Animals*. Jones, T.C., Popp, J.A., and Mohr, U. (editors), Springer Verlag, New York, pp. 101–103.

Stegelmeier, B.L., Molyneux, R.J., Asano, N., Watson, A.A., Nash, R.J., 2008. The comparative pathology of the glycosidase inhibitors swainsonine, castanospermine, and calystegines A3, B2, and C1 in mice. *Toxicologic Pathology* 36, 651–659.

Stroebel, P., Mayer, F., Zerban, H., Bannasch, P., 1995. Spongiotic pericytoma: a benign neoplasm deriving from the perisinusoidal (Ito) cells in rat liver. *American Journal of Pathology* 146, 903–913.

Strobel, O., Dor, Y., Alsina, J. et al., 2007a. In vivo lineage tracing defines the role of acinar-to-ductal transdifferentiation in inflammatory ductal metaplasia. *Gastroenterology* 133, 1999–2009.

Strobel, O., Dor, Y., Stirman, A. et al., 2007b. β cell transdifferentiation does not contribute to preneoplastic/metaplastic ductal lesions of the pancreas by genetic lineage tracing in vivo. *Proceedings of the National Academy of Sciences* 104, 4419–4424.

Su, Q, Bannasch, P., 2003. Relevance of hepatic preneoplasia for human hepatocarcinogenesis. *Toxicologic Pathology* 31, 126–133.

Swirski, F.K., Wildgruber, M., Ueno, T. et al., 2010. Myeloperoxidase-rich Ly-6C+ myeloid cells infiltrate allografts and contribute to an imaging signature of organ rejection in mice. *Journal of Clinical Investigation* 120, 2627–2634.

Takama, S., Kishino, Y., 1985. Dietary effects on pancreatic lesions induced by excess arginine in rats. *British Journal of Nutrition* 54, 37–42.

Tani, S., Itoh, H., Okabayashi, Y. et al., 1990. New model of acute necrotizing pancreatitis induced by excessive doses of arginine in rats. *Digestive Diseases and Sciences* 35, 367–374.

Tapp, R.L., 1970. Anoxic and secretory vacuolation in the acinar cells of the pancreas. *Quarterly Journal of Experimental Physiology and Cognate Medical Sciences* 55, 1–15.

Thoolen, B., Maronpot, R.R., Harada, T. et al., 2010. Proliferative and nonproliferative lesions of the rat and mouse hepatobiliary system. *Toxicologic Pathology* 38, 5S–81S.

Tsokosa, M., Erbersdobler, A., 2005. Pathology of peliosis. *Forensic Science International* 149, 25–33.

Turusov, V.S., Mikinori, T., Sills, R.C. et al., 2002. Hepatoblastoma in mice in the US National Toxicology Program (NTP) studies. *Toxicologic Pathology* 30, 580–591.

Vaccaro, M.I., 2008. Autophagy and pancreas disease. *Pancreatology* 8, 425–429.

Wachtman, L.M., Mansfield, K.G., 2008. Opportunistic infections in immunologically compromised non-human primates. *ILAR Journal* 49, 191–208.

Waites, C.R., Dominick, M.A., Sanderson, T.P., Schilling, B.E., 2007. Nonclinical safety evaluation of muraglitazar, a novel PPARalpha/gamma agonist. *Toxicological Sciences* 100, 248–258.

Walgren, J.L., Mitchell, M.D., Whiteley, L.O., Thompson, D.C., 2007a. Evaluation of two novel peptide safety markers for exocrine pancreatic toxicity. *Toxicological Sciences* 96, 184–193.

Walgren, J.L., Mitchell, M.D., Whiteley, L.O., Thompson, D.C., 2007b. Identification of novel peptide safety markers for exocrine pancreatic toxicity induced by cyanohydroxybutene. *Toxicological Sciences* 96, 174–183.

Wallig, M.A., Gould, D.H., Fettman, M.J., 1988. Selective pancreatotoxicity in the rat induced by the naturally occurring plant nitrile 1-cyano-2-hydroxy-3-butene. *Food and Chemical Toxicology* 26, 137–147.

Ward, J.M., Yoon, M., Anver, M.R. et al., 2001. Hyalinosis and Ym1/Ym2 gene expression in the stomach and respiratory tract of 129S4/SvJae and wild-type and CYP1A2-null B6, 129 mice. *American Journal of Pathology* 158, 323–332.

Warren, A., Benseler, V., Cogger, V.C., Bertolino, P., Le Couteur, D.G., 2011. The impact of poloxamer 407 on the ultrastructure of the liver and evidence for clearance by extensive endothelial and Kupffer cell endocytosis. *Toxicologic Pathology* 39, 390–397.

Wickstrom, M.L., Khan, S.A., Haschek, W.M. et al., 1995. Alterations in microtubules, intermediate filaments, and microfilaments induced by microcystin-LR in cultured cells. *Toxicologic Pathology* 23, 326–337.

Williams, G.M., Iatropoulos, M.J., 2002. Alterations of liver cell function and proliferation, differentiation between adaptation and toxicity. *Toxicologic Pathology* 30, 41–53.

Wood, F.E., Tierney, W.J., Knezevich, A.L. et al., 1991. Chronic toxicity and carcinogenicity studies of olestra in Fischer 344 rats. *Food and Chemical Toxicology* 29, 223–230.

Worley, D.R., Hottinger, H.A., Lawrence, H.J., 2004. Surgical management of gallbladder mucoceles in dogs: 22 cases (1999–2003). *Journal of the American Veterinary Medical Association* 225, 1418–1422.

Xiao, K., Li, Y., Luo, J. et al., 2011. The effect of surface charge on in vivo biodistribution of PEG-oligocholic acid based micellar nanoparticles. *Biomaterials* 32, 3435–3446.

Yamamoto, M., Otani, M., Otsuki, M., 2006. A new model of chronic pancreatitis in rats. *American Journal of Physiology—Gastrointestinal and Liver Physiology* 291, G700–G708.

Yoshioka, K., Enaga, K., Tanaguchi, U., Fukushima, U., Uechi, M., Mutoh, K., 2004. Morphological characterization of ductular reactions in canine liver disease. *Journal of Comparative Pathology* 130, 92–98.

Yoshizawa, K., Marsh, T., Foley, J.F. et al., 2005. Mechanisms of exocrine pancreatic toxicity induced by oral treatment with 2,3,7,8-tetrachlorodibenzo-p-dioxin in female Harlan Sprague–Dawley rats. *Toxicological Sciences* 85, 594–606.

Yu, F.L., Bender, W., Geronimo, I.H., 1988. The binding of aflatoxin B1 to rat liver nuclear proteins and its effect on DNA-dependent RNA synthesis. *Carcinogenesis* 9, 533–540.

Yu, W., Wan, X., Wright, J.R., Jr., Coddington, D., Bitter-Suermann, H., 1994. Heterotopic liver transplantation in rats: effect of intrahepatic islet isografts and split portal blood flow on liver integrity after auxiliary liver isotransplantation. *Surgery* 115, 108–117.

11 Respiratory System

David J. Lewis and Tom P. McKevitt

CONTENTS

11.1 GENERAL INTRODUCTION

The primary functions of the respiratory system are air conducting, olfaction, and gas exchange. Gas exchange necessitates the large internal surface area of the lung, its extensive capillary bed, and the delicately structured pulmonary parenchyma. These features allow rapid absorption of pharmaceuticals and make inhalation delivery, for either local or systemic effect, an attractive option. Although the practice of inhalation therapy can be traced back many centuries, it was the invention of the metered dose inhaler (MDI) in the 1950s that provided the first truly safe and effective means of inhalation dosing of pharmaceuticals. This led to a rapid expansion of inhalation medicine research, and asthma patients were the first to benefit with the availability of MDI salbutamol (beta agonist) in 1969. Dry powder inhalers (DPIs) and nebulizers followed, and compounds for inhalation are no longer restricted to small molecules; the first protein DPI (insulin) for the treatment of diabetes became available in 2006 (Patton and Byron 2007), and there is growing interest in inhalation delivery of vaccines (Bennett et al. 2002).

In response to these advances, the field of inhalation toxicology developed rapidly to provide data necessary for hazard identification and risk assessment. Animals are exposed to a test atmosphere designed to replicate the proposed route of clinical administration to humans; for pharmaceuticals, this usually means aerosols of either solids or liquids, that is, DPI or nebulized formulations, respectively. The total dose delivered is a function of both the concentration of the test article in the test atmosphere and the duration of exposure. Generation of the test atmosphere is closely controlled to ensure that the test article (particle or droplet) is adequately respirable. This is a function of both size and shape and is described by mass median aerodynamic diameter (OECD 2009).

Inhalation exposure systems used in pharmaceutical safety testing are ideally nose- or face-only as whole-body systems are wasteful in terms of test article and have well-documented deficiencies in yielding consistent and reproducible delivered doses, especially for group-housed animals (Wong 2007). Face-only delivery facilitates the use of plethysmography to monitor breathing during dosing; this allows better estimation of delivered dose and is preferable to empirical data (DeLorme and Moss 2001; Hartings and Roy 2001). Containment of test material is also easier with face/nose-only systems, and inadvertent exposure via other routes (e.g., orally during grooming of fur) is reduced. There are also drawbacks; despite acclimatization, the procedure is less "natural" than whole-body exposure, and in sealed rodent dosing tubes, temperature and humidity can increase, potentially affecting test atmosphere and breathing patterns. Additionally, sealed dosing tube exposures can lead to stress-related findings such as thymic atrophy, and the increased body temperature has been associated with testicular atrophy. For these reasons, the time for nose-only exposures is usually limited, that is, 2 h per exposure.

Intratracheal instillation and oropharyngeal aspiration are used, particularly in the early stages of compound development. Intratracheal instillation involves the insertion of a dosing catheter to the distal trachea under anesthesia and delivery of a bolus dose (typically 200 μl) that is aspirated into the lungs. Oropharyngeal aspiration involves the placement of a bolus dose at the base of the extended tongue in an anesthetized animal. The dose is then aspirated into the lungs. Both techniques are an efficient use of test material, and intratracheal instillation bypasses the difficulties of estimating deposited lung dose encountered upon standard inhalation delivery. Distribution of the test article in the lungs following intratracheal dosing may, however, not be uniform, with the potential for hot spots of compound deposition and associated pathology.

Of critical importance for safety testing is the understanding that deposited dose (i.e., the fraction of the inhaled dose deposited in the lungs) differs between species for the same aerosol. The fractional pulmonary deposition of 1-μm particles in the rat has been estimated to be 0.1, that is, only 10% of the inhaled dose is considered to reach the lung (Snipes et al. 1989) and compares with 0.25 in humans for the same particle size. Despite this human fraction, the Food and Drug Administration (FDA) assumes 100% deposition in the human lung and 10% deposition in the rat lung for the purpose of risk assessment (Owen 2011; Forbes et al. 2011). Thus, a deposited dose correction factor of 10 for the rat (and 4 for the dog) is currently required. This, coupled with safety margins for unmonitorable lung findings of 10 for the rat and 6 for the dog, has led to combined human safety margins of 100× for the rat and 24× for the dog. As such, very large inhaled doses are required for preclinical testing, with the inherent risk of lung overload and associated pathology (Morrow 1992).

11.2   EMBRYOLOGY OF RESPIRATORY SYSTEM

The development of the mammalian respiratory system involves interaction between epithelial cells derived from a ventral outpouching of foregut endoderm and mesenchymal cells from the splanchnic mesoderm, and it begins at embryonic day 9–9.5 in the mouse (Wan et al. 2004). Lung development is under the control of transcription factors, including multiple forkhead transcription factors, GATA-6, and thyroid transcription factor-1 (Costa et al. 2001, Wan et al. 2004). The process has been divided into five stages (embryonic, pseudoglandular, canalicular, saccular, and alveolar), all of which are potentially susceptible to modification by toxicants (Fanucchi and Plopper 1997). The first four stages occur prenatally, with only the final, alveolar stage of development occurring after term. The response to a toxicant can vary significantly, depending on which developmental stage the lung is in; this is important as the rate of prenatal development varies between species. For example, the developing human lung enters the saccular stage at 60% of full gestational age, whereas in the rat, the saccular stage does not begin until gestation is 95% complete (Fanucchi and Plopper 1997).

The majority of lung growth and development occurs postpartum. The volume of the respiratory system continues to increase in line with overall body growth and ceases only when overall growth is complete. In addition, the enzyme systems capable of producing toxic metabolites do not develop until the perinatal period, with the majority of development extending into the postnatal period. The prenatal and early postnatal respiratory system is more susceptible to known respiratory system toxicants than it is in adults of the same species, and species differences in susceptibility to a respiratory toxicant are amplified if the toxicant is tested in the developing rather than the adult respiratory system (Fanucchi and Plopper 1997).

11.3   FUNCTIONAL ANATOMY OF RESPIRATORY SYSTEM

11.3.1   Nasal Cavity

The respiratory system may be divided functionally into conductive, transitional, and gas exchange regions. The conductive system includes the nasal cavity, pharynx, larynx, trachea, and bronchi, which filter, warm, and moisten air as it moves toward the gas exchange regions. The arrangement of the conducting part of the system varies such that primates and dogs can breathe nasally or oronasally, while laboratory rodents and rabbits are obligate nasal breathers. The volume of the nasal cavity has been estimated to be 0.03, 0.4, 8, and 20 cm^3 in the mouse, rat, rhesus monkey, and beagle dog, respectively (Schreider and Rabbe 1981; Herbert and Leininger 1999), and there is marked species variation in turbinate complexity between microsmatic species, such as nonhuman primates, and macrosmatic, such as rodents, rabbits, and dogs. This anatomic variation is reflected most noticeably in the percentage of the nasal cavity lined by olfactory epithelium, estimated at 50% in the laboratory rat but only 14% in the rhesus monkey (Plopper and Harkema 2005).

11.3.2 PHARYNX

The pharynx connects the nasal and oral cavities with the laryngeal airway. Its dorsal to ventral bend along its long axis particularly in the nasopharynx is determined by the posture of the species. Hence, this angle is greater in species with an upright stance, such as the rhesus monkey (estimated at 80°), than it is in either the beagle dog (30°) or rat (15°) (Schreider and Rabbe 1981). The associated change in the direction of airflow implies that greater impaction of inhaled particulates occurs at this level in humans and nonhuman primates than in other laboratory species.

11.3.3 LARYNX

An important interspecies anatomical difference in the larynx is the arrangement of the laryngeal diverticula. In rodents, a diverticulum extends ventrally from the base of the larynx (ventral pouch), whereas in the beagle dog and laboratory primates, diverticula extend bilaterally (termed laryngeal air sacs or ventricles) from the lateral walls of the laryngeal lumen. The function of these diverticula is unclear, though in some nonhuman primate species (such as the howler monkey), laryngeal air sacs appear to act as resonance chambers for the amplification of vocalizations (Hilloowala and Lass 1978). Stratified squamous epithelium lines the anterior larynx in all laboratory species but is thicker and extends further caudally in nonrodent species. The level at which the transition to respiratory epithelium occurs is therefore different between species.

11.3.4 TRACHEA AND AIRWAYS

The trachea is lined by pseudostratified columnar (respiratory) epithelium, with the focal presence of areas of stratified squamous epithelium in the dog. In the rat, the epithelium thins distally, and there are greater numbers of ciliated cells near the tracheal bifurcation than proximally. In addition, there is a zonation of ciliated cells; cilia-rich zones are found over the tracheal ligaments, while fewer ciliated cells overlie tracheal cartilage rings (Oliveira et al. 2003). The distally located cilia are also shorter and beat faster (Jeffery and Reid 1975; Boorman et al. 1990). Goblet cells are rare in the tracheas of rats and mice; however, a substantial number are seen in nonhuman primates (Hyde et al. 2006). Migratory cells, particularly globule leucocytes, are commonly seen in all species. Mainly serous glandular tissue is found primarily in the submucosa of the upper trachea of the rat; a few glands are seen below the level of the thyroid (Boorman et al. 2003). This is in contrast to humans and nonhuman primates, which have extensive submucosal glands in both the trachea and proximal airways (Plopper and Harkema 2005).

Interspecies differences in the arrangement and epithelial lining of the airways also exist; in humans and nonhuman primates, branching is dichotomous, while in the rat and mouse, it is monopodial. In nonhuman primates, goblet cells and basal cells predominate in bronchial epithelium, whereas the Clara cell is the principal nonciliated cell seen at this level in other laboratory animals (Hyde et al. 2006). Clara cells are also common throughout the respiratory tree in mice.

The bronchioles are the most distal conducting airways, are characterized by thin walls, and, in most laboratory species, are devoid of cartilage. The bronchioles of rhesus monkeys, in addition to containing cartilage, also contain large bundles of smooth muscle that are not seen in other laboratory animals (Hyde et al. 2006). The main secretory cell at this level is the Clara cell, and goblet cells are not normally present.

A region of transition between the conducting and gas exchange areas is present in nonhuman primates and carnivores, but not other laboratory species (Plopper and Harkema 2005). These airways are termed *respiratory bronchioles* and are characterized by alveolar air spaces opening directly from their walls, such that they have a conducting function, but also contribute directly to gas exchange.

The Clara cell is a multifunctional cell, having roles in immune and inflammatory regulation, xenobiotic metabolism, airway surfactant synthesis, mucin secretion, and progenitor cell activity (Snyder et al. 2010). These cells have a very distinctive appearance, characterized by a basal nucleus and a prominent apical dome, consistent with apocrine secretion. Clara cells may be identified by immunohistochemical (IHC) staining for their major secretory protein CC10, also referred to as Clara cell secretory protein (CCSP), which is a member of the secretoglobin family (Watson et al. 2001; Singh and Katyal 2000). CC10 can bind xenobiotics and may have a role in their sequestration and clearance; additionally, it forms complexes with the protein cross-linking enzyme, transglutaminase, to reduce foreign protein antigenicity (Khoor et al. 1996; Hermans and Bernard 1999; Van Miert et al. 2005). Other Clara cell proteins with similar roles include surfactant proteins (SPs) B and D, which are described separately. CC10 may be used as a biomarker for bronchiolar damage; in rats treated with known Clara cell toxicants, decreased bronchiolar CC10 is demonstrable by IHC, and alterations in CC10 levels can also be detected in bronchiolar lavage fluid (BALF) and in serum (Hermans et al. 1999). CC10 secretion in rats may be increased by beta-agonists or increased tidal volume ventilation (Massaro et al. 1981).

Ciliated cells are the other major cell type of the airway epithelium and stain positively by IHC for β-tubulin, a major structural component of cilia (Sheppard and Thurlow 1992).

Pulmonary neuroendocrine cells (PNECs) are found individually or in clusters termed neuroepithelial bodies (NEBs) within the bronchiolar epithelium (Haworth et al. 2007). These cells may be identified by their distinctive stippled nuclear pattern in hematoxylin and eosin (H&E) sections or by IHC for Protein G product 9.5 (PGP 9.5) or calcitonin gene-related peptide.

Bronchial associated lymphoid tissue (BALT) is seen in subepithelial locations in the major airways, often showing a predilection for airway branches. The epithelium overlying BALT is modified with an apical microvillous border, providing an increased area for antigen sampling. There are significant species differences in the amount of BALT found in the lungs of healthy animals; BALT is consistently seen in rats and rabbits, while it is often absent from the lungs of commonly used mouse strains, healthy control beagle dogs, and humans (Haley 2003; Pabst and Gehrke 1990; Wardlaw et al. 2005).

11.3.5 LUNG

Striking anatomical differences are seen in lung lobation. The greatest degree of lobe separation is seen in nonhuman primates, where there is separation into six lobes—left cranial (subdivided into cranial and caudal segments) and left caudal; and right cranial, middle, caudal, and accessory lobes. In contrast, the left lung in laboratory rats and mice consists of a single lobe, while the right lung is divided into four lobes.

Gas exchange occurs within the alveoli across the thin epithelial barrier (<0.1 μm in places) of Type I pneumocytes (ATI) that cover approximately 98% of the alveolar surface and also function to regulate solute and water movement between blood and the airspace (Williams 2003; Dobbs et al. 2010). These cells are terminally differentiated and normally lack mitotic activity. Aquaporin-5 is an ATI specific marker in the lung parenchyma (Nielsen et al. 1997). Type II pneumocytes (ATII), which are located at the intersections of alveolar walls, act as progenitors for ATI cells (Evans et al. 1975), produce and secrete surfactant, and are involved in transepithelial fluid and electrolyte transport (Edelson et al. 1988). By transmission electron microscopy (TEM), ATII are characterized by the presence of cytoplasmic lamellar and multivesicular bodies, and numerous microvilli are present on their apical surface. These cells may also be highlighted by alkaline phosphatase histochemistry or IHC (Edelson et al. 1988). The other epithelial cell found lining the alveoli (and respiratory tract) in some species is the pulmonary brush cell or Type III pneumocyte. These cells have been seen in rat and hamster alveoli and may be identified by TEM, having typically up to 140 microvilli on their narrow apical surface. Their function is unknown (Reid et al. 2005).

11.3.6 ALVEOLAR MACROPHAGE

The alveolar macrophage (AM) is an important effector cell of the innate immune system, a professional antigen-presenting cell, and a regulator of host defense and homeostasis (Laskin et al. 2011). Under normal quiescent conditions, most lung macrophages will have been derived from circulating monocytes that differentiate upon entering the alveoli; however, there is evidence that they may also undergo replication *in situ*—a process previously associated with a response to an inflammatory stimulus only (Bitterman et al. 1984; Geiser 2010).

AMs in the healthy lung are reported to concentrate at alveolar septal junctions (Takaro et al. 1990) and by TEM are characterized by numerous mitochondria and secondary lysosomes. Activated macrophages have been subdivided into classically activated (M1), which have largely antiproliferative, inflammatory, and cytotoxic activity, and alternatively activated (M2), which have a generally anti-inflammatory impact and are involved in initiation of wound healing and tissue remodeling (Laskin et al. 2011). The activation state is a dynamic process; an individual macrophage may switch between states depending on its environment (Murray and Wynn 2011), and the precise profile of the AM will depend also on how it became activated (Mosser and Edwards 2008; Bowdridge and Gause 2010). Markers of an activated state include inducible nitric oxide synthase for M1 macrophages and arginase 1, Fizz1, and Ym1/2 for M2 macrophages (Misson et al. 2004). CD68 IHC is commonly used as a general marker for AM; however, antibodies to this target also bind monocytes and granulocytes in the peripheral blood (Noorman et al. 1997).

AM may leave the lung via the mucociliary escalator, or they may undergo transepithelial migration (which can also occur in the airways) and enter the lymphatic system. This second route facilities contact between particles carried by the AM and local dendritic cells, providing a critical link between innate and adaptive immunity (Gehr et al. 1996; Blank et al. 2007).

11.3.7 MUCINS AND SURFACTANT IN LUNGS AND AIRWAYS

11.3.7.1 Mucins

The mucins are the major macromolecular components of the airway mucous layer and are the combined product of the secretion of epithelial goblet cells and the submucosal glands (Heidsiek et al. 1987). Acid and neutral mucins may be detected by using combined alcian blue (pH 2.5)/ periodic acid-Schiff histochemistry, and sulfated mucins may be detected by high iron diamine histochemistry (Myers et al. 2008). The protein backbones of mucin glycoproteins may also be detected by IHC, or the *MUC* gene mRNAs that encode them may be investigated by Northern blot or *in situ* hybridization. There is evidence in rats that mucous flow in the nasal cavity of older animals is slower than it is in the young. This has implications for particle retention and susceptibility to toxicity (Gross et al. 1987). In addition to providing a physical barrier and contributing to the mucociliary escalator, mucins provide specific protection to the respiratory system via influenza virus aggregation and hemagglutinin inhibition and by reducing the respiratory burst of neutrophils (White et al. 2005a,b).

11.3.7.2 Surfactant

The SPs, SP-A, SP-B, SP-C, and SP-D, constitute approximately 10% of pulmonary surfactant, with the remainder being lipid (predominantly phospholipid), of which dipalmitoylphosphatidylcholine (DPPC) is the major contributor. The main function of surfactant is to maintain a low surface tension in the lung to prevent collapse during respiration (Rooney et al. 1994), and the small, hydrophobic SP-B and SP-C play a major role in this. SP-A and SP-D are large, hydrophilic proteins, and while they contribute to surfactant homeostasis, they also have a role in host defense. Their structure includes a carbohydrate recognition domain that interacts with carbohydrates on the surface of pathogens, leading to agglutination and enhanced macrophage and neutrophil responses (Kishore et al. 2006).

Surfactant in the airways promotes luminal patency and counteracts fluid accumulation (Christmann et al. 2009). Peripheral airways are prone to collapse at maximum expiration (Tavana et al. 2011), and surfactant deficiency can compound this tendency. There is evidence that Clara cells synthesize and secrete surfactant into the airway lumen, in addition to which a small percentage of the surfactant produced in the alveolar region reaches the bronchial tree by expiration-driven extrusion, with the rest being phagocytosed and recycled locally (Hohlfeld et al. 1997; Etherton et al. 1973; Sato and Kishikawa 2001; Aryal et al. 2003).

Surfactant and mucus in the airways may be demonstrated by osmium tetroxide in perfluorocarbon fixation (Sims and Horne 1997) or by vascular perfusion fixation (Gil and Weibel 1971).

11.4 ANCILLARY TESTS OF RESPIRATORY SYSTEM FUNCTION OR DAMAGE

In addition to routine examination of standard H&E sections, a broad range of other endpoints and ancillary tests may be used to evaluate test article–related changes in the respiratory system.

Lung weights are commonly recorded on inhalation studies. If consistent trimming practice is followed, then increased lung weight is considered to correlate well with the presence of histological findings (Michael et al. 2007). Lung weights should be normalized to either body weight or brain weight before interpretation.

Bronchoalveolar lavage (BAL) allows quantitative sampling of the cellular and biochemical responses to lung toxicants and may be used to further investigate mechanism of toxicity or to gain additional data in support of a proposed no-effect level. In normal BAL fluid (BALF), >90% of cells are AM. Increased numbers of neutrophils are a sensitive indicator of an inflammatory process, whereas increased numbers of lymphocytes and eosinophils may indicate an immune-based inflammatory response. Species differences in BALF cells occur. In nonhuman primates, up to 10% of cells may be lymphocytes, and in guinea pigs, eosinophils are routinely seen in healthy animals (Henderson 2005). Useful biochemical parameters include lactate dehydrogenase for cytotoxicity, proinflammatory cytokines such as tumor necrosis factor-alpha (TNF-α) and interleukin-1 (IL-1), chemoattractants such as macrophage inflammatory protein-2 (MIP-2) and IL-8 (neutrophil attractants in rodents and primates, respectively), and macrophage chemoattractant protein-1 (MCP-1) and IL-6. In larger species, segmental BAL (i.e., lavage of a single lobe either by bronchoscopy or lobar excision at necropsy) may be used. The excision technique can also be used in rats. A ligature allows the excision site to be sealed such that the remainder of the lungs may be inflated with fixative, allowing normal histological examination. This technique is useful as it allows comparison of BALF findings with histopathology in the same animal without compromising the lobes examined by light microscopy. Imaging techniques may also be used to assess structural changes within the lung.

Techniques such as magnetic resonance imaging (MRI) and microcomputed tomography (micro-CT) can be used to address onset and development of test article–related changes in the lung (Beckmann et al. 2003; Johnson 2007). Imaging can also be used to plan optimal sampling time for terminal endpoints in investigative studies. Imaging the lung of a living animal is technically very challenging due to movement of both the lungs and heart, particularly in rodents with rapid respiratory and heart rates. In addition, the air in the lungs has traditionally limited the resolution capability of MRI (Beckmann et al. 2003). Applications include the capability to reveal structural changes such as emphysema and fibrosis and to assess functional changes in the efficiency of gas exchange in the living animal (Driehuys and Hedlund 2007).

Lung function analysis is usually performed as part of the battery of safety pharmacology testing to support first-time-in-human dosing but is increasingly used in investigatory animal models of lung disease. These studies provide data on the efficiency of gas exchange by measuring parameters such as lung airflow, elasticity, and ventilatory patterns. Details of these techniques are reviewed elsewhere (Murphy 1994; Murphy et al. 2007; Hoymann 2006).

Quantitative analysis of test article–related effects in the respiratory system is hampered by issues of sample bias due to the nonuniform distribution and size of cells and structures. For example, the statistical probability of a particular cell type being detected on a single, thin, histological section is proportional to the size of that particular cell (specifically its height along the direction of sectioning) rather than the frequency with which it appears in the tissue. The technique of design-based stereology accounts for nonuniformity of tissue components and varying size of individual structures and may be used for nonuniform samples such as lung tissue. The technique has recently been applied to the lungs of rhesus monkeys and rats to demonstrate a method of unbiased assessment of changes to the epithelial lining of the respiratory system, down to the level of the distal airways (Hyde et al. 2006).

11.5   NON-NEOPLASTIC NASAL CAVITY FINDINGS

The epithelial lining of the nasal cavity includes squamous epithelium, which is largely restricted to the anterior nasal cavity; ciliated respiratory epithelium, a region of poorly ciliated transitional epithelium between the squamous and respiratory areas; and olfactory epithelium located in the dorsal and dorso-posterior areas (Harkema 1991). Distribution maps are available for the rat, mouse, and rhesus monkey (Mery et al. 1994; Kepler et al. 1995). These epithelia are exposed to toxicants either directly in the inhaled air stream, systemically via the blood stream, or following retrograde aspiration of refluxed material. Contact between nasal cavity epithelia and toxicants produces a spectrum of changes dependent upon the method of delivery, the nature of the toxicant, the dose, duration of exposure, and recovery time. In practice, multiple findings are often noted in the same area of epithelium.

Following inhalation of a toxicant, the pattern of findings in the nasal cavity is influenced by airflow, distribution of the nasal cavity epithelia, and deposition patterns, which vary with turbinate structure across species (Harkema 1990; Harkema et al. 2006; Schreider and Rabbe 1981). More complex turbinate structure leads to increased deviation of airflow, such that in the dog, rat, and mouse (complex turbinates), airflow is greatest through the upper half of the nasal cavity, while in higher primates and humans (simple turbinates), airflow is greatest ventrally.

Test article–related changes may also occur in the nasal cavity following systemic exposure, and, as such, it is recommended that at least one nasal cavity section (usually the posterior section) be examined in noninhalation studies (Kittel et al. 2004), although many laboratories' standard procedure is to examine three to four sections. It should also be borne in mind that nasal cavity changes in inhalation studies can be the result of systemic exposure as a consequence of swallowing a portion of the inhaled dose.

Retrograde aspiration of stomach material and/or test article can also lead to changes in the nasal cavity. Material can reach the oropharynx by emesis (in species where this occurs), passive gastro-esophageal reflux, or gavage-related reflux. From the oropharynx, material is driven into the nasal cavity during exhalation, resulting in a spectrum of changes typically including epithelial degeneration/necrosis, an acute/subacute inflammatory response, and, in some cases, turbinate fusion. In oncogenicity studies, these changes can progress to extensive hyperostosis of damaged turbinate bones and obliteration of much of the nasal cavity (Figure 11.1a). Refluxed material can also be inhaled deeper into the respiratory system. Reflux-related changes are typically most pronounced in posterior nasal sections and may be associated with increased salivation, audible respiration,

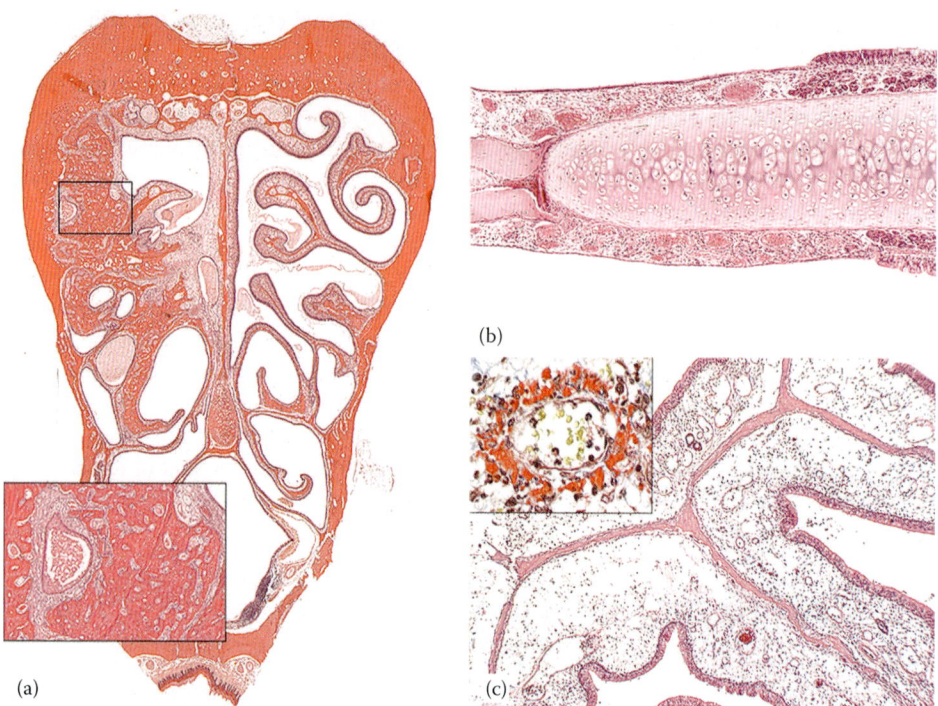

FIGURE 11.1 (a) Turbinate hyperostosis secondary to repeated nasal reflux. Nasal cavity, rat. (b) Olfactory epithelial atrophy on left of image (dorsal) with sparing of respiratory epithelium on the right. This pattern of epithelial destruction is indicative of a metabolically activated toxicant. Nasal septum, rat. (c) Vasculopathy with extensive subepithelial edema. Insert shows MSB positive material (fibrin) and neutrophil extravasation characteristic of this lesion. Inhaled PDE IV inhibitor, nasal cavity, dog.

dyspnea, and sudden death. Changes are typically restricted to animals given a test article. This is related to a variety of predisposing factors such as irritancy or viscosity of the test article formulation, pharmacology of the test article, or generalized poor clinical condition in treated animals leaving them more susceptible to reflux. Differentiating between pharmacologically driven changes and those due, for instance, to gavage procedure is essential to avoid misinterpretation of nasal cavity findings. Pharmacologically driven reflux will also be expected to occur following dosing of the test article by an alternative route (e.g., intravenous) at equivalent exposure levels. Strategies for reducing the incidence of reflux include reducing dose volume and viscosity and withholding food for several hours before dosing to allow at least partial emptying of the stomach (Damsch et al. 2011).

The pattern of findings in the nasal cavity may also give insight to the mechanism of toxicity. Local metabolism of xenobiotics can occur in the epithelial lining of the nasal cavity and in the Bowman's glands underlying the olfactory epithelium following both inhaled and systemic delivery (Harkema 1991). This is due to the presence of a wide variety of xenobiotic metabolizing enzymes, including P450 and non-P450 enzymes. The majority of this metabolic capacity resides in the respiratory and olfactory epithelia, and for most enzymes, activity is greatest in the olfactory epithelium, particularly within the sustentacular cells (Thornton-Manning and Dahl 1997). Interspecies variation in the content and activity of these enzymes exists within laboratory species; however, this is a poorly understood area. The significance of such variation is that it could be linked (via toxic metabolite formation) to pathology that is species specific and therefore not of relevance for human risk assessment. Local metabolism can also result in distinctive patterns of toxicity, such as destruction of the olfactory epithelium with relative sparing of other epithelia (Figure 11.1b). Examples of systemically delivered olfactory toxicants requiring local metabolic activation include acetaminophen (Genter et al. 1998), methimazole (Genter et al. 1995), and coumarin (Gu et al. 1997).

11.5.1 ATROPHY

Atrophy is characterized by thinning of the epithelium, with decreased cell number resulting in loss of specialized cells (e.g., goblet cells) and function (e.g., olfaction). Atrophy must be differentiated from degeneration, in which epithelial height is largely maintained, and metaplasia, which can cause thinning of the epithelium, but is due to a switch in epithelial type. Atrophy may also be associated with changes in the underlying turbinate bone, which can result in a grossly visible change in the shape of the turbinates.

A common consequence of olfactory epithelial atrophy is accompanying atrophy of the subjacent nerve bundles within the lamina propria. Olfactory cues are important in normal behavioral patterns, particularly in laboratory rodents, and thus, a subtle shift in behavior is a possible sequel to olfactory epithelial atrophy. It must be borne in mind that olfactory epithelial atrophy also occurs as a consequence of ageing, and this is most commonly noted in the dorsal meatus in rodents (Leininger et al. 1996). Atrophy of the olfactory epithelium in the mouse (preceded by apoptosis) occurred following intravenous administration of the antimicrotubule agents vincristine, vinblastine, vindesine, and paclitaxel (Jeffrey et al. 2006).

11.5.2 DEGENERATION

Degeneration is characterized primarily by loss of organization of the cell layers normally present in the epithelium, accompanied by changes such as deciliation, cytoplasmic blebbing, and increased intercellular spaces. The epithelial height is largely maintained, though individual cells may be lost, resulting in a vacuolated appearance, particularly in olfactory epithelium (Hardisty et al. 1999). Dilation of submucosal glands may also occur, with accumulation of secretory material. Physical damage during histological processing and early autolytic change can resemble epithelial degeneration.

11.5.3 NECROSIS

Mucosal necrosis is characterized by cytoplasmic eosinophilia, nuclear pyknosis/karryohexis, and cellular exfoliation. Necrosis triggers an inflammatory response, and continued exfoliation will result in erosion or ulceration of the mucosa. Repair can begin once the toxic insult is removed, but the outcome depends on the severity of the insult. All epithelium types lining the nasal cavity are capable of full repair; however, metaplasia or postnecrotic atrophy may be seen following chronic or severe injury. Regenerating surface epithelium may seal the excretory ducts of submucosal glands, blocking their outflow, leading to pressure atrophy, with hypertrophy of adjacent unaffected glands. Atrophy of the nerve bundles within the lamina propria often occurs following necrosis of olfactory epithelium. Another possible sequel to epithelial necrosis is turbinate fusion, resulting mainly from organization of the associated inflammatory exudate or from contact between denuded areas of basement membrane. Severe necrosis can extend through the submucosa to affect the underlying submucosal glands directly and the nasal septum/bone. Epithelial necrosis and suppurative inflammation were seen in the nasal cavity of rats following a 1-month inhalation study with the β-agonist tulbuterol hydrochloride (Dudley et al. 1989).

11.5.4 EOSINOPHILIC GLOBULES (INCLUSIONS, DROPLETS)

Bright eosinophilic, single or multiple globules may be seen in both the respiratory epithelium and the sustentacular cells of olfactory epithelium in rats and mice (Buckley et al. 1985). Ultrastructural examination reveals amorphous flocculent material in membrane-bound vacuoles. Eosinophilic inclusions may be seen in control animals, and their numbers increase with age (Leininger et al. 1996; St. Clair and Morgan 1992). They are considered a nonspecific response to mucosal irritation, and their significance is that they may be increased in response to a test article in chronic inhalation studies. The inclusions are considered to be cytoplasmic accumulation of protein(s) of the chitin-ase family; however, there is also evidence of carboxylesterase activity, implying a possible role in xenobiotic metabolism (Lewis et al. 1995). Similar inclusions are seen in the mouse lung (see Section 11.10.6).

11.5.5 EROSION/ULCERATION

Erosion or ulceration is a loss of epithelial continuity. Erosion does not extend through the basement membrane, while ulceration is a full-thickness defect, including the basement membrane. Erosion or ulceration that occurs in life will illicit an inflammatory response, and areas of degeneration/necrosis, or attempts at regeneration, may be seen at the margins or base of the defect. Exudation will occur in response to the loss of epithelial continuity, and this exudate, consisting of fibrin admixed with inflammatory cells, may be seen in the nasal cavity if it has not been removed during fixation. The main differential is artifactual loss of epithelium; hence, evidence of an inflammatory response or attempts at repair are useful in confirming that the change occurred during life.

11.5.6 REGENERATION

The process of epithelial repair, characterized by proliferation of undifferentiated basal cells and their subsequent organization and differentiation into a mature epithelium, is referred to as regeneration. Regeneration may return the epithelium to its original state or result in the appearance of a different epithelium type (metaplasia). Early (undifferentiated) regenerating cells are typically basophilic due to high nuclear/cytoplasm ratios and increased ribosomal content. In toxicity studies without off-dose/recovery periods, regeneration usually occurs in the face of continued epithelial damage, such that regeneration may be accompanied by other findings. The capacity for regeneration has been noted in all the types of epithelium lining the nasal cavity, including the olfactory epithelium (Farbman 1990). Whether olfactory epithelium regenerates or undergoes metaplasia/atrophy depends on the nature of the toxicant and the duration of exposure (Bergman et al. 2002). Regenerating olfactory epithelium may form rosette-like intraepithelial structures and may be mapped using GAP-43 IHC, a marker of immature neurons (Monticello et al. 1990; Bergman et al. 2002). Early regenerating epithelium appears flattened and squamoid and must be differentiated from true squamous metaplasia. Cytokeratin markers of epithelial differentiation can be used when differentiation by light microscopy is difficult (Schlage et al. 1998).

11.5.7 INFLAMMATION

A degree of background inflammation is common even in modern laboratory animal facilities and must be differentiated from test article–related change. The severity of background inflammation can be increased by high levels of ammonia in the environment, for example, as a result of infrequently changed bedding. Foreign bodies may also be a source of inflammation within the nasal cavity, though foreign bodies may be visible in section. A complication is that the incidence of foreign bodies may be increased in animals given a test article either due to a pharmacological effect on the airways or if the test article results in poor clinical condition and, therefore, a greater chance of inhaling foreign material.

Inflammation may be seen within the nasolacrimal ducts; this has been noted following inhalation exposure to a muscarinic agonist in the dog and was considered secondary to keratoconjunctivitis sicca.

11.5.7.1 Acute Inflammation (Inflammation, Neutrophilic)

Acute inflammation is characterized by a neutrophilic inflammatory cell infiltrate, local vascular congestion, edema within the lamina propria, and the variable presence of serous, fibrinous, or mucous exudates within the nasal cavity (Monticello et al. 1990). Involvement of the submucosal glands may lead to plugging of gland ducts by inflammatory cells, resulting in glandular dilatation.

11.5.7.2 Chronic Inflammation (Inflammation, Mononuclear/Lymphohistiocytic)

Chronic inflammation is characterized by the presence of a mononuclear inflammatory cell infiltrate with lymphocytes, macrophages, and plasma cells most commonly seen. Which cell predominates varies with the inciting agent. There is usually evidence of tissue necrosis and subsequent attempts at repair such as fibrosis, angiogenesis, or hyperplasia (Kumar et al. 2010).

11.5.7.3 Chronic Active Inflammation

Chronic active inflammation is used to describe a chronic inflammatory process where there is evidence of ongoing tissue damage (e.g., significant numbers of neutrophils, edema, and exudates are also variably present).

11.5.7.4 Granulomatous Inflammation

Granulomatous inflammation is a distinctive pattern of inflammation characterized by an accumulation of epithelioid macrophages (having abundant eosinophilic, often granular cytoplasm and indistinct cell boundaries), surrounded by a layer of mononuclear cells (predominantly lymphocytes and fewer plasma cells). Epithelioid macrophages may combine to form multinucleate giant cells (foreign body or Langhans type), and fibroplasia may be present, depending on the chronicity of the lesion. Granulomatous inflammation implies that the inciting agent is resistant to degradation (e.g., a foreign body) and is therefore uncommon as a test article–related change; however, a test article may alter the incidence of foreign bodies in the nasal cavities of treated animals.

11.5.8 Nasal Associated Lymphoid Tissue

Although there is considerable variation in the amount of nasal associated lymphoid tissue (NALT) visible in the nasal cavity of laboratory animals (depending both on the level of activity and section position), increased NALT cellularity is associated with chronic inflammatory change, and decreased cellularity is seen following inhalation exposure to inhaled corticosteroids (Cesta 2006).

11.5.9 Vascular Changes

Test article–related vascular changes in the nasal cavity are uncommon, unless related to an inflammatory process or severe debilitation. Administration of a Type IV phosphodiesterase inhibitor (PDE IV) to dogs either systemically (Hanton et al. 2008) or by inhalation produces an unusual vasculopathy, exclusively affecting venules subjacent to the respiratory epithelium. The lesion is characterized by a massive extravasation of neutrophils. The affected venules are often surrounded by a ring of Martius Scarlet Blue (MSB) positive fibrin (Figure 11.1c).

Animals killed in a moribund state may have angiectasis and thrombosis in the nasal cavity. Congestion may also be seen in animals killed in a moribund state due to pooling of blood in the peripheral tissues; however, this is generally a common finding in euthanized animals (Monticello et al. 1990). Hemorrhage in the nasal cavity/paranasal sinuses may be iatrogenic, indicating tissue damage during handling, or may be the result of an antemortem retro-orbital blood sample.

11.5.10 Hyperplasia

11.5.10.1 Epithelial (Squamous, Respiratory, Olfactory, Transitional)

Morphologically, simple hyperplasia represents an increase in the number of cells in a normal arrangement within any particular tissue. This results in hyperplastic epithelium having a thickened appearance. Minor changes must be interpreted with caution, as the height of a healthy epithelium varies with position in the nasal cavity, and tangential sections can also produce a thickened appearance. Hyperplastic change may be primary (i.e., directly related to the test article) or, the more common, secondary (regenerative) hyperplasia that occurs as part of the process of epithelial repair. This distinction is important in terms of human risk assessment, as a primary hyperplastic response may be relevant to a "weight of evidence" approach to carcinogenicity assessment, while this is generally not considered to be the case for secondary hyperplasia (Eustis 1989). This is because human exposure can be kept below a level that causes cytotoxicity and the associated secondary hyperplasia that goes with it. A confounding factor in the assessment of hyperplasia is the presence of cellular atypia or dysplasia within foci of hyperplasia (Boorman et al. 2003). Epithelial hyperplasia has also been reported as an age-related change in the mouse (Leininger et al. 1996).

11.5.10.2 Goblet (Mucous) Cell Hyperplasia

Goblet cell hyperplasia is considered to be an adaptive response to epithelial irritation via the production and release of increased amounts of protective mucosubstances. Hyperplastic goblet cells may form clusters within the epithelium; this has been referred to as a pseudoglandular pattern and is shown in Figure 11.2a (Gopinath et al. 1987).

11.5.10.3 Basal Cell Hyperplasia

Basal cell hyperplasia is usually focal/multifocal in distribution and represents a proliferation of the basal cell layer, often causing elevation of the overlying epithelium (Figure 11.2b). This finding often precedes metaplastic change in response to a mucosal irritant, and the overlying epithelium may be partially sloughed. Basal cell hyperplasia must be differentiated from neoplastic change. Although a small increase in mitoses may be seen with basal cell hyperplasia, cellular atypia/loss of

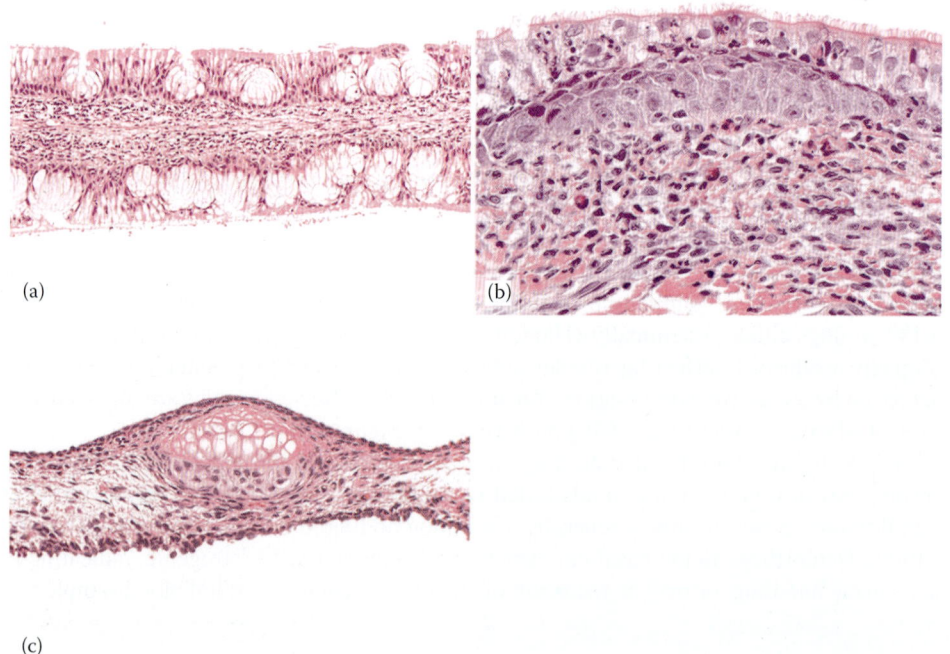

(a)

(b)

(c)

FIGURE 11.2 (a) Goblet cell hyperplasia, pseudoglandular pattern. Nasal cavity, rat. (b) Basal cell hyperplasia with early squamous metaplasia resulting in elevation of the original respiratory epithelium. Nasal cavity, rat. (c) Necrosis of the U-shaped cartilage at the level of the ventral pouch. Note cartilage regeneration ventral to the necrotic original. Larynx, rat.

polarity and other changes typical of neoplastic growth are absent. Basal cell hyperplasia affecting the olfactory epithelium of rats was seen with a PDE-IV inhibitor (Pino et al. 1999).

11.5.11 METAPLASIA

Metaplasia is the replacement of one mature type of epithelium with another. In practice, this usually means replacement with a more robust epithelium better able to resist environmental/xenobiotic challenge. Common examples in the nasal cavity include respiratory metaplasia of olfactory epithelium and squamous metaplasia of any other epithelial type. Metaplasia may be reversible depending on the nature of the inciting agent and the duration of exposure. It can be difficult to differentiate squamous metaplasia from early regenerating epithelium; however, keratinization is found only with squamous metaplasia (Brown et al. 1991). Respiratory metaplasia of olfactory epithelium has been reported as an age-related change in rats (Monticello et al. 1990).

11.6 NEOPLASTIC NASAL CAVITY CHANGES

Based on rodent carcinogenicity data, spontaneous and induced tumors of the nasal cavities are rare. The background incidence of spontaneous neoplasia in control animals is typically less than 0.4% (Chandra and Frith 1992; Maita et al. 1988; Haseman et al. 1990, 1998). A National Toxicology Program survey of 500 rodent carcinogenicity studies identified only 12 chemicals that produced nasal tumors, none of which were pharmaceuticals (Haseman and Hailey 1997). In general, rats appear more sensitive than mice to nasal carcinogens, and nasal carcinogenesis may also occur in noninhalation studies. The majority of both spontaneous and chemically induced nasal tumors are epithelial in origin (Kasahara et al. 2008; Haseman and Hailey 1997). Mesenchymal tumors, though rare in both species, are relatively more common in mice (Brown et al. 1991). Data for other laboratory species are lacking primarily due to the few chronic studies that have been conducted; however, what data exist suggests that nasal tumors in dogs and monkeys are also rare (Wilson and Dungworth 2002; Kaspareit et al. 2007). The majority of rodent nasal carcinogens are genotoxic; however, the association of nasal carcinogenesis with local cytotoxicity is less clear. Although many nasal carcinogens also cause nasal cytotoxicity, some do not, and many chemicals that produce cytotoxicity in the nasal cavity do not produce tumors there, even following chronic exposure (Ward et al. 1993; Haseman and Hailey 1997; Jeffrey et al. 2006). The importance of metabolism is emphasized by the aromatic amine 2,6-xylidine, which produces both benign and malignant nasal cavity tumors in the rat. This chemical is a metabolite of the local anesthetics lidocaine and prilocaine, implying that these compounds are potential rat carcinogens, particularly as both have been shown to be capable of producing DNA adducts in rat nasal mucosa (Duan et al. 2008).

Human nasal tumors are also rare (Bhattacharyya 2002), and identification of a rodent-only nasal carcinogen does not necessarily imply an equivalent human hazard. One reason for this is that the clinical doses given to humans do not usually cause cytotoxicity, and a second is evidence that human nasal cavity epithelium has less xenobiotic metabolizing capability than that of rodents (Jeffrey et al. 2006).

11.6.1 SQUAMOUS CELL PAPILLOMA

Squamous cell papillomas arise from the stratified squamous epithelium of the anterior nasal cavity or from the metaplastic squamous epithelium in other regions of the nasal cavity (Herbert and Leininger 1999). These masses are usually exophytic and are characterized by well-differentiated squamous epithelium, often highly keratinized, overlying a branching fibrovascular stalk. The basement membrane remains intact, and there are no cytological signs of malignancy, which allows differentiation from squamous cell carcinoma. Endophytic/"inverted" papillomas are less common and should not be confused with squamous metaplasia of the submucosal glands. Unlike papillomas, squamous cell hyperplasia and metaplasia are usually bilateral and/or multifocal. By TEM, typical features include desmosomes, tonofilaments, and, in some cases, keratohyalin granules (Brown et al. 1991).

11.6.2 Adenoma

Adenoma may arise from respiratory, transitional, or submucosal glandular epithelium. Differentiation of cell of origin is likely to be difficult and is not usually recorded. Cell morphology varies with epithelial origin, but commonly, cells are cuboidal to low columnar and are not ciliated. Cytoplasmic eosinophilic globules are often seen (Renne et al. 2009). Cells may be arranged in sheets, but pseudo-acinar and glandular formation is also typical. When glandular structures are present, these frequently contain Periodic acid-Schiff (PAS) positive mucosubstances and inflammatory and degenerate cells within their lumina and may be cystic. Adenomas are usually exophytic (polypoid). Differentials include adenocarcinoma, which may be excluded on the basis of a lack of cytological evidence of malignancy, intact basement membrane, and lack of invasion. Hyperplastic epithelium within the nasal cavity/sinuses is usually multifocal and bilateral and does not typically form the exophytic, nodular mass associated with adenoma. Spontaneous nasal cavity adenomas are rare but are reported to be more common in mice than rats (Brown et al. 1991). A spontaneous nasal cavity adenoma has also been reported in a 4-year old cynomolgus monkey (Kaspareit et al. 2007). Test article–related Bowman's gland adenoma was reported following an inhalation carcinogenicity study with a PDE-IV inhibitor in the rat (Pino et al. 1999).

11.6.3 Squamous Cell Carcinoma

Squamous cell carcinoma is most frequently seen in the anterior nasal cavity, where it originates from preexisting, stratified squamous epithelium. It can also be found in other nasal cavity locations and in the paranasal sinuses, resulting from malignant transformation of local metaplastic squamous epithelium. Neoplastic cells are frequently arranged in branching cords and may exhibit areas of anaplasia. Intercellular bridges are seen, though they may be few in number in poorly differentiated tumors (Renne et al. 2009). Keratin production is variable, and although classic "keratin pearls" occur, keratinization may be restricted to cytoplasmic keratohyalin granules or may be absent. The main differentials are adenocarcinoma with squamous metaplasia and adenosquamous carcinoma. In the former case, areas of squamous metaplasia are generally minor and well differentiated. In the latter, entrapped glandular elements within a squamous cell carcinoma can be confusing; however, in squamous cell carcinoma, only the squamous elements are neoplastic. Some poorly differentiated squamous cell carcinomas can also assume a spindloid form, which may be difficult to differentiate from sarcoma (Brown et al. 1991). IHC for cytokeratins, or TEM for tonofilaments, may be required to reach a definitive diagnosis. Nasal squamous cell carcinoma has been recorded following an oral (dietary) carcinogenicity study with phenacetin related to local bioactivation (Isaka et al. 1979; Jeffrey et al. 2006).

11.6.4 Adenocarcinoma

Nasal cavity adenocarcinomas frequently arise from respiratory epithelium (Brown et al. 1991) and also from transitional or glandular epithelium, Bowman's glands, or the epithelium of the paranasal sinuses. Cells may retain a columnar appearance or be irregular or anaplastic. Cellular patterns vary; only well-differentiated adenocarcinomas are likely to produce prominent glandular or cystic structures lined by typical secretory cells. Where glandular structures are seen, the lumina are likely to be filled by mucosubstances. Penetration of the basement membrane provides clear evidence of malignancy. Some adenocarcinomas may contain regions of squamous metaplasia. In these tumors, the squamous regions tend to be well differentiated and appear benign; this is used to differentiate from adenosquamous carcinoma that has both squamous and glandular neoplastic elements. Tumors arising from Bowman's glands must be differentiated from neuro-epithelial carcinoma by demonstration of neural elements or rosette formation in the latter. Test article–related nasal adenocarcinomas have been reported in the Bowman's gland following an inhalation carcinogenicity study with a PDE-IV inhibitor (Pino et al. 1999) and following an oral (dietary) carcinogenicity study with phenacetin (Isaka et al. 1979), both in the Sprague–Dawley rat.

11.6.5 ADENOSQUAMOUS CARCINOMA

Adenosquamous carcinomas contain both glandular and squamous neoplastic elements. There must be clear cytological evidence of malignancy in both tissue compartments to allow this diagnosis and to differentiate from squamous carcinomas, which entrap non-neoplastic glandular elements, and adenocarcinomas that have regions of well-differentiated squamous metaplasia.

11.6.6 NEUROEPITHELIAL CARCINOMA (OLFACTORY NEUROBLASTOMA)

Neuroepithelial carcinoma is a general term for malignant tumors arising within the olfactory epi-thelium and includes several possible cells of origin such as sustentacular cells, sensory cells, and basal cells (Renne et al. 2009). The neoplastic cells are round to columnar in appearance, with scant cytoplasm and round to oval, often hyperchromatic nuclei. True rosettes and/or pseudoro-settes are typically seen; however, tumors often have anaplastic areas. Tumor cells are frequently compartmentalized by a scant, fibrovascular stroma, and an intercellular plexiform, fibrillar matrix is often seen. Diagnosis may be confirmed by TEM for ultrastructural features typical of olfactory epithelium (e.g., olfactory vesicles and microvilli). IHC findings vary, but positive results have been reported for β III-tubulin and neurofilament 120/200 (Takagi et al. 2010). The main differential is adenocarcinoma; the glandular structures that may occur within adenocarcinomas must be dif-ferentiated from true rosettes, and adenocarcinomas do not form plexiform, intercellular fibrils. Test article–related neuroepithelial carcinoma was reported following an inhalation carcinogenicity study with a PDE-IV inhibitor in the rat (Pino et al. 1999) and following intraperitoneal administra-tion of procarbazine in rats and mice (Jeffrey et al. 2006).

11.7 LARYNX, TRACHEA, AND BRONCHI

The larynx is lined by stratified squamous, respiratory, and transitional epithelium. The vary-ing resistance of these epithelial types to damage, coupled with the effects of airflow and the anatomical features of the larynx, leads to some epithelial regions being particularly sensitive to damage in inhalation studies. Precise, consistent sections are therefore required for an adequate histological assessment. Standard sampling guidelines for the rodent larynx are available to aid processing (Kittel et al. 2004). Predilection sites for induced laryngeal changes in rodents are as follows.

1. *The base of the epiglottis.* The base of the epiglottis is the region most sensitive to squa-mous metaplasia in rodents. In rats, it is lined by a mix of columnar, cuboidal, and oval to flattened cells with few ciliated cells present (Renne et al. 1992). Taste buds may be seen, and focal squamous metaplasia is a normal variant (Kaufmann et al. 2009). In mice and hamsters, the epithelium is typically taller than that seen in rats, and in the hamster, more ciliated cells are present (Renne et al. 1992, 1993). In rats and mice, the seromucous glands beneath the epithelium in the ventral midline are a consistent point of reference, allowing identification of the base of the epiglottis (Renne et al. 1992). In hamsters, however, the seromucous glands extend cranially beneath the stratified squamous epithelium and cannot

be used in this way (Renne et al. 1993). The openings of the ducts of the ventral submucosal glands are sometimes included in sections cut at this level and are typically surrounded by a patch of ciliated epithelium.

2. *Inner aspect of the vocal processes of the arytenoid cartilages.* The medial surfaces of the vocal processes are lined by squamous epithelium. In rodents, this is low ventrally (two to three cells thick) and unkeratinized and becomes slightly thicker and keratinized dorsally. The degree of keratinization decreases caudally through the vocal processes.

3. *The ventral pouch region.* The epithelium found lining the ventral pouch in the rat consists of round to cuboidal cells, two to four layers thick, but this is variable and affected by distension of the pouch. This is similar to the hamster; however, in mice, more ciliated cells are seen, particularly ventrally. The pouch is supported by a U-shaped cartilage, the wings or base of which are also visible at this level. The epithelium overlying the wings is squamoid and typically one to two cells thick. The base of the cartilage varies in prominence, with hamsters > rats > mice, such that the overlying epithelium in this position is particularly sensitive in hamsters (Renne et al. 1992, 1993). In addition, the epithelium in the ventrolateral region of the larynx wall, adjacent and anterior to the ventral pouch, is another area where induced changes are commonly seen (Gopinath et al. 1987).

In nonrodents, laryngeal stratified squamous epithelium is thicker and extends further caudally; for example, the epiglottal epithelium of the beagle dog is stratified squamous throughout and is approximately seven layers thick. As a result of this, an induced change is likely to be seen more caudally in nonrodents than in rodents. In beagle dogs and nonhuman primates, the transition from stratified squamous to respiratory epithelium occurs at the level of the vocal processes of the arytenoid cartilages. This area is located just caudal to the junction of the lateral ventricles with the laryngeal lumen (can be used as a sectioning landmark) and should be examined routinely (Renne and Gideon 2006).

Laryngeal irritants typically produce a spectrum of changes, including degeneration, necrosis, ulceration and accompanying inflammation, edema, and fibrosis. Attempts at repair can include epithelial regeneration, hyperplasia, squamous metaplasia, and hyperkeratosis. Under normal circumstances, minor lymphoid aggregates are seen in the submucosa at all laryngeal levels. These are not recorded unless the extent exceeds the background level or a shift in cell type (e.g., neutrophilia) is present. The majority of the information on induced laryngeal change is based on rodent inhalation studies, reflecting both the greater number of studies conducted in rodents and the relative susceptibility of the rodent larynx to induced change. The Fischer 344 rat is particularly predisposed to laryngeal cartilage degeneration/mineralization and laryngeal inflammatory change. These changes are aggravated by gavage dosing, and this can have an effect on mortality in chronic studies, particularly in females (Germann et al. 1998).

The tracheal bifurcation is the region of the trachea most sensitive to inhaled irritants due to particle impaction at this level. For this reason, a longitudinal horizontal section, including the carina, is recommended for inhalation studies (Kittel et al. 2004). Similarly, airway bifurcations are typical sites for induced change in inhalation studies. Severe changes may also be seen in the larynx/airways in response to misdosing the upper respiratory tract on an oral gavage study. Gavage accidents can result in the death of the animal or may cause stertor, nasal discharge/hemorrhage, and subcutaneous edema. Subsequent inhalation of test article intended for gavage will lead to inflammation in the lung. The Fischer 344 rat is predisposed to degeneration of tracheal cartilage, which has been seen in animals from 6 weeks of age (Germann et al. 1995).

11.7.1 Epithelial Degeneration and Regeneration of Larynx and Airways

Epithelial degeneration is a common and often subtle response to low-grade irritancy. The minimal degenerative change seen by light microscopy is epithelial deciliation. This is particularly difficult to detect in areas of transitional epithelium, as these are normally only sparsely ciliated. Other degenerative changes include cytoplasmic blebbing, vacuolation, and pyknotic appearing nuclei. A decrease in the number of globule leukocytes in the epithelium may also be a part of the spectrum of degenerative change (Lewis 1991). Degeneration and regeneration often occur together in repeat dose studies within the larynx and airways and are as previously described for the nasal cavity.

11.7.2 Necrosis

Mucosal necrosis is characterized by cytoplasmic eosinophilia, nuclear pyknosis/karyorrhexis, and cellular exfoliation. Severe necrosis can extend into the submucosal tissues and can be accompanied by sufficient inflammatory exudate to block the airways and cause death. The underlying cartilage may also be affected. This is most commonly seen in the U-shaped cartilage, which supports the entrance to the ventral pouch in rodents, presumably due to its superficial location. Necrotic cartilage may also be noted after epithelial repair has been completed, and with sufficient recovery time, attempts at cartilage repair may also occur, usually ventral to the original necrotic cartilage (Lewis 1991) (Figure 11.2c). Procedure-related necrosis and sloughing of tracheal epithelium are a common finding in studies using intratracheal dosing, and subepithelial fibrosis may be seen as part of the process of repair.

11.7.3 Erosion/Ulceration

Erosion or ulceration is a loss of epithelial continuity. Erosion does not extend through the basement membrane, whereas ulceration is a full-thickness defect including the basement membrane. A serofibrinous or suppurative exudate usually accompanies erosion or ulceration, and submucosal inflammatory cell infiltration and edema are also usually seen. Procedure-related erosion or ulceration may be associated with misdosing on a gavage study or poor intratracheal dosing technique. In addition, the tracheal epithelium of rodents in particular is easily removed during processing, making this a common site for artifactual epithelial loss.

11.7.4 Ectasia of Submucosal Glands

Ectasia of the submucosal glands usually occurs secondary to blockage of the ducts, usually as the result of an inflammatory process, or during metaplastic repair of the surface epithelium (Lewis 1991). Back pressure then leads to gland ectasia, which may progress to atrophy.

11.7.5 Inflammation

The histological appearance of the various forms of airway inflammation is as previously described for the nasal cavity. In cases of severe airway inflammation, exudate formation can be extensive enough to block the airway lumen, particularly at the larynx. A common site for granulomatous inflammation in the airways is the laryngeal ventral pouch in rodents, as foreign material (typically fur) frequently becomes lodged there (Weber et al. 2009). Airway inflammation may also have an infectious origin, following inhalation of high doses of immunosuppressive compounds such as corticosteroids (Ullmann et al. 2007; Duong et al. 1998).

11.7.6 Hyperplasia

Common types of epithelial hyperplasia seen in the larynx and airways include squamous hyperplasia of the anterior larynx (which may include a degree of hyperkeratosis) and goblet cell hyperplasia within the respiratory epithelium of the trachea and airways. The term *squamous hyperplasia* should be restricted to areas of preexisting squamous epithelium. Goblet cell hyperplasia of the airways is part of the spectrum of changes seen with subacute and chronic inflammation. There is some debate about the relative contribution that metaplasia makes to the increased goblet cell numbers seen in inflamed airways, and some pathologists use the term *goblet cell metaplasia* synonymously with *goblet cell hyperplasia* (Curran and Cohn 2010). In severe cases, goblet cells may appear to occupy the entire epithelial surface. Goblet cell hypersecretion can be induced by systemic administration of isoprenaline and pilocarpine to rats (Sturgess and Reid 1973).

In addition to altering the amount of mucus produced, exposure to an irritant material or infection can also result in an alteration in the type of mucus synthesized and secreted, usually to a more acidic form. This may be confirmed by AB/PAS histochemistry, can also cause a subtle increase in basophilia in the affected cells, and is visible by H&E staining. This shift can also be induced by epidermal growth factor (EGF) and transforming growth factor-α (TGF-α) (Takeyama et al. 1999).

Although PNECs normally have a low rate of turnover (Fehrenbach et al. 2002), they may proliferate with hyperoxia (in weanling rats) (Shenberger et al. 1997) and in infant nonhuman primates following maternal dexamethasone (Dayer et al. 1985). Diagnosis of hyperplasia of these NEBs can be difficult due to plane of section, and a threshold of ≥ 40 nuclei has been suggested for this diagnosis (Haworth et al. 2007).

Respiratory epithelial hyperplasia is uncommon in the larynx and airways of laboratory animals.

11.7.7 Squamous Metaplasia

Squamous metaplasia may be focal or diffuse and may affect the surface epithelium and/or the ductal epithelium of submucosal glands. This change is most commonly seen in the rodent larynx, where it is characterized by the presence of at least three to four layers of flattened stratified epithelium, and can occur within 3 days of test article exposure (Lewis 1991; Kaufmann et al. 2009). Increased severity is indicated by increasing number of cell layers, degree of keratinization, and presence of desquamation. An example grade and description guide for squamous metaplasia in the rodent larynx is presented in a recent review (Kaufmann et al. 2009). Marked focal change can be seen as a spontaneous finding in ageing animals. Laryngeal squamous metaplasia is considered a nonadverse, adaptive response to irritation that typically does not progress and will recover given a suitable off-dose period (Renne and Gideon 2006). It is, therefore, not considered to be a precancerous lesion; however, the risk assessment changes if cellular atypia or dysplasia is also present. Another factor relevant for risk assessment is the susceptibility of the rat larynx to squamous metaplasia, given the large number of inhalation studies conducted using this species. The incidence of this change in rats is higher than in humans, primates, or dogs. This is likely to be related to the presence of sensitive epithelia in regions of high particle deposition in the rat larynx (Lewis 1981; Renne and Gideon 2006).

Squamous metaplasia in the trachea can also develop in dogs subjected to dry air challenge, due to desiccation and hyperventilation (Davis et al. 2003), and can be modeled in rats fed with a vitamin A–deficient diet (Renne et al. 2009).

Squamous metaplasia may be seen at the sensitive bronchioloalveolar junction or in the alveolar region and is characterized by foci of squamous epithelium lining the airway walls. The lesion may show keratinization, and may develop into cysts (Sells et al. 2007; Renne et al. 2009), and is generally seen only in rats.

11.8 BRONCHIOLES

Histological changes in bronchiolar epithelial cells can range from obvious necrosis to subtle alteration in cell size and shape, particularly in regard to the presence and prominence of the apical dome of the Clara cell. Assessment of the latter is aided by IHC demonstration of proteins such as CC10.

11.8.1 CLARA CELL CHANGES

11.8.1.1 Clara Cell Hypertrophy

Inhaled corticosteroids have been shown to cause hypertrophy of mouse Clara cells (Roth et al. 2007) and increased expression of CC10 (Hagen et al. 1990; Fengming et al. 2002; Roth et al. 2007). Intraperitoneal administration of isoprenaline to mice increased Clara cell secretion and the size of the apical cap (Aryal et al. 2003). Proliferation of smooth endoplasmic reticulum (SER) may also cause Clara cell hypertrophy, and this has been reported in mice given phenobarbital (Kitamura et al. 1987).

11.8.1.2 Clara Cell Inclusions

Kambara et al. (2009) found increased numbers of eosinophilic inclusions in rat Clara cells exposed to an inhaled corticosteroid. These cytoplasmic inclusions were large, homogenous, membrane bound, and positive by IHC for SP-D.

11.8.1.3 Clara Cell Degeneration/Necrosis

Most chemicals do not cause Clara cell toxicity directly (Delaunois 2004), but as these cells contain the enzyme systems necessary to metabolize xenobiotics, indirect toxicity involving bioactivation can occur. A diverse group of chemicals induce Clara cell necrosis in mice via metabolic activation by cytochrome P450 (Kehrer and Kacew 1985; Born et al. 1998). Species differences in metabolic activity are known to exist (Baldwin et al. 2004); hence, findings in one species will not necessarily translate to another, with implications for human risk assessment.

11.8.1.4 Mucous Cell Metaplasia

Mucous cell metaplasia is characterized by the presence of typical goblet cells in the terminal or respiratory bronchioles, usually to the exclusion of the resident Clara cells.

In recent years, Clara cells have become recognized as a major mucin-secreting cell, a role masked by the absence of any appreciable numbers of mucin granules (Davis and Dickey 2008). It is now established that under normal conditions, the rate of mucin synthesis is in balance with the rate of secretion, with little storage; however, a shift to a typical mucous cell phenotype can occur following irritant exposure (Davis and Dickey 2008).

11.8.1.5 Clara Cell Proliferation

Clara cells are the progenitor cell of the terminal and respiratory bronchioles, and following epithelial damage, they are able to both self-renew and give rise to ciliated cells. Keratinocyte growth factor is a potent Clara cell mitogen in rats (Fehrenbach et al. 2002).

11.8.1.6 Clara Cell Phospholipidosis

The involvement of Clara cells in phospholipidosis (PLO) is likely underestimated as, although vacuolation can be seen by light microscopy, detection/confirmation requires ultrastructural examination. Clara cell PLO has been reported with the hypocholesteremic drug, AY-9944 (Kikkawa and Suzuki 1972), and has been seen with chloroquine and amodiaquine.

11.8.1.7 Clara Cell Lipid Vacuolation

In dogs, an age-related Clara cell lipid vacuolation has been briefly described (Grebenskaya 1966). In some dog studies with novel inhaled corticosteroids, an increased incidence of focal Clara cell lipid vacuolation may be seen in some respiratory bronchioles. These vacuoles, which fill the Clara cell cytoplasm, are usually associated with foamy (lipid laden) macrophage aggregations and a similar vacuolation in ATII cells in immediately adjacent alveoli. The lesion can be difficult to detect with routine H&E staining, as the cells are usually closely associated with foamy macrophages, and the vacuoles are similar in appearance, at low power, to leached formalin-fixed glycogen, normally abundant in dog Clara cells. Confirmation of the diagnosis is readily achieved by adipophilin immunohistochemistry or oil red O (ORO) histochemistry. In longer duration studies, this form of Clara cell vacuolation may be associated with the development of small bronchioliths (see Section 11.8.2). The most likely explanation for the presence of this neutral lipid is that corticosteroids enhance fatty acid synthesis in nonadipose tissues (Batenburg and Haagsman 1998; Beneke and Rooney 2001; Kooistra and Galac 2010). However, other mechanisms that have been considered include eicosanoid synthesis driven by corticosteroid exposure (Dvorak et al. 1992; Ochs et al. 2004; Bozza et al. 2009), upregulation of free fatty acid (FFA) synthesis in response to the presence of infectious agents (Coonrod et al. 1984), or a switch from glyconeogenesis to lipogenesis (Floetmann et al. 2010).

11.8.2 BRONCHIOLAR MICROLITHIASIS

Inhaled corticosteroids in dogs induce Clara cell lipid vacuolation that can subsequently become associated with the development of small microliths (Figure 11.3a). Although these basophilic, calcified bodies appear to arise within the epithelium and project into the bronchiolar lumina, ultrastructural and IHC investigations show that they actually arise from thickened and folded areas of the basement membrane, subjacent to the vacuolated Clara cells. Although their etiology is

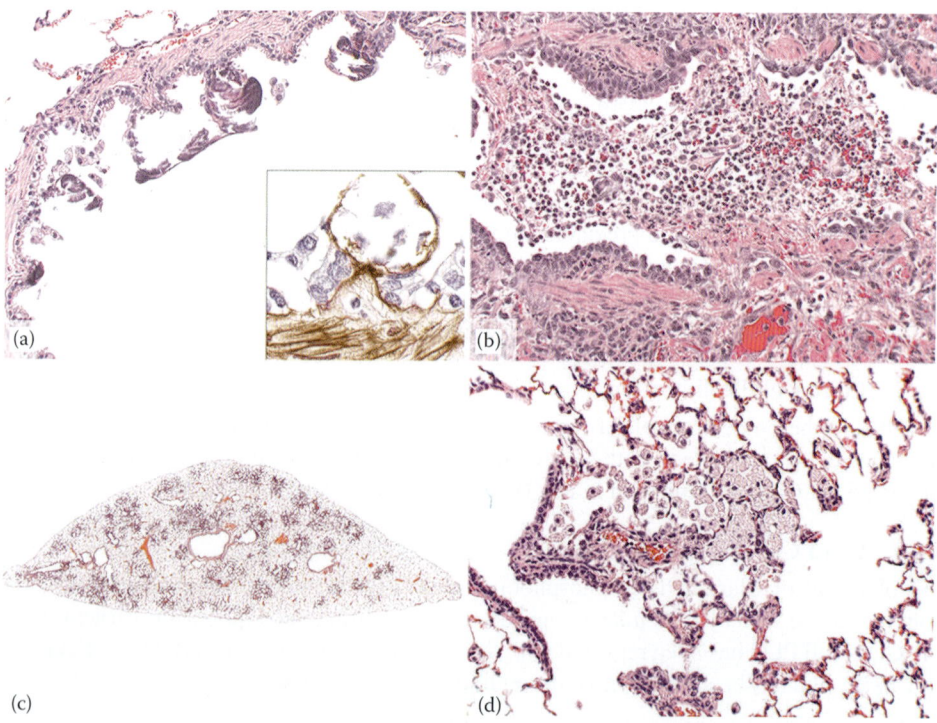

FIGURE 11.3 (a) Bronchiolar microlith formation. Insert shows positive IHC for laminin surrounding a microlith, indicating that these form within the airway epithelial basement membrane. Inhaled corticosteroid, bronchiole, dog. (b) BO following severe damage to the airway and characterized by early organization/fibrosis of inflammatory exudates. Bronchiole, dog. (c) Severe macrophage aggregation, centered on the bronchiolar–alveolar duct region and visible to the naked eye in this histological section. Distribution is typical of an inhaled lung challenge. Dog. (d) Foamy appearance of macrophage cytoplasm characteristic of macrophage aggregation secondary to an inhaled challenge to the lung. Note location at bronchiolar–alveolar duct region. Left lung lobe, rat.

uncertain, as they arise in connective tissue, it is possible that they represent a localized form of Cushingoid-type interstitial mineralization (Capen et al. 1975; Berry et al. 1994; Blois et al. 2009).

11.8.3 Airway Wall Remodeling

The term *airway wall remodeling* has become widely used to encompass the array of persistent structural changes that can occur consequent to inflammation, injury, and aberrant repair, which occur at this site in human asthma and chronic obstructive pulmonary disease (COPD) patients (Shinagawa and Kojima 2003; Ramos- Barbón et al. 2004). These changes include acute and chronic inflammation, epithelial shedding, basement membrane thickening, increased vascular cross-sectional area, airway smooth muscle hypertrophy and hyperplasia, mucous gland and goblet cell hyperplasia, squamous metaplasia, and increased collagen deposition. Most of these features are reasonably well developed in mouse models (Shinagawa and Kojima 2003) and may be reproduced by irritant compounds. The origins of asthma are now believed to lie in the epithelial mesenchymal trophic unit. Squamous metaplastic cells induce subjacent fibroblasts to secrete TGF-β and Il-1β (Araya et al. 2007; Bolton et al. 2009). Thus, although epithelial squamous metaplasia in laboratory species is generally considered an adaptive or protective change, it can have important pathologic consequences (Araya et al. 2007; Bolton et al. 2009).

11.8.4 Bronchiolitis Obliterans

Bronchiolitis obliterans (BO) develops following initial damage to the bronchiolar respiratory epithelium and is characterized by exudation and inflammation (Figure 11.3b), followed by organization, fibrosis, and gradual development of pendulous, polypoid lesions within the airway lumina. The development of these lesions is accompanied by epithelial regeneration, which extends over the new tissue, sometimes with evidence of recanalization (Gopinath et al. 1987). The lesions show focal attachments to the original bronchiolar walls.

BO is occasionally seen in dogs following inhalation of corticosteroids, muscarinic antagonists, and PDE-IV inhibitors. This is related to pathogen exposure secondary to immunosuppression, gastric reflux, and arteriopathy, respectively. BO has also been reported following accidental misdosing during oral gavage of oleic acid in dogs (Li et al. 2006).

11.8.5 Bronchiolization

The epithelial lining at the junction between the terminal airway and the alveolar duct is a prime site for induced metaplasia in inhalation studies (Renne et al. 2009), and the replacement epithelium, which is usually associated with a macrophage reaction (Renne et al. 2009), is characterized by the predominant presence of one of three cell types: Clara, ciliated, or rarely, mucus. This process represents a peripheral or lateral (Nettesheim and Szakal 1972) extension of bronchiolar epithelium; however, the factors determining which cell type predominates in the extended epithelium are unknown. The proliferation of Clara cells may reflect a need for xenobiotic metabolic capacity, while ciliated and mucous cell proliferation may allow an extension of the mucociliary escalator into the damaged area (Gopinath et al. 1987).

11.8.6 Neoplastic Changes in Larynx and Trachea and Airways

11.8.6.1 Papilloma

Papillomas in the larynx and airways may originate from squamous or respiratory epithelium. They are most commonly exophytic and are supported by a central connective tissue stalk. The surface epithelium may be hyperplastic, but cellular atypia is not a feature; furthermore, mitotic figures tend to be rare and limited to the basal epithelial layers. Papillomas must be differentiated from exophytic squamous cell carcinomas and adenocarcinomas. Invasion of the stalk by neoplastic cells is a clear sign of malignancy; however, care must be taken as a plane of the section can sometimes give a misleading impression of invasion.

11.8.6.2 Squamous Cell Carcinoma

Squamous cell carcinoma in this region may originate from a preexisting stratified squamous epithelium or from a metaplastic respiratory epithelium. Neoplastic cells can be irregular rather than squamous, and giant cells are rarely seen (Dungworth et al. 2001). Intercellular bridges are a common finding, and if keratinization occurs, it is often seen in the midst of irregular clusters of neoplastic cells (keratin pearls). Dysplastic/anaplastic areas may be seen, and invasion of the basement membrane is a clear sign of malignancy, allowing differentiation from a florid or inflamed squamous cell papilloma. Where basement membrane invasion occurs, there is often a scirrhous response. Adenocarcinomas may be differentiated by their lack of clear intercellular bridges or significant keratin production.

11.8.6.3 Adenocarcinoma

Adenocarcinomas of the airways arise from malignant transformation of the respiratory epithelium. They may contain areas of mucinous differentiation or irregular glandular structures. Invasion of the basement membrane is a clear sign of malignancy and can be used to differentiate a well-differentiated carcinoma from a papilloma. Cytological features of malignancy are also likely to be present in adenocarcinomas. These are rare tumors and must be clearly differentiated from alveolar/bronchiolar tumors that have invaded the airways.

11.9 LUNG PARENCHYMA

11.9.1 MACROPHAGE REACTIONS

As AMs not only remove foreign agents from the lung but also inhaled soluble pharmaceuticals (by pinocytosis) and relatively poorly soluble drugs (by phagocytosis), macrophage reactions are the most common findings seen in preclinical studies with inhaled pharmaceuticals (Gopinath et al. 1987). Interpretation of a marginal increase in macrophage findings in a treated group may be difficult, particularly if group sizes are small due to the variable nature of background changes seen in these cells. The interpretation is actually easier in inhalation studies, where almost inevitably, the "test article–related" macrophage reactions are localized in and around the alveolar ducts of rats and mice or the respiratory bronchioles and their evaginating alveoli (Lambert's canals) in dogs (Figure 11.3c), whereas spontaneous aggregates tend to be randomly dispersed.

Macrophage reactions may display a continuum from a simple minor increase in the numbers of diffuse macrophages, through various degrees of hypertrophy, to more solid aggregations, colocalization with hypertrophy/hyperplasia of ATIIs of the adjacent alveolar walls, association with infiltrations of neutrophils or lymphocytes, cholesterol cleft granulomas, and full granulomatous inflammation or fibrosis (Dungworth et al. 1992). There is some evidence that adhesion molecules may be involved in the development and persistence of macrophage aggregates (Sasaki et al. 2001; Brown et al. 1993).

AMs are capable of contributing to a wide range of often opposing outcomes following a challenge to the lung; they may be immunogenic or tolerogenic, proinflammatory or anti-inflammatory, and tissue destructive or tissue reparative (Stout et al. 2005).

11.9.2 FOAMY MACROPHAGE REACTIONS

There are several possible etiologies of the commonly reported foamy appearance of macrophage cytoplasm. In their simplest form, these macrophages are hypertrophic, and the foamy cytoplasmic appearance (Figure 11.3d) is usually ascribed to the predominant presence of either lysosomal lamellar bodies (LLBs) (phospholipids-surfactant) or neutral lipid (Figure 11.4a). In some studies, excessive salivation may lead to accidental inhalation of saliva and result in foamy macrophage accumulations in and around terminal airways (Gopinath et al. 1987), and laryngeal paralysis or laryngospasm, known to occur with barbiturates, increases the incidence of saliva inhalation (Gopinath et al. 1987). Diets with a high fat content can also result in foamy AMs in rats (Flodh and Magnussen 1973). Compounds contained in liposomal delivery vehicles are also phagocytosed by macrophages (Chono et al. 2006, 2008), resulting in a foamy appearance (Myers et al. 1993). In addition, misdosing on oral gavage studies can result in accidental pulmonary exposure to drug formulations and vehicles, such as methylcellulose, which can give rise to foamy macrophages (among other lesions). Inhaled antisense oligonucleotides (AONs) in nonhuman primates induce foamy macrophage accumulations, with intracytoplasmic basophilic granules that represent ingested AONs (Templin et al. 2000).

The overarching point illustrated by the preceding examples is that AMs are incredibly efficient at removing inhaled material from the lungs (Patton and Platz 1992). Therefore, it is not surprising that macrophage reactions are frequently seen following inhalation exposure to formulations composed of relatively insoluble drug particles (Davies and Feddah 2003; Klapwijk 2011; Owen et al. 2010; Owen 2011). These reactions have been ascribed to a low soluble particle effect, resulting in rapid phagocytosis (Pauluhn 2005), and can be considered a nonspecific response by macrophages

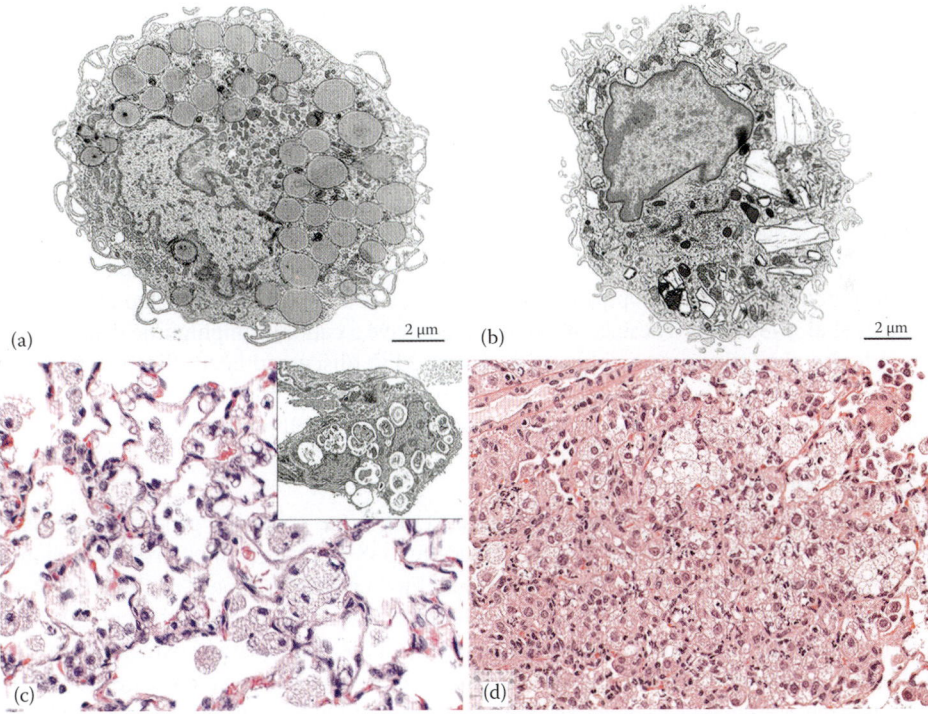

FIGURE 11.4   (a) Cytoplasmic neutral lipid droplets in an AM, demonstrating one of the causes of "foamy" macrophage cytoplasm that may be seen by H&E light microscopy. TEM, dog macrophage. (b) Crystalline material within an AM, consistent with phagocytosis of a low-solubility test article. This process also imparts a foamy appearance to macrophages by standard light microscopy. TEM, rat macrophage. (c) Foamy macrophages may also result from PLO. Main image shows a typical H&E appearance, and the insert TEM demonstrates enlarged cytoplasmic LLBs in an alveolar type II cell confirming PLO. Rat lung. (d) Inflammatory cell infiltration seen in association with severe PLO, dog lung.

to the inhalation of high concentrations of poorly soluble material with a rate of deposition that exceeds the clearance and dissolution capacity of the lung. The material therefore accumulates, leading to macrophage overload and a proinflammatory response (Owen 2011; Klapwijk 2011). In such cases, ultrastructural investigation allows demonstration of numerous cytoplasmic crystals within the macrophages (Figure 11.4b), which impart the foamy appearance seen by light microscopy (Rabinow 2004; Klapwijk 2011). Comparison with scanning electron micrographs of the crystalline form of the compound (Rasenack et al. 2003; Fults et al. 1997; Chan and Gonda 1989) allows confirmation of the etiology of the macrophage changes by TEM (Klapwijk 2011). These intracellular crystals can be seen in situ in macrophages recovered from BALF, and their induction can be replicated *in vitro*.

Pulmonary drug accumulation has been suggested as a means to extend therapeutic activity (Villetti et al. 2006; Casarosa et al. 2009); however, as poorly soluble crystalline formulations are used to achieve this aim, they are inevitably associated with macrophage reactions (Davies and Feddah 2003; Klapwijk 2011). As such, this strategy is considered to have unwittingly contributed to compound attrition (Pauluhn 2005; Forbes et al. 2011; Owen 2011). It should be noted, however, that although poorly soluble drugs may induce particle effects, this does not preclude other effects ascribable to their pharmacological actions.

Foamy macrophages due to increased numbers of cytoplasmic LLBs imply increased phagocytosis of pulmonary surfactant, synthesized and secreted by the ATIIs (Nkadi et al. 2009). Although the majority of surfactant is normally cleared and recycled by the same cell type, excess surfactant is phagocytosed and cleared by macrophages (Nkadi et al. 2009; Kramer et al. 2001). This can cause foamy macrophage accumulations following corticosteroid inhalation, as inhaled corticosteroids stimulate overproduction of surfactant by ATIIs (Young and Silbajoris 1986), which then accumulates within the macrophages as phospholipids and neutral lipid—the latter likely due to breakdown of the former (Sakagami et al. 2010). Although corticosteroids are generally poorly soluble, foamy macrophages are also seen when they are administered systemically (Okazaki et al. 1992; Owen 2011); hence, the foamy phenotype is unlikely due solely to a particle effect.

With some orally delivered drugs, multifocal foamy macrophage aggregates appear scattered throughout the parenchyma. This effect, which often becomes more evident in 2-year oncogenicity studies, has been seen in rats with peroxisome proliferator-activated receptor alpha (PPARα) agonists such as clofibrate and nafenopin, a PPARδ agonist, a p38 kinase inhibitor, and an iNOS inhibitor (Fringes et al. 1988a,b,c). These compounds do not have a cationic amphiphilic drug (CAD)-like structure; hence, the lesions were not consistent with PLO (discussed later). Similar changes were not seen in the corresponding mouse studies or the 9-month dog or nonhuman primate studies. The macrophages were not associated with any other inflammatory cell infiltration.

11.9.2.1 Phospholipidosis

A common cause of foamy macrophages (Figure 11.4c) is the condition generally referred to as phospholipidosis (PLO), which was first described in 1948 in rats given chloroquine, though the term was not introduced until much later (Nelson and Fitzhugh 1948; Zhou et al. 2011). PLO is characterized by the excessive accumulation of phospholipids in lysosomes (Piccotti et al. 2005), which are referred to as LLBs. Although macrophages are inevitably (and characteristically) affected and often the only cell type identified by routine light microscopic examination, careful observation often reveals the presence of vacuoles in ATIIs and Clara cells by light microscopy, and LLBs in endothelial cells, smooth muscle cells, and ATIs by electron microscopy.

Although most incidences of PLO are not associated with any degenerative of inflammatory changes, some clear evidence of macrophage necrosis, neutrophilic infiltration (Figure 11.4d), or even abscessation (Figure 11.5a) may be seen, particularly at very high doses or with prolonged treatment. There has been some debate whether these types of associated changes are directly due to the PLO or to some other toxic mechanism (Reasor and Kacew 2001; Anderson and Borlak 2006). For example, once a compound–phospholipid complex exceeds a certain concentration, lysosomal

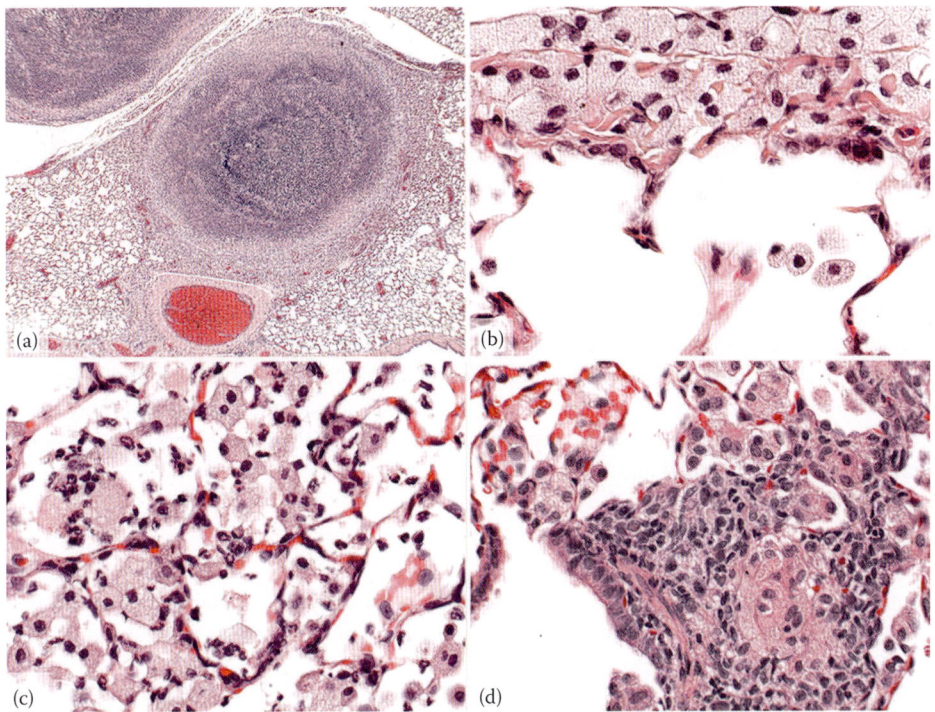

FIGURE 11.5 (a) Multiple abscessation of the lung, seen in association with PLO, rat lung. (b) Pleural macrophage aggregation. Although test article–related macrophage aggregation is usually seen in the bronchiolar–alveolar duct region, test article–related pleural/subpleural accumulation may also be rarely seen. Cynomolgus monkey lung. (c) Macrophage aggregation with neutrophil infiltration, indicative of macrophage activation, rat. (d) Macrophage accumulation admixed with a mononuclear inflammatory cell infiltrate, indicative of a chronic inflammatory reaction, rat.

fragility and leakage of proteolytic enzymes may occur, with consequent cell damage and death. This has been reported with amiodarone, which was found to exert a cytotoxic effect on ATIIs due to disruption of lysosomal membranes, release of toxic oxygen radicals, and apoptosis (Papiris et al. 2010). In its mildest form, PLO is usually reversible but suppresses macrophage clearance (Ferin 1982; Pauluhn 2005), and therefore recovery may take time. This impaired clearance in PLO leads to a self-amplifying macrophage accumulation (Pauluhn 2005), and the delayed clearance is likely to be similar to the macrophage overload phenomenon seen with inhaled particulates (Morrow 1988). In severe cases in carcinogenicity studies, the majority of alveoli may appear to be completely filled with enlarged foamy macrophages and eosinophilic material (free surfactant). Clearly, recovery periods are not practical in life-span studies, but even if they were performed (e.g., by limiting dosing to 2 years in a long-lived strain such as Han–Wistar), it is unlikely that complete recovery would take place. PLO has also been shown to accelerate the accumulation of some other pneumophilic, coadministered drugs in rat lungs (Ohmiya et al. 1983), and macrophages from amiodarone-treated rats showed a decreased ability to phagocytose Candida (Wilson et al. 1993).

The significance of PLO in terms of adversity is complex, with some authors considering it an adaptive response (Zhou et al. 2011), and, while others agree that this is primarily the case, they nevertheless conclude that it should be regarded as adverse, in view of the concomitant toxicological changes with which it is sometimes associated (Hanumegowda et al. 2010). In view of the ability of at least some CADs to form complexes with phospholipids, the administration of a CAD, particularly by the inhaled route, is clearly not without risk as any drug capable of binding to free alveolar surfactant could potentially affect its multiple homeostatic functions.

11.9.2.2 Pulmonary Alveolar Proteinosis

Foamy macrophages are also seen in lung lesions consistent with a diagnosis of PLO, but from animals treated with non-CADs. This change is histologically identical to pulmonary alveolar proteinosis (PAP) in man, with PLO and PAP being used as synonyms by some authors (Presneill et al. 2004; Seymour and Presneill 2002). PAP and PLO may be difficult to distinguish in H&E-stained lung sections. Eosinophilic intra-alveolar material is more prominent in PAP, and macrophages may be less prominent (Renne et al. 2009). ORO staining or adipophilin immunohistochemistry may help to distinguish the two conditions as the foamy macrophages in some cases of PAP staining strongly for neutral lipids (Thomassen et al. 2007; Sakagami et al. 2010; Trapnell and Whitsett 2002), whereas macrophages in PLO usually do not (Obert et al. 2007). In addition, ultrastructurally, tubular myelin is more commonly seen in PAP than in PLO (Trapnell and Whitsett 2002; Hook 1991). PAP may also be induced by inhalation of some dusts such as silica, and in man, a congenital form is recognized (Seymour and Presneill 2002). The pathogenesis of PAP may be related to effects on granulocyte/monocyte colony stimulating factor (GM-CSF) (Thomassen et al. 2007; Sakagami et al. 2010; Trapnell and Whitsett 2002).

11.9.3 PIGMENTED AM REACTIONS

Pigmented macrophages are relatively rare in most laboratory animal species but are encountered in a few specific conditions such as inhalation of compounds containing dyes resistant to histological processing (Gopinath et al. 1987).

Diffusely distributed hemosiderin-laden macrophages are classically seen secondary to cardiac failure (Greaves 2007) but also focally at sites of minor hemorrhages (Renne et al. 2009). These siderocytes appear brown with H&E and blue with Perl's Prussian Blue stain.

Macrophages containing brown pigment, believed to be derived from inhalation of fossilized diatoms and silicon, may be seen in nonhuman primates (Dayan et al. 1978).

Rarely, exposure of a tissue or cells (particularly macrophages) to a pharmaceutical can result in the development of a pigment that stains negatively for iron and is weakly positive with lipofuscin stains. It is likely that these pigments represent drug, drug metabolites, or drug bound to a tissue component such as phospholipid. These pigments tend to persist, suggesting that they are resistant to lysosomal enzymes. Recovery of pigmented macrophage reactions is dependent on lung clearance.

11.9.4 INTERSTITIAL MACROPHAGE REACTIONS

There are considerable species differences in particle clearance rates (Snipes 1996), with most rodents (without respiratory bronchioles) exhibiting rapid clearance, whereas larger species (with respiratory bronchioles), such as dogs, nonhuman primates, and humans, exhibit slower clearance (Snipes 1996; Kreyling et al. 2001). As a result of this, respiratory bronchioles, and their evaginating alveoli and alveolar ducts, are known to accumulate high particle loads (Macklin 1955; Gross et al. 1966; Johanson 2003) that may be up to 25–100 times higher than in main stem bronchi, and this can result in local sequestration within macrophages and long-term local storage of low-solubility compounds (Snipes 1989; Kuempel 2000). In these circumstances, aggregates of macrophages may be seen in the alveolar interstitium, and the peribronchiolar and perivascular connective tissues that correspond to "pulmonary dust sumps" (Macklin, 1955), and pigmented forms have been likened to a pulmonary "tattoo" (Lehnert 1992; Sorokin and Brain 1975). The potential chronicity of this effect is illustrated by persistence of vacuolated interstitial macrophages in dogs and nonhuman primates, 5 years after cessation of exposure to fluorocarbon liquids (Modell et al. 1976; Hood and Modell 2000; Tuazon et al. 1973; Calderwood et al. 1973). With these sequestered macrophages, there is a risk of subsequent damage to the lung following their death; or they may act as a reservoir of compound and are capable of unpredictably increasing local tissue and blood concentrations.

11.9.5 SUBPLEURAL/PLEURAL MACROPHAGE REACTIONS

Subpleural aggregates of macrophages may occasionally be seen as spontaneous events, particularly in rats. In addition, although most macrophage reactions to poorly soluble inhaled test articles occur in and around the terminal airways, a test article–related subpleural/pleural (Figure 11.5b) distribution may rarely be seen. Macrophage reactions at these sites are considered secondary to two possible mechanisms: peripheral lymphatic flow and translocation via the airspaces (pleural drift) (Morrow 1972; Schraufnagel 2010; Dungworth et al. 1992; Lehnert 1992; Holt 1983; Henderson et al. 1995).

Subpleural macrophage accumulations may also be seen in association with disruption of lipid homeostasis in rodents and in some diabetogenic rat strains (Kennedy et al. 2005; Bernick and Alfin-Slater 1963; Foster et al. 2010).

11.9.6 INTRAVASCULAR MACROPHAGE REACTIONS

Intravascular macrophage reactions have not been reported in nonclinical studies as a test article–related effect but have been reported in a rat surgical model of the human condition hepatopulmonary syndrome, which is associated with liver cirrhosis (Fallon 2005; Chang and Ohara 1994; Miot-Noirault et al. 2001; Nunes et al. 2001).

11.9.7 REVERSIBILITY/ADVERSITY OF MACROPHAGE REACTIONS

Loose accumulations of macrophages are usually readily reversible, but more solid aggregations are more resistant to regression. This is likely to reflect a number of features. Firstly, when the volumetric load on the macrophage cytoplasm becomes excessive, the cells become immotile, with cessation of clearance (Morrow 1988; Lehnert 1990). Secondly, the densely packed, hypertrophic macrophages are likely to have reduced deformability, and thus are physically incapable of extricating themselves from the alveolus, or to pass through the pores of Kohn. Thirdly, macrophages move by pseudopodal movement on surfaces, and the degree of adhesion to the surface is an important determinant of motility (Laplante and Lemaire 1990). Most macrophages in an aggregate have nothing to adhere to other than each other, thus restricting locomotion and clearance. Fourthly, there is no lymphatic clearance from alveoli.

The designation of adverse/nonadverse to macrophage reactions has received considerable attention in recent years, partly due to regulatory concerns as they are unmonitorable in clinical trials. In practice, this is in fact relatively straightforward. A macrophage reaction characterized by a loose accumulation of cells with evidence of reversibility, but without evidence of degeneration, neutrophil involvement, pigment accumulation, or involvement of the adjacent alveolar walls, is clearly adaptive and nonadverse, merely reflecting macrophages "doing their job" (Owen 2011).

However, in cases with associated inflammatory cell involvement, the reaction is clearly adverse. In addition, the association of ATII hypertrophy/hyperplasia with macrophage reactions, other than those explicable by pharmacology, may indicate stimulation by the macrophages and, thus, should also be considered adverse.

11.9.8 TYPE II PNEUMOCYTE HYPERTROPHY

ATII hypertrophy is often seen in conjunction with macrophage responses, as previously described. ATII hypertrophy may also be seen in situations where the total number of ATIIs has been reduced, such that the remaining cells undergo what may be regarded as compensatory hypertrophy. This phenomenon has been reported in monocrotaline-treated rats (Wilson and Segall 1990).

ATII hypertrophy may also be associated with peroxisome proliferation, as reported in rats given a number of PPARα agonists (Batenburg and Haagsman 1998; Karnati and Baumgart-Vogt 2008).

11.9.9 Type II Pneumocyte Hyperplasia

Diagnosis of ATII hyperplasia is relatively straightforward as the proliferating cells give the alveolar epithelium a cuboidal appearance. However, when associated with densely aggregated foamy macrophages and when they contain hypertrophic LLBs (giving them also a foamy appearance), distinguishing between the two cell types can be difficult and may require additional investigation such as the use of fatty acid synthase (FAS) IHC, a marker for ATII cells.

ATII hyperplasia is often regarded as secondary to adjacent macrophage reactions, but macrophage reactions may also be stimulated by chemoattractants released from the ATIIs (Koyama et al. 1997). When ATII hyperplasia occurs at the bronchioloalveolar junction, it must be distinguished from bronchiolarization (Slesinski and Turnbull 2008).

ATIIs may also proliferate in the absence of macrophage responses; intratracheal administration of keratinocyte growth factor induces ATII hyperplasia in rats without any associated increase in foamy macrophages (Ulich et al. 1994; Fehrenbach et al. 1999, 2003).

11.9.10 Surfactant Dysfunction

Although not detectable by light microscopy, the ultrastructural features of dysfunctional surfactant are readily identified, involving increased amounts of unilamellar forms, distinct from the normal LLBs and tubular myelin (Ochs et al. 1999; Schmiedl et al. 2003; Schleh et al. 2009). In addition, ultrastructural examination can readily identify alterations in LLBs, such as increased or decreased numbers, size, and configuration of the lamellae. Following ozone exposure, ATIIs produce a distinct form of LLB, which is unable to unfold during exocytosis and hence is unable to form tubular myelin (Balis et al. 1988).

The importance of surfactant dysfunction has been highlighted in recent years by the suggestion that in addition to its involvement in acute lung injuries, it may also play a major role in the pathogenesis of COPD (Zhao et al. 2010).

11.9.11 Diffuse Alveolar Damage

Diffuse alveolar damage (DAD) is a common manifestation of drug-induced pulmonary injury (Rossi et al. 2000), which is characterized histologically by extensive epithelial and endothelial destruction and flooding of the alveolar air spaces with proteinaceous material (Guidot et al. 2000). A striking feature of DAD is the appearance of hyaline membranes at the site of alveolar epithelial destruction. These "membranes" stain strongly by PAS, contain cellular debris, and undergo either resolution or fibroproliferation (Gopinath et al. 1987; Peres e Serra et al. 2006). The herbicide, paraquat, is probably the best-known chemical cause of DAD (Kehrer and Kacew 1985).

11.10 INFLAMMATORY REACTIONS IN THE LUNG

11.10.1 Acute Inflammatory Reactions

Acute inflammation may be characterized by variable degrees of serous, fibrinous, or suppurative intra-alveolar exudates. Macrophages with a classically activated phenotype release cytotoxic and pro-inflammatory cytokines and chemokines (Ma et al. 2003; Laskin et al. 2011; Gordon 2003; Duffield 2003) and are associated with neutrophilic infiltration (Figure 11.5c). In such cases, in addition to neutrophil infiltration, there is often evidence of damage to the adjacent alveolar walls, with interstitial inflammatory cells, increased alveolar wall thickness, and ATII hyperplasia.

11.10.2 Chronic Inflammatory Reactions

Excessive and inappropriate T-cell responses have been suggested to play a major role in the pathogenesis of respiratory diseases in man (Strickland et al. 1996a). Under normal conditions, T-cells are "locked" in the G_0/G_1 stage of the cell cycle, and AMs play a major role in this control (Strickland et al. 1996b). Hence, a change in macrophage phenotype could potentially lead to loss of this control. In addition, in chronic inflammatory conditions, macrophage changes are often seen in short-term studies before any detectable involvement of other cell types becomes apparent, suggesting an initiating role in chronic inflammation. Subsequently, ATII hyperplasia and infiltration of lymphoid cells (Figure 11.5d) including plasma cells in the interstitium occur. In some cases, extensive BALT develops, with perivascular lymphoid aggregates and even germinal centers with high endothelial venules appearing. By IHC, these lymphoid structures can be shown to be surprisingly well structured and reminiscent of lymph nodes (Goya et al. 2003).

In practice, marked chronic inflammatory conditions characterized by lymphocytic involvement secondary to macrophage reactions are rarely seen following inhaled or systemic administration of pharmaceuticals. However, this has been recorded in our laboratory in rats, becoming pronounced with increased study duration.

Classically activated macrophages can also stimulate MHC-dependent antigen presentation by other cell types (Byers and Holtzman 2010), and what appears to be an adaptive immune reaction may also occur in rats, characterized by a pronounced lymphoid reaction as described above, but with large numbers of plasma cells located around the peripheral pulmonary airways, vessels, and alveolar ducts. There are relatively few macrophages in these lesions, but in the initial short-duration studies, a macrophage reaction is often the only notable change.

Chronic inflammatory changes in the lung may also be induced by immunogenic proteins such as rhDNase (Clarke et al. 2008) and haptens.

11.10.3 GRANULOMATOUS INFLAMMATORY REACTIONS

Pulmonary granulomatous inflammatory conditions induced by inhaled particulates may be grouped under the generic term *pneumoconiosis* (Renne et al. 2009) and are characterized by the presence of macrophages, lymphocytes, plasma cells, with some evidence of epithelioid cell palisading, and characteristic multinucleated giant cells. The latter cells originate from the fusion of macrophages and have an enhanced capacity to degrade large particles (Helming and Gordon 2009). With silver stains, reticulin fibers may be demonstrated (Figure 11.6a), even at a relatively early stage of the developing lesion. Occasional foreign bodies, due to inhaled diet or aspiration, may be seen as an incidental finding (Innes et al. 1967; Greaves and Faccini 1984; Greaves 2007). After oral gavage dosing, reflux may occur, particularly in rodents, which can result in aspiration into the lungs inducing a range of lesions dependent on the characteristics of the dose material and the vehicle (Eichenbaum et al. 2011; Damsch et al. 2011).

Brown Norway strain rats may spontaneously develop a high incidence of granulomatous inflammation, which may be also induced in rats and mice following intravenous bacilli Calmette–Guérin (BCG) injection (Takizawa et al. 1986; Chang et al. 1986; Greaves 2007).

Granulomatous inflammation may also result from parasitic infestation, and although canine filaroidiasis is very uncommon in modern beagle colonies, a hyperinfection of *Filaroides hirthi* has been reported in corticosteroid-treated animals (Genta and Schad 1984).

11.10.4 REGIONAL LYMPH NODE/BALT REACTIONS

Initiation of an adaptive response following pulmonary exposure to an allergen requires allergen translocation to local lymph nodes rather than BALT (Haley 2003). However, in cases of a strong stimulus, there can be a marked, generalized increase in cellularity within BALT with distinct follicles, demonstrable T- and B-cell areas, and the development of a characteristic lymphoepithelium composed of cuboidal epithelial cells (Greaves 2007).

In addition, chronic pulmonary macrophage reactions can often result in changes in the local lymph nodes and, in some species, BALT. These changes usually involve the presence of

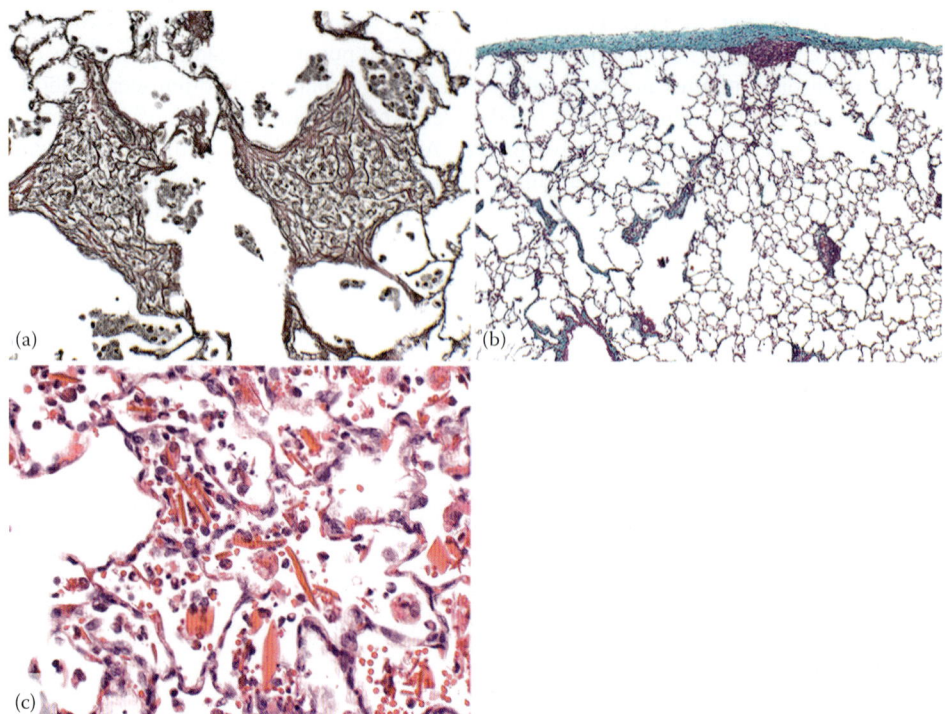

FIGURE 11.6 (a) Reticulin fibers within foci of chronic inflammation, indicating extensive early fibrosis. Silver stain, rat lung. (b) Pleural and pulmonary fibrosis following inhalation administration of a PDE-IV inhibitor. This finding was not associated with vascular damage. Trichrome stain, rat. (c) Alveolar hemorrhage with eosinophilic crystal formation (hemoglobin) and a mild acute inflammatory cell infiltrate. Increased incidence of this lesion is seen in rats following inhalation exposure to β-agonists.

macrophages of the same phenotype as those present in the lung, for example, foamy or pigmented, and their presence in this location indicates lymphatic clearance. These macrophages are often associated with a generalized increase in cellularity of the lymphoid tissue (Slesinski and Turnbull, 2008), although in some cases, the main response may be germinal center development. The reactions occur in all species and are often detected at necropsy as enlargement/discoloration. In acute inflammatory lung reactions, neutrophils may also translocate to the lymph nodes, where they may cause microabscess formation (Harmsen et al. 1987).

The main route of clearance of AMs from the lungs in the dog is via the interstitium/lymphatics, while in rats, clearance is mainly via the mucociliary escalator. This explains the increased propensity of translocation of macrophages to the regional lymph nodes of dogs compared to rats (Snipes 1989; Valberg et al. 1985).

11.10.5 PNEUMONIA

Clinically relevant pneumonia is extremely rare as a spontaneous condition in all species of laboratory animal; however, immunosuppression is known to predispose dogs to pneumonia, and, as such, this condition has been reported secondary to spontaneous canine hyperadrenocorticoidism and following chronic inhalation exposure to corticosteroids (Crowell et al. 1978; Capen et al. 1975). With pneumonia secondary to corticosteroids, the severity of infection varies considerably between animals given the same treatment and housed in the same room, with an occasional dog developing severe bronchopneumonia while its kennel mates remain unaffected.

Immunosuppression induced by corticosteroids in rats and dogs can lead to exacerbation of opportunistic *Pneumocystis carinii* infections, which may lead to pneumonia (Chandler et al. 1979; Lanken et al. 1980; Barton and Campbell 1969). Recently, *P. carinii* has been shown to be the likely cause of the problematic condition seen in immunocompetent rats and ascribed to the "rat respiratory virus" (Livingston et al. 2011). This condition is characterized by focal, perivascular lymphocytes, increased peribronchiolar lymphoid tissue, and infiltrates of macrophages and neutrophils.

Inhalation dosing of muscarinic antagonists induces low incidences of inflammatory lung lesions, usually with no dose relationship in the dog. This includes a spectrum of pathologies ranging from acute inflammation, features consistent with gastric reflux to alveolitis and even pneumonia. In addition, in some cases, chronic granulomatous lesions are seen, consistent with the inhalation of particulates such as food. These pathologies, which are often found as single foci, are considered to be related to the pharmacological properties of muscarinic antagonists in the dog, such as diminished salivary flow/dry mouth and concomitant increased risk of oropharyngeal flora aspiration (Gibson and Barrett 1992). This effect is potentiated in treated animals by reduced mucus production in the airways leading to a suboptimal mucociliary escalator (Yeates et al. 1975). In addition, dogs experience spontaneous gastroesophageal reflux (Patrikios et al. 1986), and as muscarinic antagonists reduce lower esophageal sphincter tone and delay gastric emptying, they increase the risk of reflux and aspiration of gastric contents (Hoyt 1990; Chiba et al. 2002; Wilson and Walshaw 2004). Modification of the postdosing feeding regime and a moistened diet diminishes the incidence and severity of these lesions.

11.10.6 EOSINOPHILIC CRYSTALLINE PNEUMONIA

This idiopathic, subclinical to fatal condition is seen in mice and is characterized by infiltrations of eosinophilic macrophages (some multinucleate), eosinophils, neutrophils, lymphocytes, and plasma cells. This inflammation is associated with elongated, eosinophilic crystals, which are immunoreactive with a chitinase-like protein, Yml (Hoenerhoff et al. 2006).

11.11 PULMONARY/PLEURAL FIBROSIS

Fibrosis results in disruption of the pulmonary architecture due to an increase in the amount or abnormal location of collagen (Renne et al. 2009), which may be demonstrated by use of trichrome or Van Gieson stains.

Dogs are unusual among laboratory animal species in having a relatively high incidence of spontaneous pulmonary fibrosis (Hahn and Dagle 2001). The lesion appears to begin in the respiratory bronchiolar epithelium with a process of focal squamous metaplasia, likely followed by myofibroblast formation, and progresses toward the pleura forming a wedge-shaped lesion. Pleural involvement is easily seen at necropsy. As the lesion matures, the amount of collagen increases and eventually becomes the predominant feature. The cause of this lesion is unknown, but an absence of exacerbation in immunosuppressed dogs suggests that an infectious etiology is unlikely.

Published reports of pulmonary fibrosis following administration of pharmaceuticals are rare; however, both pulmonary (alveolar duct) and pleural fibrosis have been seen in a rat study with an inhaled PDE-IVB inhibitor (Figure 11.6b). The lesions were not associated with any vascular damage.

Models of pulmonary fibrosis include bleomycin and fluorescein isothiocyanate (FITC) (Endo et al. 2003; Degryse and Lawson, 2011). FITC has the novel feature that immunofluorescence can be used to demonstrate its location relative to the development of the fibrotic change.

11.12 EMPHYSEMA

Emphysema is defined as abnormal, permanent enlargement of the airspaces distal to the terminal bronchioles (Kasahara et al. 2000). Proteolytic/antiproteolytic imbalance is an important etiological factor and can be due to either an increase in proteolytic enzyme activity, such as results from extensive neutrophil degranulation, or loss of antiproteolytic protection, such as a genetic deficiency of α-1-proteinase inhibitor PI (α-1-PI) (Abrams et al. 1981). The standard animal model for emphysema is intratracheal administration of elastase or papain to rats or dogs (Takaro et al. 1990).

A suspicion that there was a vascular component to the development of emphysema was suggested many years ago (Liebow 1959; Kasahara et al. 2000) when it was noted that alveolar septae in emphysematous patients were thin and virtually avascular. This raised the possibility that a reduction in blood supply could cause loss of alveolar septae. VEGF is known to be a survival factor for endothelial cells, and chronic administration of a VEGF receptor blocker to rats and ablation of the VEGF gene in mice are both reported to bring about emphysematous changes (Kashara et al. 2000; Tang et al. 2004).

11.13 ALVEOLAR INTERSTITIAL MINERALIZATION

Interstitial mineralization is characterized by the linear deposition of slightly basophilic material within collagen, elastin, or the basement membranes and can be demonstrated by Von Kossa stain (Renne et al. 2009). The presence of mineral often results in poor section quality as decalcification is not performed when the lesion is unsuspected. This can be alleviated to a considerable degree by decalcification of the paraffin block surface.

Administration of high doses of corticosteroids by inhalation to dogs for up to 9 months results in a Cushing's disease–like syndrome, which includes pulmonary interstitial mineralization. This occurs despite normal blood calcium and phosphorus levels (Blois et al. 2009) and has been attributed to the protein catabolic action of corticosteroids, with deposition of calcium and phosphorus into the damaged organic matrix of partially catabolized collagen and elastin proteins (Capen et al. 1975; Berry et al. 1994; Blois et al. 2009). This corticosteroid-related condition is not seen in other laboratory species and is not reported in man (Berry et al. 1994).

In laboratory animals, classic metastatic pulmonary interstitial mineralization is seen spontaneously in rats with chronic renal disease (Renne et al. 2009), although with dietary changes introduced over the years, the incidence has declined. Renal insufficiency induces secondary hyperparathyroidism, elevated hormone levels, disordered mineral metabolism with elevated Ca and P levels, and calcification of pulmonary vessels and interalveolar septae (Lopez et al. 2006). Similarly, vitamin D and its derivatives stimulate Ca mobilization from the bones, increase its absorption in the intestine, and reduce its excretion. The resulting hypercalcemia leads to precipitation of Ca salts between elastin and collagen fibers (Hilbe et al. 2000; Price et al. 2001). Diuretics such as hydrochlorothiazide and furosemide also induce severe nephropathy in rats and mice with parathyroid hyperplasia, fibrous osteodystrophy, and pulmonary interstitial mineralization (Bucher et al. 1990a,b).

11.14 ALVEOLAR MICROLITHIASIS

Microliths are rounded, slightly basophilic, laminated, "onion skin"–like concretions that stain positively with PAS (Brix et al. 1994). They occur under pathophysiological conditions, which may lead to calcification, including hypercalcemia, an alkaline local environment, tissue injury, and increased alkaline phosphatase activity (Chan et al. 2002). Following systemic dosing with a PPARδ agonist, foamy macrophage aggregates were seen in short-term rat studies, and in chronic studies, these were associated with microliths. The microliths appeared to arise from or adjacent to ATIIs.

11.15 VASCULAR LESIONS

11.15.1 PERIVASCULAR EOSINOPHIL ACCUMULATION

Spontaneous perivascular eosinophil aggregates (of unknown etiology) may occasionally be seen in rat lungs. Eosinophil accumulation may also occur in the lungs of nonhuman primates.

In short-term studies, a very late antigen-4 (VLA-4) antagonist produced increases in the severity, and incidences of eosinophilic aggregations in rats. VLA-4 is expressed on the surface of eosinophils, is up-regulated by direct contact with eotaxin (Okigami et al. 2007), and is believed to play an important role in the regulation of their transendothelial trafficking in the lung.

Intense pulmonary eosinophilia can readily be induced in rats, particularly those of the Brown Norway strain (Namovic et al. 1996), by antigen challenge or by intravenous Sephadex particles.

A perivascular eosinophilia was reported in Sprague–Dawley rats with the immunosuppressant FK-506 (Nalesnik et al. 1987).

11.15.2 Edema

Alveolar edema may be interstitial or alveolar, the former characterized by slight swelling of the alveolar walls and the latter by acellular, eosinophilic material in the alveolar air spaces. Edema may be caused by either increased pressure (cardiogenic), characterized by slow onset, lack of cellular damage, and fluid of low protein content, or increased permeability (noncardiogenic), characterized by rapid onset, cellular damage, and protein-rich fluid (Amouzadeh et al. 1991).

A mild form of interstitial edema was described in rats given ethchlorvynol intravenously, in which ultrastructural evidence of endothelial blebbing into the capillary lumina was seen. This lesion was completely reversible (Wysolmerski et al. 1984); however, once interstitial edema becomes severe, a rapid transition to alveolar edema takes place (Miserocchi 2007).

Alveolar edema induced by alloxan was characterized ultrastructurally by marked disruption of both endothelium and epithelium, with swelling and loss of cells (Cottrell et al. 1967). One of the most utilized models of edema is alpha-naphthylthiourea (ANTU), which causes endothelial damage and gaps, which allow leakage of fibrin-rich fluid (Kehrer and Kacew 1985).

Malnutrition in rats has been shown to impair normal alveolar fluid clearance via epithelial sodium channels (ENaC) (Sakuma et al. 2004).

Edema has also been induced following intravenous administration of contrast media in rats (Hayashi et al. 1994), which was shown to be exacerbated by silicon contamination (Sendo et al. 1999).

11.15.3 Embolism

Obstruction of pulmonary vessel(s) may be due to cells, bacteria, fat, fur, foreign bodies, blood clots, or platelets (Goggs et al. 2009), and major risk factors are corticosteroids, sepsis, and in laboratory animals, intravascular injections (Schneider and Pappritz 1976; Greaves and Faccini 1984; Gopinath et al. 1987, Blois 2009; Hammer 1991). Evidence of fat embolism secondary to trauma can be seen in pulmonary vessels and has been induced experimentally in dogs by medullary pressurization (Schemitsch et al. 1998).

Pulmonary capillary thrombosis, characterized by pronounced eosinophilic staining of the alveolar walls, has been seen in phenylhydrazine (PHZ)-treated rats. Cushing's disease is reported to be a predisposing factor in the development of pulmonary thromboembolism (Burns et al. 1981; Berry et al. 1994; Blois et al. 2009), and in long-term dog studies with inhaled corticosteroids, the alveolar capillaries may be distended by platelets, many of which appeared degranulated. While this may be a direct effect of the corticosteroid, it must be borne in mind that these dogs are severely immunocompromised, often with secondary infections and possible bacterial toxin production.

Gadolinium chloride used in nuclear magnetic imaging forms an insoluble hydroxide colloid at blood pH and results in multiple mineral emboli in the pulmonary capillary bed of rats and mice (Spencer et al. 1997, 1998).

11.15.4 ALVEOLAR HEMORRHAGE

In rodents euthanized by CO_2, focal, agonal alveolar hemorrhages may develop, the degree of change being roughly proportional to the CO_2 chamber concentration (Renne et al. 2009). This may be due to a period of hypoxia during the procedure that is sufficient to cause damage to the capillary endothelial cells (Larsen et al. 1986).

In laboratory species, alveolar hemorrhage is rarely seen as an isolated lesion (Gopinath et al. 1987), but it has been reported following administration of heparin to rats (Larsen et al. 1986).

Alveolar hemorrhage with elongate, eosinophilic hemoglobin (Hb) crystals, neutrophils, and macrophages is seen as a minor background lesion in rats (Renne et al. 2009); it may be associated with leakage during vascular congestion (Greaves 2007). An increased incidence of this lesion, characterized by the focal presence of erythrocytes, Hb crystals, macrophages, and neutrophils (Figure 11.6c), with evidence of erythrocyte and Hb crystal phagocytosis, has been seen in rats following inhalation of several novel beta-2 adrenergic agonists (upublished observation). This change typically shows higher incidences throughout treated groups, but with a poor dose response, and is not seen in mouse or dog studies. Hb crystals are pro-inflammatory, explaining the neutrophil involvement (Kleinig et al. 2009; Gorbunov et al. 2006). Investigations of beta-2 agonist studies revealed that its development was associated with recent isoflurane anesthesia, and the likely explanation was that both beta-2 agonists and anesthetic agents decrease RBC deformability (Allen and Rasmussen 1971; Valensi et al. 1993; Yerer et al. 2006; Aydoğan et al. 2006) and their combination could increase the risk of hemolysis and hemorrhage by this effect (Christopher et al. 1990). In addition, rat Hb is susceptible to crystallization (Andrews and Papworth 1994; Kleinig et al. 2009), and ultrastructural investigations show that induced crystallization may actually begin while the RBCs are still within the capillaries (Rygh and Selvig 1973).

11.15.5 PULMONARY ARTERIOPATHY

Vascular damage is a frequent, well-documented change associated with PDE-IV inhibitors in rats (Zhang et al. 2008; Weaver et al. 2010) but has also been reported in nonhuman primates and dogs (Losco et al. 2004; Hanton et al. 2008). Although there is a strong predilection for the mesenteric vessels, vascular lesions may also be seen in other tissues, including the lung following either oral or inhalation administration. In the lungs, it is usually confined to single large arteries in the rat but can affect small arterioles in the dog, and it is seen only at low incidences in both species. In rats, the lesion is confined to the vessels and is characterized by intramural RBCs, fibrin insudation and exudation, disruption of smooth muscle cells, perivascular/adventitial inflammation, fibrinoid necrosis, and fibrosis. These lesions are identical to those seen in vessels in other organs and are usually severe, corresponding to grades 3–5 detailed by Zhang et al. (2008). In dogs, there is extensive neutrophilic infiltration associated with the arteriolar lesions in acute studies, which extended throughout the adjacent tissues and, in its most severe form, can resemble pneumonia. In chronic studies, the lesion progressed to include fibrosis, lymphocytic infiltration, alveolar collapse, and bronchiolar ectasia.

Monocrotaline has been used for many years as a model of chronic pulmonary hypertension in rats (Meyrick 2001) and is associated with pulmonary arterial lesions, including adventitial edema, extracellular matrix secretion, smooth muscle hypertrophy, increased medial and adventitial connective tissue in muscular arteries, development of smooth muscle in normally nonmuscular arteries, and phlebitis (Wilson et al. 1992; Cui et al. 2009; Renne et al. 2009).

11.15.6 VASCULAR MINERALIZATION

Mineralization of the elastic lamellae of pulmonary arteries has been induced in rats by the vitamin K antagonist warfarin (Price et al. 2001).

11.15.7 BRONCHIAL ARTERIOPATHY

Similar lesions to those described above with PDE-IV inhibitors may occasionally be seen in the bronchiolar arteries of rats exposed by inhalation to high doses of corticosteroids. Again the incidences are relatively low, and the lesions are usually seen only in early short-term studies, in which the highest doses are used. This finding is considered to be related to corticosteroid-induced vasoconstriction (Mendes et al. 2003; Ewing et al. 2010; Wagenvoort et al. 1974; Nemes et al. 1980; Cui et al. 2009). These lesions do not appear to develop following systemic administration of corticosteroids, and, therefore, it appears probable that the effect is mediated via deposition of drug onto the epithelium of the upper airways, with subsequent penetration to the subjacent bronchial vessels.

11.16 NEOPLASTIC CHANGES IN LUNGS

The most common spontaneous and chemically induced tumors in the lungs of laboratory rodents are bronchioloalveolar adenomas and carcinomas (Dixon and Maronpot 1991). Bronchioloalveolar tumors may arise from ATII or Clara cells; hence, "bronchioloalveolar" is a reflection of uncertain histogenesis. Other lung tumors in rodents are rare, particularly in pharmaceutical testing, and are described elsewhere (Renne et al. 2009; Dungworth et al. 2001).

The incidence of bronchioloalveolar tumors is greater in mice than in rats and in males than in females, and it varies widely with strain (Haseman et al. 1998; Chandra and Frith 1992; Maita et al. 1988; Hahn et al. 2007). Research using inbred mice has shown that *Pas* (pulmonary adenoma susceptibility) genes such as the *Kras* proto-oncogene provide a genetic basis for this variability (Bauer et al. 2004). Of particular note is the A/J strain of mouse. There is a high frequency of *Kras* activation in this strain and an exceptionally high incidence and early onset of lung tumors, with first appearance at less than 1 month of age and an incidence close to 100% at 24 months (Rittinghausen et al. 1996).

Primary lung tumors are unlikely to be encountered in pharmaceutical safety testing in nonrodent species. The incidence of lung tumors in younger dogs and nonhuman primates is very low, and a few chronic/whole-life studies are conducted in these species. A survey of several hundred control beagle dogs from life-span studies and breeding animals determined that the incidence of lung cancer was less than 1% for animals less than 13 years of age (Hahn et al. 1996). A lung tumor incidence of less than 1% was also recorded over a 15-year period in a cynomolgus monkey colony (Kaspareit et al. 2007). In these studies, the youngest dog and monkey found to have lung cancer were 4.3 and 9.4 years old, respectively.

The lung is a common site for metastasis of tumors originating elsewhere in the body, though in rodents, strain variation in susceptibility to metastatic disease does exist (Sass and Liebelt 1985; Rittinghausen et al. 1996). Metastatic tumors in the lungs of rats and mice usually retain the morphologic appearance of the primary mass; however, less well-differentiated metastases may resemble primary lung tumors. In such cases, a typically multifocal, perivascular distribution aids in the identification of metastatic tumors (Rittinghausen et al. 1996). Common metastatic tumors in mouse lungs include lymphoma, histiocytic sarcoma, mammary gland, and hepatocellular carcinomas (Rittinghausen et al. 1996). In the rat, mammary, adrenal cortical, and uterine lung metastases are relatively common, particularly in Wistar rats (Rittinghausen et al. 1992).

Comparison of laboratory animal and human lung cancer reveals several important differences. Squamous differentiation is common in human lung cancer (particularly bronchogenic squamous carcinoma associated with cigarette smoking) but is rare in rats and mice, even those exposed to cigarette smoke. Neuroendocrine differentiation is common in human lung cancer but is not reported in rats or mice (Hahn et al. 2007; Nikitin et al. 2004). In addition, metastasis of rat and mouse lung tumors is rare, particularly outside the thoracic cavity, but occurs commonly and widely in human lung cancer. An assessment of 15 known human lung carcinogens in rats and mice in 2-year studies determined that rats were a better model of human lung response, based primarily on the lack of response of mice to metal or mineral compounds (Hahn et al. 2007).

Compounds with positive lung tumor findings in rodent carcinogenicity studies include metronidazole, flunisolide and furazolidone (mouse, both sexes), lovastatin and timolol (mouse single sex), and simvastatin and valproate (rat single sex) (Contrera et al. 1997).

The most common tumors seen in the lung in rodent carcinogenicity studies are described below. Other forms of lung cancer are rare in pharmaceutical safety testing and are described elsewhere (Renne et al. 2009).

11.16.1 Bronchioloalveolar Adenoma

Bronchiolo-alveolar adenomas have solid, papillary, or mixed (both solid and papillary) growth patterns, are most commonly located at the periphery of the lung lobe, and in mice, are frequently visible through the pleura at necropsy (Dungworth et al. 2001; Rittinghausen et al. 1996; Dixon and Maronpot 1991). Masses are typically well demarcated, though surrounding ATII may be hyperplastic (Dungworth et al. 2001). Tumor cells are round to oval with abundant eosinophilic, sometimes granular cytoplasm, though cells within papillary masses may have a cuboidal/low columnar phenotype (Renne et al. 2009). Foamy macrophages may also be seen in association with adenomas, particularly of the papillary type. Mitotic figures are rare. It can be difficult to differentiate adenoma from bronchioloalveolar hyperplasia, as a morphologic continuum between the two findings exists. Adenomas are more densely cellular and obscure the alveolar architecture to a greater degree than areas of hyperplasia. A hyperplastic cell population may display some variation (e.g., presence of mucous or ciliated cells) that contrasts with the uniform phenotype of adenoma. Compression and collapse of surrounding alveoli is unhelpful as a distinguishing feature, as this is likely to be an artifact of processing.

11.16.2 Cystic Keratinizing Epithelioma

This tumor has been reported in rats only and is considered to arise either from neoplastic transformation of areas of squamous metaplasia in the lung, from the alveolar epithelium, or Clara cells. It consists of an irregular cystic mass (often with abundant keratin/necrotic material at its center), with stratified squamous neoplastic growth of varying thickness, typically disorganized, and with numerous mitoses. This mass must be differentiated from squamous metaplasia (usually multifocal and lacks cytological evidence of malignancy), squamous cell carcinoma (destruction of basement membrane, hence lacks cystic appearance), and other cystic lesions of the rat lung, such as pulmonary keratinizing cyst (thin cyst wall) and nonkeratinizing epithelioma (little keratin present) (Rittinghausen and Kaspareit 1998).

11.16.3 Bronchioloalveolar Carcinoma

Bronchioloalveolar carcinoma is characterized by variable patterns of irregular, usually nodular growth, is often only moderately or poorly circumscribed, and shows cytological features of malignancy such as loss of uniformity of cell size and shape, high nuclear/cytoplasm ratio, and a raised mitotic rate. Foamy macrophages frequently infiltrate into and around bronchioloalveolar carcinomas. Invasion of blood vessels and/or lymphatics provides clear evidence of malignancy and may induce a scirrhous response; in addition, local and/or distant metastasis may be seen. Foci of squamous or mucinous metaplasia may be seen, and large tumors often contain regions of hemorrhage and necrosis indicative of rapid growth (Rittinghausen et al. 1992; Dixon and Maronpot 1991). Pleural invasion of poorly differentiated bronchioloalveolar carcinoma may be confused with malignant mesothelioma; in ambiguous cases, IHC may be used to aid differentiation (Howroyd et al. 2009).

ACKNOWLEDGMENTS

We would like to thank Sean McCawley, Jennie Woodfine, Ian Francis, Paul McGill, John Bowles, and Ann Lewis for their input and support.

REFERENCES

Abrams, W.R., Cohen, A.B., Damiano, V.V., Eliraz, A., Kimbel, P., Meranze, D.R., and Weinbaum, G., 1981. A model of decreased functional α-1-proteinase inhibitor. *J Clin Invest* 68:1132–1139.

Allen, J.E., and Rasmussen, H., 1971. Human red blood cells: Prostaglandin E_2, epinephrine, and isoproterenol alter deformability. *Science* 174:512–514.

Amouzadeh, H.R., Sangiah, S., Qualls Jr., C.W., Cowell, R.L., and Mauromoustakos, A., 1991. Xylazine-induced pulmonary edema in rats. *Toxicol Appl Pharmacol* 108:417–427.

Anderson, N., and Borlak, J., 2006. Drug-induced phospholipidosis. *FEBS Letters* 580:5533–5540.

Andrews, C.M., and Papworth, S., 1994. Rat haemoglobin crystallisation. *Comp Haematol Int* 4:244.

Araya, J., Cambier, S., Markovics, J.A., Wolters, P., Jablons, D., Hill, A., Finkbeiner, W., Jones, K., Broaddus, V.C., Sheppard, D., Barzcak, A., Xiao, Y., Erle, D.J., and Nishimura, S.L., 2007. Squamous metaplasia amplifies pathologic epithelial-mesenchymal interactions in COPD patients. *J Clin Invest* 117:3551–3562.

Aryal, G., Kimula, Y., and Koike, M., 2003. Ultrastructure of Clara cells stimulated by isoproterenol. *J Med Dent Sci* 50:195–202.

Aydoğan, S., Yerer, M.B., Çomu, F.M., Arslan, M., Güneş-Ekinci, I., Unal, Y., and Kurtipek, O., 2006. The influence of sevoflurane anesthesia on rat red blood cell deformability. *Clin Haemorheol Microcirc* 35:297–300.

Baldwin, R.M., Jewell, W.T., Fanucchi, M.V., Plopper, C.G., and Buckpitt, A.R., 2004. Comparison of pulmonary/nasal CYP2F expression levels in rodents and rhesus macaque. *J Pharmacol Exp Ther* 309:127–136.

Balis, J.U., Paterson, J.F., Haller, E.M., Shelley, S.A., and Montgomery, M.R., 1988. Ozone-induced lamellar body responses in a rat model for alveolar injury and repair. *Am J Pathol* 132:330–344.

Barton, E.G., and Campbell, W.G., 1969. *Pneumocystis carinii* in lungs of rats treated with cortisone acetate. *Am J Pathol* 54(2):209–236.

Batenburg, J.J., and Haagsman, H.P., 1998. The lipids of pulmonary surfactant: Dynamics and interactions with proteins. *Prog Lipid Res* 37(4):235–276.

Bauer, A.K., Malkinson, A.M., and Kleeberger, S.R., 2004. Susceptibility to neoplastic and non-neoplastic pulmonary diseases in mice: genetic similarities. *Am J Physiol Lung Cell Molec Physiol* 287:L685–L703.

Beckmann, N., Tigani, B., Mazzoni, L., and Fozard, J.R., 2003. Techniques: magnetic resonance imaging of the lung provides potential for non-invasive preclinical evaluation of drugs. *Trends Pharmacol Sci* 24:550–554.

Beneke, S., and Rooney, S.A., 2001. Glucocorticoids regulate expression of the fatty acid synthase gene in fetal rat type II cells. *Biochim Biophys Acta* 1534:56–63.

Bennett, J.V., de Castro, J.F., Valdespino-Gomez, J.L., Garcia-Garcia, M., Islas-Romero, R., Echaniz-Aviles, G., Jimenez-Corona, A., and Sepulveda-Amor, J., 2002. Aerosolized measles and measles-rubella vaccines induce better measles antibody booster responses than injected vaccines: randomized trials in Mexican schoolchildren. *Bull World Health Organ* 80:806–812.

Bergman, U.B., Östergren, A., Gustafson, A.-L.G., and Brittebo, E.B., 2002. Differential effects of olfactory toxicants on olfactory regeneration. *Arch Toxicol* 76:104–112.

Bernick, S., and Alfin-Slater, R.B., 1963. Pulmonary infiltration of lipid in essential fatty-acid deficiency. Progressive changes. *Arch Pathol* 75:13–20.

Berry, C.R., Ackerman, N., and Monce, K., 1994. Pulmonary mineralization in four dogs with Cushing's syndrome. *Vet Radiol Ultrasound* 35(1):10–16.

Bhattacharyya, N., 2002. Cancer of the nasal cavity: survival and factors influencing prognosis. *Arch Otolaryngol Head Neck Surg* 128:1079–1083.

Bitterman, P.B., Saltzman, L.E., Adelberg, S., Ferrans, V.J., and Crystal, R.G., 1984. Alveolar macrophage replication. One mechanism for the expansion of the mononuclear phagocyte population in the chronically inflamed lung. *J Clin Invest* 74:460–469.

Blank, F., Rothen-Rutishauser, B., and Gehr, P., 2007. Dendritic cells and macrophages form a transepithelial network against foreign particulate antigens. *Am J Respir Cell Mol Biol* 36:669–677.

Blois, S.L., Caron. I., and Mitchell, C., 2009. Diagnosis and outcome of a dog with iatrogenic hyperadreno-corticism and secondary pulmonary mineralization. *Can Vet J* 50:397–400.

Bolton, S.J., Pinnion, K., Oreffo, V., Foster, M., and Pinkerton, K.E., 2009. Characterisation of the proximal airway squamous metaplasia induced by chronic tobacco smoke exposure in spontaneously hypertensive rats. *Resp Res* 10:118.

Boorman, G.A., Morgan, K.T., and Uraih, L.C., 1990. Nose, larynx and trachea. In *Pathology of the Fischer Rat*. G. Boorman, S.L. Eustis, C. Montgomery, and M. Elwell, editors. Academic Press, San Diego, pp. 315–338.

Boorman, G., Dixon, D., Elwell, M., Kerlin, R., Morton, D., Peters, T., Regan, K., and Sullivan, J., 2003. Assessment of hyperplastic lesions in rodent carcinogenicity studies. *Toxicol Pathol* 31:709–710.

Born, S.L., Fix, A.S., Caudill, D., and Lehman-McKeeman, L.D., 1998. Selective Clara cell injury in mouse lung following acute administration of coumarin. *Toxicol Appl Pharmacol* 151:45–56.

Bowdridge, S., and Gause, W.C., 2010. Regulation of alternative macrophage activation by chromatin remodeling. *Nat Immunol* 11:879–881.

Bozza, P.T., Magalhães, K.G., and Weller, P.F., 2009. Leukocyte lipid bodies—biogenesis and functions in inflammation. *Biochim Biophys Acta* 1791:540–551.

Brix, A.E., Latimer, K.S., Moore, G.E., and Roberts, R.E., 1994. Pulmonary alveolar microlithiasis and ossification in a dog. *Vet Pathol* 31:382–385.

Brown, H.R., Monticello, T.M., Maronpot, R.R., Randall, H.W., Hotchkiss, J.R., and Morgan, K.T., 1991. Proliferative and neoplastic lesions in the rodent nasal cavity. *Toxicol Pathol* 19:358–372.

Brown, D.M., Dransfield, I., Wetherill, G.Z., and Donaldson, K., 1993. LFA-1 and ICAM-1 in homotypic aggregation of rat alveolar macrophages: organic dust-mediated aggregation by a non-protein kinase C-dependent pathway. *Am J Respir Cell Mol Biol* 9:205–212.

Bucher, J.R., Huff, J., Haseman, J.K., Eustis, S.L., and Elwell, M.R., 1990a. Toxicology and carcinogenicity studies of diuretics in F344 rats and B6C3F1 mice 1. Hydrochlorothiazide. *J Appl Toxicol* 10(5):359–367.

Bucher, J.R., Huff, J., Haseman, J.K., Eustis, S.L., and Elwell, M.R., 1990b. Toxicology and carcinogenicity studies of diuretics in F344 rats and B6C3F1 mice 1. Furosemide. *J Appl Toxicol* 10(5):369–378.

Buckley, L.A., Morgan, K.T., Swenberg, J.A., James, R.A., Hamm, T.E., and Barrow, C.S., 1985. The toxicity of dimethylamine in F-344 rats and B6C3F1 mice following a 1-year inhalation exposure. *Fundam Appl Toxicol* 5:341–352.

Burns, M.G., Kelly, A.B., Hornoff, W.J., and Howerth, E.W., 1981. Pulmonary artery thrombosis in three dogs with hyperadrenocorticism. *J Am Vet Mod Assoc* 178:388–393.

Byers, D.E., and Holtzman, M.J., 2010. Alternatively activated macrophages as cause or effect in airway disease. *Am J Respir Cell Mol Biol* 43:1–4.

Calderwood, H.W., Modell, J.H., Rogow, L., Tham, M.K., and Hood, I., 1973. Morphologic and biochemical changes in dogs after ventilation with caroxin-D fluorocarbon. *Anesthesiology* 39(5):488–495.

Capen, C.C., Belshaw, B.E., and Martin, S.L., 1975. Endocrine disorders. In: *Textbook of Veterinary Internal Medicine*. S.J. Ettinger, editor. Sanders, Philadelphia, PA, pp. 1395–1403.

Casarosa, P., Bouyssou, T., Germeyer, S., Schnapp, A., Gantner, F., and Pieper, M., 2009. Preclinical evaluation of long-acting muscarinic antagonists: comparison of tiotropium and investigational drugs. *J Pharmacol Exp Therapeutics* 330:660–668.

Cesta, M.F., 2006. Normal structure, function, and histology of mucosa-associated lymphoid tissue. *Toxicol Pathol* 34:599–608.

Chan, E.D., Morales, D.V., Welsh, C.H., McDermott, M.T., and Schwarz, M.I., 2002. Calcium deposition with or without bone formation in the lung. *Am J Respir Crit Care Med* 165:1654–1669.

Chan, H.-K., and Gonda, I., 1989. Aerodynamic properties of elongated particles of cromoglycic acid. *J Aerosol Sci* 20(2):157–168.

Chandler, F.W., Frenkel, J.K., and Campbell, W.G., 1979. Animal model: *Pneumocystis carinii* pneumonia in the immunosuppressed rat. *Am J Pathol* 95(2):571–574.

Chandra, M., and Frith, C.H., 1992. Spontaneous neoplasms in B6C3F1 mice. *Toxicol Lett* 60:91–98.

Chang, J.C., Jagirdas, J., and Lesser, M., 1986. Long-term evolution of BCG- and CFA-induced granulomas in rat lungs. Correlation of histologic features with cells in bronchoalveolar lavage samples. *Am J Pathol* 125(1):16–27.

Chang, S.-W., and Ohara, N., 1994. Chronic biliary obstruction induces pulmonary intravascular phagocytosis and endotoxin sensitivity in rats. *J Clin Invest* 94:2009–2019.

Chiba, T., Bharucha, A.E., Thomforde, G.M., Kost, L.J., and Phillips, S.F., 2002. Model of rapid gastrointestinal transit in dogs: effects of muscarinic antagonists as a nitric oxide synthase inhibitor. *Neurogastroenterol Motil* 14(5):535–541.

Chono, S., Tanino, T., Seki, T., and Morimoto, K., 2006. Influence of particle size on drug delivery to rat alveolar macrophages following pulmonary administration of ciprofloxacin incorporated into liposomes. *J Drug Target* 14(8):557–566.

Chono, S., Tanino, T., Seki, T., and Morimoto, K., 2008. Efficient drug delivery to alveolar macrophages and lung epithelial lining fluid following pulmonary administration of liposomal ciprofloxacin in rats with pneumonia and estimation of its antibacterial effects. *Drug Dev Ind Pharm* 34:1090–1096.

Christmann, U., Buechner-Mxwell, V.A., Witonsky, S.G., and Hite, R.D., 2009. Role of lung surfactant in respiratory disease: current knowledge in large animal medicine. *J Vet Intern Med* 23:227–242.

Christopher, M.M., White, J.G., and Eaton, J.W., 1990. Erythrocyte pathology and mechanisms of Heinz body-mediated hemolysis in cats. *Vet Pathol* 27:299–310.

Clarke, J., Hurst, C., Martin, P., Vahle, J., Ponce, R., Mounho, B., Heidel, S., Andrews, L., Reynolds, T., and Cavagnaro, J., 2008. Duration of chronic toxicity studies for biotechnology-derived pharmaceuticals: is 6 months still appropriate? *Regulat Toxicol Pharmacol* 50:2–22.

Contrera, J.F., Jacobs, A.C., and DeGeorge, J.J., 1997. Carcinogenicity testing and the evaluation of regulatory requirements for pharmaceuticals. *Regulat Toxicol Pharmacol* 25:130–145.

Coonrod, J.D., Lester, R.L., and Hsu, L.C., 1984. Characterisation of the extracellular bactericidal factors of rat alveolar lining material. *J Clin Invest* 74(4):1269–1279.

Costa, R.H., Kalinichenko, V.V., and Lim, L., 2001. Transcription factors in mouse lung development and function. *Am J Physiol Lung Cell Mol Physiol* 280:L823–L838.

Cottrell, T.S., Levine, O.R., Senior, R.M., Wiener, J., Spiro, D., and Fishman, A.P., 1967. Electron microscopic alterations at the alveolar level in pulmonary edema. *Circ Res* XXI(6):783–797.

Crowell, W.A., Finco, D.R., Rawlings, C.A., Barsanti, J.A., and Rao, R.N., 1978. Lesions in dogs following renal transplantation and immunosuppression. *Vet Pathol* 24(2):124–128.

Cui, B., Cheng, Y.-S., Dai, D.-Z., Li, N., Zhang, T.-T., and Dai, Y., 2009. CPU0213, A non-selective ET_A/ET_B receptor antagonist, improves pulmonary arteriolar remodelling of monocrotaline-induced pulmonary hypertension in rats. *Clin Exp Pharmacol Physiol* 36:169–175.

Curran, D.R., and Cohn, L., 2010. Advances in mucous cell metaplasia: a plug for mucus as a therapeutic focus in chronic airway disease. *Am J Respir Cell Mol Biol* 42:268–275.

Damsch, S., Eichenbaum, G., Tonelli, A., Lammens, L., Van Den Bulck, K., Feyen, B., Vandenberghe, J., Megens, A., Knight, E., and Kelley, M., 2011. Gavage-related reflux in rats: identification, pathogenesis, and toxicological implications (review). *Toxicol Pathol* 39:348–360.

Davies, N.M., and Feddah, M.R., 2003. A novel method for assessing dissolution of aerosol inhaler products. *Int J Pharmaceut* 255:175–187.

Davis, C.W., and Dickey, B.F., 2008. Regulated airway goblet cell mucin secretion. *Annu Rev Physiol* 70:487–512.

Davis, M.S., Schofield, B., and Freed, A.N., 2003. Repeated peripheral airway hyperpnea causes inflammation and remodeling in dogs. *Med Sci Sports Exerc* 35(4):608–616.

Dayan, A.D., Morgan, R.J., Trefty, B.T., and Paddock, T.B., 1978. Naturally occurring diatomaceous pneumoconiosis in sub-human primates. *J Comp Pathol* 88(2):321–325.

Dayer, A.M., Kapanci, Y., Rademakers, A., Rusy, L.M., De Mey, J., and Will, J.A., 1985. Increased numbers of neuroepithelial bodies (NEB) in lungs of fetal rhesus monkeys following maternal dexamethasone treatment. *Cell Tissue Res* 239:703–705.

Degryse, A.L., and Lawson, W.E., 2011. Progress toward improving animal models for idiopathic pulmonary fibrosis. *Am J Med Sci* 341(6):444–449.

Delaunois, L.M., 2004. Mechanisms in pulmonary toxicology. *Clin Chest Med* 25:1–14.

DeLorme, M.P., and Moss, O.R., 2001. Pulmonary function assessment by whole-body plethysmography in restrained versus unrestrained mice. *J Pharmacol Toxicol Methods* 47:1–10.

Dixon, D., and Maronpot, R.R., 1991. Histomorphologic features of spontaneous and chemically-induced pulmonary neoplasms in B6C3F1 mice and Fischer 344 rats. *Toxicol Pathol* 19:540–555.

Dobbs, L.G., Johnson, M.D., Vanderbilt, J., Allen, L., and Gonzalez, R., 2010. The great big alveolar TI cell: evolving concepts and paradigms. *Cell Physiol Biochem* 25:55–62.

Driehuys, B., and Hedlund, L.W., 2007. Imaging techniques for small animal models of pulmonary disease: MR microscopy. *Toxicol Pathol* 35:49–58.

Duan, J.D., Jeffrey, A.M., and Williams, G.M., 2008. Assessment of the medicines lidocaine, prilocaine, and their metabolites, 2,6-dimethylaniline and 2-methylaniline, for DNA adduct formation in rat tissues. *Drug Metab Dispos* 36:1470–1475.

Dudley, R.E., Patterson, S.E., Machotka, S.V., and Kesterson, J.W., 1989. One-month inhalation toxicity study of tulobuterol hydrochloride in rats and dogs. *Fundam Appl Toxicol* 13:694–701.

Duffield, J.S., 2003. The inflammatory macrophage: a story of Jekyll and Hyde. *Clin Sci* 104:27–38.

Dungworth, D.L., Ernst, H., Nolte, T., and Mohr, U., 1992. Nonneoplastic lesions in the lungs. In: *Pathobiology of the Aging Rat*. U. Mohr, D.L. Dungworth, and C.C. Capen, editors. ILSI Press, Washington, DC, pp. 141–160.

Dungworth, D.L., Rittinghausen, S., Schwartz, L., Harkema, J.R., Hayashi, Y., Kittel, B., Lewis, D., Miller, R.A., Mohr, U., Morgan, K.T., Rehm, S., and Slayter, M.V., 2001. Respiratory system and mesothelium. In: *International Classification of Rodent Tumors, The Mouse*. U. Mohr, editor. Springer, London, pp. 87–138.

Duong, M., Ouellet, N., Simard, M., Bergeron, Y., Olivier, M., and Bergeron, M.G., 1998. Kinetic study of host defense and inflammatory response to *Aspergillus fumigatus* in steroid-induced immunosuppressed mice. *J Infect Dis* 178:1472–1482.

Dvorak, A.M., Morgan, E., Schleimer, R.P., Ryeom S.W., Lichtenstein, L.M., and Weller, P.F., 1992. Ultrastructural immunogold localization of prostaglandin endoperoxide synthase (cyclooxygenase) to non-membrane-bound cytoplasmic lipid bodies in human lung mast cells, alveolar macrophages, type II pneumocytes, and neutrophils. *J Histochem Cytochem* 40:759–769.

Edelson, J.D., Shannon, J.M., and Mason, R.J., 1988. Alkaline phosphatase: a marker of alveolar type II cell differentiation. *Am Rev Respir Dis* 138:1268–1275.

Eichenbaum, G., Damsch, S., Looszova, A., Vandenberghe, J., Van den Bulck, K., Roels, K., Megens, A., Knight, E., Hillsamer, V., Feyen, B., Kelley, M.F., Tonelli, A., and Lammens, L., 2011. Impact of gavage dosing procedure and gastric content on adverse respiratory effects and mortality in rat toxicity studies. *J Appl Toxicol* 31:342–354.

Endo, M., Oyadomari, S., Terasaki, Y., Takeya, M., Suga, M., Mori, M., and Gotoh, T., 2003. Induction of arginase I and II in bleomycin-induced fibrosis of mouse lung. *Am J Physiol Lung Cell Mol Physiol* 285:L313–L321.

Etherton, J.E., Conning, D.M., and Corrin, B., 1973. Autoradiographical and morphological evidence for apocrine secretion of dipalmitoyl lecithin in the terminal bronchiole of mouse lung. *Am J Anat* 138:11–36.

Eustis, S.L., 1989. The sequential development of cancer: A morphological perspective. *Toxicol Lett* 49:267–281.

Evans, M.J., Cabral, L.J., Stephens, R.J., and Freeman, G., 1975. Transformation of alveolar type 2 cells to type 1 cells following exposure to NO2. *Exp Molec Pathol* 22:142–150.

Ewing, P., Ryrfeldt, A., Sjöberg, C.-O., Andersson, P., Edsbäcker, S., and Gerde, P., 2010. Vasoconstriction after inhalation of budesonide: A study in the isolated and perfused rat lung. *Pulm Pharmacol Therapeut* 23:9–14.

Fallon, M.B., 2005. Mechanisms of pulmonary vascular complications of liver disease. Hepatopulmonary syndrome. *J Clin Gastroenterol* 39:S138–S142.

Fanucchi, M.V., and Plopper, C.G., 1997. Pulmonary developmental responses to toxicants. In: *Comprehensive Toxicology*. I.G. Sipes, C.A. McQueen, and A.J. Gandolfi, editors. Pergamon Elsevier Science, New York, pp. 203–220.

Farbman, A.I., 1990. Olfactory neurogenesis: genetic or environmental controls? *Trends Neurosci* 13:362–365.

Fehrenbach, A., Bube, C., Hohlfeld, J.M., Stevens, P.A., Tschernig, T., Hoymann, H.G., Krug, N., and Fehrenbach, H., 2003. Surfactant homeostasis is maintained in vivo during KGF-induced rat lung type II cell hyperplasia. *Am J Respir Crit Care Med* 167(9):1264–1270.

Fehrenbach, H., Kasper, M., Tschernig, T., Pan, T., Schuh, D., Shannon, J.M., Müller, M., and Mason, R.J., 1999. Keratinocyte growth factor-induced hyperplasia of rat alveolar type II cells in vivo is resolved by differentiation into type I cells and by apoptosis. *Eur Respir J* 14:534–544.

Fehrenbach, H., Fehrenbach, A., Pan, T., Kasper, M., and Mason, R.J., 2002. Keratinocyte growth factor-induced proliferation of rat airway epithelium is restricted to Clara cells *in vivo*. *Eur Respir J* 20:1185–1197.

Fengming, L., Zengli, W., Xiaojing, L., Chuntao, L., Xiaohong, Z., and Wenzhi, W., 2002. The effect of budesonide on Clara cell secretory protein and its mRNA expression in a rat model of asthma. *Chin J Tuberculosis Respir Dis* 25(9):538–541.

Ferin, J., 1982. Alveolar macrophage mediated pulmonary clearance suppressed by drug-induced phospholipidosis. *Exp Lung Res* 4:1–10.

Flodh, H., and Magnusson, G., 1973. Genesis of foam cells: study in rats after administration of Intralipid®. *Acta Pathol Microbiol Scand* 81(5):651–656.

Floettmann, E., Gregory, L., Teague, J., Myatt, J., Hammond, C., Poucher, S.M., and Jones, H.B., 2010. Prolonged inhibition of glycogen phosphorylase in livers of Zucker diabetic fatty rats models human glycogen storage disease. *Toxicol Pathol* 38:393–401.

Forbes, B., Asgharian, B., Dailey, L.A., Ferguson, D., Gerde, P., Gumbleton. M., Gustavsson, L., Hardy, C., Hassall, D., Jones, R., Lock, R., Maas. J., McGovern, T., Pitcairn, G.R., Somers, G., and Wolff, R.K., 2011. Challenges in inhaled product development and opportunities for open innovation. *Adv Drug Del Rev* 63:69–87.

Foster, D.J., Ravikumar, P., Bellotto, D.J., Unger, R.H., and Hsia, C.C.W., 2010. Fatty diabetic lung: altered alveolar structure and surfactant protein expression. *Am J Physiol Lung Cell Mol Physiol* 298:L392–L403.

Fringes, B., Gorgas, K., and Reith, A., 1988a. Modification of surfactant metabolizing cells in rat lung by clofibrate, a hypolipidemic peroxisome proliferating agent. Evidence to suggest that clofibrate influences pulmonary surfactant metabolism. *Virchows Archiv B Cell Pathol* 54:232–240.

Fringes, B., Gorgas, K., and Reith, A., 1988b. Clofibrate increases the number of peroxisomes and of lamellar bodies in alveolar cells type II of the rat lung. *Eur J Cell Biol* 46(1):136–143.

Fringes, B., Gorgas, K., and Reith, A., 1988c. Two hypolipidemic peroxisome proliferators increase the number of lamellar bodies in alveolar cells type II of the lung. *Exp Mol Pathol* 48(2):262–271.

Fults, K.A., Miller, I.F., and Hickey, A.J., 1997. Effect of particle morphology on emitted dose of fatty acid-treated disodium cromoglycate powder aerosols. *Pharm Dev Technol* 2(1):67–79.

Gehr, P., Green, F.H.Y., Geiser, M., Hof, I.M., Lee, M.M., and Schürch, S., 1996. Airway surfactant, a primary defense barrier: mechanical and immunological aspects. *J Aerosol Med* 9(2):164–181.

Geiser, M., 2010. Update on macrophage clearance of inhaled micro- and nanoparticles. *J Aerosol Med Pulm Drug Deliv* 23(4):207–217.

Genta, R.M., and Schad, G.A., 1984. *Filaroides hirthi*: hyperinfective lungworm infection in immunosuppressed dogs. *Vet Pathol* 21:349–354.

Genter, M.B., Deamer, N.J., Blake, B.L., Wesley, D.S., and Levi, P.E., 1995. Olfactory toxicity of methimazole: dose-response and structure-activity studies and characterization of flavin-containing monooxygenase activity in the Long-Evans rat olfactory mucosa. *Toxicol Pathol* 23:477–486.

Genter, M.B., Liang, H.C., Gu, J., Ding, X., Negishi, M., McKinnon, R.A., and Nebert, D.W., 1998. Role of CYP2A5 and 2G1 in acetaminophen metabolism and toxicity in the olfactory mucosa of the Cyp1a2(–/–) mouse. *Biochem Pharmacol* 55:1819–1826.

Germann, P.G., Ockert, D., and Tuch, K. 1995. Oropharyngeal granulomas and tracheal cartilage degeneration in Fischer-344 rats. *Toxicol Pathol* 23:349–355.

Germann, P.G., Ockert, D., and Heinrichs, M., 1998. Pathology of the oropharyngeal cavity in six strains of rats: predisposition of Fischer 344 rats for inflammatory and degenerative changes. *Toxicol Pathol* 26:283–289.

Gibson, G., and Barrett, E., 1992. The role of salivary function on oropharyngeal colonization. *Spec Care Dentist* 12(4):153–156.

Gil, J., and Weibel, E.R., 1971. Extracellular lining of bronchioles after perfusion-fixation of rat lungs for electron microscopy. *Anat Rec* 169(2):185–199.

Goggs, R., Benigni, L., Fuentes, V.L., and Chan, D.L., 2009. Pulmonary thromboembolism. *J Vet Emerg Crit Care* 19(1):30–52.

Gopinath, C., Prentice, D.E., and Lewis, D.J., 1987. The respiratory system. In: *Atlas of Experimental Toxicological Pathology*. MTP Press, Lancaster, pp. 22–42.

Gorbunov, N.V., Asher, L.V., Ayyagari, V., and Atkins, J.L., 2006. Inflammatory leukocytes and iron turnover in experimental hemorrhagic lung trauma. *Exp Mol Pathol* 80:11–25.

Gordon, S., 2003. Alternative activation of macrophages. *Nat Rev Immunol* 3:23–35.

Goya, S., Matsuoka, H., Mori, M., Morishita, H., Kida, H., Kobashi, Y., Kato, T., Taguchi, Y., Osaki, T., Tachibana, I., Nishimoto, N., Yoshizaki, K., Kaware, I., and Hayashi, S., 2003. Sustained interleukin-6 signalling leads to the development of lymphoid organ-like structures in the lung. *J Pathol* 200(1):82–87.

Greaves, P., 2007. *Histopathology of Preclinical Toxicity Studies,* 3rd edition, Elsevier, Amsterdam, pp. 215–269.

Greaves, P., and Faccini, J.M., 1984. *Rat Histopathology*, Elsevier, Amsterdam, pp. 62–73.

Grebenskaya, N.I., 1966. Histochemistry of lipids in the lungs. *Bull Exp Biol Med* 64(3):1019–1021.

Gross, E.A., Patterson, D.L., and Morgan, K.T., 1987. Effects of acute and chronic dimethylamine exposure on the nasal mucociliary apparatus of F-344 rats. *Toxicol Appl Pharmacol* 90:359–376.

Gross, P., Pfitzer, E.A., and Hatch, T.F., 1966. Alveolar clearance: its relation to lesions of the respiratory bronchiole. *Am Rev Resp Dis* 94:10–19.

Gu, J., Walker, V.E., Lipinskas, T.W., Walker, D.M., and Ding, X., 1997. Intraperitoneal administration of coumarin causes tissue-selective depletion of cytochromes P450 and cytotoxicity in the olfactory mucosa. *Toxicol Appl Pharmacol* 146:134–143.

Guidot, D.M., Modelska, K., Lois, M., Jain, L., Moss, I.M., Pittet, J-F., and Brown, L.A.S., 2000. Ethanol ingestion via glutathione depletion impairs alveolar epithelial barrier function in rats. *Am J Physiol Lung Cell Mol Physiol* 279:L127–L135.

Hagen, G., Wolf, M., Katyal, S.L., Singh, G., Beato, M., and Suske, G., 1990. Tissue specific expression, hormonal regulation at 5^1-flanking gene region of the rat Clara cell 10KDa protein comparison with rabbit uteroglobin. *Nucleic Acids Res* 18:2939–2946.

Hahn, F.F., Muggenburg, B.A., and Griffith, W.C., 1996. Primary lung neoplasia in a beagle colony. *Vet Pathol Online* 33:633–638.

Hahn, F.F., Gigliotti, A., and Hutt, J.A., 2007. Comparative oncology of lung tumors. *Toxicol Pathol* 35:130–135.

Hahn, F.F., and Dagle, G.E., 2001. Non-neoplastic pulmonary lesions. In: *Pathobiology of the Aging Dog*. U. Mohr, W.W. Carlton, D.L. Dungworth, S.A. Benjamin, C.C. Capen, and F.F. Hahn, editors. Iowa State University Press, Ames, IA, pp. 57–65.

Haley, P.J., 2003. Species differences in the structure and function of the immune system. *Toxicology* 188:49–71.

Hallman, M., and Bry, K., 1996. Nitric oxide and lung surfactant. *Semin Perinatol* 20(3):173–185.

Hammer, A.S., 1991. Thrombocytosis in dogs and cats: a retrospective study. *Comp Haematol Int* 1:181–186.

Hanton, G., Sobry, C., Dagues, J.P., Provost, J.P., Le Net, J.-L., Comby, P., and Chevalier, S., 2008. Characterisation of the vascular and inflammatory lesions induced by the PDE4 inhibitor CI-1044 in the dog. *Toxicol Lett* 179:15–22.

Hanumegowda, U.M., Wenke, G., Regueiro-Ren, A., Yordanova, R., Corradi, J.P., and Adams, S.P., 2010. Phospholipidosis as a function of basicity, lipophilicity, and volume of distribution of compounds. *Chem Res Toxicol* 23:749–755.

Hardisty, J.F., Garman, R.H., Harkema, J.R., Lomax, L.G., and Morgan, K.T., 1999. Histopathology of nasal olfactory mucosa from selected inhalation toxicity studies conducted with volatile chemicals. *Toxicol Pathol* 27:618–627.

Harkema, J.R., 1990. Comparative pathology of the nasal mucosa in laboratory animals exposed to inhaled irritants. *Environ Health Perspect* 85:231–238.

Harkema, J.R., 1991. Comparative aspects of nasal airway anatomy: relevance to inhalation toxicology. *Toxicol Pathol* 19:321–336.

Harkema, J.R., Carey, S.A., and Wagner, J.G., 2006. The nose revisited: a brief review of the comparative structure, function, and toxicologic pathology of the nasal epithelium. *Toxicol Pathol* 34:252–269.

Harmsen, A.G., Mason, M.J., Muggenburg, B.A., Gillett, N.A., Jarpe, M.A., and Bice, D.E., 1987. Migration of neutrophils from lung to tracheobronchial lymph node. *J Leuk Biol* 41(2):95–103.

Hartings, J.M., and Roy, C.J., 2001. The automated bioaerosol exposure system: preclinical platform development and a respiratory dosimetry application with nonhuman primates. *J Pharmacol Toxicol Methods* 49:39–55.

Haseman, J.K., and Hailey, J.R., 1997. An update of the National Toxicology Program database on nasal carcinogens. *Mutat Res/Fundam Molec Mech Mutagen* 380:3–11.

Haseman, J.K., Arnold, J., and Eustis, S.L., 1990. Tumor incidences in Fischer 344 rats: NTP historical data. In: *Pathology of the Fischer Rat*. G. Boorman, S.L. Eustis, C. Montgomery, and M. Elwell, editors. Academic Press, San Diego, pp. 555–564.

Haseman, J.K., Hailey, J.R., and Morris, R.W., 1998. Spontaneous neoplasm incidences in Fischer 344 rats and B6C3F1 mice in two-year carcinogenicity studies: a National Toxicology Program update. *Toxicol Pathol* 26:428–441.

Haworth, R., Woodfine, J., McCawley, S., Pilling, A.M., Lewis, D.J., and Williams, T.C., 2007. Pulmonary neuroendocrine cell hyperplasia: identification, diagnostic criteria and incidence in untreated ageing rats of different strains. *Toxicol Pathol* 35:735–740.

Hayashi, H., Kumazaki, T., and Asano, G., 1994. Pulmonary edema induced by intravenous administration of contact media: experimental study in rats. *Radiat Med* 12(2):47–52.

Heidsiek, J.G., Hyde, D.M., Plopper, C.G., and St George, J.A., 1987. Quantitative histochemistry of mucosubstance in tracheal epithelium of the macaque monkey. *J Histochem Cytochem* 35:435–442.

Helming, L., and Gordon, S., 2009. Molecular mediators of macrophage fusion. *Trends Cell Biol* 19(10):514–522.

Henderson, R.F., 2005. Use of bronchoalveolar lavage to detect respiratory tract toxicity of inhaled material. *Exp Toxicol Pathol* 57:155–159.

Henderson, R.F., Driscoll, K.E., Harkema, J.R., Lindenschmidt, R.C., Chang, I.-Y., Maples, K.R., and Barr, E.B., 1995. A comparison of the inflammatory response of the lung to inhaled versus instilled particles in F344 rats. *Fundam Appl Toxicol* 24:183–197.

Herbert, R.A., and Leininger, J.R., 1999. Nose, larynx and trachea. In: *Pathology of the Mouse*. R.R. Maronpot, editor. Cache River Press, Vienna, IL, pp. 259–292.

Hermans, C., and Bernard, A., 1999. Lung epithelium-specific proteins. Characteristics and potential applications as markers. *Am J Respir Crit Care Med* 159:646–678.

Hermans, C., Knoops, B., Wiedig, M., Arsalane, K., Toubeau, G., Falmagne, P., and Bernard, A., 1999. Clara cell protein as a marker of Clara cell damage and bronchoalveolar blood barrier permeability. *Eur Respir J* 13:1014–1021.

Hilbe, M., Sydler, T., Fischer, L., and Naegeli, H., 2000. Metastatic calcification in a dog attributable to ingestion of a tacalcitol ointment. *Vet Pathol* 37:490–492.

Hiloowala, R.A., and Lass, N.J., 1978. Spectrographic analysis of laryngeal air sac resonance in rhesus monkey. *Am J Phys Anthropol* 49:129–131.

Hoenerhoff, M.J., Starost, M.F., and Ward, J.M., 2006. Eosinophilic crystalline pneumonia as a major cause of death in 129S4/SvJae mice. *Vet Pathol* 43:682–688.

Hohlfeld, J., Fabel, H., and Hamm, H., 1997. The role of pulmonary surfactant in obstructive airways disease. *Eur Respir J* 10:482–491.

Holt, P.F., 1983. Translocation of inhaled dust to the pleura. *Environ Res* 31:212–220.

Hood, C.I., and Modell, J.H., 2000. A morphologic study of long-term retention of fluorocarbon after liquid ventilation. *Chest* 118:1436–1440.

Hook, G.E.R., 1991. Alveolar proteinosis and phopholipidoses of the lungs. *Toxicol Pathol* 19:482–513.

Howroyd, P., Allison, N., Foley, J.F., and Hardisty, J., 2009. Apparent alveolar bronchiolar tumors arising in the mediastinum of F344 rats. *Toxicol Pathol* 37:351–358.

Hoymann, H.G., 2006. New developments in lung function measurements in rodents. *Exp Toxicol Pathol* 57:5–11.

Hoyt, J., 1990. Analytic reviews: aspiration pneumonitis: patient risk factors, prevention and management. *J Int Care Med* 5:S2–S9.

Hyde, D.M., Harkema, J.R., Tyler, N.K., and Plopper, C.G., 2006. Design-based sampling and quantitation of the respiratory airways. *Toxicol Pathol* 34:286–295.

Innes, J.R.M., Garner, F.M., and Stookey, J.L., 1967, Respiratory disease in rats. In: *Pathology of Laboratory Rats and Mice*. E. Cotchin and F.J.C. Roe, editors. Blackwell Scientific Publications, Oxford and Edinburgh, pp. 229–257.

Isaka, H., Yoshi, H., Otsuji, A., Koike, M., Nagai, Y., Masatoshi, K., Sugiyasu, K., and Kanabayashi, T., 1979. Tumors of Sprague–Dawley rats induced by long-term feeding of phenacetin. *Gann* 70:29–36.

Jeffrey, A.M., Iatropoulos, M.J., and Williams, G.M., 2006. Nasal cytotoxic and carcinogenic activities of systemically distributed organic chemicals. *Toxicol Pathol* 34:827–852.

Jeffery, P.K., and Reid, L., 1975. New observations of rat airway epithelium: a quantitative and electron microscopic study. *J. Anat* 120:295–320.

Johanson, G., 2003. Occupational exposure limits—approaches and criteria. Proc NIVA Uppsala, Sweden, 24–28 September 2001. Arbete och Halsa17:1–109.

Johnson, K.A., 2007. Imaging techniques for small animal imaging models of pulmonary disease: micro-CT. *Toxicol Pathol* 35:59–64.

Kambara, T., McKevitt, T.P., Francis, I., Woodfine, J.A., McCawley, S.J., Jones, S.A., Pilling, A.M., Lewis, D.J., and Williams, T.C., 2009. Eosinophilic inclusions in rat Clara cells and the effect of an inhaled corticosteroid. *Toxicol Pathol* 37:315–323.

Karnati, S., and Baumgart-Vogt, E., 2008. Peroxisomes in mouse and human lung: their involvement in pulmonary lipid metabolism. *Histochem Cell Biol* 130(4):719–740.

Kasahara, Y., Tuder, R.M., Taraseviciene-Stewart, L., Le Cras, T.D., Abman, S., Hirth, P.K., Waltenberger, J., and Voelkel, N.F., 2000. Inhibition of VEGF receptors causes lung cell apoptosis and emphysema. *J Clin Invest* 106:1311–1319.

Kasahara, K., Yamakawa, S., Nagatani, M., Tsurukame, M., and Tamura, K., 2008. Spontaneous leiomyosarcoma arising from the ethmoid turbinate of a rat. *Toxicol Pathol* 36:247–249.

Kaspareit, J., Friderichs-Gromoll, S., Buse, E., and Habermann, G., 2007. Spontaneous neoplasms observed in cynomolgus monkeys (*Macaca fascicularis*) during a 15-year period. *Exp Toxicol Pathol* 59:163–169.

Kaufmann, W., Bader, R., Ernst, H., Harada, T., Hardisty, J., Kittel, B., Kolling, A., Pino, M., Renne, R., Rittinghausen, S., Schulte, A., Wöhrmann, T., and Rosenbruch, M., 2009. 1st International ESTP Expert Workshop: "Larynx squamous metaplasia." A re-consideration of morphology and diagnostic approaches in rodent studies and its relevance for human risk assessment. *Exp Toxicol Pathol* 61:591–603.

Kehrer, J.P., and Kacew, S., 1985. Systematically applied chemicals that damage lung tissue. *Toxicology* 35:251–293.

Kennedy, M.A., Barrera, G.C., Nakamura, K., Baldan, A., Tarr, P., Fishbein, M.C., Frank, J., Francone, O.L., and Edwards, P.A., 2005. ABCG1 has a critical role in mediating cholesterol efflux to HDL and preventing cellular lipid accumulation. *Cell Metab* 1:121–131.

Kepler, G.M., Joyner, D.R., Fleishman, A., Richardson, R., Gross, E.A., Morgan, K.T., Kimbell, J.S., and Godo, M.N., 1995. Method for obtaining accurate geometrical coordinates of nasal airways for computer dosimetry modeling and lesion mapping. *Inhal Toxicol* 7:1207–1224.

Khoor, A., Gray, M.E., Singh, G., and Stahlman, M.T., 1996. Ontogeny of Clara cell-specific protein and its mRNA: their association with neuroepithelial bodies in human fetal lung and in bronchopulmonary dysplasia. *J Histochem Cytochem* 44:1429–1438.

Kikkawa, Y., and Suzuki, K., 1972. Alteration of cellular and acellular alveolar and bronchiolar walls produced by hypocholesteremic drug AY99. *Lab Invest* 26(4):441–447.

Kishore, U., Greenhough, T.J., Waters, P., Shrive, A.K., Ghai, R., Kamran, M.F., Bernal, A.L., Reid, K.B.M., Madan, T., and Chakraborty, T., 2006. Surfactant proteins SP-A and SP-D: structure, function and receptors. *Mol Immunol* 43:1293–1315.

Kitamura, H., Inayama, Y., Ito, T., Yabana, M., Piegorsch, W.W. and Kanisawa, M., 1987. Morphologic alteration of mouse Clara cells induced by glycerol: ultrastructural and morphometric studies. *Exp Lung Res* 12:281–302.

Kittel, B., Ruehl-Fehlert, C., Morawietz, G., Klapwijk, J., Elwell, M.R., Lenz, B., O'Sullivan, M.G., Roth, D.R., and Wadsworth, P.F., 2004. Revised guides for organ sampling and trimming in rats and mice—Part 2: A joint publication of the RITA and NACAD groups. *Exp Toxicol Pathol* 55:413–431.

Klapwijk, J., 2011. HESI Emerging Issues. Alveolar macrophage changes in response to inhaled drugs: factors distinguishing adaptive from adverse effects. HESI Annual Meeting, June 2011.

Kleinig, T.J., Helps, S.C., Ghabriel, M.N., Manavis, J., Leigh, C., Blumbergs, P.C., and Vink, R., 2009. Hemoglobin crystals: A pro-inflammatory potential confounder of rat experimental intracerebral haemorrhage. *Brain Res* 1287:164–172.

Kooistra, H.S., and Galac, S., 2010. Recent advances in the diagnosis of Cushing's syndrome in dogs. *Vet Clin Small Anim* 40:259–267.

Koyama, S., Sato, E., Nomura, H., Kubo, K., Nagai, S., and Izumi, T., 1997. Type II pneumocytes release chemoattractant activity for monocytes constitutively. *Am J Physiol* 272:L830–L837.

Kramer, B.W., Jobe, A.H., and Ikegami, M., 2001. Exogenous surfactant changes the phenotype of alveolar macrophages in mice. *Am J Physiol Lung Cell Mol Physiol* 280:L689–L694.

Kreyling, W.G., Takenaka, S., Schumann, G., and Ziesenis, A., 2001. Particles are predominantly transported from the canine alveolar epithelium towards the interstitial spaces and not to larynx! Analogy to human lungs. *Am J Respir Crit Care Med* 163:A166.

Kuempel, E.D., 2000. Comparison of human and rodent lung dosimetry models for particle clearance and retention. *Drug Chem Toxicol* 23(1):203–222.

Kumar, V., Abbas, A., Fausto, N., and Aster, J., 2010. Acute and chronic inflammation. In: *Pathologic Basis of Disease.* V. Kumar, A. Abbas, N. Fausto, and J. Aster, editors. Saunders Elsevier, Philadelphia, pp. 43–78.

Lanken, P.N., Minda, M., Pietra, G.G., and Fishman, A.P., 1980. Alveolar responses to experimental *Pneumocystis carinii* pneumonia in the rat. *Am J Pathol* 99:561–588.

Laplante, C., and Lemaire, I., 1990. Interactions between alveolar macrophage subpopulations modulate their migratory function. *Am J Pathol* 136:199–206.

Larsen, A.K., Newberne, P.M., and Langer, R., 1986. Comparative studies of heparin and heparin fragments: distribution and toxicity in the rat. *Fundam Appl Toxicol* 7:86–93.

Laskin, D.L., Sunil, V.R., Gardner, C.R., and Laskin, J.D., 2011. Macrophages and tissue injury: agents of defense or destruction? *Annu Rev Pharmacol Toxicol* 51:267–288.

Lehnert, B.E., 1990. Alveolar macrophages in a particle "overload" condition. *J Aerosol Med* 3(1):S9–S30.

Lehnert, B.E., 1992. Pulmonary and thoracic macrophage subpopulations and clearance of particles from the lung. *Environ Health Perspect* 97:17–46.

Leininger, J.R., Herbert, R.A., and Morgan, K.T., 1996. Aging changes in the upper respiratory tract. In: *Pathobiology of the Aging Mouse*, Volume 1. U. Mohr, D.L. Dungworth, C.C. Capen, W.W. Carlton, J.P. Sundberg, and J.M. Ward, editors. ILSI, Washington, pp. 245–328.

Lewis, D.J., 1981. Factors affecting the distribution of tobacco smoke-induced lesions in the rodent larynx. *Toxicol Lett* 9:189–194.

Lewis, D.J., 1991. Morphological assessment of pathological changes within the rat larynx. *Toxicol Pathol* 19:352–357.

Lewis, J.L., Nikula, K.J., and Sachetti, L.A., 1995. Induced xenobiotic metabolizing enzymes localized to eosinophilic globules in olfactory epithelium of toxicant-exposed F344 rats. In: *Nasal Toxicity and Dosimetry of Inhaled Xenobiotics: Implications for Human Health*. F.J. Miller, editor. Taylor & Francis, Washington, DC, pp. 422–425.

Li, X., Botts, S., Morton, D., Knickerbocker, M.J., and Adler, R., 2006. Oleic acid-associated bronchiolitis obliterans-organizing pneumonia in beagle dogs. *Vet Pathol* 43:183–185.

Liebow, A.A., 1959. Pulmonary emphysema with reference to vascular changes. *Am Rev Respir Dis* 80(1):67–93.

Livingston, R.S., Besch-Williford, C.L., Myles, M.H., Franklin, C.L., Crim, M.J., and Riley, L.K., 2011. *Pneumocystis carinii* infection causes lung lesions historically attributed to rat respiratory virus. *Comp Med* 61(1):45–52.

Lopez, I., Aguilera-Tejero, E., Mendoza, F.J., Almaden, Y., Perez, J., Martin, D., and Rodriguez M., 2006. Calcimimetic R-568 decrease extraosseous calcifications in uremic rats treated with calcitriol. *J Am Soc Nephrol* 17:795–804.

Losco, P.E., Evans, E.W., Barat, S.A., Blackshear, P.E., Reyderman, L., Fine, J.S., Bober, L.A., Anthes, J.C., Mirro, E.J., and Cuss, F.M., 2004. The toxicity of SCH 351591, a novel phosphodiesterase-4 inhibitor in cynomolgus monkeys. *Toxicol Pathol* 32(3):295–308.

Ma, J., Chen, T., Mandelin, J., Ceponis, A., Miller, N.E., Hukkanen, M., Ma, G.F., and Konttinen, Y.T., 2003. Regulation of macrophage activation. *CMLS Cell Mol Life Sci* 60:2334–2346.

Macklin, C.C., 1955. Pulmonary sumps, dust accumulations, alveolar fluid and lymph vessels. *Acta Anat* 23:1–33.

Maita, K., Hirano, M., Harada, T., Mitsumori, K., Yoshida, A., Takahashi, K., Nakashima, N., Kitazawa, T., Enomoto, A., Inui, K., and Shirasu, Y., 1988. Mortality, major cause of moribundity, and spontaneous tumors in CD-1 mice. *Toxicol Pathol* 16:340–349.

Massaro, G.D., Fischman, C.M., Chiang, M.J., Amado, C., and Massaro, D., 1981. Regulation of secretion in Clara cells: studies using the isolated perfused rat lung. *J Clin Invest* 67:345–351.

Mendes, E.S., Pereira, A., Danta, I., Duncan, R.C., and Wanner, A., 2003. Comparative bronchial vasoconstrictive efficacy of inhaled glucocorticosteroids. *Eur Respir J* 21:989–993.

Mery, S., Gross, E.A., Joyner, D.R., Godo, M., and Morgan, K.T., 1994. Nasal diagrams: a tool for recording the distribution of nasal lesions in rats and mice. *Toxicol Pathol* 22:353–372.

Meyrick, B., 2001. The pathology of pulmonary artery hypertension. *Clin Chest Med* 22(3):393–404.

Michael, B., Yano, B., Sellers, R.S., Perry, R., Morton, D., Roome, N., Johnson, J.K., and Schafer, K., 2007. Evaluation of organ weights for rodent and non-rodent toxicity studies: a review of regulatory guidelines and a survey of current practices. *Toxicol Pathol* 35:742–750.

Miot-Noirault, E., Faure, L., Guichard, Y., Montharu, J., and Le Pape, A., 2001. Scintigraphic in vivo assessment of the development of pulmonary intravascular macrophages in liver disease. Experimental study in rats with biliary cirrhosis. *Chest* 120:941–947.

Miserocchi, G., 2007. Lung interstitial pressure and structure in acute hypoxia. *Hypoxia and the Circulation*. R.C. Roach et al., editors. Springer, New York, pp. 141–168.

Misson, P., van den Brule, S., Barbarin, V., Lison, D., and Huaux, F., 2004. Markers of macrophage differentiation in experimental silicosis. *J Leukoc Biol* 76:926–932.

Modell, J.H., Calderwood, H.W., Ruiz, B.C., Tham, M.K., and Hood, C.I., 1976. Liquid ventilation of primates. *Chest* 69:79–81.

Monticello, T.M., Morgan, K.T., and Uraih, L., 1990. Nonneoplastic nasal lesions in rats and mice. *Environ Health Perspect* 85:249–274.

Morrow, P.E., 1972. Lymphatic drainage of the lung in dust clearance. *NY Acad Sci* 22:46–65.

Morrow, P.E., 1988. Possible mechanisms to explain dust overloading of the lungs. *Fundam Appl Toxicol* 10:369–384.

Morrow, P.E., 1992. Dust overloading of the lungs: update and appraisal. *Toxicol Appl Pharmacol* 113:1–12.

Mosser, D.M., and Edwards, J.P., 2008. Exploring the full spectrum of macrophage activation. *Nat Rev Immunol* 8(12):958–969.

Murphy, D.J. 1994. Safety pharmacology of the respiratory system: techniques and study design. *Drug Dev Res* 32:237–246.

Murphy, D.J., Renninger, J.P., and Coatney, R.W., 2007. A novel method for chronic measurement of respiratory function in the conscious monkey. *J Pharmacol Toxicol Methods* 46:13–20.

Murray, P.J., and Wynn, T.A., 2011. Obstacles and opportunities for understanding macrophage polarization. *J Leukoc Biol* 89:557–563.

Myers, M.A., Thomas, D.A., Straub, L., Soucy, D.W., Niven, R.W., Kaltenbach, M., Hood, C.I., Schreier, H., and Gonzalez-Rothi, R.J., 1993. Pulmonary effects of chronic exposure to liposome aerosols in mice. *Exp Lung Res* 19:1–19.

Myers, R.B., Fredenburgh, J.L., and Grizzle, W.E., 2008. Carbohydrates. In: *Theory and Practice of Histological Techniques*. J.D. Bancroft and M. Gamble, editors. Churchill Livingstone Elsevier, Philadelphia, pp. 161–186.

Nalesnik, M.A., Todo, S., Murase, N., Gryzan, S., Lee, P.-H., Makowka, L., and Starzl, T.E., 1987. Toxicology of FK-506 in the Lewis rat. *Transplant Proc* 19(5 Supp 6):89–92.

Namovic, M.T., Walsh, R.E., Goodfellow, C., Harris, R.R., Carter, G.W., and Bell, R.L., 1996. Pharmacological modulation of eosinophil influx into the lungs of Brown Norway rats. *Eur J Pharmacol* 315:81–88.

Nelson, A.A., and Fitzhugh, O.G., 1948. Chloroquine (SN-7618) pathologic changes observed in rats which for 2 years had been fed various proportions. *Arch Pathol* 45(4):454–462.

Nemes, Z., Dietz, R., Mann, J.F.E., Luth, J.B., and Gross, F., 1980. Vasoconstriction and increased blood pressure in the development of accelerated vascular disease. *Virchows Arch A Pathol Anat Histol* 386:161–173.

Nettesheim, P., and Szakal, A.K., 1972. Morphogenesis of alveolar bronchiolization. *Lab Invest* 26(2):210–219.

Nielsen, S., King, L.S., Christensen, B.M., and Agre, P., 1997. Aquaporins in complex tissues. II. Subcellular distribution in respiratory and glandular tissues of rat. *Am J Physiol Cell Physiol* 273:C1549–C1561.

Nikitin, A.Y., Alcaraz, A., Anver, M.R., Bronson, R.T., Cardiff, R.D., Dixon, D., Fraire, A.E., Gabrielson, E.W., Gunning, W.T., Haines, D.C., Kaufman, M.H., Linnoila, R.I., Maronpot, R.R., Rabson, A.S., Reddick, R.L., Rehm, S., Rozengurt, N., Schuller, H.M., Shmidt, E.N., Travis, W.D., Ward, J.M., and Jacks, T., 2004. Classification of proliferative pulmonary lesions of the mouse. *Cancer Res* 64:2307–2316.

Nkadi, P.O., Merritt, T.A., and Pillers, D.-E.M., 2009. An overview of pulmonary surfactant in the neonate: genetics, metabolism, and the role of surfactant in health and disease. *Mol Genet Metab* 97:95–101.

Noorman, F., Braat, E.A., Barrett-Bergshoeff, M., Barbe, E., van Leeuwen, A., Lindeman, J., and Rijken, D.C., 1997. Monoclonal antibodies against the human mannose receptor as a specific marker in flow cytometry and immunohistochemistry for macrophages. *J Leukoc Biol* 61:63–72.

Nunes, H., Lebrec, D., Mazmanian, M., Capron, F., Heller, J., Tazi, K.A., Zerbib, E., Dulmet, E., Moreau, R., Dinh-Xuan, A.T., Simonneau, G., and Hervé, P., 2001. Role of nitric oxide in hepatopulmonary syndrome in cirrhotic rats. *Am J Respir Crit Care Med* 164:879–885.

Obert, L.A., Sobocinski, G.P., Bobrowski, W.F., Metz, A.L., Rolsma, M.D., Altrogge, D.M., and Dunstan, R.W., 2007. An immunohistochemical approach to differentiate hepatic lipidosis from hepatic phospholipidosis in rats. *Toxicol Pathol* 35:728–734.

Ochs, M., Nenadic, I., Fehrenbach, A., Albes, J.M., Wahlers, T., Richter, J., and Fehrenbach, H., 1999. Ultrastructural alterations in intraalveolar surfactant subtypes after experimental ischemia and reperfusion. *Am J Respir Crit Care Med* 160:718–724.

Ochs, M., Fehrenbach, H., and Richter, J., 2004. Occurrence of lipid bodies in canine type II pneumocytes during hypothermic lung ischemia. *Anat Rec Part A* 277a:287–297.

OECD, 2009. OECD Environment Directorate Publications Series on Testing and Assessment No. 39—Guidance Document on Acute Inhalation Toxicity Testing.

Ohmiya, Y., Angevine, L.S., and Mehendale, H.M., 1983. Effect of drug induced phospholipidosis on pulmonary disposition of pneumophilic drugs. *Drug Metab Dispos* 11:25–30.

Okazaki, S., Yamazaki, E., Tamura, K., Hoshiya, T., Anabuki, K., Tanaka, H., and Tanaka, G., 1992. A 13-week subcutaneous toxicity study of prednisolone farnesylate (PNF) in rats. *J Toxicol Sci* 17(III):1–48.

Okigami, H., Takeshita, K., Tajimi, M., Komura, H., Albers, M., Lehmann, T.E., Rölle, T., and Bacon, K.B., 2007. Inhibition of eosinophilia in vivo by a small molecule inhibitor of very late antigen (VLA)-4. *Eur J Pharmacol* 559:202–209.

Oliveira, M.J.R., Pereira, A.S., Guimarães, L., Grande, N.R., Moreira de Sá, C., and Aquas, A.P., 2003. Zonation of ciliated cells on the epithelium of the rat trachea. *Lung* 181:275–282.

Owen, K., 2011. Regulatory toxicology considerations for the development of inhaled pharmaceuticals. *Drug Chem Toxicol.* doi:10.3109/01480545.2011.648327.

Owen, K., Beck, S.L., and Damment, S.J.P., 2010. The preclinical toxicology of salmeterol hydroxynaphthoate. *Human Exp Toxicol* 29(5):393–407.

Pabst, R., and Gehrke, I., 1990. Is the bronchus-associated lymphoid tissue (BALT) an integral structure of the lung in normal mammals, including humans? *Am J Respir Cell Mol Biol* 3:131–135.

Papiris, S.A., Triantafillidou, C., Kolilekas, L., Markoulaki, D., and Manali, E.D., 2010. Amiodarone review of pulmonary effects and toxicity. *Drug Saf* 33(7):539–558.

Patrikios, J., Martin, C.J., and Dent, J., 1986. Relationship of transient lower esophageal sphincter relaxation to postprandial gastroesophageal reflux and belching in dogs. *Gastroenterology* 90(3):545–551.

Patton, J.S., and Platz, R.M., 1992. Pulmonary delivery of peptides and proteins for systemic action. *Adv Drug Del Rev* 8:179–196.

Patton, J.S., and Byron, P.R., 2007. Inhaling medicines: delivering drugs to the body through the lungs. *Nature* 6:67–74.

Pauluhn, J., 2005. Inhaled cationic amphiphilic drug-induced pulmonary phospholipidosis in rats and dogs: time-course and dose-response of biomarkers of exposure and effect. *Toxicology* 207:59–72.

Percy, D.H., and Barthold, S.W., 2007. *Pathology of Laboratory Rodents and Rabbits*, 3rd edition, Blackwell Publishing, Ames, Iowa, USA.

Peres e Serra, A., Parra, E.R., Eher, E., and Capelozzi, V.L., 2006. Nonhomogeneous immunostaining of hyaline membranes in different manifestations of diffuse alveolar damage. *Clinics* 61(6):497–502.

Piccotti, J.R., LaGattuta, M.S., Knight, S.A., Gonzales, A.J., and Bleavins, M.R., 2005. Induction of apoptosis by cationic amphiphilic drugs amiodarone and imipramine. *Drug Chem Toxicol* 28(1):117–133.

Pino, M.V., Valerio, M.G., Miller, G.K., Larson, J.L., Rosolia, D.L., Jayyosi, Z., Crouch, C.N., Trojanowski, J.Q., and Geiger, L.E., 1999. Toxicologic and carcinogenic effects of the type IV phosphodiesterase inhibitor RP 73401 on the nasal olfactory tissue in rats. *Toxicol Pathol* 27:383–394.

Plopper, C.G., and Harkema, J.R., 2005. The respiratory system and its uses in research. In: *The Laboratory Primate*. S. Wolfe-Coote, editor. Elsevier, London, pp. 503–526.

Presneill, J.J., Nakata, K., Inoue, Y., and Seymour, J.F., 2004. Pulmonary alveolar proteinosis. *Clin Chest Med* 25:593–613.

Price, P.A., Buckley, J.R., and Williamson, M.K., 2001. The amino bisphosphonate ibandronate prevents vitamin D toxicity and inhibits vitamin-D induced calcification of arteries, cartilage, lungs and kidneys in rats. *J Nutr* 131:2910–2915.

Rabinow, B.E., 2004. Nanosuspensions in drug delivery. *Nat Rev* 3:785–796.

Ramos-Barbón, D., Ludwig, M.S., and Martin, J.G., 2004. Airway remodelling. Lessons from animal models. *Clin Rev Allergy Immunol* 27:3–21.

Rasenack, N., Steckel, H., and Müller, B.W., 2003. Micronization of anti-inflammatory drugs for pulmonary delivery by a controlled crystallization process. *J Pharm Sci* 92:35–44.

Rawlins, E.L., Okubo, T., Xue, Y., Brass, D.M., Auten, R.L., Hasegawa, H., Wang, F., and Hogan, B.L.M. 2009. The role of Scgb1a1+ Clara cells in the long-term maintenance and repair of lung airway, but not alveolar, epithelium. *Cell Stem Cell* 4:525–534.

Reasor, M.J., and Kacew, S., 2001. Drug-induced phospholipidosis: are there functional consequences. *Exp Biol Med* 226(9):825–830.

Reid, L., Meyrick, B., Antony, V.B., Chang, L.Y., Crapo, J.D., and Reynolds, H.Y., 2005. The mysterious pulmonary brush cell: a cell in search of a function. *Am J Respir Crit Care Med* 172:136–139.

Renne, R.A., and Gideon, K.M., 2006. Types and patterns of response in the larynx following inhalation. *Toxicol Pathol* 34:281–285.

Renne, R.A., Gideon, K.M., Miller, R.A., Mellick, P.W., and Grumbein, S.L., 1992. Histologic methods and interspecies variations in the laryngeal histology of F344/N rats and B6C3F1 mice. *Toxicol Pathol* 20:44–51.

Renne, R.A., Sagartz, J.W., and Burger, G.T., 1993. Interspecies variations in the histology of toxicologically important areas in the larynges of CRL:CD rats and Syrian golden hamsters. *Toxicol Pathol* 21:542–546.

Renne, R., Brix, A., Harkema, J., Herbert, R., Kittel, B., Lewis, D., March, T., Nagano, K., Pino, M., Rittinghausen, S., Rosenbruch, M., Tellier, P., and Wohrmann, T., 2009. Proliferative and nonproliferative lesions of the rat and mouse respiratory tract. *Toxicol Pathol* 37:5S–73S.

Reynolds, S.D., Zemke, A.C., Giangreco, A., Brockway, B.L., Teisanu, R.M., Drake, J.A., Mariani, T., Di, P.Y.P., Taketo, M.M., and Stripp, B.R., 2008. Conditional stabilization of β-catenin expands the pool of lung stem cells. *Stem Cells* 26:1337–1346.

Rittinghausen, S., Dungworth, D.L., Ernst, H., and Mohr, U., 1992. Primary pulmonary tumors. In: *Pathobiology of the Aging Rat*, Volume 1. U. Mohr, D.L. Dungworth, C.C. Capen, W.W. Carlton, J.P. Sundberg, and J.M. Ward, editors. ILSI, Washington, pp. 161–172.

Rittinghausen, S., Dungworth, D.L., Ernst, H., and Mohr, U., 1996. Primary pulmonary tumors. In: *Pathobiology of the Aging Mouse*, Volume 1. U. Mohr, D.L. Dungworth, C.C. Capen, W.W. Carlton, J.P. Sundberg, and J.M. Ward, editors. ILSI, Washington, pp. 301–314.

Rittinghausen, S., and Kaspareit, J., 1998. Spontaneous cystic keratinizing epithelioma in the lung of a Sprague–Dawley rat. *Toxicol Pathol* 26:298–300.

Rooney, S.A., Young, S.L., and Mendelson, C.R., 1994. Molecular and cellular processing of lung surfactant. *FASEB J* 8:957–967.

Rossi, S.E., Erasmus, J.J., McAdams, H.P., Sporn, T.A., and Goodman, P.C., 2000. Pulmonary drug toxicity: radiologic and pathologic manifestations. *RadioGraphics* 20:1245–1259.

Roth, F.D., Quintar, A.A., Echevarría, E.M.U., Torres, A.I., Aoki, A., and Maldonado, C.A., 2007. Budesonide effects on Clara cell under normal and allergic inflammatory condition. *Histochem Cell Biol* 127:55–68.

Rygh, P., and Selvig, K.A., 1973. Erythrocyte crystallization in rat molar periodontium incident to tooth movement. *Scand J Dent Res* 81:62–73.

Sakagami, T., Beck, D., Uchida, K., Suzuki, T., Carey, B.C., Nakata, K., Keller, G., Wood, R.E., Wert, S.E., Ikegami, M., Whitsett, J.A., Luisetti, M., Davies, S., Krischer, J.P., Brody, A., Ryckman, F., and Trapnell, B.C., 2010. Patient-derived granulocyte/macrophage colony-stimulating factor autoantibodies reproduce pulmonary alveolar proteinosis in nonhuman primates. *Am J Respir Crit Care Med* 182:49–61.

Sakuma, T., Zhao, Y., Sugita, M., Sagawa, M., Toga, H., Ishibashi, T., Nishio, M., and Matthay, M.A., 2004. Malnutrition impairs alveolar fluid clearance in rat lungs. *Am J Physiol Lung Cell Mol Physiol* 286:L1268–L1274.

Sasaki, M., Namioka, Y., Ito, T., Izumiyama, N., Fukui, S., Watanabe, A., Kashima, M., Sano, M., Shioya, T., and Miura, M., 2001. Role of ICAM-1 in the aggregation and adhesion of human alveolar macrophages in response to TNF-α and INF-γ. *Mediat Inflamm* 10:309–313.

Sass, B., and Liebelt, A.G., 1985. Metastatic tumors, lung, mouse. In: *Respiratory System*. T.C. Jones, U. Mohr, and R.D. Hunt, editors. Springer-Verlag, Berlin, pp. 138–159.

Sato, S., and Kishikawa, T., 2001. Ultrastructural study of the alveolar lining and the bronchial mucus layer by block staining with oolong tea extract: the role of various surfactant materials. *Med Electron Microsc* 34:142–151.

Schemitsch, E.H., Turchin, D.C., Anderson, G.I., Byrick, R.J., Mullen, J.B., and Richards, R.R., 1998. Pulmonary and systemic fat embolization after medullary canal pressurization: a hemodynamic and histologic investigation in the dog. *J Trauma* 45(4):738–42.

Schlage, W.K., Bulles, H., Friedrichs, D., Kuhn, M., and Teredesai, A., 1998. Cytokeratin expression patterns in the rat respiratory tract as markers of epithelial differentiation in inhalation toxicology. I. Determination of normal cytokeratin expression patterns in nose, larynx, trachea, and lung. *Toxicol Pathol* 26:324–343.

Schleh, C., Mühlfeld, C., Pulskamp, K., Schmiedl, A., Nassimi, M., Lauenstein, H.D., Braun, A., Krug, N., Erpenbeck, V.J., and Hohlfeld, J.M., 2009. The effect of titanium dioxide nanoparticles on pulmonary surfactant function and ultrastructure. *Respir Res* 10:90.

Schmiedl, A., Hoymann, H.-G., Ochs, M., Menke, A., Fehrenbach, A., Krug, N., Tschernig, T., and Hohlfeld, J.M., 2003. Increase of inactive intra-alveolar surfactant subtypes in lungs and asthmatic Brown Norway rats. *Virchows Arch* 442:56–65.

Schneider, P., and Pappritz, G., 1976. Hairs causing pulmonary emboli. A rare complication in long-term intravenous studies in dogs. *Vet Pathol* 13(5):394–404.

Schraufnagel, D.E., 2010. Lung lymphatic anatomy and correlates. *J Pathophys.* 17:337–343.

Schreider, J.P., and Rabbe, O.G., 1981. Anatomy of the nasal-pharyngeal airway of experimental animals. *Anat Rec* 200:195–205.

Sells, D.M., Brix, A.E., Nyska, A., Jokinen, M.P., Orzech, D.P., and Walker, N.J., 2007. Respiratory tract lesions in noninhalation studies. *Toxicol Pathol* 35:170–177.

Sendo, T., Hirakawa, M., Fujie, K., Kataoka, Y., and Oishi, R., 1999. Contrast medium-induced pulmonary edema is aggravated by silicone contamination in rats. *Radiology* 212:97–102.

Seymour, J.F., and Presneill, J.J., 2002. Pulmonary alveolar proteinosis. *Am J Respir Crit Care Med* 166:215–235.

Shenberger, J.S., Shew, R.L., and Johnson, D.E., 1997. Hyperoxia-induced airway remodelling and pulmonary neuroendocrine cell hyperplasia in the weanling rat. *Pediat Res* 42(4):539–544.

Sheppard, M.N., and Thurlow, N.P., 1992. Distribution of the cytoskeletal protein β-tubulin in normal lung, cryptogenic fibrosing alveolitis and lung tumors. *Histopathology* 20:421–425.

Shinagawa, K., and Kojima, M., 2003. Mouse model of airway remodelling. Strain differences. *Am J Respir Crit Care Med* 168:959–967.

Sims, D.E., and Horne, M.M., 1997. Heterogeneity of the composition and thickness of tracheal mucus in rats. *AJP Lung Physiol* 273(5):L1036–L1041.

Singh, G., and Katyal, S.L., 2000. Clara cell proteins. *Ann N Y Acad Sci* 923:43–58.

Slesinski, R.S., and Turnbull, D., 2008. Chronic inhalation exposure of rats for up to 104 weeks to a non-carbon-based magnetite photocopying toner. *Int J Toxicol* 27:427–439.

Snipes, M.B., 1989. Long-term retention and clearance of particles inhaled by mammalian species. *Crit Rev Toxicol* 20:3 175–211.

Snipes, M.B., 1996. Current information on lung overload of nonrodent mammals: contrast with rats. *Inhal Toxicol* 8(suppl):91–109.

Snipes, M.B., McClellan, R.O., Mauderly, J.L., and Wolff, R.K., 1989. Retention patterns for inhaled particles in the lung: comparisons between laboratory animals and humans for chronic exposures. *Health Phys* 57:69–77.

Snyder, J.C., Reynolds, S.D., Hollingsworth, J.W., Li, Z., Kaminski, N., and Stripp, B.R., 2010. Clara cells attenuate the inflammatory response through regulation of macrophage behaviour. *Am J Respir Cell Mol Biol* 42(2):161–171.

Sorokin, S.P., and Brain, J.D., 1975. Pathways of clearance in mouse lungs exposed to iron oxide aerosols. *Anat Rec* 181:581–626.

Spencer, A.J., Wilson, S.A., Batchelor, J., Reid, A., Rees, J., and Harpur, E., 1997. Gadolinium chloride toxicity in the rat. *Toxicol Pathol* 25(3):245–255.

Spencer, A., Wilson, S., and Harpur, E., 1998. Gadolinium chloride toxicity in the mouse. *Human Exp Toxicol* 17:633–637.

St. Clair, M.G.B., and Morgan, K.T., 1992. Changes in the upper respiratory tract. In: *Pathobiology of the Aging Rat*, Volume 1. U. Mohr, D.L. Dungworth, and C.C. Capen, editors. ILSI Press, Washington, pp. 111–128.

Stout, R.D., Jiang, C., Matta, B., Tietzel, I., Watkins, S.K., and Suttles, J., 2005. Macrophages sequentially change their functional phenotype in response to changes in microenvironmental influences. *J Immunol* 175:342–349.

Strickland, D., Kees, U.R., and Holt, P.G., 1996a. Regulation of T-cell activation in the lung: isolated lung T-cells exhibit surface phenotypic characteristics of recent activation including down-modulated T-cell receptors, but are locked into the G_0/G_1 phase of cell cycle. *Immunology* 87:242–249.

Strickland, D., Kees, U.R., and Holt, P.G., 1996b. Regulation of T-cell activation in the lung: alveolar macrophages induce reversible T-cell energy in vitro associated with inhibition of interleukin-2 receptor signal transduction. *Immunology* 87:250–258.

Sturgess, J., and Reid, L., 1973. The effect of isoprenaline and pilocarpine on (a) bronchial mucus-secreting tissue and (b) pancreas, salivary glands, heart, thymus, liver and spleen. *Br J Exp Pathol* 54(4):388–403.

Takagi, M., Shiraiwa, K., Kusuoka, O., and Tamura, K., 2010. A case of olfactory neuroblastoma induced in a rat by N-nitrosobis(2-hydroxypropyl)amine. *J Toxicol Pathol* 23:111–114.

Takaro, T., Chapman, W.E., Burnette, R., and Cordell, S., 1990. Acute and subacute effects of injury on the canine alveolar septum. *Chest* 98:724–732.

Takeyama, K., Dabbagh, K., Lee, H.-M., Agusti, C., Lausier, J.A., Ueki, I.F., Grattan, K.M., and Nadel, J.A., 1999. Epidermal growth factor system regulates mucin production in airways. *Proc Natl Acad Sci* 96:3081–3086.

Takizawa, H., Suko, M., Shoji, S., Ohta, K., Horiuchi, T., Okudaira, H., Miyamoto, T., and Shiga, J., 1986. Granulomatous pneumonitis induced by bacille Calmette–Guérin in the mouse and its treatment with cyclosporin A. *Am Rev Respir Dis* 134(2):296–299.

Tang, K., Rossiter, H.B., Wagner, P.D., and Breen, E.C., 2004. Lung-targeted VEGF inactivation leads to an emphysema phenotype in mice. *J Appl Physiol* 97:1559–1566.

Tavana, H., Zamankhan, P., Christensen, P.J., Grotberg, J.B., and Takayama, S., 2011. Epithelium damage and protection during reopening of occluded airways in a physiological microfluidic pulmonary airway model. *Biomed Microdevices* 13(4):731–742.

Templin, M.V., Levin, A.A., Graham, M.J., Aberg, P.M., Axelsson, B.I., Butler, M., Geary, R.S., and Bennett, C.F., 2000. Pharmacokinetic and toxicity profile of a phosphorothioate oligonucleotide following inhalation delivery to lung in mice. *Antisense Nucleic Acid Drug Dev* 10:359–368.

Thomassen, M.J., Barna, B.P., Malur, A.G., Bonfield, T.L., Farver, C.F., Malur, A., Dalrymple, H., Kavuru, M.S., and Febbraio, M., 2007. ABCG1 is deficient in alveolar macrophages of GM-CSF knockout mice and patients with pulmonary alveolar proteinosis. *J Lipid Res* 48:2762–2768.

Thornton-Manning, J.R., and Dahl, A.R., 1997. Metabolic capacity of nasal tissue: interspecies comparisons of xenobiotic-metabolizing enzymes. *Mutat Res/Fundam Molec Mech Mutagen* 380:43–59.

Trapnell, B.C., and Whitsett, J.A., 2002. GM-CSF regulates pulmonary surfactant homeostasis and alveolar macrophage-mediated innate host defense. *Annu Rev Physiol* 64:775–802.

Tuazon, J.G., Modell, J.H., Hood, C.I., and Swenson, E.W., 1973. Pulmonary function after ventilation with fluorocarbon liquid (caroxin-D). *Anesthesiology* 3(2):134–140.

Ulich, T.R., Yi, E.S., Longmuir, K., Yin, S., Biltz, R., Morris, C.F., Housley, R.M., and Pierce, G.F., 1994. Keratinocyte growth factor is a growth factor for type II pneumocytes in vivo. *J Clin Invest* 93:1298–1306.

Ullmann, A.J., Krammes, E., Sommer, S., Buschmann, I., Jahn-Muehl, B., Cacciapuoti, A., and Schmitt, H.-J., 2007. Efficacy of posaconazole and amphotericin B in experimental invasive pulmonary aspergillosis in dexamethasone immunosuppressed rats. *J Antimicrob Chemother* 60:1080–1084.

Valberg, P.A., Wolff, R.K., and Mauderly, J.L., 1985. Redistribution of retained particles. Effect of hyperpnea. *Am Rev Respir Dis* 131:273–280.

Valensi, P., Gaudey, F., Parries, J., and Attali, J.R., 1993. Glucagon and noradrenaline reduce erythrocyte deformability. *Metabolism* 42(9): 1169–1172.

Van Miert, E., Dumont, X., and Bernard, A., 2005. CC16 as a marker of lung epithelial hyperpermeability in an acute model of rats exposed to mainstream cigarette smoke. *Toxicol Lett* 159:115–123.

Villetti, G., Bergamaschi, M., Bassani, F., Bolzoni, P.T., Harrison, S., Gigli, P.M., Janni, A., Geppetti, P., Civelli, M., and Patacchini, R., 2006. Pharmacological assessment of the duration of action of glycopyrrolate vs tiotropium and ipratropium in guinea-pig and human airways. *Br J Pharmacol* 148:291–298.

Wagenvoort, C.A., Wagenvoort, N., and Dijk, H.J., 1974. Effect of fulvine on pulmonary arteries and veins of the rat. *Thorax* 29:522–529.

Wan, H., Kaestner, K.H., Ang, S.L., Ikegami, M., Finkelman, F.D., Stahlman, M.T., Fulkerson, P.C., Rothenberg, M.E., and Whitsett, J.A., 2004. Foxa2 regulates alveolarization and goblet cell hyperplasia. *Development* 131:953–964.

Ward, J.M., Uno, H., Kurata, Y., Weghorst, C.M., and Jang, J.-J., 1993. Cell proliferation not associated with carcinogenesis in rodents and humans. *Environ Health Perspect* 101:125–136.

Wardlaw, A.J., Guillen, C., and Morgan, A., 2005. Mechanisms of T cell migration to the lung. *Clin Exp Allerg* 35:4–7.

Watson, T.M., Reynolds, S.D., Mango, G.W., Boe, I.-M., Lund, J., and Stripp, B.R., 2001. Altered lung gene expression in CCSP-null mice suggests immunoregulatory roles for Clara cells. *Am J Physiol Lung Cell Mol Physiol* 281:L1523–L1530.

Weaver, J.L., Zhang, J., Knapton, A., Miller, T., Espandiari, P., Smith, R., Gu, Y.-Z., and Snyder, R.D., 2010. Early events in vascular injury in the rat induced by the phosphodiesterase IV inhibitor SCH 351591. *Toxicol Pathol* 38:738–744.

Weber, K., Germann, P.G., Iwata, H., Hardisty, J., Kaufmann, W., and Rosenbruch, M., 2009. Lesions in the larynx of Wistar RccHanTM: WIST rats. *J Toxicol Pathol* 22:229–246.

White, M.R., Crouch, E., van Eijk, M., Hartshorn, M., Pemberton, L., Tornoe, I., Holmskov, U., and Hartshorn, K.L., 2005a. Cooperative anti-influenza activities of respiratory innate immune proteins and neuraminidase inhibitor. *Am J Physiol Lung Cell Molec Physiol* 288:L831–L840.

White, M.R., Crouch, E., Vesona, J., Tacken, P.J., Batenburg, J.J., Leth-Larsen, R., Holmskov, U., and Hartshorn, K.L., 2005b. Respiratory innate immune proteins differentially modulate the neutrophil respiratory burst response to influenza A virus. *Am J Physiol Lung Cell Molec Physiol* 289:L606–L616.

Williams, M.C., 2003. Alveolar type I cells: molecular phenotype and development. *Annu Rev Physiol* 65:669–695.

Wilson, B.D., Clarkson, C.E., and Lippmann, M.L., 1993. Amiodarone causes decreased cell-mediated immune responses and inhibits the phospholipase C signalling pathway. *Lung* 170:137–148.

Wilson, D.V., and Walshaw, R., 2004. Postanesthetic esophageal dysfunction in 13 dogs. *J Am Anim Hosp Assoc* 40(6):455–460.

Wilson, D.W., and Segall, H.J., 1990. Changes in type II cell populations in monocrotaline pneumotoxicity. *Am J Pathol* 136(6):1293–1299.

Wilson, D.W., Segall, H.J., Pan, L.C., Lamé, M.W., Estep, J.E., and Morin, D., 1992. Mechanisms and pathology of monocrotaline pulmonary toxicity. *Crit Rev Toxicol* 22(5/6):307–325.

Wilson, D.W., and Dungworth, D.L., 2002. Tumors of the respiratory tract. In: *Tumors in Domestic Animals*. D.J. Meuten, editor. Blackwell, Ames, IA, pp. 365–399.

Wong, B.A., 2007. Inhalation exposure systems: design, methods and operation. *Toxicol Pathol* 35:3–14.

Wysolmerski, R., Lagunoff, D., and Dahms, T., 1984. Ethchlorvynol-induced pulmonary edema in rats. An ultrastructural study. *Am J Pathol* 115:447–457.

Yeates, D.B., Aspin, N., Levison, H., Jones, M.T., and Bryan, A.C., 1975. Mucociliary tracheal transport rates in man. *J Appl Physiol* 39(3):487–495.

Yerer, M.B., Aydoğan, S., Comu, F.M., Arslan, M., Güneş-Ekinci, I., Kurtipek, O., and Unal, Y., 2006. The red blood cell deformability alterations under desfluran anesthesia in rats. *Clin Hemorheol Microcirc* 35:213–216.

Young, S.L., and Silbajoris, R., 1986. Dexamethasone increases adult rat lung surfactant lipids. *J Appl Physiol* 60(5):1665–1672.

Zhang, J., Snyder, R.D., Herman, E.H., Knapton, A., Honchel, R., Miller, T., Espandiari, P., Goodsaid, F.M., Rosenblum, I.Y., Hanig, J.P., Sistare, F.D., and Weaver, J.L., 2008. Histopathology of vascular injury in Sprague–Dawley rats treated with phosphodiesterase IV inhibitor SCH 351591 or SCH 534385. *Toxicol Pathol* 36:827–839.

Zhao, C.-Z., Fang, X.-C., Wang, D., Tang, F.-D., and Wang, X.-D., 2010. Involvement of type II pneumocytes in the pathogenesis of chronic obstructive pulmonary disease. *Respir Med* 104:1391–1395.

Zhou, L., Geraci, G., Hess, S., Yang, L., Wang, J., and Argikar, U., 2011. Predicting phospholipidosis: a fluorescence non-cell based in vitro assay for the determination of drug-phospholipid complex formation in early drug discovery. *Anal Chem* 83:6980–6987. Downloaded from http://pubs.acs.org on August 19, 2011.

12 Urinary System

Kendall S. Frazier and John Curtis Seely

CONTENTS

12.1 KIDNEY

12.1.1 Introduction

The kidney is a common toxicologic target organ for pharmaceutical therapeutic agents, and lesions of the urinary tract are frequently encountered in preclinical toxicologic studies by pathologists. Renal injury may occur as a result of direct effects on tubules or glomeruli or indirectly via altered hemodynamics. High renal blood flow (RBF) (as much as 25% of cardiac output) and/or proportionally high renal excretion associated with many drugs, coupled with the high doses of test articles typically given in preclinical toxicity studies, often result in effectively high local compound concentrations in the kidney of animals in these studies. The inherent high metabolic activity and high oxygen consumption of renal epithelium, coupled with the ability of the kidney to concentrate drugs in the urine, all predispose this organ to toxic injury. In addition, the significant transporter activity of the renal epithelium makes the kidney further susceptible to injury through cell specific uptake of metabolites from both urinary and blood interfaces as well as from drug–drug interactions when agents are administered in combination therapies. The specific pattern of renal injury is dependent on the nature of the drug, its toxicokinetic properties, clearance profile and particular metabolic attributes, and, ultimately, the local tissue concentration of the agent and length of time of exposure.

There are several histologic findings that are commonly encountered in the kidneys of laboratory rodents, dogs, and monkeys on toxicity studies irrespective of test article treatment. Some of these are genetically linked congenital abnormalities such as hydronephrosis and polycystic kidneys and, as such, are easily differentiated from compound-induced lesions. Others such as chronic progressive nephropathy (CPN) or amyloidosis occur at very high incidence or increase with age, such that the finding is present in a significant proportion of both control and treated animals on study. In other cases, the time of onset of the background change may be hastened with drug treatment, resulting in an apparent dose response. Many agents affect glomerular filtration rate (GFR) or alter RBF, which will indirectly accelerate the development of CPN. While it is tempting to write off many or all of these background changes as not related to test article, in some instances, these "spontaneous" lesions such as CPN in rats may in fact be increased in incidence or severity following xenobiotic administration. In such cases, there may be some clinical effect on human renal physiology, despite a lack of direct relevance of the spontaneous finding to humans. For instance, exacerbation of CPN in rats by compounds that affect tubular protein absorption does not result in similar changes of tubular basophilia and basement membrane thickening in human kidneys but may occasionally be associated with slight increases in clinical urinary protein levels. Hence, exacerbation of background changes in preclinical species may lack the direct clinical importance of a nephrotoxic signal but is not necessarily without clinical relevance.

12.1.1.1 Functional Anatomy

The kidneys are classified as unilobular in all of the most common species utilized in preclinical toxicologic studies (Figure 12.1a). The functional unit of the kidney, the nephron, is divided into

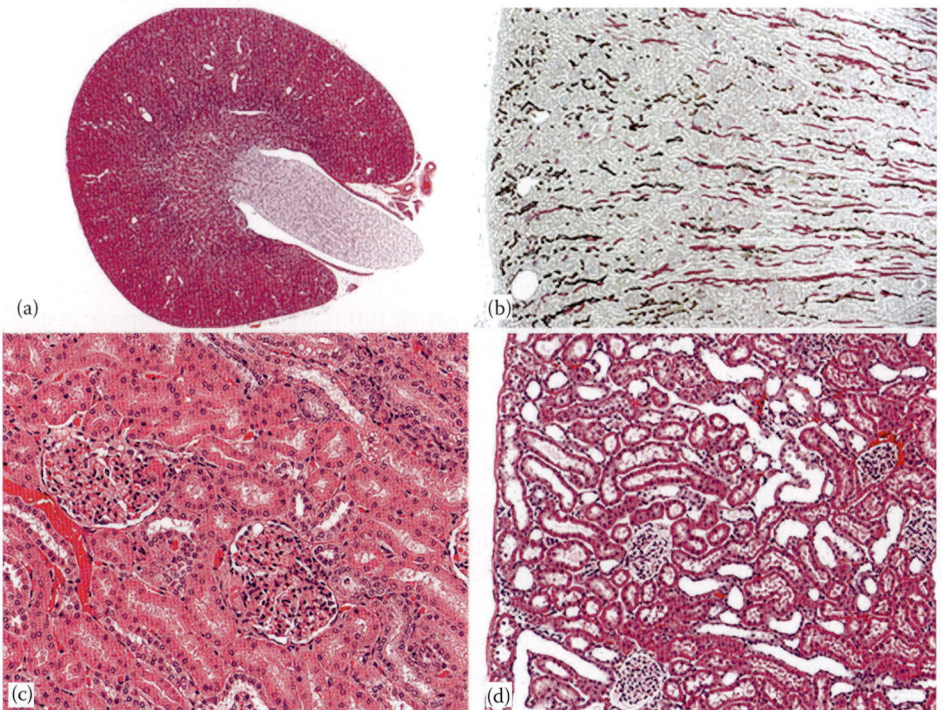

FIGURE 12.1 (a) Hematoxylin and eosin 20×. Normal rat kidney, demonstrating well-demarcated cortex and distal medulla with less defined inner and outer stripes of the outer medulla. (b) Immunohistochemical stain for aquaporin 2 (DAB) and Tamm-Horsfall protein (carmine) with hematoxylin counterstain 40×. Normal rat kidney. Aquaporin 2 stains distal convoluted tubule, connecting segment, and cortical collecting ducts in the rat. Tamm-Horsfall staining is localized to the thick ascending limb. (c) Hematoxylin and eosin 200×. Dog kidney, with evidence of drug-induced glomerulonephritis characterized by thickened basement membranes, increased cellularity and synechia within glomeruli and the presence of hyaline material within Bowman's space. (d) Hematoxylin and eosin 200×. Rat kidney, with drug-induced tubular dilation, characterized by wide tubular lumina lined by attenuated epithelium. Many tubules have intraluminal proteinic debris.

the glomerulus, proximal tubule, descending and ascending limbs of the loop of Henle, distal convoluted tubules, connecting segment, collecting ducts, interstitium, and juxtaglomerular apparatus. The kidney can also be divided into five topographic zones: cortex, outer and inner stripe of the outer medulla, inner medulla, and papilla. While the inner and outer stripes are well developed in rodents, especially rats, they are less obvious in dogs and nonhuman primates. Whenever possible, toxic renal responses should be classified on the basis of structure and topographical location. Nephrons are classified based on their topographic location or functionally by the length of their loop of Henle. This includes subcapsular (short loop) nephrons and juxtamedullary (long loop) nephrons. Subcapsular nephrons are located within the outer cortex, sending their loops of Henle into the outer medulla. Juxtamedullary nephrons, as their name implies, are situated at or near the corticomedullary junction and have very long loops, which extend into the inner medulla before bending at various levels to return to the cortex. In dogs, all nephrons are of the long-looped variety, whereas in rats and mouse, long-looped nephrons average only about 28% of the total.

The renal vascular supply arises from the renal artery, which branches into the interlobar arteries. The interlobar arteries continue as arcuate arteries that run parallel to the capsule along the corticomedullary junction. These continue as interlobular arteries and eventually to afferent arterioles and glomerular capillaries. Efferent arterioles that arise from glomeruli near the medulla give rise to interconnecting vasa recta, which supply the medulla. These vessels eventually coalesce to form arcuate veins. The distal straight (S3) segment of the proximal tubule and focal areas of the medullary thick ascending limb of the loop of Henle are the most susceptible regions of the nephron to ischemic injury (Venkatachalam et al. 1978), but this has more to do with the metabolic oxygen demand and Na^+K^+ ATPase activity of these tissues than their architectural arrangement or vascular supply. Cortical short-looped nephrons show more extensive damage with ischemia than the long-looped juxtamedullary nephrons. While the cortex receives the vast majority of RBF (>90%) as compared to the medulla (resulting in higher vascular concentrations of test article), the medullary ducts are potentially exposed to higher concentrations of compound or metabolites in the urine over time. The major lymphatic drainage follows the vasculature in all species, but an additional capsular lymphatic system has been described in humans and monkeys (Osathanondh and Potter 1966).

The glomerulus is composed of a network of capillaries, which float within Bowman's space, which is surrounded by a fibrous capsule. The glomerular tuft is attached to the capsule at its vascular pole and is lined by endothelial cells, overlying a fenestrated basal lamina and opposite a layer of podocytes. The adjacent central region of the glomerulus is composed of mesangial cells. At the vascular pole, the podocytes transition into a fourth cell type, the parietal epithelium, which lines the inner surface of Bowman's capsule. In mature male mice, and occasionally also in mature male rats, proximal convoluted tubular epithelial cells extend into Bowman's capsule, which should be considered a normal finding. The negatively charged basement membrane normally restricts passage of plasma proteins larger than 70 kD and is composed of the lamina densa, the lamina rara interna (facing the endothelium), and the lamina rara externa (adjacent to the podocytes). Glomerular size increases with age and can vary among species.

Proximal tubules make up the majority of the structural subunits of the renal cortex. In many species including rats, mice, and dogs, the proximal tubule can be subdivided into the S1 and S2 (convoluted) segments and the S3 (pars recta or straight) segment. In rats, the transition from S2 to S3 segments is well delineated, while it is more difficult to define this transition in mice, and in some species, the S2 segment encompasses the initial portion of the straight segment of the proximal tubule. Proximal convoluted tubules are tortuous and, in section, have an oval or transverse profile and a larger diameter than other segments. The S1 segment has well-developed brush borders and numerous mitochondria along its highly interdigitated basolateral border. The S2 segment has a shorter brush border with fewer mitochondria and interdigitations than those in the S1 segment, with more pronounced lysosomal bodies. The distal, straight S3 segment has fewer transverse and greater numbers of linear profiles in section. The brush border is tall, and mitochondria and lysosomes are less frequent, but peroxisomes are common. In juxtamedullary nephrons, the straight S3 segments are located within the outer stripe, while those associated with short-looped nephrons are found in both outer stripe and within medullary rays. αGST immunohistochemical stains effectively label proximal tubules including S1, S2, and S3 segments, but in practice, this is of little value since proximal tubules are relatively easy to identify through morphology alone. The S3 segment ends abruptly at the thin limb of the descending loop of Henle, which has thin tubular diameters and is lined by flattened epithelium with sparse microvilli. Luminal diameters are only slightly smaller than those of the proximal tubules. Juxtamedullary nephrons have long thin segments that can extend deep into the papilla, while short-looped nephrons have thin limbs of Henle that are shorter and distributed throughout the outer medulla. The thin ascending limb continues as the thick ascending limb past the loop of Henle and extends into the cortex within the medullary ray. The thick ascending limb is considered part of the distal nephron, which is also made up of the macula densa and distal convoluted tubules. The thick ascending limb is lined by eosinophilic, cuboidal epithelium, which tends to be shorter than those in the proximal convoluted tubules. The nucleus is often centrally located within the cell, which aids in identification. Tamm-Horsfall protein is present at the luminal surface of the apical membrane in all animals normally used in toxicology studies, and immunostains for this protein can aid in identification. The thick limb ends just past the macula densa.

The juxtaglomerular apparatus is located at one pole of the glomerulus and consists of the macula densa, efferent and afferent arterioles, granular cells of the afferent arteriole, and the extraglomerular lacis (mesangial) cells. The macula densa is composed of low columnar epithelial cells with apically placed nuclei. The juxtaglomerular apparatus is important in tubuloglomerular feedback control of renin secretion produced by the granular cells. This structure often undergoes hypertrophy with chronic administration of certain antihypertensive agents.

The distal convoluted tubules are short segments present in the cortex, near the glomeruli, which lie between the macula densa and the connecting tubules of the collecting duct system. They are typically noted in transverse or V-shaped configurations in tissue section and, especially in monkeys, tend to be lined by somewhat taller epithelium and have larger luminal diameters than proximal convoluted tubules. Calbindin D28K immunostains specifically label distal convoluted tubules in mice, rats, dogs, and monkeys, although small sections of the connecting segment may also stain positively. In mice and rats, but not monkeys or humans, the distal convoluted tubules also contain Tamm-Horsfall protein.

The connecting tubules are ill defined in the rat and mouse and represent fairly short segments in all species. They are immunostained in most species with calbindin D28 and with aquaporin-2. The collecting ducts extend from the cortex via the medullary ray through the outer and inner medulla to the tip of the papilla. The lining cells begin as low cuboidal but increase in height to low columnar in the papilla. Aquaporin-2 immunohistochemistry can be used to label collecting ducts, both in the medulla as well as those within medullary rays that extend into the cortex (Figure 12.1b). The inner medulla contains the thin loops of Henle of long-looped nephrons and collecting ducts of progressively larger diameter. The "papilla" in preclinical toxicity species usually refers to the major portion of the inner medulla, and at its tip, the ductal epithelium changes to a lining epithelium. The renal pelvis is lined by this thin layer referred to as urothelium. The urothelium of the pelvis, other than thickness, is similar to that of the ureter and bladder. As such, the toxicologic lesions noted in the renal pelvis are generally shared with those of the ureter and bladder rather than with the rest of the kidney. Urothelium can distend with changes in urine volume and, due to its impermeability, may withstand the significant fluctuations in chemical composition associated with the urinary output. The papilla is lined by a single layer of epithelium that is similar, but not equivalent, to the urothelium of the remainder of the pelvis. Although some authors refer to this tissue as transitional epithelium, "epithelium of the renal papilla" is probably a more correct term.

The renal interstitium is composed of a matrix of fibroblasts and dendritic cells and is much thicker in the medulla than in the cortex. The interstitium consists of a variety of cell types embedded within a thick extracellular matrix. In the medulla, and particularly in the papilla, this matrix is rich in mucopolysaccharides. Among the cellular components of the interstitium identified in rodents, Type I (stellate) cells are lipid-rich and associated with prostaglandin production. Type 2 (monocytic) cells are ovoid with large nuclei and scant cytoplasm. Type 3 (pericyte) cells are flattened and are often associated with the vasa recta.

Quite often, marked differences in the incidence and/or severity of renal pathology are noted between males and females administered the same dose of an agent. This is commonly associated with toxicokinetic profile differences between sexes and easily demonstrated by plasma concentration or systemic exposure differences between groups attributable to phase I or phase II hepatic metabolism. However, due to the predominance of phase II metabolic activity within the renal epithelium, local metabolic factors may also play a role. Renal cytochrome P450 enzyme differences have been noted between male and female rodents. For instance, cyp4A2 has been shown to have higher activity in male rat kidneys, and cyp2E1 likewise is higher in male mouse kidneys than in females. There are also lesions that tend to be gender specific, such as increased susceptibility to alpha-2U-globulin nephropathy, which may predispose males to secondary renal pathologies through indirect mechanisms. Finally, there are gender differences in transporter activity, which may result in greater intracellular accumulation of a toxicant or reactive metabolite within tubular epithelium. For these reasons, kidney findings from males and females may often need to be assessed separately by the toxicologic pathologist to accurately interpret histologic alterations. These differences may become even more apparent when comparing across species, such that it is quite common for xenobiotic-induced renal lesions to be present in one preclinical species and not be found in a second species tested at comparable exposure.

12.1.1.2 Embryology

The neonatal kidney in all species is smaller than the adult kidney and will increase in mass during the juvenile or pediatric growth period specific for that species. However, the number of glomeruli is constant in an individual between birth and maturity, with the increase in renal volume attributable to an increase in tubular mass. The reduced tubular mass of juvenile kidneys results in diminished capacity for fluid reabsorption and is responsible for the increased risk of dehydration in pediatric animals. In most mammals including rodents and humans, the aglomerular pronephros and functional mesonephros appear early in gestation and represent early stages of renal development, after which they undergo regression. The metanephros then develops into the eventual structures of the nephron; acid–base equilibrium and control of volume develop postnatally in all common preclinical species and humans, but there are important differences in functional maturation. For instance, concentrating ability develops prenatally in dogs but postnatally in rats and humans. In the case of laboratory rodents, maturation of both cortical and medullary elements is generally complete by 21–28 days of age. Glomerular filtration is not functionally mature until 2 years of age in humans but matures by postnatal week 6 in rats. The toxicologic pathologist should be aware of the different morphology of the pediatric kidney when examining microscopic sections for juvenile toxicity studies. The cortex in rats less than 20 days of age is thinner than those of the adult rat kidney, with many "fetal glomeruli" (characterized by small diameter, decreased matrix, and dense, peripherally placed nuclei with scant Bowman's space) and tubules with more basophilic cytoplasm and numerous mitoses. Fetal glomeruli are also noted in dogs and monkeys in the perinatal period and may be present at ages up to 1 year. The interstitium of the pediatric rodent kidney, especially in the medulla, tends to be more prominent and stain slightly basophilic as compared to the adult kidney. Toxic lesions may arise unexpectedly in the kidney in juvenile toxicity studies when no renal lesions are noted with the same compound in adults at similar doses. The reasons vary, but altered toxicokinetic profiles (due to differences in hepatic juvenile metabolism), differences in fluid dynamics, and rapid organ growth or tissue development may all be predisposing factors (Cappon and Hurt 2010).

12.1.1.3 Ancillary Tests of Renal Function or Damage

Acute kidney injury (AKI, the preferred clinical term) associated with exposure to nephrotoxicants is a primary concern in drug development. This has frequently been referred to as drug-induced kidney injury (DIKI) in animal toxicologic studies. For proper risk assessment of renal injury, histopathology should be accompanied by renal organ weight and clinical chemistry data. Irrespective of the mechanism or specific type of renal pathology, in cases where toxic injury has been noted microscopically, urinalysis with urine chemistries and sediment examination give important clues to help determine the extent of dysfunction. Changes in kidney weight are a relatively reliable correlative factor with other measures of nephrotoxicity (Kluwe 1981). Especially when combined with macroscopic observations such as parenchymal discoloration, renal organ weight changes signal the need for microscopic evaluation to further characterize potential renal lesions. Multiple pathologic processes may result in increased kidney weights including tubular degeneration, obstruction and tubulointerstitial inflammation, and, more rarely, tubular vacuolation. Mild dose-related increases in kidney weights may also occur as an adaptive phenomenon as a result of responses to pharmacologic activity of therapeutic agents. As these may occur without concomitant histomorphologic changes, uncorrelated kidney weight increases should always be interpreted with caution.

AKI has historically been diagnosed clinically by monitoring blood urea nitrogen (BUN) and serum creatinine (sCR). However, these two renal markers suffer from insensitivity, and they are elevated only when over half of renal function is compromised in humans or almost 2/3 of renal function is lost in dogs and other preclinical species (Bonventre et al. 2010). Further, interpretation of BUN and sCr elevations can be confounded by prerenal factors such as dehydration and liver dysfunction. Other serum markers of kidney function such as phosphorous or calcium may be altered only in moderately severe or chronic disease. For these reasons, there has been longstanding interest in the development of renal injury markers to enable more reliable noninvasive diagnosis and monitoring for the detection of renal injury. Urine offers an added advantage over serum as a "proximate" biofluid that can increase the specificity for monitoring renal injury such that measurement of proteins specific to either defined nephron segments or pathologic processes is being used increasingly to noninvasively characterize renal injury. These markers include serum proteins that passively enter the urine by glomerular filtration, proteins that enter the urine through glomerular and/or tubular injury, or proteins that are upregulated within the kidney in response to renal injury. The quantitative measurement of constituents excreted into urine following nephrotoxicosis has existed for several years and has included the evaluation of tubular enzymes, low molecular weight proteins, and renal-specific antigens. Among these, urinary concentrations of gamma glutamyl transpeptidase (GGT) and N-acetyl-beta-D-glucosaminidase (NAG) have historically been utilized most often. Both have some advantages over BUN and sCR, and commercial kits are available for use in preclinical species. However, neither has shown optimal selectivity, sensitivity, and predictivity that would make them advantageous additions to routine renal toxicity screening. Studies in humans with renal tubular injury led to the isolation and identification of several low molecular weight urinary proteins (<30,000 MW) including alpha$_1$ microglobulin, beta$_2$ microglobulin, and retinol-binding protein (RBP). All three proteins are readily filtered by the glomerulus and (at least in humans) almost completely resorbed and catabolized by proximal tubular epithelium. They tend to increase in concentration in response to tubular damage due to nephrotoxicosis, and commercial kits are widely available for their use. Unfortunately, there is individual variability in urine levels, and the differing proportions of both low and high molecular weight proteins in rat urine have limited their use in preclinical studies. While beta$_2$ microglobulin has been recently qualified by international regulatory agencies as an acceptable preclinical parameter in the rat, it has not been completely validated as a predictable analyte that may translate into the clinic. It is relatively unstable in acid urine with a pH below 5.5, and therefore, RBP or alpha1 microglobulin is preferred in the dog. Until further validation is performed, the value of these low molecular weight proteins as effective renal biomarkers in preclinical toxicity studies remains to be determined. Recently, a consortium of industry, academic, and regulatory nephrology experts was formed to address the need for improved nephrotoxic biomarkers in preclinical drug development to qualify a panel of these markers and to eventually translate their use into the clinical setting (Ozer et al. 2010). This panel included seven urinary biomarkers including albumin (ALB), kidney injury molecule 1 (KIM1), neutrophil gelatinase–associated lipocalin/lipocalin 2 (NGAL), beta$_1$ microglobulin (B1M), clusterin (CLU), alpha glutathione-s-transferase (αGST), and trefoil factor 3 (TFF3). In addition, they separately assessed Cystatin C and evaluated all eight parameters in a string of studies using known nephrotoxicants of various mechanisms (Ozer et al 2010; Bonventre et al. 2010). In a parallel effort, the ILSI-HESI Technical Committee on Biomarkers of Toxicity, Nephrotoxicity Working Group, evaluated the urinary biomarkers α-GST, μ-GST, CLU, and renal papillary antigen-1 (RPA-1) in rats given cisplatin, gentamicin, or N-phenylanthranilic acid (NPAA) (Harpur et al. 2011).

In separate studies performed by several different investigators, selected markers such as KIM1, CLU, and NGAL have demonstrated both sensitivity and selectivity for early renal damage in preclinical species including mice, rats, and monkeys (Ozer et al. 2010; Chiusolo et al. 2010) and have been included in many human clinical trials. It should be stressed that the primary purpose of these efforts by the consortia is to develop a validated panel of renal assays for use in humans and not to develop better preclinical assays, where DIKI can be confirmed with histopathology. However, the use of these exploratory markers may provide an earlier signal than might be expected with BUN and sCR alone. While it is premature to evaluate the long-term utility of all individual biomarkers currently under evaluation, several have been successfully adapted into first- or second-tier approaches to address renal toxicity. Urinary albumin, in particular, has become an established parameter included in many clinical and preclinical studies that can reflect both tubular and glomerular injury. Low molecular weight protein markers freely pass the glomerular filtration barrier, and their presence in urine suggests impaired tubular absorptive capacity, while intermediate or high molecular weight proteins in urine can indicate concomitant glomerular and tubular injury.

Alterations in values of urine biomarkers must be interpreted with caution. Several more years of testing will be needed before there is a consensus on the specific amplitude of elevation that is significant for each species, the combination of markers that would be adequate to assess early renal injury, and the types of renal injury that are best diagnosed by a specific marker. No single biomarker is likely to be applicable across the varied contexts and temporal presentations of all possible toxicity study designs. Although many of these biomarkers have overlapping specificity in regard to timing or localization of injury, they are generally evaluated concurrently because of differences in marker biology, species cross-reactivity, or storage stability. These differences in urinary biomarker expression patterns support a multiplex approach to analysis. For instance, αGST may be elevated in early renal injury, while KIM1 and CLU tend to be positive during the repair phases (Ozer et al. 2010). Some markers appear to be more specific for certain segments of the nephron. For instance, urinary RPA-1 and pi glutathione-s-transferase (πGST) have been used to monitor injury to the distal nephron. RPA-1 is a membrane-bound glycoprotein primarily localized to the collecting ducts in rats and is elevated with papillary necrosis, but to date, no human ortholog has been identified (Price et al. 2010). Glutathione-S-transferases are phase II detoxifying enzymes that exist in the kidney as various isoforms that vary widely between species and at different sites along the nephron. While πGST is found in high concentrations in distal tubules and collecting ducts in humans and is readily released after injury, it is less abundant than μGST in rat distal tubules and πGST has highly variable background levels in rat. Thus, the preclinical assay in rats has been disappointing. Finally, some urine analytes are constitutively expressed, while others are induced after injury. All of these factors and limitations must be considered when choosing which of the available urinary biomarkers to use and when interpreting results.

The addition of a panel of exploratory urine biomarkers may provide information on the timing, localization, and extent of drug-induced kidney damage based on constitutive versus upregulated expression of the protein biomarker, localization to specific segments of the nephron, or association with specific pathologic processes. Until these biomarkers are validated and vetted in large numbers of preclinical studies, the interpretation of alterations in their urine levels should be done in the context of concomitant changes in well-established assays such as kidney weights, histology, BUN, sCR, and urinalysis. The careful evaluation of renal morphology by the trained toxicologic pathologist is probably as sensitive as any available technique or assay for the assessment of all but the most subtle of acute renal injuries, but histopathology is not an option for monitoring AKI in the clinic. Therefore, rather than routinely including these new urine biomarkers into all preclinical toxicity studies, they are probably best employed prospectively in selected preclinical studies following the identification of drug-induced renal microscopic lesions noted in initial preclinical toxicity screens or subacute toxicity studies when their use may provide information for clinical risk assessment. When applied in this manner, findings can be put into proper context with other supporting data, and the inclusion of multiple urine analytes measured in parallel may increase the sensitivity and precision in the identification or confirmation of compound-induced renal injury. The elevation of a single exploratory parameter in isolation, while still potentially important, should not be construed as compelling evidence of renal toxicity and should not be the primary basis for clinical risk assessment.

Metabonomic approaches have also generated interest as potential renal biomarkers for several years, but review of several studies using metabonomic techniques suggests that significant additional validation work will be required to justify their widespread acceptance. There currently seems to be little advantage of metabonomic methodology over other routine approaches to assess renal injury (Gibbs 2005). However, metabonomics may provide additional data for prediction of kidney toxicity under controlled conditions and may be of value in investigational or special-use toxicologic studies (Lindon et al. 2005). Urinary cytokine levels have also been promoted as potential biomarkers of renal injury. While cytokine urinary levels increase in various types of injury (Adalsteinsson et al. 2008), recent evidence suggests that the source for the cytokines may be the systemic circulation rather than the kidney. It has been postulated that they are filtered through the glomerulus but, due to proximal tubular damage, are not reabsorbed with renal injury. This would suggest that urinary levels of cytokines would follow similar patterns to other more conventional urinary protein analytes such as urinary albumin, but with the added negative attributes of systemic background variability.

Renal safety pharmacology studies are not specifically required by worldwide regulatory guidelines for testing pharmacologic agents, but they have been utilized as adjunctive investigative activities to address the extent or mechanism of renal injury. The most commonly performed assays involve the determination of renal clearance, accurate measurement of GFR, and determination of RBF. Renal clearance of a compound can be determined by comparing the urinary excretion rate to the plasma concentration and is generally expressed in milliliters per minute. GFR has been shown to be decreased after only 20% decreases in renal function, so it potentially can demonstrate drug-induced renal damage prior to BUN or sCR alterations. GFR can be calculated or estimated (eGFR) based on the fractional excretion of creatinine or other endogenous markers such as cystatin C, but it can be more precisely determined experimentally by measuring the clearance of compounds such as inulin, iohexol, or iothalamate. Since inulin is inert, nontoxic, freely filtered through the glomerulus, and neither secreted nor reabsorbed, its measure of clearance is considered a gold standard for GFR determination. However, in human clinical nephrology practice, GFR measurement is seldom performed, and it is more often simply estimated (eGFR) via creatinine clearance. Inulin clearance can be directly measured in renal safety pharmacology studies, and therefore, accurate determination of GFR may in some cases be useful in corroborating subtle histologic lesions. RBF can be determined by a variety of imaging techniques, and its measurement can help in differentiation of renal hemodynamic effects from other pathophysiologic mechanisms of insult.

12.1.2 Glomerular Changes

The glomerulus is the initial site of exposure for a nephrotoxicant within the nephron, but glomerular changes occur much less commonly in preclinical toxicology studies than do tubular changes. However, glomerulonephritis and other related glomerular changes have been noted with somewhat greater frequency with the increasing prevalence of biopharmaceuticals and complex macromolecules during drug development. Antibody or complement-mediated injury is a frequent, but not essential, component of glomerular toxicity, and the immune response related to biopharmaceutical administration likely plays a major factor. The increased incidence of glomerular lesions appears not to be directly due to the antibody therapies themselves but to other associated factors such as anti-antibodies produced by the test animals or from the effects of biological impurities within drug substances, for example, the presence of large antibody complexes in preparations. Such complexes are able to fix complement directly at the site of the glomerular filtration barrier and podocyte/endothelial interface where they aggregate. Effects may also be due to nonhumoral immunomodulatory effects, such as the increased incidence of glomerulosclerosis noted with interferon alpha administration or glomerular changes associated with proinflammatory effects of antisense oligonucleotides in mice. Damage may result from effects on specific cell types (podocytes, mesangial cells), effects on the vascular supply, or impairment of the charge- or size-selective properties of the glomerulus.

When describing the distribution of glomerular changes, specific modifiers are used, which differs from nomenclature in the rest of the kidney. The terms "segmental" and "diffuse" are modifiers related to the distribution of lesions within an individual glomerulus. Segmental lesions are confined to only a portion of the glomerulus, whereas diffuse lesions encompass the entire glomerulus. The terms "focal" and "global" refer to distribution of glomerular lesions that involve only a small proportion and the majority of the glomeruli across the entire renal cortex, respectively. Since glomerular cells are often difficult to individually identify with routine H&E stains,

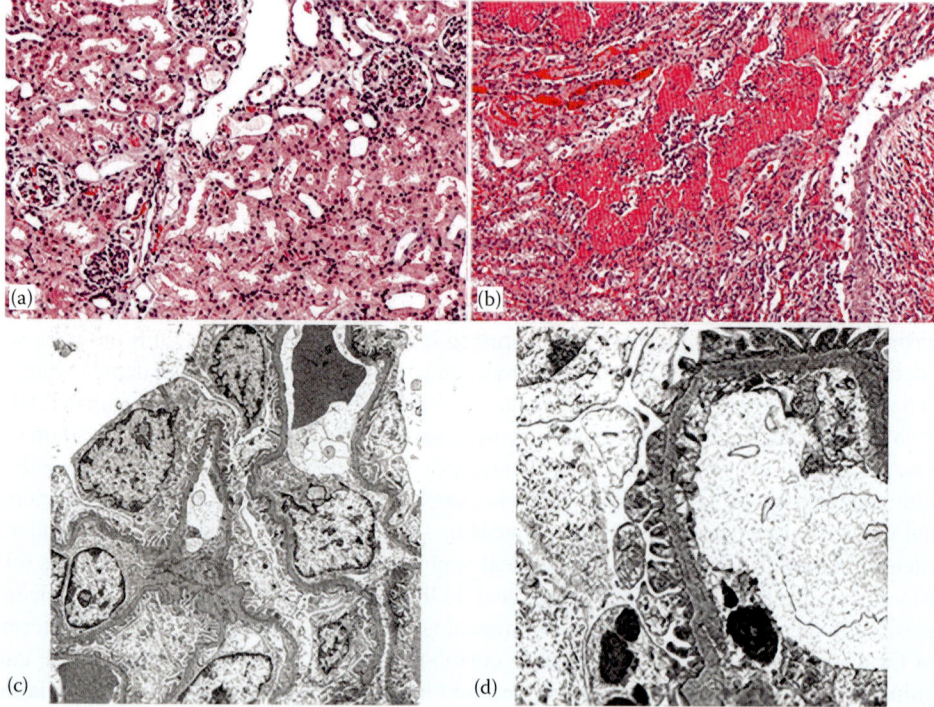

FIGURE 12.2 (a) Hematoxylin and eosin 400×. Rat kidney, with drug-induced tubular degeneration and necrosis. Note the pale tubules with slightly dilated lumina, increased cytoplasmic basophilia, and loss of nuclei. The affected tubules often have sloughed, brightly eosinophilic epithelial cells in their lumens forming cellular casts. (b) Hematoxylin and eosin 400×. Rat kidney, distal medulla at the papilla, with severe pyelonephritis. Note the multiple casts, large numbers of inflammatory cells predominated by neutrophils, and necrosis and loss of epithelium. (c) Transmission electron micrograph, osmium. Rat kidney, normal glomerulus demonstrating podocytes with their foot processes, thick basement membrane, and endothelial cells. An erythrocyte is present within a capillary at the top of the photomicrograph. (d) Transmission electron micrograph, osmium. Cynomolgus monkey kidney, glomerulus with osmiophilic inclusion bodies (presumed to be drug material) within a podocyte on left and within an endothelial cell on right.

especially in those with morphologic abnormalities, periodic acid-Schiff (PAS) stains, silver stains, or specific immunohistochemical stains may be utilized to better identify the cellular components of the glomerulus. Both PAS and silver stains delineate the mesangium, but silver stains may also help differentiate details of the basement membrane since they will specifically stain the lamina densa. PAS stains also help to delineate details of the capillary loops. Immunohistochemical stains for synaptopodin will specifically stain the podocytes, while immunostains for nephrin target the adjacent slit diaphragms of the podocytes, immunoreactivity for Von Willebrands factor identifies glomerular endothelial cells, and CD90/thy-1 immunohistochemical stains label mesangial cells in the rat. Electron microscopy is also often very useful in demonstrating ultrastructural changes within the glomerulus when alterations are noted by light microscopy (Figure 12.2c demonstrates normal ultrastructural detail of the podocytes, mesangial cells, and endothelial cells and their associated basement membranes, and Figures 12.2d and 12.3a through c demonstrate drug-induced glomerular changes). Table 12.1 demonstrates differentiating features between the various forms of glomerular injury in species common to preclinical toxicity studies.

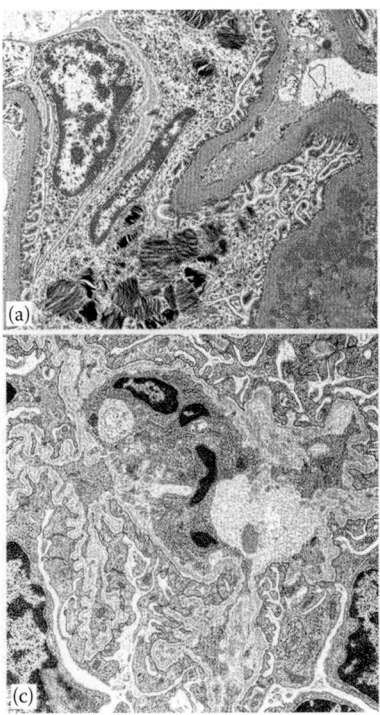
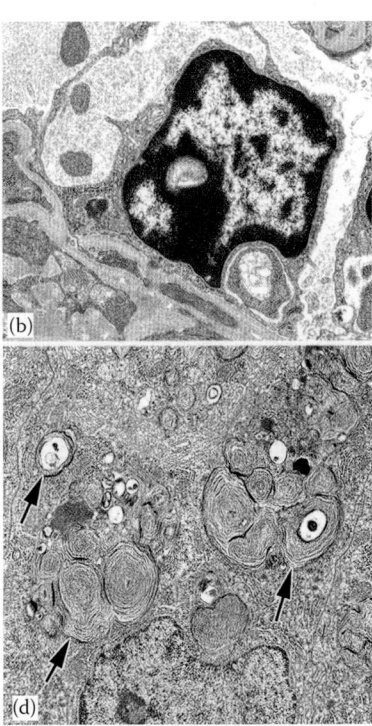

FIGURE 12.3 (a) Transmission electron micrograph, osmium. Rat kidney, glomerulus, from an animal given a chemokine antagonist. The podocytes have floccular cytoplasm and contain large membrane-bound (lysosomal) inclusion bodies with a distinct zebra stripe pattern, typical of glycoprotein accumulation. On the right-hand corner, the basement membrane appears thickened and contains accumulation of dense material, which could represent deposits of the immune system (antibodies, complement, etc.). (b) Transmission electron micrograph, osmium. Mouse kidney, glomerulus, from an animal given a phosphorothioate deoxyoligonucleotide treatment, demonstrating swelling and degeneration of an endothelial cell with alterations of the underlying basement membrane. (c) Transmission electron micrograph, osmium. Rat kidney, glomerulus with drug-induced mesangioproliferative glomerulopathy. The degenerative mesangial cell in center contains vacuoles with amorphous material and karyorhectic nuclei. The tortuous basement membranes are highly irregular and reduplicated. Some of the foot processes on adjacent podocytes are blunted and fused. (d) Transmission electron micrograph, osmium. Rat. Epithelial cell demonstrating the intracytoplasmic membrane-bound laminar concentric whorls (arrows) typical of drug-induced phospholipidosis.

TABLE 12.1

Differentiation of Preclinical Glomerular Lesions

Type of Glomerular Insult	Key Features
Glomerulonephritis	
Membranoproliferative	Thickened, reduplicated, or split basement membranes, thickened capillary walls, increased mesangium and cellular proliferation, mononuclear inflammatory cell infiltration
Crescentic	Increased visceral/parietal epithelium, synechia, adhesions and fibrosis, increased mesangial cell number, mononuclear inflammatory cell infiltration
Mesangioproliferative glomerulopathy	Increased mesangial matrix and hypertrophied/hyperplastic mesangial cells without inflammation or antibody deposits
Glomerulosclerosis	Progressive fibrosis and loss of cellularity, thickened Bowman's capsule, may be associated with CPN; usually without inflammation
Hyaline glomerulopathy	Acellular immune complex deposition of PAS-positive material resulting in thickened basement membranes without fibrosis or inflammation; progressive loss of cellularity of tufts
Glomerular atrophy	Shrinkage and contraction of glomerular tufts, with concurrent enlargement of Bowman's space
Glomerular amyloidosis	Replacement of glomerular architecture by amyloid with minimal fibrosis; progressive loss of cellularity

12.1.2.1 Glomerulonephritis

Biopharmaceutical macromolecules and some classical small molecules, such as D-penicillamine, have been associated with drug-induced glomerulonephritis in preclinical toxicity studies (Donker et al. 1984). In all of its manifestations, glomerulonephritis is characterized by cellular proliferation. Glomerulonephritis can be divided into membranoproliferative and crescentic forms in rodents, dogs, and monkeys. Both forms are associated with inflammatory cytokine involvement and potential complement activation within the glomerular capillaries. While some authors have further separated a subset of membranoproliferative glomerulonephritis in laboratory animals into a membranous form based on human classifications, this is probably unnecessary as the two are similar and there is significant overlap. In humans, membranous glomerulonephritis refers to a condition with primarily basement membrane thickening, while the syndrome of membranoproliferative glomerulonephritis involves thickened capillary walls with cellular proliferation. In laboratory animal species, lesions consistent with the human forms of membranoproliferative, crescentic, and membranous glomerulonephritis are often noted simultaneously in the same kidney when glomerulonephritis is present. Therefore, a diagnosis of glomerulonephritis is sufficiently accurate and effective in describing these particular glomerular lesions in many or most preclinical toxicity studies. Importantly, the clinical implications of crescentic or membranoproliferative glomerulonephritis are similar. A separate variety of glomerular change is noted in both preclinical species and humans that is labeled mesangioproliferative glomerulopathy. It is described separately in this text as "glomerulopathy" rather than "glomerulonephritis," as this latter form lacks significant capillary involvement or inflammation and primarily involves damage to the mesangium. Glomerulonephritis may arise secondary to antibody deposition (such as in the Heymann nephritis model in rats or in dogs with Lyme disease) but also as sequela to nephrotoxin-mediated injury to podocytes, glomerular endothelium, and/or the basal lamina. Antibodies can bind to a glomerular structural antigen or may be deposited in the glomerulus from circulating antibody complexes formed distantly. In some cases, drugs such as procainamide act as haptens (Adams et al. 1993). Cell mediated immunity may also be stimulated by some agents, and downstream effects may directly or indirectly injure glomerular components. This has been reported with cyclosporine (Remuzzi and Perico 1995).

Regardless of the morphologic pattern, glomerulonephritis can present as a diffuse or segmental change within an individual glomerulus and can be focal or global. There are seldom any gross changes evident with any form of glomerulonephritis. Thin sections stained with PAS or methanamine silver often provide better resolution than simple H&E stains.

In the membranoproliferative form of glomerulonephritis, there is thickening of the basement membrane usually with antibody or immune complex deposition along the basal lamina. These irregular, dense deposits are easily visualized with electron microscopy and sometimes appear as intermittent, linear spikes along the membrane and other times as fuzzy large ovoid structures. These occur along the capillary wall, on either the endothelial or epithelial side of the basement membrane. While there may be a slight increase in the amount of mesangial matrix, there is little or no endothelial, podocyte, or mesangial proliferation. There is generally dilation of the capillary loops with visibly thickened walls, and there is variably minimal mononuclear cell infiltration. In dogs, the basement membrane is frequently split. Glomerulonephritis has been induced in monkeys with several forms of monoclonal antibodies and in rodents by chronic low doses of mercuric chloride (Hard et al. 1999). In dogs, membranoproliferative glomerulonephritis has been found associated with other systemic conditions including heartworm disease, pyometra, and cancer, and rarely in association with drug therapy. However, the low number of published drug-related cases in dogs may be related only to the preferential use of monkeys over dogs in preclinical toxicity evaluation of biopharmaceuticals rather than to any greater resistance to the condition.

The crescentic form of glomerulonephritis is a segmental to circumferential lesion involving hyperplasia of the glomerular epithelium forming adhesions and crescents along the glomerular tufts. Bowman's space is decreased as the visceral and parietal epithelium become confluent, and there are usually slight to moderate increases in mesangial matrix. In contrast to the membranoproliferative form, there may be slight to moderate proliferation of the mesangial cells and podocytes accompanying the proliferation of parietal epithelium. Importantly, there is often mononuclear cell infiltration or accumulation within the capillary lumina. Endothelial cells swell and may become detached. Exudative glomerulonephritis of either form is associated with accumulations of neutrophils within capillary tufts due to chemokine-mediated cell recruitment, but this type of infiltrate is less common in toxicity studies than mononuclear cell involvement. Ultrastructural examination or use of PAS stains demonstrates relatively normal basement membranes but pronounced epithelial changes including parietal enlargement and blunting, effacement, and/or fusion of podocyte foot processes. In drug-associated forms of glomerulonephritis, electron microscopy often demonstrates electron-dense inclusions within podocytes, endothelial cells, or mesangial cells (Figures 12.2d and 3a). Collagen accumulation occurs over time, but fibrosis is not a central feature as it is in glomerulosclerosis and glomerular changes associated with CPN. While it may be necessary in some toxicology studies, especially investigational studies, to differentiate between subtypes of glomerulonephritis, as noted previously, in most preclinical studies, it is reasonable and generally sufficient to use the generic term of glomerulonephritis. In many cases, there is insufficient evidence or data to subclassify it further. Glomerulonephritis needs to be differentiated from hyaline glomerulopathy in mice, which lacks inflammatory infiltrates and is not associated with the epithelial proliferation or thickened basement membranes. Differentiation of glomerulonephritis from mesangioproliferative glomerulopathy is based on the lack of inflammatory cells or basement membrane deposits and predominance of mesangial matrix changes in the latter.

Glomerulonephritis has been noted as spontaneous background change in some mouse strains such as the New Zealand Black (NZB). The incidence and severity may be increased with immunostimulatory agents, but this effect should not be confused with direct toxicologic targeting of the glomerulus by a compound and may have little clinical relevance to humans. Heymann nephritis is a form of glomerulonephritis in rats that is considered an experimental model for human glomerular disease. The antigenic targets have been identified as megalin and an associated 44-kD protein called RAP. Other tubular proteins released during tubular degeneration have also been suggested as antigenic targets, but how these tubular antigens would affect glomerular antibody deposition is still unclear. The development of proteinuria in this model requires antibody complexes at the glomerulus, formation and activation of the C5b-9 membrane attack complex, and the subsequent production of reactive oxygen species in the glomerular matrix via lipid peroxidation (Kerjaschki and Neal 1996). Similar mechanistic events are likely necessary sequences in the development of drug-induced glomerulonephritis.

Glomerulonephritis is generally associated with increases in kidney weights, likely as a result of hyaline cast formation rather than due to increased glomerular size or diameter. In all forms of glomerular damage, there will be increased urinary protein loss and increased urinary albumin, but these elevations in urinary protein are likely due to secondary tubular disease from decreased reabsorption rather than increased filtration alone. Therefore, increased urinary protein should not be considered a biomarker exclusive to glomerular injury. Persistent proteinuria and secondary tubular degeneration will be associated with changes in other renal tubular biomarkers. In advanced disease, serum protein levels may fall, and urea and creatinine increase as GFR diminishes. Eventually, end-stage disease and nephrotic syndrome may ensue in the most chronic studies.

Genetic factors play an important role in the predisposition to and incidence of glomerulonephritis in animals, just as with any immune-mediated disease. Species or strain as well as specific pharmacogenomic background may all be relevant predisposing factors. Diseases associated with glomerular vascular injury or coagulopathy such as the microangiopathies may have glomerulonephritis as a secondary complication. In such situations, fibrin microthrombi may be seen concurrently with any of the forms of glomerulonephritis. More often, damage to the glomerular filtration barrier by xenobiotic agents directly, or indirectly through complement or antibody mediated effects, results in fibrin leakage into Bowman's space (Figure 12.1c).

It is often hard to predict how humans will respond to agents that produce glomerular changes in animals based on results from preclinical toxicity studies. For instance, ampicillin can produce glomerulonephritis in dogs, but similar changes have not been reported in humans. Generally, xenobiotic-associated glomerular disease in humans is present in only a small percentage of individuals given a medication, and host factors and concurrent conditions may alter this incidence further. Even when adverse glomerular effects are noted clinically, the relatively small group sizes and differences in species susceptibility associated with drug-induced glomerulonephritis make it uncertain whether changes observed in preclinical studies predict such lesions. Due to the immune-mediated pathogenesis, there may be little or no dose response, and few animals within a given study may have glomerular lesions. However, whenever glomerulonephritis is identified in a preclinical study, it is virtually always considered adverse, and a potential immunotoxicologic mechanism should be considered.

12.1.2.2 Mesangioproliferative Glomerulopathy

Mesangioproliferative glomerulopathy is characterized by thickening of the mesangial matrix, hypertrophy and hyperplasia of the mesangial cells, and increased mitoses. It lacks the inflammatory components, capillary alterations, and basement membrane involvement of glomerulonephritis, but may occasionally be associated with small antibody or complement deposits in and around mesangial cells. It is often global and diffuse and may be associated with hyaline casts depending on severity. Mesangial hyperplasia is the precursor to this lesion and is the proper diagnosis if the matrix is not thickened. As with glomerulonephritis, thin 2-μm sections, PAS, and methanamine silver stains aid in the characterization and proper classification of histologic changes. Electron microscopy may be of value in confirming mesangial injury. Mesangial proliferation may occur as a direct response to protein leakage through the glomerular filtration apparatus, and this may result in downstream changes including extracellular matrix accumulation. Therefore, drug-induced injury to other glomerular components, including podocytes or the basement membrane, may secondarily result in mesangial changes, but primary or overwhelming capillary or endothelial damage is not characteristically associated with mesangioproliferative glomerulopathy. The differential diagnosis list includes glomerulonephritis, which involves basement membrane thickening or inflammation.

In mice, it should also be differentiated from hyaline glomerulopathy, which involves loss of all cell components. There is little or no macroscopic lesion associated with mesangioproliferative glomerulopathy, but there may be small increases in kidney weights. Like glomerulonephritis, urinary protein or albumin is increased as one of the most sensitive changes, with elevations in BUN or sCr noted only in very late stages. In addition to biopharmaceutical macromolecules, changes consistent with glomerulopathy have also been associated with the administration of several antisense oligonucleotides in preclinical species. The mechanism is unclear but may be related to the proinflammatory attributes of these molecules coupled with lysosomal uptake of the material within the glomerulus. As an adverse finding, the clinical relevance of mesangioproliferative glomerulopathy mirrors that of other forms of glomerulonephritis and indicates the potential for immunotoxicologic mechanisms of injury. Mesangioproliferative glomerulopathy can be induced in the rat with the injection of anti-thy-1 antibodies, which target the mesangial cells, and so may be encountered by toxicologic pathologists in this and other early drug discovery models of human glomerular disease (Jefferson and Johnson 1999).

12.1.2.3 Hyperplasia, Mesangial

Mesangial cell hyperplasia usually precedes or may accompany glomerular scarring, as is noted in glomerulonephritis or mesangioproliferative glomerulopathy, but hyperplasia/hypertrophy may also occur as a separate entity without further progression. It is characterized histologically by increased numbers of mesangial nuclei within the glomeruli, with or without an increase in the size of the individual cells. Mesangial hyperplasia alone is rarely associated with or a cause of proteinuria. Interactions between mesangial cells, inflammatory cells, and extracellular matrix components perpetuate mesangial cell proliferation and enhance the development of glomerular fibrosis over time. Therefore, with chronic injury and stimulation, mesangial hyperplasia may be associated with an increase in the secretion of collagens, mesangial extracellular matrix proteins, and result in marked proteinuria, where the changes are more properly diagnosed as mesangioproliferative glomerulopathy. The presence of mesangial hyperplasia or hypertrophy therefore has the potential to signal further more serious and potentially less reversible changes in the glomerulus. Mesangial hyperplastic changes are not considered to be preneoplastic lesions and have not been associated with renal tumors. While diagnosis is relatively straightforward in routine H&E sections, electron microscopy may be needed to confirm that mesangial cells are the specific cell type involved in a proliferative response and ensure that there are no other significant alterations related to glomerulonephritis. With the exception of increased urine protein in more chronic cases, there are usually no clinicopathologic abnormalities, organ weight, or macroscopic changes associated with mesangial hyperplasia.

Mesangial cells share some characteristics with vascular smooth muscle cells. They increase in number, size, and cytoplasmic volume as a response to many drugs and chemicals such as cadmium (Wehner and Petri 1983; Xiao et al. 2009). Specific stimuli such as mechanical shear/stress phenomenon can induce this proliferative response, but the underlying mechanisms causing mesangial proliferation are incompletely understood. Mesangial hyperplasia occurs commonly with agents that induce hyperglycemia, including the streptozotocin-induced diabetic rat model. It may also result from phospholipidosis, where mesangial hypertrophy is accompanied by lysosomal membrane-bound whorls within mesangial cells as well as podocytes and/or endothelial cells (Wehner and Petri 1983). Other drugs, such as growth factor inhibitors or anticancer agents, result in the development of inclusion bodies within mesangial cells that may also be associated with mesangial hyperplasia. Morphine sulfate has long been associated with mesangial cell proliferation, and these effects appear to be dependent on specific opioid receptors and STAT3 signaling (Weber et al. 2008). Elevated serum ammonia levels or administration of NH_4Cl also induces hypertrophy (but not hyperplasia) in mesangial cells resulting from a completely different mechanism and signaling pathway (Ling et al. 1998). Cell culture studies have shown that mesangial cells produce cytokines and react to various cytokines. Therefore, mesangial cells have the potential for autocrine and paracrine stimulatory effects on themselves as well as from recruited inflammatory cells (Sterzel et al. 1993). This suggests that mesangial cell proliferation and/or stimulation may occur via many routes that eventually affect the cell cycle.

12.1.2.4 Glomerulosclerosis

Glomerulosclerosis is a common finding in nonclinical safety studies, as it is a component of advanced CPN in rats and chronic nephropathy in mice. It is also a frequent finding in diabetic nephropathy, so it may be encountered in early discovery efficacy studies, such as in the streptozotocin-induced rat model. Glomerulosclerosis is rare in dogs but has been noted in preclinical studies involving growth hormone and progesterone therapies in beagles (Prahalada et al. 1998). In nonhuman primates, it can result from longstanding hypertension and has been commonly noted in the spontaneous hypertensive rat (SHR) model. As such, glomerulosclerosis may be a common downstream consequence of a large number of glomerular insults affecting capillary tuft hemodynamics. It is characterized by progressive loss of glomerular podocytes, increased numbers of myofibroblasts, contraction of glomerular tufts, and enlargement of Bowman's space. Glomeruli are usually enlarged, associated with consistently increased mesangial matrix. There is eventual replacement and loss of glomerular architecture by fibrosis and/or amorphous hyaline material, but the earliest changes are limited to thickened basement membranes (Hard and Seely 2005). Synechia and crescent formation due to adhesions of visceral and parietal epithelium may be present, but unlike glomerulonephritis, there is little or no hypercellularity of glomerular elements, and antibody or complement deposition is absent. Inflammation is variable, but hyaline casts are usually numerous. Bowman's capsule may be thickened, and there is often periglomerular fibrosis. The mesangial matrix stains positively for PAS and intermittently with methanamine silver, and there is usually a concurrent increase in collagen staining by Masson's trichome. Ultrastructurally, podocytes are often swollen and enlarged, and a matrix of collagen fibers can be identified intermixed with homogenous amorphous material. Myofibroblasts can be identified adjacent to thickened basement membranes. Macroscopically, the kidney may be enlarged, pale, pitted, or scarred on gross exam, and white spots may be evident on the cut surface. Kidney weights are often increased due to matrix accumulation and casts but may be decreased in chronic stages due to scarring and infarction. Urine protein and albumin are increased early, but as with most glomerular injuries, BUN, sCr, and other markers remain unchanged until GFR is significantly reduced or secondary damage to tubules occurs from persistent proteinuria. Glomerular atrophy is a differential diagnosis for glomerulosclerosis as they both share features of tuft contraction, but atrophy lacks significant fibrosis or matrix accumulation.

Focal segmental glomerulosclerosis may be noted in a small number of glomeruli in normal control rats, generally as a consequence of CPN, and in this context, the lesion has no real clinical relevance. In such a context, it is advisable not to separate out glomerulosclerosis from CPN. Some xenobiotic agents such as omeprazole will increase the incidence of, or accelerate the onset of, CPN in rats and hence will demonstrate an apparent drug-induced increase in glomerulosclerosis incidence in preclinical studies (Ekman et al. 1985). However, many or most of these drugs are devoid of nephrotoxic potential in humans, so this effect should have little or no clinical implications. While CPN-associated glomerulosclerosis will be associated with increased numbers of renal tumors in carcinogenicity studies due to effects on cellular proliferation, this has also been shown to pose no significant cancer risk in humans (Hard et al. 2009b). When glomerulosclerosis presents in a global pattern, particularly in young rats or in subacute studies, this could suggest a toxicologic effect. This is particularly true when glomerulosclerosis is noted in nonrodents. While glomerulosclerosis may result from any number of glomerular insults, it is less commonly associated with antibody- or macromolecule-mediated pathogenesis than glomerulonephritis. Classic glomerulotoxins such as puromycin and streptozotocin have been utilized to explore the pathogenesis of glomerulosclerosis. The site of initial injury varies with the toxin. Puromycin and doxorubicin directly damage podocytes, whereas toxins such as streptozotocin target mesangial cells via hyperglycemic effects (Mizuno et al. 2004). There are a number of initiating factors that can induce the cascade of events necessary for chronic glomerular injury. Persistent elevation of GFR, associated with single nephron hyperfiltration or increased glomerular capillary hydraulic pressures, can result in protein overload at the glomerular filtration barrier and institute glomerular injury. In the case of drug-induced injury, intracellular drug accumulation with potential binding to subcellular elements may occur in the glomerulus due to high RBF, resulting in high local drug/metabolite concentrations achieved at the filtration interface on either side of the basement membrane. This can result in direct injury to the basement membrane or podocytes, as in the case of penicillamine or puromycin, respectively. Reactive oxygen species and oxidative stress generated from drugs such as doxorubicin can initiate caspase-dependent apoptotic pathways as well as mitochondrial damage, or cell swelling due to toxin-mediated injury, which may progress to necrosis or loss of specific cellular elements. Drugs such as cyclosporine may instead directly perturb glomerular hemodynamics through a vasoconstrictive effect. Once degenerative changes in the glomerulus occur, regardless of initiating cause, inflammatory cascades are invoked, leading to cytokine activation and release of IL-1 and TNF-alpha. In parallel, a complex sequence of SMAD- and cAMP-dependent events, mediated by TGF-beta and CTGF, is initiated within the mesangium, endothelium, and podocytes that include cytoskeletal alterations, integrin upregulation, and paracrine signaling. The end results of these changes are myofibroblast proliferation, collagen formation with extracellular matrix deposition, and eventual glomerular contraction (Lee and Song 2009).

12.1.2.5 Hyaline Glomerulopathy

Hyaline glomerulopathy has historically been described as a background glomerular change in control mice, but it has recently been identified as a response to chronic pulegone exposure in both rats and mice and is noted occasionally in preclinical studies as a test article–induced response to other agents. It is characterized by diffuse, global loss of cellularity of the glomerular capillary tufts, with replacement by a faintly to brightly eosinophilic homogenous matrix. Often, the remaining nuclei will be clustered centrally and have an abnormal appearance. There is extracellular deposition of immunoglobulin and proteinaceous material that thickens basement membranes and stains positively with PAS, only minimally with Masson's Trichrome, and negatively for amyloid with Congo red or SAA immunostains. Electron microscopy reveals finely granular, amorphous material and/or immune complex deposition embedded within the mesangial matrix and in subendothelial deposits composed of bundles and whorls of parallel fibrils. Hyaline glomerulopathy is associated with proteinuria and, in chronic studies, can result in morbidity. Kidney weights are generally increased. It can be differentiated from glomerulosclerosis by the presence of collagen in the latter and from amyloidosis by negative congo red staining. Hyaline glomerulopathy appears to be an uncommon sequel to other chronic degenerative changes of the glomerulus associated with immune complex deposition in rodents. The mechanism for its development remains unclear. There is probably little direct clinical relevance of hyaline glomerulopathy to humans other than the implication for an immune-mediated effect of a xenobiotic agent and therefore the possibility of clinical glomerular effects; thus, its importance is more in identification as a potential background change in mouse preclinical studies. In human nephrology, hyaline glomerulopathy appears to be a distinct and unrelated entity and, rather than immune deposits, is characterized ultrastructurally by organized microtubular structures within the mesangium (D'Agati et al. 2005).

12.1.2.6 Mesangiolysis

Mesangiolysis refers to the partial or complete dissolution of mesangial cells and their associated matrix. It is a degenerative lesion that is usually associated with primary endothelial cell injury, subsequent complement activation, and eventual loss of capillary wall patency. The glomerular lobules stain poorly due to edema within the tuft. The dissolving mesangial cells therefore become difficult to identify and lose their borders, eventually leading to dilated or cystic capillaries. There is often proteinaceous fluid within Bowman's space, fibrin deposition, and/or glomerular hemorrhage.

Mesangiolysis can be a feature of glomerulonephritis, such as in the anti-thy-1 rat model (Kriz et al. 2003), and can occur with widespread complement activation, particularly involving activation of the common terminal pathway and formation of C5b-9. In dogs and rats, mesangiolysis has also been associated with sustained hypertension. It is uncommonly encountered in preclinical toxicity studies but, due to the nature of the lesion, should suggest the potential for an agent to target glomeruli or the vasculature. In humans, mesangiolysis may occur with hemolytic uremic syndrome and in some cases with transplant glomerulopathy. Mesangiolysis is usually associated with significant morbidity and/or mortality. If the animals survive or are put on drug holiday, glomerulosclerosis or glomerular atrophy may be sequela. PAS stains are helpful in the diagnosis, as is electron microscopy, and to identify the vascular changes and primary effect on mesangial cells. Differentials would include other glomerulopathies, but the key features of mesangial dissolution and edema are not present in other glomerular lesions.

12.1.2.7 Amyloidosis

Amyloidosis is commonly encountered in chronic mouse toxicity studies and in studies involving the Syrian hamster. It is particularly common in CD-1 mice where the age of onset is generally between 8 and 12 months. It is a spontaneous disease in mice, characterized by the extracellular deposition of defective serum proteins within the glomerulus and interstitium. In severe cases, there may be involvement of the tubules or collecting ducts. Glomeruli appear hypocellular and contain amorphous pale pink deposits of amyloid protein that stain positively with Congo red and show apple green birefringence. Confirmation of amyloid deposition may also be confirmed using immunohistochemical stains. Amyloid must be differentiated from glomerulonephritis, glomerulosclerosis, and hyaline glomerulopathy and is best accomplished with Congo red and trichrome stains. The kidney tends to be one of the organs preferentially involved in amyloidosis, although the intestine, mesenteric lymph node, and ovary are also commonly affected by 8 months of age. Other organs including heart, adrenal gland, spleen, and liver as well as many others may also be affected in older mice. Renal amyloidosis may be a major cause of morbidity and mortality in carcinogenicity studies in mice. Amyloidosis of the spleen and intestine are noted occasionally in both rhesus and cynomolgus macaques, but the kidney is rarely affected in these species. Older beagle dogs have occasionally been noted with renal amyloidosis, but rats tend to be quite resistant to amyloid development.

AA amyloid is derived from circulating serum amyloid A (SAA) proteins, and these are acute-phase apolipoproteins that are associated with high-density lipoprotein (HDL) particles. Amyloid may also be a result of apolipoprotein A-II (ApoAII) fibril deposition and self-aggregation but is generally limited to experimental models (Gruys et al. 1996) and less common than amyloidosis due to SAA in mice. In most preclinical species, amyloid may also occur via deposition of polypeptide fragments of serum immunoglobulins. In contrast, human renal amyloidosis shows a wide diversity of biochemical types and is due to an even wider variety of causes including myeloma, chronic inflammatory disorders, or inherited factors. By electron microscopy, amyloid is characterized by randomly arranged, long, nonbranching 7 to 10 nm diameter fibrils. Amyloid fibrils demonstrate characteristic β-pleated structure and may ablate the normal glomerular architecture and replace mesangial cells, podocytes, endothelium, and basement membranes. As amyloidosis is progressive, it often appears in greater incidence and severity in recovery groups than in animals at the end of the treatment phase. Amyloid will often be deposited in the interstitium as well as in the glomeruli, but may be more difficult to delineate without Congo red stain. Deposition in the medulla has been associated with secondary papillary necrosis in mice due to disruption of the blood supply to the distal papilla and has also been associated with urothelial hyperplasia in the pelvis. Drug-induced amyloidosis is extremely rare in any species. In a few cases, the incidence and/or severity of amyloid may be increased in preclinical toxicity studies, or the age of onset may be hastened by drug administration. In particular, immunomodulatory compounds may have this effect in mice such as with new generation immunostimulatory therapies. Antisense oligonucleotides have been shown to upregulate SAA in mouse serum (Heikenwalder et al. 2004), and this as well as their effects on toll-like receptor activation may be responsible for the high incidence of renal amyloid with these compounds in chronic mouse studies. Since SAA is a major acute-phase protein in humans as well as mice, and prolonged elevation of plasma SAA levels may be associated with organ effects in people, any effects on the incidence of amyloid in mice cannot be dismissed outright as clinically irrelevant. However, there are few, if any, examples where an amyloidogenic compound administered to mice has resulted in similar effects in humans at therapeutic doses. Some xenobiotic agents such as colchicines may decrease, rather than increase, the incidence or severity of amyloid development in humans or animals (Zemer et al. 1986).

12.1.2.8 Glomerular Atrophy

Glomerular atrophy may be a sequela to virtually any or all chronic degenerative changes that occur in the glomeruli and is a hallmark of end-stage kidney disease (Hard et al. 1999). Atrophy is commonly noted in glomeruli associated with polycystic kidney disease (ADPKD) rats (Tanner et al. 2002) and with streptozotocin-induced diabetes rat models in the latter stages of these chronic nephropathies (Menini et al. 2007). It is characterized by contraction of the glomerular capillary tufts, generally with coincidental enlargement of Bowman's space. While the presence of concurrent fibrosis is variable, nuclei are often retained. The distribution of the change may be focal, diffuse, segmental, or global. The primary differential is glomerulosclerosis, in which fibrosis is prominent and cellular detail is lost, without significant glomerular contraction.

12.1.2.9 Bowman's Space Enlargement

Enlargement or dilation of Bowman's space may occur as a consequence of increased hydrostatic pressure within Bowman's capsule due to glomerular hyperfiltration or as a consequence of shrinkage of the adjacent glomerular capillary tufts due to atrophy. It can also result from retrograde intratubular reflux and has been noted in virtually all of the species used in preclinical toxicity testing. The change is characterized by an increased width of Bowman's space and increased diameter of Bowman's capsule but without a concomitant increase in the size of the glomerular tuft. This change is commonly associated with chronic renal disease involving advanced interstitial fibrosis and contraction of adjacent renal parenchyma (Hard and Seely 2005, 2006). Due to its pathogenesis involving altered glomerular fluid pressures, the widespread presence of this change in a kidney without a close association with parenchymal infarction or interstitial fibrosis suggests a fluid hemodynamic mechanistic effect of an administered agent. Eventually, Bowman's space enlargement will lead to degenerative sequelae in the glomeruli and accompanying tubules, resulting in changes in renal clinical biomarkers. Enlargement of a majority of glomerular spaces should be considered an adverse change that may be only partially reversible with cessation of test-article administration, so the extent of involvement has important clinical implications at relevant drug exposures.

12.1.2.10 Metaplasia and Hyperplasia of Bowman's Capsule

The cells of the parietal epithelium of Bowman's capsule are typically lined by thin squamous epithelium, but tall cuboidal epithelium may be present in male mice and rats, depending on the strain. These cells are under hormonal influence in mature males, and changes in circulating levels of testosterone may affect their morphology. Agents that affect the androgenic pathways have the potential to produce this lesion, which involves both an increase in cell number and changes in morphology. Metaplasia of Bowman's capsule may occur in female mice, and a similar change to cuboidal epithelium occurs in older rats, more commonly in males (Hard et al. 1999). Parietal epithelium may also undergo hyperplasia with advanced glomerular disease, particularly in rat CPN or severe glomerulonephritis, and has been reported commonly in SHRs (Peter et al. 1986). The lesion does not occur in monkeys, minipigs, or dogs. This change should be differentiated from fixation artifact resulting from extrusion of proximal tubular epithelium into the capsular space, where the epithelium not only resembles, but also is indistinguishable from, PCT epithelium. It is not associated with any organ weight or clinicopathologic alterations. These metaplastic/hyperplastic changes are not considered to be preneoplastic lesions, and the clinical relevance to humans is probably negligible other than the hormonal implications.

12.1.3 TUBULAR CHANGES

The proximal tubules make up a significant percentage of the cortical parenchyma, perform diverse regulatory and endocrine functions, and are the segment where numerous receptors and transporter functions are located. Normally, greater than two thirds of filtered salt and water is reabsorbed in the proximal tubules. These structures also act as immune responders to a wide range of immuno-logic and toxicologic insult, such that they represent the most common location for renal injury in nonclinical toxicology studies. They also undergo frequent secondary damage following primary chronic glomerular injury through protein overloading via megalin/cubilin–mediated endocytosis. Due to their ancillary roles in vitamin D synthesis (through 1-alpha-hydroxylase activity) and red blood cell generation (as the site of erythropoietin synthesis), persistent damage to the proximal tubules in chronic studies can also contribute to disorders of bone mineralization and anemia.

12.1.3.1 Tubular Degeneration and Tubular Basophilia

Degeneration refers to a spectrum of cellular insults and morphologic changes in tubular epithelial cells including vacuolation, attenuation, and tinctorial changes such as basophilia. When a particular component of degeneration is the overwhelming feature of a pathologic process in the kidney or within a majority of the kidneys of a study, more specific morphologic or descriptive diagnoses should be used. When there is a range of processes present, degeneration is an appropriate morphologic description to use, which characterizes this spectrum of findings. These may represent reversible injury to the renal epithelium or early manifestations of an irreversible phenomenon leading to necrosis. Changes in tinctorial characteristics of the proximal tubules represent some of the initial and earliest evidence of nephron injury. As such, tubular basophilia is one of the most frequently encountered manifestations of toxic damage in preclinical toxicity studies. It may be a consequence of degenerative changes or represent excessive cellular turnover. As one of the hallmark features of CPN, tubular basophilia occurs spontaneously in a large percentage of control rodents and increases in incidence and severity with age. Tubular basophilia may also occur as a minimal focal lesion in up to 40% of control beagles in studies. In most cases where there is a dose responsive compound-related effect, tubular basophilia probably represents persistent low-grade toxic injury. Tubular regeneration also may be reflected by an increase in basophilia, but because basophilia may reflect biochemical perturbations without evidence of concurrent repair processes, the terms "tubular regeneration," "tubular hyperplasia," and "tubular basophilia" should not be used interchangeably, and other features of hyperplasia (nuclear crowding, flattened profiles, hypertrophy, mitoses, etc.) or aspects of regeneration (appearance in recovery period) should be identified in order to distinguish between processes. In some forms of degeneration, the cytoplasm may take on an eosinophilic or granular or even floccular appearance.

Other types of degeneration such as vacuolation and dilatation are described below, but in all forms, there may be alterations in urinary biomarkers or occasionally the presence of urinary casts on sediment examination. BUN and sCr must be elevated in the more severe or longstanding cases. A number of ultrastructural alterations may be visualized with electron microscopy including loss of microvilli and cytoplasmic glycogen, vesiculation, swelling or clumping of the endoplasmic reticulum, and condensation of the nuclei. Any nephrotoxicant can induce degenerative changes, and there are a myriad of different mechanisms of cellular injury including hypoxia, ATP depletion, mitochondrial damage, free radical formation, or lipid peroxidation.

12.1.3.2 Vacuolation

Vacuolation of tubules is a largely reversible, degenerative change associated with a large number of toxicants. It can represent an early-stage preceding necrosis but more often accompanies specific types of tubular injury involving intracellular accumulation of lipids, glycogen, or fluid. Tubular vacuolation can result from cytoplasmic accumulation of excipients such as cyclodextrin-mediated vacuolation, phospholipidosis, or aminoglycoside-associated nephropathies. A vacuolated appearance can be normal in some tubular segments of some species, such as proximal tubules in the outer cortex of CD-1 mice, the distal tubules of beagles, or the collecting ducts of cynomolgus monkeys (Johnson et al. 1998). Xenobiotic induced vacuolation is characterized by clear to translucent, often ovoid, variably sized spaces within pale or granular cytoplasm. Cells may be swollen, and nuclei may be displaced. Accumulation of lipid within tubules usually occurs as a consequence of disrupted cellular metabolism due to toxicity involving biochemical pathways but in some cases can also be due to direct accumulation of intravenously administered lipid material (Cherdwongcharoensuk et al. 2005; Killary et al. 2009). Special stains such as oil red O, Sudan black, or osmium can be used to visualize lipid within cytoplasm, but these may require frozen or specially prepared specimens to observe as lipid leaches out of tissues with routine paraffin processing. Cyclodextrin vehicles have frequently been associated with vacuolation of the straight segment of the proximal tubules in rodents (Luke et al. 2010), but more severe secondary degenerative changes and/or necrosis occurs only with very high doses of these types of dextran vehicles. This vacuolar change can hinder toxicologic assessment of the tubules and make it more difficult to distinguish drug-related versus vehicle-related lesions where high concentrations of such vehicles are utilized. A similar lesion occurs following the intravenous administration of several other osmotically active compounds, which in the human nephrology literature has been labeled "osmotic nephrosis." Dextrans and some sugars are typically absorbed from the urine filtrate via apical membrane pinocytosis and are stored in phagolysosomes. Unless cellular machinery is disrupted, there are generally few systemic effects and no alterations in serum or urine chemistries from these vacuolar changes. The most common histologic presentation with phospholipidosis is vacuolation of the tubular epithelium, which can be limited to specific segments within the proximal or distal tubules (described below).

12.1.3.3   Renal Phospholipidosis

Phospholipidosis may be associated with administration of a large number of cationic amphiphilic substances, and renal phospholipidosis is noted relatively frequently in rats, mice, dogs, and occasionally monkeys (Halliwell 1997). Most cationic amphiphilic compounds share a hydrophobic aromatic/aliphatic ring structure and a hydrophilic domain containing a charged cationic substituted nitrogen group. The hydrophobic ring is usually substituted with one or more halogen moieties. The aminoglycosides are somewhat unique among phospholipidogenic substances because they lack the typical hydrophobic moieties but retain the cationic structures and, for unknown reasons, tend to have lesions centered in the kidney. Phospholipidosis may be produced by the direct interaction of xenobiotic agents with intracellular phospholipids or by effects on phospholipid synthesis and metabolism. The specific mechanism for the development of phospholipidosis for most cationic amphiphiles involves lysosomal binding, complexing with phospholipids, and inhibition of phospholipases. There is also evidence that these molecules may actually increase the synthesis or sequestration of phospholipids within the cell (Reasor et al. 2006). In H&E sections of kidney, phospholipidosis usually appears as vacuolation of the proximal tubular cytoplasm. By electron microscopy, phospholipidosis consists of membrane-bound lysosomal densities composed of lamellar bodies, concentric whorls, or, more rarely, smooth reticular membranes or crystalline aggregates of darkly osmiophilic material (Figure 12.3d). Generally, the inducing test article or a metabolite may be identified in association with the phospholipid accumulations. Cellular alterations tend to reverse or disappear after discontinuance of the test article, taking from weeks to months depending on the agent. While the kidney may be the only organ affected (depending on disposition or clearance of the drug), more often multiple organs including the liver, adrenal glands, epididymes, and many others will also contain phospholipid inclusion bodies. In fact, with the exception of some antibiotics, the kidney appears to be less sensitive to phospholipidosis than other organs. Multiple factors affect the ability of cationic amphiphilic agents to produce renal phospholipidosis including species, strain, tissue affinity, and pharmacokinetic properties, and these variables must be taken into account when extrapolating to the human during risk assessment. Only a small number of the compounds shown to produce phospholipidosis in rodents or dogs have also resulted in similar organ damage in humans, but the aminoglycoside antibiotics are an important exception in the kidney (Hruban 1984; Halliwell 1997; Quiros et al. 2011). Importantly, there is no evidence to date that the presence of renal phospholipidosis by itself is detrimental to animals or humans, and the prevailing theory suggests that it is primarily an adaptive response to exposure of cationic amphiphilic agents. In those cases where tubular damage is associated with phospholipidosis, such as with aminoglycoside or macrolide antibiotics, there appear to be concurrent mechanisms of cellular injury operating in parallel (Reasor et al. 2006).

The prototypical renal response to phospholipid accumulation occurs with gentamicin, an aminoglycoside. Very quickly after administration, gentamicin is filtered in the glomerulus and binds to the brush border of proximal tubule cells through an electrostatic interaction between its polycationic surface and the negative charge of the membrane phospholipids. It is then transported into the cell by megalin- and cubilin-mediated endocytosis. It accumulates in the endosomal compartment, as well as the Golgi and endoplasmic reticulum. Gentamicin directly inhibits enzymes that are responsible for the degradation of lipid-rich membranes, resulting in significant lysosomal accumulation and the formation of characteristic intracytoplasmic inclusion bodies, known as myelin figures or myeloid bodies, which are easily observed ultrastructurally. The lysosomal membrane is eventually perturbed by these effects, and leakage throughout the cytosol is likely responsible for the ensuing cellular necrosis and tubular injury (Quiros et al. 2011). Thus, cytotoxicity of the aminoglycosides appears to be due to cytosolic effects rather than from lysosomal accumulation. Gentamicin results in oxidative stress injury to the endoplasmic reticulum and destabilizes intracellular membranes facilitating redistribution of the drug throughout the cytosol. Gentamicin can directly act on mitochondria to produce oxidative stress and reduce ATP. In combination with release of lysosomal cathepsins, these effects will result in activation of apoptotic pathways or, if in significant concentrations, result in massive proteolysis and cellular necrosis. Gentamicin also activates the extracellular calcium-sensing receptor, which may be another factor in cell death of the tubular epithelium. Separate effects of gentamicin and other aminoglycosides have been demonstrated on the glomerulus, including charge-mediated alterations in glomerular ultrastructure and permeability as well as impaired tubular reabsorption and intracellular protein catabolism, suggesting that the mechanism of injury with this class of compounds is extremely complex (Quiros et al. 2011).

12.1.3.4 Diabetic Nephropathy and Tubular Glycogenosis

Toxicologic pathologists may evaluate drug discovery or efficacy studies involving rodent models of diabetes such as the streptozotocin rat or diabetic mouse. Pharmaceutical agents such as AKT or PI3 kinase inhibitors have also been associated with sustained hyperglycemia and hyperglucosuria associated with renal epithelial changes. Alterations in the tubules vary with severity of the glucosuria, but cytoplasmic rarefaction and clearing, vacuolation, and single cell necrosis have all been described (Nogueira et al. 1989). These degenerative changes have been assigned several morphologic diagnoses including "cell swelling," "clear cell, tubule," "cytoplasmic alteration," and "microvesicular vacuolation." As these morphologies imply, there are cytoplasmic fluid accumulation and, in many or most cases, accumulation of glycogen. Accumulation of glycogen in diabetic nephropathy occurs from distal tubular absorption of sugars or can occur similarly with other administered hypertonic substances (Monserrat and Chandler 1975). When glycogen has been definitively demonstrated via the use of special stains (PAS-diastase or Best's carmine stains), it is more appropriate to diagnose the lesion as "accumulation, glycogen." These tubular lesions associated with persistent renal glucosuria have important clinical implications because of their potential in rodents to eventually progress to clear cell adenomas and renal cell carcinomas (Dombrowski et al. 2007). Renal carcinogenesis in diabetic rats is thought to result from an adaptive metabolic response via altered growth factor signaling associated with sustained hyperglycemia and prolonged proliferative signals in tubular epithelial cells. In addition to the tubular changes, significant glomerular pathology can occur in parallel due to glycation of glomerular proteins. Mesangial proliferation, thickening of basement membranes, and sclerosis are common, and expansion of the interstitial extracellular matrix by fibrosis and increased cellularity, as well as increased cortical tubular lipid content, may also occur. Cellular alterations in tubules are generally reversible with normalization of blood sugar, but the glomerular and interstitial changes associated with persistent hyperglycemia may not recover quickly or may even be progressive. Urine glucose levels will be elevated once serum glucose hovers above 200 μg/dl and overwhelms the SGLT1/2 transporter system (which is responsible for glucose/sugar reabsorption) in the proximal tubule (Saboli et al. 2006). Hyperglucosuria in these cases will be accompanied by a large increase in urine volume.

12.1.3.5 Tubular Dilation and Cystic Tubules

Dilation of the tubular luminal diameter can be a consequence of necrosis or loss of individual renal epithelial cells and a common manifestation of acute nephrotoxicant-induced kidney injury. Tubules with expanded lumina are lined by normal to flattened epithelium (Figure 12.1d). With loss of epithelium, adjacent cells stretch to fill the defect and cover exposed basement membrane. They may become thin and attenuated, and hyperfiltration can result in greater intratubular pressure differences, especially when combined with thinner tubular walls, resulting in subsequent dilation. Mechanical strain forces appear to result in proliferative responses by the tubular epithelium, and dilated epithelium can release a variety of proinflammatory cytokines, which may result in changes in the adjacent interstitium. Dilated tubules are often clustered together in a radial pattern and represent segments along the same or adjacent nephron segments. In other cases, where there is necrosis involving a particular segment (e.g., the pars recta or thick ascending limb), tubular dilation may have a zonal distribution along the entire region adjacent to the corticomedullary junction. There may be hyaline or granular casts or other cellular debris within the affected lumen. When associated with microabscessation or pyelonephritis, suppurative or mononuclear inflammation may also be present. Tubular dilatation may be associated with increases in BUN, sCR, serum phosphorus, and urine biomarkers. Albuminuria may be increased due to decreased absorption in the more severe cases, and kidney weights may also be increased. Like other nephrotoxicants, the offending agent should be considered to have the potential for AKI in humans at relevant exposures, regardless of the preclinical species.

While tubular dilation most often accompanies other forms of renal degeneration, it can occur as a primary toxic response to a variety of xenobiotic agents including corticosteroids, lithium, and ACE inhibitors (Christensen and Ottosen 1986; Macdonald et al. 1987; Schetz et al. 2005). Tubular dilation may also occur as a consequence of obstruction from crystalluria or distal urolithiasis. This has been seen with a number of drugs such as sulfonamide or quinolone antibiotics, which tend to precipitate out of solution under the local concentrating conditions and pH changes associated with the filtrate in the distal nephron (Schetz et al. 2005). Altered hemodynamic forces from outflow obstruction distally then result in increases in intratubular pressure and/or fluid stasis in proximal segments of the nephron.

Cystic tubules are a more severe manifestation of tubular dilation and are found commonly in end-stage kidney disease and in the later stages of rodent CPN. However, in preclinical studies, cystic tubules most often appear as solitary, congenital cysts unrelated to drug treatment. They tend to have much larger luminal diameters than in tubular dilatation and are occasionally encapsulated. They are usually empty but may contain cellular debris, sloughed epithelium, or even crystals. The Sprague–Dawley IGS strain seems particularly prone to this type of spontaneous cyst development, which tends to be localized to the medulla and can be solitary or multiple. Cysts can be differentiated from large arcuate veins by the lack of endothelial lining. Rarely, multiple large cysts are noted in kidneys, with atrophy and/or hyperplasia of remaining renal parenchyma as a result of congenitally acquired polycystic kidney disease (Tanner et al. 2002). Polycystic lesions in both kidney and liver are noted in Caroli's disease, which is an autosomal recessive syndrome that is occasionally observed as a spontaneous lesion in rat strains used in preclinical studies (Nakanuma et al. 2010). Polycystic kidney disease has also been described in dogs, cats, and several other species, including humans. Since it is not related to xenobiotic administration, the presence of a polycystic kidney in an individual animal in a preclinical study has no clinical relevance.

12.1.3.6 Casts

Casts represent the accumulation of fluid and/or cell breakdown products filling the tubular lumina. While intratubular casts are morphologically a tubular alteration, they more commonly represent a defect in glomerular function, resulting in tubular proteinosis. Casts manifest as one of a few general types including hyaline casts (the most common), hemoglobin casts due to erythrocyte breakdown, or granular casts that may include cellular elements. Tubular profiles containing hyaline casts contain proteinaceous material derived from increased permeability of the glomeruli. Histologic evidence of glomerulonephritis is only rarely present, but when glomerular damage is microscopically visible, hyaline casts are usually present. Hyaline casts stain pink and homogenous with H&E stain, while hemoglobin casts tend to stain a much brighter red. Intact red blood cells may be present within the tubules mixed with acicular crystals of hemoglobin casts. Similarly staining casts composed of myoglobin have been noted in renal tubules following administration of agents that cause muscle damage. Granular casts tend to be less homogeneous than hyaline casts and have particulate matter or cellular debris mixed with the pink luminal fluid. In alpha-2u-globulin nephropathy, granular casts are frequently noted in the outer and inner stripes of the outer medulla in rats. Both hyaline and granular casts occur frequently in advanced CPN in association with glomerulosclerosis, and they can occur in several types of advanced tubular disease due to necrosis and the lack of absorption of albumin and other urinary proteins (Alden 1986; Hard and Khan 2004). Casts may also be present with xenobiotic agents that produce tubular dilatation. Pyelonephritis may result in casts that are composed largely of leukocytes and debris. A few casts are normally found in the outer medulla of control rodents, and their incidence increases with age. Casts should be differentiated from crystals and fluid accumulation that occurs as a postmortem autolytic artifact. Casts may be associated with increased urinary protein if severe enough but are more often clinically silent. Urine sediment examination is probably the diagnostic test of choice for cellular casts, and urinary protein is a good diagnostic test for hyaline casts. The clinical relevance depends on the severity and initiating cause.

12.1.3.7 Necrosis

Nephrotoxic agents often selectively target specific regions of the nephron. Acute test article–related injury will invariably be associated with some degree of tubular degeneration and necrosis. This can take various forms including single cell necrosis, cellular sloughing into tubular lumina, or overt coagulative or ischemic necrosis of renal epithelium. Necrotic epithelial cells are characterized by eosinophilic cytoplasm and pyknotic or karyorrhectic nuclei. Loss of cellular attachments leads to exfoliation into the lumen and thinning of the residual neighboring epithelium during attempts to bridge and repair the area of attenuation (Figure 12.2a). This often results in tubular dilation and the formation of tubular casts containing swollen or condensed cells and cellular debris in the affected segment. There may be a mild acute mixed inflammatory infiltrate in the tubular lumina or in the interstitium associated with the area of cell damage, but this is inconsistent in many nonclinical toxicity studies. Surrounding tubular epithelium is generally normal in appearance, but there may be an accompanying increased mitotic rate. With chronic injury, the basement membrane will be disrupted, and this can result in tubular atrophy and the initiation of interstitial fibrosis. It is common to see a mixed pattern of necrosis with other forms of renal degeneration or regeneration in the same kidney, such as vacuolation, pigmentation, tubular basophilia, dilation, or hyperplasia as various nephrons may be undergoing different stages of injury and repair. Electron microscopy may show various forms of subcellular injury, but it is usually not very helpful in elucidating pathophysiologic mechanisms of tubular injury. Necrosis needs to be differentiated from postmortem autolysis, in which the tinctorial changes are more uniform throughout the section and there is loss of cellular detail without any changes in tissue organization. The degree of damage and timing of injury are important factors in whether there will be evidence of alterations in serum biochemical or urine biomarkers. BUN and sCr will not be elevated without and until there is significant nephron loss or damage. Almost 2/3 of renal function must be compromised in preclinical species prior to alterations in these serum parameters (Bonventre et al. 2010). While the nephron may recover, in many or most cases with significant necrosis involving multiple tubular profiles, the nephron will become dysfunctional and will be lost.

The mildest form of kidney necrosis is single cell necrosis. It involves apoptosis or loss of random or solitary tubular epithelial cells scattered across the cortex or medulla and is generally associated with low-grade or at least low doses of nephrotoxicants. Careful examination of the entire microscopic field may be necessary as affected cells may be relatively few in number. While cytoplasmic eosinophilia and cell shrinkage are hallmarks, nuclear changes can be variable and include pyknosis, condensation, or karyorrhexis of individual cells. Single cell necrosis associated with inflammation is considered oncotic necrosis, while single cell necrosis in the absence of inflammation represents apoptosis. As with apoptosis in other organs, there is an absence of inflammation. Rare apoptotic cells may also be found in normal control kidneys, so their presence should not automatically trigger a diagnosis of single cell necrosis in treated animals, and a threshold approach including assessment of dose response is warranted (Davis and Ryan 1998; Short 1998). Although apoptosis predominates, there may be a mixture of both apoptosis and oncotic necrosis in the same section. Increasing doses often increases the percentage of oncotic necrosis, and this phenomenon is commonly encountered with several agents including gentamicin or anticancer chemotherapeutics (Quiros et al. 2011). Since apoptosis requires ATP, cell energy status may also affect the mode of cell death. Apoptotic epithelial cells can be positively identified by TUNEL, caspase 3, or Annexin V immunostaining, although this is rarely necessary in routine toxicology studies (Short 1998).

With higher doses or longer duration of administration, single cell necrosis may progress to more pronounced areas of necrosis involving the entire tubule or cluster of tubules. This can occur via a direct nephrotoxic effect of the test article or may result from effects on the renal vascular supply. The proximal tubules tend to be more commonly affected by necrosis following xenobiotic administration than distal convoluted tubules or medullary collecting ducts, but any or all segments may be affected simultaneously depending on the agent. This predilection for proximal tubular injury may be due to the selective accumulation of xenobiotic compounds within the proximal segments. The proximal tubule has greater permeability to ions and chemical flux than the distal tubule due to the tight intracellular junctions and high electrical resistance found in distal tubules. The proximal tubules are the site of most of the membrane-bound active transport activity within the kidney. With more severe insult or longer duration of exposure, the area of injury expands from the initial site of damage. This is due to the tendency for the entire individual nephron to respond to localized injury and the compensatory hyperfiltration response in adjacent nephron segments. For instance, acute damage to the proximal convoluted tubules has been associated with single cell necrosis of the distal tubules (Bucci et al. 1998). Ischemic necrosis tends to follow a zonal distribution involving the corticomedullary junction in the case of diffuse organ hypoperfusion or in the form of wedge-shaped infarcts when occlusion of specific branches of the arcuate arteries occurs. The distal straight segment of the proximal tubules and the thick ascending limb are particularly sensitive to anoxia due to their high metabolic and transporter activity. Many drugs such as cyclosporine or amphotericin B can directly affect the vascular endothelium of the kidney, resulting in afferent or efferent vasoconstriction, reduced renal plasma flow, and/or decreased GFR (Remuzzi and Perico 1995). This can result in both glomerular and tubular damage.

The pathogenesis of renal tubular necrosis varies with the inducing agent, but common factors include oxidative stress, ion channel flux, cytoskeletal injury, lysosomal accumulation, mitochondrial injury, and inactivation of signaling kinases (Choudhury and Ahmed 2006; Lameire 2005). Necrosis follows a rather predictable cascade of events, depending on the initial site of subcellular damage. The sequence and specifics of reversible injury can be identified ultrastructurally and include an initial loss of glycogen in the cytoplasm, blunting and exfoliation of the apical microvilli, vesicle formation along the membrane, followed by swelling of the endoplasmic reticulum. Irreversible ultrastructural damage follows and is characterized by clumping or dissolution of the nuclear chromatin, mitochondrial swelling and loss of cristae, and, eventually, cell swelling and loss of lysosomal and plasma membrane integrity with digestion of intracellular contents. Nephrotoxic agents tend to produce tubular necrosis and AKI through a variety of mechanisms. For instance, exposure of tubular cells to cisplatin (a widely used chemotherapeutic agent with nephrotoxic potential) activates complex signaling pathways that lead to tubular cell injury involving cell death promotion via p53, MAP kinase, and reactive oxygen species and through metabolic activation of a variety of other cellular factors (Pabla and Dong 2008). Simultaneously, inflammatory responses and cytokines such as TNFα are stimulated, further exacerbating renal tissue injury, and parallel damage to renal vasculature results in decreased blood flow and ischemia (Pabla and Dong 2008). It is therefore clear that the pathophysiologic damage associated with most toxicants in the kidney is incredibly complex and that necrosis involves an interplay among multiple factors.

Autophagy is a normal physiologic process in cell biology and is associated with apoptosis and necrosis in some types of renal injury. During autophagy, a portion of cytoplasm is enveloped in double membrane-bound structures called autophagosomes, which undergo maturation and fusion with lysosomes for degradation, and these processes appear to be dependent on the upregulation of a specific family of genes called Atg (Periyasamy-Thandavan et al. 2008). Autophagy is a general cellular response to stress and has been demonstrated with cisplatin and cyclosporine toxicity in the kidney. Depending on experimental conditions, autophagy can directly produce cell death or act as a mechanism of cell survival and actually be cytoprotective against further injury, in association with other cell survival genes such as p21. The eventual cellular outcome in AKI (necrosis versus regeneration) is therefore dependent on whether these and other pro-survival cytoprotective pathways can counterbalance the coincidental cellular signals promoting cell death, and this may depend on whether there is further exposure to the toxicant.

12.1.3.8 Infarction

Renal infarcts are encountered occasionally in preclinical toxicity studies in association with partial or complete obstruction of the renal vasculature. This may occur as a result of thrombosis or due to hemodynamic effects of xenobiotic agents. Subcapsular infarcts are noted as a frequent background lesion in some strains of rodents without any evidence of initiating cause. Infarcts are also a common downstream effect of chronic renal disease and can be downstream ischemic effects from metastatic tumors or leukemia. Infarction is characterized by well-demarcated, wedge-shaped areas of coagulative necrosis and tubular loss within the cortex, corresponding to the blood supply associated with arcuate arteries. The central necrotic area is homogenous and eosinophilic and lacks cellular detail. There is often nuclear karyorrhexis. The central zone is bordered by a peripheral zone or band of mixed inflammation. Recent infarcts tend to have an intervening marginal zone of congestion and hemorrhage, and the peripheral zone is predominated by neutrophils. With time, the peripheral inflammation becomes more mononuclear in character, and chronic infarcts will have marked interstitial fibrosis throughout all zones and marked tubular loss or atrophy with collapse of the parenchyma and replacement by collagen scarring and dystrophic mineralization. This results in a characteristic depression in the capsule, which can be noted grossly as discoloration and pitting of the capsular surface. Recent infarcts may exhibit only a reddened wedge-shaped area on the capsule and cut surface. Kidney weights may initially be slightly increased, but chronic infarcts will most often be associated with decreased organ weights. Alterations in clinical pathology parameters are uncommon and depend greatly on the size and chronicity of the infarct as with other necrotic lesions. Infarcts are easily differentiated from interstitial fibrosis from other causes of kidney disease by the characteristic wedge-shaped pattern of injury. The clinical implications of infarction vary tremendously with the cause. Thrombosis may occur in preclinical studies as a consequence of prolonged intravenous infusion procedures, and in this context, they are independent of test article. However, many other agents, including those that produce renal efferent or afferent vasoconstriction or anti-thrombolytic agents, may result in drug-related vascular occlusion, which may have a pharmacologic basis and signal the potential for a clinical effect on the renal vasculature.

12.1.3.9 Tubular Atrophy

One of the hallmarks of end-stage kidney disease is tubular atrophy. Irreversible damage to a majority of nephrons will eventually result in dysfunction and decompensation of the kidney and atrophy of many or most of the remaining tubules. However, tubular atrophy may also occur in individual tubules with loss of other portions of that individual nephron such as the glomerulus or distal structures. Tubular atrophy is therefore frequently noted in areas of infarction or associated with hydronephrotic kidneys, and it is a consistent feature of advanced CPN in rodents. Tubular atrophy is characterized by shrunken, collapsed basophilic tubules with little or no visible lumina. There are often thickened, wrinkled basement membranes and prominent peritubular and interstitial fibrosis. Cortical tubules are usually more involved than the medullary ducts. The atrophic tubule is no longer functional and is irretrievably lost, with accompanying loss of the entire nephron to which it is attached. Adjacent tubules may be somewhat hypertrophied or hyperplastic due to compensation or single nephron hyperfiltration phenomenon. Tubular atrophy may be a consequence of a wide range of nephrotoxicants and may be seen in both subacute and chronic studies. Alterations in clinical biochemistries largely depend on the distribution and severity of the change, but urine biomarkers are unlikely to be very helpful.

12.1.3.10 Tubular Regeneration

Regeneration refers to the morphologic alterations associated with reparative processes following injury to the tubular epithelium. After acute necrotic tubular injury, regenerative cells spread over the basement membrane in areas where epithelium has been shed into the lumina (Cuppage and Tate 1967). Increased mitotic activity in the lower part of the nephron may be responsible for the migration of cells from adjacent portions of the nephron to cover the defect. For restoration of normal function, the basement membrane must remain intact. Tubular basophilia is the most obvious microscopic feature of tubular regeneration, but the two terms are not synonymous. Tinctorial basophilia of the proximal tubular cytoplasm may also result from very early or very mild degeneration without the presence of any real regenerative physiological phenomenon in the cell. Regeneration as a diagnosis should also be associated with increased mitoses, flattening of the lining tubular profiles associated with cell spreading to cover defects from cell loss, and potentially an increase in cell numbers within a tubular profile and/or nuclear crowding. There may be heterogeneity in cell size and shape with a higher nuclear-to-cytoplasmic ratio in individual cells. There should not be alterations or thickening of the basement membrane, as this change is usually associated with ongoing degeneration and is a feature of CPN rather than regeneration. There may be some dilation of affected tubular lumina, but frank tubular dilatation suggests ongoing injury rather than regeneration. However, when the two conditions are overlapping, diagnosis can be problematic. The diagnosis of tubular regeneration is often used in preclinical studies at the end of recovery phases where there were previous minimal to mild degenerative tubular changes, and thus, the regenerative morphologic alterations are indicative of partial or active recovery. However, regeneration may also be noted during the treatment phases of studies, where a low-grade perturbation of function is induced by a xenobiotic agent without significant necrosis or basement membrane damage or occurs at an earlier timepoint not assessed histologically. Therefore, tubules may be in various states of injury and repair in cyclic phases within the same section of kidney. This has led to the frequent diagnosis of "degeneration/regeneration" with some of these low-grade nephrotoxicants in preclinical studies. Regeneration should be differentiated from mild degeneration (tubular basophilia alone), as well as mild tubular hyperplasia. Tubular hyperplasia may contain areas of regeneration but is characterized by an area of increased cellularity within tubular profiles rather than thinned individual profiles and may or may not show stratification of layers. Regeneration without concurrent necrosis generally does not result in serum clinicopathologic changes, especially in BUN or sCr, but clusterin and KIM-1 may be increased in the urine (Yang et al. 2007). In fact, regeneration is not usually considered an adverse finding, as it implies an attempt at restoration of function. However, the original degenerative or necrotic process may be considered adverse. Along with increased Ki67, PCNA, and other markers of proliferation, regeneration is also accompanied by elevated expression of intracellular osteopontin and vimentin (Yang et al. 2007). While the time required for tubular repair varies with the agent and degree of initial injury, proximal tubular epithelium can usually be restored to relatively normal numbers and function within 5–7 days if the toxicologic insult is withdrawn. This is evident as basophilic, flattened, and elongated cells with very little microvilli gradually become more cuboidal by day 5 when they form a rudimentary brush border. By 10–14 days, the regenerative cells have a more normal morphology, which in an additional 7 to 14 days is reflected in normal function. If necrosis or dilation is severe enough, there may be permanent damage to the basement membrane, in which case fibrosis may ensue and the tubules and accompanying nephron segments may undergo atrophy.

12.1.3.11   Karyomegaly

Toxic insult occasionally results in a specific alteration in cortical tubules and medullary ducts, which is characterized by nuclear enlargement. Karyomegaly is likely due to nuclear divisions without associated cytokinesis, resulting in increased nuclear size. It is noted with xenobiotic treatment most often in rats, but enlarged nuclei or multinucleated cells may occasionally be noted in the medullary ducts of control rhesus and cynomolgus monkeys as a normal finding. The nuclei may have slightly irregular profiles and may contain vesicular chromatin with multiple nucleoli or hyperchromatic staining patterns. In most cases, the pathogenesis is uncertain. Karyomegaly in proximal tubule cells has been noted in chronic studies with renal carcinogens such as ochratoxin and aflatoxin, as well as with a few specific agents such as some antineoplastic compounds affecting cell division (Adler et al. 2007; Dortant et al. 2001). However, there is no direct correlation between karyomegaly and neoplastic potential, and karyomegaly is therefore not regarded as necessarily a preneoplastic trait (Montgomery and Seely 1990). Karyomegaly may also accompany other more common forms of degeneration and necrosis in the kidney as a consequence of nephrotoxicant exposure, as occurs in monkeys given antiretroviral drugs or in rodents administered with trichloroethylene (Adler et al. 2007; Lacy et al. 1998).

12.1.3.12   Tubular Hypertrophy

Tubular epithelium may undergo compensatory hypertrophy with chronic injury, irrespective of cause. It is noted with frequency in the tubules of rodent remnant kidney models of renal failure such as the 5/6 nephrectomized rat (Dube et al. 2004). It often accompanies other morphologic alterations of acute or chronic tubular insult, such as the degeneration, regeneration, or atrophy associated with cadmium, chlorpyrifos, or lysine nephrotoxicity (Asanuma et al. 2006; Tripathi and Srivastav 2011), and is occasionally noted in the proximal convoluted tubules of rats with long-standing CPN (Hard and Khan 2004). Hypertrophy may also be a hallmark of specific toxic insult by some agents such as alterations in the collecting ducts associated with hypokalemia, chronic diuretic administration, or salt loading (Ellison et al. 1989; Evan et al. 1980). Hypertrophic tubules are lined by tall cuboidal to columnar cells that may completely occlude the lumen. Nuclei are often placed along the apical margin. The cytoplasm is often pale or eosinophilic, rather than the basophilic cytoplasm associated with regeneration or mild degeneration. There is no increase in cell number and generally no nuclear crowding or stacking. Hypertrophy must be differentiated from tubular hyperplasia, in which epithelia lose their ordered arrangement and where proliferation rates (as assessed by PCNA or Ki67) are much higher. Hypertrophic tubules are not proliferative and are not considered preneoplastic lesions. Rather, hypertrophy is considered an adaptive response to an increase in active transcellular transport capacity (Ellison et al. 1989; Hard et al. 1999). There also seems to be a relationship of hypertrophy to persistent or sustained increases in GFR (Fine and Bradley 1985). Hypertrophy does not in itself result in clinicopathologic alterations, but as it accompanies chronic tubulointerstitial injury, there may be concomitant changes from associated tubular necrosis, atrophy, or chronic degeneration. In cases where hypertrophy is noted in the collecting ducts, checking for systemic electrolyte abnormalities may be warranted due to the association with adaptive responses to altered ion flux across tubular cell membranes.

12.1.3.13 Chronic Progressive Nephropathy

CPN is undoubtedly the most commonly encountered entity in rodent toxicity studies. It has many synonyms including chronic progressive nephrosis, glomerulonephrosclerosis, spontaneous nephrosis, old rat nephropathy, and dietary nephritis. It is a spontaneous, age-related disease entity that occurs in high incidence in the strains of rats commonly used in preclinical toxicity studies. CPN occurs in both male and female rats, but at a higher incidence and severity in males. CPN is both a degenerative and regenerative condition. The spectrum of changes includes basophilic cortical tubules, thickened basement membranes, crowded nuclei, and/or the presence of hyaline casts (Hard and Khan 2004). There are also concurrent changes of glomerulosclerosis that become progressive with age. Incipient lesions of CPN are detectable as early as 2 months of age in some strains of rats and are generally identified as thickened basement membranes, particularly of Bowman's capsule (Gray et al. 1982), or surrounding a single profile of a basophilic proximal tubule (Hard and Khan 2004). With time, single affected tubular profiles progress to larger foci of basophilic proximal tubules within the same nephron, and some may contain casts. Tubular hyperplasia is a consistent feature of the lesion early on, but tubular atrophy is a common sequel. There is a variably mild mononuclear inflammatory response, which is often centered around interstitial vessels. Progressive expansion of the interstitium occurs, with only minimal or mild fibrosis by 12 months of age (Abrass 2000). Hyperplasia of the pelvic urothelium and/or of the epithelium lining the papilla may be present. In even older rats, almost the entire cortex may be affected, with cystic tubules, severe casts, and widespread interstitial fibrosis and mineralization. This chronic change may be accompanied by increased BUN and sCR, renal secondary hyperparathyroidism, and fibrous osteodystrophy. Proteinuria/albuminuria has been the best correlate of disease progression and occurs early in the onset of CPN. Other serum abnormalities including hypercholesterolemia and, to a lesser extent, hypoalbuminemia are also seen.

Administration of several chemicals and drugs can be associated with an increase in the incidence or earlier age of onset of the disease in rats without other evidence of nephrotoxicity. This effect likely represents the rat response to a low-grade chronic renal insult and is a minimal indication of chronic nephrotoxicity. However, in some cases, exacerbated CPN potentially might reflect a nonspecific but persistent effect on other renal functional parameters such as GFR. For instance, a few of the ACE inhibitors and related agents that pharmacologically target the kidney clearly exacerbate CPN incidence or severity, without resulting in any other evidence of renal toxicity. Many chemicals that induce hyaline droplet nephropathy in rats are also associated with increased CPN (Hard et al. 1993). There is no human counterpart for CPN, so an increased incidence or exacerbation of this condition by a xenobiotic agent in rats must be interpreted with extreme caution when extrapolating to humans, particularly in the absence of evidence of nephrotoxic signal in another species (Hard et al. 2009c). At worst, hazard assessment would conclude that there is a potential for slight nephrotoxicity at relevant exposures. CPN has both degenerative and regenerative components and therefore may be associated with an increased incidence of tumors of the renal tubules in chronic studies. Florid tubule profiles in advanced CPN disease are not considered preneoplastic and need to be discriminated from atypical tubular hyperplasia associated with carcinogenesis (Hard and Seely 2006). Some agents can interact with CPN to increase the incidence of renal tumors and CPN-related proliferative lesions via robust stimulation of regeneration and hyperplasia (Hard and Khan 2004). These effects should be considered a secondary, nongenotoxic mechanism for renal tumor development and a mode of action with minimal or no relevance to humans (Hard and Seely 2005).

While the etiology of CPN is still largely controversial, the incidence of the condition is influenced by various physiological factors such as caloric intake, protein content of diet, and male hormones. The total amount of ingested food over a long period seems to be a major determinant of the severity of spontaneous damage (Keenan et al. 2000). Castration is protective in the male but has no effect in females, and chronic androgen administration will accelerate damage in females, suggesting an important androgen influence (Baylis 1994). Neither vascular lesions nor immune complexes are associated with the pathogenesis of the lesion. While there are concurrent glomerular lesions associated with the tubular changes and glomerular hyperfiltration is involved to some degree in the development of glomerulosclerosis, the historical hypothesis that the pathogenesis of CPN-mediated tubular injury is also related to glomerular hyperfiltration is controversial. There is no established causal relationship between glomerular capillary pressure and degree of glomerular or tubular damage in studies of CPN (Baylis 1994). Albuminuria associated with advanced CPN may be due more to failure of postglomerular cellular processing of albumin by tubules rather than to changes in glomerular permeability, since albumin is more freely filtered than once thought (Russo et al. 2002). Rather than a primary glomerular lesion, the primary pathogenesis of CPN is now thought to involve changes in the basement membranes throughout the kidney. Alterations in the amino acid composition, hydroxylation, and glycosylation of basal lamina surrounding tubules are noted in some of the earliest lesions of CPN (Abrass 2000). The thickened basal lamina likely disturbs epithelial attachments to the basement membrane leading to cytoskeletal and functional alterations provoking cytoplasmic basophilia in the proximal tubules and altered filtration in the glomeruli. Changes in tinctorial characteristics of the PCTs are an initial and nonspecific hallmark of the nephron's response to injury, so basophilia is one of the earliest microscopic lesions that can be noted by the pathologist, but thickened basement membranes are visualized soon thereafter.

While the classical and most studied presentation of CPN occurs in the rat, a similar but pathologically distinct renal lesion also occurs in the mouse. This condition is not as well characterized as CPN in the rat, and while a similar constellation of changes occurs progressively over time, it has unique features and appears to have a separate pathogenesis. The incidence in mice is significantly less than in rat, and the age of onset is later, with the earliest evidence of lesions usually appearing only after 4 months of age. Tubular basophilia and nuclear crowding are noted, but thickening of the basal lamina is harder to appreciate except in the more chronic cases. Hyaline casts increase in number over time. Mononuclear inflammatory infiltrates are more prominent in mice than in rats with CPN and tend to expand the interstitium. Dilation of the glomerular space is often present, but glomerulosclerosis occurs only in the later stages of the disease. The clinical relevance of CPN in the mouse is thought to mirror CPN in rats, including a relationship to increased tubular epithelial proliferation in the kidney in chronic studies.

12.1.3.14 Hyaline Droplets and α-$_{2U}$-Globulin Nephropathy

Hyaline droplets are frequently found in the cytoplasm of proximal tubules in male rats, generally localized to the S2 segment, and are characterized by variably sized, refractile, brightly eosinophilic ovoid droplets consisting of lysosomal accumulations of α-$_{2U}$-globulin. There are a large number of agents (d-limonene, hydrocarbon or petroleum products, decalin) that will result in α-$_{2U}$-globulin nephropathy, characterized by an increase in droplet number and distribution, and/or altered pattern of droplet distribution (Dill et al. 2003). Although the hyaline droplets are most often not associated with any other visible evidence of tubular injury, in more severe cases, there may be occasional single cell necrosis, sloughed luminal epithelial cells, or increased mitoses of tubules, and the distribution may include all segments of the proximal tubules. In chronic cases, granular casts may form at the junction of the inner and outer medullary stripes, and linear medullary and papillary mineralization has been described (Hard et al. 1993). In carcinogenicity studies using compounds that induce α-$_{2U}$-globulin nephropathy, tubular hyperplasia and increased incidence of renal tumors have also been described (Hard et al. 1999). The change is frequently accompanied by exacerbation of the incidence or severity of spontaneous CPN (Dill et al. 2003). While test article administration can result in an increase in α-$_{2U}$-globulin accumulation, some xenobiotic agents may cause an accumulation of hyaline droplets within secondary lysosomes of proximal tubules in rats that consist of other low-molecular-weight (LMW) proteins, or of drug–protein complexes (Hard and Snowden 1991). Prominent eosinophilic droplets also occur in the cytoplasm of proximal tubules in rats with systemic histiocytic sarcoma and, in this syndrome, are composed of lysozyme. Hyaline droplets occur rarely in mice and have been noted only extremely rarely after compound administration in other species. "Hyaline droplet nephropathy" is the preferred term to use as a morphologic diagnosis in a toxicity study when there is some question of whether the accumulated material making up the droplets is α-$_{2u}$-globulin or not. This can be determined by the use of special procedures such as Mallory Heidenhain, Martius scarlet blue, or chromotrope-aniline-blue stains, or by using immunohistochemical stains directed toward α-$_{2U}$-globulin (De Rijk et al. 2003). Special stains are particularly useful in cases where the presentation is atypical for α-$_{2u}$-globulin, such as a high incidence in females, presence in a nonrodent, or where there are irregularly shaped or sized droplets. Hyaline droplets need to be distinguished from intratubular hemorrhage or hemoglobin, which will be multifocal rather than diffuse and stain brick-colored rather than pink with H&E. Although structurally similar LMW proteins have been found in the urine filtrate of other species, including humans, the characteristic lesions of α-$_{2U}$-globulin nephropathy do not occur except in rats. Moreover, compounds that produce α-$_{2U}$-globulin nephropathy or hyaline droplet nephropathy in rats have generally not resulted in other significant renal pathology in humans either. Based on cancer bioassays, hormonal studies, and gene knockout experiments, the increase in renal tumors and hyperplasias associated with this condition appears to be due to a compensatory increase in cell proliferation and turnover coupled with cytotoxicity and is not considered to pose any significant risk for human carcinogenesis since this hyaline droplet-mediated effect is rat specific and therefore not relevant to humans (Hard et al. 1993).

The pathogenesis of α-$_{2U}$-globulin nephropathy has been studied extensively. Alpha-2u-globulin is a freely filtered, androgen-regulated protein synthesized in the liver of male rats, becoming the major excreted urinary protein in this gender and species (Short et al. 1989). The amount of protein in the diet can greatly influence tubular protein reabsorption (including α-$_{2U}$-globulin) and hence affect the incidence of the condition (Neuhaus et al. 1981). The rate-determining step in the development of drug-induced forms of α-$_{2U}$-globulin nephropathy is reversible, noncovalent binding of the agent to the protein. While the binding site in rats forms a large cavity, in the homologous LMW urinary proteins of other species such as mouse and human, the cavity is shallow and does not easily accommodate ligand binding (Chaudhuri et al. 1999). The resulting complex is more resistant to hydrolytic degradation in the lysosomal compartment of the proximal tubule than the native protein. Persistence of the material may eventually result in cytoplasmic leakage and initiation of degenerative pathways, including apoptosis. Hyaline droplets other than α-$_{2U}$-globulin probably have a similar pathogenic mechanism due to lysosomal accumulation of LMW proteins or protein complexes associated with increased filtered loads or increased absorption related to xenobiotic administration (Alden 1986).

12.1.3.15 Crystalluria, Obstructive Nephropathy, and Retrograde Nephropathy

Crystals occur frequently in the lumina of tubules of both rodents and nonrodents in toxicology studies, and perhaps even more frequently in the renal pelvis and lower urinary tract. Tubular calculi are most often localized to the cortex and outer medulla. They usually appear clear to light brown in tissue sections and are birefringent under polarized light, which makes crystals easy to differentiate from mineralized deposits or casts. However, many calculi formed in the urine dissolve or eventually are voided, leaving no sign of their presence except for secondary degenerative effects (Cohen et al. 2002). Crystalluria will often be associated with a constellation of morphologic features known as obstructive nephropathy that occurs from outflow obstruction. These changes include tubular dilation, degeneration, or necrosis in the affected tubules or those immediately preceding them. Occasionally, obstructive nephropathy will also be accompanied by the presence of mononuclear or granulomatous inflammatory infiltrates as a result of secondary damage (Chevalier 2006). In the renal pelvis, crystalluria is frequently associated with urothelial hyperplasia and may result in hydronephrosis or pyelonephritis. Urolithiasis in the bladder, or as far distally as the urethra, may result in the same secondary degenerative renal tubular changes due to obstruction of the filtrate. Obstructive nephropathy can result in acute elevations of BUN, sCr, and serum potassium and can result in oliguric renal failure and be an important cause of mortality in some studies. Crystals may be identifiable by examination of urine sediments, but fresh samples are often necessary for the best assessment.

Due to the potential for concentration of drugs or metabolites in the tubular urinary filtrate, especially in the thick ascending limb and distal convoluted tubules, agents with low solubility or high renal clearance can precipitate out of solution within tubular lumina (Yarlagadda and Perazella 2008). Sulfonamides and fluoroquinolones are classic examples of such drugs with the potential for crystalluria in the dog and monkey. Agents that affect urinary pH, such as carbonic anhydrase inhibitors, may predispose coadministered drugs to form crystals, and decreased intravascular volume, as in dehydration, will also increase the potential for urolithiasis. Some agents or their metabolites, such as oxalic acid produced by alcohol dehydrogenase-mediated metabolism of ethylene glycol, will complex with minerals and become sequestered within tubules (Li and McMartin 2009). Renal tubular apoptosis is a major factor leading to tubular atrophy after obstructive damage. Proapoptotic signals and increased reactive oxygen species contribute to necrosis, loss of nephrons, and chemokine-mediated inflammatory cell recruitment and eventually lead to stimulation of paracrine growth factor/cell cycle signaling and fibrotic cascades (Chevalier 2006; Truong et al. 2011).

Due to differences in pH and solute and protein compositions of the urine filtrate between species, as well as often quite variable renal excretion profiles from one species to another, crystalluria may be confined to one or a limited number of preclinical species, and its presence does not automatically imply that similar obstructive changes may occur at relevant human exposures. However, careful examination of the pharmacokinetic and biochemical profiles of an agent and its metabolites may provide some prediction and useful extrapolation of the potential for crystalluria in humans. Analysis of the composition of crystals is often very helpful in considering their pathogenesis, particularly when drug product is identified.

Obstructive nephropathy can occasionally be noted in nonclinical studies due to factors other than crystalluria. It has been encountered in rodents with proteinaceous plugs (mouse urologic syndrome) and in cynomolgus monkeys treated with some small molecules and biopharmaceutical agents. In the latter cases, intratubular casts identified as Tamm-Horsfall protein result in tubular dilatation, interstitial inflammation and edema, and lesions indistinguishable from other forms of obstructive nephropathy (Guzman et al. 2008). Cast material was strongly PAS positive. Cytokines, urinary crystals, and even immunoglobulins may all bind with affinity to Tamm-Horsfall protein. The mechanism is therefore thought to be related to microcrystal formation acting as a nidus for aggregation or coprecipitation of the Tamm-Horsfall protein and, in the case of small molecules, may be related to a carboxylic acid moiety shared between most of the inciting agents. As drug-induced obstructive nephropathy has not been identified in humans or other nonclinical species with these agents, the clinical relevance of the monkey protein cast obstructive nephropathy is uncertain.

Certain other compounds resulting in tubular crystalluria, such as melamine in rodents, result in a specific pattern of radiating, acute, and chronic renal changes known as retrograde nephropathy (Hard et al. 2009a,b). Rather than dilation or degenerative lesions limited to the immediately adjacent and preceding tubules associated with crystalluria, retrograde nephropathy results in a spectrum of degenerative changes extending from the papilla to the cortex. There are clusters of basophilic or dilated tubules traversing the inner and outer medullary stripes and extending axially into the cortex involving some of the same nephron segments. These tend to be more common at the periphery of the papilla. Mild peritubular fibrosis and tubular atrophy will occur chronically, resulting in linear scarring. Collecting ducts may remain dilated and hyperplastic in chronic cases, but cortical tubules are more often compressed or atrophic (Hard et al. 2009a,b). While there are usually features of hyperplasia (mitoses, nuclear crowding), the lack of conspicuously thickened basement membranes or hyaline casts and the radial pattern, one can easily differentiate this lesion from CPN. Inflammatory cells are usually limited in number, which allows differentiation from pyelonephritis and other more common forms of obstructive nephropathy. The mechanism for the renal changes associated with retrograde nephropathy appears to be different from obstructive damage directly attributable to crystalluria and outflow obstruction. It has been proposed that melamine precipitation transiently alters tubular pressure and results in increased reflux, but how this differs from effects of other crystals is unclear (Hard et al. 1999). There are species differences in susceptibility to retrograde nephropathy, with mice less so than rats. In 2007, renal failure was reported worldwide in humans and many domestic animal species as a result of food formulated with triazine-contaminated wheat gluten in milk supplements and pet food from China. However, the renal changes in dogs, cats, humans, and pigs resulting from exposure to melamine and cyanuric acid actually represent a different spectrum of changes that more closely resemble obstructive nephropathy (Brown et al. 2007; Nilubol et al. 2009).

12.1.4 PAPILLARY CHANGES

Among toxic insults to the inner medulla and renal papilla, papillary necrosis and pyelonephritis are by far the most commonly encountered in nonclinical studies. The renal medulla and papilla are vulnerable to ischemic necrosis because of the unique arrangement of their blood supply and the local interstitial hypertonicity. Hydrodynamic effects may also be reflected in marked changes in the papilla, such as the medullary atrophy that occurs with hydronephrosis or necrosis associated with distal outflow obstruction. There may be marked differences in papillary responses to toxins between unipapillate kidneys of rodents or dogs and multipapillate species such as the pig. It should be noted that there are also differences between species of monkeys, with cynomolgus monkey kidneys representing unipapillate types and rhesus monkeys representing the multipapillate type, and agents may affect these species much differently.

12.1.4.1 Papillary Necrosis

Due to its association with non-steroidal anti-inflammatory drugs (NSAIDs) and analgesic nephropathy, papillary necrosis is a well-recognized entity in preclinical toxicology studies. Drugs and metabolites often reach their highest concentrations within the filtrate of the papilla predisposing this region to injury. Both pyelonephritis and obstruction due to crystalluria are important factors in the development of spontaneous papillary necrosis. In its earliest morphologic form, there are loss of cellular definition, decreased extracellular matrix glycosaminoglycans, and interstitial edema in the distal papillary tip. These progress proximally with medullary ductular and tubular necrosis, capillary degeneration, and interstitial hemorrhage. The interstitium becomes acellular and is replaced by an eosinophilic or sometimes lightly basophilic matrix. There may be secondary mixed inflammation, mineralization, and nuclear debris, especially at the abscission zone (the linear transitional region between necrotic and viable renal parenchyma). In cases where pyelonephritis is an inciting cause, the inflammatory infiltrate may contain predominantly neutrophils. Dilation of the more proximal collecting ducts or cortical tubules may be secondary changes. In the most severe cases, the entire inner medulla may be affected, resulting in sloughing of the papilla and urothelial re-epithelialization. Alterations in urinary concentrating ability as reflected in lower or isosthenuric urine specific gravity are a consistent if not particularly sensitive parameter to monitor. RPA-1 has been increased in rodents with papillary necrosis, but there is currently no commercially available ortholog for humans (Price et al. 2010). In advanced cases, there are usually elevations in BUN, sCr, and peripheral leukocyte counts, and serum phosphorus is also often elevated. Papillary necrosis may also be demonstrated antemortem by imaging modalities such as contrast radiography, computed tomography, or ultrasonography when blunting of the papilla is present. Medullary blood flow, urine concentrating capacity, pyramidal papillary morphology, and cyclooxygenase (COX) isoform distribution are all factors important in these species differences in susceptibility. Humans tend to be more resistant to papillary necrosis than dogs or especially rats. Likely due to similarities in renal anatomy and physiology, the pig is similarly resistant as humans and has been suggested as a better choice of nonrodent species for NSAIDs and other agents with a great potential for inducing papillary necrosis in preclinical toxicology studies (Swindle et al. 2012). Although there are pronounced species differences in susceptibility, many agents that result in papillary necrosis in rodents or dogs may induce the lesion in a small percentage of humans given sufficient exposure or time. Therefore, the identification of the lesion has important relevance to clinical risk assessment. In addition to NSAIDs, several other drugs and chemicals have been associated with papillary necrosis, including 2-bromoethanamine hydrobromide, cyclophosphamide, and radiocontrast media. In chronic rodent carcinogenicity studies, agents that produce papillary necrosis often result in an increased incidence of urothelial carcinoma due to proliferative responses of the urothelium. Dehydration tends to exacerbate the lesions, and decreased urine flow appears to be an important contributing factor in the pathogenesis. While there may be some differences among agents and the involved pathways are complex, the pathophysiology tends to involve the inhibition of renal vasodilatory prostaglandins and subsequent redistribution of medullary blood flow. Prostaglandin synthetases and prostaglandin hydroperoxidase activity are localized to the medullary interstitium. COX mediates the synthesis of prostaglandins through the enzymatic conversion of arachidonate to prostaglandin H2 (PGH2) and then through further metabolism to other biologically active prostanoids. Both COX1 and COX2 are constitutively expressed in the renal interstitium, with COX1 also found in the collecting duct and COX2 within the macula densa and cells of the thick ascending limb (Breyer et al. 2001). NSAIDs and other analgesics compete with arachidonate for binding to the catalytic site of cyclooxygenase, thereby blocking prostaglandin synthesis. Since medullary capillaries have abundant prostaglandin receptors responsible for vasoactivity, COX or PG inhibition can result in local vasoconstriction, and when combined with reduced urinary filtrate flow, chemical concentration in the medulla, and the innate nephrotoxic potential of a compound, the tip of the papilla is subjected to conditions of ischemia and potential direct cytotoxicity. The initial cellular targets include the medullary interstitial cells and capillaries, but this is quickly followed by changes in the epithelium of the loops of Henle and collecting ducts and the progressive loss of tissue proximally (Schnellman 1998). Other compounds such as 2,3-di-phosphoglyceric acid or phenacetin, which do not directly inhibit prostaglandin synthesis, may result in papillary necrosis by affecting the oxygen carrying capacity of the blood or inducing methemoglobinemia, respectively (Sabatini 1996). The end result of local anoxic conditions in the medulla and ischemic necrosis mimics those of the COX inhibitors. A similar mechanism is postulated for papillary necrosis that is associated with sickle cell anemia in humans. Urolithiasis and amyloidosis also produce papillary necrosis probably via secondary effects on the medullary vasculature and result in local ischemia. Amyloidosis-associated papillary necrosis is often encountered in mice in chronic studies and is thought to result from compression of vessels, which disrupts the distal medullary blood supply. Urolithiasis may produce distal medullary ischemia by both vascular compromise and blockage of urine flow.

12.1.4.2 Pyelonephritis

Pyelonephritis refers to suppurative or mixed inflammation of the medulla, pelvis, and distal nephron, involving the interstitium and tubular/collecting duct lumina, which may extend into the cortex (Figure 12.2b). There may be tubular basophilia and evidence of hyperplasia, especially in the outer stripe or cortex, and secondary tubular degeneration or necrosis. The lining epithelium, especially at the tip of the papilla, may become ulcerated. Over time and with chronicity, the lesion progresses from acute inflammation (multifocal microabscessation, discrete clusters of neutrophils) to chronic infiltrates of mononuclear cells accompanied by fibrosis. Pyelonephritis may result from extension of interstitial nephritis beginning as a cortical lesion, but more commonly, the inflammation begins in the medulla and extends radially into the cortical interstitium. Hyperemia or discoloration of the medulla is the most common presentation grossly, but in severe cases, there may be dilation of the pelvis from secondary hydronephrosis. BUN, sCr, and phosphorus are often elevated, and urine specific gravity may also be lowered, eventually reaching isosthenuric ranges. Sediment examination usually reveals both increased leukocyte counts and granular or leukocytic casts. Urine protein and albumin excretion are generally increased. Rats and mice frequently have evidence of spontaneous medullary inflammatory foci, which are usually due to ascending or embolic bacterial infections. Spontaneous vesicoureteral reflux with coincidental bacterial cystitis is considered a major predisposing factor, but other factors such as regional hypoperfusion also make the medulla more prone to infection. Differentiating spontaneous from test article–induced pyelonephritis when small numbers of animals are affected can present a diagnostic dilemma. There are many agents that may increase the incidence of pyelonephritis in animals in toxicity studies. Compounds that produce papillary injury (e.g., NSAIDs) and those that are associated with pelvic crystalluria (sulfonamides) are notable examples (Bach and Thanh 1998). Drug-induced pyelonephritis, without evidence of papillary injury, is occasionally encountered in toxicity studies with immunosuppressive compounds such as cyclosporine (Miller and Findon 1988). The clinical significance of the lesion varies with pathophysiology, but the potential for effects on immune function or urolithiasis should always be considered.

12.1.5 Interstitial and Vascular Changes

12.1.5.1 Interstitial Inflammation and Interstitial Nephritis

Focal mononuclear inflammatory cell infiltrates are noted extremely commonly as clusters within the interstitium of the renal cortex, and less commonly in the medulla, of rodents, dogs, and monkeys. These are most often of no toxicologic significance, unless they are accompanied by degenerative tubular or glomerular changes and/or show significant increase in dose responsive incidence or severity. The number of inflammatory cell foci increases in these spontaneous lesions with age and is often associated with the presence of CPN and other chronic kidney lesions in rodents. These focal to multifocal cellular aggregates most often consist of lymphocytes but may be admixed with macrophages or small numbers of plasma cells or neutrophils. Interstitial inflammation may occur in toxicologic studies with agents that affect several components within the interstitial extracellular matrix, including those associated with antibodies against the basement membrane as well as drugs that affect interstitial cells.

Xenobiotic agents may also produce a more intense and widespread, primary inflammatory reaction in the interstitium that has been labeled "interstitial nephritis." Test article–induced primary interstitial disease occurs in dogs and monkeys at least as commonly as in rodents. Persistent low-grade chronic renal toxicity in rats is more likely to be expressed as exacerbated CPN rather than as chronic interstitial nephritis, although CPN may be associated with mild interstitial inflammation. Interstitial nephritis is characterized by generalized mononuclear or mixed inflammation with variable degrees of edema or fibrosis and can be either acute or chronic. It is not synonymous with pyelonephritis, which is more severe in the medulla and especially the papilla and which is predominated by neutrophils. Pyelonephritis and other forms of acute drug-induced inflammation, such as the microabscesses of tubulitis, often have large numbers of inflammatory cells and debris within tubular lumina, which is generally lacking in interstitial nephritis. Chronic interstitial nephritis may present grossly as pale streaks within the kidney, and severe acute interstitial nephritis can appear grossly as pale enlarged kidneys due to edema, but most inflammation is not visible macroscopically. In the more severe cases of interstitial inflammation, there are often elevations in BUN and sCR, and there may be increases in urinary protein and albumin excretion. Interstitial nephritis has been associated clinically with administration of drugs such as the succinimides, lithium, methicillin, and allopurinol, and the lesion therefore has significant human relevance (Linton et al. 1980). The pathogenic mechanism responsible for the development of interstitial nephritis has not been determined in most cases, and preclinical lesions are not always predictive of a similar response in humans.

Microabscesses may form in the interstitium as a response to xenobiotic treatment. They may be either solitary or multifocal and may be found within glomeruli or tubular lumina as well as in the interstitium. They may be associated with cellular casts or surround a central focus of exfoliated cells or necrotic debris. Affected tubules are often basophilic and filled with degenerating neutrophils. Microabscessation may result from septic bacterial infection, especially when associated with intravenous test article administration secondary to the formation of infected thromboemboli. Pyelonephritis of the renal pelvis is often associated with concurrent microabscessation of the adjacent corticomedullary tubules (Duprat and Burek 1986) and is usually caused by ascending bacterial infection or crystalluria or secondary to agent-induced papillary necrosis. Solitary proximal tubules affected with microabscessation often occur in advanced stages of CPN. Grossly, the cut surface of the kidney may demonstrate yellow stippling or yellow foci within the cortex or medulla. Changes in serum biochemical data are not frequent in most cases of microabscesses, but leukocytic or granular casts may be found in the urine on sediment exams. Gram stains may be helpful in identifying bacteria if present, and from a risk assessment perspective, it is important to decide whether apparent test article–related microabscessation is a potential result of depression of immune function or related to other factors. Interstitial edema may accompany several forms of acute inflammation including microabscessation or pyelonephritis but, in some instances, can also occur independently as a xenobiotic-related response. Interstitial inflammation and edema can accompany tubular degeneration in the nephrotoxicity associated with NSAIDs independently of papillary necrosis (Hard and Neal 1992).

12.1.5.2 Interstitial Fibrosis

Interstitial fibrosis is a common feature of virtually all chronic kidney diseases, regardless of cause. Following tubular damage, fibroblasts in the adjacent interstitium proliferate, change to a myofibroblast phenotype, and increase their collagen production, resulting in interstitial fibrosis. This should be considered a reparative process in the kidney and a normal response to injury. Fibrosis is observed microscopically as an increase in extracellular matrix accumulation, usually surrounding or in association with degenerate, basophilic tubules. Typically, the cellularity of the interstitium is increased, with greater numbers of myofibroblasts and inflammatory cells. There is an abundant increase in collagen, which can be better visualized with Masson's trichrome stains or collagen immunostains. Chronically, contraction of the fibrous scar may distort the surrounding parenchymal architecture and result in depression of the renal capsular surface. Interstitial fibrosis always accompanies infarction and is a frequent feature of advanced CPN. Interstitial fibrosis as the primary or sole effect of compound-induced kidney injury is rare; however, marinobufagenin (MBG) is one such compound that appears to selectively target several fibrogenic intracellular molecules affecting collagen production and fibroblast proliferation (Federova et al. 2009). Anticancer agents such as cisplatin are often associated with cortical peritubular fibrosis but virtually always result in proximal tubular necrosis as the primary lesion. Lithium or thiazide diuretics result in fibrosis surrounding the distal tubules, but there is usually also some degree of tubular damage (Zhu et al. 1996). At least in the early phases, interstitial fibrosis may be partially reversible due to the presence of intrarenal matrix-degrading enzyme cascades (Eddy 1996).

The interstitial reaction is stimulated by changes in the tubules, with the production of cytokine and paracrine growth factor signals, including TGF-β and CTGF (Wang et al. 2000). While the majority of myofibroblasts likely arise from proliferation and differentiation of resident fibroblasts, at least a portion are now thought to be generated through epithelial–mesenchymal transition (EMT) of tubular epithelial cells or even from pluripotent precursor populations derived from the bone marrow (Frazier et al. 2000; Guarino et al. 2009; Kaissling and Le Hir 2008). The EMT process is produced by several signaling pathways and involves disruption of the basement membrane followed by the loss of intercellular cohesion and translocation of tubular epithelial cells into the interstitium, where they lose epithelial morphology and assume a mesenchymal phenotype. During EMT, TGF-β induces isoform switching of FGF receptors, causing cells to become

sensitive to FGF-2, and there are further interactions with PDGF and CTGF to initiate the transition to myofibroblastic morphology. It is still undetermined whether interstitial fibrosis can lead
to progressive tubular damage and nephron loss in vivo or whether, barring further tubular injury,
fibrosis is a self-perpetuating progressive process. In the majority of chronic renal diseases, tubular
or glomerular injury is accompanied by some degree of fibrosis, but in such cases, it is difficult or
impossible to gauge whether collagen accumulation is the cause or the consequence of tubular damage. Regardless, interstitial fibrosis is considered the strongest morphologic predictor of clinical
outcome and most tightly linked to progression in human renal disease (Barnes and Glass 2011).

12.1.5.3 Periarteritis and Vasculitis

Vascular changes are noted quite commonly in the arterioles and interlobular arteries of the kidney
in preclinical toxicity studies. Most commonly, one or a few focal arterioles are affected in a limited number of animals on study. A more diffuse form of vascular pathology, which may be found
in multiple organs including the kidney, is also encountered as a spontaneous syndrome in the
rat known as polyarteritis or periarteritis nodosa. Periarteritis nodosa is characterized by fibrinoid
necrosis of the arterial media, with disruption or duplication of the internal elastic lamina. There is
often a mixed inflammatory infiltrate of neutrophils, lymphocytes, macrophages, and occasionally
eosinophils in the adventitia, and karyorrhexis is noted transmurally in the arteriolar wall (Hard
et al. 1999). With time and chronicity, the arteriolar wall becomes thickened, and the vascular
lumina narrows due to transmural fibrosis. Thrombosis may also occur. Generally, in these focal
or diffuse forms of spontaneous vascular disease in rats, small- and medium-sized muscular arteries are most often affected. Spontaneous lesions are encountered in the arteries and arterioles in
the kidneys of mice, and focal lesions, usually limited to a solitary vessel, are very rarely noted
spontaneously in the kidneys of dogs and monkeys. The pathogenesis is unknown, but autoimmune mechanisms are thought to be involved in some inbred mouse strains, and hormonal effects
have been postulated to be associated with the etiology of this condition in rats. Food restriction
and dietary levels of fat and protein may affect the incidence of polyarteritis in both rats and mice
(Tucker 1985; Yu et al. 1982). Severe vascular changes in a renal vessel may result in local ischemia,
tubular necrosis, and infarction, particularly when multiple vessels are involved. More often, vascular lesions in the kidney are limited in distribution and severity to focal changes in a solitary vessel.
This type of vascular injury is clinically silent and not associated with any macroscopic or other
microscopic changes, differences in kidney weights, or alterations in clinicopathologic parameters.
Such changes may also be seen occasionally in control animals (particularly rodents) as spontaneous findings and are therefore unlikely to be considered adverse. In some cases, vascular lesions
may be limited to medial hypertrophy alone. This commonly occurs with agents that produce renal
hypertension and is a consistent feature in the kidneys of SHRs, but medial hypertrophy may also
occur following test article–induced vasodilation without alterations in systemic blood pressure
(Olzinski et al. 2005). Medial hypertrophy is considered an adaptive response of the vessel wall to
increases in intramural stressor responses (Limas et al. 1980), and it may lead to further vascular
wall injury and changes consistent with compound-induced vasculitis or remain as a static lesion.

It may be difficult to distinguish between compound-induced and spontaneous forms of vascular
injury, except on the basis of a dose response. Spontaneous vascular lesions in the kidney should
be observed only in a small number of random animals on study, so an increased incidence, especially in high-dose animals, suggests a possible test article effect. For instance, with drugs such as
fenoldopam, the severity and extent of damage correlate with dose and time (Dalmas et al. 2008).
Hence, the more pronounced the local vasoactive effect, the greater the incidence and severity of
medial injury. There is a predisposition in medium-sized arteries in the rat for drug-induced vascular changes, and renal vessels, as well as those in the pancreas and intestine, are also more prone to
injury than those in other organs (Nemes et al. 1980). Marked vasculitis and perivasculitis in renal
arterioles have been noted in chronic monkey toxicity studies with antisense deoxyoligonucleotide
administration, and the pathogenesis is thought to involve systemic immune stimulation rather than

be due to any hemodynamic effects. Renal biomarkers are generally not helpful until downstream ischemic necrosis affects adjacent tubules.

12.1.6   LESIONS OF RENAL PELVIS

The renal pelvis shares many features in common with the lower urinary tract, including its lining urothelium, a tendency toward urolith deposition, and responses to toxic injury. The proliferative lesions of the renal pelvis also tend to be similar to those of the ureter and bladder rather than the renal cortex or medulla. In particular, urothelial hyperplasia may occur spontaneously in rodents or other preclinical toxicity species in response to pyelonephritis, urolithiasis, or papillary necrosis (Figure 12.4a). It may also occur with chronic administration of agents that alter the pH of the urinary filtrate. Due to its similarity to urothelial hyperplasia of the ureter and bladder, urothelial hyperplasia will be discussed as part of the lower urinary tract. The pelvis is a common location for crystalluria, and variably sized uroliths may be found frequently in studies as a test article–induced change resulting in secondary urothelial hyperplasia, ulceration, and inflammation. Pelvic ulceration may also occur as a direct cytotoxic effect of a nephrotoxin, and its pathogenesis and progression mirror that of ulceration in the urinary bladder. Obstruction of the more distal lower urinary tract may result in retention and increased concentration of xenobiotic agents or their metabolites

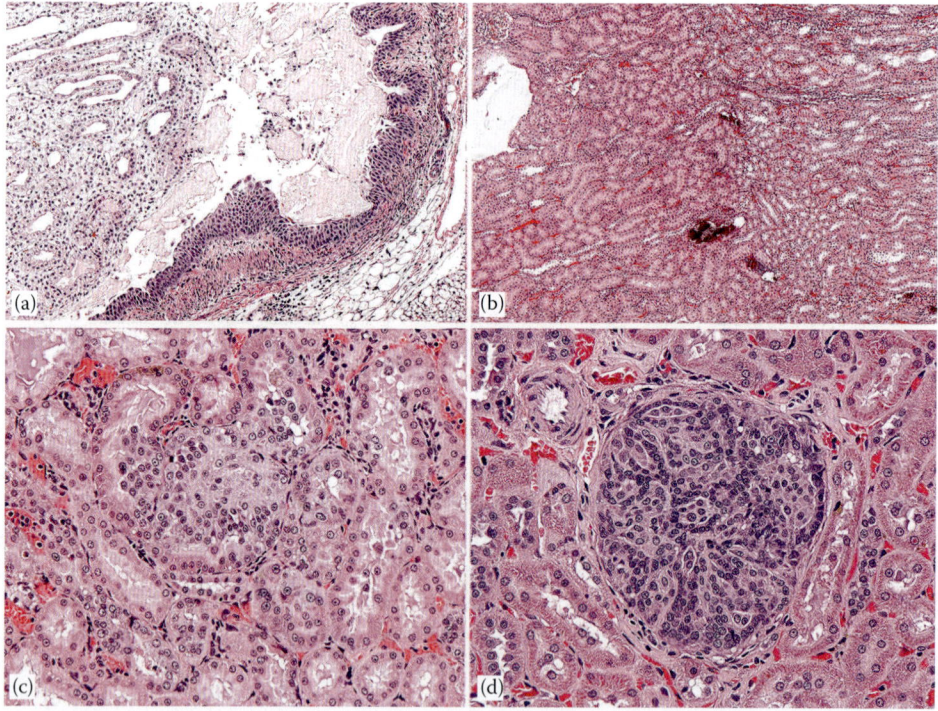

FIGURE 12.4   (a) Hematoxylin and eosin 400×. Rat kidney, Renal pelvis and distal medulla at the papilla, with crystals precipitating into the pelvic lumen (light pink glassy material) and marked urothelial hyperplasia and ulceration of the pelvic epithelium after drug administration. (b) Hematoxylin and eosin 200×. Rat kidney, untreated control, with mineralization of tubules at the corticomedullary junction. (c) Hematoxylin and eosin 32×. Rat kidney, with minimal tubule (atypical) hyperplasia characterized by cellular proliferation within the confines of a single tubule, slight tubule expansion, and lack of significant membrane thickening, and containing well-developed basophilic cytoplasm. (d) Hematoxylin and eosin 40×. Rat kidney, with renal tubule adenoma composed of a circumscribed, solid focus of basophilic cells with slight pleomorphism. Note the slight tubule differentiation and fibrovascular ingrowth near the capsule of the tumor.

within the pelvis resulting in potential injury to this area. Degenerative alterations in the pelvis are frequently encountered when agents cause compound-induced papillary necrosis or with the syndrome of papillary mineralization, which is occasionally noted in rodents in toxicity studies. Inflammatory infiltrates are commonly noted in the submucosa of the renal pelvis in rodents as a spontaneous background finding of no biological significance. Severe inflammation of the renal pelvis usually results from ascending lesions of the urinary bladder and ureter but occasionally occurs from descending pyelonephritis of the medulla.

12.1.6.1 Hydronephrosis

Hydronephrosis is a condition in which there is pelvic dilation caused from urine outflow obstruction and back pressure of urine resulting in pelvic distention. Marked dilation of the renal pelvis is a common finding in rodents and may occur as a spontaneous or test article–induced change. Congenital renal pelvic dilation refers to the often inconsequential form that may be noted in both juvenile and older rats, mice, and hamsters. Iatrogenic pelvic dilation is the term sometimes ascribed to the more severe drug-induced form, which can be associated with outflow obstruction and cortical atrophy. Hydronephrosis is the macroscopic term for either form, while pelvic dilation is the correct microscopic morphologic diagnosis. Typically, the kidney looks grossly enlarged and is soft to the touch. The condition can be unilateral or bilateral but in rats is more often observed on the right side. In early lesions, there may be no secondary histologic changes other than increased pelvic diameter and corresponding decreases in the size of the medullary parenchyma. With time, urothelial hyperplasia develops, with the accumulation of inflammatory infiltrates, hemorrhage, or hemosiderin pigments within the mesenchymal tissue underlying the pelvis and the progressive appearance of scattered to diffuse tubular dilation. In chronic or severe cases, there may be changes consistent with obstructive nephropathy, including compression atrophy of cortical and medullary tubules, degeneration or necrosis of entire nephron segments, interstitial fibrosis, and glomerulosclerosis. Clinical pathologic alterations vary widely with the stage and severity of pelvic dilation. In the most chronic cases, end-stage disease with chronic renal failure may be present, particularly if the condition is bilateral. Spontaneous or incidental dilation may be clinically silent. The pathogenesis of most cases noted in preclinical toxicity studies involves obstructive urolithiasis, so the clinical implications are similar to obstructive nephropathy. Some congenital forms likely also involve transient outflow obstruction during the late prenatal period. However, several transgenic mice strains have high rates of hydronephrosis, and this has led to the identification of several key proteins that are critical for differentiation of the renal pelvic mesenchyme and proper development of this portion of the kidney. Calcineurin is one such factor, responsible for important peristalsis of the pelvis and ureter required for normal morphologic development of these structures (Chang et al. 2004). COX-2 is another important factor involved in normal development and function of the perinatal suburothelial ureteral mesenchyme and is the specific target in hydronephrosis associated with the administration of dioxin (TCDD) (Nishimura et al. 2008).

12.1.7 Miscellaneous Lesions of Kidney

12.1.7.1 Mineralization

Renal mineralization, also referred to as calcification or nephrocalcinosis, is an extremely common finding in preclinical studies in rodents as well as occasionally in dogs and monkeys. It takes several forms, depending on the location within the kidney and the specific pathogenesis, including mineralization of the tubular cytoplasm, tubular lumina, basement membrane, and interstitium. In H&E sections, it appears as dense, blue to purple concretions filling the lumen. Alternatively, it can appear as granules or solid deposits replacing the tubular epithelial cytoplasm or linear circumferential deposits surrounding tubular or glomerular profiles (Figure 12.4b). It may occur in a zonal pattern along the corticomedullary junction or may occur randomly in small foci throughout the cortex and medulla, including the papilla. It may precede and be accompanied by degeneration or necrosis of the involved tubules or may be a consequence of tubular degeneration. Special stains such as Alizarin Red S or Von Kossa's stains can be used for confirmation. In the most severe cases, mineralization may be visible macroscopically as white stippling on the cut surface of the kidney. Renal weights are increased only with the more diffuse lesions. In the most severely affected kidneys, all renal markers may be increased including BUN, sCr, and phosphorus as well as urinary biomarkers, but in most cases, there are no clinicopathologic abnormalities. In cases of drug-induced mineralization, there may be alterations in serum calcium or phosphorus that may provide some insight into mechanism. Bacterial colonies may sometimes appear similar to mineralization, but they can be differentiated with special stains such as Gram stains. Spontaneous renal mineralization in preclinical studies has no clinical significance, but the identification of test article–related renal mineralization in preclinical studies should signal the potential need for calcium and phosphorus monitoring in human trials.

Mineralization generally occurs either as dystrophic calcification in the renal tubules and collecting ducts or as metastatic calcification in the tubules and interstitium and along basement membranes as a result of systemic calcium/phosphorus imbalance. The deposits in rodents are typically composed of calcium salts, phosphorus, and glycoprotein with trace amounts of magnesium. A similar composition has been described in other species. Dietary imbalances of calcium and phosphorus may predispose this condition in rodents. While mineralization may occur as a background change lacking clinical consequence, especially in the rat, many drugs and agents such as cholecalciferol-containing rodenticides can affect calcium, phosphorus, or parathyroid hormone regulation (Ritskes-Hoitinga and Beynen 1992). Agents affecting urinary pH such as carbonic anhydrase inhibitors may also predispose animals to luminal mineralization (Nicoletta and Schwartz 2004). Mineralization may occur spontaneously in female rats along the junction of the outer and inner stripes of the outer medulla, and it increases in incidence and severity with age. In this spontaneous tubular form, ultrastructural examination has demonstrated that the deposits are related to shedding of microvilli and microvesicles from S1 proximal tubules with accumulation at the end of the straight segment (S3) at the transition to the thin loop (Nguyen and Woodard 1980). In the chronic stage of alpha-$_{2\mu}$-globulin nephropathy in male rats, mineralization may also occur along the thin loop of Henle in the medulla and in the papilla, and this has been identified as consisting of calcium hydroxyapatite. Renal pelvic mineralization may also occur in rats and mice along the pelvic fornix. Adjacent urothelium may be ulcerated or hyperplastic and associated with mixed neutrophilic inflammation. While papillary mineralization is considered a spontaneous change in rats, some agents have increased its incidence through an undetermined mechanism. Mineralization can also be an early secondary consequence of renal failure from other causes and as a chronic effect of any number of nephrotoxins that result in significant renal impairment. A deficit of calcitriol and an abnormality in the calcium-sensing receptor may be the important factors initially, while later in advanced renal failure, hyperphosphatemia becomes an additional important pathogenic factor in mineral formation and its tubular or interstitial deposition.

12.1.7.2 Pigmentation

Pigment deposits within the renal cortical tubules are commonly noted in rats, mice, dogs, and monkeys. In beagles, light brown granular deposits of bilirubin are sometimes noted in the cortex and outer medullary tubules, and females seem to be more commonly affected than males.

In rodents, yellow to light brown stippled pigments are extremely common in the proximal convoluted tubules and generally represent lipofuscin. As a wear-and-tear pigment, the incidence increases with age. While more often a background change, several drugs and agents may result in increased renal pigmentation in rodents, including 5HT3r antagonists and the benzodiazepines (Bendele et al. 1994; Owen et al. 1970). Anticancer agents or other drugs such as thrombolytic agents that induce anemia or hemolysis may result in accumulation of hemoglobin pigments in the proximal tubules. Bilirubin accumulation in kidneys may be potentiated by drugs that inhibit transporters or enzymes involved in hepatic uptake or biliary conjugation such as organic anion transporter 1B1 or UDG glucuronosyltransferase 1, respectively. Pigmentation is rarely associated with significant renal tubular degeneration or necrosis. The determination of the specific nature of pigments may be aided by the use of special stains, such as Prussian blue for iron/hemosiderin, Hall's stain for bilirubin, or Schmorl's method for lipofuscin. Diagnosis of drug-related pigmentation should be based upon careful comparison with the amount of pigment noted in controls on any given study. Corollary changes such as serum or urine bilirubin increases may help confirm tubular bilirubin accumulation. The functional significance of pigmentation varies with the type of pigment. Renal lipofuscinosis has no real functional or clinical significance, while the presence of hemoglobin or iron pigments may indicate intravascular or extravascular hemolysis and lead to severe secondary renal damage (Ikeda et al. 1999).

12.1.7.3 Inclusion Bodies

Nuclear and cytoplasmic inclusions are frequently encountered in the renal tubules of animals in toxicity studies, and their pathogenesis may be quite diverse. Inclusion bodies in the cytoplasm may represent lysosomal membrane aggregates, protein precipitates, giant mitochondria, or proliferating endoplasmic reticulum (Pfister et al. 2005). Tubular inclusions vary from eosinophilic to basophilic and can be observed both in the nucleus and cytoplasm of affected cells. Depending on the pathogenesis and location, inclusions may be associated with degeneration or necrosis, as in the case of phospholipidosis with gentamicin, but are often not associated with any significant effects on cellular function. Inclusion bodies have been noted with a wide spectrum of presentations and an even wider variety of causative agents. They have been described in the proximal convoluted tubules with lead intoxication as well as with compounds that adversely affect iron metabolism (Navarro-Moreno et al. 2009; Donnadieu-Claraz et al. 2007). Lysosomal inclusions consisting of membranous whorls are particularly prominent in renal phospholipidosis, and these can be easily visualized using toluidine blue stains and acid phosphatase immunohistochemistry (Schneider 1992), although with routine H&E stains, phospholipidosis appears more often as large vacuoles within tubules. Inclusions may be associated with viral infections, but this is not frequently encountered in the relatively pathogen-free laboratory animals typically used in preclinical toxicity studies. Inclusion bodies need to be distinguished from more common cytoplasmic changes, such as hyaline droplet nephropathy in rats, or the basophilic granules noted in proximal tubules in animals given antisense deoxyoligonucleotides. PAS stains may accentuate the appearance of some types of inclusion bodies in histologic sections, but electron microscopy is often necessary to ascertain their origin and makeup. The clinical implications of inclusion bodies vary with their type and intracellular localization, and their presence may or may not be associated with other biologic or clinicopathologic effects.

12.1.7.4 Adipose Aggregates

While the renal interstitium normally contains small numbers of adipocytes and lipid droplets, accumulations of well-differentiated, mature adipocytes known as adipose aggregates or lipomatosis are occasionally noted in the kidneys of rats and mice. These lesions are confined to the interstitium and are more common in the medulla than the cortex. Histologically, they consist of unencapsulated foci of fat cells that may slightly compress adjacent tubules or replace normal parenchyma. While the lesion is most often considered a spontaneous change, it may increase in frequency after treatment with some drugs and agents, particularly those that affect lipid metabolism. The change can usually be diagnosed on routine H&E sections without the need for special stains, but it needs to be delineated from lipoma or liposarcoma, which tends to be larger and more invasive with less cellular differentiation. Adipose aggregates are not associated with ancillary clinicopathological abnormalities and do not adversely affect renal function. They may arise from resident adipocytes through normal proliferation, or they may result from the differentiation of pluripotent stem cells present within the renal interstitium. They are not considered preneoplastic lesions and hence have little clinical significance other than as potential harbingers for possible effects on fat metabolism.

12.1.7.5 Juxtaglomerular Hyperplasia

Juxtaglomerular cells are responsible for renin secretion. They are modified arteriolar smooth muscle cells and may show adaptive responses to reduced RBF and efferent vasoconstriction. Hyperplasia and hypertrophy of the juxtaglomerular cells may be encountered in many species used in preclinical toxicity studies with agents that are associated with vasoactive effects in the kidney such as the angiotensin I converting enzyme (ACE) inhibitors and angiotensin II antagonists (Doughty et al. 1995). Microscopic examination may demonstrate increased size and granularity of juxtaglomerular cells that surround afferent and/or efferent arterioles, thickened basal lamina, and mild mononuclear cell infiltrates. The vessels may have visibly reduced lumina and thickened walls. Immunostains often demonstrate increased renin secretion and/or increased cell proliferation with Ki67. Electron microscopy demonstrates hypertrophied cells with increased endoplasmic reticulum and free ribosomes, as well as abundant coated vesicles within the cytoplasm (Dominick et al. 1990). Juxtaglomerular cell granules are increased in number with hyperplasia and demonstrate significant structural heterogeneity (Jackson and Jones 1995). The mechanism is thought to be related to continual stimulation of renin secretion from increased demand and lack of feedback inhibition by angiotensin II. Normally, renin is localized to the media of afferent arterioles, but with increased demand, renin expression can be upregulated in efferent arterioles and even interlobular arteries. Juxtaglomerular hyperplasia is reversible with cessation of dosing, but this may take many weeks (Owen et al. 1994). Since similar juxtaglomerular changes may be present in humans with chronic administration of ACE inhibitors, these alterations have clinical significance. However, as the changes are adaptive, they are often not considered adverse but instead classified as expected pharmacology. In rare cases in rats and monkeys, juxtaglomerular hyperplasia has been associated with concomitant tubular degeneration, but the pathogenesis or relationship of these alterations to juxtaglomerular effects remains unclear (Jackson and Jones 1995). Acute renal failure has been described as an uncommon adverse reaction in humans given chronic ACE inhibitor therapy, and a similar ischemic pathogenesis has been proposed in animals with juxtaglomerular hyperplasia–associated degenerative renal tubular changes.

12.1.7.6 Congenital Lesions

Several background changes have been described that may occasionally be noted as rare congenital lesions in laboratory animals in preclinical studies, including renal agenesis, renal hypoplasia, renal dysplasia, and adrenal rests. Renal agenesis and renal hypoplasia refer to defects in renal parenchyma resulting from a reduced mass of metanephric blastema or incomplete induction of nephron formation by the ureteral bud. Renal agenesis refers to the complete lack of one kidney. Bilateral agenesis is an embryonic lethal trait. Renal hypoplasia refers to a quantitative deficit in the amount of parenchyma and is also usually unilateral. Either agenesis or hypoplasia may result in hypertrophic tubular changes in the contralateral kidney. The diagnosis is straightforward and noted macroscopically as absent or very small kidneys on gross examination. Since animals can function and thrive on only one kidney, there may be no changes in clinicopathologic parameters, but the animals will be more sensitive to the effects of nephrotoxins than normal controls on the same study due to a limited nephron functional reserve. The incidence of these anomalies varies markedly with strains. While rare in most breeds/strains used in preclinical testing, it has been noted sporadically in beagle dogs, mice, and occasionally rats. Drugs or teratogenic agents such as the ret kinase or syk kinase inhibitors that inhibit metanephros differentiation have been associated with agenesis of the kidneys in rodents (Clemens et al. 2009; Suzuki et al. 2007). Double renal pelvis is a condition occasionally encountered in some mouse strains in which there are twin papillae extending into their own pelvis and draining into a single ureter. It has no clinical significance. Adrenal rests are small foci of ectopic but well-differentiated accessory adrenocortical tissue that are found along the capsule or subcapsular cortex of the kidney in rats and mice as well as along the extracapsular tissue adjacent to the adrenal gland. They represent a developmental abnormality that is due to disturbed embryonic cell migration during organogenesis. While adrenal rests in humans have rarely been reported as preneoplastic and able to undergo malignant transformation, this has never been conclusively demonstrated in rodents (Goren et al. 1991). The lesion is not invasive and therefore easily distinguished from renal neoplasia, and it has no clinical or toxicologic significance.

Renal dysplasia refers to disorganized development of renal parenchyma associated with anomalous differentiation of renal tissue elements. Renal dysplasia has been identified in mice, rats, pigs, and dogs and is most often congenital. However, due to maturation changes occurring in the early postnatal period in these species, it is possible that dysplasia may also be associated with disease or teratogen-induced perturbation of organogenesis in the postnatal period. For instance, neonatal infection with canine herpesvirus can produce renal dysplasia in puppies. Familial forms have been described in pigs and in several breeds of dogs, including most recently in laboratory beagles used in toxicity studies (Bruder et al. 2010). Microscopically, the kidney exhibits persistent primitive mesenchyme, persistence of ectodermal structures resembling metanephric ducts, asynchronous differentiation of nephrons, and/or atypical tubular epithelium. Increased numbers of fetal or immature glomeruli and renal cysts are often noted, but inflammation and fibrosis of the adjacent corticomedullary parenchyma are variable. Metanephric ducts can be identified by the presence of pseudostratified to columnar, slightly basophilic epithelium lining the lumina (Picut and Lewis 1987). Secondary degenerative changes in adjacent tubules may extend radially from medulla to cortex and are considered due to vascular obstruction or infarction. Grossly, the dysplastic kidneys are frequently decreased in size, and they may be misshapen, and therefore, kidney weights are usually decreased. Diagnosis and differentiation from other congenital anomalies and familial renal diseases depend on the presence of anomalous structures or morphologic changes inconsistent with the animal's stage of development. In many cases, there are no clinicopathologic alterations, but if the condition is bilateral and chronic, renal dysplasia can result in signs of uremia and mortality. In addition to congenital forms, intrauterine ureteral obstruction has been implicated as a factor in the pathogenesis of some forms of renal dysplasia and is the most common form in humans.

12.1.8 Hyperplastic and Neoplastic Changes

Spontaneous preneoplastic hyperplastic and neoplastic findings of the kidney are infrequently encountered in preclinical toxicity studies involving the commonly used rodent strains. Proliferative lesions of the kidney of dogs and monkeys are rare because of the generally younger age of these test animals (Yoshizawa et al. 1996; Robinson et al. 1997; Asahina et al. 2000; Bryan et al. 2006; Kaspareit et al. 2007). Compared to humans, where neoplasms of the kidney represent 1%–3% of all visceral tumors and where 85% are carcinomas, renal tumors in rodents have an incidence of 1% or less and are generally adenomas (Alpers 2010; Beckwith 1999; Wolf 2002; Tsuda and Krieg 1992). However, some strains have a much higher incidence of a specific tumor type, such as nephroblastoma or urinary bladder neoplasms (Mesfin and Breech 1996; Hard and Noble 1981; Boorman and Hollander 1974). The incidence of renal tumors in mice is less than in rats. Malignant renal neoplasms are uncommon spontaneous tumors in both rats and mice. Females of both species tend to have fewer renal tumors than males. In rodent species, most spontaneous and induced renal proliferative lesions are of epithelial origin involving tubular epithelium. In general, non-epithelial tubule tumors are infrequent. Therefore, in the kidney, any increase in the number of tumors in a preclinical toxicity study is cause for concern. The overall incidence of spontaneous hyperplastic and neoplastic lesions of the lower urinary tract is also uncommon, tending to be less than the incidence of renal tumors. Bladder neoplasms in humans have an overall higher incidence than in rodent species and, like renal tumors, are generally malignant (Johansson and Cohen 1997; Jacobs et al. 2010; Epstein 2010). The spontaneous historical control database for neoplastic lesions reported in the urinary tract system for the more commonly used rat and mouse species has been extensively reported (Hirouchi et al. 1994; Iwata et al. 1991; Walsh and Poteracki 1994; Tamano et al. 1988; Goodman et al. 1979; Ward et al. 1979; Chandra and Frith 1992; Ando et al. 2008; Brix et al. 2005; Chandra et al. 1992; Nakazawa et al. 2001; Maita et al. 1988; McMartin et al. 1992; Haseman et al. 1998; Tsuda and Kreig 1992; Kunze 1992; Wolf and Hard 1996; Bomhard 1992; Kurata and Shibata 1996). In addition, most laboratories maintain their own historical control database. This historical control database is generally more useful since this information is continuously updated, reflects consensus diagnostic nomenclature that is commonly used within that particular laboratory, and represents data that have generally been peer reviewed. Published historical control information regarding urinary tract tumors in young animals contains little data as most renal and urinary bladder tumors generally occur later in life (Son and Gopinath 2004; Son et al. 2010). Incidence data for hyperplastic lesions are less commonly reported and are generally study specific. The published literature on treatment-related renal hyperplastic and neoplastic lesions is large and diverse and reflects the role of the urinary tract in the detoxification, metabolism, and excretion of administered compounds. It is beyond the scope of this chapter to go into depth regarding the many known and suspected mechanisms involving renal carcinogenesis other than to note that these mechanisms have been linked to species, strain, diet, and hormones, just to mention a few. Hard (1988c) summarized renal carcinogenic mechanisms as being associated with one of the following broad categories: (1) direct DNA reactivity, (2) tumor induction linked to oxidative stress, (3) sustained regenerative cell proliferation, either from direct or indirect cytotoxicity, (4) chemicals interacting with spontaneous CPN, or (5) unknown. A few mechanisms of renal carcinogenesis are linked to unique factors within the test animal and bear no risk for the development of human renal tumors. For instance, the relationship of advanced CPN as a risk factor for tumor development is based on numerous retrospective studies and seems well accepted among pathologists (Hard et al. 1997; Seely et al. 2002; Hard and Kahn 2004; Travlos et al. 2011). Since CPN is a rodent-specific disease, particularly in male rats, and there is no similar disease in humans, it can be argued that an exacerbated CPN–tumor relationship bears no relevance for extrapolation in human risk assessment (Hard et al. 2009b). Another rat-specific renal mechanism of tumor development includes $\alpha_{-2\mu}$-globulin-associated renal tubule carcinogenesis (Swenberg and Lehman-McKeeman 1999). Most likely, there will be other species-specific mechanisms as new varieties of compound are investigated. There are many excellent reviews that discuss experimental or chemically induced renal tumors (Hiasa and Ito 1987; Lipsky and Trump 1988; Barrett and Huff 1991; Konishi and Hiasa 1994; Lock and Hard 2004; Wolf 2002). The list of renal carcinogens is lengthy and includes many different chemicals. In addition, the role of experimental animal models of kidney neoplasm to improve and help understand the nature and development of renal tumors in man has been substantial (Nogueira et al. 1993). In both humans and in some rodent species, familial tumors of the kidney have been reported. Hereditary renal adenomas and carcinomas have been well characterized for the Eker rat model (Eker et al. 1981; Everitt et al. 1992; Urakami et al. 1997; Monks and Lau 2005) and the Nihon rat model (Hino et al. 2003; Kouchi et al. 2006; Okimoto et al. 2000). In these models, preneoplastic lesions and tumors develop early in life and have been associated with genetic mutations that have proved useful in understanding renal carcinogenesis. Evidence of additional suspected familial renal tumors has been reported in a number of case reports and reviews of histopathological cases. Many of these tumors also appeared in younger animals or from studies of less than 90 days' duration. The recognition and knowledge of reported familial tumor phenotypes are important when interpreting data from studies (Hard et al. 1994, 2008; Lanzoni et al. 2007; Thurman et al. 1995; Hall et al. 2007). Molecular genetics of animal models of renal tumors and human cases have shown some similarities with gene alterations (Zambrano et al. 1999; Walker 1998). Furthermore, molecular or genetic expression (signatures) has been demonstrated to identify subtypes of tumor phenotypes that have important diagnostic and therapeutic implications (Takahashi et al. 2003). Genomic alterations have also been investigated in renal cell carcinomas induced by N-ethyl-N-hydroxyethylnitrosamine (Konishi et al. 2001). Spontaneous and induced proliferative lesions of the lower urinary tract are usually reported more frequently for the urinary bladder than the ureters and urethra as the latter are in contact with urine for a shorter time and may not always be examined during routine toxicity testing. Though the urothelium is normally a quiescent tissue, it can proliferate rapidly when stimulated. Urinary bladder neoplasms may be induced by a variety of processes and chemicals, including DNA-reactive genotoxic and nongenotoxic carcinogens that increase cell replication (Cohen 1989). It is known that rats and mice can react differently to known bladder carcinogens. Most lower urinary tract neoplasms arise from the urothelium, and rodents share similarities to the disease in humans (Cohen 1998a,b, 2002; Frith et al. 1994a,b). Anatomical and/or physiological differences between humans and rats, such as bladder positioning and the presence of urinary precipitates and/or crystals, suggest that these differences are a confounding factor when assessing the human relevance of rodent bladder tumors (DeSesso 1995). The association between bladder calculi, crystalluria, and other physical factors is well known in rodent studies and, in some cases, may act as promoters (Fukushima and Murai 1999; Clayson et al. 1995; Cohen et al. 2000). The examination of urine and bladders is essential when studying bladder carcinogenesis, and guidelines have been published to provide information for the proper collection and examination of both (Cohen et al. 2007).

12.1.8.1 Hyperplastic Lesions

Hyperplastic lesions can be observed anywhere along the nephron, collecting ducts, renal pelvis, ureter, urinary bladder, and urethra. However, in this section, hyperplasia will be discussed as one part of the sequential development to neoplasia and important in the "weight of evidence" for carcinogenic assessment (Boorman et al. 2003). Hyperplasia in the urinary tract must be determined to be either a direct effect or secondary to compound administration as hyperplasia often results from regeneration or reaction to cytotoxicity or an injurious stimulus. It is recognized that hyperplasia in the kidney and urinary bladder leads to adenomas/papillomas, and consequently, these benign lesions may develop foci of carcinoma in rodents (Ward 2004). Therefore, it is necessary to accurately identify, categorize, and relate these changes to hazard identification and potential human risk (Boorman et al. 2003). Hyperplastic lesions must be differentiated from small adenomas. In some cases, this differentiation is difficult since size alone is not always a reliable criterium. The study pathologist needs to develop criteria based on the published literature and personal experience and apply these criteria in a consistent manner throughout the study.

12.1.8.2 Renal Tubule Hyperplasia

Most hyperplastic lesions involve the renal tubule cells of the nephron, more specifically, those of the proximal convoluted tubule. There are generally two diagnostic terms in current use for describing hyperplastic lesions of the renal tubule that are considered preneoplastic, "hyperplasia, renal tubule" and "atypical tubule hyperplasia." There does not appear to be a consensus term since both are used interchangeably. Hard et al. (1995) proposed "atypical tubule hyperplasia" (ATH) for those lesions that are clearly preneoplastic and reserved the term "simple tubule hyperplasia" for those nonneoplastic proliferative tubule lesions lined by a single layer of epithelial cells. However, not all pathologists use ATH routinely because it seems that laboratory lexicons may still promote the usage of "hyperplasia, renal tubule" or some other diagnostic term. If important to the study, pathologists should reference and discuss ATH to clearly indicate the potential neoplastic aspects of ATH in their narrative report. Differentiating hyperplastic lesions into clear, basophilic, or other does not appear to be meaningful in most routine preclinical studies. The main criterion for ATH is the proliferation of tubular epithelial cells within the confines of a single tubule where the growth of the lesion does not exceed one tubule or multiple cross sections of one tubule. ATH may be either focal or multifocal and is usually noted in the cortex and outer medulla. More often, these lesions appear solid but may be cystic or papillary. Generally, there is slight pleomorphism of the cell components, and the nuclear–cytoplasmic ratio is increased. The epithelial cells often have a glassy, basophilic sheen with clear cytoplasmic borders. Careful examination of the border of the lesion generally shows some circumferential expansion with the identification of fibroblasts or a small amount of fibrovascular tissue encircling the lesion. There is usually an absence of thickened CPN basement membrane. Mitotic figures may or may not be seen within the lesion. Vascular ingrowth into the lesion is not present in ATH. Tubular lesions representing a number of morphological changes associated with advanced CPN may be mistaken for ATH and must be distinguished from the latter (Figure 12.4c). Recommendations have been published for the interpretation of these lesions (Hard and Seely 2005). Although size must be considered when interpreting hyperplastic lesions, the above criteria seem better suited to diagnose hyperplasia than size alone. Occasionally in rat studies, a monomorphic population of cells with lightly eosinophilic and finely granular cytoplasm having centrally located nuclei may be seen. These lesions represent oncocytic hyperplasia. Currently, there are no reliable criteria, other than using size (larger than threefold the size of glomeruli) or well-delineated foci, for differentiating oncocytic hyperplasia from oncocytoma. Oncocytic hyperplasia and/or oncocytoma do not progress to malignant tumors and should not be categorized with ATH or other spontaneous tubule neoplasms. Oncocytic cells stain positively for cytochrome-c-oxidase and contain numerous atypical mitochondria on ultrastructural examination (Mayer et al. 1989; Krech et al. 1981). A type of tubular hyperplasia termed "amphophilic-vacuolated," because of its characteristic appearance, is consistent with the reported familial cases in rats. Tubular hyperplasia of this phenotype has shown progression from hyperplasia to adenoma to carcinoma in the same kidney.

12.1.8.3 Renal Pelvis

Preneoplastic hyperplastic lesions of the renal pelvis are uncommon findings in rodent studies, particularly in the mouse. Nonneoplastic hyperplastic lesions are commonly observed as a response to various stimuli such as infection, calculi, or chemical toxicity. If the inciting stimulus is removed, these hyperplastic lesions tend to regress. Small papillary projections along the renal papillae are noted in more severe cases of CPN in male rats. Preneoplastic urothelial hyperplasia occurs as uniform and multicellular growths of small fronds, cords, or solid sheets of epithelial cells. Hyperplastic areas may appear as simple (focal to diffuse linear thickening of the urothelium), nodular (solid round to oval nests), or papillary (small fronds with little supporting fibrovascular tissue and that project into the lumen). Slight cellular pleomorphism, squamous metaplasia, and dysplasia may be present. However, cellular atypia is generally absent, except in cases associated with administration of a renal pelvic carcinogen (Hard et al. 1995). Mitotic activity is variable.

12.1.8.4 Neoplastic Lesions of Kidney

A simplified classification of renal and lower urinary tract neoplasms is presented in Table 12.2. The morphological spectrum of spontaneous renal neoplasms has been well described and illustrated in rats (Chandra et al. 1992; Montgomery and Seely 1990; Hard 1990; Hard et al. 1995; Tsuda and Krieg 1992; Zwicker et al. 1992; Greaves 2007; Alden et al. 1992; Sugimoto et al. 1998) and mice (Frith et al. 1994a,b; Seely 1999; Wolf and Hard 1996; Chandra and Frith 1992; Hard et al. 2001). Neoplasms of the renal pelvis, ureter, urinary bladder, and portions of the urethra should be regarded as urothelial neoplasms and not as transitional cell epithelial tumors, although the two terms are still used interchangeably. It is more commonly accepted to refer to these neoplasms as being urothelial in origin. The incidence of renal pelvic tumors is generally uncommon to rare in both rats and mice. The morphological spectrum of spontaneous lower urinary tract neoplasms has been well described and illustrated in rats (Jokinen 1990; Kunze and Chowaniec 1990; Kunze 1992; Frith et al. 1995) and mice (Gaillard 1999; Boorman et al. 1994; Hard et al. 2001; Kurata and Shibata 1996). Tumors of the ureters and urethra are rare, and one partial reason may be that they are often not examined in routine preclinical toxicology studies. Urethral hyperplasia and carcinomas have been reported in mice exposed to 3,3,4,4-tetrachloroazobenzene (Singh et al. 2010).

TABLE 12.2

Classification of Renal and Lower Urinary Tract Neoplasms

Renal tubule neoplasms
Adenoma/oncocytoma
Carcinoma
Connective tissue neoplasms
Lipoma/liposarcoma
Renal mesenchymal tumor
Fibrosarcoma/sarcoma
Embryonal neoplasms
Nephroblastoma
Hematogenous/metastatic neoplasms
Renal pelvic tumors
Papilloma
Carcinoma
Squamous cell carcinoma
Lower urinary tract neoplasms
Papilloma/squamous cell papilloma
Carcinoma/squamous cell carcinoma
Adenocarcinoma
Mesenchymal proliferative lesion
Connective tissue neoplasms

12.1.8.5 Renal Tubule Neoplasms

12.1.8.5.1 Adenoma

Adenomas are generally focal, solitary lesions that are circumscribed to irregular and occur in the cortex or outer medulla. Although larger adenomas may be seen grossly as nodular lesions, most are recognized only upon microscopic examination. Most adenomas appear basophilic but may be clear, eosinophilic, amphophilic, or chromophobic or have mixtures in staining qualities. Tinctorial qualities of adenomas have been ascribed to the origin of the affected tubular segment (Tsuda et al. 1998). Small adenomas are diagnostically challenging when differentiating from larger areas of ATH, but larger adenomas usually present no such difficulties. They tend to be well demarcated with compression of the surrounding parenchyma and are generally not encapsulated. Typically, adenomas are solid, but cystic, tubular, papillary, or mixed patterns can be observed (Figure 12.4d). Adenomas of mice tend to be more cystic to cystic-papillary in appearance (Hard et al. 2001). Tumor cells vary from well differentiated to having slight pleomorphism. Usually, few mitoses are observed, and foci of necrosis are not evident. However, single cell necrosis can be occasionally observed. Proliferation exceeding the confines of one tubule and vascular to fibrovascular in growth are the defining characteristics that separate small borderline adenomas from ATH (Frazier et al. 2012; Bannasch et al. 1998a,b; Sass 1998). Oncocytoma, a variant of adenoma, is characterized by the presence of a solid mass of monomorphic cells with conspicuous cytoplasm containing faintly eosinophilic granules and a central nucleus. Oncocytomas are uncommon tumors in rats; their biological behavior suggests that they do not progress to carcinomas, and metastases have not been reported (Bannasch et al. 1998a,b). Current opinion recommends not including oncocytomas with tumors of other renal tubules because of morphological differences and their presumed lack of significance during risk assessment (Frazier et al. 2012). In rats, adenomas representing the suspected familial amphophilic-vacuolar (A-V) phenotype can also be seen as part of the spectrum of hyperplasia, adenoma, and carcinoma observed for this distinctive morphologic renal tumor (Hard et al. 2008). These neoplasms are lobulated, with a delicate fibrovascular stroma and an amphophilic, vacuolated cytoplasm. At present, A-V neoplasms should not be included with other neoplasms of renal tubule origin when considering human risk assessment or determining relationship with chemical administration.

12.1.8.5.2 Carcinoma

Spontaneous tubule carcinomas are uncommon to rare in long-term, chronic, or carcinogenicity studies. In a review of renal tumors from NTP bioassay studies, some reported that carcinomas appeared as the A-V type of familial tumor (Figure 12.5a). These carcinomas appeared similar to A-V adenomas except for their much larger size and areas of degeneration. Carcinomas tend to be grossly recognized as pale, solid to cystic masses with evidence of hemorrhagic necrosis and capsular invasion. They are generally poorly circumscribed, infiltrative, and poorly encapsulated. As with most malignant tumors, tubular carcinomas may have a variable morphology based on their degree of cellular differentiation. Therefore, carcinomas may be well differentiated to highly anaplastic. Tumor cell growth patterns may be solid, tubular, cystic, papillary, or a mixture. Staining tinctorial qualities are also variable as basophilic, eosinophilic, clear, or mixed type variants may

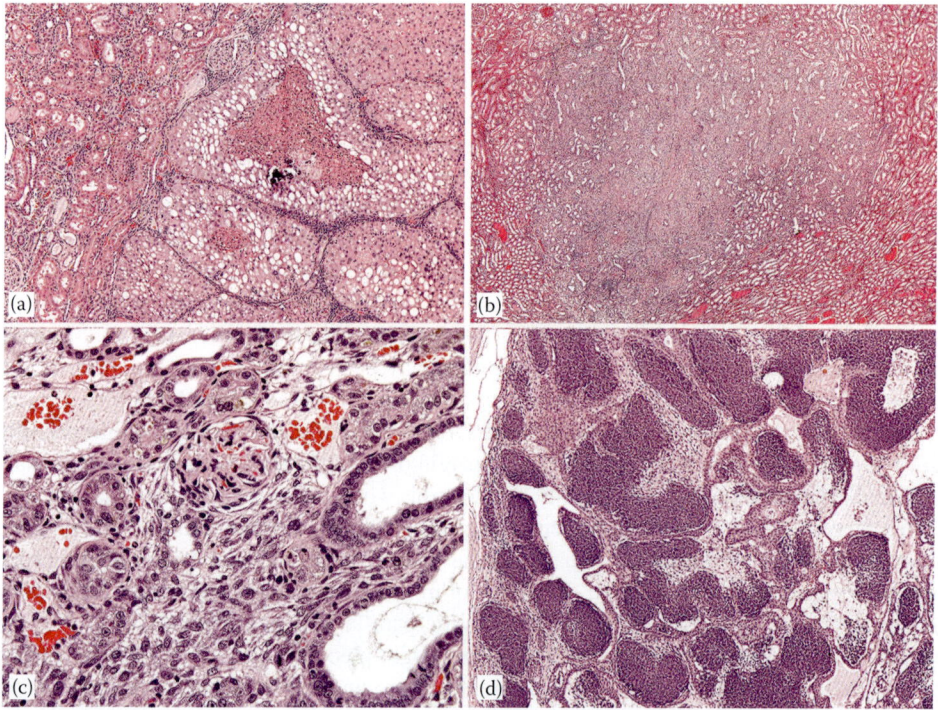

FIGURE 12.5   (a) Hematoxylin and eosin 10×. Rat kidney, with the amphophilic-vacuolar (A-V) variant of a renal tubule carcinoma now considered to represent a familial type of renal tumor in the rat. The tumor comprised a lobular growth pattern of essentially amphophilic and vacuolated cells separated by a delicate fibrovascular stroma with central degeneration/necrosis as a predominant feature. (b) Hematoxylin and eosin 4×. Rat kidney. RMTs can become progressively quite large, appearing infiltrative rather than invasive, and lacking a capsule. They are challenging for the pathologist to diagnose. The presence of heterogenous mesenchymal (connective tissue) cell types aids in their diagnosis. (c) Hematoxylin and eosin 40×. Rat kidney. RMT demonstrating the infiltrative nature of the basic spindle cell of origin around preexisting renal tubules and glomeruli. Note the metaplastic to hyperplastic epithelial lined renal tubules often seen with RMTs. (d) Hematoxylin and eosin 16×. Rat kidney, demonstrating a nephroblastoma, which is characterized by the presence of deeply basophilic blastemal cells, which other renal tumors lack. Differentiation into primitive (organoid) structures such as tubule and glomeruloid forms may often be appreciated.

be observed. Hemorrhage and necrosis can be prominent. Most carcinomas have considerable cellular pleomorphism to anaplastic features. Mitotic figures are variable. As carcinomas become more malignant, the tumor stroma becomes more scirrhous, particularly if invasion of the renal capsule has occurred. Metastases are seldom reported as renal tubule carcinomas are generally regarded as having a low metastatic potential. Abdominal seeding of tumor cells may also occur with capsular invasion (Frazier et al. 2012).

12.1.8.6 Connective Tissue Neoplasms

12.1.8.6.1 Lipoma/Liposarcoma

Lipomas and liposarcomas are neoplasms of lipocytes that are occasionally observed in rats. Small lipomas have to be differentiated from adipocytic infiltrates, although the distinction between the two is somewhat arbitrary and based on typical features of tumor morphology. They are single, usually well delineated to irregular neoplasms noted near the corticomedullary junction. Lipomas are distinguished by their uniform population of monomorphic, mature lipocytes. They tend to be infiltrative in nature and can become larger while maintaining their benign appearance. Mitoses, hemorrhage, and necrosis are absent (Gordon 1986; Hard 1998b). Larger lipomas may approach but do not infiltrate the capsule.

12.1.8.6.2 Liposarcoma

Liposarcomas are generally much larger than lipomas and are detected grossly as poorly demarcated tumors with cystic areas of hemorrhage and necrosis. Like lipomas, they are infiltrative in nature and not encapsulated. Large cystic areas of hemorrhagic necrosis may be present. Some cystic spaces represent tubule or ductal dilatation. Liposarcomas are composed of variable cell morphologies including mature lipocytes, lipoblasts, or undifferentiated spindle cells. Mitoses are more frequently observed in more malignant tumors. Spindle cell foci are more common in anaplastic tumors. They may infiltrate and penetrate the capsule. Metastases are rarely reported (Gordon 1986; Hard 1998b,c).

12.1.8.6.3 Renal Mesenchymal Tumor

Renal mesenchymal tumor (RMT) is a rat-specific tumor that poses a diagnostic challenge to pathologists because of some overlapping morphological features with nephroblastoma. The cell of origin is a stellate fibroblast-like cell that infiltrates around and entraps preexisting epithelial tubules and glomeruli. Whorls of spindle cells may encircle tubules. RMTs represent a malignant tumor as tumor growth is continuous and malignant features become progressively apparent as the tumor grows (Figure 12.5b). Large tumors can be easily recognized at gross necropsy as cystic, gelatinous, and hemorrhagic masses. They tend to be irregular and poorly demarcated tumors. RMTs represent a heterogenous mix of primitive mesenchyme or myxomatous tissue. Besides the predominant stellate-appearing cell, RMTs may present foci of fibrous tissue, smooth muscle, striated muscle, cartilage, osteoid, and hemangiomatous areas (Figure 12.5c). Occasionally, dense islands of fibrosarcomatous tissue may be seen. Hypertrophic to metaplastic tubules and/or ducts are often present. Mitoses are variable. RMTs can invade the capsule and seed the abdominal cavity and can react positively for vimentin. Collision or mixed tumors involving RMTs and carcinomas have been reported (Hard 1998a; Seely 2004).

12.1.8.7 Embryonic Primordial Neoplasia

12.1.8.7.1 Nephroblastematosis/Nephroblastoma

Nephroblastematosis (nephrogenic rests) appears as small, basophilic foci of blastemal cells that may have organoid differentiation and are presumed to have the potential to develop into nephroblastomas (Mesfin 1996; Beckwith 1998; Jackson and Kirkpatrick 2002). They are uncommon findings in the rat kidney. They usually appear in the outer medulla, are somewhat infiltrative, and have to be differentiated from lymphocytic infiltrates. The foci of nephroblastematosis are more discrete and contain a population of monomorphic cells. The presence of larger, generally well-circumscribed, pseudoencapsulated, and distinct foci of deeply basophilic blastemal cells is pathognomonic for nephroblastoma (Hard and Grasso 1976; Iida et al. 1981; Chandra and Carlton 1992; Mesfin and Breech 1992; Cardesa and Ribalta 1998; Mesfin and Breech 1996). Nephroblastomas have been reported in young rats in 90-day toxicity studies. Blastemal cells may appear as nests, cords, or islands of poorly differentiated cells. However, organoid differentiation into primitive glomeruli, tubules, or ducts is relatively common (Figure 12.5d). Blastemal cells have scant, poorly defined cytoplasm. Mitoses are often frequent in areas of blastema or primitive tubules. The stroma may vary from delicate to well developed. Triphasic nephroblastomas contain stroma, which is considered part of the neoplastic process. Metastases are rare but have been reported in the lungs and regional lymph nodes. Nephroblastomas are infrequent tumors in rats and are exceedingly rare in mice (Liebelt et al. 1989).

12.1.8.7.2 Fibrosarcoma/Sarcoma

Rats, and less commonly mice, also have a unique and rare spontaneous renal tumor that differs from RMT and resembles a highly anaplastic fibrosarcoma or sarcoma. These tumors have been experimentally induced by the polyoma virus or via chemical induction (Frazier et al. 2012). These tumors are well demarcated, densely fibrous, or sarcomatous. The tumor itself is composed of slightly basophilic, anaplastic, and monomorphic fibroblastic-like spindle cells in which collagen is scarce or absent. These aggressive tumors are infiltrative, replacing the parenchyma as they grow.

12.1.8.7.3 Hematogenous/Metastatic Neoplasms

The kidneys of rodents are often a site of hematogenous neoplastic infiltration. The most commonly observed hematogenous tumors in rats are large granular lymphoma (mononuclear cell leukemia or Fischer rat leukemia) and, in mice, lymphoma. Histiocytic sarcoma occurs in both rats and mice. Hyaline droplets, representing lysozyme, may be observed in association with the presence of histiocytic sarcoma. However, this finding is variable, strain-dependent, and affected by staining methods (Hard and Snowden 1991; Luz and Murray 1991). Hyaline droplets containing lysozyme have been identified in other tumors (Yamate et al. 1998). Kidneys are also the site of metastatic neoplasms. Commonly reported metastases are from the respiratory and gastrointestinal tracts. A helpful observation to aid in the differentiation of a primary versus metastatic tumor is the infiltrative behavior of metastatic tumor proliferations, which appear as infiltrates in the renal parenchyma, entrapping preexisting epithelial structures. Renal tubule neoplasms do not usually contain preexisting epithelial structures within the tumor; however, this observation may not be useful when considering sarcomatous metastases since RMT shows a similar pattern of growth.

12.1.8.8 Neoplasms of the Renal Pelvis

12.1.8.8.1 Papilloma

Papillomas are uncommon tumors in the renal pelvis. The differentiation between larger areas of urothelial hyperplasia and urothelial papillomas depends upon the presence of a more exophytic growth pattern, pedunculation, with pronounced fibrovascular papillary fronds or stalks. Generally, the cells are well differentiated and slightly basophilic with minimal pleomorphism. Foci of squamous or glandular metaplasia may also be present. Mitotic figures are uncommon. Inverted papillomas are less frequently observed. On rare occasions, proliferative lesions that resemble polyps have been seen in the renal pelvis.

12.1.8.8.2 Carcinoma

Urothelial carcinomas tend to be larger neoplasms with irregular growth patterns that often proliferate within the renal pelvic cavity and later invade the surrounding pelvic tissue and kidney.

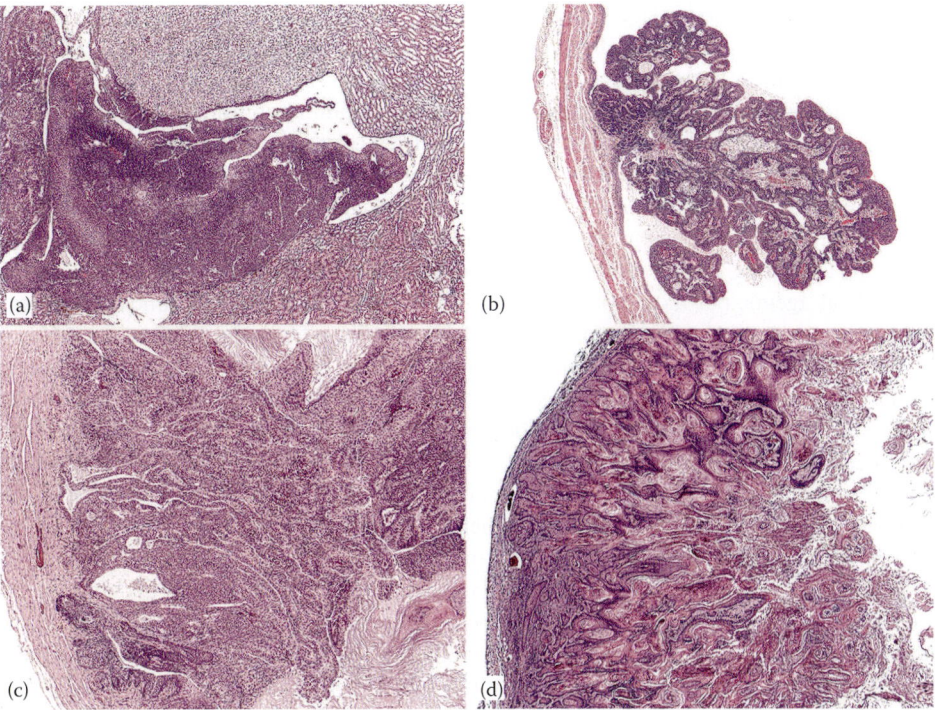

FIGURE 12.6 (a) Hematoxylin and eosin 10×. Rat kidney, with a renal pelvis urothelial carcinoma showing the typical growth pattern where tumor cells proliferate in solid sheets of pleomorphic to anaplastic cells within the renal pelvis. Invasion is often seen with larger tumors. (b) Hematoxylin and eosin 4×. Rat urinary bladder, with an exophytic urothelial papilloma. Fortuitous sections often demonstrate the fibrovascular stalk connection to the bladder epithelium. (c) Hematoxylin and eosin 10×. Rat urinary bladder, with a large and poorly demarcated urothelial carcinoma nearly filling the bladder lumen. Note the presence of anaplastic cells, necrosis, squamous metaplasia, and invasion into the bladder wall. (d) Hematoxylin and eosin 5×. Rat urinary bladder, with a highly invasive and malignant squamous cell carcinoma of the urinary bladder demonstrating the predominant features of anaplastic squamous cells and abundant keratinization.

Typically, they are solid tumors forming sheets or cords with well-differentiated to anaplastic cellular morphology. Extension of carcinoma growth can be recognized along the pelvic urothelium (Figure 12.6a). Acute to chronic inflammation usually accompanies necrosis and tumor invasion. Tumor stroma is not pronounced in most cases, and some tumors may have prominent vascularization. Mitoses are increased with increased malignancy. Foci of squamous metaplasia may be observed. Metastases to the lungs have been reported (Chandra et al. 1991). Carcinomas of the renal pelvis have to be differentiated from renal tumors that have invaded the pelvic cavity, and invasive pelvic carcinomas have to be differentiated from malignant renal tumors.

12.2 URINARY BLADDER, URETERS, AND URETHRA

12.2.1 Nonneoplastic Lesions of Lower Urinary Tract

Congenital lesions are uncommon in the lower urinary tract in rodents, dogs, and nonhuman primates but are occasionally encountered in toxicity studies as background lesions. Ureteral aplasia or agenesis is unilaterally observed in rats and mice in association with renal aplasia. Hydroureter may also be noted as a congenital lesion but is more commonly associated with obstructive uropathy resulting from urolithiasis, in which case the renal pelvis usually manifests hydronephrosis.

Inflammation is commonly noted in the submucosa throughout the lower urinary tract in both rodents and nonrodents and is usually subclinical and of no biological significance. When severe, the etiology is usually bacterial and can result from ascending infections from the urethra or descending infections from pyelonephritis (Seely 1999). Inflammation in the urinary bladder and ureters is a frequent complication of urolithiasis, even without obstruction. Hemorrhage, erosion, and ulceration are often noted concomitantly, and there may be hyperplasia of the urothelium. Infestation with the roundworm *Trichosomoides crassicauda* in the rat may result in inflammation in the urethra, bladder, or ureters and occasionally results in complete obstruction. Erosion/ ulceration of the lining urothelium in the bladder, pelvis, and ureter has been noted with some pharmaceutical agents, but more commonly following administration of chemical toxicants. Test articles that are associated with increased crystalluria or calculi formation such as the sulfonamide may result in ulcers, but other agents, particularly those with high renal clearance and concentration in the urine filtrate, may directly target urothelium and produce necrosis with loss of cell layers. Some compounds, such as acetazolamide, may result in only suburothelial inflammation and/ or mild hyperplasia (Molon-Noblot et al. 1992), and other ulcer-inducing agents may have similar limited inflammatory effects when administered at lower doses or for shorter duration as a result of low-grade irritation. Vacuolation of the urothelium may also be noted as a common response to toxicologic injury related to direct epithelial cytotoxicity. Similar to vacuoles in the renal tubules, the clear spaces represent swollen cytostructural elements such as lysosomes or endoplasmic reticulum and may contain fluid, lipid, or drug metabolites. Rarely, a compound or agent will cause the urothelium to undergo focal hypertrophy. This cytoplasmic expansion can be devoid of evidence of hyperplasia, but more commonly, both hypertrophy and hyperplasia occur together, as in the case of the peroxisome proliferator-activated receptor agonist (PPARα/PPARγ) drugs in rats where the lesions are considered to be preneoplastic (Egerod et al. 2010).

Calculi in the urinary bladder may be formed by precipitation of normal urinary constituents when drugs alter the composition and physiology of the urine (Cohen 2002). Composition of calculi in the lower urinary tract mirrors that of crystals in the kidney and may be variable from individual to individual or between species. In rodents, uroliths are typically composed of calcium phosphates or calcium carbonates, with or without magnesium components. While bladder calculi are commonly noted in some breeds of dogs, beagles tend to be less commonly affected, and, when present in a dose-responsive fashion, a test article effect on crystal formation should be considered. Spontaneous calculi are rare in the bladder of cynomolgus monkeys. Hematuria as a result of hemorrhage in the lower urinary tract is most often a reflection of ulceration and/or calculi, but some agents that inhibit clotting mechanisms such as the fibrinolytic or anti-thrombotic agents, or drugs such as the coumarins, may result in hemorrhage into the urine filtrate without overt evidence of ulceration. Urinalysis is diagnostic with discolored urine and the presence of large numbers of intact erythrocytes in sediment exams. Catheterization of the urinary bladder may result in mucosal lesions and have to be differentiated from possible effects of test article.

Proteinaceous plugs, composed of androgen-related secretions mixed with desquamated cells, sperm, and inflammatory cells, may rarely occlude the urethra in rodents, especially as part of the mouse urologic syndrome, but more commonly are a postmortem or agonal change in the bladder. Proteinaceous plugs have no clinical relevance and are not considered to form a nidus for calculi formation. Eosinophilic inclusion bodies have been encountered in the urothelial cytoplasm of rodents, primarily in the bladder. They are most commonly observed in the outer layers but may also be present in the intermediate and basal layers of the transitional epithelium. These inclusions may appear as pink droplets or as clear spaces (washed out during tissue processing) and are a nonspecific response to a variety of agents that are toxic to the urothelium. In mice, they can occur commonly as a background lesion unrelated to test article administration. They are thought to represent degradation products of cellular machinery and in some cases have been identified as intramitochondrial deposits (Suzuki et al. 2008).

12.2.2 Hyperplastic Lesions of Lower Urinary Tract

Urothelial hyperplasia in the lower urinary tract appears morphologically similar to renal pelvic hyperplasia with minor differences. Excellent reviews on the spectrum of hyperplastic lesions have been published by Kunze (1998), Cohen (2002), and Frith et al. (1995). Hyperplasia may be focal, multifocal, or diffuse. In the bladder, hyperplasia is also differentiated into simple, nodular, or papillary types. In addition, regression of hyperplastic lesions has been shown by comparing experimental and spontaneous types of bladder hyperplasia (Shinohara and Frith 1981). Handling of the animal may also result in urothelial hyperplasia (Cohen et al. 1996).

12.2.3 Neoplastic Lesions of Lower Urinary Tract

12.2.3.1 Papilloma

Urothelial papillomas are similar to those appearing in the renal pelvis and are uncommon. Typically, exophytic papillomas are seen, but inverted papillomas are also recognized (Shirai and Takahashi 1998). Bladder papillomas usually pose no problem for the pathologist when a stalk is present with a prominent fibrovascular core (Figure 12.6b). However, sectioning may create a diagnostic challenge for the pathologist in determining the biological behavior of papillomas since some carcinomas are well differentiated. On rare occasions, proliferative lesions that resemble polyps have been seen in the urinary bladder (Jokinen 1990).

12.2.3.2 Carcinoma

Urothelial carcinomas are rarely reported as spontaneous tumors but have been associated with test article administration (Hard 1990). Usually carcinomas are solitary tumors, which may become large and are poorly demarcated. They tend to be invasive, with well-differentiated to anaplastic cellular morphology. The growth pattern may be papillary to solid with a broad base. Highly malignant tumors have considerable anaplastic features (Figure 12.6c). Mitoses are variable in some abnormal forms, and the stroma is sparse. Both squamous and glandular metaplasia may be observed, and metastases have been reported (Frith 1998; Frith et al. 1995; Pauli et al. 1998). Spindle cell or undifferentiated carcinomas are positive for cytokeratin (Sykes and Stula 1989). Uroplakins, transmembrane proteins found in umbrella cells, have proved useful as a marker in detecting urothelial lineage in tumors (Moll et al. 1995; Ramos-Vara et al. 2003; Romih et al. 2005). However, Ogawa et al. (1999) reported an induced carcinoma tumor model in which the number of uroplakin-positive cells decreased relative to tumor differentiation. Urothelial carcinomas, particularly of the prostatic urethra, have been reported in a colony of beagle dogs (Nikula et al. 1989).

12.2.3.3 Squamous Cell Carcinoma

Squamous cell carcinoma represents a highly malignant tumor. They are exceedingly rare as spontaneous tumors but have been induced (Hard 1990). The main diagnostic criterion distinguishing between carcinoma and squamous cell carcinoma is the predominance of anaplastic squamous cells with pronounced keratinization and "pearl" formation (Figure 12.6d). Squamous cell carcinomas have an irregular growth pattern and are invasive. Tumors tend to be solid with sheets or islands of highly pleomorphic to anaplastic cellular morphology. Atypia may be present, and the stroma is well developed. Mitoses are increased as malignancy increases, and metastases are common. Inflammation accompanies invasive tumors (Hirose and Shirai 1998).

12.2.3.4 Adenocarcinoma

Adenocarcinomas have been observed following administration of agents but are either exceedingly rare or nonexistent as spontaneous tumors. Principal histological features include the presence of glandular elements and/or tubules, lined by pleomorphic to anaplastic cuboidal cells, which may contain mucous (Stula and Sykes 1998).

12.2.4 Connective Tissue and Smooth Muscle Neoplasms

The lower urinary tract, particularly the bladder, may be a site for connective tissue tumors. Generally, these tumors represent either benign or malignant fibrous or lipomatous tumors. Benign and malignant smooth muscle tumors may also be seen.

12.2.5 Mesenchymal Proliferation Lesion

Mesenchymal proliferative lesion, reported in mice, is discussed with neoplasia as the histogenesis of this interesting lesion was originally thought to represent a neoplastic condition (Chandra and Frith 1991; Frith et al. 1994b; Halliwell 1998). But more recently, mesenchymal proliferative lesions have been shown to be similar to decidual-like lesions occurring in male accessory sex glands of older mice (Karbe et al. 1998, 2000; Karbe 1999). Most pathologists believe that these lesions do not represent neoplasms (Frazier et al. 2012). Most lesions are noted in the caudal half of the bladder or near the bladder trigone. Lesions tend to be solitary, although multifocal lesions have been reported. Lesions are well demarcated but not encapsulated. Growth is solid or polypoid and often protrudes into the bladder lumen. Typically, the lesion contains both large pleomorphic epithelioid cells and spindle cells. Epithelioid cells have distinct cytoplasm borders and homogenous eosinophilic cytoplasm, and the spindle cells resemble either fibrocytes or smooth muscle cells. Invasion into either the urothelium or overlying serosa is occasionally seen, and mitoses are variable. Mesenchymal proliferative lesions have been reported to be cytochrome-negative with slight desmin positivity. This lesion appears to be strain-specific, common in Swiss Webster mice but absent in B6C3F1 mice. Induction of mesenchymal proliferative lesions by chemicals is presently unknown (Frazier et al. 2012).

12.2.6 Hematogenous/Metastatic Neoplasms

The urinary bladder of rodents is often a site of hematogenous neoplastic infiltration, similar to the kidneys. Most commonly observed hematogenous tumors in rats are large granular lymphoma (mononuclear cell leukemia) and, in mice, lymphoma. Foci of histiocytic sarcoma may also be observed.

REFERENCES

Abrass, C.K. 2000. The nature of chronic progressive nephropathy in aging rats. *Adv Renal Replacement Ther* 7:4–10.

Adalsteinsson, V., Parajuli, O., Kepics, S., Gupta, A., Reeves, W.B., and Hahm, J.-I. 2008. Ultrasensitive detection of cytokines enabled by nanoscale ZnO arrays. *Analyt Chem* 80:6594–601.

Adams, L.E., Roberts, S.M., Donovan-Brand, R., Zimmer, H., and Hess, E.V. 1993. Study of procainamide hapten-specific antibodies in rabbits and humans. *Int J Immunopharmacol* 15:887–97.

Adler, M., Muller, K., Rached, E., Dekantz, W. and Mally, A. 2007. Modulation of key regulators of mitosis linked to chromosomal instability is an early event in ochratoxin A carcinogenicity. *Carcinogenesis* 30:711–9.

Alden, C.L. 1986. A review of unique male rat hydrocarbon nephropathy. *Toxicol Pathol* 14:109–11.

Alden, C.L., Hard, G.C., Krieg, K., Takahashi, M., and Turusov, V.S. 1992. Urinary system. In: *International Classification of Rodent Tumours Part I: Rat*, ed Mohr, U., pp. 1–39. Lyon: IARC Scientific Publ No. 122.

Alpers, C.E. 2010. The kidney. In: *Robbins and Cotran Pathologic Basis of Disease*, eds. Kumar, V., Abbas, A.K., Fausto, N., and Aster, J.C., pp. 905–69. Philadelphia, PA: Sanders Elsevier.

Ando, R., Nakamura, A., Nagatani, M. et al. 2008. Comparison of past and recent historical control data in relation to spontaneous tumors during carcinogenicity testing in Fischer 344 rats. *J Toxicol Pathol* 21:53–60.

Asahina, M., Ohmachi, Y., Yasosima, A., Iwasaki, H., and Kawai, Y. 2000. A case of renal mesenchymal tumor in a young Beagle dog. *J Toxicol Pathol* 13:45–7.

Asanuma, K., Adachi, K., Sugimoto, T., and Chiba, S. (2006). Effects of lysine-induced acute renal failure in dogs. *J Toxicol Sci* 31:87–98.

Bach, P.H., and Thanh, N.T.K. 1998. Renal papillary necrosis-40 years on. *Toxicol Pathol* 26:73–91.

Bannasch, P., Zerban, H., and Ahn, Y.S. 1998a. Renal cell adenoma and carcinoma, rat. In: *Monographs on Pathology of Laboratory Animals. Urinary System 2nd ed.*, eds. Jones, T.C., Hard, G.C., and Mohr, U., pp. 79–118. Berlin: Springer-Verlag.

Bannasch, P., Zerban, H., Ahn, Y.S., and Hacker, H.J. 1998b. Oncocytoma, kidney, rat. In: *Monographs on Pathology of Laboratory Animals. Urinary System 2nd ed.*, eds. Jones, T.C., Hard, G.C., and Mohr, U., pp. 64–79. Berlin: Springer-Verlag.

Barnes, J.L., and Glass II, W.F. 2011. Renal interstitial fibrosis: A critical evaluation of the origin of myofibroblasts. *Contrib to Nephrol* 169:73–93.

Barrett, J.C., and Huff, J. 1991. Cellular and molecular mechanisms of chemically induced renal carcinogenesis. *Renal Failure* 13:211–25.

Baylis, C. 1994. Age-dependent glomerular damage in the rat. Dissociation between glomerular injury and both glomerular hypertension and hypertrophy. Male gender as a primary risk factor. *J Clin Invest* 94:1823–9.

Beckwith, J.B. 1998. Nephrogenic rests and the pathogenesis of Wilms tumor. *Am J Med Genet* 79:268–73.

Beckwith, J.B. 1999. Human renal carcinoma—pathogenesis and biology. In: *Species Differences in Thyroid, Kidney and Urinary Bladder Carcinogenesis*, eds. Capen, C.C., Dybing, E., Rice, J.M., and Wilbourn, J.D., pp. 81–93. Lyon: IARC Scientific Publications No. 147 International Agency for Scientific Cancer.

Bendele, A.M., Buenger, D.A., Mcgrath, J.P., Schmalz, C.A., and Hanasono, G.K. 1994. Chronic toxicity, metabolism, and pharmacokinetics of the 5-HT3 receptor antagonist zatosetron (LY277359) in Fischer 344 rats. *Tox Sci* 22:494–504.

Bomhard, E. 1992. Frequency of spontaneous tumors in Wistar rat in 30-month studies. *Exp Toxic Pathol* 44:381–92.

Bonventre, J.V., Vaidya, V.S., Schmouder, R., Feig, P., and Dieterle, F. 2010. Next-generation biomarkers for detecting kidney toxicity. *Nat Biotech* 28:436–40.

Boorman, G.A., and Hollander, C.F. 1974. High incidence of spontaneous urinary and ureter tumors in the Brown Norway rat. *J Natl Cancer Inst* 52:1005–8.

Boorman, G.A., Wood, M., and Fukushima, S. 1994. Tumours of the urinary bladder. In: *Pathology of Tumours in Laboratory Animals, Vol 2. Tumours of the Mouse, 2nd ed.*, eds. Turusov, V.S., and Mohr, U., pp. 383–406. Lyon: IARC Scientific Publications No. 111.

Boorman, G., Dixon, D., Elwell, M. et al. 2003. Assessment of hyperplastic lesions in rodent carcinogenicity studies. *Toxicol Pathol* 31:707–10.

Breyer, M.D., Hao, C.-M., and Qi, Z. 2001. Cyclooxygenase-2 selective inhibitors and the kidney. *Curr Opin Crit Care* 7:393–400.

Brix, A.E., Nyska, A., Haseman, J.K., Sells, D.M., Jokinen, M.P., and Walker, N.J. 2005. Incidences of selected lesions in control female Harlan Sprague–Dawley rats from two-year studies performed by the National Toxicology Program. *Toxicol Pathol* 33:477–83.

Brown, C.A., Jeong, K.S., Poppenga, R.H. et al. 2007. Outbreaks of renal failure associated with melamine and cyanuric acid in dogs and cats in 2004 and 2007. *J Vet Diagn Invest* 19:525–31.

Bruder, M.C., Shoieb, A.M., Shirai, N., Boucher, G.G., and Brodie, T.A. 2010. Renal dysplasia in beagle dogs: four cases. *Toxicol Pathol* 38:1051–7.

Bryan, J.N., Henry, C.J., Turnquist, S.E. et al. 2006. Primary renal neoplasia of dogs. *J Vet Intern Med* 20:1155–60.

Bucci, T.J., Howard, P.C., Tolleson, W.H., Laborde, J.B., and Hansen, D.K. 1998. Renal effects of fumonisin mycotoxins in animals. *Toxicol Pathol* 26:160–4.

Cappon, G.D., and Hurtt, M.E. 2010. Developmental toxicity of the kidney. In: *Reproductive Toxicology. 3rd ed.*, eds. Kapp, R.W., and Tyl, R.W., pp. 193–204. New York: Informa Health Care.

Cardesa, A., and T. Ribalta. 1998. Nephroblastoma, kidney, rat. In: *Monographs on Pathology of Laboratory Animals. Urinary System 2nd ed.*, eds. Jones, T.C., Hard, G.C., and Mohr, U., pp. 129–38. Berlin: Springer-Verlag.

Chandra, M., and Carlton, W.W. 1992. Incidence, histopathologic, and electron microscopic features of spontaneous nephroblastomas in rats. *Tox Lett* 62:179–90.

Chandra, M., and Frith, C.H. 1991. Spontaneously occurring leiomyosarcoms of the mouse urinary bladder. *Toxicol Pathol* 19:164–7.

Chandra, M., and Frith, C.H. 1992. Spontaneous neoplasms in B6C3F1 mice. *Tox Lett* 60:91–8.

Chandra, M., Riley, M.G, and Johnson, D.E. 1991. Incidence and pathology of spontaneous renal pelvis transitional cell carcinomas in rats. *Toxicol Pathol* 19:287–9.

Chandra, M., Riley, M.G.I., and Johnson, D.E. 1992. Spontaneous neoplasms in aged Sprague–Dawley rats. *Arch Toxicol* 66:496–502.

Chang, C.P., McDill, B.W., Neilson, J.R. et al. 2004. Calcineurin is required in urinary tract mesenchyme for the development of the pyeloureteral peristaltic machinery. *J Clin Invest* 113:1051–6.

Chaudhuri, B.N., Kleywegt, G.J., Bjorkman, J., Lehman-McKeeman, L.D., Oliver, J.D., and Jones, T.A. 1999. The structures of alpha 2u-globulin and its complex with a hyaline droplet inducer. *Acta Crystallogr D Biol Crystallogr* 55:753–62.

Cherdwongcharoensuk, D., Henrique, R., Upatham, S., Pereira, A.S., and Aguas, A.P. 2005. Tubular kidney damage and centrilobular liver injury after intratracheal instillation of dimethyl selenide. *Toxicol Pathol* 33:225–9.

Chevalier, R.L. 2006. Pathogenesis of renal injury in obstructive uropathy. *Curr Op Pediatr* 18:153–60.

Chiusolo, A., Defazio, R., Zanetti, E. et al. 2010. Kidney injury molecule-1 expression in rat proximal tubule after treatment with segment-specific nephrotoxicants: a tool for early screening of potential kidney toxicity. *Toxicol Pathol* 38:338–45.

Choudhury, D., and Ahmed, Z. 2006. Drug-associated renal dysfunction and injury. *Nat Clin Pract Nephrol* 2:80–91.

Christensen, S., and Ottensen, P.D. 1986. Lithium-induced uremia in rats. Survival and renal function and morphology after one year. *Acta Pharmacol Toxicol (Copenhagen)* 58:339–47.

Clayson, D.B., Fishbein, L., and Cohen, S.M. 1995. Effects of stones and other physical factors on the induction of rodent bladder cancer. *Food Chem Toxic* 33:771–84.

Clemens, G.R., Schroeder, R.E., Magness, S.H. et al. 2009. Developmental toxicity associated with receptor tyrosine kinase ret inhibition in reproductive toxicity testing. *Birth Defects Res A—Clin Molec Teratol* 85:130–6.

Cohen, S.M. 1989. Toxic and nontoxic changes induced in the urothelium by xenobiotics. *Tox Appl Pharmacol* 101:484–98.

Cohen, S.M. 1998a. Induction of cancer in the rat bladder: pathogenesis, role of cell proliferation, and relevance to human disease. In: *Monographs on Pathology of Laboratory Animals. Urinary System, 2nd ed.*, eds. Jones, T.C., Hard, G.C., and Mohr, U., pp. 420–6. Berlin: Springer-Verlag.

Cohen, S.M. 1998b. Urinary bladder carcinogenesis. *Toxicol Pathol* 26:121–7.

Cohen, S.M. 2002. Comparative pathology of proliferative lesions of the urinary bladder. *Toxicol Pathol* 30:663–71.

Cohen, S.M., Cano, M., Anderson, T., and Garland, E.M. 1996. Extensive handling of rats leads to mild urinary bladder hyperplasia. *Toxicol Pathol* 24:251–7.

Cohen, S.M., Arnold, L.L., Cano, M., Ito, N., Garland, E.M., and Shaw, R.A. 2000. Calcium phosphate-containing precipitate and the carcinogenicity of sodium salts in rats. *Carcinogenesis* 21:783–92.

Cohen, S.M., Johansson, S.L., Arnold, L.L., and Lawson, T.A. 2002. Urinary tract calculi and thresholds in carcinogenesis. *Food Chem Toxicol* 40:793–9.

Cohen, S.M., Ohnishi, T., Clark, N.M., He, J., and Arnold, L.L. 2007. Investigations of rodent urinary bladder carcinogens: Collection, processing, and evaluation of urine and bladders. *Toxicol Pathol* 35:337–47.

Cuppage, F.E., and Tate, A. 1967. Repair of the nephron following injury with mercuric chloride. *Am J Pathol* 51:405–29.

Dalmas, D.A., Scicchitano, M.S., Chen, Y. et al. 2008. Transcriptional profiling of laser capture microdissected rat arterial elements: fenoldopam-induced vascular toxicity as a model system. *Toxicol Pathol* 36:496–519.

Davis, M.A., and Ryan, D.H. 1998. Apoptosis in the kidney. *Toxicol Pathol* 26:81–5.

D'Agati, V.D., Jennette, J.C., and Silva, F.G. 2005. *Non-Neoplastic Kidney Diseases. An Atlas of Nontumor Pathology*. American Registry of Pathology and Armed Forces Institute of Pathology, Washington DC. ARP Press, Silver Spring, M.D. AFIP Fascide 4, first series, Chapter 9, pp. 225–30.

De Rijk, E.P.C.T., Ravesloot, W.T.M., Wijnands, Y., and Van Esch, E. 2003. A fast histochemical staining method to identify hyaline droplets in the rat kidney. *Toxicol Pathol* 31:462–4.

DeSesso, J.M. 1995. Anatomical relationships of urinary bladders compared: their potential role in the development of bladder tumors in human and rats. *Food Chem Toxicol* 33:705–14.

Deszo, B., Rady, P., Morocz, I. et al. 1990. Morphological and immunohistochemical characteristics of dimethylnitrosamine-induced malignant mesenchymal renal tumor in F-344 rats. *J Cancer Res Clin Oncol* 116:372–8.

Dill, J.A., Lee, K.M., Renne, R.A. et al. 2003. Alpha 2u-globulin nephropathy and carcinogenicity following exposure to decalin (decahydronaphthalene) in F344/N rats. *Toxicol Sci* 72:223–34.

Dinse, G.E., Peddada, S.D., Harris, S.F., and Elmore, S.A. 2010. Comparison of NTP historical control tumor incidence rates in female Harlan Sprague–Dawley and Fischer 344/N rats. *Toxicol Pathol* 38:765–75.

Dombrowski, F., Klotz, L., Bannasch, P., Evert, M. 2007. Renal carcinogenesis in models of diabetes—metabolic changes are closely related to neoplastic development. *Diabetologia* 50:2580–90.

Dominick, M.A., Bobrowski, W.F., Metz, A.L., Gough, A.W., and MacDonald, J.R. 1990. Ultrastructural juxtaglomerular cell changes in normotensive rats treated with quinapril, an inhibitor of angiotensin-converting enzyme. *Toxicol Pathol* 18:396–406.

Donker, A.J., Venuto, R.C., and Vladutiu, A.O. 1984. Effects of prolonged administration of D-penicillamine or captopril in various strains of rats. Brown Norway rats treated with D-penicillamine develop autoantibodies, circulating immune complexes, and disseminated intravascular coagulation. *Clin Immunol Immunopathol* 30:142–5.

Donnadieu-Claraz, M., Bonnehorgne, M., Dhieux, B. et al. 2007. Chronic exposure to uranium leads to iron accumulation in rat kidney cells. *Radiat Res* 167:454–64.

Dortant, P.M., Peters-Volleberg, G.W.M., Van Loveren, H. et al. 2001. Age-related differences in the toxicity of ochratoxin A in female rats. *Food Chem Toxicol* 39:55–65.

Doughty, S.E., Ferrier, R.K., Hillan, K.J., and Jackson, D.G. 1995. The effects of ZENECA ZD8731, an angiotensin II antagonist, on renin expression by juxtaglomerular cells in the rat: comparison of protein and mRNA expression as detected by immunohistochemistry and in situ hybridization. *Toxicol Pathol* 23:256–61.

Dube, P.H., Almanzar, M.M., Frazier, K.S. et al. 2004. Osteogenic Protein-1: gene expression and treatment in rat remnant kidney model. *Toxicol Pathol* 32:384–92.

Duprat, P., and Burek, J.D. 1986. Suppurative nephritis, pyelonephritis, rat. In: *Monographs on Pathology of Laboratory Animals. Urinary System*, eds. Jones, T.C., Mohr, U., and Hunt, R.D., pp. 219–24. Berlin: Springer-Verlag.

Eddy, A.A. 1996. Molecular insights into renal interstitial fibrosis. *J Am Soc Nephrol* 7:2495–508.

Egerod, F.L., Brünner, N., Svendsen, J.E., Oleksiewicz, M.B. 2010. PPARα and PPARγ are co-expressed, functional and show positive interactions in the rat urinary bladder urothelium. *J Appl Toxicol* 30:151–62.

Eker, R., Mossige, J., Johannessen, J.V., and Aars, H. 1981. Hereditary adenomas and adenocarcinomas in rats. *Diag Histopathol* 4:99–110.

Ellison, D.H., Velazquez, H., and Wright, F.S. 1989. Adaptation of the distal tubule of the rat. Structural and functional effects of dietary salt intake and chronic diuretic infusion. *J Clin Invest* 83:113–26.

Evan, A., Huser, J., Bengele, H.H., and Alexander, E.A. 1980. The effect in alterations in dietary potassium on collecting system morphology in the rat. *Lab Invest* 42: 668–75.

Everitt, J.I., Goldsworthy, T.L., Wolf, D.C., and Walker, C.L. 1992. Hereditary renal cell carcinoma in the Eker rat: A rodent familial cancer syndrome. *J Urol* 148:1932–6.

Federova, L.V., Raju, V., El-Okdi, N. et al. 2009. The cardiotonic steroid hormone marinobufagenin induces renal fibrosis: implication of epithelial-to-mesenchymal transition. *Am J Physiol Renal Physiol* 296:F922–34.

Fine, L.G., and Bradley, T. 1985. Adaptation of proximal tubular structure and function: insights into compensatory renal hypertrophy. *Fed Proc* 44:2723–7.

Frank, A.A., Heidel, J.R., Thompson, D.J., Carlton, W.W., and Beckwith, J.B. 1992. Renal transplacental carcinogenicity of 3,3-dimethyl-1-phenyltriazine in rats: relationship of renal mesenchymal tumor to congenital mesoblastic nephroma and intralobar nephrogenic rests. *Toxicol Pathol* 20:313–22.

Frazier, K.S., Dube, P., Paredes, A., and Styer, E. 2000. Connective tissue growth factor expression in the rat remnant kidney model and association with tubular epithelial cells undergoing transdifferentiation. *Vet Pathol* 37:328–35.

Frazier, K.S., Seely, J.C., Hard, G.C. et al. 2012. Proliferative and nonproliferative lesions in the rodent urinary system. *Toxicol Pathol* 40 (4 suppl.):14–86.

Frith, C.H. 1998. Transitional cell carcinoma, urinary tract, mouse. In: *Monographs on Pathology of Laboratory Animals. Urinary System.* eds. Jones, T.C., Mohr, U., and Hunt, R.D. pp. 393–9. Berlin: Springer.

Frith, C.H., Greenman, D.L., and Cohen, S.M. 1994a. Urinary bladder carcinogenesis in the rodent. In: *Carcinogenesis*, eds. Waalkes, M.P., and Ward, J.M. pp. 161–97. New York: Raven Press.

Frith, C.H., Terracini, B., and Turusov, V.S. 1994b. Tumours of the kidney, renal pelvis and ureter. In: *Pathology of Tumours in Laboratory Animals, Vol 2. Tumours of the Mouse, 2nd ed.*, eds. VS Turusov, U Mohr, pp. 357–81. Lyon: IARC Scientific Publications No. 111.

Frith, C.H., Eighmy, J.J., Fukushima, S., Cohen, S.M., Squire, R.A., and Chandra, M. 1995. Proliferative lesions of the lower urinary tract (urinary bladder, urethra and ureters) in rats. In: *Guides for Toxicologic Pathology*. Washington, DC: STP/ARP, AFIP.

Fukushima, S., and Murai, T. 1999. Calculi, precipitates and microcrystalluria associated with irritation and cell proliferation as a mechanism of urinary bladder carcinogenesis in rats and mice. In: *Species Differences in Thyroid, Kidney and Urinary Bladder Carcinogenesis*. eds. Capen, C.C., Dybing, E., Rice, J.M., and Wilbourn, J.D. pp. 159–74. Lyon: IARC Scientific Publications No. 147 International Agency for Scientific Cancer.

Gaillard, E.T. 1999. Ureter, urinary bladder and urethra. In: *Pathology of the Mouse. Reference and Atlas*. eds. Maronpot, R.R., Boorman, G.A., and Gaul, B.W. pp. 235–58. Vienna: Cache River Press.

Gibbs, A. 2005. Comparison of the specificity and sensitivity of traditional methods for assessment of nephrotoxicity in the rat with metabonomic and proteomic methodologies. *J Appl Toxicol* 25:277–95.

Goodman, D.G., Ward, J.M., Squire, R.A., Chu, K.C., and Linhart, M.S. 1979. Neoplastic and nonneoplastic lesions in aging F344 rats. *Toxicol Appl Pharmacol* 48:237–48.

Gordon, L.R. 1986. Spontaneous lipomatous tumors in the kidney of the Crl:Cd (Sd) BR rat. *Toxicol Pathol* 14:175–82.

Goren, E., Engelberg, I., and Eidelman, A. 1991. Adrenal rest carcinoma in hilum of kidney. *Urology* 38:187–90.

Gray, J.E., van Zwieten, M.J., and Hollander, C.F. 1982. Early light microscopic changes of chronic progressive nephrosis in several srains of aging laboratory rats. *J Gerontol* 37:142–50.

Greaves, P. 2007. *Histopathology of Preclinical Toxicity Studies, 3rd ed*, pp. 591–2. Amsterdam: Elsevier.

Gruys, E., Tooten, P.C., and Kuijpers, M.H. 1996. Lung, ileum and heart are predilection sites for AApoII amyloid deposition in CD-1 Swiss mice used for toxicity studies. Pulmonary amyloid indicates AApoAII. *Lab Anim* 30:28–34.

Guarino, M., Tosoni, A., and Nebuloni, M. 2009. Direct contribution of epithelium to organ fibrosis: epithelial-mesenchymal transition. *Hum Pathol* 40:1365–76.

Guzman, R.E., Datta, K., and Khan, N.K. 2008. Obstructive protein cast nephropathy in cynomolgus monkeys treated with small organic molecules. *Vet Pathol* 45:945–8.

Hall, W.C., Elder, B., Walker, C.L. et al. 2007. Spontaneous renal tubular hyperplastic and neoplastic lesions in three Sprague–Dawley rats from a 90-day toxicity study. *Toxicol Pathol* 35:233–41.

Halliwell, W.H. 1997. Cationic amphiphilic drug-induced phospholipidosis. *Toxicol Pathol* 25:53–60.

Halliwell, W.H. 1998. Submucosal mesenchymal tumors of the mouse urinary bladder. *Toxicol Pathol* 26:128–36.

Hard, G.C. 1998a. Mesenchymal tumor, kidney, rat. In: *Monographs on Pathology of Laboratory Animals. Urinary System 2nd ed.*, eds. Jones, T.C., Hard, G.C., and Mohr, U. pp. 118–29. Berlin: Springer-Verlag.

Hard, G.C. 1998b. Lipomatous tumors, kidney, rat. In: *Monographs on Pathology of Laboratory Animals. Urinary System 2nd ed.*, eds. Jones, T.C., Hard, G.C., and Mohr, U. pp. 139–46. Berlin: Springer-Verlag.

Hard, G.C. 1998c. Mechanisms of chemically induced renal carcinogenesis in the laboratory rodent. *Toxicol Pathol* 26:104–12.

Hard, G.C. 1990. Tumours of the kidney, renal pelvis and ureter. pathology of tumours. In: *Laboratory Animals, Vol 1. Tumours of the Rat, 2nd ed.*, eds. Turusov, V.S., and Mohr, U. pp. 301–44. Lyon: IARC Scientific Publications No. 99.

Hard, G.C., and Grasso, P. 1976. Nephroblastoma in the rat: histology of a spontaneous tumor, identity with respect to renal mesenchymal neoplasms, and a review of the previously recorded cases. *J Natl Cancer Inst* 57:323–9.

Hard, G.C., and Khan, K.N. 2004. A contemporary overview of chronic progressive nephropathy in the laboratory rat, and its significance for human risk assessment. *Toxicol Pathol* 32:171–80.

Hard, G.C., and Neal, G.A. 1992. Sequential study of the chronic nephrotoxicity induced by dietary administration of ethoxyquin in Fischer-344 rats. *Fund Appl Toxicol* 18:278–87.

Hard, G.C., and Noble, R.L. 1981. Occurrence, transplantation, and histological characteristics of nephroblastoma in the NB hooded rat. *Investig Urol* 18:371–6.

Hard, G.C., and Seely, J.C. 2005. Recommendations for the interpretation of renal tubule proliferative lesions occurring in rat kidneys with advanced chronic progressive nephropathy (CPN). *Toxicol Pathol* 33:641–9.

Hard, G.C., and Seely, J.C. 2006. Histological investigation of diagnostically challenging tubule profiles in advanced chronic progressive nephropathy (CPN) in the Fischer 344 rat. *Toxicol Pathol* 34:941–8.

Hard, G.C., and Snowden, R.T. 1991. Hyaline droplet accumulation in rodent kidney proximal tubules: an association with histiocytic sarcoma. *Toxicol Pathol* 19:88–97.

Hard, G.C., Rodgers, I.S., Baetcke, K.P., Richards, W.L., McGaughy, R.E., and Valcovic, L.R. 1993. Hazard evaluation of chemicals that cause accumulation of alpha2u-globulin, hyaline droplet nephropathy, and tubule neoplasia in the kidneys of male rats. *Environ Health Perspect* 99:313–49.

Hard, G.C., Long, P.H., Crissman, J.W., Everitt, J.I., Yano, B.L., and Bertram, T.A. 1994. Atypical tubule hyperplasia and renal tubule tumors in conventional rats on 90-day toxicity studies. *Toxicol Pathol* 22:489–96.

Hard, G.C., Alden, C.L., E.F. Stula, and Trump, B.F. 1995. Proliferative lesions of the kidney in rats. In: *Guides for Toxicologic Pathology*, pp. 1–19. STP/ARP/AFIP.

Hard, G.C., Whysner, J., English, J.C., Zang, E., and Williams, G.M. 1997. Relationship of hydroquinone-associated rat renal tumors with spontaneous chronic progressive nephropathy. *Toxicol Pathol* 25:132–43.

Hard, G.C., Alden, C.L., Bruner, R.H. et al. 1999. Non-proliferative lesions of the kidney and lower urinary tract in rats. In: *Guides for Toxicologic Pathology*, pp. 1–32. Washington, DC: STP/ARP/AFIP.

Hard, G.C., Durchfeld-Meyer, B., Short, B. et al. 2001. Urinary system. In: *International Classification of Rodent Tumors. The Mouse*, ed. Mohr, U., pp. 139–62. Berlin: Springer-Verlag.

Hard, G.C., Seely, J.C., Kissling, G.E., and Betz, L.J. 2008. Spontaneous occurrence of a distinctive renal tubule tumor phenotype in rat carcinogenicity studies conducted by the National Toxicology Program. *Toxicol Pathol* 36:388–96.

Hard, G.C., Flake G.P., and Sills, R.C. 2009a. Re-evaluation of kidney histopathology from 13-week toxicity and two-year carcinogenicity studies of melamine in the F344 rat: morphologic evidence of retrograde nephropathy. *Vet Pathol* 46:1248–57.

Hard, G.C., Johnson, K.J., and Cohen, S.M. 2009b. A comparison of rat chronic progressive nephropathy with human renal disease-implications for human risk assessment. *Crit Rev Toxicol* 39:332–46.

Harpur, E., Ennulat D., Hoffman D. et al. 2011. Biological qualification of biomarkers of chemical-induced renal toxicity in two strains of male rat. *Toxicol Sci* 122:235–52.

Haseman, J.K., Hailey, J.R., and Morris, R.W. 1998. Spontaneous neoplasm incidences in Fischer 344 rats and B6C3F1 mice in two-year carcinogenicity studies: A National Toxicology Program update. *Toxicol Pathol* 26:428–41.

Heikenwalder, M., Polymenidou, M., Junt, T. et al. 2004. Lymphoid follicle destruction and immunosuppression after repeated CpG deoxyoligonucleotide administration. *Nat Med* 10:187–92.

Hiasa, Y., and Ito, N. 1987. Experimental induction of renal tumors. *CRC Crit Rev Toxicol* 17:279–343.

Hino, O., Kobayashi, T., Momose, S., Kikuchi, Y., Adachi, H., and Okimoto, K. 2003. Renal carcinogenesis: Genotype, phenotype and dramatype. *Cancer Sci* 94:142–7.

Hirose, M., and Shirai, T. 1998. *Monographs on Pathology of Laboratory Animals. Urinary System 2nd ed.*, eds. Jones, T.C., Hard, G.C., and Mohr, U. pp. 403–8. Berlin: Springer-Verlag.

Hirouchi, Y., Iwata, H., Yamakawa, S. et al. 1994. Historical data of neoplastic and non-neoplastic lesions in B6C3F1 (C57BL/6CrSlc x C3H/HeSlc) mice. *J Toxicol Pathol* 7:153–77.

Hruban, Z. 1984. Pulmonary and generalized lysosomal storage induced by amphiphilic drugs. *Environ Health Perspect* 55:53–76.

Iida, M., Yasub, M., and Itakur, C. 1981. Spontaneous nephroblastoma in Sprague–Dawley rats. *Exp Anim* 30:31–4.

Ikeda, H., Tauchi, H., Shimasaki, H. 1999. Age and organ difference in amount and distribution of autofluorescent granules in rats. *Mech Ageing Dev* 31:139–46.

Iwata, H., Hirouchi, Y., Koike, Y. et al. 1991. Historical control data of non-neoplastic and neoplastic lesions in F344/Ducrj Rats. *J Toxicol Pathol* 4:1–24.

Jackson, C.B., and Kirkpatrick, J.B. 2002. Nephrogenic rest in a Crl:CD (SD) IGS rat. *Vet Pathol* 39:588–9.

Jackson, D.G., and Jones, H.B. 1995. Histopathological and ultrastructural changes in the juxtaglomerular apparatus of the rat following administration of ZENECA ZD6888 (2-ethyl-5,6,7,8-tetrahydro-4-[(2′-(1H-tetrazol-5-yl)biphenyl-4-yl)- methoxy]quinoline), an angiotensin II antagonist. *Toxicol Pathol* 23:256–61.

Jacobs, B.J., Lees, C.T., and Montie, J.E. 2010. Bladder cancer in 2010. *CA: Cancer J Clin* 60:244–72.

Jefferson, J.A., and Johnson, R.J. 1999. Experimental mesangial proliferative glomerulorephritis (the anti-thyl-1 model). *J Nephrol* 12:297–307.

Johansson, S.L., and Cohen, S.M. 1997. Epidemiology and etiology of bladder cancer. *Sem Surg Oncol* 13:291–8.

Johnson, R.C., Dovey-Hartman, B.J., Syed, J. et al. 1998. Vacuolation in renal tubular epithelium of Cd-1 mice. An incidental finding. *Toxicol Pathol* 26:789–92.

Jokinen, M.P. 1990. Urinary bladder, ureter, and urethra. In: *Pathology of the Fisher Rat. Reference and Atlas*, ed. Boorman, G.A., Eustis, S.L., Elwell, M.R., Montgomery, C.A., and MacKenzie, W.F. pp. 109–26. San Diego: Academic Press.

Kaissling, B., and Le Hir, M. 2008. The renal cortical interstitium: morphological and functional aspects. *Histochem Cell Biol* 130:247–62.

Karbe, E. 1999. "Mesenchymal tumor" or "decidual-like reaction." *Toxicol Pathol* 27:354–62.

Karbe, E., Hartman, E., George, C., Wadsworth, P., Harleman, J., and Geiss, V. 1998. Similarities between the uterine decidual reaction and the "mesenchymal lesion" of the urinary bladder in aging mice. *Exp Toxicol Pathol* 50:330–40.

Karbe, E., Schaetti, P., Hartmann, E., Wadsworth, P., Brander Weber, P., and Zeller, G. 2000. Mesenchymal proliferation with decidual-like morphology in seminal vesicles of aging mice. *Exp Toxicol Pathol* 52:465–72.

Kaspareit, J., Friderichs-Gromoll, S., Buse, E., and Haberman, G. 2007. Spontaneous neoplasms observed in cynomolgus monkeys (*Macca fascicularis*) during a 15-year period. *Exp Toxicol Pathol* 59:163–9.

Keenan, K.P., Coleman, J.B., McCoy, C.L., Hoe, C.M., Soper, K.A., and Laroque, P. 2000. Chronic nephropathy in ad libitum overfed Sprague-Dawley rats and its early attenuation by increasing degrees of dietary (caloric) restriction to control growth. *Toxicol Pathol* 28:788–98.

Kerjaschki, D., and Neale, T.J. 1996. Molecular mechanisms of glomerular injury in rat experimental membranous nephropathy (Heymann nephritis). *J Am Soc Nephrol* 7:2518–26.

Killary, K., Diaz, D., Argentieri, G., Dugyala, R., and Bowenkamp, K. 2009. Kidney changes after daily slow-bolus IV injection of Polyoxyl 35 Castor oil/ethanol in 5% Dextrose for 2 weeks to Wistar rats. *Microsc Microanal* 15(Suppl S2):968–9.

Kluwe, W.M. 1981. Acute toxicity of 1,2-dibromo-3-chloropropane in the F344 male rat. II. Development and repair of the renal, epididymal, testicular, and hepatic lesions. *Toxicol Appl Pharmacol* 59:84–91.

Konishi, N., and Hiasa, Y. 1994. Renal carcinogenesis. In: *Carcinogenesis*, eds. Walkes, M.P., and Ward, J.M. New York: Raven Press. pp. 123–59.

Konishi, N., Nakamura, M., Ishida, E. et al. 2001. Specific genomic alterations in rat renal cell carcinomas induced by N-ethyl-N-hydroxyethylnitrosamine. *Toxicol Pathol* 29:232–6.

Kouchi, M., Okimoto, K., Matsumoto, I., Tanaka, K., Yasuba, M., and Hino, O. 2006. Natural history of the Nihon (Bhd gene mutant) rat, a novel model for human Birt-Hogg-Dube syndrome. *Virchows Arch* 448:463–71.

Krech, R., Zerban, H., and Bannasch, P. 1981. Mitochondrial anomalies in renal oncocytes induced in rat by N-nitrosomorphine. *Eur J Cell Biol* 25:331–9.

Kriz, W., Hahnel, B., Hosser, H., Ostendorf, T., Gaertner, S., Kranzlin, B., Gretz, N., Shjimizu, F., and Floege, J. 2003. Pathways to recovery and loss of nephrons in anti-Thy-1 nephritis. *J Am Soc Nephrol* 14:1904–26.

Kunze, E. 1992. Nonneoplastic and neoplastic lesions of the urinary bladder, ureter, and renal pelvis. In: *Pathobiology of the Aging Rat.* eds. Mohr, U., Dungworth, C.C., and Capen, C.C. pp. 259–84. Washington, DC: ILSI Press.

Kunze, E. 1998. Hyperplasia, urinary bladder, rat. In: *Monographs on Pathology of Laboratory Animals. Urinary System 2nd ed.*, eds. Jones, T.C., Hard, G.C., and Mohr, U. pp. 332–66. Berlin: Springer-Verlag.

Kunze, E., and Chowaniec, J. 1990. Tumours of the urinary bladder. pathology of tumours. In: *Laboratory Animals, Vol 1. Tumours of the Rat, 2nd ed.*, eds. Turusov, V.S., and Mohr, U. pp. 345–97. Lyon: IARC Scientific Publications No. 99.

Kurata, Y., and Shibata, M.-A. 1996. Aging changes in the urinary bladder. In: *Pathobiology of the Aging Mouse*, eds. Mohr, U., Dungworth, D.L., Capen, C.C., Carlton, W.W., Sundberg, J.P., and Ward, J.M. pp. 345–57. Washington, DC: ILSI Press.

Lacy, S.A., Hitchcock, M.J.M., Lee, W.A., Tellier, P., and Cundy, K.C. 1998. Effect of oral probenecid coadministration on the chronic toxicity and pharmacokinetics of intravenous cidofovir in cynomolgus monkeys. *Toxicol Sci* 44:97–106.

Lameire, N. 2005. The pathophysiology of acute renal failure. *Crit Care Clin* 21:197–210.

Lanzoni, A., Piaia, A., Everitt, J. et al. 2007. Early onset of spontaneous renal neoplastic lesions in young conventional rats in toxicity studies. *Toxicol Pathol* 35:589–93.

Lee, H.S., and Song, C.Y. 2009. Differential role of mesangial cells and padocytes in TGF-beta-induced mesangial matrix synthesis in chronic glomerular disease. *Histol Histopathol* 24:901–8.

Li, Y., and McMartin, K.E. 2009. Strain differences in urinary factors that promote calcium oxalate crystal formation in kidney in ethylene glycol treated rats. *Am J Physiol Renal Physiol* 296: F1080–7.

Liebelt, A.G., Sass, B., Sobel, H.J., and Werner, R.M. 1989. Spontaneous nephroblastoma in a strain CE/J mouse. A case report. *Toxicol Pathol* 17:57–61.

Limas, C., Westrum, B, and Limas, C.J. 1980. The evolution of vascular changes in the spontaneously hypertensive rat. *Am J Pathol* 98:357–84.

Lindon, J.C., Keun, H.C., Ebbels, T.M. et al. 2005. The consortium for metabonomic toxicology (COMET): aims, activities and achievements. *Pharmacogenomics* 6:691–9.

Linton, A.L., Clark, W.F., Driedger, A.A., Turnbull, D.I., and Lindsay, R.M. 1980. Acute interstitial nephritis due to drugs. Review of the literature with a report of nine cases. *Ann Intern Med* 93:735–41.

Ling, H., Ardjomand, P., Samvakas, S. et al. 1998. Mesangial cell hypertrophy induced by NH_4Cl: Role of depressed activities of cathepsins due to elevated lysosomal pH. *Kid Int* 53:1706–12.

Lipsky, M.M., and Trump, B.F. 1988. Chemically induced renal epithelial neoplasia in experimental animals. *Int Rev Exp Path* 30:357–83.

Lock, E.A., and Hard, G.C. 2004. Chemically induced renal tubule tumors in the laboratory rat and mouse: review of the NCI/NTP database and categorization of renal carcinogens based on mechanistic information. *Crit Rev Toxicol* 34:211–99.

Luke, D.R., Tomaszewski, K., Damle, B., and Schlamm, H.T. 2010. Review of the basic and clinical pharmacology of sulfobutylether-beta-cyclodextrin (SBECD). *J Pharm Sci* 99:3291–301.

Luz, A., and Murray, A.B. 1991. Hyaline droplet accumulation in kidney proximal tubules of mice with histiocytic sarcoma. *Toxicol Pathol* 19:670–1.

Macdonald, J.S., Bagdon, W.J., Peter, C.P. et al. 1987. Renal effects of enalapril in dogs. *Kid Int* 31 Suppl 20:S148–53.

Maita, K., Hirano, M., Harada, T. et al. 1988. Mortality, major cause of moribundity, and spontaneous tumors in CD-1 mice. *Toxicol Pathol* 38:292–6.

Mayer, D., Weber, E., Kadenbach, B., and Bannasch, P. 1989. Immunocytochemical demonstration of cytochrome-c-oxidase as a marker for renal oncocytes and oncocytomas. *Toxicol Pathol* 17:46–9.

McMartin, D.N., Sahota, P.S., Gunson, D.E., Hsu, H.H., and Spaet, R.H. 1992. Neoplasms and related proliferative lesions in control Sprague–Dawley rats from carcinogenicity studies. Historical data and diagnostic considerations. *Toxicol Pathol* 20:212–25.

Menini, S., Iacobini, C., Oddi, G. et al. 2007. Increased glomerular cell (podocyte) apoptosis in rats with streptozotocin-induced diabetes mellitus: role in the development of diabetic glomerular disease. *Diabetologia* 50:2591–9.

Mesfin, G.M. 1999. Intralobar nephroblastemosis: precursor lesions of nephroblastoma in the Sprague–Dawley rat. *Vet Pathol* 36:379–90.

Mesfin, G.M. and Breech, K.T. 1992. Rhabdomyocytic nephroblastoma (Wilm's tumor) in the Sprague–Dawley rat. *Vet Pathol* 29:564–566.

Mesfin, G.M., and Breech, K.T. 1996. Heritable nephroblastoma (Wilms' tumor) in the Upjohn Sprague–Dawley rat. *Lab Anim Sci* 46:321–26.

Miller, T.E., and Findon, G. 1998. Exacerbation of experimentally induced infection by cyclosporine. *Transplantation Proc* 20(suppl. 3):913–19.

Mizuno, S., Wen, J., and Mizuno-Horikawa, Y. 2004. Repeated streptozotocin injections cause early onset of glomerulosclerosis in mice. *Exp Anim* 53:175–80.

Moll, R., Wu, X.-R., Lin, J.-H., and Sun, T.-T. 1995. Uroplakins, specific membrane proteins of urothelial umbrella cells, as histological markers of metastatic transitional cell carcinomas. *Am J Pathol* 147:1383–97.

Molon-Noblot, S., Boussiquet-Leroux, C., Owen, R.A. et al. 1992. Rat urinary bladder hyperplasia induced by oral administration of carbonic anhydrase inhibitors. *Toxicol Pathol* 20:93–102.

Monks, T.J., and Lau, S.S. 2005. Chemical-induced nephrocarcinogenicity in the eker rat: a model of chemical-induced renal carcinogenesis. In: *Toxicity of the Kidney 3rd ed.*, eds. Tarloff, J.B., and Lash, L.H. pp. 343–74. Boca Raton: CRC Press.

Monserrat, A.J., and Chandler, A.E. 1975: Effects of repeated injections of sucrose in the kidney: histologic, cytochemical and functional studies in an animal model. *Virchows Arch B* 19:77–91.

Montgomery, C.A., and Seely, J.C. 1990. Kidney. In: *Pathology of the Fischer Rat. Reference and Atlas.*, eds. Boorman, G.A., Eustis, S.L., Elwell, M.R., Montgomery, C.A., and MacKenzie, W.F. pp. 127–53. San Diego: Academic Press.

Nakanuma, Y., Harada, K., Sato, Y., and Ikeda, H. 2010. Recent progress in the etiopathogenesis of pediatric biliary disease, particularly Caroli's disease with congenital hepatic fibrosis and biliary atresia. *Histol Histopathol* 25:223–35.

Nakazawa, M., Tawaratani, T., Uchimoto, H. et al. 2001. Spontaneous neoplastic lesions in aged Sprague–Dawley rats. *Exp Anim* 50:99–103.

Navarro-Moreno, L.G., Quintanar-Escorza, M.A., Gonzalez, S. et al. 2009. Effects of lead intoxication on intercellular junctions and biochemical alterations of the renal proximal tubule cells. *Toxicol In Vitro* 23:1298–1304.

Nemes, Z., Dietz, R., Mann, J.F.E., Luth, J.B., and Gross, F. 1980. Vasoconstriction and increased blood pressure in the development of accelerated vascular disease. *Virchows Arch A* 386:161–73.

Neuhaus, O.W., Flory, W., Biswas, N., and Hollerman, C.E. 1981. Urinary excretion of alpha 2 mu-globulin and albumin by adult male rats following treatment with nephrotoxic agents. *Nephron* 28:133–40.

Nicoletta, J.A., and Schwartz, G.J. 2004. Distal renal tubular acidosis. *Curr Opin Pediat* 16:194–8.

Nikula, K.J., Benjamin, S.A., Angleton, G.M., and Lee, A.C. 1989. Transitional cell carcinomas of the urinary tract in a colony of Beagle dogs. *Vet Pathol* 26:455–61.

Nguyen, H.T., and Woodard, J.C. 1980. Intranephronic calculosis in rats: an ultrastructural study. *Am J Pathol* 100:39–56.

Nilubol, D., Pattanaseth, T., Boonsri, K., Pirarat, N., and Leepipatpiboon, N. 2009. Melamine- and cyanuric acid-associated renal failure in pigs in Thailand. *Vet Pathol* 46:1156–9.

Nishimura, N., Matsumura, F., Vogel, C.F.A. et al. 2008. Critical role of cyclooxygenase-2 activation in pathogenesis of hydronephrosis caused by lactational exposure of mice to dioxin. *Toxicol Appl Pharmacol* 231:374–83.

Nogueira, E., Klimek, F., Weber, E., Bannasch, P. 1989. Collecting duct origin of rat renal clear cell tumors. *Virchows Arch B Cell Pathol Incl Mol Pathol* 57:275–83.

Nogueira, E., Cardesa, A., and Mohr, U. 1993. Experimental models of kidney tumors. *J Cancer Res Clin Oncol* 119:190–8.

Ogawa, K., St. John, M., Luiza de Oliveira, M. et al. 1999. Comparison of uroplakin expression during urothelial carcinogenesis induced by N-Butyl-N-(4-Hydroxybutyl) Nitrosamine in rats and mice. *Toxicol Pathol* 27:645–51.

Okimoto, K., Kouchi, M., Kikawa, E. et al. 2000. A novel "Nihon" rat model of a mendelian dominantly inherited renal cell carcinoma. *Jpn J Cancer Res* 91:1096–9.

Olzinski, A.R., McCafferty, T.A., Zhao, S.Q. et al. 2005. Hypertensive target organ damage is attenuated by a p38 MAPK inhibitor: Role of systemic blood pressure and endothelial protection. *Cardiovasc Res* 66:170–8.

Osathanondh, V., and Potter, E.L. 1966. Development of the human kidney as shown by microdissection. V. Development of tubular portions of nephrons. *Arch Pathol* 82:403–9.

Owen, G., Smith, T.H.F., and Agersborg Jr., H.P.K. 1970. Toxicity of some benzodiazepine compounds with CNS activity. *Toxicol Appl Pharmacol* 16:556–70.

Owen, R.A., Molon-Noblot S. Hubert, M.F., Kindt, M.V., Keenan, K.P., and Eydelloth, R.S. 1994. The morphology of juxtaglomerular cell hyperplasia and hypertrophy in normotensive rats and monkeys given an angiotensin II receptor antagonist. *Toxicol Pathol* 23:606–19.

Ozer, J.S., Dieterle, F., Troth, S. et al. 2010. A panel of urinary biomarkers to monitor reversibility of renal injury and a serum marker with improved potential to assess renal function. *Nat Biotech* 28:486–97.

Pabla, N., and Dong, Z. 2008. Cisplatin nephrotoxicity: mechanisms and renoprotective strategies. *Kid Int* 73:994–1007.

Pauli, B.U., Gruber, A.D., and Weinstein, R.S. 1998. *Monographs on Pathology of Laboratory Animals. Urinary System 2nd ed.*, eds. Jones, T.C. Hard, G.C. and Mohr, U. pp. 381–92. Berlin: Springer-Verlag.

Periyasamy-Thandavan, S., Jiang, M., Wei, Q., Smith, R., Yin, X.-M., and Dong, Z. 2008. Autophagy is cytoprotective during cisplatin injury of renal proximal tubular cells. *Kid Int* 74:631–60.

Peter, C.P., Burek, J.D., and Van Zwieten, M.J. 1986. Spontaneous nephropathies in rats. *Toxicol Pathol* 14:91–100.

Pfister, T., Atzpodien, E., Bohrmann, B., and Bauss, F. 2005. Acute renal effects of intravenous bisphosphonates in the rat. *Basic Clin Pharmacol Toxicol* 97:374–81.

Picut, C.A., and Lewis, R.M. 1987. Microscopic features of canine renal dysplasia. *Vet Pathol* 24:156–63.

Prahalada, S., Stabinski, L.G., Chen, H.Y. et al. 1998. Pharmacological and toxicological effects of chronic porcine growth hormone administration in dogs. *Toxicol Pathol* 26:185–200.

Price, S.A., Davies, D., Rowlinson, R. et al. 2010. Characterization of renal papillary antigen 1 (RPA-1), a biomarker of renal papillary necrosis. *Toxicol Pathol* 38:346–58.

Quiros, Y., Vicente-Vicente, L., Morales, A.I., Lopez-Novoa, J.M., and Lopez-Hernandez, F.J. 2011. An integrative overview on the mechanisms underlying the renal tubular cytotoxicity of gentamicin. *Toxicol Sci* 119:245–56.

Ramos-Vara, J.A., Miller, M.A., Boucher, M.M., Roudabush, A., and Johnson, G.C. 2003. Immunohistochemical detection of uroplakin III, cytokeratin 7, and cytokeratin 20 in canine urothelial tumors. *Vet Pathol* 40:55–62.

Reasor, M.J., Hastings, K.L., and Ulrich, R.G. 2006. Drug-induced phospholipidosis: issues and future directions. *Exp Opin Drug Saf* 5:567–83.

Remuzzi, G., and Perico, N. 1995. Cyclosporine-induced dysfunction in experimental animals and humans. *Kid Int Suppl* 52:S70–4.

Ritskes-Hoitinga, J., and Beynen, A.C. 1992. Nephrocalcinosis in the rat: a literature review. *Prog Food Nutr Sci* 16:85–124.

Robinson, R.L., Grosenstein, P.A., and Argentieri, G.J. 1997. Mixed mesenchymal tumor in the kidney of a young Beagle dog. *Toxicol Pathol* 25:326–8.

Romih, R., Korosec, P., de Mello, W., and Jezernik, K. 2005. Differentiation of epithelial cells in the urinary tract. *Cell Tissue Res* 320:259–68.

Russo, L.M., Bakris, G.L., and Comper, W.D. 2002. Renal handling of albumin: A critical review of basic concepts and perspective. *Amer J Kidney Dis* 39:899–919.

Sabatini, S. 1996. Pathophysiologic mechanisms in analgesic-induced papillary necrosis. *Am J Kid Dis* 28(Suppl 1):S34–8.

Saboli, I., Skarica, M., Gorboulev, V. et al. 2006. Rat renal glucose transporter SGLT1 exhibits zonal distribution and androgen-dependent gender differences. *Am J Physiol Renal Physiol* 290:F913–26.

Sass, B. 1998. Adenoma, adenocarcinoma, kidney, mouse. In: *Monographs on Pathology of Laboratory Animals. Urinary System 2nd ed.*, eds. Jones, T.C., Hard, G.C., and Mohr, U. pp. 146–59. Berlin: Springer-Verlag.

Schetz, M., Dasta, J., Goldstein, S., and T. Golper. 2005. Drug-induced acute kidney injury. *Curr Opin Crit Care* 11:555–65.

Schnellman, R.G. 1998. Analgesic nephropathy in rodents. *J Toxicol Environ Health B* 1:81–90.

Seely, J.C. 1999. Kidney. In: *Pathology of the Mouse*, eds. Maronpot, R.R., Boorman, G.A. and Gaul, B.W. pp. 207–34. Vienna: Cache River Press.

Seely, J.C. 2004. Renal mesenchymal tumor vs nephroblastoma: revisited. *J Toxicol Pathol* 17: 131–36.

Seely, J.C., Haseman, J.K., Nyska, A., Wolf, D.C., Everitt, J.I., and Hailey, J.R. 2002. The effect of chronic progressive nephropathy on the incidence of renal tubule cell neoplasms. *Toxicol Pathol* 30:681–6.

Shinohara, Y., and Frith, C.H. 1981. Comparison of experimental and spontaneous bladder urothelial hyperplasias occurring in BALB/c mice. *Invest Urol* 18:233–8.

Shirai, T., and Takahashi, S. 1998. Papilloma, urinary bladder, rat. In: *Monographs on Pathology of Laboratory Animals. Urinary System*, eds. Jones, T.C., Mohr, U., and Hunt, R.D. pp. 399–403. Berlin: Springer.

Short, B.G. 1998. Apoptosis in the kidney: a toxicologic pathologist's perspective. *Toxicol Pathol* 26:826–7.

Short, B.G., Burnett, V.L., and Swenberg, J.M. 1989. Elevated proliferation of proximal tubule cells and localization of accumulated α2u-globulin in F344 rats during exposure to unleaded gasoline or 2,2,4-trimethylpentane. *Toxicol Appl Pharmacol* 101:414–31.

Singh, B.P., Nyska, A., Kissling, G.E. et al. 2010. Urethral carcinoma and hyperplasia in male and female B6C3F1 mice treated with 3,3′,4, 4′-tetrachloroazobensene (TCAB). *Toxicol Pathol* 38:373–83.

Son, W.-C., and C. Gopinath. 2004. Early occurrence of spontaneous tumors in Cd-1 mice and Sprague–Dawley rats. *Toxicol Pathol* 32:371–4.

Son, W.-C., Bell, D., Taylor, I., and Mowat, V. 2010. Profile of early occurring spontaneous tumors in Han Wistar rats. *Toxicol Pathol* 38:292–6.

Sterzel, R.B., Schulze-Lohoff, E., and Marx, M. 1993. Cytokines and mesangial cells. *Kid Int Suppl* 39:S26–31.

Stula, E.F., and Sykes, G.P. 1998. *Monographs on Pathology of Laboratory Animals. Urinary System 2nd ed.*, eds. Jones, T.C., Hard, G.C., and Mohr, U. pp. 409–16. Berlin: Springer-Verlag.

Sugimoto, K., Harada, T., and Maita, K. 1998. Case report on lipomatous tumors in the rat. *Toxicol Pathol* 26:171.

Suzuki, H., Yagi, M., Saito, K., and Suzuki, K. 2007. Embryonic pathogenesis of hypogonadism and renal hypoplasia in hgn/hgn rats characterized by male sterility, reduced female fertility and progressive renal insufficiency. *Congen Anomal* 47:34–44.

Suzuki, S., Arnold, L.L., Muirhead, D. et al. 2008. Inorganic arsenic-induced intramitochondrial granules in mouse urothelium. *Toxicol Pathol* 36:999–1005.

Swenberg, J.A., and Lehman-McKeeman, L.D. 1999. Alpha-urinary globulin-associated nephropathy as a mechanism of renal tubule cell carcinogenesis in male rats. In: *Species Differences in Thyroid, Kidney and Urinary Bladder Carcinogenesis.*, eds. Capen, C.C., Dybing, E., Rice, J.M., and Wilbourn, J.D. pp. 95–118. Lyon: IARC Scientific Publications No. 147 International Agency for Scientific Cancer.

Swindle, M.M., Larkin, A., Herron, A.J., Clubb, F., and Frazier, K.S. 2012. Swine as models in biomedical research and toxicologic testing. *Vet Pathol* 49:344–56.

Sykes, G.P., and Stula, E.F. 1989. *Monographs on Pathology of Laboratory Animals. Urinary System 2nd ed.*, eds. Jones, T.C., Hard, G.C., and Mohr, U. pp. 416–20. Berlin: Springer-Verlag.

Takahashi, M., Yang, X.J., Sugimura, J. et al. 2003. Molecular subclassification of kidney tumors and the discovery of new diagnostic markers. *Oncogene* 22:6810–8.

Tamano, S., Hagiwara, A., Shibata, M., Kurata, Y., Fukushima, S., and Ito, N. 1988. Spontaneous tumors in again (C57BL/6N x C3H/HeN)F1 (B6C#F1) mice. *Toxicol Pathol* 16:321–6.

Tanner, G.A., Tielker, M.A., Connors, B.A., Phillips, C.L., Tanner, J.A., and Evan, A.P. 2002. Atubular glomeruli in a rat model of polycystic kidney disease. *Kid Int* 62:1947–57.

Thurman, J.D., Hailey, J.R., Turturro, A., and Gaylor, D.W. 1995. Spontaneous renal tubular carcinoma in Fischer-344 rat littermates. *Vet Pathol* 32:419–22.

Travlos, G.S., Hard, G.C., Betz, L.J., and Kissling, G.E. 2011. Chronic progressive nephropathy in male F344 rats in 90-day toxicity studies: its occurrence and association with renal tubule tumors in subsequent 2-year bioassays. *Toxicol Pathol* 39:381–9.

Tripathi, S., and Srivastav, A.K. 2011. Cytoarchitectural alterations in kidney of Wistar rat after oral exposure to cadmium chloride. *Tissue Cell* 43:131–6.

Truong, L.D., Gaber, L., and Eknoyan, G. 2011. Obstructive uropathy. *Contrib Nephrol* 169:311–26.

Tsuda, H., and Krieg, K. 1992. Neoplastic lesions in the kidney. In: *Pathobiology of the Aging Rat*, eds. Mohr, U., Dungworth, C.C., and Capen, C.C. pp. 227–40. Washington, DC: ILSI Press.

Tsuda, H., Iwase, T., Matsumoto, K. et al. 1998. Histogenetic stereological reconstruction of rat basophilic, clear, and oncocytic neoplastic renal cell lesion using carbonic anhydrase type II-PAS double-stained sections. *Toxicol Pathol* 26:769–76.

Tucker, M.J. 1985. Effect of diet on spontaneous disease in the inbred mouse strain C57Bl/10J. *Toxicol Lett* 25:131–5.

Urakami, S., Tokuzen, R., Tsuda, H., Igawa, M., and Hino, O. 1997. Somatic mutation of the tuberous sclerosis (Tsc2) tumor suppressor gene in chemically induced rat renal carcinoma cell. *J Urol* 158:275–8.

Venkatachalam, M.A., Bernard, D.B., Donohoe, J.F., and Levinsky, N.G. 1978. Ischemic damage and repair in the rat proximal tubule: differences among the S1, S2 and S3 segments. *Kid Int.* 14:31–6.

Walker, C. 1998. Molecular genetics of renal carcinogenesis. *Toxicol Pathol* 26:113–20.

Walsh, K.M., and Poteracki, J. 1994. Spontaneous neoplasms in control Wistar rats. *Fund Appl Toxicol* 22:65–72.

Ward, J.M. 2004. Preneoplastic and precancerous lesions in rodents: Morphologic and molecular characteristics. *J Toxicol Pathol* 15:123–8.

Ward, J.M., Goodman, D.G., Squire, R.A., Chu, K.C., and Linhart, M.S. 1979. Neoplastic and nonneoplastic lesions in aging C57BL/6N x C3H/HeN(F1) (B6C3F1) mice. *J Natl Cancer Inst* 63:849–54.

Weber, M.L., Farooqui, M., Nguyen, J. et al. 2008. Morphine induces mesangial cell proliferation and glomerulopathy via kappa-opioid receptors. *Am J Physiol Renal Physiol* 294:F1388–97.

Wehner, H., and Petri, M. 1983. Glomerular alterations in Experimental diabetes of the rat. *Pathol Res Pract* 176:145–57.

Wolf, D.C., and Hard, G.C. 1996. Pathology of the Kidneys. In: *Pathobiology of the Aging Mouse.*, eds. Mohr, U., Dungworth, D.L., Capen, C.C., Carlton, W.W., Sundberg, J.P., and Ward, J.M. pp. 333–44. Washington, DC: ILSI Press.

Wolf, J.C. 2002. Characteristics of the spectrum of proliferative lesions observed in the kidney and urinary bladder of Fischer 344 rats and B6C3F1 mice. *Toxicol Pathol* 30:657–62.

Xiao, W., Liu, Y., and Templeton, D.M. 2009. Pleiotropic effects of cadmium in mesangial cells. *Toxicol Appl Pharmacol* 238:315–26.

Yamate, J., Iwaki, M., Nakatsuji, S., Kuwamura, M., Kotani, T., and Sakuma, S. 1998. Lysozyme-containing renal tubular hyaline droplets in F344 rats bearing a rat fibrosarcoma-derived transplantable tumor. *Toxicol Pathol* 26:699–703.

Yang, A., Trajkovic, D., Illanes, O., and Ramiro-Ibanez, F. 2007. Clinicopathological and tissue indicators of para-aminophenol nephrotoxicity in Sprague–Dawley rats. *Toxicol Pathol* 35:521–32.

Yarlagadda, S.G., and Perazella, M.A. 2008. Drug-induced crystal nephropathy: An update. *Exp Opin Drug Saf* 7:147–58.

Yoshizawa, K., Oishi, Y., Makino, N. et al. 1996. Congenital mesoblastic nephroma in a young Beagle dog. *J Toxicol Pathol* 9:101–5.

Yu, B.P., Masoro, E.J., Murata, I., Bertrand, H.A., and Lynd, F.T. 1982. Life span study of SPF Fischer 344 male rats fed ad libitum or restricted diets: longevity, growth, lean body mass and disease. *J Gerontol* 37:130–41.

Zambrano, N.R., Lubensky, I.A., Merino, M.J., Linehan, W.M., and Walther, M.M. 1999. Histopathology and molecular genetics of renal tumors: toward unification of a classification system. *J Urol* 162:1246–58.

Zemer, D., Pras, M., Sohar, E., Modan, M., Capbill, S., and Gafni, J. 1986. Colchicine in the prevention and treatment of amyloidosis of familial Mediterranean fever. *N Engl J Med* 314:1001–5.

Zhu M.-Q., De Broe, M.E., and Nouwen, E.J. 1996. Vimentin expression and distal tubular damage in the rat kidney. *Experimental Nephrology* 4:172–83.

Zwicker, G.M., Eyster, R.C., Sells, D.M., and Gass, J.H. 1992. Spontaneous renal neoplasms in aged Crl:Cd BR rats. *Toxicol Pathol* 20:125–30.

13 Hematopoietic System

Kristin Henson, Glenn Elliott, and Gregory S. Travlos

CONTENTS

13.1 INTRODUCTION

Alterations in the circulating blood cell (erythrocyte or leukocyte) or platelet (thrombocyte) mass in animals or humans exposed to agents of environmental or therapeutic importance are a key consideration when assessing potential toxicity and hazard of the agent. Since an agent may directly or indirectly affect the circulating blood cell mass or production of blood cells, evaluations of the whole blood and the hematopoietic system (i.e., the bone marrow) are essential to understand agent-induced alterations in the erythron, leukon, or thrombon.

Hematopoiesis is the process by which the cellular components of blood are produced. The primary site of hematopoiesis in adult domestic and laboratory animals and humans is the bone marrow. The spleen also retains hematopoietic capability, and, in adult rats and large laboratory animals under conditions of hematopoietic stress, active splenic hematopoiesis (extramedullary hematopoiesis) may be seen. In mice, the spleen is hematopoietically active during the postnatal period and throughout adult life (Jain 1993). To meet the demands of oxygenation, hemostasis, and microbial defense, the hematopoietic population of the bone marrow is constantly dividing and undergoing differentiation in a coordinated and highly regulated manner. A dynamic process, hematopoietic activity involves the production of erythrocytes, granulocytes, monocytes, lymphocytes, and platelets at a high rate of production. For example, in humans, hematopoietic cells are turned out at approximately 6×10^9 cells/kg body weight/day (Abboud and Lichtman 2001). Consequently, hematopoiesis may be adversely affected by compounds targeting rapidly dividing cells or by alterations in cytokines, growth factors, or bone marrow microenvironment. Responsive changes related to peripheral disturbances, such as inflammation or red blood cell loss, are also observed. Clinical findings of hematopoietic toxicity include lethargy secondary to anemia, clotting deficiencies or overt hemorrhage, or increased susceptibility to infection. These defects may be life threatening depending on the severity of the hematopoietic deficit. Due to the bone marrow's susceptibility to toxic insult, and the potential for serious consequences of hematopoietic toxicity, peripheral blood and bone marrow evaluation is an integral part of nonclinical toxicological assessments.

As the relationship between the circulating blood cell mass and hematopoiesis is complex, appropriate assessment of compound-related effects on the hematopoietic system must include integration/ review of clinical pathology data and histopathological evaluation, as well as in-life findings, toxicokinetic data, genomics, and other molecular or investigative assessments. Based upon the study findings, discussions between the clinical and anatomic pathologist become essential in the determination if additional hematopoietic assessments, for example, cytological examination of the bone marrow, are needed. This chapter will review the development of the hematopoietic system, hematopoietic processes, structure, function, gross and microscopic appearance of the hematopoietic system, and alterations in hematopoiesis as an understanding of these areas is essential in the evaluation of hematotoxicity.

13.2 ONTOGENY

During prenatal development, primitive hematopoiesis (hematopoiesis occurring from progenitor cells that produce erythrocytes containing embryonic hemoglobin) gives way to definitive hematopoiesis (hematopoiesis in the adult animal that occurs from progenitor cells capable of repopulating the bone marrow and producing all cell lineages) in a coordinated, sequential pattern. The location and chronology of the emergence of hematopoietic progenitors and developed blood cells have been recorded and summarized for mouse embryos (Speck et al. 2002). Detailed reviews regarding ontogeny of the hematopoietic system can be found elsewhere (Speck et al. 2002; Baron 2003; Badillo and Flake 2006).

In the developing embryo, hematopoiesis initially occurs within the extra-embryonic blood islands of the visceral yolk sac. Blood cells first appear in the blood islands at embryonic day (ED) 7.0 in the mouse and human gestation day 16, and they consist of a synchronously maturing wave of large erythroblasts (Lux et al. 2008; Oberlin et al. 2010; Palis et al. 2010). This initial phase of blood cell formation between ED7.5 and ED9.0 in the mouse is referred to as primitive hematopoiesis and includes production of megakaryocytes from bipotential megakaryocyte-erythroid progenitor (MEP) cells, as well as nonmonocyte derived primitive macrophages (Shepard and Zon 2000; Tober et al. 2007). Primitive erythroid cells, large embryonic platelets, and primitive macrophages begin to circulate around ED8.5 in the mouse and ED21 in humans after the onset of cardiac contractions. These cells provide for early post-implantation survival and growth and, in the case of primitive macrophages, tissue remodeling in the developing embryo (Palis 2008; Shepard and Zon 2000; Tober et al. 2007). Primitive nucleated immature erythroid cells are the predominant cell type produced during this phase of yolk sac hematopoiesis and are extremely large (400–700 fL). As these cells mature and divide within the embryonic circulation, morphological changes typical for adult erythroid maturation are observed, including a decrease in cell size and volume, nuclear condensation, increasing amounts of hemoglobin, and, ultimately, loss of nuclei (reviewed in Palis et al. 2010). In addition to low levels of adult α- and β-hemoglobins, murine primitive erythroid cells contain embryonic hemoglobins (BH1-globin, ζ-globin, and εγ-globin), which have a high oxygen affinity to promote placental oxygen exchange (reviewed in Palis 2008; Palis et al. 2010).

The second phase of embryonic hematopoiesis, referred to as definitive hematopoiesis, also occurs within the yolk sac and is characterized by the appearance of highly proliferative, myeloid/erythroid hematopoietic progenitor cells (HPCs) at murine ED8.25, followed by the production of smaller erythroid cells with adult hemoglobin between ED8.25 and ED10.5 (reviewed in Palis 2008). By murine ED10.5 and approximately human gestation day 42, definitive hematopoiesis, including myeloid and lymphoid lineages, is also occurring in the fetal liver (Valli and Jacobs 2010). In addition to the appearance of multilineage hematopoietic progenitors in the yolk sac, intraembryonic hematopoietic stem cells (HSCs) first appear within the intraembryonic aorta–gonad–mesonephros (AGM) region at murine ED10.5 and between human gestation days 27 and 40 (Boyd and Bolon 2010; Tavian et al. 2010). HSCs are self-replicating, multilineage producing hematopoietic progenitor cells. Hematopoietic cells also appear in the major umbilical and vitelline vessels and placenta (Samokhvalov et al. 2007). Tracing experiments have shown that definitive hematopoietic precursors, including adult HSC, are derived from progenitors produced within intraembryonic sites and the yolk sac (Lux et al. 2008; Palis 2008; Samokhvalov et al. 2007). Hematopoiesis occurs primarily in the liver from ED11 in the mouse and approximately gestation day 42 in humans (Valli and Jacobs 2000), followed by a mixed distribution between liver, spleen, thymus, and bone marrow, and predominantly in the bone marrow by postnatal day 4 in the mouse and during the latter half of gestation in humans (Bloom and Brandt 2008; Boyd and Bolon 2010).

Yolk sac blood islands and intraembryonic sites of hematopoiesis, such as the AGM, are thought to be formed from the hemangioblast, a mesodermal vascular and hematopoietic progenitor cell found transiently in the posterior primitive streak at approximately 12–18 h of mouse gestation (Huber et al. 2004; Lancrin et al. 2010; Park et al. 2005). Hemangioblasts migrate to the sites of extraembryonic and intraembryonic hematopoiesis to form the endothelial and hematopoietic cells of these sites and produce hematopoietic precursors through a hemogenic endothelial intermediate cell expressing both endothelial (Tie2) and hematopoietic (c-kit) markers (Lancrin et al. 2009, 2010; Oberlin et al. 2010; Zovein et al. 2008). A complex and interrelated system of growth factors, hormones, and transcription factors is involved in the initiation, direction, and regulation of embryonic and fetal hematopoiesis, beginning with the hemangioblast (Boyd and Bolon 2010; Chen et al. 2009; Lancrin et al. 2009, 2010; Yokomizo et al. 2008). Key transcription factors include stem cell leukemia (Scl)/T-cell acute lymphocytic leukemia 1 (Tal1), which is critical for initial generation of all blood cells, primitive and definitive, and Runx1/acute myeloid leukemia 1 (AML1) that is essential for definitive hematopoietic progenitor and HSC production (Lancrin et al. 2009, 2010). Wnt proteins, a group of secreted cysteine-rich signaling proteins important for embryonic development and self-renewal of HSCs, have been shown to be involved in primitive erythropoiesis; Notch receptors, single-pass Type I transmembrane proteins used to select between preexisting developmental programs, have a positive role in definitive hematopoiesis (Kopan and Ilagen 2009; Kumar et al. 2005; reviewed in Lancrin et al. 2010; Wodarz and Nusse 1998). Disruptions or toxic exposures occurring at various critical windows of hematopoietic development may result in embryo or fetal lethality or bilineage or multilineage cytopenias with the potential for anemia, increased risk for infection or hemorrhage, or altered response to neoantigens or autoantigens.

13.3 ANATOMY AND PHYSIOLOGY

13.3.1 SITES AND MACROSCOPIC APPEARANCE

The bone marrow is the primary site of hematopoiesis in adult animals and is a primary lymphoid organ. Bone marrow is a diffuse organ and comprises approximately 3% of the body mass in rats, 2% in dogs, and 5% in humans (reviewed in Travlos 2006a). In young animals and humans, most bone marrow is active. However, marrow activity decreases with age, with adult hematopoiesis occurring primarily within the central cavities of axial and long bones. In young animals with active hematopoiesis, the marrow appears red, and, as activity decreases, the adipocyte content of the marrow space increases resulting in pale or yellow-appearing marrow. If there is increased demand for blood cells, marrow activity will increase and regain the red appearance; however, the conversion from fat (yellow marrow) to red marrow is slow. The presence of red marrow in adult animals and humans is indicative of increased demand for blood cells of several months' duration (Valli and Jacobs 2000). Sudden increases in demand, such as occurs during hemorrhage or acute infection, result in contraction of the hematopoietic cords with dilation of the venous sinuses causing the marrow to appear red, which may not necessarily indicate increased blood cell production if underlying defects in hematopoiesis are present (Valli and Jacobs 2000). The spleen is a site of active hematopoiesis in the mouse and in other laboratory animals. Extramedullary sites of hematopoiesis may be found in the splenic red pulp and, less commonly, liver under conditions of hematopoietic stress.

13.3.2 MICROSCOPIC STRUCTURE AND CELLULAR COMPOSITION

Bone marrow tissue consists of a sinusoidal system, hematopoietic cells, adipose tissue, supporting reticular cells, and extracellular matrix contained within a boney cortex and supported by a meshwork of trabecular bone (Sharkey and Hill 2010). The vascular supply to the marrow is provided by the nutrient arteries that enter via one or more nutrient canals. The arteries bifurcate and coil around the main venous channel and central longitudinal vein forming arterioles and capillaries that penetrate the endosteal surface. The capillaries communicate with cortical capillaries from arteries supplying local muscle tissue, facilitating communication between bone and hematopoietic cells (Sharkey and Hill 2010; Travlos 2006a). Near the bone, arterioles anastomose with medullary venous sinuses, which drain blood into the central venous sinus and, subsequently, peripheral circulation from the emissary vein exiting via the nutrient foramen. Thus, blood flow in the bone marrow is circular from the center to the periphery and back to the center (Travlos 2006a). The marrow is innervated via myelinated and nonmyelinated nerves that enter through the nutrient foramen. Nerve bundles follow the arterioles and innervate the smooth muscle of the blood vessels or terminate within the hematopoietic cell compartment (Travlos 2006a). There is no lymphatic drainage of the marrow (Travlos 2006a).

Endosteal cells with a thin layer of connective tissue line the inner surface of the bone cavities and the trabecular meshwork or spicules in the cavities (Sharkey and Hill 2010). Osteoblasts and osteoclasts are found in the endosteal layer in close proximity to hematopoietic stem cells and are thought to influence the endosteal microenvironment and play a role in regulation of hematopoietic stem cell proliferation and movement (Frisch et al. 2008; Kollet et al. 2007; Lorenzo et al. 2008). Spindloid to stellate stromal cells extend from the endosteal surface into the hematopoietic space and produce factors involved in hematopoiesis in addition to providing a supporting network for hematopoietic cells, adipocytes, and blood vessels via production of structural fibrils (collagen, reticulin, laminin, fibronectin) (Sharkey and Hill 2010). Adipocyte tissue within the marrow consists of both brown and white types, likely providing both structural and hematopoietic support (Sharkey and Hill 2010).

The hematopoietic compartment is extravascular and located in the spaces between the marrow venous sinuses. In adults, hematopoiesis is closely associated with bone tissue and cells (osteoblasts

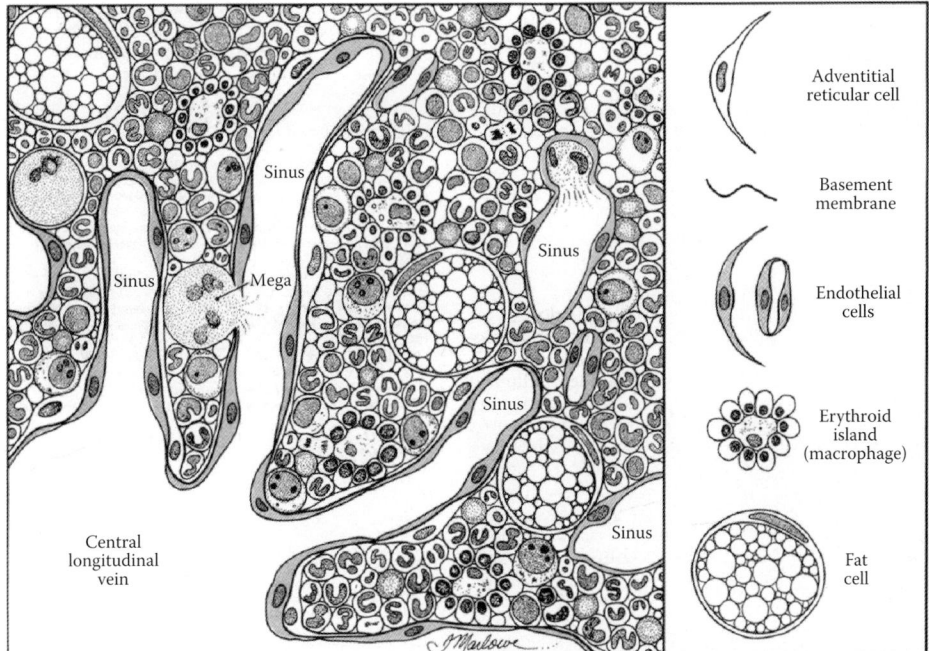

FIGURE 13.1   Schematic depiction of the hematopoietic compartment of the medullary cavity. Hematopoiesis occurs in cords composed of differentiating hematopoietic cells, stromal cells, adventitial reticular cells, adipocytes, and endothelial cells. Megakaryocytes (Mega) are located near venous sinuses, shedding platelets directly into the sinus. Erythropoiesis occurs around macrophages, termed "erythroid islands." Some evidence suggests structural variation in the location of primitive versus differentiated cells, with more primitive cells located nearer the bone surface. (Reprinted with permission from Sieff, C. and D. Williams, Hemopoiesis, in *Blood: Principles and Practice of Hematology*, Philadelphia: JB Lippincott, 1995.)

and osteoclasts) and occurs within 200 μm of bone (Valli and Jacobs 2000). There is also a close relationship between the hematopoietic cells and the venous lining cells, including the flat endothelial cells and the reticular outer layer. The basement lamina between the sinusoids and hematopoietic cells is thin and interrupted. The endothelial cells do not have tight junctions, a specialization of marrow endothelial cells facilitating passage of blood cells into the vascular space (Lichtman 1981). Within the hematopoietic compartment, the erythroid and megakaryocytic cells are adjacent to the venous sinuses, while the myeloid cells (granulocytes, monocytes/macrophages) and lymphocytes are located near the endosteum and arterioles (Sharkey and Hill 2010). Figure 13.1 is a schematic depiction of the hematopoietic compartment within the marrow cavity. The histological appearance of normal bone marrow is shown in Figure 13.2.

13.3.3   CYTOLOGICAL APPEARANCE OF HEMATOPOIETIC CELLS

The erythroid lineage is characterized by cells with round, deeply basophilic, centrally located nuclei with basophilic cytoplasm. The first identifiable erythroid precursor is the rubriblast, followed by the prorubricyte, basophilic rubricyte, polychromatophilic rubricyte, metarubricyte, reticulocyte, and erythrocyte. During the maturation process, erythroid cells decrease in size with condensation of the nucleus resulting in a decreased nuclear-to-cytoplasm ratio. Additionally, erythroid cells lose cytoplasmic organelles, acquire hemoglobin resulting in decreased cytoplasmic basophilia, and undergo nuclear pyknosis, with eventual extrusion of the nucleus to form a reticulocyte. Erythropoiesis occurs

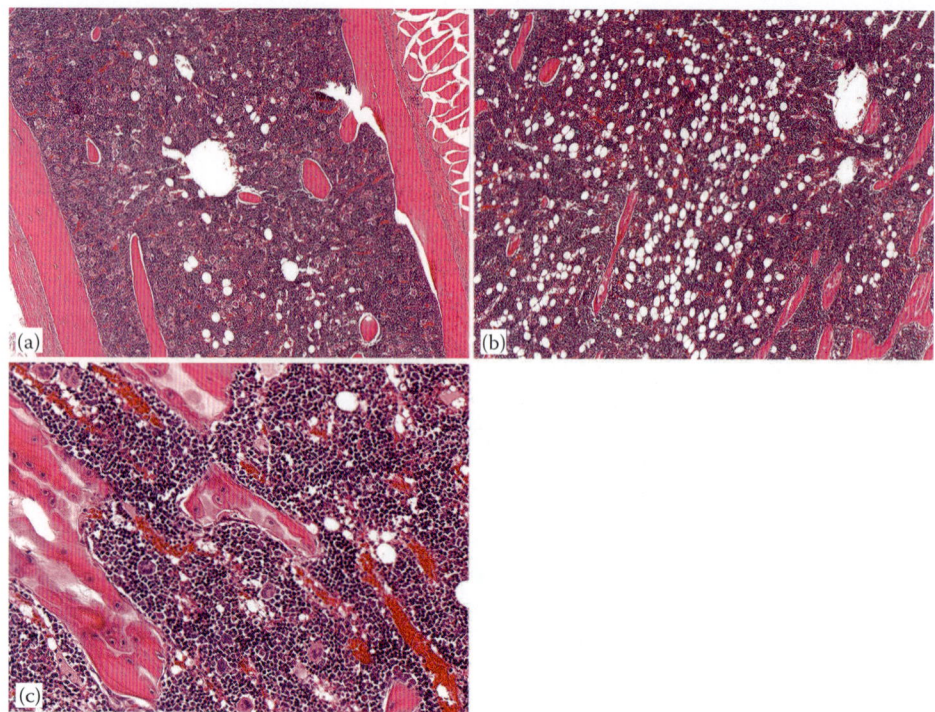

FIGURE 13.2 Longitudinal sections of bone marrow from male Wistar Hannover rat dosed with vehicle control for 2 weeks. (a) Sternum. Note central vein in center of section. In young animals, marrow cellularity relative to fat may approach 80%. In adult animals, marrow cellularity to fat is approximately 50%. (b) Femur. Lipid is more apparent compared to sternal section. The morphological appearance of marrow may vary by anatomical site. (c) Higher magnification of femoral section showing hematopoietic compartment with trabecular bone and venous sinuses. In normal marrow, the proportion of myeloid (paler-staining cells) to erythroid (darkly staining cells) is approximately 1:1 with predominantly mature megakaryocytes distributed throughout the compartment.

within erythroblastic islands featuring maturing erythroid cells surrounding a central macrophage. Myeloid precursors display round to indented to segmented, eccentrically located nuclei and moderately basophilic cytoplasm. The first identifiable myeloid precursor is the myeloblast, followed by the promyelocyte/progranulocyte, myelocyte, metamyelocyte, band forms, and mature segmented neutrophils, eosinophils, and basophils. Similar to the erythroid series, as myeloid cells mature, there is a decrease in size with a concomitant decrease in the nuclear-to-cytoplasmic ratio. Myeloblasts and promyelocytes feature cytoplasmic primary granules. As maturation progresses, secondary granules appear consistent with the granulocytic cell type, that is, neutrophilic, eosinophilic, or basophilic granules. In rats and mice, as myeloid cells mature from the promyelocyte stage, the cells may develop as "ring forms" characterized by a generally round nucleus with a central "hole." As the cells continue to mature, the nuclear hole increases in diameter with only a thin rim of nucleus remaining at the band stage (Provencher Bolliger 2004). In marrow preparations, the myeloid ring forms are found together with the typical indented to band-shaped myeloid cells. Monocytes mature from monoblasts, which are similar in appearance to the early myeloid/granulocytic precursor cells. Immature lymphoid cells are larger and more basophilic than the mature lymphocytes, which are uniformly distributed within the hematopoietic compartment. Differentiation between erythroid and lymphoid cells is difficult upon examination of routine histological sections.

Platelet production begins with the megakaryoblast, which is a large, single-nucleated cell with deeply basophilic cytoplasm. The megakaryoblast undergoes endomitosis resulting in a larger

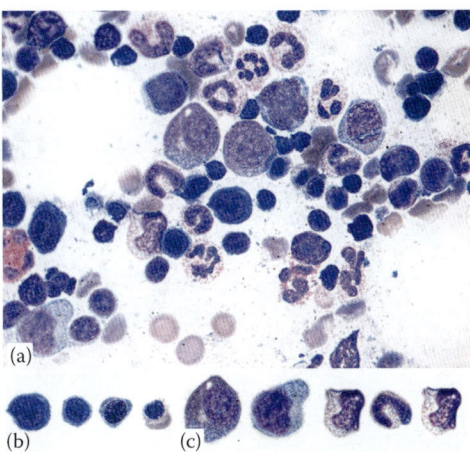

FIGURE 13.3 (a) Bone marrow cytology. Marrow smears prepared from male cynomolgus monkey dosed with vehicle control for 4 weeks. Romanowsky-type stain. Mixture of mature and immature erythroid and myeloid cells. Myeloid cytoplasmic granulation is more apparent in nonhuman primates compared to rodent or dog. (b) Progression of erythroid maturation (left to right): prorubricyte, basophilic rubricyte, polychromatophilic rubricyte, metarubricyte. (c) Progression of myeloid maturation (left to right): promyelocyte/progranulocyte, myelocyte, metamyelocyte, band neutrophil, segmented neutrophil.

multinucleated cell with increased amounts of moderately basophilic cytoplasm. As maturation progresses, the megakaryocyte cytoplasm develops numerous eosinophilic granules. Emperipolesis, the movement of blood cells (neutrophils, erythrocytes, lymphocytes) within megakaryocytes, is fairly common with up to 5% of megakaryocytes containing blood cells in normal bone marrow from humans (Centurione et al. 2004; Harvey 2001). Emperipolesis differs from phagocytosis in that the blood cells exist temporarily within the megakaryocyte (Harvey 2001). Emperipolesis has been described as a random process, although other proposed explanations include facilitation of cell traffic across the marrow–blood barrier, particularly with high demand for blood cells, or as a sanctuary for normal granulocytes in an unfavorable marrow environment (reviewed in Tanaka et al. 1997). Tanaka et al. (1997) showed that emperipolesis in Sprague–Dawley rats was associated with interactions between neutrophil leukocyte function-associated antigen 1 (LFA-1) (Cd11a/CD18) and megakaryocytic intercellular adhesion molecule 1 (ICAM-1), and emperipolesis was increased following administration of lipopolysaccharide. Interestingly, these findings are similar to that reported for transmigration of neutrophils through the blood–CSF barrier associated with C11b/CD18 and ICAM-1 interactions, and involving formation of a cytoplasmic funnel-like structure, as well as transmigration of neutrophils through endothelial cells (Engelhardt and Wolburg 2004; Wewer et al. 2011). The cytological appearance of erythroid, myeloid, and megakaryocytic cells, including examples of rodent ring forms, is found in Figures 13.3 and 13.4.

13.3.4 HEMATOPOIESIS

Hematopoiesis is a complex process involving pluripotential hematopoietic stem cell replication and differentiation into the various erythroid, myeloid, and megakaryocytic lineages. Stem cells have two defining characteristics: capability for self-renewal and capacity to form differentiated or specialized cell types (Overmann et al. 2010). When HSCs divide, one daughter cell is a replica of the parent stem cell, and the other daughter cell is programmed to differentiate. This asymmetric cell division allows for the maintenance of a pool of undifferentiated stem cells and development of lineage-specific hematopoietic precursors (Overmann et al. 2010). HSCs may be identified by their

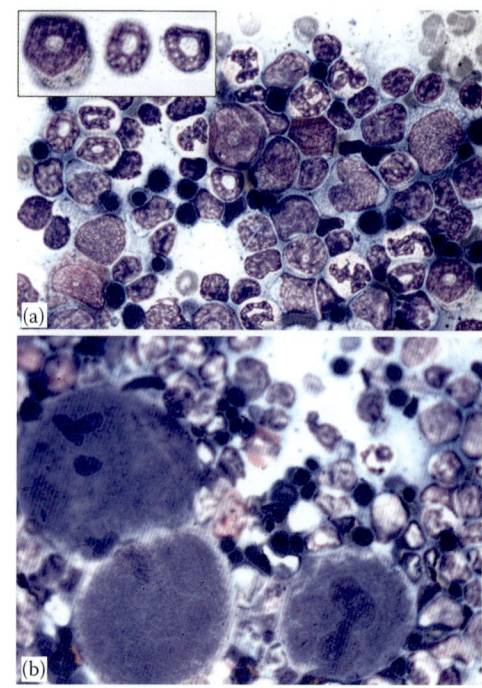

FIGURE 13.4 (a) Bone marrow cytology. Marrow smears prepared from male Wistar Hannover rat dosed with vehicle control for 2 weeks. Romanowsky-type stain. Mixture of immature and mature erythroid and myeloid cells with ring forms and lower numbers of small lymphocytes (note two lymphocytes in upper right corner of field). Inset photos show progression of ringed metamyelocytes with widening of central hole. Ring forms in the myeloid series are a normal finding in rodent marrow smears but are considered a dysplastic change in other laboratory animal species. (b) Three mature megakaryocytes with lobulated nuclei and granular cytoplasm.

positivity for cell surface markers, including CD34 (regulator of stem cell adhesion), c-kit (CD117, receptor for stem cell factor), and stem cell antigen-1 (Sca-1); expression of certain transcription factors, namely, Oct-4, Nanog, and Sox-2; and negativity for lineage-specific markers (Lin⁻) (Alison et al. 2006; Bradfute et al. 2005; Darr and Benvenisty 2006; Healy et al. 1995). Additionally, some CD34-negative cells, referred to as side population (SP) cells, are able to efflux fluorescent dye and are thought to be among the most undifferentiated HSCs (Overmann et al. 2010).

During fetal development, HSCs migrate to niches within hematopoietic tissues, including bone marrow, that are able to maintain and regulate stem cells via physical contact, cell-to-cell interactions, and production of soluble mediators (Morrison and Spradling 2008). These local microenvironments, consisting of adventitial reticular cells, endothelial cells, macrophages, adipocytes, osteoblasts, and extracellular matrix, are located adjacent to the endosteum and bone marrow sinusoids (Gasper 2000; Morrison and Spradling 2008; Travlos 2006a). Both extrinsic factors (cytokines) and intrinsic factors (transcription factors, microRNAs) are involved in HSC stem cell survival and maintenance of pluripotency (Arai et al. 2004; Darr and Benvenisty 2006; Houbaviy et al. 2003; Kaushansky 2006; Overmann et al. 2010).

Based upon tissue demand, the bone marrow niche microenvironment and growth factors stimulate the HSCs to differentiate into multipotential progenitor cells (MPPs) with limited self-renewal, followed by lineage committed progenitors with minimal ability to self-replicate, and then to lineage-specific precursors without self-renewing capability (Car 2010; Radin and Wellman 2010). Stem and progenitor cells appear cytologically as small lymphocytes, and precursor cells are the first cells cytologically identifiable as to lineage (Car 2010). Multipotential progenitors differentiate into two types of progenitor cells: a common myeloid progenitor (CMP) responsible for formation of granulocytes, erythroid cells, monocytes, and megakaryocytes (colony forming unit-GEMM); and a common lymphoid progenitor (CLP) (Car 2010; Kaushansky 2006; Travlos 2006a). In mice, a common myelolymphoid progenitor cell (CMLP) has also been identified (Lu et al. 2002). CMP, under appropriate stimulation from cytokines and growth factors, will divide to form bipotential granulocyte-monocyte progenitors (GMPs) and megakaryocyte-erythroid progenitors (MEPs) (Kaushansky 2006; Radin and Wellman 2010). Neutrophilic and eosinophilic unipotential progenitors (NeuPs, EoPs) and basophil/mast cell bipotential progenitors (BMCPs) are derived from the GMP, although mast cells may also be derived directly from the MPP (Radin and Wellman 2010). Basophils derived from unipotential BaPs mature in the bone marrow, whereas mast cell progenitors leave the marrow, enter circulation, and mature in peripheral tissues (Radin and Wellman 2010). The bipotential and unipotential progenitor cells will continue to differentiate into the morphologically identifiable rubriblast, megakaryoblast, myeloblast, or monoblast precursor cells. The precursor cells will continue to divide and differentiate to form mature erythrocytes, platelets, granulocytes, or monocytes. The multipotential lymphoid stem cell, CLP, will produce B-lymphocyte and T-lymphocyte progenitor cells. B-lymphopoiesis continues in the marrow, whereas T-lymphocyte stem cells migrate to the thymus (Kaushansky 2006; Overmann et al. 2010; Travlos 2006a). This process of division and differentiation of lineage-specific progenitor cells into mature blood cells is controlled by a variety of growth factors, including stem cell factor, IL-7, erythropoietin and thrombopoietin, IL-3, IL-5, granulocyte monocyte–colony stimulating factor (GM-CSF), G-CSF, M-CSF, and IL-2 (Kaushansky 2006), and is produced from a variety of cells and tissues. Figure 13.5 illustrates the progression of hematopoietic stem cell and progenitor cell differentiation and the cytokines and growth factors involved at the various steps.

Within the bone marrow compartment, erythropoiesis occurs in erythroblastic islands, which are composed of erythroid cells and a central macrophage located adjacent to the venous sinuses. The central macrophage assists with erythropoiesis by providing iron for hemoglobin synthesis and probably other nutrients and cytokines. The central macrophage is also important in the removal of the erythroid nucleus during maturation and phagocytosis of defective cells (Abboud and Lichtman 2001; Chasis and Mohandas 2008; Sharkey and Hill 2010). Erythroblastic islands contain erythroid cells in the same stage of development and have been shown to migrate toward sinusoids as they mature (Chasis and Mohandas 2008; Yokoyama et al. 2003). Granulopoiesis occurs in less distinct foci, and megakaryocytopoiesis occurs adjacent to the sinus endothelium (Travlos 2006a). Mature erythroid and myeloid cells migrate through the venous sinuses to enter the bloodstream, whereas platelets are released directly into the bloodstream through cytoplasmic projections of the megakaryocytes into the venous sinuses (Gasper 2000; Travlos 2006a). The identifiable erythroid and myeloid precursor cells, rubriblasts and myeloblasts, undergo approximately four cell divisions to form the first mature erythroid or myeloid cell that is no longer capable of cell division, the metarubricyte and metamyelocyte, respectively (Harvey 2001; Olver 2010). These cells then undergo one to three maturation steps to produce mature erythrocytes and granulocytes (neutrophil, eosinophil, or basophil) (Harvey 2001). Reticulocytes, immature erythrocytes containing cytoplasmic RNA (reticulin), are released from the bone marrow in the laboratory species (dogs, pigs, rodents, and nonhuman primates), unlike other veterinary species, such as ruminants and horses. Following release from the bone marrow, reticulocytes mature to erythrocytes within 24 to 48 h in the blood or spleen (Fernandez and Grindem 2000). Red blood cell production is complete within 4 days, granulocyte production is complete within 6 days, and thrombopoiesis is completed in 4 days (Valli et al. 2002). Mature red blood cell life span is approximately 30 days in mice, 50 days in rats, and 120 days in dogs and humans (Valli et al. 2002). Mature granulocytes are replaced three to four times a day with a peripheral circulation time of 6 to 8 h, and they do not reenter blood circulation following egress into the tissues. Platelet life span is approximately 3 to 5 days in rabbits and rats and 7 to 9 days in larger species (Valli et al. 2002).

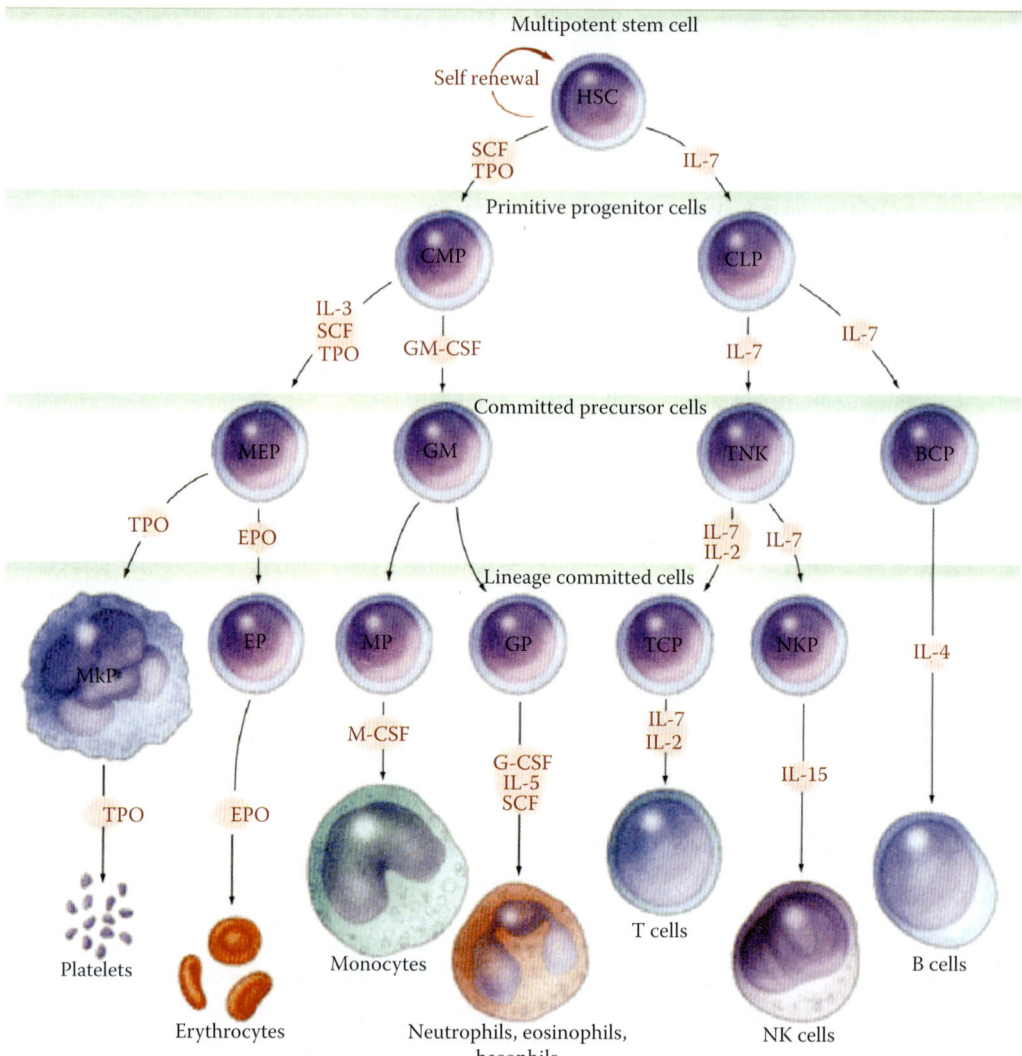

FIGURE 13.5 General model of hematopoiesis. Blood cell development progresses from a hematopoietic stem cell (HSC), which can undergo either self-renewal or differentiation into a multilineage committed progenitor cell: a CLP (common lymphoid progenitor) or CMP (common myeloid progenitor). These cells then give rise to more differentiated progenitors, comprising those committed to two lineages that include T cells and natural killer cells (TNKs), granulocytes and macrophages (GMs), and megakaryocytes and erythroid cells (MEPs). Ultimately, these cells give rise to unilineage committed progenitors for B cells (BCPs), NK cells (NKPs), T cells (TCPs), granulocytes (GPs), monocytes (MPs), erythrocytes (EPs), and megakaryocytes (MkPs). Cytokines and growth factors that support the survival, proliferation, or differentiation of each type of cell are shown in red. For simplicity, the three types of granulocyte progenitor cells are not shown: in reality, distinct progenitors of neutrophils, eosinophils, and basophils or mast cells exist and are supported by distinct transcription factors and cytokines (e.g., interleukin-5 in the case of eosinophils, stem-cell factor [SCF] in the case of basophils or mast cells, and G-CSF in the case of neutrophils). IL denotes interleukin, TPO thrombopoietin, M-CSF macrophage colony stimulating factor, GM-CSF granulocyte-macrophage CSF, and EPO erythropoietin. (Reprinted from Kaushansky, K., *N Engl J Med* 354:2034–2045, 2006. With permission.)

13.4 BONE MARROW EVALUATION

Recently, best practices for bone marrow evaluation in nonclinical studies were published providing recommendations for the preparation and evaluation of bone marrow histopathological and cytological specimens (Reagan et al. 2011). Nonclinical toxicological assessment of the hematopoietic system begins with evaluation of hematology results and histopathological examination of bone marrow. In most instances, information derived from in-life findings, toxicokinetic and hematological data, and bone marrow histopathological evaluations are sufficient for determination of compound-related effects on hematopoiesis. If needed, cytological evaluation of bone marrow smears may also be performed. The decision to perform cytological examination of bone marrow smears should be made on a case-by-case basis following discussions between the anatomic and clinical pathologist and in consultation with the study director and project team safety expert. Additional considerations for performing marrow smear examinations include dose response, tolerability, severity, and reversibility of compound-related findings, as well as stage of compound development and impact or usefulness of cytological evaluation on the clinical safety plan (Reagan et al. 2011). If smear assessments are performed in early toxicity studies, cytological examinations may not be needed for later studies, although this should be decided on a case-by-case basis. Routine bone marrow smear evaluations are not recommended for carcinogenicity studies (Reagan et al. 2011). Additional evaluations of bone marrow tissue include flow cytometric analysis, which may be performed in conjunction with bone marrow smear evaluation or as a stand-alone assay, and electron microscopy and clonogenic assays for mechanistic information on compound-related changes in hematopoiesis (Reagan et al. 2011). Flow cytometry and additional bone marrow assays will be discussed later in this section.

Histopathological examination of bone marrow is used to assess marrow cellularity, megakaryocyte numbers and morphology, presence of focal lesions, such as inflammation or necrosis, estimation of myeloid and erythroid proportions, and assessment of iron stores, especially in conjunction with iron staining. Structural changes to the hematopoietic compartment, including the endosteum, bone, interstitium, adipose tissue, and vasculature, are also assessed by histopathology (Reagan et al. 2011). Cytological examination of bone marrow smears may be performed to evaluate effects on early progenitor cells, changes in hematopoietic cell maturation or morphology, unexplained increases or decreases in peripheral erythrocyte, leukocyte, or platelet counts, differentiation of effects on erythroid or lymphoid cell lineages, and evaluation of changes in peripheral red blood cell indices or morphology, or to further characterize changes in peripheral leukocyte morphology, that is, presence of Döhle bodies (retained aggregates of rough endoplasmic reticulum appearing as blue cytoplasmic inclusions), cytoplasmic basophilia or vacuolation in leukocytes, and reactive lymphocytes (Harvey 2012; Reagan et al. 2011). Bone marrow cytological examination is not needed for evaluation of appropriate changes in erythroid or myeloid cells and/or megakaryocytes in response to increased erythrocyte turnover, inflammation, or platelet destruction/consumption, or if increases in peripheral neutrophils and/or decreases in eosinophils are appropriately attributable to stress (Reagan et al. 2011). As peripheral blood lymphocyte counts are not reflective of altered lymphopoiesis, alterations in lymphocyte counts do not necessitate marrow smear evaluation (Reagan et al. 2011). Additionally, as decreases in bone marrow cellularity have been shown to be proportional to decreased food consumption or food restriction, changes in bone marrow cellularity, concurrent with decreased food consumption or decreased body weight or body weight gain, may not require cytological evaluation (Reagan et al. 2011).

13.4.1 HISTOPATHOLOGIC COLLECTION, PROCESSING, AND EVALUATION

Accurate histopathological assessment of bone marrow requires collection and preparation of good-quality tissue samples. As reviewed by Reagan et al. (2011), a few key points for histopathology sample collection, processing, and preparation should be noted. Samples should be collected within 20 min of euthanasia to provide good-quality specimens; however, shorter collection times (i.e., within 5 min) are needed if cytological specimens are also to be prepared. For rodents and other small laboratory animals, samples for hematopoietic evaluation should be collected from bones with active marrow, such as the sternum, rib, humerus, and femur, with the sternum and distal femur most routinely collected. In rats, the distal tibia should be avoided for marrow collection as this site has a lack of active hematopoiesis (Cline and Maronpot 1985). For large laboratory animals, sites of active hematopoiesis that may be collected include rib, sternum, vertebrae, proximal humerus/femur, and ilium. The central (diaphyseal) portion of the marrow cavity in large animals should not be collected as these areas are usually composed primarily of fat. Bone marrow core biopsy may be obtained from large animals if an in-life evaluation of hematopoiesis is needed. In dogs and nonhuman primates, the iliac crest and humerus have been recommended for bone marrow biopsy and aspiration with a perfusion method has been described for nonhuman primates to facilitate collection of marrow samples for flow cytometry (Kushida et al. 2002; Penny and Carlisle 1970).

Paraffin-embedded, decalcified sections of marrow tissue fixed in 10% neutral buffered formalin are recommended for routine nonclinical toxicology studies. For routine studies, decalcification by immersion in a chelating agent, such as ethylenediaminetetraacetic acid (EDTA), or weak organic acid such as formic or acetic acid, is recommended (Reagan et al. 2011). For routine evaluation, approximately 5-μm, hematoxylin and eosin (H&E)-stained slides are sufficient, although additional stains may be used for identification of erythroid precursors, plasma cells, and mast cells, differentiation of neutrophil and eosinophil granules (Giemsa), and evaluation of iron stores (Perls) (Reagan et al. 2011). As acid decalcification results in loss of basophilic staining with Giemsa stain, use of a chelator, such as EDTA, may be used to improve Giemsa staining (Reagan et al. 2011).

As best practice, histopathological evaluation of marrow tissue should be performed in a systematic manner with marrow from dosed animals compared to concurrent controls, and these results correlated with in-life and clinical pathology findings. Initially, the bone marrow section is scanned at low magnification (40×) for staining quality, composition of cortical bone and associated marrow, and the presence or absence of crush artifact. Also at low magnification, marrow cellularity should be estimated relative to marrow fat, megakaryocyte numbers and morphology assessed, any focal lesions (granulomas or inflammatory foci, necrosis, metastatic infiltrates) identified, and the presence of myelofibrosis determined (Reagan et al. 2011). Examination at 100× to 400× for focal lesions and hematopoietic and stromal elements, as well as iron stores (hemosiderin), should be performed. If the bone marrow section is to be the only bone tissue to be evaluated, trabecular bone thickness and presence and numbers of osteoblasts, osteoclasts, and Howship's lacunae should also be evaluated (Reagan et al. 2011). A general estimate of myeloid to erythroid cell proportions (estimated myeloid/erythroid [M/E] ratio) or, in rodents, myeloid to erythroid/lymphoid ratio, should be determined, followed by evaluation of the myeloid and erythroid cell lines. Megakaryocytes are evaluated for location, presence of cell clusters, and morphology, including abnormalities such as increased emperipolesis and asynchrony of nucleus-to-cytoplasmic ratio (dwarf megakaryocytes). Within the myeloid and erythroid cell lines, the maturation and proliferation pools are evaluated for relative proportions, the presence of increased numbers of immature cells or increased numbers of mature cells, synchrony of maturation, evidence of morphological changes, and neoplasia. Some stages of myeloid and erythroid cells, adipocytes, macrophages, and megakaryocytes are readily identifiable. However, hematopoietic stem cells, early myeloid and erythroid precursors, mast cells, lymphocytes, monocytes, and stromal cells may be difficult to identify (Reagan et al. 2011). If needed, cytological examination may be appropriate, though cytology may also not be able to readily identify stem cells or differentiate between myeloid, monocytic, lymphoid, or erythroid progenitor cells, and additional tests may be considered, including flow cytometry, immunohistochemistry, or cytochemistry (Reagan et al. 2011). Differentiation between lymphocytes and erythroid cells is difficult on H&E sections; however, lymphoid follicles are readily identifiable and may be seen in healthy dogs and nonhuman primates (Ito et al. 1992; Weiss 1986).

Test article–related changes should be recorded using descriptive or semiquantitative terminology, such as decreased hematopoietic cellularity, rather than interpretive terms, that is, hyperplasia, hypoplasia, or aplasia (Elmore 2006; Haley et al. 2005; Reagan et al. 2011). This is particularly important as differentiation between relative versus absolute changes in hematopoietic populations may be difficult on initial histological examination. For instance, an apparent increase in the estimated M/E ratio may be due to an absolute increase in the myeloid compartment or absolute decrease in the erythroid compartment. As the cause of the change in the M/E ratio requires correlation with in-life findings, hematology, and examination of other tissues, the histological findings should be recorded as increased myeloid cellularity and/or decreased erythroid cellularity. The interpretation of the apparent change in the M/E ratio, such as myeloid hyperplasia or erythroid hypoplasia, should be reserved for the interpretative portion of the pathology narrative. The narrative should summarize, describe, and interpret changes in correlation with in-life findings, clinical pathology, and any additional testing, including flow cytometry, immunohistochemistry, or electron microscopy (Reagan et al. 2011).

13.4.2 Cytologic Sample Collection, Processing, and Evaluation

Bone marrow smears for cytological examination should be the first samples obtained at necropsy and ideally collected within 5 min of euthanasia. Due to the rapid loss of cytological detail following death, collection of bone marrow smears from animals found dead is not appropriate. Collection of smears from moribund animals is of questionable value, and, if done, smears should be evaluated and interpreted with caution (Reagan et al. 2011). The presence of shrunken and condensed megakaryocytic nuclei is an early and easily identifiable sign of autolysis (MacKenzie and Eustis 1990). Bone marrow for cytological examination should be collected from the same sites as for histopathological evaluation to aid in the correlation of observed findings (Reagan et al. 2011). As noted in the previous section, smears may be prepared from marrow of the femur and sternum in small laboratory animals and from active (red) marrow of the proximal femur or, due to more uniform hematopoietic activity, preferably from the rib or sternum of large laboratory animals (Reagan et al. 2011). After the marrow cavity is exposed, the bone is squeezed with forceps or pliers to extrude marrow, and slides are prepared immediately using appropriate slide preparation techniques (Reagan et al. 2011). Use of the paintbrush technique is generally preferred as this method consistently produces slides of good quality, especially in small laboratory animals. In this method, a clean natural-bristle (sable) paintbrush dipped into a small amount of protein (5% bovine serum albumin [BSA], heterologous serum, or fetal calf serum) mixed 2:1 with 7.5% EDTA is used to obtain marrow from the exposed cavity (Reagan et al. 2011). It is important that a fresh brush is used for each animal or the brush is cleaned thoroughly with distilled water between each animal to prevent cross-contamination. Other slide preparation methods include the push slide method (also used to prepare blood smears), the squash or pull prep technique similar to that used for diagnostic cytology specimens, and the cytocentrifuge method. In the cytocentrifuge method, marrow from mice and young rats is collected by flushing the marrow from the femur or humerus. The proximal and distal ends of the bone are removed, and a needle attached to a syringe with appropriate buffer is used to flush the marrow into a collection tube. After resuspension, the sample is cytocentrifuged for cytological examination, and absolute counts of the hematopoietic cells can be performed using a hematology analyzer or flow cytometer (Provencher Bolliger 2004; Valli et al. 2002). Slides for cytological examination should be kept separately from formalin containers to prevent loss of staining quality secondary to exposure to formalin fumes. Air-drying of smear slides and staining within a few days of preparation will provide good-quality specimens for cytological staining. If slides are not to be stained immediately following air-drying, they should be kept in a slide holder or slide tray to prevent exposure to light and dust that may adversely affect staining. Bone marrow smears do not need fixation in methanol prior to staining, unless a delay of weeks to months is anticipated prior to staining (Reagan et al. 2011). Modified Wright-Giemsa stain, commonly used in automated hematology analyzers, is preferred for smear staining and evaluation, although other types of Romanowsky-type stains, such as Giemsa or May-Grunwald, may be used (Reagan et al. 2011). Staining time should be increased over that used for routine hematology smears due to the thickness of the smear preparations. Infrequently, bone marrow for cytological evaluation may be obtained from live animals (dogs, nonhuman primates) and is typically collected from the ilial crest or proximal humerus (Harvey 2001; Kushida et al. 2002).

Cytological evaluation of bone marrow smears should be performed by a qualified clinical pathologist, with results in dosed animals compared to concurrent control animals. Bone marrow smears should be of adequate cellularity and uniform preparation (i.e., cells with good staining arranged in a monolayer) with minimal squash artifact and an appropriate number of intact cells for evaluation. Initial examination should consist of a low-magnification (100× to 200×) scan to assess staining, cell arrangement, and adequacy of sample. Megakaryocytes are noted at these low magnifications, and their morphology may also be assessed. At higher magnification (500× to 1000×), myeloid, erythroid, monocytoid, and lymphoid cells and megakaryocytes are evaluated for proportions, morphology, and evidence of changes in maturation or dysplasia. The relative proportions of the myeloid and erythroid maturation and proliferation pools are assessed qualitatively. Qualitative assessments are often sufficient to evaluate observed histological change(s), morphological abnormalities, alterations in synchrony of maturation, and an estimate of the M/E ratio (Reagan et al. 2011). Increases in other cell types, such as mast cells, monocytes, plasma cells, or macrophages, should be described. Quantitative assessments provide additional information regarding cellular proportions and calculation of the M/E ratio and are particularly useful when compound-related changes in cellular proportions are subtle or affect multiple cell lines. Differential counts should be based upon a minimum of 200 cells and, preferably, 300 to 500 cells. A basic quantitative assessment involves categorizing hematopoietic cells as myeloid, erythroid, and lymphoid and calculating the M/E ratio. Although generally not necessary, a complete differential classifying the myeloid and erythroid cells into each identifiable maturation stage allows for the most detailed evaluation of each lineage. For myeloid cells, the identifiable stages are myeloblasts, promyelocytes, myelocytes (immature/proliferating pool) and metamyelocytes, band neutrophils, and mature neutrophils (maturation pool). It is not necessary to differentiate the stages for eosinophils or basophils. For erythroid cells, the identifiable stages are rubriblasts, prorubricytes, basophilic rubricytes (immature/proliferating pool) and polychromatophilic rubricytes, and metarubricytes (maturation pool). A modified differential categorizing the myeloid and erythroid cells into immature/proliferating and maturation pools and lymphoid cells is less time consuming while still allowing for calculation of the M/E ratio and myeloid and erythroid maturation indices (MMI and EMI), which are the total mature percentage divided by the total immature percentage for each lineage (Hoff et al. 1985). The maturation index may be used to semiquantitatively assess shifts in myeloid or erythroid maturation. Similar to the histopathology report, descriptive terms, such as decreased mature myeloid cells or increased immature erythroid cells, are preferable to diagnostic terminology, for example, myeloid hypoplasia or erythroid hyperplasia.

13.4.3 ADDITIONAL BONE MARROW EVALUATIONS

Flow cytometric analysis of bone marrow may be used to provide cellular differentials in place of bone marrow smear examination and has the advantage of evaluating many more cells (i.e., 10,000 to 50,000 versus 200 to 500) and providing results more rapidly. For flow cytometry, the forward and side-scatter properties of the cells, with or without staining for the cell surface marker CD45, can be used to categorize cells as immature and mature erythroid cells, immature granulocytic cells, metamyelocytes, band/segmented neutrophils, and megakaryocytes (Weiss et al. 2000; Weiss 2004). Fluorochrome-labeled antibodies to cell surface markers may also be used to differentiate hematopoietic cells and provide additional differentiation of lymphoid cells into T-lymphocytes and B-lymphocytes (Kakiuchi et al. 2004; Kurata et al. 2007; Kushida et al.

2002; Schomaker et al. 2002). However, as flow cytometry does not provide durable specimens, will not provide morphological assessment, and cannot differentiate all the microscopically identifiable stages of myeloid and erythroid lineages, bone marrow smears should be prepared in addition to the flow cytometry analysis. Additionally, the decision to perform bone marrow flow cytometry must be made prior to necropsy as the samples must be collected and analyzed at the time of sample collection. Thus, retrospective analysis of bone marrow using flow cytometry is not possible.

Specialized techniques for evaluating mechanisms of compound-related changes in hematopoiesis include clonogenic assays and electron microscopy, as recently reviewed by Reagan et al. (2011). Clonogenic assays have previously been used to evaluate multilineage or single-lineage precursors (colony-forming units) in cultures promoting proliferation and differentiation of the hematopoietic cells. The intracellular ATP (iATP) concentration, which varies proportionately with proliferation, or incubation of purchased stem cells with lanthanide-conjugated antibody may also be used to evaluate marrow cell populations in various stages of maturation. Electron microscopy, typically transmission electron microscopy (TEM), may be used to evaluate bone marrow cytological or histopathological specimens or cell culture samples. As with all electron microscopy sampling and evaluation, the decision to evaluate marrow using TEM is ideally made *a priori* to allow for appropriate sample collection and processing.

13.5   ALTERATIONS IN HEMATOPOIESIS

Alterations in hematopoiesis may be the result of primary injury to cellular elements or bone marrow microenvironment and/or vascular supply, or a secondary response to peripheral hematological changes, tissue injury, or metabolic disturbances. Alterations in endogenous hematopoietic growth factors or cytokines or administration of biological compounds with direct or indirect effects on hematopoiesis may result in pharmacological or unintended changes in hematopoietic tissue. For hematopoietic injury, the severity and recoverability are dependent on the type of injured cell. For example, chemotherapeutics toxic to proliferating progenitor and differentiated precursor cells result in dose-dependent peripheral neutropenia and thrombocytopenia. Due to the longer life span of erythrocytes, peripheral red blood cell decreases develop slowly or may not be apparent depending on the duration of the toxic exposure (Weiss 2010a). Peripheral cytopenias are generally reversible following withdrawal of the myelotoxic agent, and an exuberant rebound response may be seen with bone marrow hypercellularity and increased numbers of immature precursors (Rebar 1993). The consequences of toxic insult to pluripotent stem cells or the hematopoietic microenvironment are more unpredictable, and recovery is uncertain (Weiss 2010a).

Histopathologic or cytologic findings related to primary injury or compensatory responses may be classified as quantitative, involving changes in erythroid, myeloid, megakaryocytic numbers, or qualitative, encompassing morphological changes in immature or mature cells (dysplasia, cytoplasmic toxicity), marrow reactivity or inflammation, or necrosis and/or fibrosis (Rebar 1993). In most instances, histopathological examination of bone marrow, in conjunction with evaluation with other tissues, clinical pathology data, and clinical signs, is sufficient to categorize compound-related effects on hematopoiesis and perform appropriate risk assessment for clinical administration. If maturation abnormalities or dysplastic changes are suspected because of a disparity in hematology parameters or between hematology and histopathology findings, or if changes in marrow cellularity are subtle or affecting only one cell line, cytological evaluation of bone marrow smears may be needed. Flow cytometry can also be used to provide quantitative analysis of marrow cellular increases or decreases.

The quantitative and qualitative changes occurring in individual cell lines associated with marrow toxicity along with the expected histological, cytological, and hematological findings are described in the following sections. Hematopoietic neoplasia is a relatively uncommon finding, particularly in short- and medium-term nonclinical studies.

13.5.1   Generalized Hematopoietic Cell Increases or Decreases

Increases (hypercellularity) or decreases (hypocellularity) in marrow cell numbers are determined by comparing the percentage of marrow space occupied by hematopoietic cells to the percentage of marrow space occupied by fat. Generally, marrow cellularity in rodents and large laboratory animal species is considered increased if the marrow cavity is occupied by more than 75% cells, while cellularity is considered decreased if the cavity is occupied by 25% or fewer cells (Cline and Maronpot 1985; Harvey 2001; MacKenzie and Eustis 1990). As marrow cellularity can vary with age and location, cellularity in dosed animals should be compared to appropriate concurrent controls (MacKenzie and Eustis 1990). In rats with marked hypercellularity, hematopoietic cells fill the marrow and may extend through the nutrient foramina into adjacent adipose tissue (MacKenzie and Eustis 1990). Changes in marrow cellularity may involve all cell lineages (pan-hyper or hypo-cellularity) or one or two lineages and should be categorized according to the lineage(s) involved.

Marrow hypercellularity is often a secondary response to increased tissue demand for blood cells, although increased cellularity can be seen with primary marrow disorders, including myelodysplastic or myeloproliferative disorders, alterations in maturation, or as a rebound response to previous myelotoxicity. Peripherally, marrow hypercellularity may be associated with increased or decreased peripheral blood cell counts, depending on the cause of the hypercellularity (primary disorder versus compensatory response), timing of sample collection, and effectiveness of the marrow response. Marrow hypocellularity may be associated with direct toxicity involving one or more cell lineages or indirect toxicity secondary to immune-mediated destruction of mature and/or immature cells, decreased food consumption, or systemic disorders such as high fever and

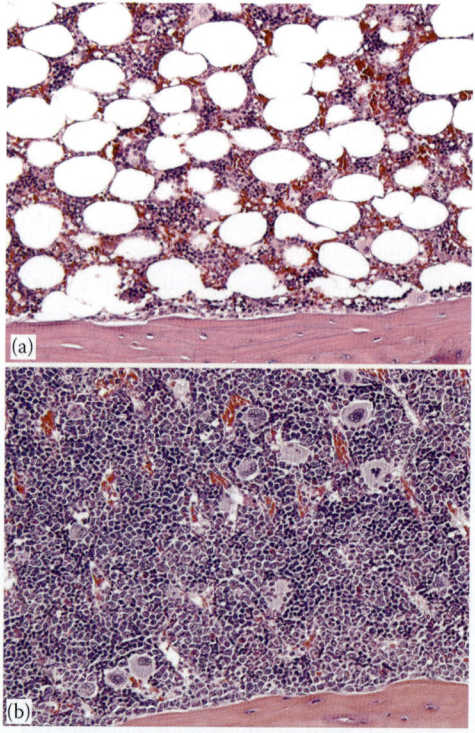

FIGURE 13.6   (a) Section from femur of male Fischer 344 rat dosed with vehicle control for 2 years. Note the predominance of fat in the marrow of this older adult animal. (b) Section from femur of male Fischer 344 rat administered compound for 2 years. Compared to concurrent control sample in a, there is a generalized increase in cell density affecting the erythroid, myeloid, and megakaryocytic lineages. (Reprinted from Travlos, G., *Toxicol Pathol* 34:566–598, 2006. With permission.)

viral infections (Levin et al. 1993; Lowenstine 2003; Rebar 1993; Weiss 1986). Decreased marrow cellularity is frequently associated with peripheral cytopenias, such as a nonregenerative anemia, leukopenia (granulocytopenia, monocytopenia), and/or thrombocytopenia. Severe marrow hypoplasia or aplastic anemia is characterized by peripheral pancytopenia and bone marrow hypoplasia, without evidence of primary marrow disease (Weiss 1986). In aplastic anemia, marrow cellularity is severely decreased with multiple cell lines affected and has been associated with estrogen toxicosis, administration of phenylbutazone, chemotherapeutics, sulfadiazines, and ionizing radiation (Weiss 1986, 2010a; Harvey 2001). In young adult and aging rats, a finding of focal or multifocal "atrophy" of bone marrow of unknown etiology has been described, characterized by relatively well-defined areas of reduced hematopoietic cells and adipocytes with a more prominent stroma (MacKenzie and Eustis 1990; Travlos 2006b). An increase in macrophage numbers has been noted with these lesions suggestive of an inflammatory component to the cellular loss (MacKenzie and Eustis 1990; Travlos 2006b). An indirect cause of pan-marrow hypocellularity and decreased hematopoiesis that should be considered in the context of nonclinical safety studies is decreased food consumption. In rodents, a dose-dependent decrease in marrow cellularity was associated with food restriction of 25% to 50% (Levin et al. 1993). Severe food restriction of 75% was associated with marked marrow hypocellularity, ablation of marrow fat, marrow necrosis and degeneration, and thymic atrophy and lymphopenia (Levin et al. 1993). The marrow changes were reflected peripherally as decreases in granulocytes and monocytes in the severely restricted group and decreases in platelets in all restricted groups. Decreases in hematopoiesis have also been reported in dogs with food restriction (Hill et al. 2005; Lawler et al. 2006). Figures 13.6 and 13.7 depict the histological appearance of increased and decreased marrow cellularity, respectively.

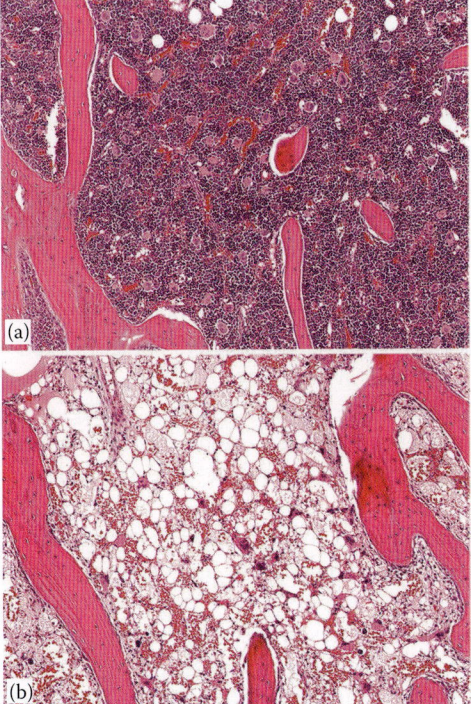

FIGURE 13.7   (a) Sections from sternum of male Wistar Hannover rat dosed with vehicle control by intravenous infusion on four occasions over 2-week dosing period. (b) Section from sternum of male Wistar Hannover rat administered mid-dose of compound by intravenous infusion on four occasions over 2-week dosing period. Note the generalized decrease in marrow cellularity (hypoplasia). Leukogram characterized by dose-dependent decreases in granulocytes, monocytes, and lymphocytes.

13.5.2 INCREASES IN ERYTHROID, MYELOID, AND MEGAKARYOCYTIC NUMBERS

An increase in erythroid cells (erythroid hyperplasia) is the expected and appropriate response of the marrow to increased tissue demand for red blood cells due to blood loss or decreased erythrocyte life span. In nonhuman primates, a common cause for blood loss in nonclinical studies is iatrogenic due to blood collection for toxicokinetics, clinical pathology, and other endpoints. The most common test article–related causes for blood loss are gastrointestinal lesions (Lund 2000). Decreased erythrocyte life span (increased destruction) may result from immune-mediated destruction or oxidant damage, alterations in erythrocyte membrane stability, or intravascular damage (coagulopathy, immune-complex deposition) (Rebar 1993; Lund 2000; Weiss 2010a). Hemoparasitism is a significant cause of responsive (regenerative) anemia in veterinary medicine. In nonhuman primates originating from malaria endemic areas, although low-level plasmodium parasitemia occasionally occurs, responsive anemia is uncommon but may occur when animals are immunosuppressed. The marrow erythroid response to blood loss or decreased erythrocyte life span is characterized by increases in immature and mature erythroid cells, with a predominance of the maturation pool (i.e., polychromatophilic rubricytes and metarubricytes). A few atypical cells, such as binucleated rubricytes or Howell–Jolly bodies, may be present due to the increased production (Weiss 1986). Iron stores are normal to increased (Harvey 2001). In rodents, extramedullary hematopoiesis (erythropoiesis) may also be seen in the spleen and, on occasion, in the liver. The marrow has only a small reticulocyte reserve compartment, which is rapidly released. Thus, the response to increased demand for red blood cells is dependent upon increased production, resulting in a 3- to 4-day latency period for appropriate peripheral reticulocytosis. The peripheral increase in reticulocytes is considered the most efficient and clinically relevant measure of marrow erythroid response (Hoff et al. 1985) and, in conjunction with histological examination of the marrow, is usually sufficient to assess the regenerative response. Changes in peripheral erythrocyte parameters (red blood cell count, hemoglobin concentration, and hematocrit) are dependent on the species, length of the study, timing of sample collection, and severity of the blood loss or destruction. In an effective erythroid response, the calculated M/E ratio should be decreased, unless there is a concurrent increase in the myeloid compartment. Additionally, the marrow erythroid maturation index (EMI), if calculated, should be low and, in conjunction with a high reticulocyte count, is indicative of synchronous maturation and effective erythropoiesis (Hoff et al. 1985). A mild increase in reticulocytes with low to increased EMI, in the presence of erythroid hypercellularity, would be indicative of an ineffective erythroid response and/or asynchronous maturation, for example, chronic blood loss resulting in iron deficiency (Hoff et al. 1985). Erythroid hyperplasia is also associated with absolute polycythemia (i.e., increased peripheral red cell parameters not associated with dehydration). Absolute polycythemia can be nonerythropoietin dependent (primary myeloproliferative disorder) or erythropoietin dependent (secondary). In the nonclinical safety setting, secondary polycythemia related to administration of erythropoietin, increased erythropoietin production due to chronic hypoxia or renal disorders resulting in local tissue hypoxia, or erythropoietin-secreting tumors are more commonly seen as compared to primary polycythemia (Meyer and Harvey 2004; Travlos 2006b). Iron stores are decreased to absent, presumably related to increased erythrocyte production (Weiss 1986). Examples of extramedullary hematopoiesis and erythroid hyperplasia are found in Figures 13.8 and 13.9, respectively.

In nonclinical safety studies, increases in the myeloid compartment (myeloid hyperplasia) are most often due to increased tissue demand or utilization of leukocytes related to inflammation or tissue injury. The degree and appearance of the response are dependent on the type, duration, and severity of inflammation and timing of marrow collection (Rebar 1993). Direct stimulation of myelopoiesis is also possible via administration of granulopoietic growth factors or cytokines or chemicals, such as lithium, all of which stimulate stem cell differentiation into the granulopoietic pathway (Lund 2000). The time course of the marrow myeloid response to inflammation is characterized by an early depletion of the neutrophil storage pool with a concurrent peripheral neutrophilia

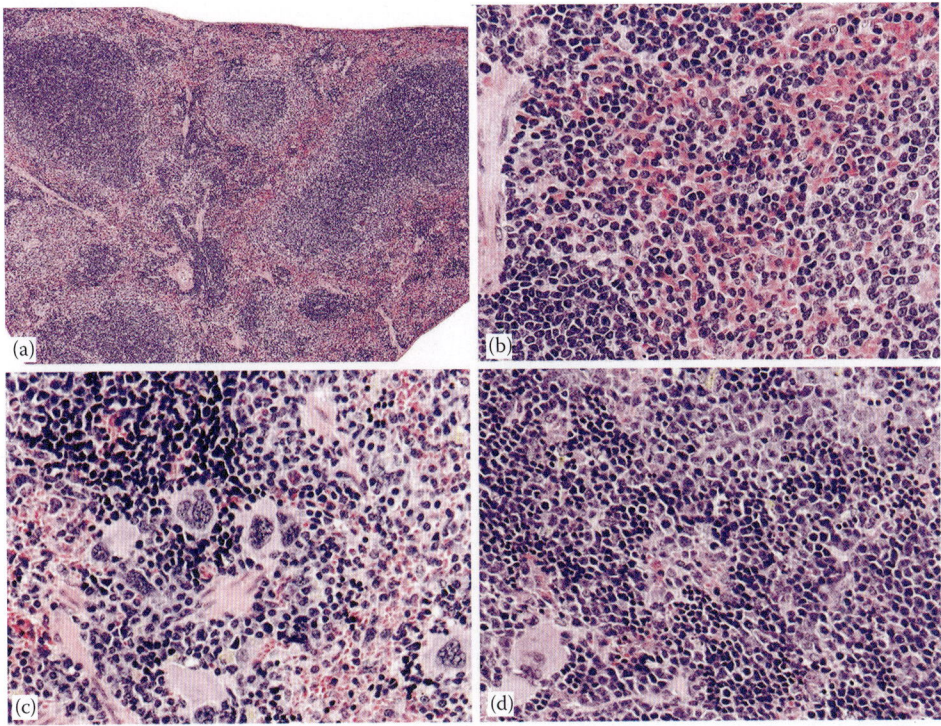

FIGURE 13.8 (a) Section of spleen from mouse dosed with vehicle control. (b) Higher magnification of section in a. Note mixed hematopoietic population (extramedullary hematopoiesis) in splenic red pulp. In mice, the spleen is hematopoietically active throughout adult life. (c) Section of spleen from mouse administered compound. Note the increased number of hematopoietic cells, especially erythroid precursors and megakaryocytes (grade 2). (d) Section of spleen from mouse administered compound. Note the significantly increased number of darkly staining erythroid precursors (grade 4). (Photos courtesy of Dr. Kristen Hobbe, Integrated Laboratory Systems, Inc.)

consisting of segmented and band neutrophils or, if acute inflammation is severe, a neutropenia with leukopenia (Rebar 1993; Lund 2000; Weiss 1986). The decrease or absence of mature marrow neutrophils resulting from storage pool depletion should not be interpreted as a maturation arrest. Due to increased production rates in the acute response, atypical cells including giant cells or, in the dog, ring forms may also be noted (Travlos 2006b). If the inflammation is severe, changes may be observed in the cytoplasm of neutrophils, including increased cytoplasmic basophilia, Döhle bodies, and atypical granulation and vacuolation (Rebar 1993). With continued inflammation, immature neutrophils appear in the circulation, and increased numbers of immature myeloid cells are seen in the marrow. With an appropriate myeloid response to continued inflammatory stimulus, the myeloid compartment expands with restoration of the maturation pool, increased M/E ratio, and peripheral leukocytosis (Rebar 1993). In chronic inflammation, the proliferation and mature myeloid storage pools are expanded, the M/E ratio is high, and the marrow is hypercellular, but due to equilibrium between tissue demand and marrow production, the peripheral leukocyte counts may be only slightly elevated (Rebar 1993). Histological evaluation of the marrow, correlated with hematology and clinical signs, is generally sufficient to identify the cause of the myeloid hyperplasia. If no source of an inflammatory response is noted or the myeloid response appears asynchronous or ineffective, marrow smears may be evaluated with calculation of the M/E ratio and cytological evaluation for dysplastic changes. In dogs, calculation of the myeloid maturation index (MMI) was shown to be highly variable with different disease processes and likely due to the variability in

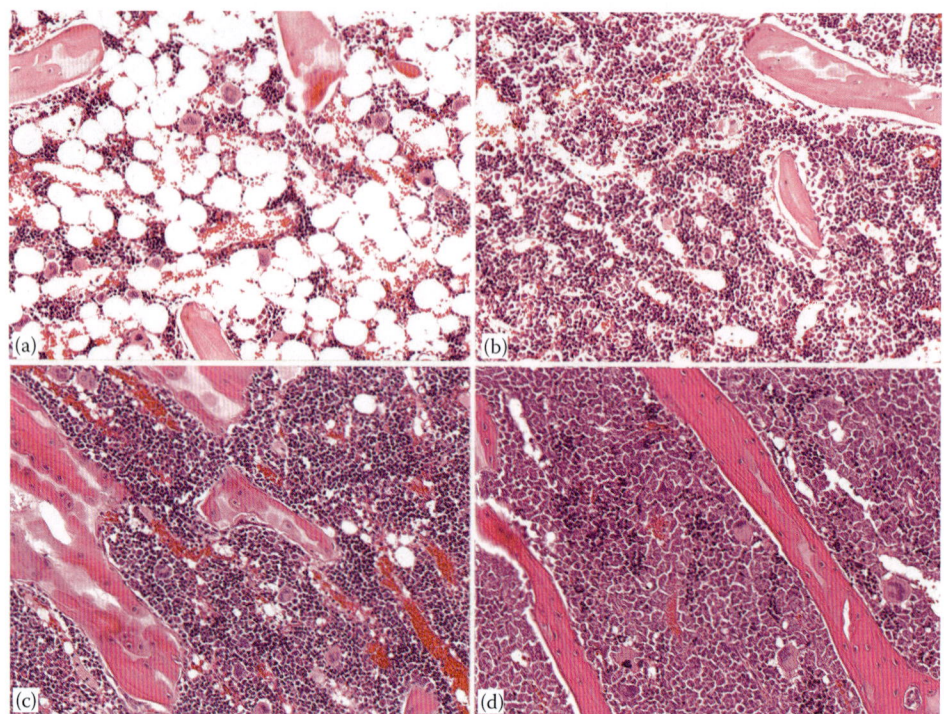

FIGURE 13.9 (a) Section from femur of female Fischer 344 rat dosed with vehicle control for 90 days. (b) Section from femur of female Fisher 344 rat administered compound for 90 days. Increased numbers of small, darkly staining erythroid precursor cells (erythroid hyperplasia) are present as compared to the concurrent control. (c) Sections from femur of male Wistar Hannover rat dosed with vehicle control by intravenous infusion on four occasions over 2-week dosing period. (d) Section from sternum of male Wistar Hannover rat administered low dose of compound by intravenous infusion on four occasions over 2-week dosing period. Note increased myeloid cell numbers (myeloid hyperplasia) with decrease in darkly staining erythroid cells. Leukogram characterized by dose-dependent decreases in granulocytes, monocytes, and lymphocytes. (a and b reprinted from Travlos, G., *Toxicol Pathol* 34:566–598, 2006. With permission.)

release of granulocytes from the storage pool (Hoff et al. 1985). However, the MMI could be used to characterize an ineffective myeloid response (peripheral neutropenia with marrow myeloid hyperplasia) or asynchronous maturation (Hoff et al. 1985). Figure 13.9 shows the histological appearance of myeloid hyperplasia.

Increased megakaryocyte numbers (megakaryocytic hyperplasia) are the expected marrow response to decreases in circulating platelets. The most common causes of thrombocytopenia in nonclinical studies are immune-mediated platelet destruction and consumptive coagulopathy (Rebar 1993). Megakaryocytic hyperplasia may also occur following stimulation with erythropoietin or thrombopoietin, that is, administration of exogenous growth factors or as part of marrow response to peripheral erythrocyte decreases (Rebar 1993; Travlos 2006b; Weiss 1986). Megakaryocyte numbers are best evaluated on histopathological examination at low magnification.

Evaluation of other marrow cellular components, such as lymphocytes, plasma cells, mast cells, and macrophages, is part of the qualitative assessment; however, lymphocytes are typically included on marrow smear differentials and may be assessed by flow cytometry. Increased lymphocyte percentages or numbers, as compared to concurrent controls, may indicate reactivity or immune stimulation, or lymphoproliferative disease. Lymphocyte increases should be correlated with other hematological and histological findings for the most accurate interpretation.

13.5.3 DECREASES IN ERYTHROID, MYELOID, AND MEGAKARYOCYTIC NUMBERS

Decreases in erythroid numbers (erythroid hypoplasia) may be the result of direct damage to erythroid cells or indirect decreases in erythropoiesis secondary to systemic or metabolic disorders. Compounds associated with direct toxicity to erythroid cells include estrogen, chloramphenicol, antiviral agents, and cytotoxic agents (Harvey 2001; Travlos 2006b; Weiss 1986, 2010a). Indirect erythroid hypoplasia may occur secondarily to chronic inflammation, chronic blood loss, chronic renal disease, endocrine deficiencies, and neoplasia (Harvey 2001; Rebar 1993; Travlos 2006b; Weiss 1986). Administration of human recombinant erythropoietin in dogs (Cowgill et al. 1998) as well as rats and nonhuman primates (G. Elliott, personal communication) has been associated with immuonogenicity and development of cross-reactive antibodies that neutralize endogenous erythropoietin, resulting in marked erythroid hypoplasia. Peripherally, decreased erythropoiesis is associated with decreased reticulocyte counts or counts that are similar to or slightly increased as compared to control animals (nonregenerative to poorly regenerative response). Red blood cell parameters may be decreased or normal, depending on the duration of the study and species. Rodents with erythrocyte life spans of 30 to 50 days would more likely demonstrate decreases in red cell parameters as compared to dogs and nonhuman primates with erythrocyte life spans of approximately 120 days. With decreased erythropoiesis, the marrow may appear hypocellular with an increase in the calculated M/E ratio and shift to more mature or normocellular forms, especially in studies of short duration (Travlos 2006b). In anemia of chronic inflammation/disease, the marrow is often normocellular, with slight to absent erythroid hyperplasia and an often increased M/E ratio due to concurrent myeloid hyperplasia (Harvey 2001; Weiss 1986). Iron stores are adequate to increased with a predominance of coarse hemosiderin in macrophages consistent with decreased erythrocyte turnover and increased iron availability (Hoff et al. 1985; Harvey 2001; Weiss 1986). The mechanism for decreased erythropoiesis in chronic inflammation/disease is multifactorial and may include elaboration of inflammatory mediators inhibitory to erythropoiesis, decreased serum iron, shortened erythrocyte life spans, and blunted response to erythropoietin (reviewed in Harvey 2001). In anemia of chronic blood loss, marrow cellularity and erythroid numbers are dependent on duration of the blood loss and may vary from hypocellular to normocellular to hypercellular, with erythroid hypoplasia or hyperplasia (Weiss 1986). As the mechanism of blood loss anemia is external loss of iron resulting in decreased hemoglobin production with subsequent erythrocyte maturation defects, marrow iron stores are decreased to absent (Harvey 2001; Weiss 1986). Selective decreases in myeloid cells (myeloid hypoplasia) occur less commonly than decreases in erythroid lineages, but compound-related myeloid hypoplasia has been observed with administration of chemotherapeutics, chloramphenicol, cephalosporins, sulfonamides, antihypertensives, phenobarbital, and griseofulvin (Harvey 2001; Travlos 2006b; Weiss 1986, 2010a). Some instances of drug-induced myeloid hypoplasia may be secondary or immune-mediated (phenylbutazone and sulfonamides); however, primary defects on myelopoiesis have been postulated for phenylbutazone, cephalosporins, and captopril (Harvey 2001; reviewed in Weiss 2010a). The marrow may be hypocellular or normocellular, depending on the severity of the myeloid decreases, with a decrease in the M/E ratio and synchronous or asynchronous maturation. The MMI may be useful to further assess potential maturation abnormalities within the myeloid lineage. Peripheral granulocytopenias (neutrophils, eosinophils), with or without monocytopenias, would be expected.

Peripheral thrombocytopenias associated with decreased bone marrow megakaryocytes are more often associated with bi-cytopenias or pancytopenias and generalized marrow hypoplasia. Idiopathic amegakaryocytopenic thrombocytopenia has been reported rarely in dogs and cats and is thought to be immune mediated (reviewed in Harvey 2001). Selective decreases in megakaryocytic numbers (megakaryocytic hypoplasia) associated with drug or compound exposure are infrequent, although decreases have been reported with dapsone treatment in dogs (Harvey 2001; Lees et al. 1979). Examples of anemia of chronic inflammation/disease and myeloid decreases are shown in Figure 13.10.

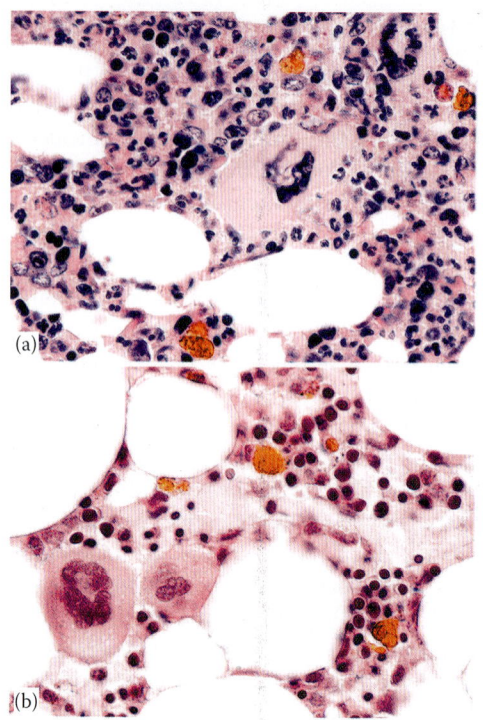

FIGURE 13.10 (a) Anemia of chronic inflammation in a dog. Erythroid cellularity is decreased with increased iron stores (hemosiderin) apparent as orange-staining material. (b) Granulocytic hypoplasia in a dog 6 days following chemotherapeutic administration (vincristine, L-asparaginase, prednisone). Note the predominance of darkly staining erythroid precursors and two mature megakaryocytes. Hemosiderin is also present. (Reprinted from *Veterinary Hematology: A Diagnostic Guide and Color Atlas*, Harvey, J.W. Copyright 2012, with permission from Elsevier.)

13.5.4 HEMATOPOIETIC CELL DYSPLASIA

Dysplastic changes in erythroid, myeloid, or megakaryocytic lineages are the result of maturation defects resulting in abnormal nuclear and/or cytoplasmic morphology. If significant, the alteration in maturation may be associated with ineffective hematopoiesis with concomitant peripheral cytopenias in affected cell line(s). Red blood cell indices may be indicative of erythrocyte macrocytosis or microcytosis. Marrow cellularity may be decreased, normal, or increased depending on the causative agent or inciting event, with increased numbers of precursors related to ineffective hematopoiesis often observed. Hematopoietic cell dysplasia is best identified on cytological preparations, although changes in megakaryocytes can be seen in histological sections. Dysplasia, while a characteristic feature of myelodysplastic syndrome (MDS) and other myeloproliferative disorders, has also been associated with drug or chemical exposure, nutritional deficiencies, chronic blood loss, and recovery from previous hypoplasia with increased cell production.

Cytological changes observed with dyserythropoiesis include abnormal nuclear shapes (peanut-shaped nuclei), asymmetrical binucleation, premature pyknosis, nuclear fragmentation, nuclear to cytoplasmic maturation asynchrony (immature nuclei with hemoglobinized cytoplasm), maturation arrest, and iron-positive basophilic stippling (Harvey 2001). Erythrodysplasia is often associated with megaloblastic change or macrocytic response due to interference with DNA synthesis. For example, folate or cobalamin deficiencies, or administration of compounds that inhibit folate absorption from the intestines (ethanol, barbiturates, diphenylhydantoin) or inhibit cellular uptake of folate (methotrexate), result in megaloblastic anemia, with ineffective erythropoiesis due to inhibition of DNA synthesis and arrest of nuclear maturation and cell division (MacKenzie and Eustis 1990; Rebar 1993). Erythroid dysplastic changes following administration of the chemotherapeutic drug vincristine include increased mitoses, abnormal nuclear configurations, and fragmented nuclei due to binding of tubulin and inhibition of the mitotic spindle (Alleman and Harvey 1993). Iron deficiency, most commonly related to chronic blood loss, is associated with decreased heme synthesis resulting in an extra cell division and smaller-than-normal metarubicytes and erythrocytes (microcytosis). The cytoplasm of hemoglobin-deficient metarubricytes appears shaggy with poorly defined margins (Rebar 1993). Lead toxicosis also interferes with heme synthesis resulting in iron accumulation in erythroid precursors, which can be detected using iron stains such as Perls Prussian blue. The lesion is referred to as sideroblastic change, and the affected erythroid cells are called siderocytes/sideroblasts (Travlos 2006b).

Dysgranulopoiesis is characterized by accumulation of myeloid precursors due to ineffective granulopoiesis, maturation arrest at myelocyte–metamyelocyte stage, giant mature myeloid cells (metamyelocytes, band cells, segmented granulocytes), multinucleated cells, large primary granules or granules surrounded by vacuoles, hyposegmented nuclei (pseudo-Pelger Huet anomaly), hypersegmented nuclei, and abnormal shapes (Harvey 2001). Administration of cephalosporin has been associated with dysgranulopoiesis in dogs (Harvey 2001). Cytological features of dysmegakaryopoiesis include asynchrony of maturation with formation of dwarf granular megakaryocytes containing single or multiple nuclei and large megakaryocytes with nuclear hypolobulation, hyperlobulation, or multiple round nuclei (Harvey 2001). Rarely reported with drug therapy, megakaryocyte dysplasia is most often associated with MDS and acute myelocytic leukemias (Harvey 2001). Examples of erythroid, myeloid, and megakaryocytic dysplastic changes are found in Figure 13.11.

13.5.5 REACTIVITY AND INFLAMMATION

Compound-related acute and chronic inflammation of bone marrow in laboratory animals is an infrequent finding. Acute inflammation of the bone marrow has been described in dogs consisting of an exudative lesion that may not contain inflammatory cells (fibrinous exudate) or that contains neutrophils (acute myelitis) (Weiss 1986). Focal granulomatous inflammation, consisting of macrophage aggregates separated by dense accumulations of mononuclear cells, has been observed in the marrow and spleen of young adult and aged rats, predominantly in females (MacKenzie and Eustis 1990). Granulomatous inflammation has also been observed in rat bone marrow, spleen, lymph nodes, and liver with administration of certain compounds (MacKenzie and Eustis 1990). In dogs, granulomatous inflammation, characterized by a mixed infiltrate of macrophages, giant cells, small lymphocytes, or plasma cells, has been associated with disseminated histoplasmosis and mycobacterial infections as well as discrete granulomas consisting primarily of macrophages (some epithelioid) (Weiss 2010b). Of note, bone marrow granulomas have been reported in humans with a variety of drug hypersensitivities, including phenytoin, procainamide, phenylbutazone, chlorpropamide, sulfasalazine, ibuprofen, indomethacin, allopurinol, and carbamazepine (reviewed in Weiss 2010b).

Hematopoietic reactivity refers to increases in lymphocytes, plasma cells, or macrophages associated with antigenic stimulation, marrow injury, or necrosis. Diffuse increases in lymphocytes and/or plasma cells are indicative of increased immune or antigenic stimulation. Although discrete lymphoid follicles may be seen in histological sections of bone marrow from healthy dogs and nonhuman primates, the presence of follicles may also be considered indicative of immune-mediated hematologic disorders and immune stimulation when observed in dogs and retroviral infections in nonhuman primates (Ito et al. 1992; Lowenstine 2003; Weiss 1986, 2010b). Increased numbers of macrophages are associated with cleanup of necrotic debris or, less likely in the context of nonclinical studies, removal of infectious agents (Rebar 1993; Weiss 2010b). Macrophage reactivity with increased erythrophagocytosis has been observed with immune-mediated red cell destruction or hemoparasitism (Weiss 1986). An example of lymphoid reactivity in bone marrow is shown in Figure 13.12.

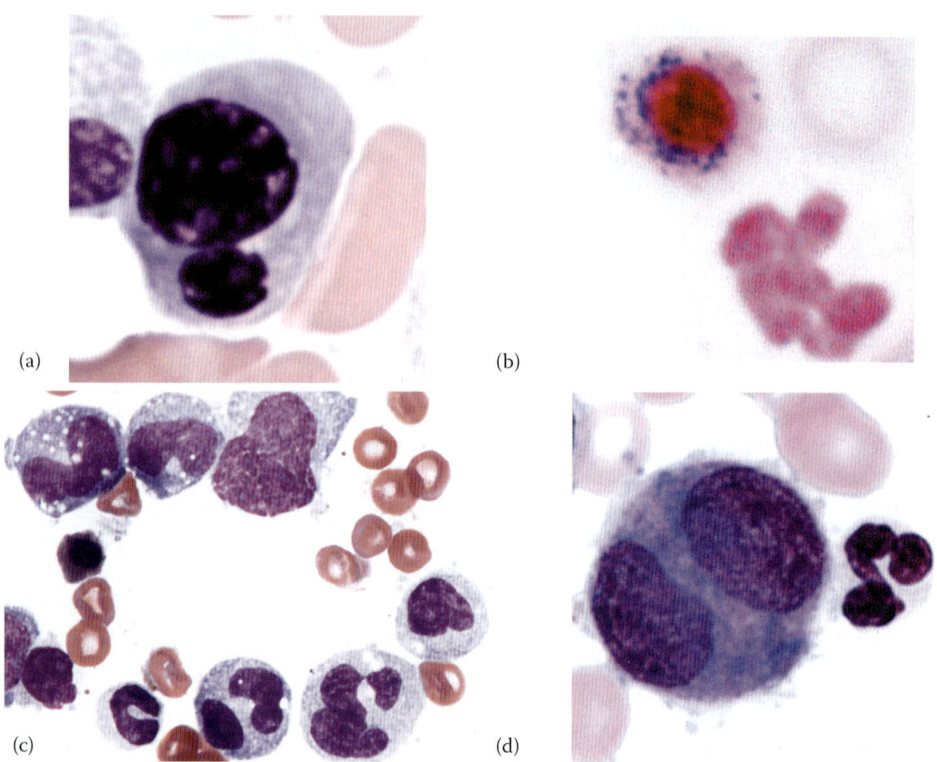

FIGURE 13.11   (a) Lobulated polychromatophilic rubricyte in a dog with mild erythrodysplasia. Wright-Giemsa stain. Dog was not treated with vincristine. (b) Ringed sideroblast (iron-positive metarubricyte) in a dog following chloramphenicol administration. Prussian blue stain. Chloramphenicol blocks the final step of heme synthesis resulting in iron accumulation (Lund 2000). Erythrocytes containing iron-positive (siderotic) inclusions are called siderocytes. (c) Myeloid dysplasia in a dog with idiopathic dysgranulopoiesis. Giant metamyelocytes are present with abnormal nuclear segmentation and cytoplasmic vacuoles. (d) Dwarf megakaryocyte in a dog with myeloproliferative disorder (chronic myeloid leukemia). Note the small size with binucleation and granular cytoplasm resulting from asynchronous maturation. Wright-Giemsa stain. (Reprinted from *Veterinary Hematology: A Diagnostic Guide and Color Atlas*, Harvey, J.W. Copyright 2012, with permission from Elsevier.)

13.5.6   Necrosis

Bone marrow necrosis may be primary, due to direct toxic injury to hematopoietic cells, or secondary, related to severe infectious or degenerative disease, extreme hyperthermia, or ischemia/infarction of the marrow blood supply (MacKenzie and Eustis 1990; Rebar 1993; Weiss 1986). Necrosis is best identified histologically and should be differentiated from autolysis associated with the release of lysosomal enzymes from the resident leukocytes or decreased penetration of fixatives due to presence of bone (MacKenzie and Eustis 1990). Shrinkage and condensation of megakaryocytic nuclei are an early and easily identifiable sign of autolysis (MacKenzie and Eustis 1990). Marrow necrosis may be patchy, focal, multifocal, or diffuse and characterized initially by nuclear pyknosis and karyorrhexis, which is most prominent in the erythroid cells, followed by cytoplasmic vacuolation and lysis with subsequent replacement of the affected areas by amorphous, granular, eosinophilic debris (MacKenzie and Eustis 1990; Rebar 1993; Weiss 1986). Hemorrhage may also be present, and increased numbers of macrophages containing phagocytic debris are apparent (MacKenzie and Eustis 1990; Weiss 1986). In chronic stages, variable degrees of fibrosis may be present (Weiss 1986). Smears prepared from necrotic marrow are difficult to interpret with low

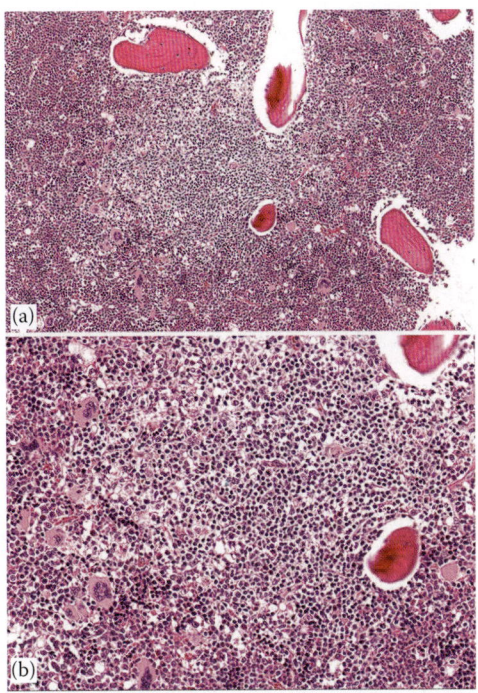

FIGURE 13.12   (a) Section from sternum of male cynomolgus monkey administered high dose of compound once daily by oral gavage for 4 weeks. Multifocal lymphoid aggregates were present with myeloid hyperplasia—note lymphoid aggregate in center of field. Test article–related lymphoid hyperplasia and inflammation were observed in other organs, and the hemogram was consistent with systemic inflammation. (b) Higher magnification of lymphoid aggregate.

numbers of precursor cells showing a loss of nuclear and cellular detail, with granular cellular debris and nuclear fragments in the background (Rebar 1993).

13.5.7   STROMAL ALTERATIONS, PROLIFERATIONS, AND FIBROSIS

Stromal cell hyperplasia and proliferations have been described in Fischer 344 (F344) rats. A focal hyperplasia of stromal, possibly adventitial cells, categorized as focal stromal hyperplasia, has been described as small lesions with cells containing round vesicular nuclei, single nucleoli, and pale vacuolated cytoplasm, which is a very similar description to myelostromal proliferation (MacKenzie and Eustis 1990; Travlos 2006b). As described by MacKenzie and Eustis (1990), myelostromal proliferation in F344 rats is rarely observed. It occurs in marrow from multiple axial and appendicular bones and is characterized by a diffuse cellular proliferation of either stromal reticular cells or histiocytes with oval or slightly irregular vesicular nuclei, single prominent nucleoli, and abundant finely vacuolated cytoplasm containing occasional iron-positive granules and with indistinct cell borders. Cellular atypia is absent to minimal, mitotic figures are infrequent, and a few multinucleated cells that may be megakaryocytes are present. The lesion is associated with anemia and compensatory extramedullary hematopoiesis in the spleen and, less frequently, the liver. Although myelostromal proliferation was not considered to be a form of histiocytic sarcoma involving the bone marrow, it has been reported that histological differentiation of myelostromal proliferation from histiocytic sarcoma by several experienced pathologists was difficult, and, in fact, these lesions may represent a spectrum of neoplastic proliferation (Travlos 2006b). Examples of focal stromal hyperplasia and myelostromal proliferation are shown in Figure 13.13.

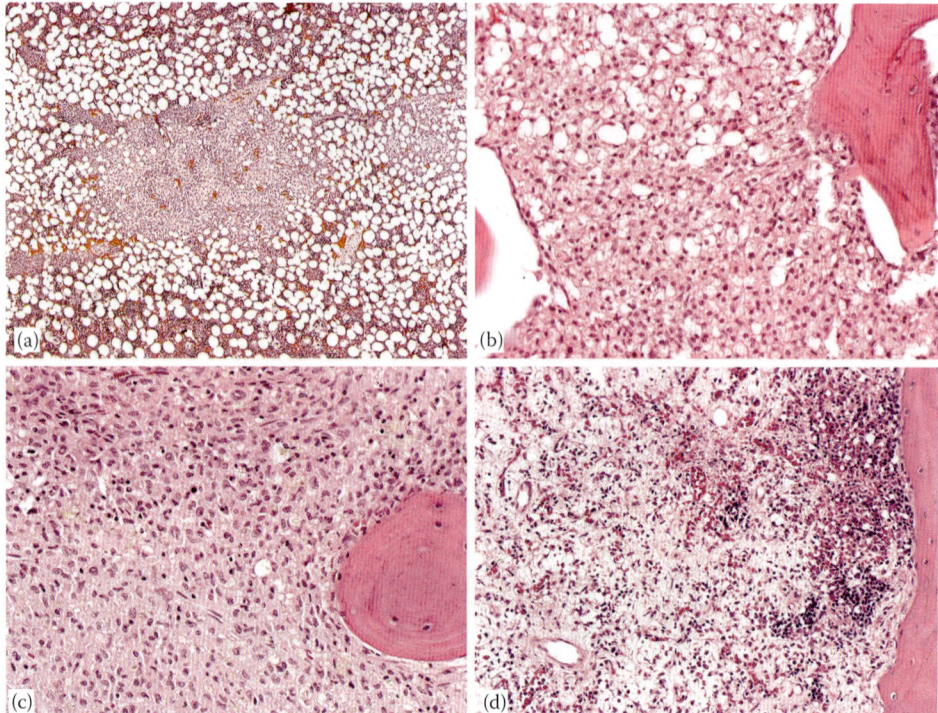

FIGURE 13.13 (a) Section from Fischer 344 rat administered vehicle control. Focal stromal hyperplasia is apparent in center of field characterized by cells with pale vacuolated cytoplasm and round vesicular nuclei. (b) Section of bone marrow from male Fischer 344 rat dosed with vehicle control. Myelostromal proliferation is apparent and characterized by displacement of the hematopoietic population by a diffuse proliferation of cells, presumably of stromal reticular origin. (c) Section from bone marrow of male Fischer 344 rat dosed with vehicle control. Histiocytic sarcoma. In comparison to myelostromal proliferation, the neoplastic cells in histiocytic sarcoma display greater cytoplasmic and nuclear pleomorphism, less cytoplasmic vacuolation, and multinucleation (not apparent in this figure). Typically, there is multiorgan involvement in histiocytic sarcoma. (d) Section of bone marrow from Fischer 344 rat dosed with vehicle control. Fibrosis. There are decreased numbers of hematopoietic cells (hypocellularity) with most of the bone marrow space occupied by an early fibrous proliferation with a loose and almost myxomatous appearance. (Photos b, c, and d reprinted from Travlos, G., *Toxicol Pathol* 34:566–598, 2006. With permission.)

13.5.8 FIBROSIS/MYELOFIBROSIS

The term myelofibrosis has been used in human and veterinary medical literature to describe an excess of collagen and/or reticulin in bone marrow produced by reactive or proliferating fibroblasts (Harvey 2001). In humans, myelofibrosis is associated with a primary myeloproliferative disorder, also called idiopathic myelofibrosis (IMF) or agnogenic myeloid metaplasia, associated with a malignant event originating in a pluripotent stem cell resulting in a cytokine-mediated, secondary fibroblast proliferation and fibrosis (reviewed in Chagraoui et al. 2002). In addition to the intramedullary fibrosis, there is a distinct syndrome of hematological disturbances, including extramedullary hematopoiesis, thrombocytosis, increased numbers of circulating hematopoietic precursors, and splenomegaly (Schmitt et al. 2000; Yan et al. 1996). Increased erythrocyte poikilocytosis, consisting primarily of teardrop-shaped cells called dacryocytes, is also observed (Reagan 1993). An idiopathic, myelofibrosis-like syndrome with similar clinical features has been described in mice that over express thrombopoietin or have a deletion in the megakaryocytic-specific regulatory sequences of the transcription factor GATA-1 (Centurione et al. 2004; Chagraoui et al. 2002; Schmitt et al. 2000; Yan et al. 1996). Bone marrow fibrosis or myelofibrosis may also occur in humans and animals as a secondary response to marrow injury, including necrosis, vascular injury, inflammation, whole-body irradiation, myeloproliferative disorders, chronic hemolytic anemia, and neoplasia of either marrow or nonmarrow origin (Courtney et al. 1991; Harvey 2001; MacKenzie and Eustis 1990; Reagan 1993; Yan et al. 1996). In rodents, focal marrow fibrosis may be seen in aging rats and is likely related to marrow injury, inflammation, or necrosis (MacKenzie and Eustis 1990). The term "myelofibrosis" has been used to describe lesions following infection with murine leukemia virus and in rodents receiving whole-body irradiation (MacKenzie and Eustis 1990). In the context of compound-related myelotoxic injury, secondary myelofibrosis would be an expected healing response to previous injury, much like production of fibrous tissue or scarring in other organs, and is one of the most important endpoints in nonclinical safety studies (Rebar 1993).

Hematological changes have been described in dogs with secondary myelofibrosis and are dependent on the severity and duration of the fibrosis. The replacement of hematopoietic elements (myelophthisis) by fibrous tissue is often associated with nonregenerative anemia and leukopenia, whereas platelets may be decreased, normal, or increased (Reagan 1993; Rebar 1993). Poikilocytosis does not appear to be as prominent a feature of myelofibrosis in dogs as in humans with IMF; however, shape abnormalities of erythrocytes, including dacryocytes, ovalocytes, and schistocytes, have been described (Reagan 1993; Rebar 1993). In rats, hematological changes associated with histological lesions similar to those seen in humans with idiopathic myelofibrosis, mice with IMF-like syndrome, or dogs with secondary myelofibrosis, have not been described (MacKenzie and Eustis 1990). Thus, in rats, it is preferable to avoid the diagnostic term "myelofibrosis" and refer to the lesion as "fibrosis" (Travlos 2006b).

In primary myelofibrosis, IMF-like syndrome in mice, and injury-related myelofibrosis, the fibroplasia and subsequent production of excess matrix are a secondary, reactive process. Courtney et al. (1991) suggested that new bone formation and marrow fibrosis associated with nonclinical dosing of anticancer compounds were mediated by release of inflammatory and growth factors. Several studies have demonstrated that the mechanism of fibroplasia, and increased collagen and reticulin production, is related to the release of megakaryocyte-associated growth factors (i.e., platelet-derived growth factor [PDGF] and transforming growth factor-1 beta [TGF-1β]), resulting in increased fibroblastic activity (Chagraoui et al. 2002; Centurione et al. 2004; Schmitt et al. 2000; Yan et al. 1996). Specifically, in mice overexpressing thrombopoietin and displaying IMF-like syndrome, high circulating levels of PDGF and TGF-1β were observed with megakaryocytes shown to be the primary source of the increased growth factors (Chagraoui et al. 2002; Yan et al. 1996). Chagraoui et al. (2002) also demonstrated the pivotal role of TGF-1β in the development of fibrosis. Additionally, the association of neutrophil emperipolesis with the development of myelofibrosis has been demonstrated. While increased emperipolesis may occur in patients with extreme thrombocytosis, either myeloproliferative or reactive, it is not necessarily associated with fibrosis (Centurione et al. 2004). However, in all cases of human IMF or murine IMF-like syndrome with thrombocytosis and fibrosis, emperipolesis is observed (Centurione et al. 2004). In studies of murine models of IMF and *in vitro* studies utilizing human bone marrow cells from IMF patients, pathological emperipolesis of neutrophils and, on occasion, eosinophils was noted within megakaryocytes (Centurione et al. 2004; Schmitt et al. 2000, 2002). The emperipolesis was considered pathological as the megakaryocytes displayed cytological abnormalities compatible with cytotoxic damage (Centurione et al. 2004). Abnormal localization of P-selectin was noted on the megakaryocytic demarcation membrane system (DMS) and was associated with an increased incidence of emperipolesis (Centurione et al. 2004; Schmitt et al. 2000, 2002). Thus, interaction of granulocyte P-selectin ligand 1 (PSGL-1) with the abnormally located P-selectin, followed by sequestration of granulocytes within the DMS and subsequent release of granulocyte proteolytic enzymes, disruption of megakaryocytic alpha-granules, and release of PDGF and TGF-1β, was proposed as the mechanism of myelofibrosis (Centurione et al. 2004; Schmitt et al. 2000, 2002). Granulocytic proteases may also cleave adhesion receptors from the surface of hematopoietic precursors, leading to egress of the precursors from the marrow with subsequent circulation and extramedullary hemato-poiesis (Centurione et al. 2004). In the context of nonclinical safety studies, it is likely that marrow fibrosis associated with myelotoxic injury is related to the release of growth factors from damaged megakaryocytes and that alterations in megakaryocytic–neutrophil interactions may play a role in the development of the fibrosis. The histological appearance of fibrosis in bone marrow is depicted in Figure 13.13.

13.5.9 Fibro-Osseous Proliferations

Excessive and unorganized production of trabecular bone and increased production of collagenous matrix (fibrosis) have been noted in mice, rats, and dogs. These lesions may result in decreased hematopoiesis related to invasion of the marrow cavity by new bone and collagen. Fibro-osseous proliferations have been classified using a variety of different terminology. Osteosclerosis (myelo-sclerosis) refers to excessive new trabecular bone formation with increased bone density and is almost always associated with severe myelofibrosis (Weiss 2010b). Histologically, osteosclerosis appears as spurs of bone containing increased numbers of osteoblasts and osteoclasts and extend-ing from the trabeculae into the intramedullary space (Weiss 2010b). Osteopetrosis is a congenital condition of dogs and humans, characterized by severe nonregenerative anemia or pancytopenia and generalized increased bone density (Weiss 2010b).

Fibrous osteodystrophy is characterized by formation of new bone with thickened trabeculae that encroach into the marrow cavity and fibrosis that is especially prominent near the endosteal surface of cortical bone (MacKenzie and Eustis 1990; Travlos 2006b). Fibrous osteodystrophy is a characteristic feature of primary or secondary hyperparathyroidism and may also be a drug-induced lesion (Travlos 2006b). Lesions with an appearance similar to fibrous osteodystrophy were seen in rats administered myelotoxic anticancer compounds. These lesions were characterized by new bone formation consisting of immature woven bone occurring either as metaphyseal and diaphyseal islands with associated plump osteoblasts or adjacent to the endosteum and encroaching centrip-etally into the marrow cavity (Courtney et al. 1991). The new bone formation was also associated with increased numbers of intramedullary spindle-shaped cells. These changes were classified as proliferative new bone formation with myelostromal proliferation (Courtney et al. 1991).

In mice, fibro-osseous lesion (FOL) has been described as a fibroproliferative lesion of bone eventually invading and crowding the marrow cavity, but without associated hematological changes (Travlos 2006b). FOL is associated with accelerated osteoclastic bone resorption and proliferation of fibrovascular stroma, thereby resembling fibrous osteodystrophy on histological examination. However, there is no association with primary or secondary hyperparathyroidism (Travlos 2006b). FOL is most frequently reported in the sternebrae, long bones, and vertebrae and is a common spontaneous lesion of female B6C3F1 mice, male mice being much less affected. The etiology is uncertain, but a hormonal component is likely (Travlos 2006b).

13.5.10 Focal Lipomatosis

Well-circumscribed foci of adipocytes have been described as spontaneous lesions of unknown significance in the bone marrow of young adult and aged F344 rats and are referred to as focal lipomatosis (MacKenzie and Eustis 1990; Travlos 2006b). The focus of adipocytes is in the center of the marrow with hematopoietic cells concentrated around the periphery of the cavity, adjacent to the cortical bone (MacKenzie and Eustis 1990).

13.5.11 Serous Atrophy of Fat/Gelatinous Transformation

Serous atrophy of fat/gelatinous transformation of the bone marrow is a condition associated with starvation or cachexia where bone marrow hematopoietic cells and adipocytes are replaced by ground substance. The marrow is hypocellular to aplastic, with atrophy of fat and the presence of amorphous eosinophilic granular material (Weiss 2010b). In bone marrow samples from affected humans, the granular material has been shown to stain strongly positive for alcian blue at pH 2.5 consistent with acid mucopolysaccharides (Bohm 2000).

13.5.12 NEOPLASIA

Neoplasia of hematopoietic tissue may occur as primary leukemias of hematopoietic cells, (erythroid, myeloid, lymphoid, mast cells, monocytes), tumors of stromal cells (fibrosarcoma, histiocytic sarcoma), or tumors of vascular elements (hemangioma, hemangiosarcoma) (Travlos 2006b). Secondary neoplasia involving metastases from distant organs, invasion from local tissues, or multicentric neoplasms (lymphoma, histiocytic) may also occur in hematopoietic tissue, including the spleen and bone marrow. Identification of the tumor type relies on evaluation of light microscopic features and ancillary tests as appropriate, including immunohistochemistry, immunocytochemistry, and flow cytometry.

   Primary neoplasms of the bone marrow are considered rare in F344 rats (MacKenzie and Eustis 1990). Additionally, there are no reported incidences of primary bone marrow neoplasia, including multicentric tumors, in the NTP database (Travlos 2006b). Histiocytic sarcomas were reported to be a primary bone marrow neoplasm in Donryu rats with an approximate incidence of 4.5% and possibly a primary bone marrow neoplasm in F344 rats with an approximate incidence of 1.5% (Ogasawara et al. 1993; Travlos 2006b). A review of neoplasms identified in Crl:CD-1 mice noted that lymphoma was the most common cause of death in carcinogenicity studies; however, no neoplasms were specifically identified as originating in the bone marrow (Bradley and Petersen-Jones 2011). In the NTP database, bone marrow hemangiosarcoma was reported with an incidence of approximately 1% for male and 0.5% for female B6C3F1 mice (Travlos 2006b). Benign and malignant mast cell tumors were reported in bone marrow, also from B6C3F1 mice, with an incidence of 0.04% and 0.24%, respectively, and with an incidence of 0.04% for malignant mast cell tumors in the females (Travlos 2006b).

REFERENCES

Abboud C.N. and M.A. Lichtmann. 2001. Structure of the marrow and the hematopoietic microenvironment. In *William's Hematology*, 6th ed. eds. E. Beutler, B.S. Coller, M.A. Lichtman, T.J. Kipps, and U. Seligsohn. pp. 29–51. New York: McGraw-Hill.

Alison M.R., Brittan M., Lovell M.J. et al. 2006. Markers of adult tissue-based stem cells. *Handb Exp Pharmacol* 174:185–227.

Alleman A.R. and J.W. Harvey. 1993. The morphologic effects of vincristine sulfate on canine bone marrow cells. *Vet Clin Pathol* 22:36–41.

Arai F., Hirao A., Ohmura M. et al. 2004. Tie2/Angiopoietic-1 signaling regulates hematopoietic stem cell quiescence in the bone marrow niche. *Cell* 188:149–161.

Badillo A.T. and A.W. Flake. 2006. The regulatory role of stromal microenvironments in fetal hematopoietic ontogeny. *Stem Cell Rev* 2:241–246.

Baron M.H. 2003. Embryonic origins of mammalian hematopoiesis. *Exp Hematol* 31:1160–1169.

Bloom J. and J. Brandt. 2008. Toxic responses of the blood. In *Casarett and Doul's Toxicology: The Basic Science of Poisons*. pp. 455–484. New York: McGraw Hill.

Bohm J. 2000. Gelatinous transformation of the bone marrow. *Am J Surg Pathol* 24:56–65.

Boyd K.L. and B. Bolon. 2010. Embryonic and fetal hematopoiesis. In *Schalm's Veterinary Hematology*, 6th ed. eds. D.J. Weiss and K.J. Wardrup. pp. 3–7. Ames, IA: Wiley-Blackwell.

Bradfute S.B., Graubert T.A., and M.A. Goodell. 2005. Roles of Sca-1 in hematopoietic stem/progenitor cell function. *Exp Hematol* 33:836–843.

Bradley A. and M. Petersen-Jones. 2011. Spontaneous pathology of the lymphoid and hematopoietic system of Crl:CD-1 mice. Continuation Education Course: Histopathology of the rodent lymphoid and hematopoietic systems. Society of Toxicologic Pathology 30th Annual Symposium, Denver.

Car B.D. 2010. The hematopoietic system. In *Schalm's Veterinary Hematology*, 6th ed. eds. D.J. Weiss and K.J. Wardrup. pp. 27–35. Ames, IA: Wiley-Blackwell.

Centurione L., Di Baldassarre A., Zingariello M. et al. 2004. Increased and pathogenic emperipolesis of neutrophils within megakaryocytes associated with marrow fibrosis in GATA-1^{low} mice. *Blood* 104:3573–3580.

Chagraoui H., Komura E., Tulliez M. et al. Prominent role of TGF-1β in thrombopoietin-induced myelofibrosis in mice. 2002. *Blood* 100:3495–3503.

Chasis J.A. and N. Mohandas. 2008. Erythroblastic islands: niches for erythropoiesis. *Blood* 112:470–478.

Chen M., Yokomizo T, Zeigler B. et al. 2009. Runx1 is required for the endothelial to haematopoietic cell transition but not thereafter. *Nature* 457:887–892.

Cline M.J. and R.R. Maronpot. 1985. Variations in the histologic distribution of rat bone marrow cells with respect to age and anatomic site. *Toxicol Pathol* 13:349–355.

Courtney C., Kim S., Walsh K., et al. 1991. Proliferative bone lesions in rats given anti-cancer compounds. *Toxicol Pathol* 19:184–188.

Cowgill L., James K., Levy J. et al. 1998. Use of recombinant human erythropoietin for the management of anemia in dogs and cats with renal failure. *J Am Vet Med Assoc* 212:521–528.

Darr H. and N. Benvensity. 2006. Factors involved in self-renewal and pluripotency of embryonic stem cells. *Handb Exp Pharmacol* 174:1–19.

Elmore S.A. 2006. Enhanced histopathology of the bone marrow. *Toxicol Pathol* 34:666–686.

Engelhardt B. and H. Wolburg. 2004. Transendothelial migration of leukocytes: through the front door or around the side of the house? *Eur J Immunol* 34:2955–2963.

Fernandez F.R. and C.B. Grindem. 2000. Reticulocyte response. In *Schalm's Veterinary Hematology*, 5th ed. eds. B.F. Feldman, J.G. Zinkl, and N.C. Jain. pp. 110–116. Philadelphia: Lippincott Williams & Wilkins.

Frisch B.J., Porter R.L., and L.M. Calvi. 2008. Hematopoietic niche and bone meet. *Curr Opin Support Palliat Care* 2:211–217.

Gasper P.W. 2000. Hemopoietic microenvironment. In *Schalm's Veterinary Hematology*, 5th ed. eds. B.F. Feldman, J.G. Zinkl, and N.C. Jain, pp. 74–78. Philadelphia: Lippincott Williams & Wilkins.

Haley P., Perry R., Ennulat D. et al. 2005. STP position paper: best practice guideline for the routine pathology evaluation of the immune system. *Toxicol Pathol* 33:404–408.

Harvey J.W. 2001. *Atlas of Veterinary Hematology*. Philadelphia: W.B. Saunders.

Harvey J.W. 2012. *Veterinary Hematology: A Diagnostic Guide and Color Atlas*. St. Louis, Missouri: Elsevier.

Healy L., May G., Gale K. et al. 1995. The stem cell antigen CD34 functions as a regulator of hemopoietic cell adhesion. *Proc Natl Acad Sci USA* 92:12240–12244.

Hill R., Lewis D., Randell S. et al. 2005. Effect of mild restriction of food intake on the speed of racing Greyhounds. *Am J Vet Res* 66:1065–1070.

Hoff, B., Lumsden J.H., and V.E.O. Valli. 1985. An appraisal of bone marrow biopsy in assessment of sick dogs. *Can J Comp Med* 49:34–42.

Houbaviy H.B., Murray M.F., and P.A. Sharp. 2003. Embryonic stem cell-specific microRNAs. *Dev Cell* 5:531–358.

Huber T.L., Kouskoff V., Fehling H.J. et al. 2004. Haemangioblast commitment is initiated in the primitive streak of the mouse embryo. *Nature* 432:625–630.

Ito T., Fumio C., Sasaki S. et al. 1992. Spontaneous lesions in cynomolgus monkeys used in toxicity studies. *Exp Anim* 41:455–469.

Jain N.C. 1993. Hematopoiesis. In *Essentials of Veterinary Hematology*. pp. 72–81. Philadelphia: Lea & Febiger.

Kakiuchi S., Ohara S., Ogata S. et al. 2004. Flow cytometric analyses on lineage-specific cell surface antigens of rat bone marrow to seek potential myelotoxic biomarkers: status after repeated dose of 5-fluorouracil. *Toxicol Sci* 29:101–111.

Kaushansky K. 2006. Lineage-specific hematopoietic growth factors. *New Engl J Med* 354:2034–2045.

Kollet O., Dar A., and T. Lapidot. 2007. The multiple roles of osteoclasts in host defense: bone remodeling and hematopoietic stem cell mobilization. *Annu Rev Immunol* 25:51–69.

Kopan R. and M. Ilagan. 2009. The canonical notch signaling pathway: unfolding the activation mechanism. *Cell* 137:216–233.

Kumar V., Abbas A., and N. Fausto. 2005. Neoplasia. In *Robbins and Cotran Pathologic Basis of Disease*. pp. 269–342. Philadelphia: Elsevier.

Kurata M., Idaka T., Hamada Y. et al. 2007. Simultaneous measurement of nucleated cells counts and cellular differentials in rat bone marrow examination using flow cytometer. *Toxicol Sci* 32:289–299.

Kushida T., Inaba M., Ikebukuro K. et al. 2002. Comparison of bone marrow cells harvested from various cynomolgus monkeys at various ages by perfusion or aspiration methods: a preclinical study of human bone marrow transplantation. *Stem Cells* 20:155–162.

Lancrin C., Sroczynska P., Stephenson C. et al. 2009. The haemangioblast generates haematopoietic cells through a haemogenic endothelium stage. *Nature* 457:892–896.

Lancrin C., Sroczynska P., Serrano A. et al. 2010. Blood cell generation from the hemangioblast. *J Mol Med* 88:167–172.

Lawler D., Ballam J.M., Meadows R. et al. 2006. Influence of lifetime food restriction on physiological variables in Labrador retriever dogs. *Exp Geron* 42:204–214.

Lees G., McKeever P., and G. Ruth. Fatal thrombocytopenic hemorrhagic diathesis associated with dapsone administration to a dog. 1979. *J Am Vet Med Assoc* 175:49–52.

Levin S., Semler D., and Z. Ruben. 1993. Effects of two weeks of feed restriction on some common toxicologic parameters in Sprague–Dawley rats. *Toxicol Pathol* 21:1–14.

Lichtman M.A. 1981. The ultrastructure of the hemopoietic environment of the marrow: a review. *Exp Hematol* 9:391–410.

Lorenzo J., Horowitz M., and Y. Choi. 2008. Osteoimmunology: interactions of the bone and immune system. *Endocr Rev* 29:403–440.

Lowenstine L.J. 2003. A primer of primate pathology: lesions and nonlesions. *Toxicol Pathol* 31 (Suppl.):92–102.

Lu M., Kawamoto H., Katsube Y. et al. 2002. The common myelolymphoid progenitor: a key intermediate stage in hemopoiesis generating T and B cells. *J Immunol* 169:3519–3525.

Lund J.E. 2000. Toxicologic effects on blood and bone marrow. In *Schalm's Veterinary Hematology*, 5th ed. eds. B.F. Feldman, J.G. Zinkl, and N.C. Jain. pp. 44–50. Philadelphia: Lippincott Williams & Wilkins.

Lux C.T., Yoshimoto M., McGrath K. et al. 2008. All primitive and definitive hematopoietic progenitor cells emerging before E10 in the mouse embryo are products of the yolk sac. *Blood* 111:3435–3438.

MacKenzie W.F. and S.L. Eustis. 1990. Bone marrow. In *Pathology of the Fischer Rat*. eds. G.A. Boorman, S.L. Eustis, M.R. Elwell, C.A. Montgomery, and W.F. MacKenzie. pp. 394–403. San Diego: Academic Press, Inc.

Meyer D.J. and J.W. Harvey. 2004. *Veterinary Laboratory Medicine*, 3rd ed. St. Louis: Saunders.

Morrison S.J. and A.C. Spradling. 2008. Stem cells and niches: mechanisms that promote stem cell maintenance throughout life. *Cell* 132:598–611.

Oberlin E., El Hafny B., Petit-Cocault L. et al. 2010. Definitive human and mouse hematopoiesis originates from the embryonic endothelium: a new class of HSCs based on VE-cadherin expression. *Int J Dev Biol* 54:1165–1173.

Ogasawara H., Mitsumori K., Onodera H. et al. 1993. Spontaneous histiocytic sarcoma with possible origin from the bone marrow and lymph node in Donryu and F-344 rats. *Toxicol Pathol* 21:63–70.

Olver C.S. 2010. Erythropoiesis. In *Schalm's Veterinary Hematology*, 6th ed. eds. D.J. Weiss and K.J. Wardrup, pp. 36–42. Ames, IA: Wiley-Blackwell.

Overmann J.A., Modiano J.F., and T.O. O'Brien. 2010. Stem cell biology. In *Schalm's Veterinary Hematology*, 6th ed. eds. D.J. Weiss and K.J. Wardrup. pp. 14–19. Ames, IA: Wiley-Blackwell.

Palis J. 2008. Ontogeny of erythropoiesis. *Curr Opinion Hematol* 15:155–161.

Palis J., Malik J., McGrath K.E. et al. 2010. Primitive erythropoiesis in the mammalian embryo. *Int J Dev Biol* 54:1011–1018.

Park C., Ma Y., and K. Choi. 2005. Evidence for the hemangioblast. *Exp Hematol* 33:965–970.

Penny R.H. and C.H. Carlisle. 1970. The bone marrow of the dog: a comparative study of biopsy material obtained from the iliac crest, rib, and sternum. *J Small Anim Pract* 11:727–734.

Provencher Bolliger A. 2004. Cytological evaluation of bone marrow in rats: indications, methods, and normal morphology. *Vet Clin Pathol* 33:58–67.

Radin M.J. and M.A. Wellman. 2010. Granulopoiesis. In *Schalm's Veterinary Hematology*, 6th ed. eds. D.J. Weiss and K.J. Wardrup. pp. 43–49. Ames, IA: Wiley-Blackwell.

Reagan W. 1993. A review of myelofibrosis in dogs. *Toxicol Pathol* 21:164–169.

Reagan W.J., Irizarry-Rovira A., Poitout-Belissent F. et al. 2011. Best practices for evaluation of bone marrow in nonclinical toxicity studies. *Toxicol Pathol* 39:435–448.

Rebar A.H. 1993. General responses of the bone marrow to injury. *Toxicol Pathol* 21:118–129.

Samokhvalov I.M., Samokhvalova N.I., and S. Nishikawa. 2007. Cell tracing shows the contribution of the yolk sac to adult hematopoiesis. *Nature* 446:1056–1061.

Schmitt A., Joualult H., Guichard J. et al. 2000. Pathologic interaction between megakaryocytes and polymorphonuclear leukocytes in myelofibrosis. *Blood* 96:1342–1347.

Schmitt A., Drouin A., Masse J.M. et al. 2002. Polymorphonuclear neutrophil and megakaryocyte mutual involvement in myelofibrosis pathogenesis. *Leuk Lymphoma* 43:719–724.

Schomaker S.J., Clemo F.A.S., and D. Amacher. 2002. Analysis of rat bone marrow by flow cytometry following in vivo exposure to cyclohexane oxime or daunomycin HCl. *Toxicol Appl Pharmacol* 185:48–54.

Sharkey L.C. and S.A. Hill. 2010. Structure of bone marrow. In *Schalm's Veterinary Hematology,* 6th ed. eds. D.J. Weiss and K.J. Wardrup. pp. 8–13. Ames, IA: Wiley-Blackwell.

Shepard J.L. and L.I. Zon. 2000. Developmental derivation of embryonic and adult macrophages. *Curr Opin Hematol* 7:3–8.

Speck N., Peeters M. and E. Dzierzak. 2002. Development of the vertebrate hematopoietic system. In *Mouse development patterning, morphogenesis, and organogenesis.* eds. J. Rossant and P.P.L. Tam. pp. 191–210. San Diego: Academic Press.

Tanaka M., Aze Y., and T. Fujita. 1997. Adhesion molecule LFA-1/ICAM-1 influences on LPS-induced mega-karyocytic emperipolesis in the rat bone marrow. *Vet Pathol* 34:463–466.

Tavian M., Biasch K., Sinka L. et al. 2010. Embryonic origin of human hematopoiesis. *Int J Dev Biol* 54:1061–1065.

Tober J., Koniski A., McGrath K.E. et al. 2007. The megakaryocyte lineage originates from hemangioblast precursors and is an integral component both of primitive and of definitive hematopoiesis. *Blood* 109:1433–1441.

Travlos G. 2006a. Normal structure, function, and histology of the bone marrow. *Toxicol Pathol* 34:548–565.

Travlos G. 2006b. Histopathology of bone marrow. *Toxicol Pathol* 34:566–598.

Valli V.E. and R.M. Jacobs. 2000. Structure and function of the hemopoietic system. In *Schalm's Veterinary Hematology*, 5th ed. eds. B.F. Feldman, J.G. Zinkl, and N.C. Jain. pp. 225–239. Philadelphia: Lippincott Williams & Wilkins.

Valli V.E., McGrath J.P., and I. Chu. 2002. Hematopoietic system. In *Handbook of Toxicologic Pathology*, 2nd ed. eds. W.M. Haschek, C.G. Rousseaux, and M.A. Wallig. pp. 647–677. San Diego: Academic Press.

Weiss D. 1986. Histopathology of canine nonneoplastic bone marrow. *Vet Clin Pathol* 15:7–11.

Weiss, D. 2004. Flow cytometric evaluation of canine bone marrow based on intracytoplasmic complexity and CD45 expression. *Vet Clin Pathol* 33:96–101.

Weiss D. 2010a. Drug-induced blood cell disorders. In *Schalm's Veterinary Hematology*, 6th ed. eds. D.J. Weiss and K.J. Wardrup. pp. 98–105. Ames, IA: Wiley-Blackwell.

Weiss D. 2010b. Chronic inflammation and secondary myelofibrosis. In *Schalm's Veterinary Hematology*, 6th ed. eds. D.J. Weiss and K.J. Wardrup. pp. 112–117. Ames, IA: Wiley-Blackwell.

Weiss D., Blauvelt M., Sykes J., and D. McCenahan. 2000. Flow cytometric evaluation of canine bone marrow differential counts. *Vet Clin Pathol* 29:97–104.

Wewer C., Seibt A., Wolburg H. et al. 2011. Transcellular migration of neutrophil granulocytes through the blood-cerebrospinal fluid barrier after infection with *Streptococcus suis. J Neuroinflam* 8:51. http://www.jneuroinflammation.com/content/8/1/51.

Wodarz A. and R. Nusse. 1998. Mechanisms of wnt signaling in development. *Annu Rev Cell Dev Biol* 14:59–88.

Yan X., Lacey D., Hill D. et al. 1996. A model of myelofibrosis and osteosclerosis in mice induced by over-expressing thrombopoietin (mpl ligand): reversal of disease by bone marrow transplantation. *Blood* 88:402–409.

Yokomizo T., Hasegawa K., Ishitobi H. et al. 2008. Runx1 is involved in primitive erythropoiesis in the mouse. *Blood* 111:4075–4080.

Yokoyama T., Etoh T., Kitagawa H. et al. 2003. Migration of erythroblastic islands toward the sinusoid as ery-throid maturation proceeds in rat bone marrow. *J Vet Med Sci* 65:449–452.

Zovein A.C., Hofmann J.J., Lynch M. et al. 2008. Fate tracing reveals the endothelial origin of hematopoietic stem cells. *Cell Stem Cell* 3:625–636.

14 Lymphoid System

Patrick J. Haley

CONTENTS

14.1   INTRODUCTION

Histomorphologic assessment of the immune system is a recognized cornerstone in the identification of immunotoxicity. Broad-based scientific forums have culminated in the generation of an International Conference on Harmonization (ICH) guidance and "Best Practices" for evaluation of the immune system (ICH S8 2006; Haley et al. 2005). Additionally, multiple excellent manuscripts and book chapters provide detailed methods to assist in the accurate and consistent characterization of intended and unintended drug-induced alterations of the immune system (Jones et al. 1990; Kuper et al. 1991, 1992, 1995; Greaves 2000; Gopinath et al. 1987; Sternberg 1997), and the reader is encouraged to obtain and regularly refer to these and the numerous excellent articles that are presented in the work of Maronpot (2006).

This chapter is intended to assist anatomic pathologists in the identification and categorization of changes to the immune system, both subtle and obvious. Careful and thoughtful histopathologic examination of lymphoid organs, accompanied by integration of clinical pathology and organ weight data, is essential in identifying biological meaningful effects on the lymphoid system and determining "how much immunosuppression or immunomodulation is too much."

In addition, this chapter focuses some discussion on relevant molecular and cellular biology of the lymphoid system because identifying the histomorphologic alterations of the lymphoid organs is the easy part; understanding the pathobiological implications of these changes is the real challenge. As bench pathologists, it is essential that we not only identify compound-induced tissue changes but also be able to put these changes into a sound immunobiological context.

14.2   REVIEW OF THE *BEST PRACTICE GUIDELINE FOR THE ROUTINE PATHOLOGY EVALUATION OF THE IMMUNE SYSTEM* AND IMPORTANCE OF COMPARTMENTAL ANALYSIS OF LYMPHOID ORGANS

According to *ICH S8: Immunotoxicity Studies for Human Pharmaceuticals,* all new investigational drugs should be evaluated for potential immunotoxicity. Standard toxicity studies (STSs) are designated as a first step, with additional immunotoxicity studies conducted as deemed appropriate. A cause for concern for potential immunotoxicity should be determined using a weight-of-evidence review of all data from STS observations, including the following: clinical pathology endpoints (standard hematology, with an emphasis on the white blood cell [WBC] count with differential cell count, and clinical chemistry with emphasis on globulin and A/G ratios); gross pathology observations of the lymphoid organs/tissues; organ weights of the thymus and spleen; and a compartmental histological analysis of the thymus, spleen, bone marrow, Peyer's patches (PPs), draining lymph nodes, and at least one additional node.

The Society of Toxicologic Pathology (STP) Working Group (WG) on the Best Practices for the Routine Pathology Evaluation of the Immune System identified and debated a number of relevant points including the definition of enhanced histopathology (Haley et al. 2005). First, it was agreed that enhanced histopathology does not require tissue immunohistochemistry, blind scoring of lymphoid tissues, morphometry of lymphoid tissues, or flow cytometry of lymphoid tissue cell suspensions.

Such specialized techniques are useful but need not be used on a routine basis and should be performed only to answer a specific scientific question(s) after effects on the immune system are suggested by observations made during the STS.

Secondly, all lymphoid tissues have a limited number of possible responses to tissue damage or stimuli that include, but are not limited to, hyperplasia, hypertrophy, atrophy, necrosis, inflammation, and neoplasia. In addition, some lymphoid tissue changes may merely reflect the normal function of that particular lymphoid tissue, that is, filtering lymph, and, while possibly appearing different than controls as a result, may not be abnormal (pathologic) per se. For example, sinus erythrocytosis (the accumulation of red blood cells [RBCs]) in a lymph node draining from a distant site of vascular damage is not the same as nodal hemorrhage in which there should be evidence of vascular compromise. Antigens translocated to lymph nodes may lead to normal immune stimulation and follicular hyperplasia, or particulates may be translocated and accumulate in lymph nodes, leading to nonspecific reactive lymphoid hyperplasia (RLH). Lymphoid tissues, especially lymph nodes and spleen, are not static organs and have resident as well as transient cell populations that include cells migrating through the tissue on a normal basis and cells being translocated to the lymphoid tissue from distant sites of tissue damage or from sites of antigen exposure. Recognizing which cell population within the lymphoid tissue is being affected is essential to understanding the significance of the observed histomorphological changes.

As to the utility of obtaining lymphoid organ weights, the Best Practice Guideline for the Routine Pathology Evaluation of the Immune System makes the following points: (1) recording and evaluating thymic and splenic weights should be done routinely; (2) interpretation of these organ weights requires consideration of all other clinical, histopathological, and clinical pathological data from the study; (3) alterations of spleen and thymus weights (along with histopathology) are reasonable indicators of systemic immunomodulation; and (4) spleen and thymus weights are likely to be more reliable indicators of lymphoid tissue effects than are changes in the weight of peripheral lymph nodes. In fact, weighing of lymph nodes is not recommended because of difficulties in consistent tissue collection and processing and the lack of historical databases for such data.

The normal histology of peripheral lymph nodes can be highly variable and often overlaps with that of pathologically altered nodes. Minor differences in collection, embedding, and sectioning combined with high intrinsic variability make consistent histologic characterization of peripheral lymph nodes problematic (Haley 2008). Other than the mandibular and mesenteric lymph nodes, it is not recommended to collect and examine peripheral lymph nodes unless they drain the site of xenobiotic application or show macroscopic changes. Lymph nodes that drain the site of drug administration represent a site of high, first-pass drug exposure of lymphoid tissue and may therefore provide clues to potential effects on the immune system. The gut-associated lymphoid tissue (GALT), including the PPs and mesenteric lymph nodes, should be collected in any standard necropsy and is considered the lymphoid tissue most proximal to exposure by oral administration. Similarly, the bronchus-associated lymphoid tissue (BALT) is appropriate for examination following intrapulmonary administration of agents. Tracheobronchial lymph nodes, which are not routinely collected in most STSs, should also be included in studies evaluating pulmonary exposure. The nasal-associated lymphoid tissue (NALT) should be considered if the nasal route of exposure is used.

The semiquantitative description of lymphoid tissue changes is considered central to best practices for lymphoid tissue microscopic examination and is a core element of enhanced histopathology. This approach is based on the following concepts: (1) each lymphoid organ has separate compartments that support specific immune functions; (2) these compartments can and should be evaluated individually for changes; and (3) descriptive, rather than interpretative, terminology should be used to characterize changes within these compartments. Careful compartmental assessment of tissue changes can provide useful insight into the pathobiology and biological consequence of the lesions. It is essential that age and sex-matched controls are included in each study to ensure accuracy of this determination. In addition, observations should be made for specific compartments only if an abnormality is identified within that compartment. An entry indicating normal status should be made for the entire organ if all tissue compartments are considered to be within the normal range of variability and separate observations for each compartment are not necessary. If all compartments are affected to a similar degree, then terms such as "decreased lymphocytes, generalized severity grade, lymph node (specify)" Are acceptable. See Figure 14.10b and d for examples of nodes that would fit the description of a generalized decrease in lymphocytes.

Harmonization of histopathology terminology is particularly challenging for the immune system. At this writing, the STP INHAND WG continues to work toward finalizing the terminology of pathology descriptors for the immune system. In their consideration of terminology, the STP WG recognized that the application of the same terms for macroscopic and microscopic changes can be confusing and that some terms carried a greater emphasis for diagnostic interpretation than description. Some terms such as "atrophy" or "hypertrophy" are more appropriately used in a macroscopic context. With the view that clarity of communication of pathology findings is a preeminent goal of the Best Practices Guideline, the STP WG suggested some basic principles. Descriptive terms (i.e., increased or decreased cells with the cell type specified if at all possible) are emphasized over interpretative terms to provide a more objective, semiquantitative description for a given change. For example, a descriptive term would be "decreased cells," whereas interpretative terms might include "atrophy," "involution," or "hypoplasia." Another example might be "lymphocytes, decreased, cortex, lymph node," rather than "lymphoid hypoplasia." Additional examples of descriptive terms can be found within the Best Practices Guideline as well as throughout the "A Monograph on Histomorphologic Evaluation of Lymphoid Organs" (Maronpot 2006).

When beginning the assessment of the immune system, the pathologist should start with some basic questions: (1) Is the lymphoid organ grossly larger or smaller than normal: is it macroscopically *increased or decreased in size*? (2) Does the shape, weight, color, or texture differ from normal background and/or control group tissues macroscopically? (3) Is the change in size of the organ because of microscopically evident changes in components (e.g., cells, stroma, edema fluid) of a particular compartment? (4) Is this change in size due to a change in cell numbers in one or more compartments, that is, microscopically *increased or decreased number of cells, and if so, which cells are involved* (lymphocytes, macrophages, stromal cells, etc.)? (5) Which compartment(s) is specifically involved? (6) Are the changes because of resident cells within the compartment or the result of cells migrating through the compartment? By following this simplified approach, it is possible to demystify the histomorphology of these complex and highly plastic tissues. Greater detail is provided in subsequent sections of this chapter on an organ-by-organ basis.

14.3 THYMUS

14.3.1 THYMUS STRUCTURE: HISTORICAL PERSPECTIVE

The macroscopic presentation of the thymus is similar across species, and descriptive terminology has remained relatively unchanged over time. For example, in 1918, Gray stated in describing the human thymus:

"Each lateral lobe is composed of numerous lobules held together by delicate areolar tissue; the entire gland being enclosed in an investing capsule of a similar but denser structure. The primary lobules vary in size from that of a pin's head to that of a small pea, and are made up of a number of small nodules or follicles, which are irregular in shape and are more or less fused together, especially toward the interior of the gland" (Gray 1918).

14.3.2 THYMUS STRUCTURE: SPECIES DIFFERENCES

In more contemporary terminology, the thymus has a thin connective tissue capsule that surrounds the tissue and penetrates and divides the organ into multiple lobules that are most easily identified in larger species such as dog or monkey; mice, however, have no such lobular separation (see Figure 14.1a through d). In most mammals, including humans, dogs, and nonhuman primates, the thymus is recognized as a bilobed lymphoid organ that is located in the anterior thoracic cavity just cranial to the heart and cardiac vessels. However, rats have a variable extension of one or both lobes into the cervical region, the thymus of guinea pigs is located

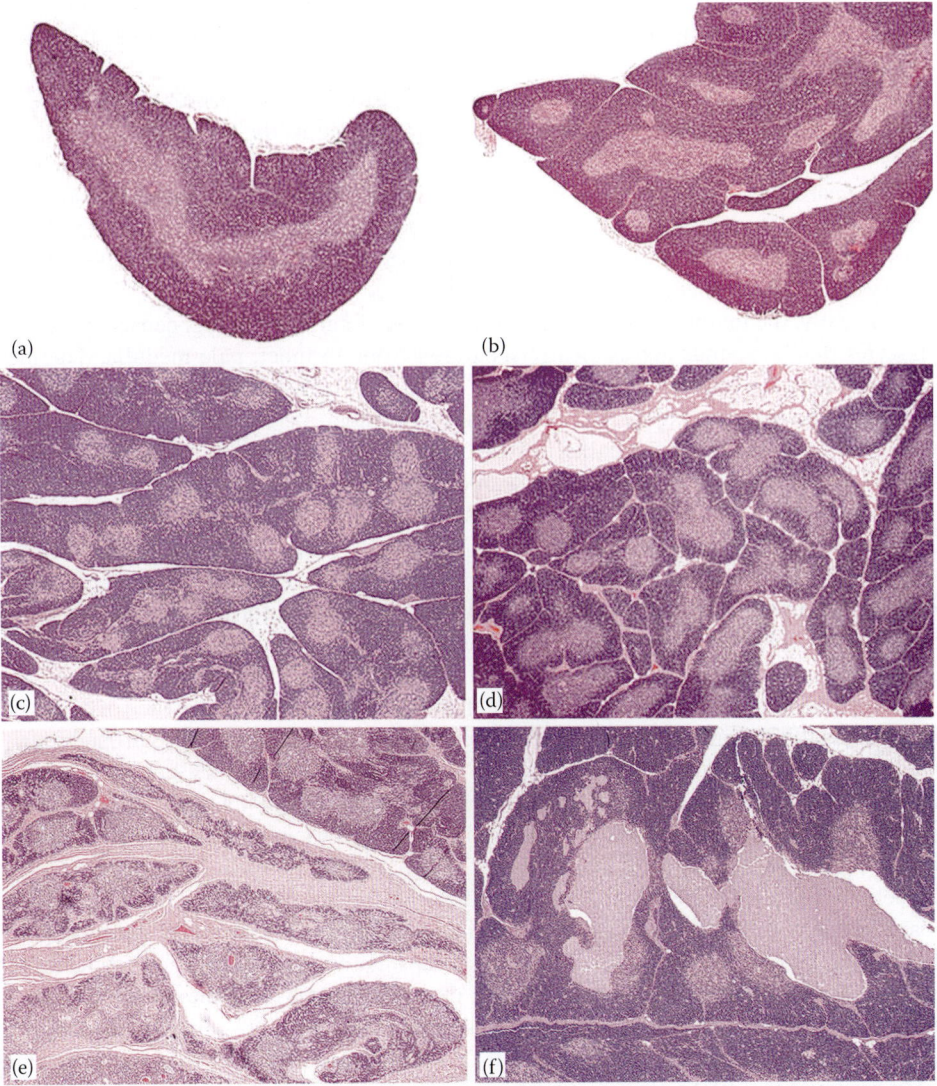

FIGURE 14.1 Photomicrographs of thymus from four species. Note the increasing amount of lobulation of the thymus of dogs (c) and monkeys (d) versus mice (a) and rats (b). (a) Mouse thymus shows a continuous medulla without lobulation. (e) Normal involution of a control dog thymus seen in a 3-month toxicity study. (f) Persistent embryonic remnants forming cysts in the thymic medulla of a normal cynomolgus monkey.

more anteriorly in the neck region (Dijkstra and Sminia 1990), and a cervical thymus has been reported in mice (Terszowski et al. 2006). In swine, the thymus is also located in the thoracic cavity and lies over the pericardium with extension into the thoracic inlet. As in other species, it is bilobed; however, the two lobes continue along the left and right jugular grooves in close association with the carotid artery up to the pharyngeal region, where it is referred to as the "cervical thymus" (Haley 2012).

14.3.3 Thymus: Growth and Development

The thymus increases in size in most species until the time of sexual maturity and then begins to regress, a change that is most apparent in dogs, monkeys, and humans (Figure 14.1e). As animals age, functional thymic tissue becomes replaced by adipose tissue, referred to as atrophy or involution, and epithelial structures (cords, tubules, cysts), especially of the medulla, become more prominent.

In rodents, the thymus is robust at the ages at which most acute and subchronic repeat-dose toxicity studies are performed; however, in humans, the thymus begins the process of involution in the first 10 years of life and largely consists of fat and connective tissue by the time a human reaches the age of 30. Because the human thymus is essentially absent in adults, the relevance of observations of compound-induced decreased thymic cellularity may appear questionable. However, in nonclinical safety assessment, alterations of the thymus in laboratory species remain a reasonable indicator of possible systemic effects on the immune system.

Histologically, the thymus consists of an outer cortex of darkly staining, densely packed small lymphocytes that surrounds and is clearly separated from an inner, pale medulla. The medulla is continuous between adjacent lobules but may appear as distinct islands surrounded by cortex, depending on the section (Figure 14.1a through d). Eosinophilic concentric whorls of flattened reticular cells of epithelial origin called Hassall's corpuscles are present within the medulla and contain keratohyalin and bundles of cytoplasmic filaments. These may be significantly keratinized in dogs, swine, and monkeys but are less so in rats and are not in mice (Figure 14.2c and d). In rats, the keratinization is limited in young animals (150–200 g) but increases with age and may be accompanied by cystic changes as the organ undergoes involution. Epithelial cells other than Hassall's corpuscles provide the structural framework for the thymus as well as the source of important thymic hormones that include thymic humoral factor, thymulin, thymosin, and thymopoietin that are essential in the growth, maturation, and differentiation of the cells of the thymus (Anderson et al. 1996; van Ewijk et al. 1994). In humans, the presence of cystic degeneration of Hassall's corpuscles has been attributed to an exaggerated response of medullary duct epithelium-derived structures of the thymus to underlying inflammatory processes (Sternberg 1997). Cystic structures of the medulla that are infrequently encountered in rats and dogs, but are frequently seen in cynomolgus monkeys, may be the consequence of persistent embryonic remnants (Figure 14.1f).

Epithelium-free areas (EFAs) or "holes" within the thymus have been described by Pearse (2006a) and others in some strains of rats, and abundant large EFAs have been frequently seen in normal beagle dogs (Figure 14.2a and b). These subcapsular accumulations of lymphocytes appear darker than the adjacent cortex due to the lack of epithelial cells. As they often contain many tingible-bodied macrophages (macrophages containing "tingible" or stainable apoptotic debris within their cytoplasm), they should not be mistaken for areas of increased cortical apoptosis. It has been proposed that EFAs are areas in which lymphocytes move between the medulla and cortex without epithelial cell contact, thereby bypassing stromal cell–mediated selection processes (Bruijntjes et al. 1993).

A number of studies suggest that detectable weight changes of the thymus frequently precede histomorphologic changes (ICICIS 1998; Savino et al. 2002). However, as with all lymphoid

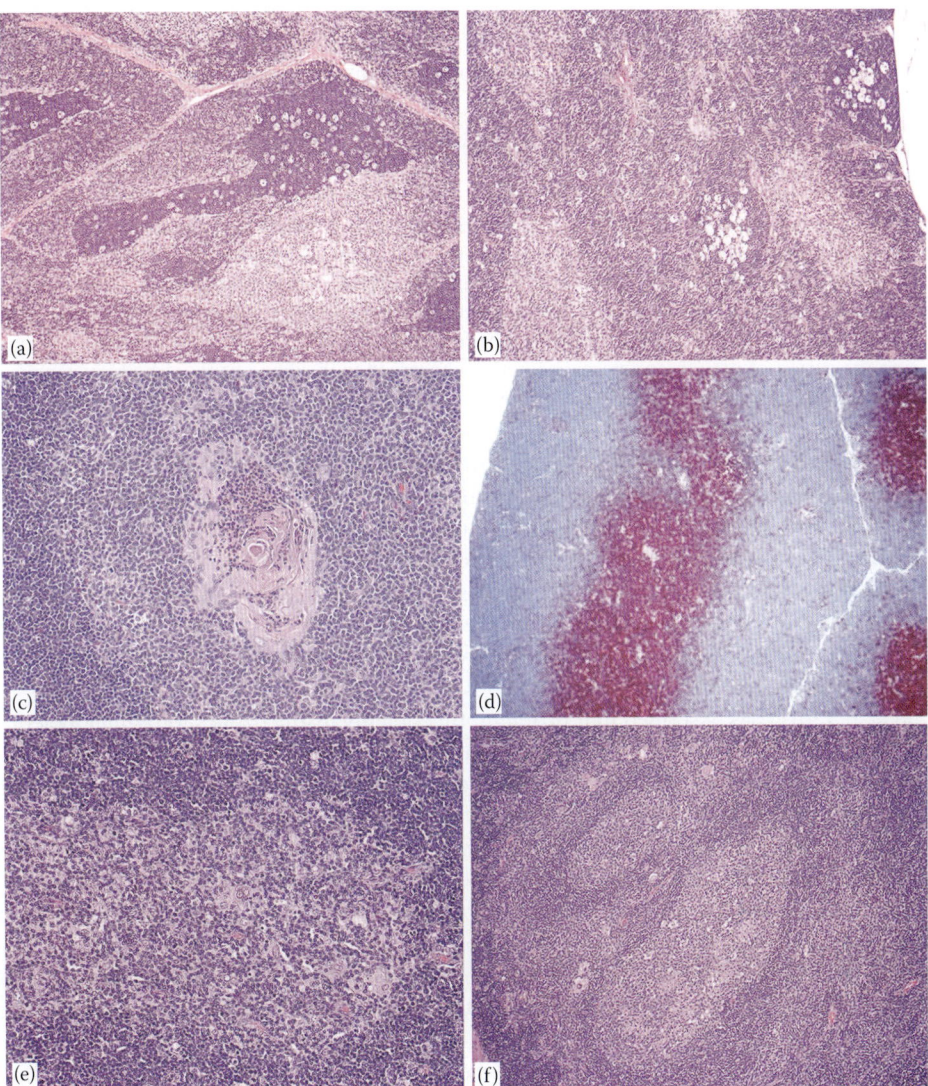

FIGURE 14.2 EFAs of a thymus from a Sprague–Dawley rat (a) and from a dog (b). Note the many darkly stained lymphocytes accompanied by apoptosis and tingible-bodied macrophages. (c) Large keratinized Hassal's corpuscle infiltrated by neutrophils in a normal miniature swine. (d) Intense CD3+ staining of the medulla of a rat. (e) Thymic medulla of a normal rat showing small and indistinct Hassal's corpuscles. (f) Two large lymphoid follicles with germinal centers in the thymus of a control beagle dog.

organs, weights can be problematically variable. Some of the variability around thymic weights, as well as for the spleen, can be addressed by developing consistent collection techniques employed by well-trained staff. A historical database of lymphoid organ weights should be developed and maintained for each species and strain of laboratory animal used, along with the age, weight, and sex of the animals from which the data are collected. Even under such conditions, the median thymic weight of a sexually mature normal male or female Sprague–Dawley rat may vary by as much as 70% or more, and that for a normal male or female beagle dog by approximately 120%–170%.

14.3.4 THYMUS: FUNCTION

Thymus function has puzzled medical researchers for many years and has resulted in some very creative and fascinating perceptions of the organ:

> "Watney has made the important observation that hemoglobin is found in the thymus, either in cysts or in cells situated near to, or forming part of, the concentric corpuscles. This hemoglobin occurs as granules or as circular masses exactly resembling colored blood corpuscles. He has also discovered, in the lymph issuing from the thymus, similar cells to those found in the gland, and, like them, containing hemoglobin in the form of either granules or masses. From these facts he arrives at the conclusion that the gland is one source of the colored blood corpuscles. More recently Schaffer has observed actual nucleated red-blood corpuscles in the thymus. The function of the thymus is obscure. It seems to furnish during the period of growth an internal secretion concerned with some phases of body metabolism, especially that of the sexual glands" (Gray 1918).

Since the time of Watney, many advances have been made in the understanding of thymus biology. It is now known that the thymus is a primary lymphoid organ in which T-cell precursors, derived from the bone marrow, go through a number of maturational changes that culminate in the generation and release of mature T-cells (Anderson et al. 1996). Central to this understanding is the recognition of the pivotal role of the thymus in T-cell maturation and in the initiation of cell-mediated systemic immune responses. This core function of the thymus does not appear to vary across species, and the reader is encouraged to review any of the many texts on the subject (Lind et al. 2011; Anderson et al. 1996; Capone et al. 2001).

Lind et al. (2011) has described four different, functionally distinct zones for lymphopoietic precursor development in the thymus. Briefly, thymus progenitor cells originating in the bone marrow migrate to the thymus, and they enter via the blood vessels at the corticomedullary junction. They then proceed through four stages of maturation that include proliferation and differentiation with T-cell receptor gene rearrangement, surface T-cell receptor expression, and interleukin receptor expression. This is accomplished as the lymphocytes move from the subcapsular region through the cortex and into the medulla, during which positive and negative selection steps via interaction with major histocompatibility complex (MHC)/peptide complexes occur, with the final release of mature TCR^{high} CD4$^-$CD8$^+$and TCR^{high} CD4$^+$ and CD8$^-$ T-cells into the circulation (Anderson et al. 1996; Capone et al. 2001). Immunohistochemical staining of the thymus shows large numbers of CD3$^+$ T-cells within the medulla (Figure 14.1e). Maturation of lymphocytes is supported by interaction with thymic epithelial cells (TECs) within the cortex via humoral factors such as thymulin and thymopoietin or through direct contact. It has been demonstrated that TEC-derived Stat3 is pivotal for thymic lymphocyte survival and the maintenance of thymic architecture, and that elimination of Stat3 from TEC results in acceleration of thymic aging and involution (Sano et al. 2001). It is concluded that Stat3 suppresses specific genes that induce apoptosis of thymic lymphocyte in response to stress and aging.

Growth hormone (GH) is critical to the successful growth and development of the thymus via lymphocyte trafficking to thymic nurse cells, T-cell engraftment of new emigrants into the thymus, enhancement of thymic lymphocyte proliferation, and adhesion of thymic lymphocyte with TEC (Savino et al. 2002). GH and insulin-like growth factor (IGF-1) both play a role in thymulin secretion.

A special subpopulation of epithelial cells designated as nurse cells simultaneously engulfs numerous T-cells and thereby provides a specialized microenvironment for maturation, differentiation, and selection. Other stromal cells that interact with T-cells during maturation include macrophages, dendritic cells (DCs), and fibroblasts. Thus, while the cortical lymphocytes are the first that come to our attention when evaluating the histopathology of the thymus, the stromal elements of the cortex and medulla are also vital for thymic health based on the two-way interaction between stroma and thymic lymphocyte (van Ewijk et al. 1994).

Distinct lymphoid nodules with well-developed germinal centers within the medulla of normal beagle dogs and nonhuman primates (NHP) may also be encountered (Figure 14.2f). The role these reactive lymphoid nodules play in systemic immunity is unknown.

14.3.5 THYMUS: CONUNDRUM OF INVOLUTION VERSUS PATHOBIOLOGY

Involution is the biologically programmed physiologic elimination of thymic lymphocytes that is coordinated via a number of hormones, especially sex hormones that change over the life span with most species experiencing commencement of involution at the time of sexual maturity (Sano et al. 2001). The process of thymic involution is mediated by the microenvironment of the thymus via TEC and thymic lymphocyte signaling (Mackall et al. 1998). The decline in thymic lymphocytes is achieved through apoptosis and phagocytic removal of cell debris from the cortex, the trademark of which is a "starry-sky" appearance as a result of increased numbers of tingible-bodied macrophages. It is important to consider the age, strain, sex, and species of the animal being tested. In rodent studies especially, comparisons should be made primarily within a sex as female rats appear to have more prominent epithelial structures as compared to males (Pearse 2006b). The thymuses of aged Wistar and WAG female rats show lymphocyte masses accompanied by limited epithelial components, whereas aging Brown Norway female rats have thymuses that consist predominantly of cords and tubules with few lymphocytes. Background apoptosis of cortical thymic lymphocytes is part of the normal involution process and may increase significantly between the beginning and end of a subchronic or chronic study in rats, thus making the careful examination of study controls essential for identification of test article–induced effects.

Dogs may develop highly variable degrees of thymic involution as they undergo sexual maturity, and it is not uncommon to see a wide range of thymic development and atrophy in normal dogs at 9–12 months, making identification of test article effects difficult (Figure 14.1e).

Nonhuman primates also demonstrate significant thymic variability, but this may be due to the source of the animals (wild-caught versus purpose bred) as well as age and degree of sexual maturity. Increased numbers of adipocytes and more obvious interlobular stroma become apparent in dogs and NHP as involution progresses. Even under the best of purpose-bred conditions, cynomolgus monkeys may still harbor helminths, malaria, or viral infection, which in turn can have significant effects on lymphoid tissue presentation secondary to chronic antigenic stimulation or stress that may contribute to variable thymus morphology.

The classic histologic presentation of the thymic cortex in toxicity studies, whether as a direct (test article–induced) or indirect (stress-induced) effect, is characterized by decreased cells of thymic cortex accompanied variably by increased lymphocyte apoptosis and increased numbers of tingible-bodied macrophages within the cortex (starry-sky appearance), increased keratinization of Hassall's corpuscles, and decreased delineation between cortex and medulla (Figures 14.3 and 14.4). As these changes progress, the thymus may become tattered, and if severe, the relative cellularity of the cortex and medulla may appear to be reversed. However, because histomorphologic examination essentially looks at the tissue in a snapshot in time, not all of the changes described above will necessarily be present at the time of tissue collection. Identifying tissue changes as mediated by test article is reinforced if a dose–response relationship can be identified. Making interpretation of microscopic changes more difficult is the recognition that the intensity and duration of the insult and/or stressor and the time between the insult and tissue collection affect the morphological presentation. If the insult is acute and severe following a single dose of compound, but the tissue is collected days later, apoptosis may occur suddenly throughout the organ and be rapidly cleared, leaving behind only the appearance of decreased cells but without significant numbers of apoptotic bodies or tingible-bodied macrophages. In contrast, if the insult is persistent and intense, or if the tissue is collected soon after the insult, the lesion may be characterized by the presence of numerous

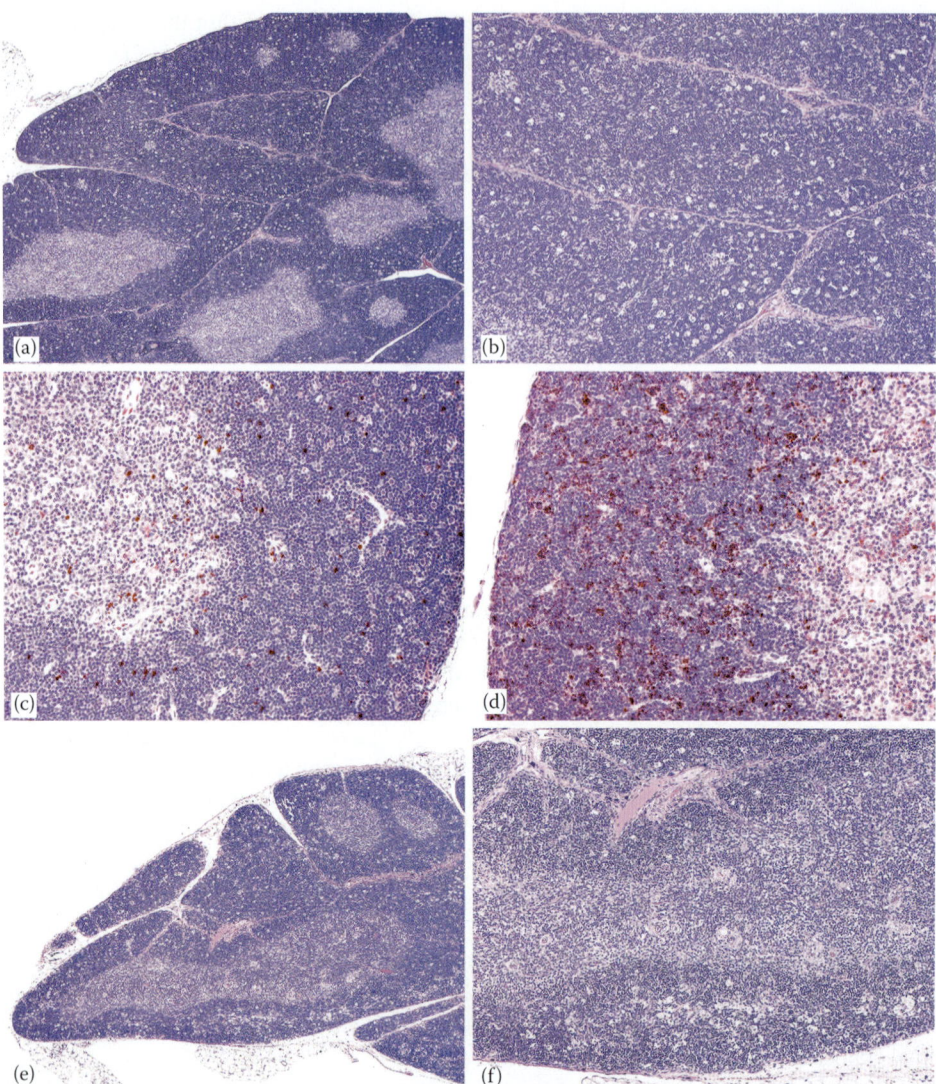

FIGURE 14.3 H&E-stained section of a normal thymus from a mature control Sprague–Dawley rat (a). (b) Higher magnification of a showing typical low-grade background apoptosis of cortical lymphocytes. (c) Caspase 3–stained thymus of a control Sprague–Dawley rat showing normal low level of background apoptosis. (d) Caspase-stained thymus of a rat given an immunomodulatory compound that targets T-cells showing a significant increase in apoptotic cells. (e) Thymus of a rat given an immunomodulatory drug. Note thin but otherwise well-ordered cortex and increased keratinized Hassall's corpuscles. (f) Higher magnification of (e) showing irregular patches of apoptotic cells resulting in a thin and tattered cortex.

and distinct tingible-bodied macrophages (Figure 14.4a through c). The thymus is a highly regenerative organ and, in rodents, given enough time, can undergo complete recovery even when the initial insult is severe (personal observation).

Other changes are generally similar across species, including humans, and include cystic dilatation of Hassall's corpuscles with accumulation of cellular debris, dystrophic calcification, and the accumulation of foamy macrophages. Increased numbers and size of keratinized Hassall's corpuscles in rats can be striking and accompany cortical changes of increased lymphocyte apoptosis and cellular depletion (Figure 14.4f).

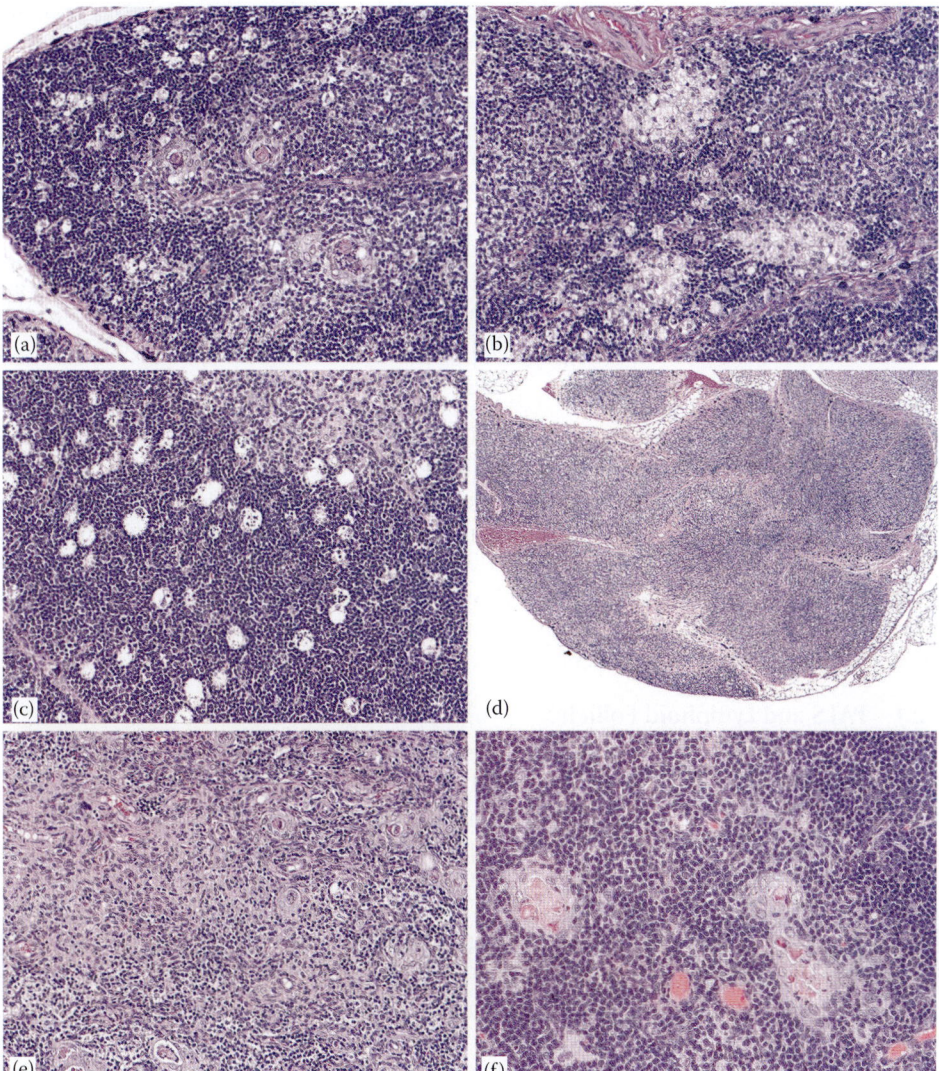

FIGURE 14.4 Thymus from a rat given an immunomodulatory drug at a high dose. Note significant decrease in cortical thickness, decreased cortical cells, and extensive apoptosis resulting in a tattered appearance (a). (b) Higher magnification of a showing numerous tingible-bodied macrophages in the cortex resulting in confluent patches of cell loss and increased cellular debris. (c) Example of less severe apoptosis of cortical cells with many distinct and well-formed tingible-bodied macrophages. (d) Severe loss of cortical cells after repeated dosing of a Sprague–Dawley rat with a potent immunosuppressive compound. Tingible-bodied macrophages were not seen at high magnification. (e) Medulla of a rat thymus with increased visibility of Hassel's corpuscles. (f) Higher magnification of e showing increased keratinization of enlarged Hassel's corpuscles, a change that frequently accompanies the loss of cortical cells regardless of cause.

14.4 SPLEEN

14.4.1 SPLEEN: HISTORICAL PERSPECTIVE

The Functions of the Spleen
(A paper written in October, 1923, and delivered before the Bexar County Medical Society on February 21, 1924.)

At a regular meeting of the Bexar County Medical Society held on October 23rd, 1919, at the suggestion of the author (not specified), the following memorandum was entered in the minutes of the Society: "It has been my good fortune to make a discovery, which, coupled with my experience in malaria, has led me to the following conclusions: That the spleen, which has so long baffled and been a puzzle to the physiologist, is given to man primarily as a defense against malaria. In other words, the spleen contains the defensive agent or hormone hostile to the malarial parasite, which enables it, first, to resist the initial invasion, thus accounting for immunization; and, second, to resist the influence of the continued residence of the parasite in the body."

We have come a long way from relegating the spleen solely to the defense against malaria, and we now appreciate the spleen's central role in immunological defense, but we have also come to recognize that there are functional variations that are reflective of structural differences.

14.4.2 Spleen: White Pulp

The identification and histological evaluation of the white pulp compartments consisting of periarteriolar lymphoid sheaths (PALSs), primary and secondary lymphoid follicles, marginal zone (MZ), and mantle zone are essential but can be challenging in the evaluation of the spleen (Figure 14.6a and c). Nevertheless, a careful comparison of treated versus control animals, with accurate characterization of the relative size and cellularity of the PALSs, the size and maturation of lymphoid follicles, the presence or absence of the MZ cells, and the relative number of smaller lymphoid aggregates scattered throughout the spleen can assist in understanding the specific immunological impact of a test article.

14.4.2.1 PALS and Lymphoid Follicles

The classical description of the white pulp focuses on the PALS with its dense accumulation of CD3+ lymphocytes that extend along central arteries accompanied by lymphoid follicles, which blend with the PALS at the bifurcation of central arterioles (see Figure 14.5c). The white pulp is most obvious and extensive in the mouse but lacks the clear anatomical organization and demarcation seen in rat white pulp, and while both species have clearly developed PALS, the lymphoid follicles can be difficult to identify in mice versus rats (Ward et al. 1999). The PALSs have a T-cell–dependent inner zone that consists mostly of CD4+ T-cells accompanied by low numbers of CD8+ T-cells and interdigitating DCs, whereas the darker H&E staining outer PALS is made up of small T-cells, B cells, macrophages, and occasional plasma cells (Van Rees et al. 1996). The white pulp of the dog spleen has less distinctive PALS structures as compared to that of the rat spleen (Figure 14.5d), which is limited to scattered lymphoid follicles of various sizes. The spleen in nonhuman primates appears similar to that of dogs, with the exception of a greater number of lymphoid follicles, which in some cases can be large, irregular, and bizarre (Figure 14.5e and f).

14.4.2.2 Marginal Zone, Mantle Zone, and Marginal Sinus

Three components of the splenic white matter that may be confusing when comparing species include the mantle zone or corona, the marginal sinus, and the MZ. The mantle zone is a ring of darkly staining small lymphocytes that surround the germinal centers of secondary follicles in dogs, nonhuman primates, and humans (Sternberg 1997), whereas, in rats, the mantle zone is poorly identifiable or lacking and, as a result, is often not mentioned in rodent literature (Figure 14.6a). In those species that have one, the mantle zone is then surrounded by the medium-sized lymphocytes of the MZ (Figure 14.6c). In rats, the follicle is separated from the MZ by a distinct marginal sinus. A marginal sinus is not visible in humans, mice, dogs, or nonhuman primates by standard microscopy (Cesta 2006b; Han et al. 1997).

The MZ, an insufficiently appreciated lymphoid compartment of the spleen, is a highly ordered and functionally distinct region consisting of a reticular network and the termination of splenic arteries that separates the red pulp from PALS and follicles. The MZ is composed primarily of B cells and MZ macrophages (MZMs). MZMs are located at the outer side of the MZ, and a second

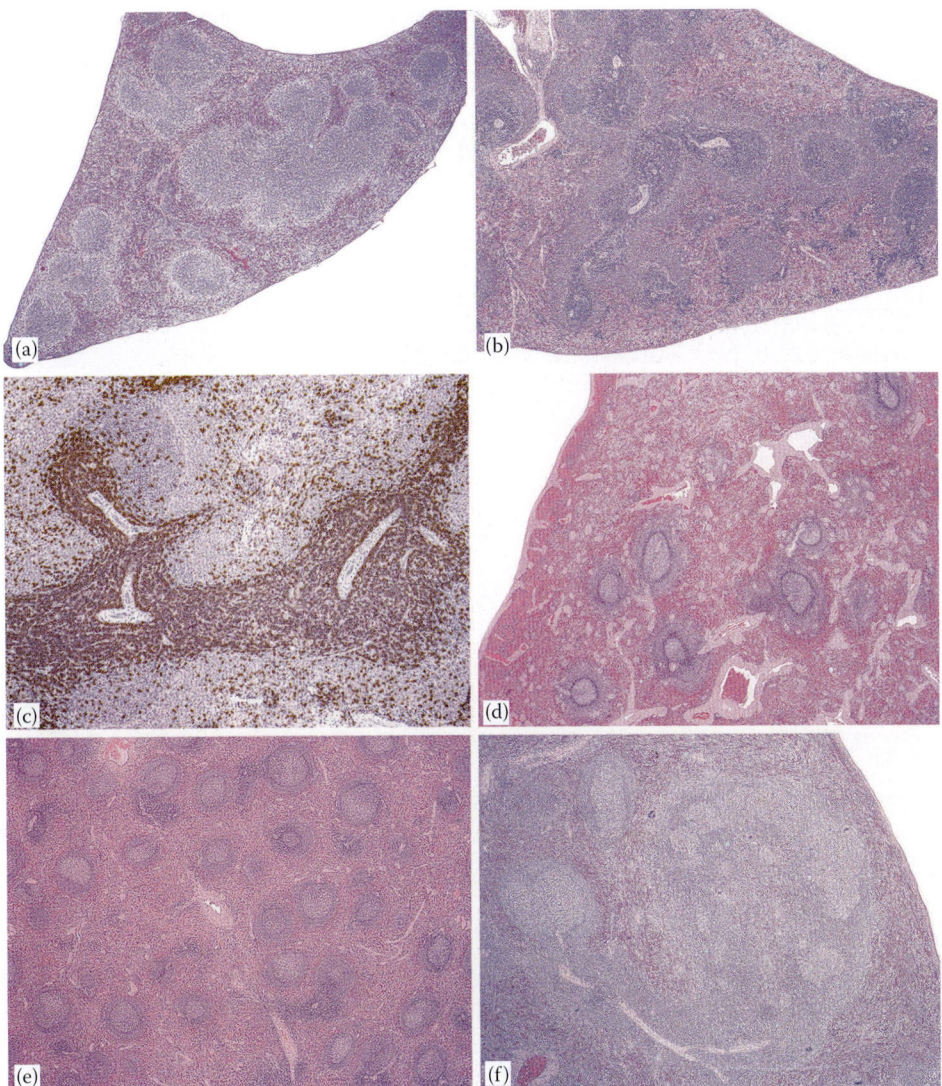

FIGURE 14.5 (a) Spleen from a control mouse showing extensive white pulp with poorly delineated follicles and indistinct margins between red and white pulp. (b) Normal rat spleen with well-developed and sharply delineated white pulp (PALS, lymphoid follicles) of a defensive spleen. (c) Higher magnification of a rat spleen showing abundant CD3+ cells located in the PALS. Distinct but unstained lymphoid follicle can be seen arising from a branch of the PALS. (d) Spleen from a normal dog showing less developed white pulp in comparison to the rat and greater muscular trabeculae consistent with a storage spleen. (e) Defensive spleen of an NHP with well-developed lymphoid follicles but without distinct PALS. (f) Spleen from a control purpose-bred cynomolgus monkey showing large, well-developed secondary follicles and an irregular large and complex lymphoid follicle with an extensive germinal center. Such complex lymphoid nodules are not infrequently encountered in purpose-bred cynomolgus monkeys. The secondary follicles show a distinct mantle (corona) and MZ like that described in man.

specialized macrophage, the marginal metallophilic macrophage (MMM), is found at the inner side of the MZ (Guo et al. 2007). The MZ may become prominent in aging rats because of lymphoid atrophy, histiocytosis, plasmacytosis, or reticuloendothelial hyperplasia (Losco 1992).

Through a sequence of complex steps, bone marrow cells committed to the B-cell lineage translocate to the spleen, become transitional B cells, and then mature into either follicular B cells or, while still in red pulp venules, into MZ B precursors (MZP). These MZP cells then migrate to the

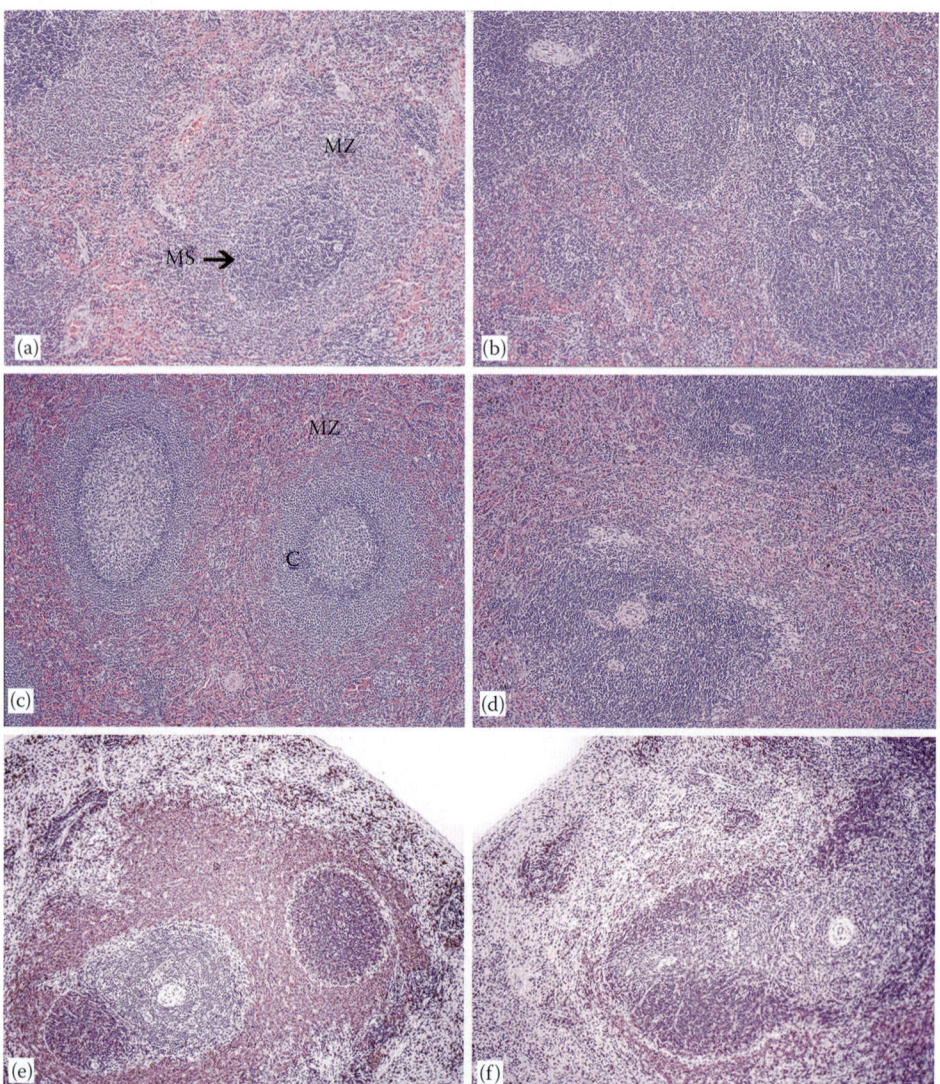

FIGURE 14.6   Labeled images of the spleen of a rat (a) and a cynomolgus monkey (c) show the MZ (MZ), marginal sinus (MS), mantle or corona (C), and red pulp (RP). (b and d) Loss of MZ in both species after dosing with a potent immunomodulatory drug. (e) (control) and (f) (treated) use CD20 staining for B cells to confirm the selective effects on B cells observed in (a) and (b).

MZ where, depending on subsequent signaling, they develop into MZ B cells (Feng et al. 2007; Pillai and Cariappa 2009). The marginal B cells in rodents are identified as being IgD⁻ and IgM⁺, whereas follicular B cells are IgD⁺ and IgM⁺ (Van Rees et al. 1996). In contrast to follicular B cells that recirculate and home to B-cell follicles in secondary lymphoid organs, MZ B cells are a relatively sessile population that do not recirculate, but can be induced to migrate into the white pulp, and transition to lymphoid follicles after exposure to bacterial products, such as lipopolysaccharide (LPS). In this manner, the MZ B cells contribute to natural immune responses and act primarily in initial antibody responses against blood-borne antigens (Martin and Kearney 2000). Naïve MZ B cells intrinsically have properties similar to memory cells (Pillai and Cariappa 2009). MZMs are known to participate in the clearance of microorganisms and viruses and are positive for toll-like receptors (TLRs) (Cesta 2006b). Thus, the lymphocytes in this zone support T-cell–independent humoral immune responses and are vulnerable to the effects of immunomodulatory compounds, including cellular depletion. Malaria and other infections can rapidly deplete MZ B cells of the spleen of mice (Achtman et al. 2003). Marked decreases in the cellularity of MZ lymphocytes have been seen in rodents, NHPs, and dogs following dosing with immunomodulating compounds, but without consistent evidence of immunological compromise (Figure 14.6a through f). Additional work such as that of Guo et al. (2007) is needed to further characterize the function and significance of this frequently impacted lymphoid cell population.

14.4.3 Spleen: Red Pulp

The red pulp in all species is characterized by a three-dimensional meshwork of splenic cords and venous sinuses (Cesta 2006b). The reticular cells and associated fibers, along with macrophages, make up the splenic cords that provide the filtration function of the spleen by trapping effete RBCs and blood-borne particulates. Variable and sometimes considerable amounts of iron pigment (hemosiderin) present in macrophages in the red pulp are indicative of RBC recycling and may increase in conditions of increased RBC removal. Ceroid and lipofuscin are also often encountered within macrophages of the red pulp and within the MZ, especially in NHP. The red pulp is also the location of extramedullary hematopoiesis in rodents. Because of the passage of blood through the red pulp, other circulating cell types can be found therein. In cases of lymphoid depletion, indigenous and/or transient cell populations may become more visible and incorrectly suggest an increase of a particular cell population.

14.4.3.1 Blood Flow and Filtration

The vasculature of the spleen is complicated and demonstrates species differences. Generically, the blood flows in at the hilus and through the spleen via the following sequential steps: splenic artery → trabecular arteries → small arteriole branches → red pulp → central arterioles → small arteriole branches → white pulp capillary beds, with termination at the marginal sinus in the MZ or in the red pulp. Blood moves through the MZ toward the red pulp via penicillar arteries and small arterioles and into either the venous sinuses (90%) or the reticular meshwork, where it encounters macrophages that phagocytize effete RBCs and particulates (Dijkstra and Veerman 1990; Schmidt et al. 1993; Mebius and Kraal 2005). Rats and mice have numerous capillaries in the PALS, while dogs have few. The pig spleen has poorly developed or no sinuses and therefore is considered to be nonsinusal, whereas dogs and rats have a sinusal spleen. True sinusoidal lining cells are lacking in mice (Snook 1950). The venous sinuses of rats are larger and more easily identified than those of mice, which are sometimes referred to as pulp venules (Schmidt et al. 1985).

14.4.4 Spleen: Structure Recapitulates Function

There are three functional variations of splenic architecture, which include defensive, storage, and intermediate types (Banks 1986). While all three forms perform the necessary function of blood filtration, the role of the lymphoid components varies.

14.4.4.1 Defensive Spleen

The defensive type of spleen, best seen in rodents, is characterized by extensive PALS, numerous lymphoid follicles, and a thin capsule and thin trabeculae that have limited contractile capability (Figure 14.5b). The predominantly lymphoid architecture of the defensive spleen reflects a focus on immunologic defense rather than blood filtration or storage and can be found in humans, NHPs, mice, rats, and rabbits (Figure 14.5a, b, and e). Because most bench pathologists will frequently encounter the rat spleen in toxicology studies, consideration of Cesta (2006b) is encouraged for an exceptional and detailed review of the microanatomy of the rodent spleen.

Accessory spleens sometimes referred to as ectopic spleens or splenic nodules are occasionally seen in cynomolgus monkeys. These may be embedded in or attached to the pancreas. Such ectopic spleens have been seen in up to 15% of cynomolgus monkeys used in toxicology studies. Similar structures are seen in humans and have been called "splenculi" and, according to Han et al. (1997), can be found in 25% of human autopsies.

14.4.4.2 Storage Spleen
The storage spleen, as found in dogs, is characterized by the presence of a thick capsule with many trabeculae of well-developed smooth muscle (Figure 14.5d). The smooth muscle allows the spleen to be contractile so that in addition to functioning as a blood filtering organ by trapping and removing effete erythrocytes, it can store up to 1/3 the circulating blood volume and can be rapidly emptied. Lymphoid tissue is comparatively sparse (versus rodents) as indicated by the relatively small PALS and few, poorly formed follicles.

14.4.4.3 Intermediate Spleen
The intermediate type of spleen is characterized by trabecular and lymphoid development intermediate to the other two types and is found in ruminants and swine; however, the spleen of swine shares many traits with that of dogs, both macroscopically and microscopically (Haley 2012). In both species, the spleen is long, narrow, and highly variable in size. It has a thick capsule of interwoven smooth muscle and elastic fibers with a moderate number of similarly heavy muscular trabeculae penetrating deep into the parenchyma. The lymphoid components of the pig spleen have small, less distinct lymphoid follicles as compared to dogs but well-developed PALS. For pigs, branches of pulp arteries identified as sheathed capillaries are derived from the central arteries, and these are surrounded by concentric layers of periarterial macrophage sheaths (ellipsoids) and can be readily seen in the MZ. These can be quite large and numerous. Ellipsoids are also seen in dogs but not rats. As mentioned earlier, the pig spleen has poorly developed or no sinuses and therefore is considered to be nonsinusal. In pigs, there are wisps of smooth muscle throughout the red pulp (Bacha and Wood 1990).

14.4.4.4 Hematopoiesis
The spleen is a major source of hematopoietic activity throughout life in mice as evidenced by large numbers of myeloid and erythroid precursors in the mature mouse spleen. Comparatively, splenic hematopoiesis is much reduced in rats, whereas humans and rabbits have little hematopoietic activity in the embryonic spleen and essentially none in the adult, except under pathologic conditions (Dijkstra and Veerman 1990); however, under conditions of increased demand, the adult rat spleen can significantly increase extramedullary hematopoiesis (EMH) activity. EMH is not seen in larger species such as dogs or NHPs in toxicology studies, even when the bone marrow is a target organ for toxicity (Irons 1991). EMH frequently occurs in rodents, and is more likely seen in younger untreated animals, but is also encountered under conditions of bone marrow toxicity, systemic inflammation, neoplasia, or anemia (Losco 1992).

14.4.4.5 Lymphopoiesis
Lymphopoiesis, as compared to hematopoiesis, is recognized as the major function of the adult spleen in most species (Dellman and Brown 1987), but spleens of humans over the age of 20 only rarely have active germinal centers (Han et al. 1997). In most mammals, lymphocytes produced in the spleen migrate to multiple lymphoid organs and bone marrow. Migration of newly formed lymphocytes from the spleen to bone marrow and to T- and B-cell areas of PPs, lymph nodes, and tonsils, as well as to the intestinal lamina propria and within intestinal epithelium (intraepithelial lymphocytes), has been demonstrated using radiolabeled spleen cells (Pabst and Nowara 1982). Splenic lymphocytes that migrate to bone marrow transform into plasma cells. Bone marrow and spleen receive the largest number of recirculating lymphocytes (Binns and Pabst, 1994). Recirculating lymphocytes enter the spleen by way of marginal sinuses and cross a barrier of sinus lining cells that express MAdCAM-1 (Kraal et al. 1995).

Lastly, it should be pointed out that much of what is known concerning the molecular biology of the spleen has been derived from mice. However, it has been established that humans and mice differ significantly with regard to B-cell populations, including the ontogeny of MZ B cells, and general spleen anatomy. Moreover, even less is known about species differences, other than mice, with regard to such details. Therefore, extrapolating changes in spleen histomorphology to functional outcomes, based on observations of mice, must be done with caution.

14.4.5 SPLEEN: HISTOPATHOLOGY

As for most organs, the spleen has limited morphologic expressions of response to an insult. These include decreased cellularity of the PALS, MZ, and follicles (white pulp), with or without increased apoptosis and tingible-bodied macrophages; increased cellularity (hyperplasia) of the PALS or white pulp; age-related atrophy; fibrosis of the capsule; decreased or increased EMH; infarction; inflammation; and necrosis (Figure 14.7c through e). Other possible histomorphologic changes include amyloidosis (Figure 14.7f), phospholipidosis, lipidosis (adipocyte infiltration), and pigmentation. Recognition of these changes is no different than for other tissues, but a few additional notes are warranted. Hyperplasia of the white pulp may be diffuse, or nodular and marked, resulting in compression of the surrounding tissue. Focal white pulp hyperplasia, also called nodular hyperplasia or lymphohistiocytic (a mixture of lymphocytes and macrophages) hyperplasia, can occur spontaneously in F344 rats or secondary to treatment with xenobiotics (Stefanski et al. 1990).

As indicated above, NHPs have defensive spleens and usually present with many well-formed secondary lymphoid follicles (Figure 14.5e). In some follicles, the centers may contain an amorphous eosinophilic material, possibly a result of persistent antigenic stimulation and the deposition of putative antigen–antibody complexes. It is not uncommon to also observe large and often variably shaped lymphoid follicles with irregular and bizarre germinal centers (Figure 14.5f) that may be the result of chronic parasitic (including malaria), bacterial, or viral infection, which occur in both wild-caught and purpose-bred cynomolgus monkeys (Lowenstine 2003).

A major challenge when evaluating changes in the spleen of any species is that all compartments may sometimes be similarly involved rather than just a single compartment. As a result, the spleen may look histologically similar to controls but appear macroscopically smaller. Careful evaluation of organ weights is beneficial, as in most cases, at least a 25%–35% decrease in organ weight is needed before a histological correlate can be identified in the spleen. Placing the histology slides of both controls and dosed animals side by side on a white piece of paper to make a subgross assessment of the relative size and shape is also helpful, followed by these questions: (1) Are the dosed spleens obviously smaller than those in the controls? (2) Are the edges round or sharp when looking at a cross section? (3) Is the surface concave, flat, or distended (bulging)? Answers to these questions will help to determine if there has been an effect on the spleen and if the effect is focal or diffuse.

Excessive macrophage pigmentation from either hemosiderin (confirmed by Prussian blue staining) or ceroid/lipofuscin (by acid fast staining) should be carefully compared between controls and dosed animals. Focally intense or diffuse nuclear and cellular debris without significant presence of tingible-bodied macrophages is suggestive of direct cellular necrosis (Figure 14.7e).

Splenic weight, especially relative to the brain, is an important component in the analysis for immunotoxicity, and decreased spleen weight has been found to be a reliable indicator of systemic immunotoxicity in rodents, especially when combined with histomorphology. However, in dogs, incomplete exsanguination of the spleen can result in erroneously high spleen weights, making their utility problematic. Incomplete exsanguination can also give the appearance that the lymphoid compartment is depleted, as the abundant RBCs crowd and compress the white pulp. Careful histologic examination can help determine if exsanguination has been complete and if a histological artifact is present that must be accounted for.

The reader is strongly encouraged to review the manuscript by Suttie (2006) for excellent photographic examples of spleen lesions of rodents and for additional descriptions and discussion.

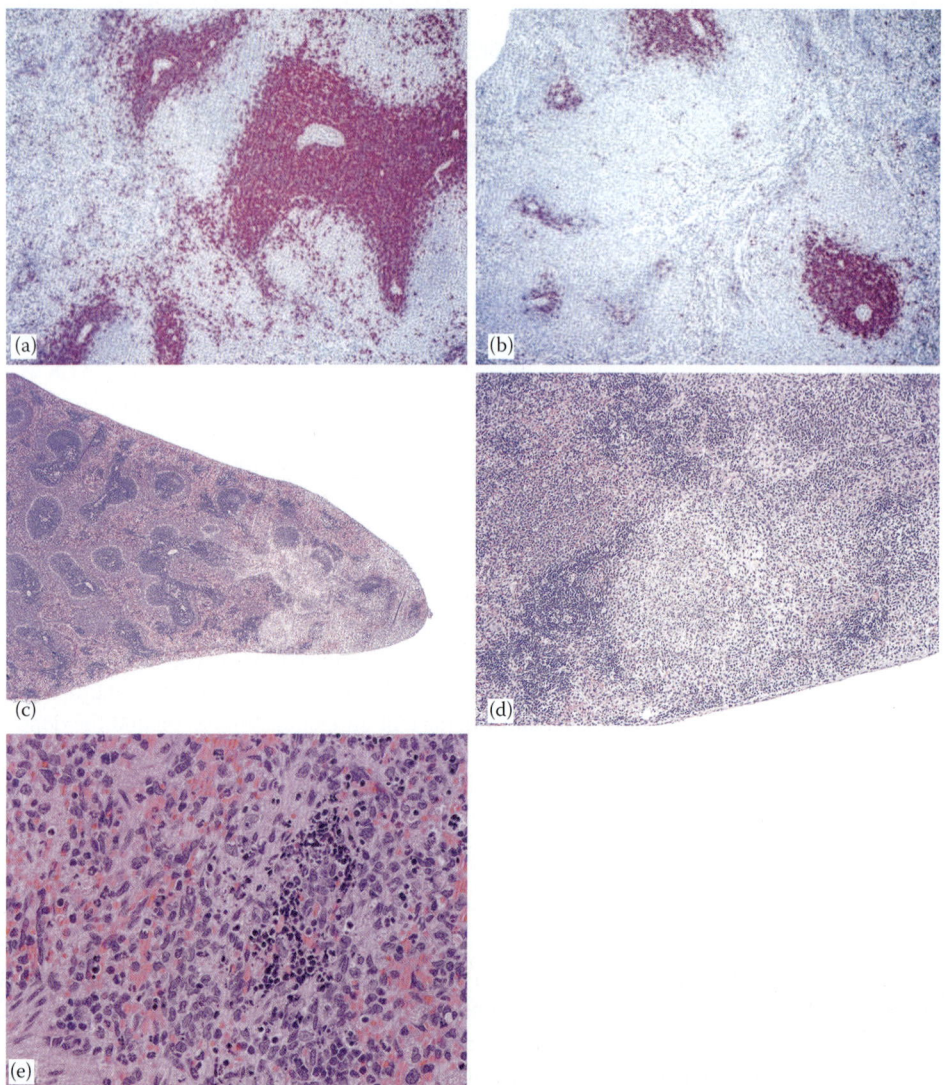

FIGURE 14.7 Rat spleen showing CD3 staining of PALS (a) that is markedly decreased (b) following treatment with an immunosuppressive compound. (c) Example of splenic infarction and localized necrosis. (d) Higher magnification of (c). (e) Small area of discrete cellular necrosis in a spleen; note the absence of tingible-bodied macrophages, suggesting that this lesion is necrosis and not apoptosis.

14.5 LYMPH NODES

14.5.1 LYMPH NODES: HISTORICAL PERSPECTIVE

Lymph glands (lymphoglandulæ): "The lymph glands are small oval or bean-shaped bodies, situated in the course of lymphatic and lacteal vessels so that the lymph and chyle pass through them on their way to the blood.... The stream of lymph in its passage through the lymph sinuses is much retarded by the presence of the reticulum, hence morphological elements, either normal or morbid, are easily arrested and deposited in the sinuses. Many lymph corpuscles pass with the efferent lymph stream to join the general blood stream" (Gray 1918).

14.5.2   LYMPH NODES: STRUCTURE AND SPECIES DIFFERENCES

Classical biomedical anatomy suggests that lymph nodes of all species are similar to that of mice and can be characterized as being relatively simple, bean-shaped, and uniform, with a peripherally located, continuous cortex that surrounds the medulla (Job 1915; Dunn 1954; Ioachim 1994). Over the years, there have been changes in the perception of lymph nodes from being small universally simple structures, such as the description of the mouse lymph node, to nodes that display a significant range of distinctly different architectures that vary within an animal and across species. Therefore, while the basic premises of nodal histomorphology and function might remain the same for lymph nodes in general, the pathologist must be prepared to factor in a number of variables depending on which specific lymph nodes are examined as well as the age, species, and strain of animals from which the nodes are collected. An accurate knowledge of the number, location, and anatomy of draining lymph nodes and their regional lymphatics is essential to accurately assess potential xenobiotic damage to the lymphoid system.

In comparison to other species, the lymph nodes of mice are relatively few (approximately 22) and organized into simple chains (Dunn 1954). Conversely, as species get larger, lymph nodes become more numerous (approximately 450 in humans) and are organized into more complex chains that individually drain proportionately smaller areas of tissue. For example, the lung of rats is drained by two posterior mediastinal nodes (Tilney 1971), while in dogs, this is achieved by three to five tracheobronchial nodes (Hare 1975) and in humans, 35 or more tracheobronchial nodes separated into five groups.

The increased number of smaller nodes in larger species is accompanied by an increased number of anastomoses of afferent lymphatic vessels within lymph node chains compared to that in smaller species. Sainte-Marie et al. (1982) have shown that this difference in degree of lymphatic anastomosis translates into a fundamental difference in the processing of particles or antigens delivered to a node. The rat, having a relative lack of lymphatic anastomoses, translocates small amounts of material to subportions of the node, rather than the entire node. Extensive anastomosis of lymphatic channels in larger species results in the mixing of lymph arising from a specific site that culminates in lymph nodes with a more uniform drainage pattern and simultaneous exposure of more nodal compartments to the lymph.

Elegant work by Bélisle and Sainte-Marie (1981a,b,c) has delineated the complexities of lymph nodes wherein, while some nodes have a continuous subcapsular sinus and peripheral cortex, most have highly variable segmentation by extension of the medullary sinus into the subcapsular sinus. Understanding this variability is key to recognizing the limitations of histologic examination in identifying subtle alterations in lymph nodes following test article administration. Bélisle and Sainte-Marie were the first to describe "functional complexes" within the node that are composed of semirounded structures with a dense lymphocyte population in the center surrounded by a loose population of lymphocytes, reticulum network, postcapillary venules, and lymphatic sinuses. These complexes may be single or multiple and fused into large units composed of multiple follicles with a single expansive bulge of lymphocytes that extends into the medullary space and essentially constitutes the paracortical zone (Figure 14.8a through d). Lymph nodes from mice, guinea pigs, hamsters, rabbits, dogs, and humans share similar tridimensional architecture (Bélisle and Sainte-Marie 1981d), but in larger species, there is an increase in the number of functional units rather than an increase in the size of individual units. Thus, the microscopic complexity seen in large versus small animals recapitulates what is seen grossly.

Variation of lymph node microanatomy can be seen within an individual depending on the location of the node (i.e., central versus peripheral) and among animals within the same species. The conditions under which laboratory animals are maintained impact the appearance of lymph nodes as those from specific pathogen-free (SPF) rats and mice display the architecture of a resting node with small numbers of primary follicles and few secondary follicles (Figure 14.9a) as compared to larger species. Exceptions to this are nodes that drain tissues with high exposure to external

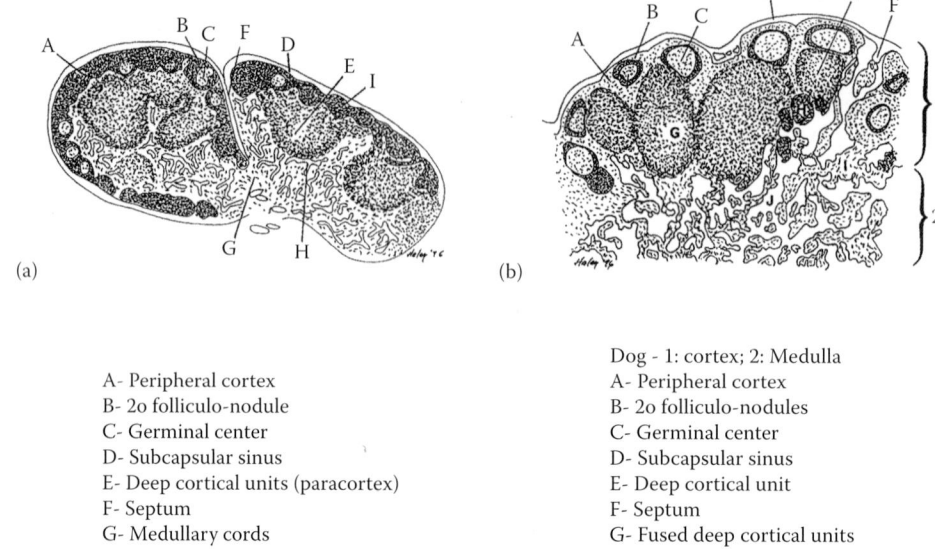

A- Peripheral cortex
B- 2o folliculo-nodule
C- Germinal center
D- Subcapsular sinus
E- Deep cortical units (paracortex)
F- Septum
G- Medullary cords
H- Medullary sinuses

Dog - 1: cortex; 2: Medulla
A- Peripheral cortex
B- 2o folliculo-nodules
C- Germinal center
D- Subcapsular sinus
E- Deep cortical unit
F- Septum
G- Fused deep cortical units
H- Small 1o folliculo-nodule
I- Medullary cords

(c)

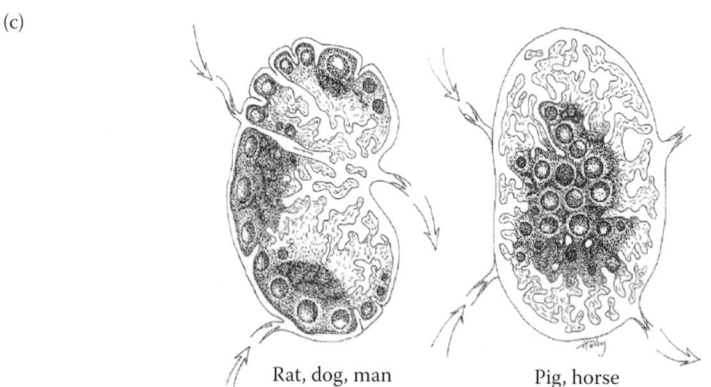

FIGURE 14.8 Stylized drawing of the microscopic anatomy of lymph nodes from rat (a) and dog (b). Note similarity of deep cortical units. (c) Diagram showing the anatomical difference of nodes of swine from dogs and rats. Note the centrally located cortical tissue in the lymph node of swine.

microbes and pathogens, such as the mandibular and mesenteric nodes, and as a result, frequently contain large secondary follicles with germinal centers together with wider medullary cords filled with plasma cells (e.g., mandibular nodes; Figure 14.9b), accompanied by sinuses filled with macrophages (sinus histiocytosis, e.g., mesenteric nodes; Figure 14.9c and d). The peripheral lymph nodes of normal dogs maintained in kennels or in cages usually have numerous, well-developed secondary follicles with large, reactive germinal centers that may extend into the deep cortex. Likewise, NHPs often have large numbers of well-developed germinal centers throughout their lymph nodes. Age-related variations in all species, including humans, can be profound as the node atrophies and become replaced by fibrous connective tissue and fat. Residual hematopoietic activity can be found in rodent but not human, dog, or NHP lymph nodes.

Remarkable variability can be encountered when sampling the same node from different animals. It is this variability that continues to challenge the anatomic pathologist when attempting to

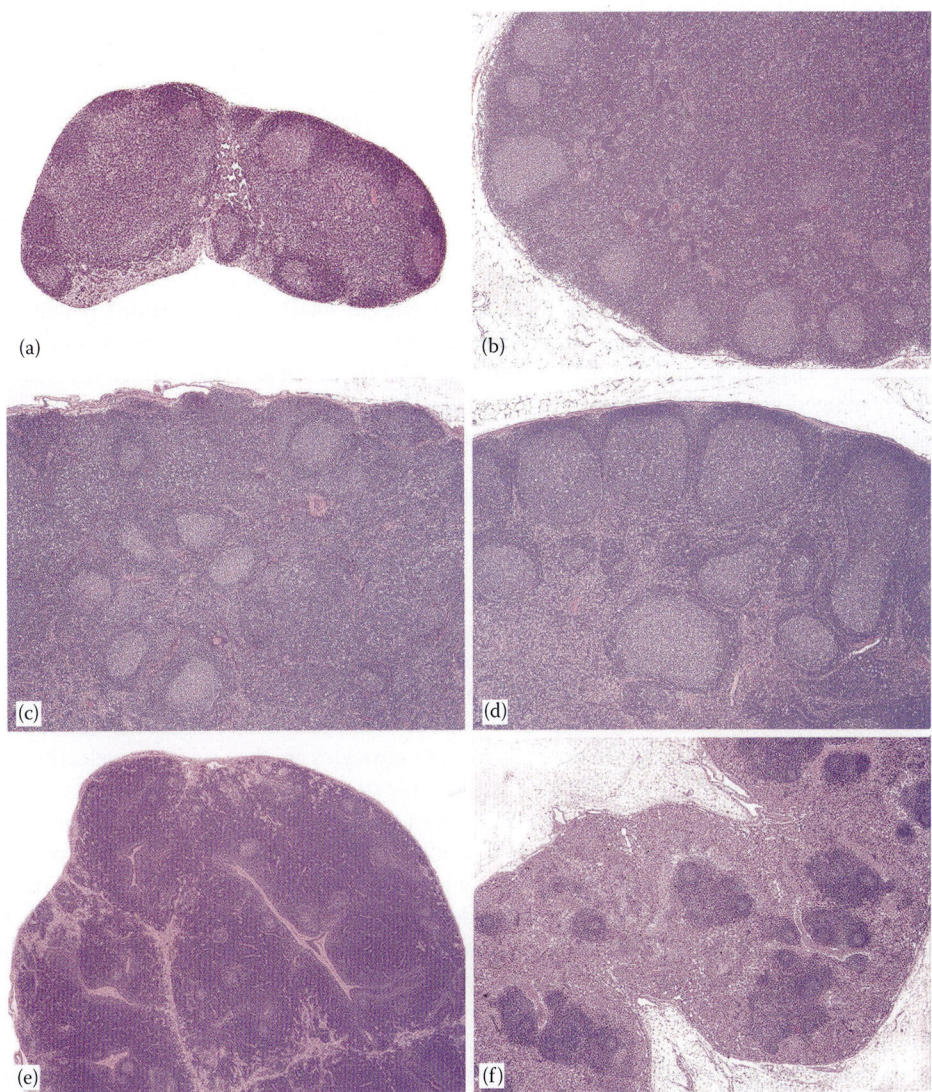

FIGURE 14.9 (a) Mandibular lymph node of a CD-1 mouse. (b) Mandibular node from an SD rat. (c) Mandibular node from purpose-bred beagle dog. (d) Mesenteric node of a purpose-bred cynomolgus monkey. Note numerous and large lymphoid follicles in each of the species that is characteristic of a lymph node draining mucosal sites. (e) Mandibular lymph node from a Sinclair miniature swine. Node is almost entirely composed of cortical tissue with only a small rim of medullary tissue immediately under the capsule. (f) Section of a mesenteric lymph node from control Sinclair miniature swine showing small centrally located islands of cortical tissue. Surrounding medullary sinuses and cords are filled with macrophages.

determine test article–induced changes to specific lymph nodes. This inherent structural variability can be further exaggerated by variable collection and sectioning techniques (Haley 2008). Stepwise serial sections through a node can reveal areas of markedly different proportions of cortex and medulla. Careful judgment is needed when an inadequate piece of lymph node is collected and recuts do not improve section quality. To determine the significance of diminished lymph node tissue, it is helpful to consider the histomorphology of other lymphoid tissues in the same animal.

In swine, there is an anatomical reversal of the classical cortical and medullary components in lymph nodes (Dellmann and Brown 1987). The paracortical T-cell–dependent areas and the lymphoid follicles with their B cell–dependent areas are located centrally within the node, whereas the medullary sinusoids and cords tend to be located peripherally (Figure 14.9e and f). However, even this presentation is highly variable, and medullary sinusoids may penetrate irregularly into the center or occupy the majority of one pole of the node. In pigs, lymph usually flows into the node centrally and leaves the node through efferent vessels located on the capsular surface.

14.5.3   Lymphoid Follicle: Functional Anatomical Dynamics

The cortex of the lymph node contains lymphoid follicles designated as primary and secondary follicles. Primary follicles are distinct, rounded aggregates of small, densely staining lymphocytes. The presence of secondary follicles, heralded by the formation of germinal centers composed of immunoblasts (large, pale-staining, activated B lymphocytes), indicates that antigen has been presented by antigen-presenting cells such as follicular DCs (FDCs) or T lymphocytes. Subsequent mitoses and differentiation into plasma cells or small memory B lymphocytes ensue. The memory B lymphocytes ultimately locate to the mantle zone of secondary follicles and are long lived. T lymphocytes migrate to and locate in the paracortical zone of the node, while the remaining cortical cells are predominantly B lymphocytes. The medullary cords are composed of packed lymphocytes and numerous plasma cells. Around the cords are medullary sinuses that join efferent lymphatic vessels that conduct lymph away from the node.

When examining a lymphoid follicle, it is possible to clearly identify the light zone composed of large, light-staining centrocytes and FDCs, the dark zone composed of darkly stained centroblasts, and the surrounding mantle zone composed of small, dark B lymphocytes. The Ig variable genes of centroblasts diversify by somatic hypermutation, exit the cell cycle, and re-express B-cell receptors as they become centrocytes located in the light zone. Centrocytes are then subject to selection based on the ability to bind antigens presented by FDC. Centrocytes with low-level affinity pass back into the dark zone and undergo apoptosis, whereas higher-affinity cells survive in the germinal center and differentiate and proliferate into antibody-forming cells and memory B cells. Background low-grade apoptosis of lymphocytes with a starry-sky appearance occurs most frequently in the dark zone of the follicle in resting lymph nodes, but as demand increases for antibody production, greater cell turnover, accompanied by tingible-bodied macrophages in the pale germinal center, becomes apparent. B-cell maturation and differentiation result in the formation of early-stage plasma cells, which translocate to the medullary cords where, after further maturation, they produce and release antibodies.

As described in the section on the thymus, T-cells originate in the bone marrow and migrate to the thymus, where they undergo a series of complex maturational steps that culminate in the release of mature T-cells. These T-cells locate within secondary lymphoid organs, such as lymph nodes, where they participate in both cell-mediated and humoral-mediated immune responses. However, once in the lymph node, the functional dynamics of T-cells are not as morphologically obvious as those of the B cells described above. T-cells enter the lymph node either from the vasculature via high endothelial venules (HEVs) or from locally draining lymph via afferent lymphatics. A thorough description of the role of HEV in lymph node dynamics is beyond the scope of this chapter, and the reader is encouraged to review Gretz et al. (2000), Ohtani et al. (2003), and Yang et al. (2007). Once in the node, T-cells migrate to the interfollicular cortical areas or to the paracortex, where they encounter antigen-presenting DCs. DCs actively sample antigen at distant sites, that is, the skin, and translocate to regional lymph nodes where they seek out and present antigen to T-cells within the paracortex (Basketter et al. 1999).

14.5.4   Lymph Nodes: Histopathology

As mentioned, the lymph node has a limited number of morphologic expressions associated with either functional activity or disease states, and these include increased or decreased lymphocytes, inflammation, necrosis, apoptosis, and neoplasia. Remember that many of the changes identified in lymph nodes in toxicology studies reflect normal function and not pathology per se such as follicular hyperplasia, sinus histiocytosis, sinus erythrocytosis, or accumulation of particulates (Losco and Harlemen 1992). A commonly encountered change in lymph nodes is RLH. RLH can be specific (e.g., antigen driven by viruses or bacteria) or nonspecific (e.g., driven by chemical pollutants, particulates, or tissue damage) and can display complex changes involving one, several, or all of its anatomic subunits and thereby display a follicular, sinus, diffuse, or mixed pattern (Ioachim 1994). RLH may involve one or more resident cell populations and/or migrating cell populations and can be indicative of not only local lesions but also systemic conditions. Peripheral lymph nodes draining cutaneous or mucosal sites such as the mandibular or popliteal nodes, as compared to deeper lymph nodes (e.g., hepatic), will often show marked RLH as a response to exposure to either antigens or nonspecific irritants encountered through the skin and/or mucocutaneous surfaces. Not surprisingly, RLH, especially involving peripheral nodes, is more often encountered in larger outbred animals that are not kept under SPF conditions. Because cage sores and pododermatitis are often encountered in caged beagles, inflammatory infiltrates and RLH of the popliteal and/or axillary nodes are not uncommon (Kovacs et al. 2005). Follicular hyperplasia, as indicated by increased size and number of secondary lymphoid follicles, is suggestive of a humoral immune response. Highly enlarged and coalescing lymphoid follicles may be seen following prolonged antigen stimulation and are not infrequent in dogs or in NHPs. Diffuse lymphoid hyperplasia can result in the loss of clear delineation of nodal architecture and is commonly associated with viral lymphadenitides (Ioachim 1994).

Mixed granulomatous and pyogranulomatous lesions can be seen in cases of bacterial, fungal, or parasitic infection/infestation of lymph nodes with part or all of the nodal architecture being effaced and/or destroyed by the inflammatory response. Translocation of microbes or parasites such as demodectic mites in dogs can result in severe destructive changes to the afferent lymphatics and regional draining lymph node, including but not limited to abscess formation, diffuse suppurative inflammation, or pyogranulomatous and/or granulomatous inflammation. Granulomatous inflammation in this context may be localized and sometimes nodular with accumulation of enlarged and frequently epithelioid macrophages (with or without multinucleated giant cells) within the stroma and medullary cords of the lymph node. This should not be confused with sinus histiocytosis, which is the accumulation of vacuolated/foamy-appearing macrophages within sinusoids, and is considered a normal finding for mesenteric lymph nodes (Elmore 2006); however an increase in incidence and severity can indicate a treatment effect by a test article. Plasma cell hyperplasia of the medullary cords can accompany any of these patterns but can also be present independently as often observed in the mandibular node of rodents.

Amyloidosis characterized by the accumulation of a homogenous pale eosinophilic material in the subcapsular sinus and paracortex of mice (especially CD-1) and on rare occasions in NHP can be confirmed with congo red stain. Amyloidosis is a systemic condition, and other tissues such as the spleen may also contain similar deposits. Amyloidosis is rare in purpose-bred beagle dogs but may be associated with juvenile polyarteritis including involvement of the spleen (Snyder et al. 1995). Its presence in mice is genetically driven, but in NHPs, chronic antigen–antibody responses and/or chronic inflammation are suspected.

During a review of lymph nodes in beagle dogs by this author, large numbers of eosinophils were identified in the peripheral (mandibular, axillary, popliteal), but not central (mesenteric, hepatic), lymph nodes. The basis for this specific distribution of eosinophils is presumed to be clinically silent, demodectic mange mite infestation that is common in most dogs, including purpose-bred beagle dogs. In fact, occasional demodectic mange mite granulomas have been identified in the peripheral nodes of control dogs with no clinical evidence of demodicosis. Thus, the eosinophil infiltrates within peripheral nodes reflect the functional aspect of a regional draining node and are not an indication of nodal pathology per se (i.e., eosinophilic lymphadenitis). Recording the observation as "eosinophil, infiltrate, *severity*, *designated* node" with a short discussion in the pathology narrative is appropriate to place such observations in the proper context.

In each case, it is best to describe the changes as specifically as possible with regard to the compartment involved, such as "decreased cells or decreased lymphocytes, cortex" if the change is limited to the cortex or "decreased cells, lymphoid follicles, cortex" if the follicles are clearly involved (Webb et al. 2010). If all compartments are similarly affected, it is acceptable to simply describe "decreased, lymphocytes, generalized, lymph node (location)" (Figure 14.10b and d).

Even when the overall cellularity of a node appears to be within normal limits at low magnification, lymph nodes need to be examined at high magnification so as to confirm that the normal resident cells have not been replaced by other cells but without disturbance of the usual anatomy. Just as in the previous example with eosinophils in canine lymph nodes, if a lymph node contains increased numbers of neutrophils, it is important to determine if they are present because of migration from a

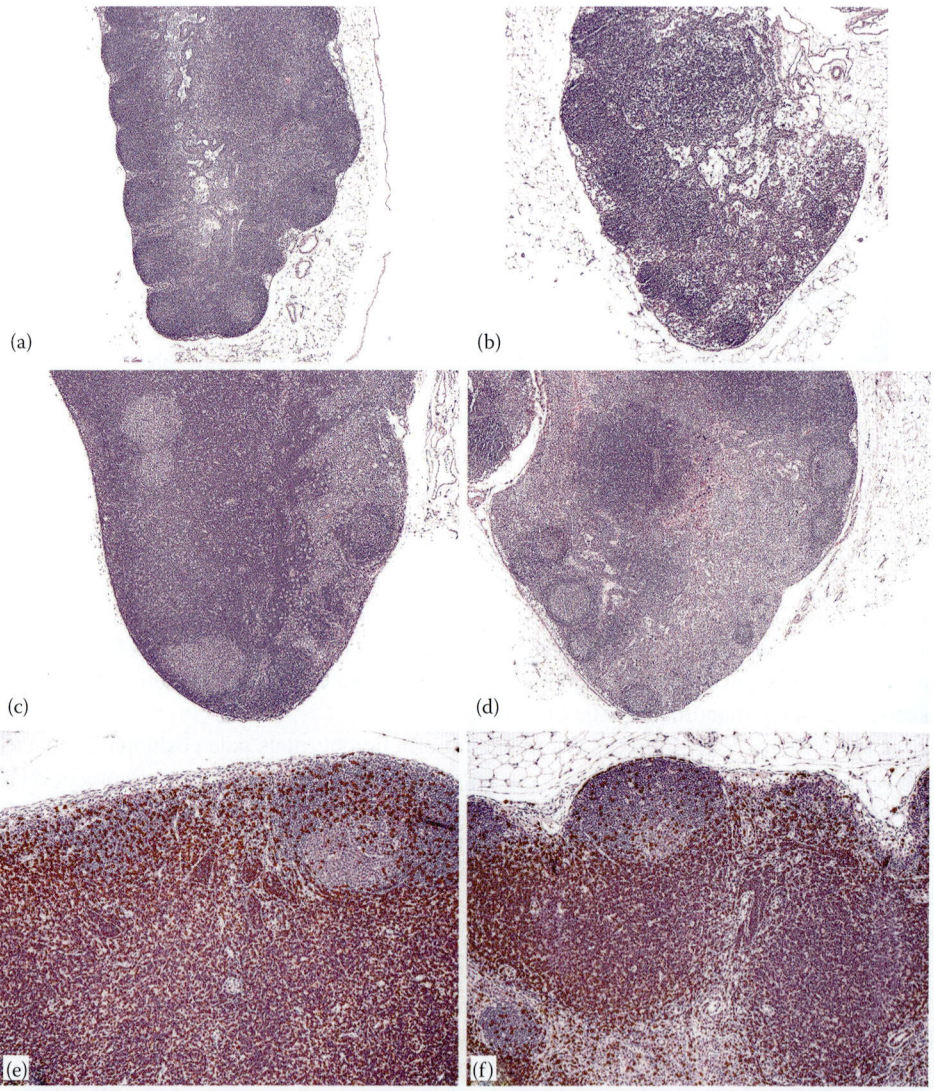

FIGURE 14.10 Images of rat mesenteric (b) and mandibular (d) lymph nodes that show generalized loss of lymphocytes from all compartments following exposure to a potent immunosuppressive compound in the same study. Their respective controls are shown in (a) and (c) and provide a reference for the magnitude and extensiveness of the cellular loss. (e) shows extensive CD3+ staining of cortical and paracortical lymphocytes in a control rat that is markedly diminished after dosing with the same immunosuppressive compound (f).

site of other tissue inflammation, or because of active inflammation of the node itself, or both. The identification of active necrosis and/or microorganisms within the node is conclusive proof that the node is directly involved.

14.6 MUCOSAL-ASSOCIATED LYMPHOID TISSUE

A central component of the lymphoid system, both functionally and anatomically, is the mucosal-associated lymphoid tissue (MALT). MALT is composed of dispersed aggregates of nonencapsulated lymphoid tissue within the mucosa that are essential in maintaining local immune responses at mucosal surfaces and are functionally integrated to form the common mucosal immune system. MALT has numerous subcomponents, the most predominant being the BALT, the NALT, and the GALT. Additional representatives of MALT include conjunctiva-associated lymphoid tissue (CALT), larynx-associated lymphoid tissue (LALT), and salivary duct–associated lymphoid tissue (DALT), with more being added to the list as thorough morphological and functional evaluations continue (Cesta 2006a).

Cesta (2006a) describes how MALT can be further subdivided based on functional attributes of being either inductive sites (sites of MALT that show IgA class switching and B-cell expansion and T-cell activation) or effector sites that receive B and T-cells derived from inductive MALT. At effector sites of MALT, secretory IgA molecules are linked by J-chains to a secretory component that is then released across mucosal epithelium (Pabst 1987).

The histomorphology of the BALT, GALT, and NALT shares anatomic and functional attributes that include distinct lymphoid follicles, interfollicular areas, a subepithelial dome, and an overlying follicle-associated epithelium (FAE or lymphoepithelium), with or without M cells or microfold cells (Figure 14.11a and b). M cells are responsible for sampling luminal antigen from the mucosal surface and transferring it to antigen-presenting cells within the lymphoid tissue. Other than M cells and FAE, MALT is home to the typical cells of other lymphoid tissues, including B cells, CD4+ and CD8+ T-cells, and DCs. MALT does not have afferent lymphatics, but HEVs are present.

14.6.1 Bronchus-Associated Lymphoid Tissue

BALT was initially described by Bienenstock et al. (1973a,b) as organized bronchial lymphoid aggregates or follicles that are morphologically similar to other components of MALT. BALT is located within the bronchial submucosa of rabbits, rats, guinea pigs, mice, dogs, pigs, chickens, and humans, often at the bifurcations of airways. Pabst and Gehrke (1990) have found that not all species have significant amounts of BALT. They suggest that rabbits and rats have the most BALT, mice and guinea pigs have an intermediate amount, while humans have little to none. The refinement of SPF conditions has resulted in marked decreases in BALT of normal healthy rodents, and as a result, the BALT in rodents is limited and difficult to consistently collect using routine methods.

14.6.2 Nasal-Associated Lymphoid Tissue

NALT is defined as focal submucosal aggregates of lymphoid cells within the nasal cavity. Similar to PPs, NALT has FAE and M cells. Specific surface markers are expressed by M cells that act as antigen sampling sites within the nose (Takata et al. 2000; Jeong et al. 2000). While NALT in rats appears to be restricted to the ventral aspects of the lateral walls at the opening of the nasopharyngeal duct, NALT in NHPs is more prominent and is located on both lateral and septal walls of the proximal nasopharynx (Harkema 1991). The pharyngeal tonsil (adenoid) of humans is part of NALT together with less prominent collections of submucosal lymphoid follicles on the nasopharyngeal surface of the soft palate, in the lateral and posterior wall of the nasopharynx, and around the orifice of the eustachian tube (Mills and Fechner 1997).

The NALT of mice, rats, and hamsters is functionally and structurally similar (Giannasca et al. 1997: Wu and Russell 1997; Asanuma et al. 1997: Asakura et al. 1998; van der Ven and Sminia

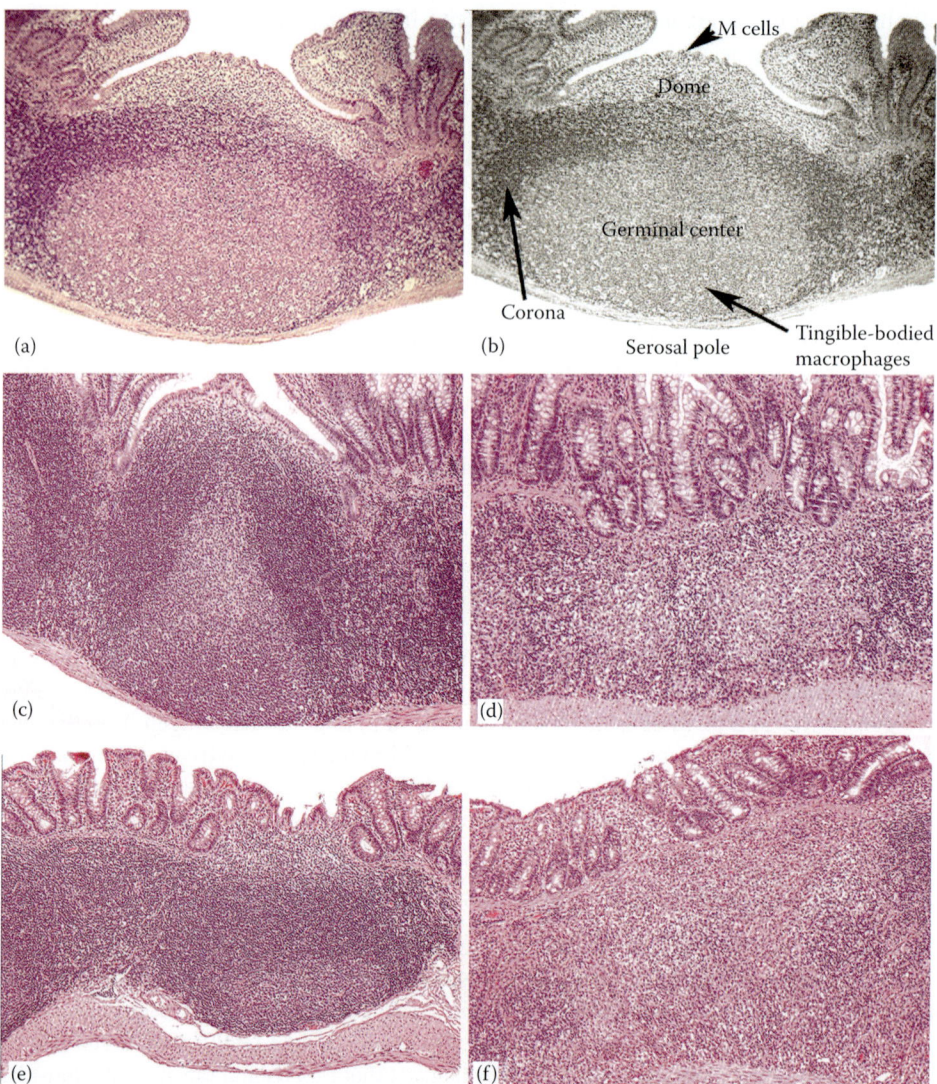

FIGURE 14.11 (a and b) Unlabeled and labeled images of a mouse PP showing the basic structures. (c) PP from a normal rat and shows a very similar structure to that of the mouse; however, while the PPs of mice tend to be either singular or in small patches of 2 or 3, those of the rat tend to be more numerous and extensive. Loss of follicular and interfollicular lymphocytes from a rat PP following dosing with an immunomodulatory compound is seen in (d). (e) Normal-appearing lymphoid nodule in the cecum of a control rat; (f) loss of lymphocytes from a similar cecal lymphoid nodule in a treated rat.

1993; Kuper et al. 1990; Hameleers et al. 1989). NALT is present in normal dogs, and reduction of NALT cellularity has been identified following the nose-only inhalation of corticosteroids by dogs (Nasonex, Summary Basis of Approval for NDA, 20-762, 1997).

14.6.3 GUT-ASSOCIATED LYMPHOID TISSUE

GALT is probably one of the more commonly recognized forms of MALT in laboratory animals. It is characterized by discrete follicles of lymphocytes called PPs located within the mucosa along the free wall of the small intestine, but GALT also includes lymphocytes scattered throughout the lamina propria (LPL), intraepithelial lymphocytes (IEL), cryptopatches in the small intestine, and lymphoglandular complexes in the colon (Figures 14.11 and 14.12). A specialized overlying epithelium (FAE) covers PP and includes M cells (Bockman and Cooper 1973) that actively sample antigen from intestinal luminal contents and transfer antigenic material to lymphoid cells within the follicle (Bockman and Stevens 1977). Approximately 50% of the overlying cells in rabbits are M cells, whereas only 5%–10% of the overlying cells are M cells in rats and humans, the biological significance of which is unknown. Follicular B cells and adjacent T-cell areas lie beneath the FAE.

LPLs are numerous and may be equivalent to the spleen in overall mass. They synthesize IgA and can recirculate back to the point of origin. This underappreciated lymphoid tissue may play a central role in primary mucosal tissue immune defenses and should be carefully inspected especially when evaluating the effects of orally administered novel immunomodulatory compounds (Figure 14.12).

GALT varies in location, size, and appearance depending upon the species, especially PP, but corresponding differences in function have not been determined. For example, the follicles of mice and rats are of uniform size throughout the small intestine, with 6–12 follicles present in an aggregate (Pospischil 1989), whereas those of pigs, dogs, and ruminants have two distinct types of PP. These two types present as discrete patches in the jejunum and upper ileum and as long continuous patches in the terminal ileum. Microbial exposure is not required for growth of jejunal or ileal PP in the pig, and the numbers and size of follicles increase with age, accounting for their increase in the length in the jejunum and ileum. The number of follicles in pigs may reach 75,000 by approximately 1 month of age, with the majority of them located in the ileum. The ileal PPs regress to a few small scattered follicles in older animals (Pabst et al. 1988). The proximal PP of dogs, humans, and rodents are similar in appearance (HogenEsch and Felsburg 1992). Unlike pigs, the presence of bacteria is needed for development of PP in rodents (Cornes 1965). In humans, PP follicles increase in size and number with age until puberty, after which there is a uniform decrease in the number of patches in all parts of the small intestine. Duodenal patches in humans are small and contain few follicles, but follicles increase in size and number distally in the gut, achieving the largest size at the ileocecal valve. At maturity, the terminal ileal PP in humans may contain 900–1000 individual follicles (Cornes 1965).

The PP is the source of IgA-positive lymphocytes. The domes of PP in pigs are devoid of IgA plasma cells, and few IgA-positive cells are found in the PP of humans or rats (Sminia et al. 1983). The domes of the human appendix and the dome region of all dog PPs have many IgG plasma cells, but far fewer are present in the domes of rodent PP (HogenEsch and Felsburg 1992). In rats, both T-cells and IgA-, IgG-, and IgM-positive B cells are present at birth, as are Ia+ cells. The sacculus rotundus is a distinctive hypertrophied PP that encircles the terminal ileum in humans. Both humans and rabbits have a large aggregation of lymphoid nodules at the ileocecal valve called the appendix. While an appendix is absent in mice and rats, these latter species have large aggregations of lymphocytes in the walls of the cecum.

The colon and rectum have many single and aggregate lymphoid nodules that are especially prominent in dogs. Histologic changes in those near the rectum must be interpreted with caution as self-induced trauma and/or pathology of the adjacent anal glands can result in considerable localized damage and inflammation.

14.6.4 GALT: Histopathology

Orally administered immunomodulatory and immunotoxic compounds can have dramatic effects on GALT as indicated by decreased lymphocytes within the interfollicular zone and/or within lymphoid follicles. The presentation of increased numbers of apoptotic cells and tingible body macrophages is similar to that of other lymphoid tissues (Figures 14.11b through e and 14.12a and b). Thorough documentation of such changes to GALT is an important part of characterizing the effects of immunotoxic or immunomodulatory compounds, and every study design should include the identification and collection of PP for histological examination.

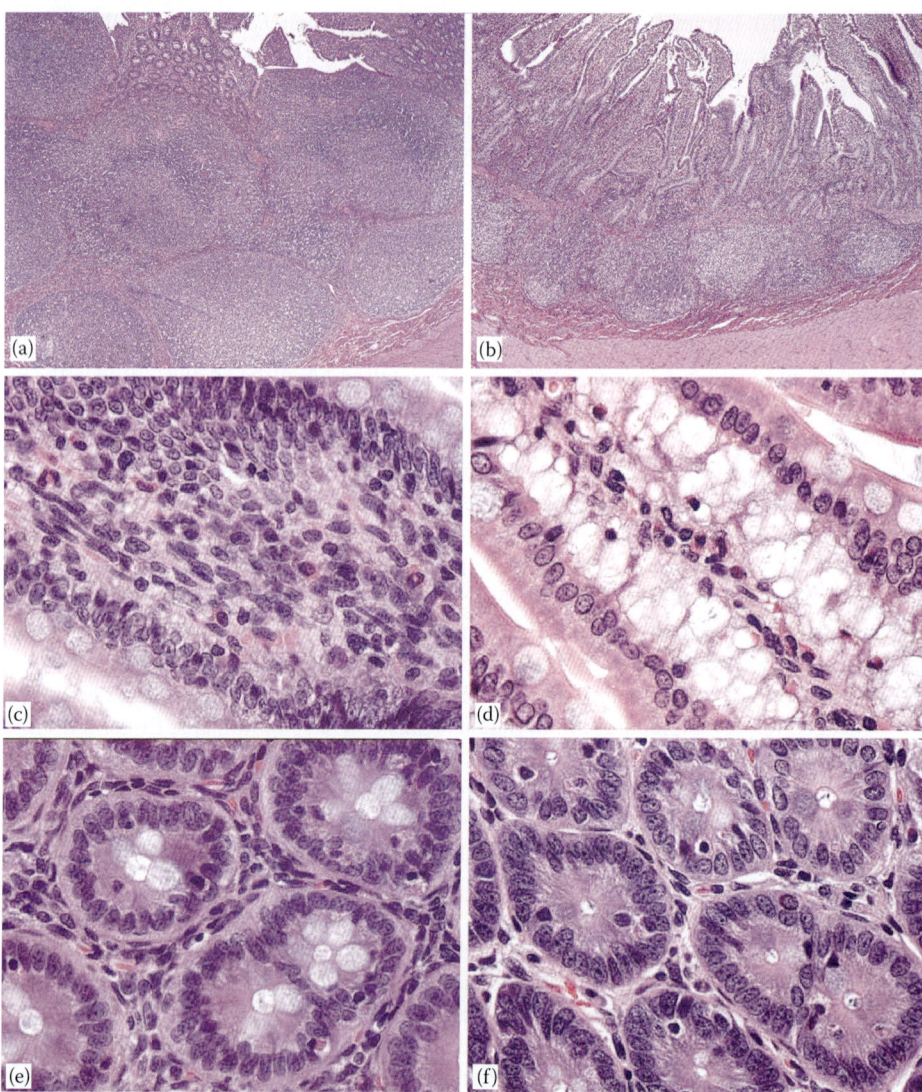

FIGURE 14.12 Large and complex PP of a normal dog is shown in a; marked loss of follicular and interfollicular lymphocytes is seen in b after treatment with the same compound that was given to rats in d. (c) Control SD rat duodenum showing robust numbers of lamina propria lymphocytes (LPLs). (d) Duodenum of a treated rat with loss of LPL after 9 days of dosing with a potent immunosuppressive drug. (e) Cross section of ileum of the same control in c and shows numerous LPLs nestled between villi that are markedly decreased after treatment (f). Changes in LPL are often overlooked when evaluating the impact of systemic immunosuppression.

Decreases in GALT lymphocytes may be associated with the mucosal invasion by opportunistic microbes and/or parasites in dogs and monkeys that, when unchecked, may culminate in overt gastrointestinal pathology, local mucosal erosion and ulceration, and systemic dissemination of pathogens. Even small foci of acute inflammation in PP may allow the entrance of microbes to regional draining mesenteric lymph nodes. In such cases, the mesenteric lymph node should be carefully examined for correlating evidence of inflammation. This is a particular risk for the NHP as captive macaques have a high incidence of chronic gastritis and enterocolitis because of the presence of opportunistic and/or obligate parasites and bacteria. Recurring diarrhea from a number of bacterial species that include *Campylobacter* spp., *Shigella flexneri*, *Yersinia enterocolitica*, adenovirus, and

Strongyloides fuelleborni is the leading cause of NHP morbidity requiring veterinary care (Sestak et al. 2003). Background levels of infestations/infections can be worsened secondary to the stress of being put on study and/or treatment with immunomodulatory compounds. Because the gastro-intestinal submucosa of dogs and NHPs usually has a high background of mixed inflammatory cell infiltrates, it can be very difficult to differentiate between normal levels of background inflammation and early low-grade effects of a test article. Distinct GALT of the stomach (GGALT) may be particularly prominent in dogs and NHP if *Heliobacter* sp. is present (Lowenstine 2003).

14.7 BONE MARROW: LYMPHOPOIESIS

The bone marrow plays a pivotal role in the development and maintenance of immune responses, and it is recommended that it be evaluated in any study testing for immunotoxicity. However, a detailed review of considerable literature on the anatomy and complex biology of the bone marrow is beyond the scope of this chapter. Two excellent references that should be consulted are Travlos (2006a,b). The hematopoietic attributes of the bone marrow are addressed in Chapter 13.

Simply stated, bone marrow is comparable across species. The marrow cavity contains cancellous bony trabeculae that are lined by endosteum, a single layer of cells resting on a delicate layer of reticulum, accompanied by aggregates of osteoclasts and osteoblasts. Microvasculature is obvious within the marrow, but there are no lymphatic channels present. Normally, the marrow has a limited network of fine, branching reticulum fibers located between the parenchyma of erythroid, myeloid, and lymphoid precursors and maturing cell types.

The bone marrow is the site of origin of pluripotent stem cells, which give rise to lymphoid stem cells that then go on to produce B-cell and T-cell progenitors. B cells mature via a sequence of antigen-independent steps within the nurturing microenvironment of the marrow, replete with growth factors and numerous cytokines, after which they are released and migrate to the B-cell zones of the peripheral lymphoid tissues. Bone marrow–derived T-cells and related stem cells are translocated to the thymus, where they also undergo an antigen-independent selection process, surface marker changes, and self-selection deletion steps. They then migrate systemically to T-cell–dependent areas of peripheral lymphoid tissues. T-cells play a role in the maturation and development of erythroid and myeloid precursors via the production and release of burst promoting activity (BPA) and IL-3, along with a variety of colony stimulating factors, including B-cell growth factor, B-cell differentiation factor, and most other interleukins (Travlos 2006a).

While the structure of the bone marrow is generally the same across species, this simplification can lead the unprepared pathologist to misinterpret changes, or lack thereof, in bone marrow specimens. There are histological differences in the appearance of bone marrow depending on the age, species, strain, and specific bone used for the evaluation and the particular bone that is being examined (i.e., femur versus sternum). For example, rodents used in acute and subchronic studies have abundant hematopoietic tissue in the femoral head, femoral shaft, sternum, and rib; however, dogs and nonhuman primates tend to have little hematopoietic tissue in the head of the femur and distal femoral shaft.

The first impression an anatomic pathologist makes during the microscopic evaluation of a bone marrow section is its cellularity or, in the case of toxicity, the lack thereof. Unfortunately, clear differentiation of lymphoid cells from other bone marrow cells using H&E-stained sections is very difficult. Bone marrow toxicities run the gamut of typical tissue lesions that include decreases or increases in all cells or specific cell subtypes, adipocyte infiltration (lipidosis), necrosis, infarction, fibrosis, and hemorrhage. Complicating the determination of compound effects in long-term studies are age-related changes in rat bone marrow that include hyperplastic and atrophic changes, as well as stromal proliferative changes including myelofibrosis, myelosclerosis, fibrosis, osteosclerosis, osteopetrosis, and osseous metaplasia (Stromberg 1992). The amount of lymphopoietic tissue declines noticeably in normal rodents over a 3- to 6-month period, thereby making it mandatory to only use age-matched controls for evaluating xenobiotic-induced alterations. Dogs and NHPs are known to occasionally have variably organized lymphoid aggregates, with and without follicular development, within the bone marrow. It has been suggested that such lymphoid aggregates in NHPs are related to type D retrovirus infection, as is the generalized lymphoid hyperplasia within the spleen that was discussed earlier (Lowenstine 2003). Frith et al. (2000) have described similar lymphoid cell aggregates with well-developed germinal centers in bone marrow of rats given a test article.

Decreases in lymphoid populations of the bone marrow typically parallel and reinforce observations of test article effects in other lymphoid tissues such as the spleen and thymus. Early or low-level decreases in bone marrow cellularity are accompanied by the apparent increase in number and size of adipocytes that are variably accompanied by small, scattered aggregates of apoptotic bodies. However, in addition to direct toxic effects on the marrow (as induced by several cytotoxic antineoplastic agents), decreased cellularity, including the lymphoid compartment, can be seen in conditions of marked decreased caloric intake, chronic inflammation, neoplasia, hypothyroidism, hypoadrenocorticism, and chronic renal or hepatic disease (Travlos 2006b). Outright bone marrow necrosis is seen with severe caloric restriction of 25% of control for at least 2 weeks (Levin et al. 1993), and bone marrow depletion has been reported with cachexia or in severely debilitated animals (MacKenzie and Eustis 1990).

Whenever possible, the anatomic pathologist should make an attempt to identify the affected cell population, whether it is erythroid, myeloid, or lymphoid. Once an effect is apparent, it is recommended that an experienced clinical pathologist perform an evaluation of bone marrow smears to determine the myeloid-to-erythroid ratio as well as for the presence of any cytological abnormalities.

14.8 IMMUNOTOXICANTS VERSUS STRESS, THE HOBGOBLIN OF TOXICOLOGIC PATHOLOGY

Few topics have caused as much confusion and consternation in lymphoid pathology as the differentiation of stress-induced effects from direct lymphoid toxicity. The literature supports the premise that stress-induced endogenous corticosteroid release may drive thymic lymphocyte apoptosis, and it has been suggested that the thymus is the most stress-sensitive organ in the body, with massive thymic lymphocyte death seen as one of the main responses to acute stress (Savino et al. 2002; Pearse 2006a). Chemical, psychological, and physical stressors have all been observed to activate the hypothalamic–pituitary–adrenal axis, culminating in increased levels of endogenous glucocorticoids and subsequent apoptosis of thymic lymphocytes (Crabtree et al. 1979; Tecoma and Huey 1985). Therefore, thymic changes induced by increased endogenous or applied corticosteroids appear to be scientifically valid (Greaves 2000; Everds et al. 2012).

The International Committee of Harmonization (ICH) guidelines stipulate that if alterations of the immune system are thought to be attributable to stress, evidence to support this interpretation must be provided. In addition, the ICH S8 Immunotoxicity Studies for Human Pharmaceuticals guidance states that evidence of immunotoxicity in nonclinical safety assessments may dictate the need for additional evaluations of immunotoxicity. Thus, it is essential to determine if the effects seen are direct immunotoxic effect or indirect stress-related effect.

Hallmarks of stress effects include decreased body weights, decreased feed consumption, decreased thymic weights, increased adrenal gland weights, and increased neutrophils and monocytes accompanied by decreased lymphocytes and eosinophils (stress leukogram). Additional findings that are particularly helpful in identifying stress are clearly identifiable systemic changes or lesions of nonimmune organs that contribute to moribundity. If the animal is showing definitive evidence of systemic toxicity, as described in Figure 14.13a through f, then alterations of the lymphoid histomorphology are likely to be secondary rather than primary effects (Smialowicz et al. 1985). Stress-induced alterations of leukocytes may last for hours to days in nonhuman primates because of their sensitivity to external stimuli and conditions (Everds et al. 2012).

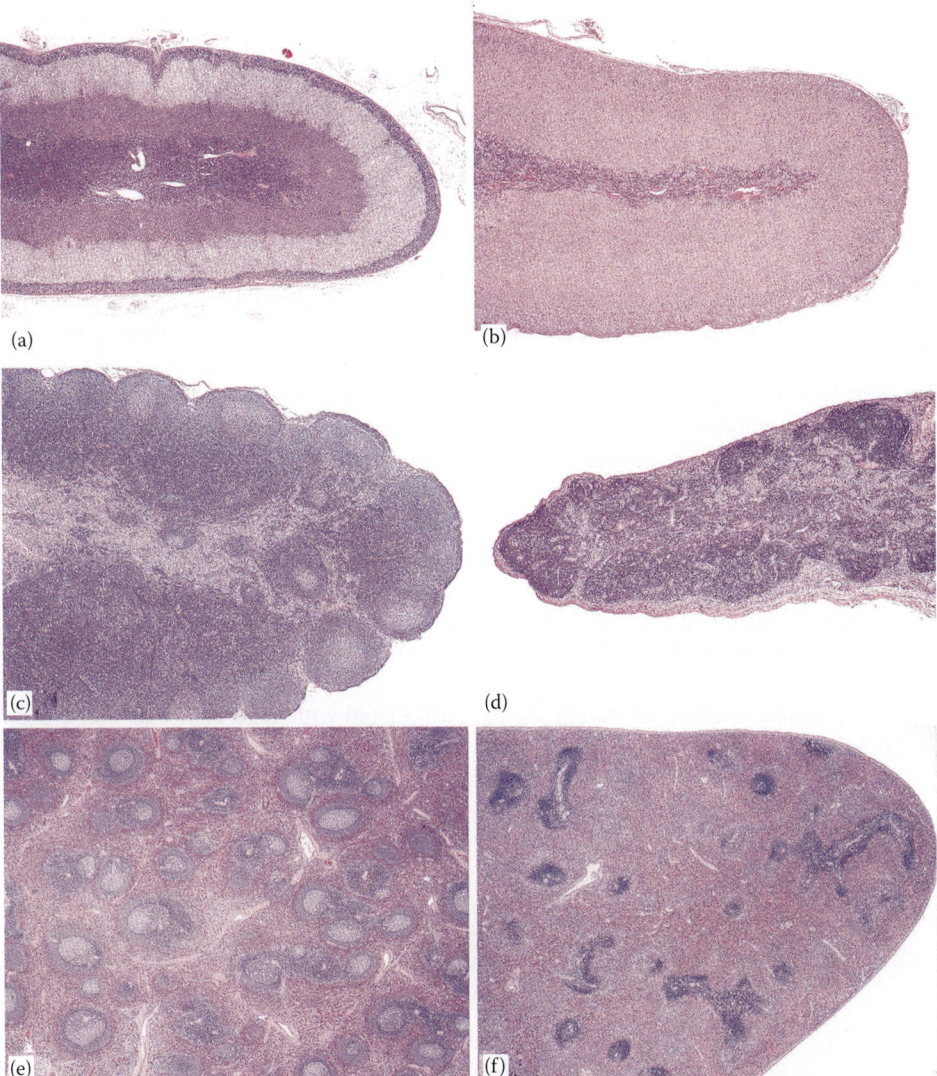

FIGURE 14.13   (a–f) Comparison of tissues from a control cynomolgus monkey (a, c, e) with those of a monkey that experienced severe esophageal trauma during dosing (b, d, f) at a mid-dose level. The trauma resulted in esophageal rupture and subsequent severe bacterial esophagitis and endocarditis that precipitated euthanasia. The compound that was administered in this study had no known immunological effects, and no other monkey on study developed alterations of the immune system. (b) Marked adrenal cortical hyperplasia; severe lymphoid depletion of (d) lymph nodes and (f) spleen. These changes are consistent with severe stress-induced, glucocorticoid-mediated alterations of lymphoid tissue.

The relationship among glucocorticoids, stress, and immunosuppression is well accepted and supported by the molecular basis of glucocorticoid action. Glucocorticoids diffuse through the cell membrane and bind to glucocorticoid receptors, after which they undergo nuclear translocation, followed by repression of cytokine gene expression. Molecular-driven outcomes manifest as altered leukocyte traffic, apoptosis of eosinophils and T-cells, inhibited expression of adhesion molecules, suppressed cytokine production, suppressed Th1 function, potentiation of acute phase reactions, and extension of lymphocyte pseudopods (Chrousos 1995; Almawi and Melemedjiian 2002; Fukuda et al. 2004). It has been suggested that glucocorticoids may also exert their effects via a direct interaction between glucocorticoid receptors and the T-cell receptor complex through nontranscriptional pathways (Lowenberg et al. 2007).

Exogenous glucocorticoid effects have been the benchmark for evaluating immunosuppressive effects of new chemical entities and characteristically induce increased lymphocyte apoptosis, generalized decreased lymphoid tissue cellularity, and decreased lymphoid organ weights that ultimately culminate in increased susceptibility to viral, bacterial, and parasitic infections (Figure 14.14a through d). But even in the case of endogenous glucocorticoids, the magnitude and duration of the glucocorticoid induction (via stressors) can produce variable histologic pictures that bridge the entire span of low-grade chronic loss of lymphocytes (with limited visibility of apoptosis) to acute, severe, and widespread lymphocyte apoptosis. However, stress effects are not limited to the effects of increased endogenous corticosteroids but also include changes secondary to increased catecholamines. For a thorough and rigorous review of the complex pathobiology of stress and its effects on the immune system, the reader is encouraged to review the work of Everds et al. (2012).

In addition to immunotoxicity and stress, the consequences of excessive pharmacology must be recognized so as to accurately identify no observed adverse effect levels (NOAELs) and establish appropriate therapeutic margins for humans. Multilymphoid organ decreases in cellularity seen following treatment with the classic broad-spectrum, small molecule immunosuppressants have been thoroughly described. However, with the advent of newer and highly selective immunomodulatory drugs, the pathologist is increasingly challenged to recognize the difference between immunotoxicity, dose-related pharmacological effects, and lesions induced by dose-related increased endogenous corticosteroids secondary to stress. The histopathology of a number of known immunotoxicants is presented herein.

Cyclophosphamide, a DNA alkylating agent, is associated with general T- and B-cell depletion of lymphoid tissues, such as splenic PALS, when given at high doses, but with B-cell zones being

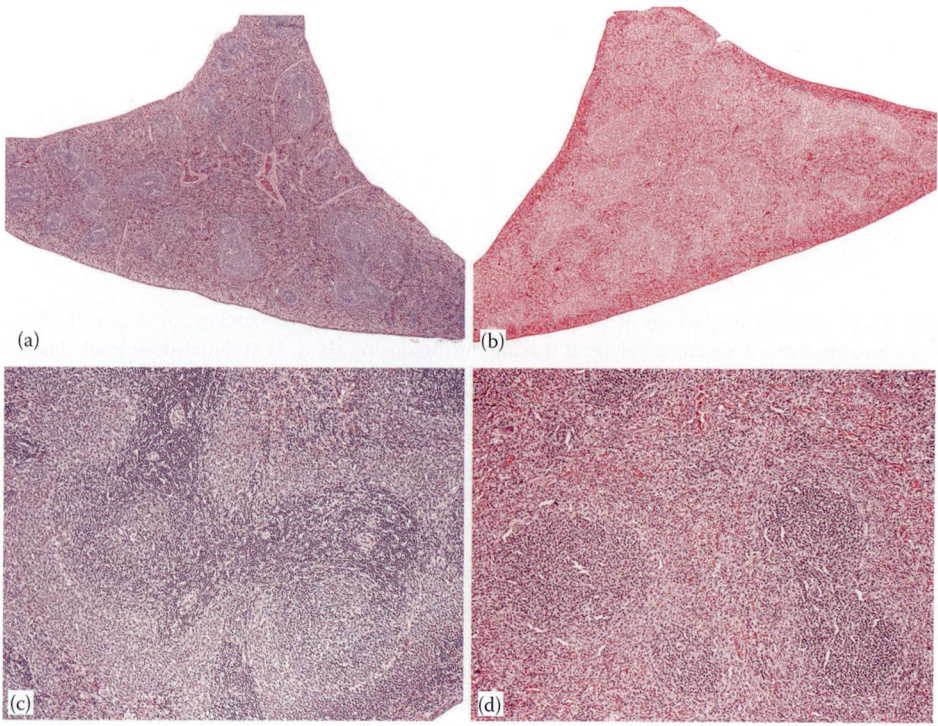

(a)   (b)   (c)   (d)

FIGURE 14.14   (a and c) Spleen of a control SD rat. (b and d) Spleen from a rat given dexamethasone resulting in severe generalized lymphoid depletion of all compartments.

more affected than T-cell zones at intermediate doses; depletion of suppressor T-cells is seen at very low doses (Gopinath et al. 1987).

Another classic immunosuppressive drug, cyclosporine A (CycA), is a cyclic polypeptide derived from the fungus *Beauvaria nivea* that directly interferes with normal T-cell function. B cells are not directly inhibited, but humoral responses are reduced secondary to altered Th function. Histologically, there is a marked reduction of the thymic medulla, decrease in MHC-II expression in medullary stroma, a loss of DCs, and blocked thymic cortical cell apoptosis that prevents the clonal elimination of thymic cortical cells (Greaves 2000). Epithelial reticular cells in the cortex show ultrastructural signs of severe degeneration and lysis. The single-positive medullary thymocytes are greatly depleted, while the immature CD4$^+$8$^+$ double-positive cortical lymphocytes remain. CD4$^+$ cells are decreased in proportion to CD8$^+$ cells in the medulla but not the cortex. Medullary B cells appear to be increased, and there is a loss of Hassall's corpuscles. The cytokeratin net of the medulla is decreased and focally shrunken in the cortex (Rossmann et al. 1997). This results in the unusual appearance of a thymus as having a well-formed cortex but with no apparent medulla. CycA also induces depletion of splenic lymphocytes of PALS and MZs in rats.

FK-506 (Tacrolimus, Prograf, Advagraf, Protopic) is an immunosuppressive drug produced from the fermentation broth of *Streptomyces tsukubaensis* that is primarily used to reduce organ transplant rejection. FK-506 has a similar spectrum of activity to CycA despite being structurally dissimilar. Rats given FK-506 orally for 13 weeks had dose-related decreased thymus cellularity with cortical lymphocytolysis, but after 52 weeks, a reduction of the thymic medulla was also identified. Baboons given FK-506 for 13 weeks had decreased thymic weights as a result of decreased numbers of medullary lymphocytes. However, lymph nodes demonstrated a proliferation of large lymphocytes in the paracortical region, reduced germinal centers, and reduced cellularity of PP follicles. FK-506 ointment, a possible treatment for atopic dermatitis, when administered dermally to rats for 26 weeks, caused a reduction in cellularity of the thymic medulla accompanied by increased cortical lymphocyte apoptosis. Lymph node germinal centers were diminished in cervical lymph nodes with and without increased apoptosis of germinal center cells. Likewise, PALS lymphocytes of the spleen were decreased as were circulating WBCs (NDA 50-777).

Rapamycin, an antifungal element derived from *Streptomyces hygroscopicus* and structurally similar to FK-506, causes marked reduction in thymic weight secondary to a reduction in medullary areas along with a transient reduction in cortical CD4$^+$ and CD8$^+$ lymphocytes (Zheng et al. 1991).

In the laboratory, histological alterations of the thymus have been seen following administration of adriamycin, gemcitabine, or paclitaxel to rats in which the cortex is markedly depleted of lymphocytes and increased numbers of small darkly staining lymphocytes appear to fill the medulla. However, the spleen and lymph nodes in these same studies appear to be within normal limits (Figure 14.15a through d).

Numerous contemporary immunomodulatory drugs that target specific kinases, such as PI3Kδ, are being pursued. Inhibition of PI3Kδ in rats is associated with a dose-related decrease in lymph node and PP secondary follicles and a distinct decrease in MZ B lymphocytes in the spleen (Webb et al. 2010). As with many selective kinase inhibitors, selectivity may be reduced or lost in toxicity studies as exposures are increased in pursuit of maximally tolerated doses (MTDs) and pharmacological IC50 values are exceeded. In the case of PI3Kδ inhibitors, T-cell populations begin to be affected at higher doses.

Other less selective kinase inhibitors are associated with off-target toxicities that include effects on the lymphoid system. The tyrosine kinase inhibitors sorafenib, imatinib, dasatinib, gefitinib, and lapatinib have all been associated with lymphoid necrosis and/or atrophy, and dasatinib has induced mineralization of multiple organs including the spleen. A species-specific immunotoxicity has been described for p38 kinase inhibitors, which cause acute lymphoid necrosis of B cells of lymph nodes and spleen but only in dogs. This effect was found to be a result of a species-specific difference in p38 protein expression in dog B cells (Morris et al. 2010).

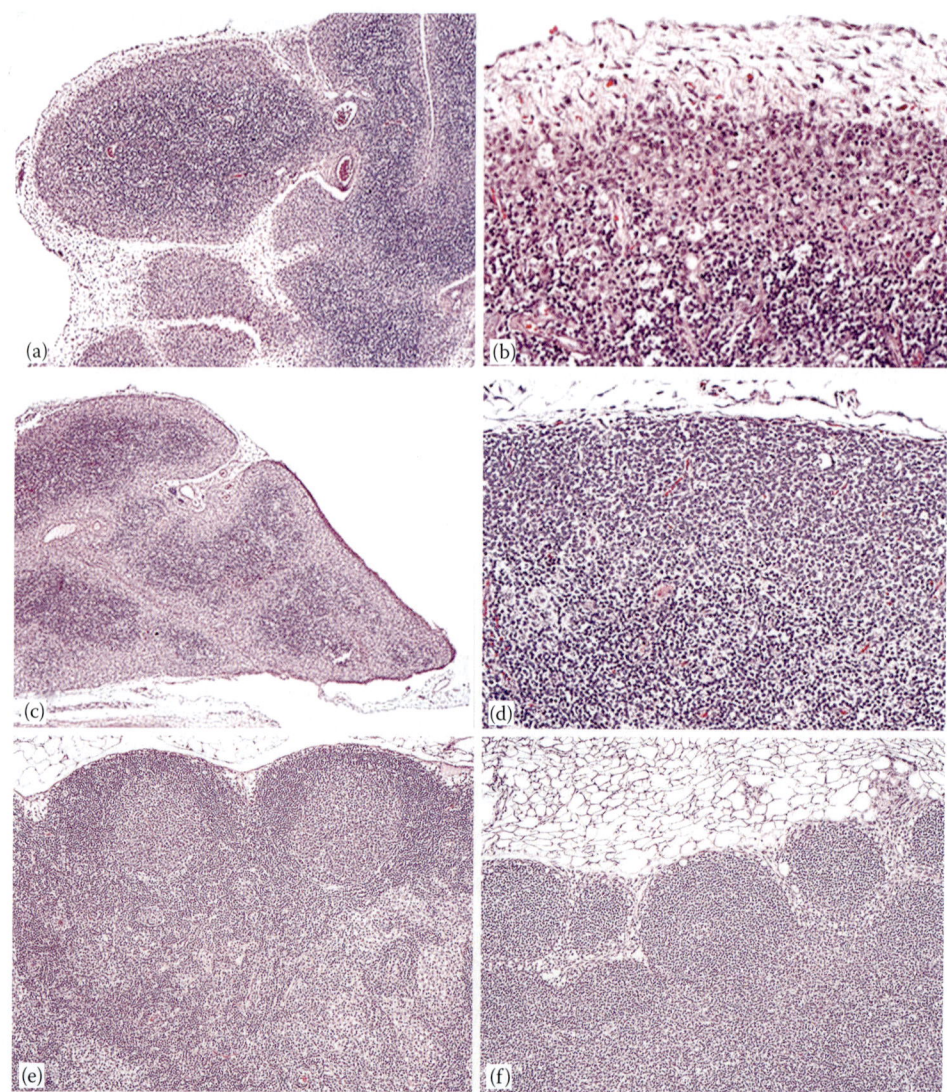

FIGURE 14.15   Two examples of acute severe loss of cortical lymphocytes in rats resulting in the apparent "reversal" of cortical versus medullary cellular density. (a) Thymus from a rat given adriamycin. (b) Image from the same rat at a higher magnification. (c) Thymus from a rat given paclitaxel. (d) Higher magnification of the image from the same rat as in c. In both cases, cortical lymphocytes are virtually absent, and apoptotic bodies and tingible-bodied macrophages are rare. (e) Mesenteric node from a control SD rat. (f) Mesenteric node from a rat given adriamycin. Note the loss of darkly staining T-cells and absence of germinal centers.

14.9   LYMPHOID NEOPLASIA OF MICE AND RATS

The author extends sincere appreciation to J. Ward for his thorough review and editing of this section.

The complex field of lymphoid neoplasia in rodents continues to change, and numerous manuscripts detailing the evolution of lymphoid tumor nomenclature are available. For a more detailed description of rodent lymphoid neoplasms and a thorough review of the history leading up to the current terminology, the reader is encouraged to obtain the following essential references: (1) STP Guidelines for lymphomas (Frith et al. 1996); (2) "Lymphomas and Leukemia in Mice" (Ward 2006);

(3) "Bethesda Proposal for Classification of Lymphoid Neoplasms in Mice" (Morse III et al. 2002); (4) "The Morphology, Immunohistochemistry, and Incidence of Hematopoietic Neoplasms in Mice and Rats" (Frith et al. 1993); and (5) "Morphologic Classification and Incidence of Hematopoietic Neoplasms in the Sprague–Dawley Rat" (Frith 1988). Additional valuable references include the adaptation of the 2001 WHO terminology for mouse tumors (Frith et al. 2001), the review of classification of mouse lymphoid cell neoplasms by Pattengale (1990), and manuscripts by Kunder et al. (2007), Ward et al. (2006), Hao et al. (2010), and Thomas et al. (2007).

It is important that pathologists have a good understanding of the incidence, the tumor type, and the typical organ of origin for spontaneously arising tumors in the particular strain of rodents they are working with (Frith et al. 1993). This information will aid in the accurate differentiation of background neoplasia from compound-induced neoplasia. Several strains of mice (CD-1; C57BL/6; B6C3F1) that are often used in carcinogenesis bioassays are known to commonly, and spontaneously, develop lymphomas. C58 and AKR mice are also known to have a high incidence of leukemia and lymphomas. Sprague–Dawley rats have been reported to spontaneously develop lymphomas, but to a much lesser extent (<1%) than in mice, and large granular cell lymphoma/leukemia (LGL) is very frequently encountered in aging Fischer 344 rats (Frith 1988).

The following will provide a basic guide to rodent lymphoid neoplasms based on the references given above. In some cases, it may be of interest to relate such rodent neoplasms in perspective to human lymphoid tumors. For this, the reader is encouraged to review the work of Morse III et al. (2002) and the Mouse Models for Human Cancers Consortium (http://emice.nci.nih.gov).

Table 14.1 lists spontaneous rodent lymphoid neoplasms based on multiple references.

TABLE 14.1
Categories and General Species Association of Hematopoietic Tumors in Rodents

Morphologic Type	Mice	Rat
Malignant Lymphomas		
Small lymphocyte: B or T-cell	√	
Follicular/pleomorphic (B cell)	most common lymphoma in most strains	√
Marginal Zone	√ - low incidence	
Immunoblastic (B cell)	√	√
Plasma cell (B cell)/plasmacytic	√	√
Lymphoblastic (lymphocytic) (B or T-cell)	√	rare
LGL lymphoma (leukemia) (non-T, non-B, or null cell)		√; common in F344; less common in SD rat
Myelogneous leukemia		
Granulocytic	√	√
Erythoid	rare	not spontaneous
Monouclear phagocytic system		
Histiocytic sarcoma	reticulum cell sarcoma type A; histiocytic lymphoma and sarcoma	malignant fibrous histiocytoma; histocytic sarcoma
Thymoma		
Lymphocytic predominant	√	√
Epithelial predominant	√	√
Carcinoma	√	√
Sarcoma	√	√
Other		
Mast cell tumor	rare	

Table adapted from similar tables in Frith 1988; Frith et al. 1993; Frith et al. 2001; and Ward 2006.

14.9.1 Small Lymphocyte: B- or T-Cell Origin

This uncommon spontaneous neoplasm of mice is characterized by uniform, small- to medium-sized and well-differentiated cells similar to typical circulating lymphocytes. The cytoplasm is scant and presents as a narrow rim; the nuclear chromatin is densely clumped, and mitotic figures are infrequent. The noncohesive cells may infiltrate multiple organs, such as the spleen, liver, or lymph nodes, resulting in effacement of normal architecture, especially in cases that include leukemia (Morse III et al. 2002).

14.9.2 Follicular/Pleomorphic Lymphoma

Follicular lymphomas are best identified in the mouse and originate predominantly in the spleen as well as in the mesenteric lymph node and/or ileal PP from germinal center B cells. These tumors may be single or multicentric and either follicular or diffuse, with a particularly pronounced multinodular presentation when occurring in the spleen. As indicated by the name, these tumors may be variably pleomorphic with small to medium to large lymphocytes, the latter being suggestive of centrocytes and centroblasts. These tumors may consist predominantly of either small or large cells, or a mixture of both. The larger cells can have scant or abundant cytoplasm, and the nuclei may be cleaved, or uncleaved and vesicular; nucleoli are often prominent. Originally, these tumors were classified as reticulum cell sarcoma, type B, or pleomorphic/mixed cell lymphoma, but recognition that this tumor produces immunoglobulins, stains positively for IgM, B220, and CD19, and is morphologically similar to human lymphoma led to its reclassification (Frith et al. 1993; Ward 2006). Follicular lymphomas are extremely rare in Sprague–Dawley rats but represent the most common form of spontaneous lymphoma in some strains of mice (Morse III et al. 2002).

14.9.3 MZ Lymphoma

The MZ lymphoma, first described by Ward et al. (1999), is a less common tumor of mice with an incidence of 1%–2% in strains other than p53 KO mice, in which it is most commonly found. As indicated by its name, it originates in the mantle zone of the spleen, and its growth pattern results in widening of the MZ and local invasion of the red pulp. Tumor cells tend to be homogenous medium-sized cells that may evolve to larger cells as the MZs coalesce. The nuclei are round to ovoid with stippled to vesicular chromatin; nucleoli are not prominent, and mitotic figures are few. Being clones of mature B cells, they stain positively for IgM, B220, and CD19 (Morse III et al. 2002). The PALS and the red pulp may be completely obliterated in more advanced tumors. Other than splenic nodes, lymph nodes are usually not involved.

14.9.4 Immunoblastic Lymphoma

Immunoblastic lymphomas arise from germinal center or postgerminal center B cells and are characterized by large noncohesive cells with abundant, amphophilic cytoplasm; large rounded and sometimes vesicular nuclei; a single, prominent nucleoli; and frequent mitotic figures. Plasma cells and plasmacytoid cells are seen in some cases. The molecular phenotype is consistent with mature clonal B cells (Morse III et al. 2002). This highly invasive tumor demonstrates a growth pattern similar to follicular lymphomas but with a more aggressive infiltration of the lungs (along the vascular tree), liver, kidney, and ovaries (Frith et al. 2001). Immunoblastic lymphomas are rare in most strains of mouse and rat.

14.9.5 Plasma Cell/Plasmacytic Lymphoma

An uncommon spontaneous tumor of both rats and mice, plasma cell lymphomas display morphology consistent with their heritage. Large, mature noncohesive plasma cells with abundant amphophilic cytoplasm have round nuclei with a classic cartwheel appearance. A small perinuclear halo (Golgi apparatus) may be present. Mitotic figures are rare.

14.9.6 LYMPHOBLASTIC/LYMPHOCYTIC LYMPHOMA

A very common tumor in mice, but less so in rats, lymphoblastic lymphoma is the archetype of rodent lymphomas and may be of T- or B-cell origin. Lymphoblastic lymphomas are characterized by homogenous sheets of variably (usually medium) sized but uniform noncohesive cells with scant cytoplasm; round, distinct, and often multiple nucleoli; and intermediate to high numbers of mitotic figures. These tumors can be found in lymph nodes, thymus, bone marrow, and kidneys. Leukemia may accompany the solid tumor along with invasion of the central nervous system. T-cell lymphoblastic tumors may develop as early as 1 month of age in some mouse strains, and the incidence increases with age. T or B lymphoblastic lymphomas may also be induced by chemicals, irradiation, or retroviruses.

14.9.7 LGL LYMPHOMA (LEUKEMIA)

Most commonly encountered in F344 rats, less so in Sprague–Dawley rats, and not in mice, LGL lymphoma was first identified as a mononuclear cell leukemia. Distinct clinical manifestations are frequently noted and include depression, pallor, icterus, weight loss, splenomegaly, hemolytic anemia, and tumor cell erythrophagocytosis (Ward and Reynolds 1983). Small pleomorphic cells have irregular to reniform nuclei, a small amount of cytoplasm, and characteristic pink to red-purple cytoplasmic granules (seen with Romanovski-stained peripheral blood). While originating in the splenic MZ, this tumor can rapidly spread to other tissues, especially the liver, where accumulation of tumor cells is reminiscent of lymphoblastic lymphoma. When F344 rats are used in life span studies, the incidence of LGL leukemia may reach 30%–50% or greater (Losco and Ward 1984; Thomas et al. 2007), thus potentially complicating treatment-related survival data from such studies.

14.9.8 HISTIOCYTIC SARCOMA (MONONUCLEAR PHAGOCYTE SYSTEM)

The terminology for this tumor has evolved over time as can be seen in Table 14.1. Murine forms of this tumor have been referred to as reticulum cell sarcoma type A, histiocytic lymphoma, or histiocytic sarcoma. In the rat, the tumors have been classified as malignant fibrous histiocytoma or histiocytic sarcoma. For consistency, this chapter recommends the term "histiocytic sarcoma" (according to Frith et al. 1993, 2001). These tumors are distinct from lymphomas by virtue of having a fibrous structure with and without large multinucleated foreign body giant cells. The cytoplasm is abundant and eosinophilic, and the nuclei are large and basophilic. The tumor rarely displays a conventional lymphoid pattern and can originate retroperitoneally, in mesenteric lymph nodes, uterus (most common site in female mice), or liver (most common site in male mice). Other sites include the spleen, bone marrow, lung, kidney, skin, subcutaneous tissue, and ovaries. The cell of origin has been determined to be histiocytic cells derived from the mononuclear phagocytic system. Neoplastic histiocytes stain positively for mononuclear antigens and lysozymes but not with T- or B-cell markers.

14.9.9 MYELOGENOUS LEUKEMIA

14.9.9.1 Granulocytic Leukemia

Rare as a spontaneous tumor in rodents, the development of granulocytic leukemia has been attributed to retroviruses and some chemicals. Circulating leukemic cells may be large, blastic immature forms or smaller mature cells with lobed and segmented nuclei. Circulating cells may be characterized by either the mature or immature forms or a blend of each. Granulocytic leukemia is usually associated with a very high WBC count and marked involvement of the spleen. The liver, lymph nodes, and bone marrow may also be involved.

14.9.9.2 Erythroid Leukemia

Erythroid leukemia is a spontaneous neoplasia of the erythroid lineage (erythroblasts) that is rare in mice and has not been described in rats. When present, erythroblastic cells may be found in the bone marrow, spleen, thymus, lymph nodes, liver, and kidney. Erythroid leukemia can be induced in mice with Friend leukemia virus or Rauscher virus, and it has been described in rats following radiation or trimethylbenz[a]anthracene exposure.

14.9.10 THYMOMA

1. Thymomas are neoplasms of TECs that are typically subdivided into three general categories depending on their relative cellular composition. For example, Kuper et al. (1986) classified tumors of the thymus in Wistar rats as being thymoma with medullary differentiation, thymoma without differentiation, and lymphoma. In comparison, Frith et al. (1993) described tumors of the rodent thymus as being predominantly derived from epithelial cells or Hassall's corpuscles, with varying degrees of neoplastic lymphocytes. Greaves (2000) references Rosai and Levine (1976) when he separates thymomas into epithelial type, mixed epithelial and lymphoid cell type, and predominantly lymphoid cells (lymphoid type). Thymomas may present as either benign tumors or malignant carcinomas and sarcomas; however, metastasis is rare. The degree of reticular tissue in these tumors can be quite variable. Thymomas in conventional rat and mouse strains are rare with the exception of Buffalo and Wistar/Neuherberg rats.
2. Thymic lymphomas are distinct from thymoma-lymphoid type and have large numbers of lymphocytes and lymphoblasts that develop into multinodular tumors with little to no epithelial or medullary components. Large tumors may have irregular and extensive areas of necrosis and sometimes invade into the surrounding mediastinal fat. Thymic T-cell lymphomas are common in AKR mice late in life and have been used extensively in this strain as models of chemical-induced T-cell tumors.

Despite the relatively consistent literature-based description of four basic presentations of thymomas, additional morphologies may be encountered that include epidermoid nodules of nonkeratinizing squamous epithelium, cystic papillary forms, forms with ribbons, cords or tubules, endocrine or adenoid forms, neuroendocrine forms, and myoid (with skeletal muscle differentiation) forms (Pearse 2006b).

14.9.11 MAST CELL TUMOR

Spontaneous, benign, and malignant mast cell tumors have been described rarely in mice but not in rats. The tumors are typically disseminated in the skin, liver, spleen, and kidneys. Staining for metachromasia will usually show definitive cytoplasmic granules.

Keep in mind that the prevalence of leukemia and lymphoma in safety assessment studies in rodents is influenced by additional factors such as cage size and shelf level, population density, quantity of diet (caloric intake), amino acid deficiencies, mineral deficiencies, hormone status, and immunosuppression. Numerous chemicals have been associated with the development of tumors of the rodent lymphoid tissue (hematopoietic system), and the reader is encouraged to read the work of Greaves (2000) and Gold et al. (2001) for detailed reviews.

ACKNOWLEDGMENT

The author would like to express his sincere thanks to Denise Hertel and Rebecca Stewart for their continued support and consistent production of the many high-quality histological preparations used to support this chapter.

REFERENCES

Achtman, A.H., Khan, M., Maclennan, I.C., Langhorne, J. 2003. *Plasmodium chabaudi* infection in mice induces strong B cell responses and striking but temporary changes in splenic cell distribution. *J. Immunol.* 171:317–324.

Almawi, W.Y., Melemedjiian, O.K. 2002. Molecular mechanisms of glucocorticoid antiproliferative effects; antagonism of transcription factor activity by glucocorticoid receptor. *J. Leukoc. Biol.* 71:9–15.

Anderson, G., Moore, N.C., Owen, J.J., Jenkinson, E.J. 1996. Cellular interactions in thymocyte development. *Annu. Rev. Immunol.* 14:73–99.

Asanuma, H., Thompson, A.H., Iwasaki, T., Sato, Y., Inaba, Y., Aizawa, C., Kurata, T., Tamura, S. 1997. Isolation and characterization of mouse nasal-associated lymphoid tissue. *J. Immunol. Methods* 202:123–131.

Asakura, K., Saito, H., Hata, M., Kataura, A. 1998. Antigen-specific IgA response of NALT and cervical lymph node cells in antigen-primed rats. *Acta Oto-Laryngol.* 118:859–863.

Bacha, W.J. Jr., Wood, L.M. 1990. Color *Atlas of Veterinary Histology*. Philadelphia: Lea & Febiger.

Banks, W.J. 1986. *Applied Veterinary Histology*, 2nd cd., Baltimore: Williams and Wilkins.

Basketter, D., Gerberick, F., Kimber, I., Willis, C. 1999. *Toxicology of Contact Dermatitis: Allergy, Irritancy, and Urticaria*. Current Toxicology Series. New York: John Wiley & Sons.

Bélisle, C., Sainte-Marie, G. 1981a. Tridimensional study of the deep cortex of the rat lymph node. I. Topography of the deep cortex. *Anat. Rec.* 199:45–59.

Bélisle, C., Sainte-Marie, G. 1981b. Tridimensional study of the deep cortex of the rat lymph node. II. Relation of deep cortex units to afferent lymphatic vessels. *Anat. Rec.* 199:61–72.

Bélisle, C., Sainte-Marie, G. 1981c. Tridimensional study of the deep cortex of the rat lymph node. III. Morphology of the deep cortex units. *Anat. Rec.* 199:213–226.

Bélisle, C., Sainte-Marie, G. 1981d. Topography of the cortex of the lymph nodes of various mammalian species. *Anat. Rec.* 201:553–561.

Bienenstock, J., Johnston, N., Percy, D.Y.E. 1973a. Bronchial and lymphoid tissue. I. Morphologic characteristics. *Lab. Invest.* 28:686–692.

Bienenstock, J., Johnston, N., Percy, D.Y.E. 1973b. Bronchial and lymphoid tissue. II. Functional characteristics. *Lab. Invest.* 28:693–698.

Binns, R.M., Pabst, R. 1994. Lymphoid tissue structure and lymphocyte trafficking in the pig. *Vet. Immunol. Immunopathol.* 43:79–87.

Bockman, D.E., Cooper, M.D. 1973. Pinocytosis by epithelium associated with lymphoid follicles in the bursa of Fabricius, appendix and Peyer's patches. An electron microscopic study. *Am. J. Anat.* 136:455–477.

Bockman, D.E., Stevens, W. 1977. Gut-associated lymphoepithelial tissue: bidirectional transport of tracer by specialized epithelial cells associated with lymphoid follicles. *J. Reticuloendothel. Soc.* 21:245–254.

Bruijntjes, J.P., Kuper, C.F., Robinson, J.E., Schuurman, H. 1993. Epithelium-free area in the thymic cortex of rats. *Dev. Immunol.* 3:113–122.

Capone, M., Romagnoli, P., Beerman, F., MacDonald, H.R., van Meerwijk, J.P. 2001. Dissociation of thymic positive and negative selection in transgenic mice expressing major histocompatibility complex class I molecules exclusively on thymic cortical epithelial cells. *Blood* 97:1336–1342.

Cesta, M.F. 2006a. Normal structure, function and histology of mucosa-associated lymphoid tissue. *Toxicol. Pathol.* 34:599–608.

Cesta, M.F. 2006b. Normal structure, function and histology of the spleen. *Toxicol. Pathol.* 34:455–465.

Chrousos, G.P. 1995. The hypothalamic-pituitary-adrenal axis and immune-mediated inflammation. *N Engl J Med*. May 18;332(20):1351–1362.

Cornes, J.S. 1965. Number, size and distribution of Peyer's patches in the human small intestine. I. The development of Peyer's patches. *Gut* 6:225–229.

Crabtree, G.R., Gillis, S., Smith, K.A., Munck, A. 1979. Glucocorticoids and immune responses. *Arthritis Rheum.* 22:1246–1256.

Dellmann, H.D., Brown, E.M. 1987. *Textbook of Veterinary Histology*, pp. 174–175. Philadelphia: Lea & Febiger.

Dijkstra, C.D., Sminia, T. 1990. Thymus: normal anatomy, histology, ultrastructure, rat. In *Monographs on Pathology of Laboratory Animals, Hematopoietic System*, eds. T.C. Jones, J.M. Ward, U. Mohr, R.D. Hunt, pp. 249–256. Berlin: Springer-Verlag.

Dijkstra, C.D., Veerman, A.J.P. 1990. Spleen: normal anatomy, histology, ultrastructure, rat. In *Monographs on Pathology of Laboratory Animals, Hematopoietic System*, eds. T.C. Jones, J.M. Ward, U. Mohr, R.D. Hunt, pp. 185–193. Berlin: Springer-Verlag.

Dunn, T.B. 1954. Normal and pathologic anatomy of the reticular tissue in laboratory mice. *J. Natl. Cancer Inst.* 14:1303–1395.

Elmore, S. 2006. Lymph node histopathology. *Toxicol. Pathol.* 34:425–454.

Everds, N.E., Snyder, P.W., Bailey, K.L., Bolon, B., Creasy, D.M., Foley, G.L., Rosol, T.J., Sellers, T. 2012. Interpreting Stress Responses during Routine Toxicology Studies: A Review of the Biology, Impact, and Assessment. Accepted for publication ToxPath.

Feng, G., Debra, W., Elke, M., Falk, W. 2007. Constitutive alternative NF-κB signaling promotes marginal zone B-cell development but disrupts the marginal sinus and induces HEV-like structures in the spleen. *Blood* 110:2381–2389.

Frith, C.H. 1988. Morphologic classification and incidence of hematopoietic neoplasms in the Sprague–Dawley rat, *Toxicol. Pathol.* 16:451–457.

Frith, C.H., Ward, J.M. and Chandra, M. 1993. The morphology, immunohistochemistry, and incidence of hematopoietic neoplasms in mice and rats, *Toxicol. Pathol.* 21:206–218.

Frith, C.H., Ward, J.M., Chandra, M., and Losco, P. 2000. Non-proliferative lesions of the hematopoietic system in rats, HL-1. In *Guides for Toxicologic Pathology*, pp. 1–22. Washington, DC: STP/ARP/AFIP.

Frith, C.H., Ward, J.M., Harleman, J.H., Stromberg, P.C., Halm, S., Inoue, T., Wright, J.A. 2001. Hematopoietic system. In *International Classification of Rodent Tumors. The Mouse*, ed. U. Mohr, pp. 417–451. Berlin: Springer.

Frith, C.H., Ward, J.M., Fredrickson, T., Harleman, J.H. 1996. Neoplastic lesions of the hematopoietic system. In *Pathobiology of aging mice*, eds. U. Mohr, D.L. Dungworth, C.C. Capen, W.W. Carlton, J.P. Sundberg, J.M. Ward, pp. 219–235. Washington, DC: ILSI Press.

Fukuda, S., Mitsuoka, H., Schmid-Schonbein, G.W. 2004. Leukocyte fluid shear response in the presence of glucocorticoid. *J. Leukoc. Biol.* 75:664–670.

Gretz, J.E., Norbury, C.C., Anderson, A.O., Proudfoot, A.E.I., Shaw, S. 2000. Lymph-borne chemokines and other low molecular weight molecules read high endothelial venules via specialized conduits while a functional barrier limits access to the lymphocyte microenvironments in lymph node cortex. *J. Exp. Med.* 192:1425–1439.

Giannasca, P.J., Boden, J.A., Monath, T.P. 1997. Targeted delivery of antigen to hamster nasal lymphoid tissue with M-cell directed lectin. *Infect. Immunol.* 65:4288–4298.

Gold, L.S., Manley, N.B., Slone, T.H., Ward, J.M. (2001). Compendium of chemical carcinogens by target organs: results of chronic bioassays in rats, mice, hamsters, dogs, and monkeys. *Toxicol. Pathol.* 29:639–652.

Gopinath C., Prentice, D.E., Lewis, D.J. 1987. *Atlas of Experimental Toxicological Pathology*, vol. 13. Lancaster, UK: MTP Press Limited.

Gray, H. 1918. *Anatomy of the Human Body*, 20th ed. Philadelphia: Lea & Febiger.

Greaves, P. 2000. *Histopathology of Preclinical Toxicity Studies; Interpretation and Relevance in Drug Safety Evaluation*, 2nd ed., New York: Elsevier.

Guo, F., Weih, D., Meier, E., Weih, F. 2007. Constitutive alternative NK-κB signaling promotes marginal zone B-cell development but disrupts the marginal sinus and induces HEV-like structures in the spleen. *Blood* 110(7): 2381–2389.

Haley, P. 2008. Histomorphology of the immune system: a basic step in assessing immunotoxicity. In *Immunotoxicology Strategies for Pharmaceutical Safety Assessment*, eds. D.J. Herzyk and J.L. Bussiere, pp. 27–44. Hoboken, NJ: Wiley and Sons, Inc.

Haley, P. 2012. The immune system of pigs: structure and function. In *The Minipig in Biomedical Research*, eds. P.A. McAnulty, A.D. Dayan, N.-C. Ganderup, K. Hastings, pp. 343–356. Boca Raton: CRC Press, Taylor and Francis Group.

Haley, P., Perry, R., Ennulat, D., Frame, S., Johnson, C., Lapointe, J.-M, Nyska, A., Snyder, P.W., Walker, D., Walter, G. 2005. STP Position Paper: Best Practice Guideline for the Routine Pathology Evaluation of the Immune System. *Toxicol. Pathol.* 33:404–407.

Hameleers, D.M., van der Ende, M., Biewenga, J., Sminia, T. 1989. An immunohistochemical study on the postnatal development of rat nasal-associated lymphoid tissue (NALT). *Cell & Tissue Research* 256(2):431–438.

Han, J., van Krieken, J.M., te Velde, J. Spleen, Chapter 29. 1997. In *Histology for Pathologists,* 2nd edition, ed. S.S. Sternberg. Philadelphia: Lippincott-Raven.

Hare, W.C.D. 1975. Carnivore respiratory system. In: *Sisson and Grossman's The Anatomy of the Domestic Animals*, vol. 2, 5th ed., ed. Getty, R., p. 1573. Philadelphia: W.B. Saunders Company.

Harkema, J.R. 1991. Comparative aspects of nasal airway anatomy: relevance to inhalation toxicology. *Toxicol. Pathol.* 19:321–336.

Hao, X., Fredrickson, T.N., Chattopadhyay, S.K., Han, W., Qi, C.F., Wang, Z., Ward, J.M., Hartley, J.W., Morse, H.C. 3rd. 2010. The histopathologic and molecular basis for the diagnosis of histiocytic sarcoma and histiocyte-associated lymphoma of mice. *Vet. Pathol.* May;47(3):434–445.

HogenEsch, H., Felsburg, P.J. 1992. Immunohistochemistry of Peyer's patches in the dog. *Vet. Immunol. Immunopharmacol.* 30:147–160.

ICICIS Group Investigators Report of validation study of assessment of direct immunotoxicity in the rat. 1998. *Toxicology* 125(2–3):183–201.

International Conference on Harmonization (ICH). 2006. *Guidance for Industry. S8 Immunotoxicity Studies for Human Pharmaceuticals.*

Ioachim, H.L. 1994. *Lymph Node Pathology,* 2nd ed. Philadelphia: J.B. Lippincott Company.

Irons, R., 1991. Chapter 16; Blood and bone marrow. In *Handbook of Toxicologic Pathology*, eds. W.M., Hashcek, C.G. Rousseau, pp. 389–419. San Diego, Academic Press.

Jeong, K.I., Suzuki, H., Nakayama, H., Doi, K. 2000. Ultrastructural study on the follicle-associated epithelium of nasal-associated lymphoid tissue in specific pathogen-free (SPF) and conventional environment-adapted (SPF-CV) rats. *Journal of Anatomy* 196(Pt 3):443–51.

Job, T.T. 1915. The adult anatomy of the lymphatic system in the common rat (*Epimy norvegicus*). *Anat. Rec.* 9:447–458.

Jones, T.C., Ward, J.M., Moher, U., Hunt, R.D. 1990. *Monographs on Pathology of Laboratory Animals. Hematopoietic System*, p. 270. New York: Springer-Verlag.

Kovacs, M.S., McKiernan, S., Potter, D.M., Chilappagari. S. 2005. An epidemiological study of interdigital cysts in a research Beagle colony. *Contemp. Top Lab. Animal Sci.* 44:17–21.

Kraal, G., Schomagel, K., Streeter, P.R., Holzman, B., Butcher, E.C. 1995. Expression of the mucosal vascular addressing, MAdCAM-1 on sinus-lining cells in the spleen. *Am. J. Pathol.* 147:763–771.

Kunder, S., Calzada-Wack, J., Holzlwimmer, G., Muller, J., Kloss, C., Howat, W., Schmidt, J., Hofler, H., Warren, M., and Quintanilla-Martinez, L. 2007. A comprehensive antibody panel for immunohistochemical analysis of formalin-fixed, paraffin-embedded hematopoietic neoplasms of mice: analysis of mouse specific and human antibodies cross-reactive with murine tissue. *Toxicol. Pathol.* 35:366–375.

Kuper, C.F., Beems, R.B., Hollanders, V.M.H. 1986. Spontaneous pathology of the thymus in aging Wistar (Cpb:WU) rats. *Vet. Pathol.* 23:270–277.

Kuper, C.F., Hameleers, D.M., Bruijntjes, J.P., van der Ven, I., Biewenga, J., Sminia, T. 1990. Lymphoid and non-lymphoid cells intranasal-associated lymphoid tissue (NALT) in the rat. An immuno- and enzyme–histochemical study. *Cell Tissue Res.* 259:371–377.

Kuper, C.F., deHeer, E., Van Loveren, H., Vos, J.G. 1991. Chapter 39, Immune system. In *Handbook of Toxicologic Pathology*, 2nd ed. eds. W. Hascheck, C.G. Rousseaux, M.A. Wallig, vol. 2, pp. 585–646, San Diego: Academic Press.

Kuper, C.F., Beems, R.B., Bruijntnes, J.P., Schuurman, H.J., Vos, J.G. 1992. Normal development, growth, and aging of the thymus. In *Pathobiology of the Aging Rat*, vol. 1, eds. U. Mohr, D.L. Dungworth, C.C. Capen, pp. 25–48. Washington, DC: ILSI Press.

Kuper, C.F., Schuurman, H.-J., Vos, J.K.G. 1995. Pathology in immunotoxicology. In *Methods in Immunotoxicology*, eds. G.R. Burleson, J.H. Dean, A.E. Munson, vol. 1, pp. 378–436. New York: Wiley-Liss.

Levin, S., Semle, R.D., Ruben, Z. 1993. Effects of two weeks of feed restriction on some common toxicologic parameters in Sprague–Dawley rats. *Toxicol. Pathol.* 21:1–14.

Lind, E.F., Prockop, S.E., Porritt, H.E., Petrie, H.T. 2011. Mapping precursor movement through the postnatal thymus reveals specific microenvironments supporting defined stages of early lymphoid development. *J. Exp. Med.* 194:127–134.

Losco, P.E., Ward, J.M. 1984. The early stage of large granular lymphocyte leukemia in the F344 rat. *Vet. Pathol.* 21:286–291.

Losco, P., Harlemen, H. 1992. Normal development, growth, and aging of the lymph node. In: *Pathobiology of the Aging Rat*, vol. 1, eds. U. Mohr, D.L. Dungworth, C.C. Capen, pp. 49–73. Washington, DC: ILSI Press.

Losco, P. 1992. Normal development, growth, and aging of the spleen. In: *Pathobiology of the Aging Rat*, vol. 1, eds. U. Mohr, D.L. Dungworth, C.C. Capen, pp. 75–94. Washington, DC: ILSI Press.

Lowenberg, M., Verhaar, A.P., van der Brink, G.R., Hommes, D.W. 2007. Glucocorticoid signaling: a non-genomic mechanism for T-cell immunosuppression. *Trends Mol. Med.* 13:158–163.

Lowenstine, L.J. 2003. A primer of primate pathology: lesions and nonlesions. *Toxicol. Pathol.* 31: 92–102.

Mackall, C.L., Punt, J.A., Morgan, P., Farr, A.G., Gress, R.E. 1998. Thymic function in young/old chimeras: substantial thymic T-cell regenerative capacity despite irreversible age-associated thymic involution. *Eur. J. Immunol.* 28:1886–1893.

MacKenzie, W.F., Eustis, S.L. 1990. Bone marrow. In *Pathology of the Fischer* Rat. eds. G.A. Boorman, S.L. Eustis, M.R. Elwell, C.A. Montgomery, and W.F. MacKenzie. pp. 395–403. San Diego, CA: Academic Press, Inc.

Maronpot, R.R. 2006. A monograph on histomorphologic evaluation of lymphoid organs. *Toxicol. Pathol.,* 34(5):409–696.

Martin, F., Kearney, J.F. 2000. B-cell subsets and the mature preimmune repertoire: marginal zone B1 B cells as part of the "natural immune memory." *Immunol. Rev.* 175:70–79.

Mebius, R.E., Kraal, G. 2005. Structure and function of the spleen. *Nat. Rev. Immunol.* 5:606–616.

Mebius, R.E., Nolte, M.A., Kraal, G. 2004. Development and function of the splenic marginal zone. *Crit. Rev. Immunol.* 24:449–464.

Mills, S.E., Fechner, R.E. 1997. Chapter 16. Larynx and pharynx. In *Histology for Pathologists*, 2nd ed., ed. S.S. Sternberg, pp. 391–404. Philadelphia: Lippincott-Raven.

Morris, D.L., O'Neil, S.P., Devraj, R.V., Portanova, J.P., Gilles, R.W., Gross, C.J., Curtiss, S.W., Komocsare, W.J., Garner, D.S., Happa, F.A., Kraus, L.J., Nikula, K.J., Monahan, J.B., Selness, S.R., Galluppi, G.R., Shevlin, K.M., Kramer, J.A., Walker, J.K., Messing, D.M., Anderson, D.R., Mourey, R.J., Whitely, L.O., Daniels, J.S., Yang, J.Z., Rowlands, P.C., Alden, C.L., Davis II, J.W., and Sagartz, J.E. 2010. Acute lymphoid and gastrointestinal toxicity induced by selective p38α Map kinase and Map kinase-activated protein kinase-2 (MK-2) inhibitors in the dog. *Toxicol. Pathol.* 38:606–618.

Morse III, H.C., Anver, M.R., Fredrickson, T.N., Haines, D.C., Harris, A.W., Harris, N.L., Jaffe, E.S., Kogan, S.C., MaLennan, I.C.M., Patttengale, P.K., Ward, J.M. 2002. Bethesda Proposal for Classification of Lymphoid Neoplasms in mice. *Blood* 100:246–258.

Nasonex. 1997. Summary basis of approval for NDA 20-762, SCH 32088, Mometasone furoate monohydrate.

Ohtani, O., Ohtani, Y., Carati, C., Gannon, B.J. 2003. Fluid and cellular pathways of rat lymph nodes in relation to lymphatic labyrinths and Aquapori-1 expression. *Arch. Histol. Cytol.* 66:261–272.

Pabst, R., Nowara, E. 1982. Organ distribution and fate of newly formed splenic lymphocytes in the pig. *Anat. Rec.* 202:85–94.

Pabst, R. 1987. The anatomical basis for the immune function of the gut. *Anat. Embryol.* (Berl). 176: 135–144.

Pabst, R., Gehrke, I. 1990. Is the bronchus-associated lymphoid tissue (BALT) an integral structure of the lung in normal mammals, including humans? *Am. Respir. Cell Mol. Biol.* 3:131–135.

Pabst, R., Geist, M., Rothkotter, H.J., Fritz, F.J., 1988. Postnatal development and lymphocytes production of jejunal and ileal Peyer's patches in normal and gnotobiotic pigs. *Immunology* 64:539–544.

Pattengale, P.K. 1990. Classification of mouse lymphoid cell neoplasms. In *Monographs on Pathology of Laboratory Animals, Hemopoietic System*, eds. T.C. Jones, J.M. Ward, U. Mohr, R.D. Hunt, pp. 137–143. New York: Springer-Verlag.

Pearse, G. 2006a. Normal structure, function and histology of the thymus. *Toxicol. Pathol.* 34:504–514.

Pearse, G. 2006b. Histopathology of the thymus. *Toxicol. Pathol.* 34:515–547.

Pillai, S., Cariappa, A. 2009. The follicular versus marginal zone B lymphocyte cell fate decision. *Nat. Rev. Immunol.* 9:767–777.

Pospischil, A. 1989. Struktur und funktion von Peyerschen platen im darm verschiedener tierarten. *Schweiz. Arch. Teirhekik.* 131:595–603.

Renoux, G. 1985. Immunomodulatory agents. In *Immunotoxicology and Immunopharmacology*, eds. J.H. Dean, M.L. Luster, A.E. Munson, H. Amos, pp. 193–205. New York: Raven Press.

Rosai, J., Levine, G.D. 1976. Tumors of the thymus, Fasc 13, 2nd series, pp. 34–37. Washington, DC: Armed Forces Institute of Pathology.

Rossmann, P., Ríhová, B., Strohalm, J., Ulbrich, K. 1997. Morphology of rat kidney and thymus after native and antibody-coupled cyclosporin A application (reduced toxicity of targeted drug). *Folia Microbiol (Praha)* 42(3):277–287.

Sack, W.O. 1982. *Essentials of Pig Anatomy.* New York: Veterinary Textbooks.

Sainte-Marie, G., Peng, F.S., Belisle, C. 1982. Overall architecture and pattern of lymph flow in the rat lymph node. *Am. J. Anat.* 164:275–309.

Sano, S., Takahama, Y., Sugawara, T., Kosaka, H., Itami, S., Yoshikawa, K., Miyazaki, J. Van Ewijk W., Takeda, J. 2001. Stat3 in thymic epithelial cells is essential for postnatal maintenance of thymic architecture and thymocytes survival. *Immunity* 15:261–273.

Savino, W., Postel-Vinay, M.C., Smaniotto, S., Dardenne, M. 2002. The thymus gland: a target organ for growth hormone. *Scand. J. Immunol.* 55:442–458.

Schmidt, E.E., MacDonald, I.C., Groom, A.C. 1985. Microcirculation in mouse spleen (nonsinusal) studied by means of corrosion casts. *J. Morphol.* 186:17–29.

Schmidt, E.E., MacDonald, I.C., Groom, A.C. 1993. Comparative aspects of splenic microcirculatory pathways in mammals: the region bordering the white pulp. *Scanning Microsc.* 7:613–628.

Sestak, K., Merritt, C.K., Borda, J., Saylor, E., Schwamberger, S.R., Cogswell, F., Didier, E.S., Didier, P.J., Plauche, G., Bohm, R.P., Aye, P.P., Alexa, P., Ward, R.L., Lackner, A.A. 2003. Infectious agent and immune response characteristics of chronic enterocolitis in captive rhesus macaques. *Infect. Immun.*, 71, 4079–4086.

Smialowicz, R.J., Luebke, R.W., Riddle, M.M., Rodgers, R.R., Rowe, D.G. 1985. Evaluation of the immunotoxic potential of chlordecone with comparison of cyclophosphamide. *J. Toxicol. Environ. Health* 15:561–574.

Sminia, T., Janse, E.M., Plesch, B.E.C. 1983. Ontogeny of Peyer's patches of the rat. *Anat. Rec.* 207:309–316.

Snook, T. 1950. A comparative study of the vascular arrangements in mammalian species. *Am. J. Anat.* 87:31–77.

Snyder, P.W., Kazacos, E.A., Scott-Moncrieff, J.C., HogenEsch, H., Carlton, W.W., Glickman, L.T., Felsburg, P.J. 1995. Pathologic features of naturally occurring juvenile polyarteritis in beagle dogs. *Vet. Pathol.* 32(4):337–345.

Stefanski, S.A., Elwell, M.R., Stromberg, P.C. 1990. Spleen, lymph node, and thymus. In *Pathology of the Fischer Rat*, Eds. G. Boorman, C.A. Montgomery, W.F. MacKenzie. San Diego, CA: Academic Press.

Sternberg, S.S. 1997. *Histology for Pathologists*, 2nd ed. Philadelphia: Lippincott-Raven.

Stromberg, P.C. 1992. Changes in the hematologic system. In *Pathobiology of the Aging Rat*, vol. 1. eds. U. Mohr, D.L. Dungworth, C.C. Capen, pp. 15–24. Washington, DC: ILSI Press.

Suttie, A.W. 2006. Histopathology of the spleen. *Toxicol. Pathol.* 34:466–503.

Takata, S., Ohtani, O., Watanabe, Y. 2000. Lectin binding patterns in rat nasal-associated lymphoid tissue (NALT) and the influence of various types of lectin on particle uptake in NALT. *Arch. Histol. Cytol.* 63:305–312.

Tecoma, E.S., Huey, L.Y. 1985. Minireview: psychic distress and the immune response. *Life Sci.* 36:1799–1812.

Terszowski, G. Muller, S.M., Bleul, C.C., Blum, C., Schirmbeck, R., Reimann, J., Du Pasquier, L., Amagai, T., Boehm, T., Rodewald, H.R. 2006. *Science* 312:284–287.

Teske, E. 1994. Canine malignant lymphoma: a review and comparison with human non-Hodgkin's lymphomas. *Vet. Quat.* 4:209–219.

Thomas, J., Haseman, J.K., Goodman, J.I., Ward, J.M., Loughran, T.P. Jr., Spencer, P.J.A. 2007. Review of large granular lymphocytic leukemia in Fischer 344 rats as an initial step toward evaluating the implication of the endpoint to human cancer risk assessment. *Toxicol. Sci.* Sep;99(1):3–19.

Tilney, N.L. 1971. Patterns of lymphatic drainage in the adult laboratory rat. *J. Anat.* 109:369–383.

Travlos, G.S. 2006a. Normal structure, function and histology of the bone marrow. *Toxicol. Pathol.* 34:548–565.

Travlos, G.S. 2006b. Histopathology of bone marrow. *Toxicol. Pathol.* 34:566–598.

Valli, V.E., SanMyint, M., Barthel, A., Bienzle, D., Caswell, J., Colbatzky, F., Durham, A., Ehrhart, E.J., Johnson, Y., Jones, C., Kiupel, M., Labelle, P., Lester, S., Miller, M., Moore, P., Moroff, S., Roccabianca, P., Ramos-Vara, J., Ross, A., Scase, T., Tvedten, H., Vernau, W. 2011. Classification of canine malignant lymphomas according to the World Health Organization criteria. *Vet. Pathol.* 48(1):198–211.

van der Ven, I., Sminia, T. 1993. The development and structure of mouse nasal-associated lymphoid tissue: an immuno- and enzyme histochemical study. *Reg. Immunol.* 5:69–75.

van Ewijk, W., Shores, E.W., Singer, A. 1994. Crosstalk in the mouse thymus. *Immunol. Today* 15:214–217.

Van Rees, E.P., Sminia, T., Dijkstra, C.D. 1996. Structure and development of the lymphoid organs. In *Pathobiology of the Aging Mouse*. eds. U. Mohr, D.L. Dungworth, C.C. Capen, W.W. Caldron, J.P. Sundberg. J.M. Ward, vol. 1, pp. 173–187. Washington, DC: ILSI Press.

Ward, J.M. 2006. Lymphomas and leukemia in mice, experiment. *Toxicol. Pathol.* 57:377–381.

Ward, J.M., Reynolds, C.W. 1983. Large granular lymphocyte leukemia. A heterogenous lymphocytic leukemia of F344 rats. *Am. J. Pathol.* 111:1–10.

Ward, J.M., Mann, P.C., Morshima, H., Firth, C.H. 1999. Thymus, spleen and lymph nodes. In *Pathology of the Mouse*, ed. R.R. Maronpot. Vienna, IL: Cache River Press.

Ward, J.M., Erexson, C.R., Faucette, L.J., Foley, J.F., Dijkstra, C., Cattoretti, G. 2006. Immunohistochemical markers for the rodent immune system. *Toxicol. Pathol.* 34:616–630.

Webb, H.K., Ulrich, R.G., Puri, K.D., Chen, H., Sutherland, J.E., Hall, W.C. 2010. Effects of CAL-101, a selective inhibitor of the class 1 PI3K p110delta, on lymphocytes in spleen and lymph nodes. SOT abstract 1060. Presented at the 2010 SOT Annual Meeting, Salt Lake Utah.

Wu, H.Y., Russell, M.W. 1997. Nasal lymphoid tissue. Intranasal immunization and compartmentalization of the common mucosal immune system. *Immunol. Res.* 16:187–201.

Yang, B.-G., Tanaka, T., Ho Jang, M., Bai, Z., Hayasaka, H., Miyasaka, M. 2007. Binding of lymphoid chemo-
     kines to collagen IV that accumulates in the basal lamina of high endothelial venules: its implications in
     lymphocyte trafficking. *J. Immunol.* 179:4376–4382.
Zheng, B., Shorthouse, R., Masek, M.A., Berry, G., Billingham, M.E., Morris, R.E. 1991. Effects of the new
     and highly active immunosuppressant rapamycin on lymphoid tissues and cells in vivo. *Transplanta.
     Proc.* 23:851–855.

15 Bone, Muscle, and Tooth

*John L. Vahle, Joel R. Leininger, Philip H. Long,
D. Greg Hall, and Heinrich Ernst*

CONTENTS

15.1 BONE AND JOINT

15.1.1 FUNCTIONAL ANATOMY

Bone and cartilage are highly specialized connective tissues that together make up the skeleton. The skeleton has multiple functions including (1) locomotion, by providing a structure and attachment sides for muscle; (2) protection, by encasing vital organs and tissues; and (3) metabolism, by serving as a reserve of mineral ions such as calcium and phosphorus. The following section provides a brief overview of the anatomy of the skeleton. Comprehensive reviews of structure and function of the skeleton are provided in review articles and reference texts (Marks and Popoff 1988; Bullough 2011).

It is useful for the toxicologic pathologist to have an understanding of the various regions or subcomponents of bones to aid in accurate identification and description of alterations. Structurally, the skeleton consists of two types of bone: flat bones, such as the calvarium, scapula, or ileum, and long bones, such as the humerus or tibia. The typical long bone consists of two wide ends referred to as the epiphyses joined by a central, cylindrical area referred to as the diaphysis. Joining the epiphyses to the diaphysis is the metaphysis. In the growing skeleton, the epiphysis is separated from the metaphysis by the physis or growth plate. The physis is an anatomically complex tissue, which, together with the metaphysis, is responsible for longitudinal bone growth. In the diaphysis, the bone consists of a dense layer referred to as cortical or compact bone, which surrounds a central medullary cavity containing the hematopoietic bone marrow. In the metaphysis, the cortical bone layer becomes thinner, and the central portions of the bone contain a complex network of interconnecting bony rods, plates, and arches, which are variably referred to as trabecular, cancellous, or spongy bone. This chapter will use the terms *cortical* and *trabecular bone*. The relative proportions of trabecular and cortical bone vary throughout the skeleton to accommodate the biomechanical forces a given bone is subjected to. For example, to give the femur the rigidity it needs to function as a mechanical lever during locomotion, it has a cylindrical shape, and the diaphysis is composed primarily of cortical bone. In contrast, the vertebrae require the ability to absorb compressive forces without cracking and are therefore rich in trabecular bone with only a relatively thin cortical shell. In routine toxicity studies, the most commonly examined bones are a long bone (typically femur and/or tibia) and the sternum. The long bones should be trimmed and embedded such that a proximal or distal end is evaluated to allow examination of both the trabecular bone in the metaphysis and the cortical bone in the diaphysis.

Both cortical and trabecular bone consist primarily of lamellar bone in which the collagen fibers are highly organized and arranged in parallel layers. In contrast to lamellar bone, woven bone refers to immature bone in which the collagen fibers are randomly oriented and lacks the structural organization of lamellar bone. Woven bone is rapidly formed, often in response to injury and, in the normal setting, is replaced by more structurally sound lamellar bone. The simple use of transmitted polarized light in routine, decalcified, paraffin-embedded sections of bone is an effective way for the bench pathologist to visualize the orientations of collagen fibers. In dogs and nonhuman primates, the cortical bone is organized in concentric layers around a central channel. This unit is referred to as an osteon or Haversian system. In contrast, rats and mice lack or have poorly developed Haversian systems.

The cell types in bone include bone lining cells, osteoblasts, osteocytes, and osteoclasts. The bone lining cells are thought to be osteoprogenitor cells and morphologically appear as flattened, quiescent cells on the bone surface. Osteoblasts are most commonly associated with bone formation; however, these cells also have complex communications with other bone cells and play roles in both bone formation and resorption. Morphologically "active" osteoblasts appear as plump, round to oval cells on bone surfaces. Osteocytes are small cells residing in lacunae within the mineralized bone matrix. Although these cells are small and nondescript on histologic examination, they possess long processes that radiate through a bone canalicular system and have important functions in sensing mechanical load and triggering local bone turnover. Osteoclasts are readily detected in histologic sections and are essentially multinucleated macrophages and function in the resorption of bone matrix. These cells can occur singly or in small clusters within depressions (resorption pits, Howship's lacunae) on bone surfaces. When osteoclastic activity is increased, these resorption pits give the bone surface a scalloped appearance that can be observed with routine light microscopy. Bone matrix is composed of a complex mixture of inorganic mineral ions such as calcium and phosphorus, various types of collagen, and glycoproteins. For the toxicologic pathologist, it is important to recognize that the initial deposition of matrix is an unmineralized material referred to as osteoid that consists primarily of collagen and glycosaminoglycans. Osteoid is subsequently mineralized by incorporation of calcium phosphates and carbonates, and the interface where this process occurs is referred to as the mineralization front. The external surfaces of the bone are covered by the periosteum. The inner layer of the periosteum consists of the osteoblasts, which function to deposit osteoid on the bone surface, resulting in increased bone diameter (appositional bone growth). The middle layer of the periosteum is a fibrocellular matrix, which is thought to contain osteoprogenitor cells. The outer layer consists of dense fibrous connective tissue, which connects to the surface of the bone through numerous projections known as Sharpey's fibers.

The physis (growth plate) is responsible for the increases in diaphyseal length that occur postnatally through a process called endochondral ossification. Because many routine toxicity studies are conducted in rodents that are rapidly growing, it is not uncommon to detect alterations in the structure of the physis. The normal physis has an orderly structure with distinct zones that have different functions. The zone nearest the epiphysis is the reserve zone that consists of flattened chondrocytes, which are in a resting state. In the proliferating zone, the chondrocytes undergo cell divisions, organize into distinct columns, and synthesize substantial amounts of matrix. As the chondrocytes move distally, they lose their capacity for replication, begin to increase in size, and become part of the hypertrophic zone. Within the hypertrophic zone, chondrocytes are large and round in appearance and begin to have increases in intracellular calcium. Oxygen tension is low in this zone, which stimulates new blood vessels from the adjacent primary spongiosa of the metaphysis. The chondrocytes mineralize, undergo apoptosis, and leave behind a calcified cartilage scaffold. Capillary invasion into the empty chondrocyte lacunae brings in osteoblast and osteoclasts. The osteoblasts lay down a delicate layer of new bone on the surface of the calcified cartilage, resulting in the primary spongiosa of the metaphysis. As endochondral ossification proceeds, the primary spongiosa is modeled into larger secondary spongiosa. A more detailed description of the structure of the physis and the process of endochondral ossification can be found in reviews by Kronenberg (2003) and Hall et al. (2006).

A synovial joint consists of a joint cavity lined by synovial cells, the underlying fibrous joint capsule, the articular cartilage, and ligaments. Synovial cells are often one to three cell layers thick and are supported by variable amounts of fibrous connective tissue and adipose tissue. In routine toxicity studies with standard sectioning, only limited amounts of synovium may be present. If changes in joints are anticipated, standard trimming and embedding measures will need to be modified to ensure that the joints are thoroughly examined. Hyaline cartilage is present not only on the articular joints but in the physis and larynx as well. Healthy articular cartilage is a firm yet pliable tissue composed of large amounts of extracellular matrix with relatively few cells. Chondrocytes are located within well-defined lacunae and, in the articular cartilage, occur in a series of four layers. Near the surface is a zone of oval or elongate chondrocytes and collagen fibers. In the intermediate transitional zone, the cells are round to oval, and the collagen forms an open meshwork. The deeper radiate zone contains large, round chondrocytes, which may be arranged in short columns. The deepest zone is the mineralized zone, which is adjacent to the subchondral bone. A distinct basophilic tidewater mark separates the mineralized zone from the radiate zone. Water is a large component by weight of hyaline articular cartilage, and Type II and Type IX collagen, along with various proteoglycans, compromise much of the matrix.

15.1.2 Species Differences

Similar to other organ systems, there are important differences across species in various aspects of bone anatomy and physiology. In particular, endochondral bone growth is very rapid in the young growing rat, the age used in most toxicity studies. For example, 6-week-old rats have been reported to grow up to 300 µm per day at the tibial growth plate (Hansson et al. 1972). Although longitudinal growth begins to slow after 8 weeks of age in rats, some degree of growth continues, and rats are not considered skeletally mature until 10 months of age (Lelovas et al. 2008). The rapid growth of the rodent skeleton is one of the reasons that compound-induced morphologic changes in the physis are often detected in rodents, but not the nonrodent species, in a pharmaceutical safety testing program. Another variable to be aware of is that closure of the physis varies widely across bone sites within a species and between species. For example, in male rats, some physes remain open up to 30 months of age, whereas the distal tibial physis closes at approximately 3 months of age. In dogs, rapid bone growth ceases at approximately 5 months of age (Yonamine et al. 1980), and in monkeys, fusion of the growth plate occurs between 5 and 6 years of age (Zoetis et al. 2003).

Another species difference to be aware of are differences between the rodent and nonrodent skeleton with respect to how bone, particularly cortical bone, is formed. These differences have been characterized most extensively for the rat and nonhuman primate skeleton due to their common use in the nonclinical development of osteoporosis therapies. In rats, particularly in young growing rats used in traditional toxicity studies, the predominant activity is modeling. Modeling refers to a process in which bone formation and bone resorption occur independent of each other. In nonhuman primates, similar to humans, the predominant process is remodeling, in which bone formation is closely coupled to bone formation at a specific site. This coupled process results in a cycle of activation–resorption–formation (Parfitt 1984; Eriksen 2010; Jerome and Peterson 2001; Lelovas et al. 2008).

15.1.3 Evaluation Methods

In the vast majority of routine toxicity studies, formalin-fixed, decalcified, paraffin-embedded bone sections stained with hematoxylin and eosin (H&E) are adequate for histologic evaluation. The standard sections of bone vary between laboratories but most often include the sternum and a long bone, most often the distal femur and/or proximal tibia. The most commonly encountered technical issues are excessive decalcification resulting in poor staining quality, inconsistency in the plane of section, and fragmentation and distortion of the section. The toxicologic pathologist is assessing the relative amounts of various components such as the quantity of metaphyseal bone or thickness of the physis in comparison with study control sections, and therefore, consistent orientation and trimming are important to allow an accurate assessment. The trimming of the long bone should allow for evaluation of an articular surface, the epiphysis, physis, metaphysis, and a region of diaphyseal bone. Obtaining sections of all of these regions on a single slide is not an issue for rodent species but can be more challenging in dogs and nonhuman primates. During the primary evaluation, the pathologist should be attentive to ensure that the section provides an adequate representation of each of these regions.

In addition to the routine histologic processing, a variety of methods are available to more thoroughly characterize bone structure. These techniques are best conducted in specialized laboratories that have specific expertise in this unique area of histotechnology. It should also be recognized that many of these procedures are time and resource intensive. These techniques include the following:

1. *Undecalcified sections:* If there is a need to assess the mineralization status, undecalcified sections prepared by embedding the specimen in a plastic such as methyl methacrylate are required. In these undecalcified sections, alizarin red (stains calcium components) or von Kossa (stains phosphate components) is often used.
2. *Histochemical stains:* Special stains are not commonly employed in routine paraffin-embedded sections; however, collagen can be demonstrated by a trichrome stain, and proteoglycans can be demonstrated with Alcian blue or toluidine blue. The use of these stains is more common in the evaluation of articular cartilage and is often used in evaluation of animal models of arthritis.
3. *Fluorochrome labeling:* Agents such as tetracycline, alizarin red, or calcein have affinity for mineralization surfaces and serve as a supravital dye when administered to the animals at defined intervals prior to necropsy. The sections are examined via fluorescence to highlight regions of bone formation.
4. *Histomorphometry:* Bone histomorphometry yields important quantitative information for a diverse array of measured and derived parameters such as trabecular bone volumes, cortical area, bone formation rate, and activation frequency. The nomenclature and practice of bone histomorphometry are relatively standardized and should be conducted according to established criteria (Parfitt et al. 1987). When combined with fluorescent labels, morphometry is referred to as dynamic histomorphometry. When performed on non-fluorochrome-treated sections, it is referred to as static histomorphometry.

In addition to the above histology-based methods, it is useful for the toxicologic pathologist to be aware of other methods that can provide important insights into bone structure and function. Blood-based biomarkers of bone formation and resorption such as amino-terminal propeptide of Type I procollagen (P1NP), bone-specific alkaline phosphatase, and N-telopeptides are available in several preclinical species and are readily translatable to clinical trials (Allen 2003). Another important tool is the use of imaging modalities such as dual energy x-ray absorptiometry (DEXA) or quantitative computed tomography (QCT) to provide a quantitative assessment of bone mass. Common parameters include bone mineral content (BMC) and bone mineral density (BMD). These methods can be employed either as in vivo scans during the conduct of an animal study or as an ex vivo analysis on excised bone specimens (Sato et al. 2002; Smith et al. 2009). A clear advantage of in vivo measurements is the ability to characterize the time course of change, and each animal can serve as its own control, enabling greater sensitivity to detect changes. Because the skeleton is covered by muscle and other soft tissues, focal lesions may not be detected at necropsy, and therefore, plain film radiographs can be useful in specialized studies. Finally, if there are concerns regarding the structural integrity of the bone, carefully excised and prepared bone specimens can be subjected to biomechanical testing to characterize the material properties of the tissue (Turner and Burr 2007).

Similar to bone, a variety of specialized techniques are available to detect and characterize changes in joint structure. While not commonly used in routine toxicity studies, they are widely used in a variety of animal models of arthritis (Bendele 2011). In many of the models, the use of a frontal trimming plane is preferred to allow for examination of both the medial and lateral components of the joint. The most commonly used stains are H&E for a routine evaluation of overall joint histology and the cationic stain toluidine blue to evaluate the hyaline cartilage, including detection of changes in proteoglycan content. Safranin O and other special stains, as well as immunohistochemical techniques to evaluate various collagen types, can be employed.

15.1.4 Nonproliferative Lesions of Bone

15.1.4.1 Hyperostosis

One of the most common bone changes detected in toxicity studies is an increased amount of bone. This change may be either congenital or induced by xenobiotics that affect bone formation or resorption. The change is most commonly detected as a diffuse increase in mature lamellar bone in the metaphysis that can be recognized in tissue sections as increased trabecular number and thickness with a subsequent reduction in marrow spaces (Figures 15.1a and b). In the case of congenital conditions (e.g., osteopetrosis), or following treatment with potent anabolic bone agents, there may

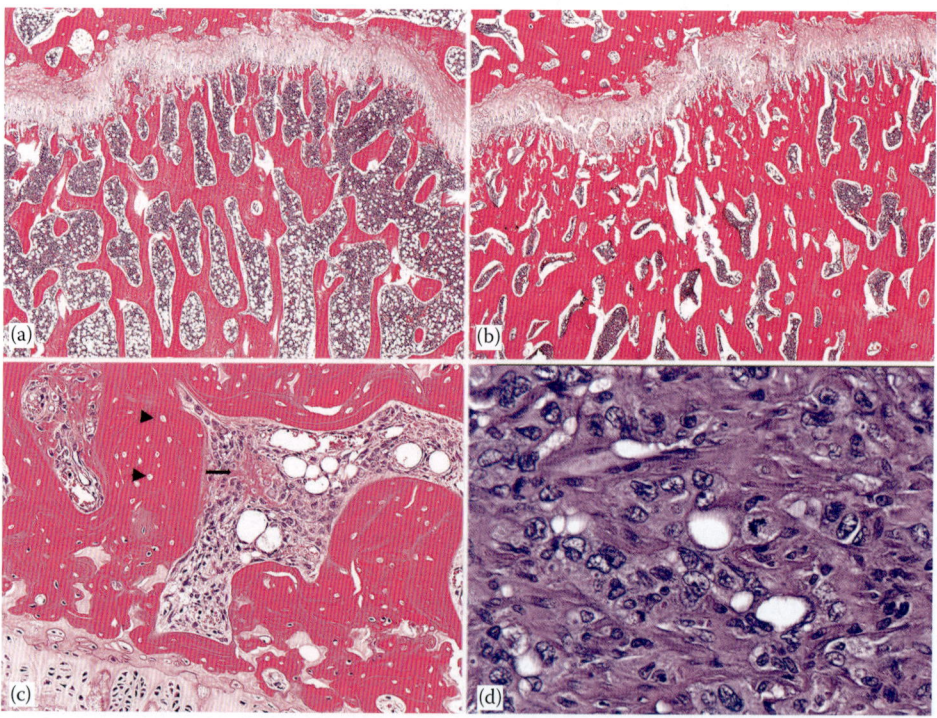

FIGURE 15.1 (a) Physis and metaphysis from a control cynomolgus monkey, demonstrating the normal appearance of the metaphyseal trabecular bone. (b) Physis and metaphysis from a monkey treated with a bone anabolic agent, demonstrating increased thickness of the trabeculae warranting a diagnosis of hyperostosis or increased trabecular bone. Note the commensurate reduction in marrow space. (c) Proximal femoral epiphysis from an untreated control Sprague–Dawley rat, 12 weeks of age. Osteonecrosis is present. Note the empty lacunae (arrowheads) and the formation of new woven bone within the marrow space (arrow). The changes in the marrow space support the conclusion that the empty lacunae represent osteonecrosis and are not an artifact. In more advanced lesions, greater evidence of osteoclastic resorption would be present. (d) Osteosarcoma from an F344 rat in a 2-year carcinogenicity study. Note the highly cellular and pleomorphic appearance with only small spicules of tumor osteoid. If tumor osteoid is not identified, some of these neoplasms may be diagnosed as sarcoma, not otherwise specified. In general, the diagnostic features of osteosarcoma in rodents are similar to those in other species.

be near-complete filling of epiphysis, metaphysis, and diaphysis resulting from continual deposition of bone. While changes are initially detected in the metaphysis, they can also be observed in the epiphysis and diaphysis. Typically, the structure of the physis is not affected. With routine evaluation methods, it is not possible to determine if the increased bone is due to inhibited bone resorption or increased bone formation. Differentiating increased bone due to hyperostosis from neoplastic bone is straightforward as there is a lack of cellular (osteoblast) proliferation and the matrix is mature lamellar bone rather than tumor osteoid. The presence of mature, mineralized bone aids in differentiating hyperostosis from conditions such as hyperosteoidosis in which there is an abnormal increase in unmineralized osteoid. When of sufficient severity, hyperostosis may be suspected at necropsy as the bones may be notably harder and more difficult to transect.

As a spontaneous entity, hyperostosis is most commonly reported in aging rodents, particularly female rats in 2-year carcinogenicity studies. In these instances, the change is readily detected in sections of sternum but can also be noted in the femur and tibia sections. Focal increases in trabecular bone may also occur spontaneously in any species, but these are most often a component of a reaction to an old fracture, osteonecrosis, or other condition, and they generally do not warrant a separate diagnosis. As an induced change, hyperostosis or generalized increases in bone have been reported for agents that inhibit osteoclastic bone resorption, such as bisphosphonates (Movsowitz et al. 1990), and for bone anabolic agents such as parathyroid hormone and related peptides (Vahle et al. 2002; Jolette et al. 2006) or inhibitors of sclerostin (Ominsky et al. 2010). Sodium fluoride was reported to cause osteosclerosis in 2-year rat carcinogenicity studies; however, the increased trabecular bone occurred in conjunction with increased endosteal resorption and areas of periosteal proliferation (Bucher et al. 1991). For quantitative changes in trabecular and cortical bone, histopathology provides useful qualitative data; however, it is often valuable to incorporate more sensitive and quantitative measures of bone mass and structure (densitometry, histomorphometry) if pharmacologically induced bone changes are anticipated.

15.1.4.2 Bone Atrophy (Osteopenia)

Less commonly observed than hyperostosis, a generalized or local decrease in the relative quantity of bone is referred to as bone atrophy or osteopenia. In most cases, using a descriptive term such as "trabecular bone, decreased" in the histology lexicon is most appropriate, and reserve the term osteopenia for those cases in which bone mass has been characterized by more quantitative methods such as densitometry. Atrophy should be reserved for those cases in which the composition of the bone matrix appears histologically normal but is decreased in quantity. This change will be most readily detected within the metaphyseal trabecular bone; however, the toxicologic pathologist should use caution in interpreting subtle decreases in the relative amounts of trabecular bone, as small differences in orientation of the section can be misleading. Atrophy or osteopenia has been reported as a spontaneous, age-related finding (Kiebzak et al. 1988) but is not typically recorded or observed as a common background finding in aging rodents in carcinogenicity studies. Older reports of processes inducing generalized decreases in bone mass include diminished feed intake, cortisone toxicity, thyrotoxicosis, pyridoxine deficiency, heparin, B-aminoproprionitrile, and dextran sulfate. Osteopenia can be induced by a variety of experimental manipulations such as ovariectomy or limb immobilization; however, more quantitative measures, rather than routine histology, are generally employed in these settings.

15.1.4.3 Increased Resorption

Bone formation and resorption are normal components of bone turnover; however, in some cases, sites of increased resorption are recognized at microscopic examination by the presence of increased numbers of osteoclasts (osteoclast hyperplasia) along a bone surface, and the presence of surface excavations gives the bone surface an irregular, serrated appearance. In many cases, increased bone resorption is a component of a process such as fibrous osteodystrophy or as a response to cleaning up necrotic bone. If increased resorption is suspected as a primary test article–induced effect, specialized studies to quantify osteoclasts and various aspects of bone formation and resorption may be needed.

15.1.4.4 Necrosis

Microscopically, the hallmarks of bone necrosis are lack of osteocytes in lacunae and lack of osteoblasts on bone surfaces (Figure 15.1c). Early in the process, the lack of bone cellular elements may be the only detectable change; however, in most cases, there is also necrosis of the adjacent marrow elements. At low magnification, the lack of osteocytes may not be readily apparent, and the loss of marrow elements may be the first feature recognized by the pathologist. As the process enters the repair phase, several features, including increased numbers of mesenchymal cells and capillaries on the bone surface, peritrabecular and/or marrow fibrosis, or deposition of woven bone on the surface of the dead bone at the margin of dead bone, may be observed. Other features may include a focal increase in density of the adjacent bone (sclerosis), and, in some cases, the fragment of necrotic bone may become isolated as a sequestrum.

Mechanistically, bone necrosis is most often attributed to ischemia and has been most widely studied in the context of animal models of aseptic necrosis of the femoral head (Boss and Misselevich 2003). The femoral head is not routinely examined in the majority of toxicity studies, and bone necrosis, regardless of location, is not a common spontaneous event in strains of animals typically used in toxicology. Femoral head necrosis is reported in the Wistar Kyoto (WKR) and spontaneously hypertensive (SHR) rat strains (Naito et al. 2009; Hirano et al. 1988). Small foci of bone necrosis have been observed in the femoral head in untreated, young (6-8 weeks of age) Sprague–Dawley rats in routine toxicity studies (Figure 15.1d, personal observations). Corticosteroids and bisphosphonates can cause osteonecrosis in humans and a number of animal species (Jones and Allen 2011). Osteonecrosis and physeal alterations subsequent to thrombosis have been described following administration of 2-butoxyethanol (Nyska et al. 1999).

15.1.4.5 Fracture and Callus Formation

Mechanical injury may occur during a toxicity study and result in gross and/or microscopic evidence of a fracture with subsequent callus formation. If observed in the early stages, hemorrhage, fibrin, and necrosis will be predominant. As the response progresses, mesenchymal cells with enlarged nuclei and increased mitotic figures appear. It is important to note that these cytologic features are a normal response to injury and do not represent a preneoplastic condition. Depending on whether or not the periosteum is intact, the maturing callus can form either through a cartilage model or via woven bone. As the repair process completes, the woven bone is replaced by lamellar bone, and the fracture site is remodeled. In routine studies, histologic evidence of fracture and/or callus formation are not common entities; however, they are reported as one of the few background lesions of bone in nonhuman primate toxicity studies (Chamanza et al. 2010).

15.1.4.6 Bone Cyst

Microscopically, bone cysts are a discrete cavity of variable size and shape, often in the metaphysis of the long bone. They are typically lined by a thin fibrous membrane; however, the lining cells may be indistinct. In diagnostic human and veterinary pathology, various subtypes have been characterized. The most distinctive subtype that may be observed in toxicity studies is the aneurysmal bone cyst, which consists of multiple cystic spaces of variable size that contain blood but are not clearly lined with vascular endothelium. In the epiphysis, subchondral bone cysts may be detected. These are not true cysts in that they lack a discrete cellular lining and are most often associated with degenerative changes in the joint. Differential diagnoses are limited as these are typically distinct structures. In some cases, irregular spaces may be observed in lytic bone lesions; however, these structures are less well demarcated, lack a cellular lining, and would not warrant a separate diagnosis. The origin of bone cysts is typically not known. Simple bone cysts are generally thought to represent a focal developmental defect. Aneurysmal bone cysts appear to arise due to a disturbance in blood flow in the bone marrow. Subchondral bone cysts are regarded as pseudo-cysts and arise secondary to an inflammatory or degenerative process of the joint.

In routine toxicity studies, true bone cysts appear to be relatively rare based on published reports. An online review of the National Toxicology Program Pathology Database revealed sporadic reports of cysts in a variety of bone sites in both male and female rats and mice in rodent bioassays. Examples of xenobiotic-induced bone cysts appear to be even rarer. Rats administered with aminopropionitrile developed aneurysmal-like bone cysts in the mandible (Baden 1987). In humans, bone cysts can arise in the context of fibrous osteodystrophy secondary to hyperparathyroidism (osteitis fibrosa cystica); however, this manifestation is not common in rodents.

15.1.4.7 Fibrous Osteodystrophy

Fibrous osteodystrophy is characterized by increased osteoclastic bone resorption combined with an increase in fibrous connective tissue. The increased bone resorption is recognized in histologic sections as increased osteoclast numbers and increased number and size of surface excavations on both trabecular and cortical surfaces. In some cases, the process may dissect into existing trabecular or cortical bone. Increased marrow fibrous connective tissue (peritrabecular fibrosis) may be limited to a thin layer covering the endosteal surface or be a more prominent component with thicker bands of fibrosis within the marrow space. When the histologic features of fibrous osteodystrophy are present in bone, it is important to look for morphologic or biochemical evidence of primary or secondary hyperparathyroidism (advanced renal disease, parathyroid gland hyperplasia, diffuse tissue mineralization, etc.). In mice, an important differential diagnosis is fibro-osseous lesion (described below). Marrow fibrosis, a relatively nonspecific entity, can be differentiated by the lack of prominent increases in osteoclastic bone resorption.

In toxicology studies, fibrous osteodystrophy is most often encountered in 2-year studies in the setting of chronic renal failure with renal secondary hyperparathyroidism. While increased circulating parathyroid hormone is an important part of the pathogenesis, other factors such as metabolic acidosis likely contribute to the stimulation of bone resorption. Experimental manipulations that result in advanced renal disease, such as administration of cadmium (Uchida et al. 2010) or hydrochlorothiazide (Bucher et al. 1990) or nephrectomy models (Mandalunis and Ubios 2005), result in an increased incidence of fibrous osteodystrophy. In humans with hyperparathyroidism, large lytic lesions resembling neoplasia (brown tumor of hyperparathyroidism) may be present in advanced cases; however, this is not a typical feature in rodents.

15.1.4.8 Fibro-Osseous Lesions

Fibro-osseous lesions are a specific entity that occurs as both a spontaneous and induced lesion in a variety of strains of mice. The lesions occur primarily in females and can occur in a variety of skeletal sites. In affected animals, the marrow spaces contain a fibrocellular infiltrate with abundant eosinophilic matrix. Small spicules of osteoid and/or focal areas of woven or lamellar bone formation may occur. In severe lesions, there is more extensive lamellar bone formation, which can produce a hyperostotic or sclerotic appearance. The microscopic appearance of these lesions is similar to fibrous osteodystrophy. Fibrous osteodystrophy is typically diagnosed if there is concurrent renal disease or evidence of parathyroid hyperplasia and/or an increase in osteoclastic bone resorption. The toxicologic pathologist will most likely encounter this lesion as a spontaneous background finding in mice in 2-year carcinogenicity studies. The best characterized cause of an increased incidence of fibro-osseous lesions in mice is the administration of estrogens (Highman 1981). If a treatment-related exacerbation of the change is observed, an investigation into a potential estrogen-like effect may be warranted.

15.1.4.9 Physeal Dysplasia

Physeal dysplasia has been used to describe drug-induced alterations in the physis, particularly in young growing rats. "Physeal dysplasia," "physeal hypertrophy," and "endochondral hypertrophy" are terms that have been used to encompass a spectrum of changes that vary, depending on the nature of the pharmacologic properties of the molecule and the degree of modulation of the molecular target or pathway. Agents that inhibit angiogenesis are a well-known cause of physeal changes (see excellent review by Hall et al. 2006) due to the important role of vascular invasion in the process of endochondral ossification. In these cases, the physis is thickened, primarily due to an expansion of the zone of hypertrophic chondrocytes, and a similar change can be observed in the epiphyseal growth cartilage subjacent to articular surfaces. The trabeculae of the primary and secondary spongiosa may also be decreased in number and thickness, and there is an inappropriate retention of hypertrophic chondrocytes within the primary spongiosa. While most commonly observed in growing rodents, the physeal effects of angiogenesis inhibitors have also been described in nonhuman primates (Ryan 1999). Perturbation of other pathways important in endochondral ossification such as bFGF (Brown et al. 2005), ALK5 (Frazier et al. 2007), and hedgehog (Kimura

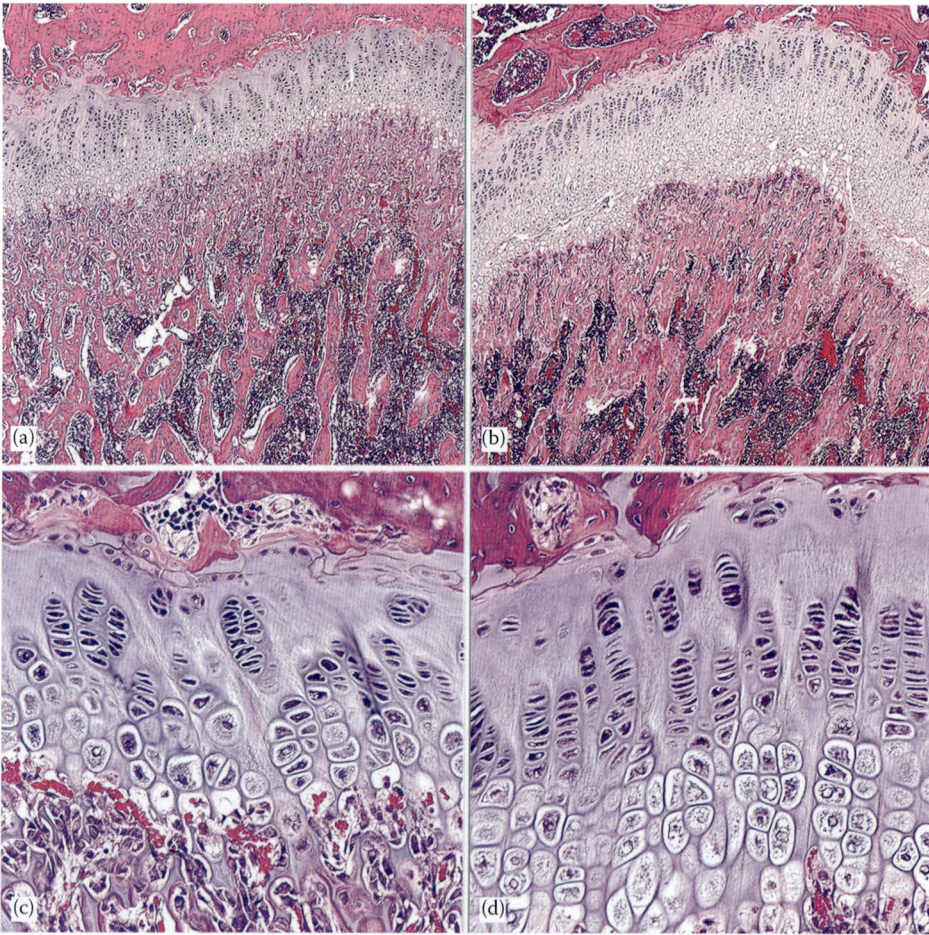

FIGURE 15.2 Proximal femoral physis of Sprague–Dawley rats. In 10-week-old rats, treatment with an ALK5 inhibitor (b) results in marked thickening of the physis and an increase in submetaphyseal trabecular bone compared to the concurrent control animal (a). Similar lesions have been reported with a variety of xenobiotics, which affect signaling pathways important in endochondral ossification. These effects are most prominent in the young growing rat. The effect of age is demonstrated in c and d. Both 9-month-old (c) and 10-week-old (d) rats were treated with an ALK5 inhibitor. Note the marked increased in physeal thickness in the young rat compared to the older rat. (Reprinted from Frazier, K. et al., *Toxicologic Pathology*, 35:284–295, 2007. With permission.)

et al. 2008) has been shown to produce physeal dysplasia. Although generally characterized by an increased thickness of the physis, other characteristics such as effects on the primary and secondary spongiosa and age dependency of the lesion appear to vary depending on the signaling pathway that has been interrupted. The morphology of physeal effects of pharmaceutical agents that inhibit ALK5 (Frazier et al. 2007) and FGF (Brown et al. 2005) has been especially well characterized (see Figures 15.2a through d). In addition to these pharmacologic agents that directly impact cell signaling, physeal and/or articular cartilage lesions have been induced by other agents as well. Semicarbazide administration results in a spectrum of osteochondral lesions of both physeal and articular cartilage (Takahashi et al. 2010). In addition to thickening of the growth plate, there is degeneration of hypertrophic chondrocytes and deformation and fissures of the articular cartilage. Marimastat, a broad-spectrum matrix metalloproteinase inhibitor (MMP), has been shown to cause prominent thickening of the physeal cartilage in rats, primarily due to an increase in the zone of chondrocyte maturation and hypertrophy (Renkiewicz et al. 2003). The metaphyseal bone immediately subjacent to the physis becomes thickened and disorganized. Thickening of the articular cartilage does not occur, but there are soft tissue changes, including formation of a vascular pannus and thickening of the synovial lining of the joint. These findings are thought to represent a model of the musculoskeletal syndrome that has been observed in patients administered with MMP inhibitors.

As a spontaneous change, physeal abnormalities appear to be relatively uncommon. In aging F344 rats, focal degenerative changes and fissures between the physis and epiphysis have been described (Yamasaki and Inui 1985). Chamanza et al. (2010) described a low incidence of metaphyseal abnormalities in a survey of control cynomolgus monkeys from routine toxicity studies. In dog toxicity studies, focal defects and/or overt necrosis of physeal cartilage can be observed (Yamasaki 1995).

15.1.5 PROLIFERATIVE LESIONS OF BONE

15.1.5.1 Osteoblast Hyperplasia

Osteoblast hyperplasia is an unusual focal lesion that was described in rat 2-year carcinogenicity studies of parathyroid hormone or related peptides (Jolette et al. 2006; Vahle et al. 2002). Osteoblast hyperplasia was characterized by single or multiple foci of well-differentiated osteoblast-like cells. The focal lesions may fill enlarged trabecular spaces but lack significant disruption of the adjacent bone.

15.1.5.2 Osteoma

Microscopically, these lesions arise from the periosteal surface of cortical bone and consist of dense, sclerotic bone that is primarily lamellar. The interior of the lesion has a paucity of cells, and lacunae may lack cells all together. At the periphery of the lesion, there are often more delicate trabeculae covered by a layer of osteoblasts. The external surface of the neoplasm is smooth, and there is no evidence of invasion. Osteoma occurs at a low incidence in control rats and mice in 2-year carcinogenicity studies, and increased incidences have been observed following glucocorticoid (Zwicker and Eyster 1996) and parathyroid hormone fragment administration (Vahle et al. 2002; Jolette et al. 2006). In mice, retroviral-induced osteoma has been extensively studied (Gimbel et al. 1996).

15.1.5.3 Osteoblastoma

Osteoblastoma is a well-characterized benign bone tumor in humans but, in toxicity studies, has been reported only in association with administration of bone anabolic agents (Jolette et al. 2006; Vahle et al. 2002). Microscopically, the lesion is characterized by an intramedullary pattern of disorganized trabeculae of immature bone, often accompanied by a fibrovascular stroma. There are typically moderate numbers of large, well-differentiated osteoblasts arranged along trabecular surfaces. There is typically minimal cytologic atypia, and low numbers of mitotic figures may be present. In studies where osteoblastoma has been observed, the lesion was often first recognized at a lower magnification as a focus of disorganized trabeculae.

15.1.5.4 Osteosarcoma

Although all bone proliferative lesions are rare as a background finding, osteosarcomas appear to be the most common of the bone tumors observed in rodent carcinogenicity studies. In rodents, the morphology of the lesions are similar to that in other species in they are a highly invasive lesion composed of pleomorphic spindle cells with cytologic atypia and the presence of tumor osteoid (Figure 15.1d). The presence of tumor osteoid is the essential diagnostic feature and may be limited to small amounts of wispy, eosinophilic matrix within a highly cellular lesion. While there are various subtypes recognized in various diagnostic schemes (e.g., osteoblastic, fibroblastic, telangiectatic), subclassification is not particularly informative in most toxicology studies. Due to their often large and destructive nature, osteosarcomas are often visible at necropsy and often have gross or microscopic metastasis to the lung. While most frequently affecting the appendicular skeleton, they may arise at a variety of sites and, although rare, may occur as an extraskeletal osteosarcoma (Pace et al. 1995). Osteosarcomas have been induced in rodents by a variety of agents, including radiation, viruses, glucocorticoids (Zwicker and Eyster 1996), and parathyroid hormone (Vahle et al. 2002; Jolette et al. 2006).

15.1.5.5 Chondroma and Chondrosarcoma

Chondromas are occasionally observed in the nasal turbinate in rodents and are a well-demarcated and expansile lesion composed of relatively mature hyaline cartilage (Wadsworth 1989; Jori and Cooper 2001). The chondrocytes are well differentiated and are sparsely populated throughout an abundant matrix. Chondrosarcomas are the malignant counterpart. These neoplasms are highly cellular and composed of generally well-differentiated, large basophilic cells within lacunae, surrounded by variable amounts of cartilaginous matrix. Lesions may contain multinucleated chondrocytes with nuclear atypia. These tumors are described as being minimally invasive but readily metastasize to the lung (Gregson and Offer 1981).

15.1.5.6 Osteochondroma

Although a distinct entity in diagnostic pathology practice, osteochondromas are not common as either a spontaneous or induced change in toxicity studies (Ernst et al. 1992; Iwata et al. 1995). Osteochondromas are focal proliferations of lamellar bone covered by a cap of cartilage that consists of irregularly arrayed, hypertrophic chondrocytes. These lesions are to be differentiated from osteophytes, which form in the epiphysis in the setting of degenerative joint disease. Historically, these lesions have been induced by radiation and vinyl chloride.

15.1.5.7 Primary Bone Fibrosarcoma

Although not previously included in most rodent classification schemes, fibrosarcoma of bone has been observed in both control and treated rodents in 2-year bioassay studies conducted by the National Toxicology Program and has been reported as an induced lesion in rats (Jolette et al. 2006).

Histologically, the neoplasm is characterized by pleomorphic-shaped cells, intermixed with variable amounts of collagenous matrix. Similar to fibrosarcoma in other locations, the mitotic index is increased, and cytologic features include significant nuclear and cellular pleomorphism. Cells are often arranged in an interlacing pattern. A key feature is expansion with lysis of adjacent trabecular or cortical bone. If possible, it is important to obtain adequate sections to clarify if the lesion truly represents a primary tumor of bone, rather than an extension of a soft tissue fibrosarcoma. A key differential is the occurrence of osteosarcomas, which have a primarily fibroblastic component; however, these lesions would contain at least a limited amount of tumor osteoid.

15.1.6 Nonproliferative Lesions of Joint/Articular Cartilage

15.1.6.1 Osteoarthritis (Degenerative Joint Disease)

Osteoarthritis, or degenerative joint disease, is a disease complex that can include a wide array of histologic features. In the early stages, a reduction or lack of uniformity of staining of the articular cartilage can be detected. Although this can be detected in routinely stained H&E sections as a focal loss of basophilia, early changes are best characterized via special stains such as toluidine blue. The lesion progresses to include fibrillation, irregularities, erosions, and ulcerations of the articular surface, and clusters or nests of chondrocytes (chondrones) in the adjacent cartilage. As the cartilage is progressively damaged, biomechanical forces begin to directly impact the subchondral bone, resulting in an increased thickness and density of the subchondral bone plate. In some cases, a cyst-like space (subchondral bone cyst) will develop subjacent to the region of articular cartilage damage. Additional sequelae can include the formation of osteophytes on the periarticular bone surface, synovial cell hyperplasia, and joint capsule fibrosis and ossification. Due to the wide spectrum of histologic features that may occur, the nomenclature used to tabulate the findings in toxicity studies could include either a general term of osteoarthritis or a listing of specific components of the lesion. The decision on which terms to use depends on the nature and severity of the particular change. In studies supporting osteoarthritis research, it is typical to score various components of the lesion (Glasson et al. 2010; Gerwin et al. 2010).

As a spontaneous change, the frequency of osteoarthritis varies with the age and species but can be observed in any of the commonly used laboratory species used in toxicology studies. Multiple strains of mice have age-related spontaneous cartilage degeneration that most often affects the medial compartment of the knee joint and can be quite severe. In rats, spontaneous lesions generally develop by 13 months of age. In dogs and cynomolgus monkeys in routine toxicity studies, spontaneous cases are not common; however, they have been observed in older populations (8–16 years) of cynomolgus monkeys.

15.1.6.2 Chondromucinous Degeneration

In rodents, chondromucinous degeneration is a relatively common spontaneous background lesion in routine toxicity studies and affects the synarthroses of the sternum and physeal, as well as articular cartilage of long bones. The lesion increases in incidence and severity with increasing age. The lesion is most prominent in the sternum, and histologic features include a focal region of necrosis with loss of chondrocytes, fragmentation of the matrix, nest of proliferating chondrocytes adjacent to the lesion, and, in some cases, distinct areas of cavitation. In severe cases, the lesions are large enough to be noted at necropsy. Caloric restriction is reported to decrease the severity of the change (Kawahara et al. 2002); however, examples of compound-induced changes in the incidence or severity of the lesion do not appear to be common based on published reports.

15.1.6.3 Cartilage Degeneration

Distinct from osteoarthritis and chondromucinous degeneration is degeneration of the articular cartilage associated with various xenobiotics. Often referred to as drug-induced arthropathies, these entities are primarily characterized by degeneration of the articular cartilage and lack a significant inflammatory component. One of the most well-characterized articular cartilage toxicities is quinolone-induced arthropathy (Burkhardt et al. 1990, 1992). In severe cases, the changes are associated with lameness during the in-life evaluation, and at necropsy, affected animals may have gross lesions of vesiculation and detachment of the superficial layer of cartilage in multiple joints. The intermediate zone of cartilage in the articular–epiphyseal complex appears to be particularly sensitive, and the histologic lesions include focal loss of matrix, cavitation, and erosion of the cartilage. It has been suggested that the pathogenesis is due to an inhibition of proteoglycan synthesis (Yabe et al. 2004). Semicarbazide administration results in a spectrum of osteochondral lesions including chondrocyte degeneration and deformation and fissures of the articular cartilage (Takahashi et al. 2010).

15.1.6.4 Inflammation

Inflammatory conditions of the joint are not common in toxicity studies but have been intensely studied and well-characterized in a number of animal models of rheumatoid and osteoarthritis (Bendele 2011). Infections within the joint typically present as the presence of edema, congestion, and an infiltrate of inflammatory cells of varying composition within the synovium and may expand the periarticular soft tissues. The joint space often contains a fibrinosuppurative exudate. With time, inflammation of the joint leads to synovial hyperplasia, pannus formation, fibrosis, and, ultimately, erosion or ulceration of the articular cartilage with loss of subchondral bone. In the case of degenerative joint disease (see above), inflammatory lesions are typically limited to mild infiltrates of lymphocytes and macrophages within the synovium and lack the exudation noted in cases of infection.

15.1.7 Proliferative Lesions of Joint/Articular Cartilage

15.1.7.1 Synovial Hyperplasia

Hyperplasia of the synoviocytes is a commonly observed component of various degenerative or inflammatory conditions and is not typically a primary component. An increased thickness of the synovium has been reported in conjunction with a spectrum of joint and physeal lesions in rodents administered with a matrix metalloproteinase inhibitor (Renkiewicz et al. 2003).

15.1.7.2 Synovial Sarcoma

A rare tumor in rats in toxicologic pathology, synovial sarcomas are morphologically similar to human synovial sarcomas in that they can display both epithelial cell-like and mesenchymal cell-like differentiation. Mesenchymal areas consist of dense, cellular bundles of spindle cell, whereas the epithelial areas are composed of cuboidal to columnar cells forming solid cords. These lesions may be visible at necropsy and impart a roughened or frond-like appearance to synovial lining surfaces. Both spontaneous and induced sarcomas appear to be rare. A search of an online National Toxicology Program database did not reveal any instances of synovial sarcoma in control animals.

15.2 SKELETAL MUSCLE

15.2.1 Basic Histology

Skeletal muscle is primarily represented by striated muscle that originates and inserts on the skeleton. There are isolated nonskeletal sites including the esophagus, tongue, and the retrobulbar muscle of the eye. The predominant cell type is the myocyte (synonym: myofiber), which is derived from the fusion of individual myoblasts to result in long, cylindrical, multinucleated cells. A single myofiber may only be 10–120 μm in diameter but may course the entire length of a muscle fascicle. The primary components of a myofiber are the highly organized contractile elements composed of the interleaved myofilaments actin and myosin and additional linking, anchoring, and regulatory proteins. Myofilaments are organized in a highly structured manner, resulting in the characteristic striated light microscopic appearance and the distinctive bands and zones observed ultrastructurally. Small groups of myofilaments constitute myofibrils, and individual myofibrils within the sarcoplasm are surrounded by a highly specialized smooth endoplasmic reticulum, the sarcoplasmic reticulum. The plasma membrane of the myocyte, the sarcolemma, includes an extensive network of membranous invaginations within the cytoplasm (the T-tubules). Depolarization of this membranous network allows movement of calcium into the sarcoplasm, triggering the contractile process. Although variable in number across species and muscle types, mitochondria are a key subcellular organelle in myocytes given the energy demands involved in muscle contraction. Ribosomes adjacent to the nucleus and scattered throughout the sarcoplasm are responsible for the extensive protein synthesis requirements involved in myocyte hypertrophy and regeneration. The nuclei within fully mature skeletal myocytes are flat to oval and peripherally located adjacent to the sarcolemma. Adjacent to the myocyte cell membrane, but within its basement membrane, are the normally small and nondescript satellite cells containing a small, dark, flat nucleus within an indistinct cytoplasm. With tremendous capacity to proliferate and differentiate into myocytes, satellite cells play an important role in myofiber repair.

Muscle fiber types are usually classified using either histochemical methods, which demonstrate activities of different energy-producing enzymes under various conditions of pH (e.g., myosin ATPase), or immunohistochemical labeling of the different myosin heavy-chain isotypes. In general, Type I refers to slow-twitch/slowly fatiguing, myoglobin-rich fibers with many mitochondria, and ATP production is primarily via oxidative metabolism. Type IIB fibers are fast-twitch/rapidly fatiguing cells with less myoglobin and fewer mitochondria and are dependent upon glycolytic energy production. The intermediate type IIA fibers are fast-twitch/rapidly fatiguing cells capable of generating energy with a combination of oxidative and glycolytic processes. The relative proportions of the different fiber types vary between different muscle groups (e.g., biceps femoris compared to soleus) and also across species (Schiaffino and Reggiani 2011). In addition, these distinct phenotypes can contribute to different susceptibilities of muscle groups to xenobiotic-induced injury. For example, slow-twitch oxidative fibers are thought to be particularly sensitive to peroxisome proliferator-activated receptor alpha (PPARα)–mediated toxicity (De Souza et al. 2006), and fast-twitch glycolytic fibers are more sensitive to statin-induced toxicity (Westwood et al. 2005, 2008).

In routine toxicity studies, a limited number of muscles such as the biceps femoris, pectoralis, and/or quadriceps are collected; however, in some cases, it may be useful to collect additional muscles such as the diaphragm, soleus, and/or gastrocnemius to provide a more extensive survey with more complete representation of fiber types. In routine studies, standard H&E-stained sections are usually sufficient for recognition of important treatment-related effects on muscle; however, special stains may be employed, such as periodic acid-Schiff (PAS) to detect glycogen or phosphotungstic acid-hematoxylin (PTAH) to highlight cross-striations that may be helpful in classifying some neoplasms. Transmission electron microscopy (TEM) of muscle may be appropriate in some situations, particularly if there is a need to better characterize vacuolation of the sarcoplasm, accumulations of material noted during light microscopic evaluation, or myofilament structure. TEM is also essential if there is a need to characterize potential mitochondrial abnormalities (see rosuvastatin example in Westwood et al. 2008).

An important consideration in the design of toxicity studies to detect and characterize myotoxicity is the application of serum biomarkers. While classic diagnostic panels have long relied on analytes such as creatine kinase (CK), aspartate aminotransferase (AST), and, to a lesser extent, alanine aminotransferase (ALT), there has been significant progress in the development of novel markers that may provide more specific and/or sensitive detection of myotoxicity across species. Potentially useful markers include skeletal muscle troponin I (fsTnI), myosin light chain 3 (Myl3), urinary myoglobin, and fatty acid binding protein 3 (Fabp3) (Pritt et al. 2008; Vassallo et al. 2009). While these investigative markers are not currently standard in routine toxicity studies, they can be employed on a case-by-case basis.

15.2.2 LESIONS IN MUSCLE

15.2.2.1 Degeneration, Necrosis, and Regeneration

The prototypical and probably the most commonly encountered response to a myotoxic agent is myofiber degeneration and necrosis with subsequent regeneration. The histologic features of muscle degeneration and regeneration proceed through a predictable sequence of stages (Figures 15.3a through d). Following a single inciting event, such as focal trauma or a single exposure to a myotoxic xenobiotic, the histologic changes in most examined fields will be monophasic, with affected

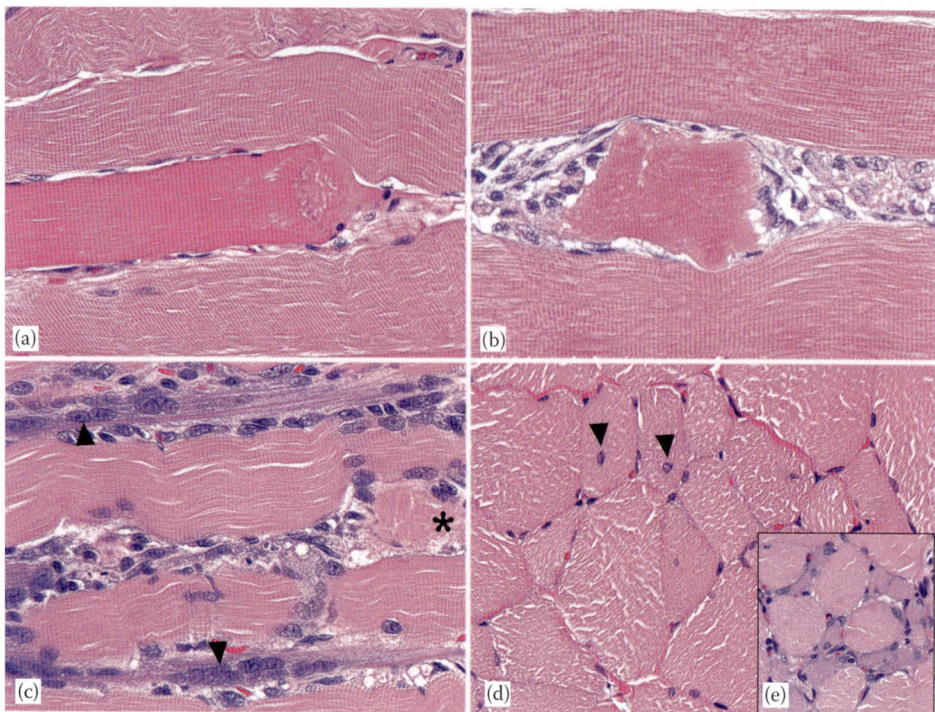

FIGURE 15.3 Histologic features of various stages of muscle degeneration and regeneration following a single dose of a myotoxicant are presented. One day postdosing (a), the acute changes are noted as increased eosinophilia and hyalinization of the sarcoplasm. At two days postdosing (b), infiltrates of macrophages are apparent. The lesion becomes more cellular (arrows) during the regenerative phase on day 4 (c); however, degenerative changes (*) are still present. As shown in the inset (e), examination of cross section of myofibers on day 8 demonstrates the small, angular, and basophilic nature of regenerating myofibers. By day 15 (d), there is near-complete resolution of the lesion; however, centrally located nuclei (arrows) are present.

myocytes at similar chronologic stages in the process. In repeat-dose toxicity studies and many cases of compound-related muscle injury, the presentation is often polyphasic, with myocytes in different chronologic stages of the degenerative/regenerative process present within histologic sections. While this process is discussed here as a continuum, the toxicologic pathologist may record observations of degeneration, necrosis, and myofiber regeneration either separately or by use of a combination term depending on the presentation in any given study or the study purpose. Because myocytes are multinucleated syncytial cells running the entire length of a muscle, the entire cell is almost never in view in a histologic section, and it is, therefore, difficult or impossible to discern whether morphologic changes affect individual myocytes segmentally or entirely and whether an entire cell is indeed dead. Additionally, it is typical for myocyte profiles exhibiting early (potentially prelethal) or later (necrotic) phases to be present in histologic sections. For both of these reasons, the terms "degeneration/necrosis" are frequently combined. Another characteristic of myotoxicity is that the multifocal nature of most induced injuries, combined with the repeated dosing pattern of toxicity studies, results in a polyphasic presentation of degeneration and regeneration at any given time, meaning that morphologic changes ranging from peracute through chronic are frequently observed in the same muscle. In these frequently encountered situations, individually recording the various features of degeneration/necrosis and concurrent features of regeneration will result in unnecessarily complex histopathology incidence tables.

In the initial phases of injury, myofibers frequently become rounded and hyalinized cells with pyknotic nuclei. At this early stage, it can be difficult to distinguish test article–induced injury from the occasional hypereosinophilic fibers that may be observed as a spontaneous or even as an artifactual change. As the injury progresses, myofibers begin to exhibit focal or segmental necrosis with loss of striations and fragmentation of the sarcoplasm. Necrotic fibers may be accompanied by variable amounts of hemorrhage and edema. In cases in which there is mitochondrial mineralization, sarcoplasmic basophilic granules may be present. As the fibers become fragmented, one of the early signs of the response to injury is the presence of macrophages within the myofiber. The macrophages become more prominent as the lesion progresses and are eventually joined by myoblasts, which can form long chains of nuclei. As the repair response begins to predominate, regenerative fibers are readily recognized by their intensely basophilic cytoplasm. As these fibers mature, they enlarge and regain the typical myocyte phenotype. In some cases, retention of a centralized nucleus may be apparent. A wide variety of agents have been demonstrated to induce myotoxicity (Greaves 2000). In addition to classical myotoxicants such as monensin and selenium, myotoxicity has been an important consideration when evaluating lipid-lowering therapeutic agents such as statins and PPARα (Westwood et al. 2008; De Souza et al. 2006).

15.2.2.2 Hypertrophy

Myocyte hypertrophy, which is an expansion of sarcoplasm due to the addition of contractile proteins and supporting organelles, is usually most convincingly recognized as an increased myocyte cross-sectional area. However, because the cellular enlargement may be difficult to detect with routine light microscopy when diffusely present at a low level, quantitative methods (morphometry) may be needed to confidently identify this change. With appropriate and consistent dissection techniques, muscle wet weights can provide a useful and sensitive endpoint for muscle hypertrophy. Muscle hypertrophy is an expected physiologic response to exercise. Xenobiotic-induced muscle hypertrophy has long been recognized following treatment with growth factors and hormones, such as growth hormone (Prysor-Jones and Jenkins 1980) and, more recently, inhibitors of myostatin (Whittemore et al. 2003). Reports of hypertrophy as an unexpected or off-target toxicity are seldom observed.

15.2.2.3 Atrophy

Atrophy of skeletal muscle is recognized histologically as a reduction in myofiber diameter in the absence of other sarcoplasmic changes such as vacuolation. Unless robust, changes in myocyte caliber, whether increased (hypertrophy) or decreased (atrophy), may be difficult to recognize microscopically and may require quantitative morphometric assessment. The pathogenesis of muscle atrophy may be either primary via direct injury to the myocytes or secondary due to immobilization, cachexia, or loss of innervation. Although marked reductions in body weight or food consumption often occur in high-dose toxicity testing, histologic observations of muscle atrophy are not a commonly recognized sequela. As a spontaneous effect, muscle atrophy is noted in aging rats; however, the mechanism of this change is not known (Yarovaya et al. 2002). If a test article–induced atrophy is detected, close examination of the peripheral nerves to rule out a primary neuropathy is warranted. Denervation atrophy is classically recognized by groups of small, angular myofibers. Regeneration is possible following reinnervation, with muscle fiber type driven by the nerve fiber that reestablishes contact with the myocyte.

15.2.2.4 Vacuolation

Although vacuolation may occur as a component of myofiber degeneration; the term is used in this section to denote instances in which vacuolation of the sarcoplasm occurs in the absence of other histologic changes, suggesting degenerative injury. In pharmaceutical toxicologic pathology, phospholipidosis is one of the most common causes of cytoplasmic vacuolation of a variety of cell types. Depending on the magnitude of the response, the presentation of phospholipidosis can vary from low numbers of small vacuoles scattered throughout the sarcoplasm to larger numbers of variably sized vacuoles. Typically appearing devoid of contents in routinely processed H&E-stained

sections, in toluidine blue–stained plastic embedded sections, the vacuoles stain dark blue, and TEM examination reveals lamellated membranous lysosomal inclusions. Cationic amphophilic drugs (Halliwell 1997) have long been known to produce phospholipidosis, and for many of these tissues, the skeletal muscle is a prominently affected tissue (Vonderfecht et al. 2004). Molecules with these physicochemical characteristics are thought to bind to membrane phospholipids, and the resulting membrane complex tends to accumulate and sequester within lysosomes.

15.2.2.5 Inflammation

As a primary process, diffuse inflammatory lesions of muscle are not common spontaneous or induced findings in toxicity studies. However, localized muscle inflammation occurs commonly at intramuscular and subcutaneous injection sites. The severity and cellular characteristics of the inflammatory infiltration vary depending on the nature of the inciting substance. It is, therefore, important that the study pathologist be aware of experimental procedures involving parenterally administered substances. For example, intramuscular administration of sedatives or anesthetics required to conduct various experimental protocols may result in an inflammatory process in the muscle specimen collected for histologic evaluation. Because the injections may not be consistently or precisely located among animals, the incidence of injection site lesions may not be equally distributed among treatment groups and could lead to an erroneous appearance of a test-article effect in muscle. It is also important to recognize that focal muscle degeneration and inflammation can be induced by relatively innocuous procedures such as repeated needle insertion or injections of saline.

15.2.2.6 Rhabdomyosarcoma

Although a variety of soft tissue neoplasms may infiltrate skeletal muscle, primary muscle tumors (rhabdomyosarcomas) are rare spontaneous tumors in the toxicologic pathology setting (Chang et al. 2008). These highly pleomorphic neoplasms are composed of a heterogeneous population of spindle cells with variable amounts of eosinophilic cytoplasm. When identified, the presence of elongate cells (strap cells) or oval cells (racket cells), especially when containing discernible cytoplasmic cross-striations, can confirm the diagnosis. However, the pathologist should be aware that entrapped and regenerating nonneoplastic myocytes can have similar features. Rhabdomyosarcomas are infiltrative and frequently metastasize to distant sites. For poorly differentiated lesions, various diagnostic aids can be considered including a phosphotungstic acid-hematoxylin (PTAH) stain, which may aid in identifying cytoplasmic cross-striations and immunohistochemical procedures to label myoglobin or actin. Rhabdomyosarcomas have been induced by injections of chemical carcinogens or a murine sarcoma virus; however, induction following parenteral administration of a xenobiotic appears to be extremely rare.

15.3   TEETH

15.3.1   Functional Anatomy

The embryology and early postnatal growth of teeth vary among mammalian species and the particular type of tooth being studied. This section deals with mouse and rat incisors, the most commonly examined tooth in toxicology studies. A detailed review of rodent incisor changes in toxicologic pathology can be found in the article by Kuijpers et al. (1996) and in other book chapters and guides for toxicologic pathology terminology (Long and Leininger 1999; Long et al. 1993; Brown and Hardisty 1990).

Figure 15.4a shows the structure of a fully developed rat incisor on an H&E slide. Ameloblasts, the cells that produce enamel, consist of a single row of columnar epithelial cells at the outer area of the tooth section. External to the ameloblasts is a layer of stratified epithelium, which is the remainder of the embryonic dental organ. Internal to the ameloblasts is enamel, but it may appear as a clear space in decalcified tooth sections; it is often lost during decalcification. The periodontal

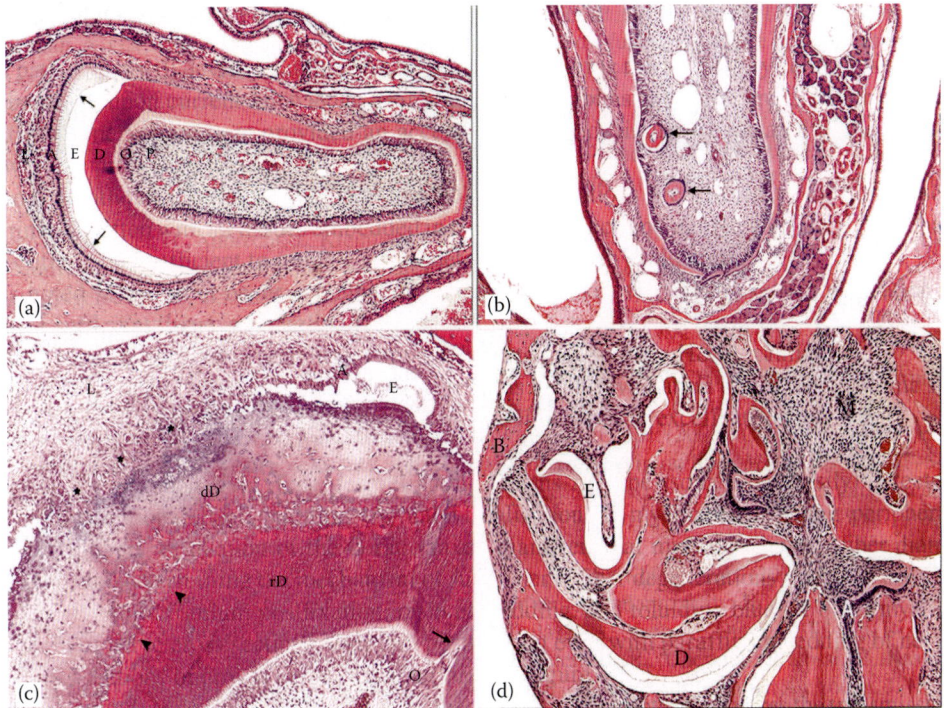

FIGURE 15.4 (a) Transverse section of normal mouse incisor (neck region). From left to right: periodontal ligament (L), enamel-producing ameloblasts (A), enamel layer/space (E), dentin layer (D), dentin-producing odontoblast (O), and pulp mesenchyme (P). Dentin shows a well-mineralized outer zone and a less-mineralized inner zone (= predentin) adjacent to the odontoblasts. Note the narrowing of enamel layer (arrows) due to tissue shrinking and enamel dissolution during tissue processing. (b) Mouse incisor showing multiple intrapulpal denticles (arrows). Such lesions develop from pathological projections of ameloblastic epithelium into the pulp tissue with subsequent induction of surrounding mesenchymal cells into dentin-producing odontoblasts. (c) Incisor from rat treated with an angiogenesis inhibitor. The inner layer of dentin is mostly regular (rD) and distinct from the outer layer (dD), which exhibits severe degeneration and irregular mineralization (arrowheads mark transition zone). Focal degeneration of odontoblasts (O) has resulted in formation of a dentin niche (arrow). Due to degeneration of ameloblasts (A), the enamel space (E) has focally collapsed, and the periodontal ligament (L), which shows inflammatory cell infiltration, is focally continuous with the dysplastic dentin (asterisks). (d) Odontoma (complex variety) of upper incisor in a mouse. The lesion shows a characteristic poor morphodifferentiation with little resemblance to normal tooth structure. Haphazardly arranged dentin trabeculae (D) intermingle with pulp-like mesenchyme (M) and small areas of normal-appearing ameloblastic epithelium (A), which is consistently associated with crescents of enamel (E). The maxillary bone (B) is largely atrophic due to compression of the tumor. (Note: Figures 15.4b and c kindly provided by the US National Toxicology Program—NTP, NIEHS, NIH.)

ligament, a connective tissue area well supplied with blood vessels and nerves, lies just external to the cementum-covered dentin. The periodontal ligament also contains the cells responsible for formation of cementum, the avascular bone-like material that helps anchor the tooth in its socket (alveolus). Cementum is present only on the concave/lingual aspect of rodent incisors.

Dentin is the more eosinophilic, acellular material internal to the enamel or the vacant space left by decalcification of the enamel. Dentin and predentin (the unmineralized material internal to the dentin, closest to the odontoblasts) are formed by odontoblasts, which are columnar, derived from pulp mesenchymal cells, and located at the peripheral surface of the pulp/pulp cavity.

The pulp consists of connective tissue, blood and lymphatic vessels, and nerves. The pulp cavity of molar teeth progressively decreases in size with age.

Enamel does not cover the tip or the lingual/internal surface of rodent incisors. Only the labial/ outer portion has an enamel surface, where a film of iron is deposited between the dentin and enamel, giving rodent incisors a yellow appearance. Dentin (and new dentin) covers the incisor tips; it is continually produced by odontoblasts in rodents to account for the wear and tear that incisors encounter in these species. Rodent molars have enamel on all but the cusps (elevated ridges), which, like the tips of incisors, are also covered by dentin.

15.3.2 Nonproliferative Lesions of Teeth

15.3.2.1 Inflammation

Inflammation may involve the entire tooth or only certain parts, such as the pulp cavity or periodontium, which consists of cementum, periodontal ligament, alveolar bone, and part of the gingiva. Inflammation of the entire tooth is common following fracture/traumatic injury and subsequent infection, especially in incisors that have been trimmed because of overgrowth. Inflammation of the pulp cavity usually occurs secondary to fracture and/or inflammation in the adjacent nasal tissues or bone. Periodontitis is most commonly caused by an accumulation of bacteria on the surface of the tooth and under the gingiva. Dental plaque refers to masses of bacteria adhering to the tooth. As the bacterial plaque mineralizes, it forms what is called calculus or tartar. As the periodontal ligament is destroyed and the alveolar bone is resorbed, the gingival epithelium migrates down along the root surface to form what are called periodontal pockets. Dietary factors such as fiber type and processing methods have been shown to influence the incidence and severity of periodontal disease in rats (Robinson et al. 1991). Fibrosis in and around the tooth may occur as a sequela to long-standing inflammation.

15.3.2.2 Degeneration

Loss or degeneration of ameloblasts may be diffuse or focal, resulting in irregularities in the ameloblast layer. Enamel formation (or lack thereof) mirrors the changes in the ameloblast layer and, therefore, may also appear irregular in contour. In chronic fluorosis (US National Toxicology Program 1996), loss of ameloblasts may be accompanied by flattening of the underlying stratum intermedium, herniation of ameloblasts into the enamel, and inclusions of enamel within the ameloblastic layer (Maurer et al. 1990).

Basophilic granules noted in teeth from fluoride-treated rats are reported to represent calcium fluoride crystal formation that occurs during decalcification of tooth/bone specimens (Lindemann et al. 1979). Degenerative changes in ameloblasts have been described in rats following administration of puromycin and tetracycline hydrochloride (Weinstock 1970; Westergaard 1980). In addition, colchicines (which disrupt microtubule formation) are reported to disrupt enamel formation and pigmentation (Hashimoto 1984). Hexachlorobenzene-induced incisor degeneration has been described in Sprague–Dawley rats (Long et al. 2004).

Degeneration of odontoblasts may be subtle with minimal irregularity in dentin formation (see Section 15.3.2.4), or it may be more pronounced (see Section 15.3.2.5) with displacement of odontoblasts to the pulp, along with displaced dentin production within the pulp. Infarction/coagulative necrosis of odontoblasts and failure to form dentin may also be encountered in toxicology studies.

15.3.2.3 Necrosis

Tooth necrosis can affect all cells; however, it is most often seen within the pulp cavity/chamber. Inflammation may accompany necrosis. Common causes include fracture and infection. Coagulative necrosis is secondary to thrombosis of pulp vessels (Nyska et al. 1999).

15.3.2.4 Dentin Niches

Odontoblast degeneration and subsequent failure to form dentin are typically focal or multifocal and may result in the formation of recesses within the dentin (Figure 15.4b). The recommended terminology for tabulating such alterations is "dentin niche(s)."

15.3.2.5   Dentin, Decreased (Generalized)

A generalized decrease in odontoblast activity may result in decreased dentin formation resulting in a tooth (usually an incisor) in which the entire tooth wall is abnormally thin, as opposed to focal thinning with dentin niches. A generalized decrease in dentin renders teeth susceptible to fracture. A form of dioxin has been associated with defective dentin formation (Alaluusua et al. 1993).

15.3.2.6   Dentin Matrix Alteration

Odontoblast degeneration and subsequent attempts at repair may result in alterations in the appearance of dentin and may contain trapped cellular inclusions. Such alterations, although secondary, may be noteworthy.

15.3.2.7   Dysplasia

Incisors grow throughout life in rodents. This characteristic, coupled with infection, chronic inflammation, nutritional/metabolic/vascular alterations, and injury/fracture, can result in abnormal development of odontogenic tissues (Losco 1995). A version of dental dysplasia and degeneration is associated with exposure to angiogenesis-inhibitor drugs (Fletcher et al. 2010; Hall 2005). Figure 15.4c is one example of the type of dysplastic lesion that can result from angiogenesis inhibition.

Dysplastic lesions can vary considerably, depending on the nature and extent of injury, the tissues affected, and the plane of section. Alveolar bone, cementum, dentin, enamel, and/or connective tissue resembling that of the dental papilla may develop in various combinations and abnormal patterns. In some cases, the tooth socket becomes filled with large irregular masses of osteodentin surrounded by fragments of the original tooth. Tooth-like structures (denticles), with tissue resembling the dental papilla, may also form but tend to remain relatively small and solitary. Dental dysplasia needs to be carefully considered as an alternative diagnosis to a dental neoplasm. Dental dysplasia (abnormal development) may give rise to fractures, which are sometimes difficult to see microscopically due to histological processing/sectioning in areas of the tooth not containing the fracture. Dysplasia and fractures may also lead to ankylosis, which is fusion of alveolar bone with the tooth.

15.3.2.8   Resorption

Resorption of dental hard tissues (cementum, dentin, and/or bone) is characterized by loss of these tissues, which is mediated by osteoclasts. Some initiating factors include malocclusion, infection/inflammation, and trauma/injury. Resorption may progress to complete loss of the tooth and replacement with fibrous connective tissue. It may also be accompanied by abnormal development of remaining viable odontogenic tissue (dental dysplasia).

15.3.2.9   Denticle(s)

Denticles may be seen in rodent incisors (Long and Herbert 2002). They form from buds that pinch off from the epithelial sheat (Figure 15.4b). They are round to slightly oval and are composed of dentin with dentin tubules. The center appears hollow but may contain ameloblasts or fragments of ameloblasts. The outer margin may or may not be lined with odontoblasts. Some denticles may collide with the inner wall of the tooth, where they may be associated with irregularities in the contour of the dentin along the inner margin of the pulp cavity. In some cases, the denticles may become incorporated into the wall of the tooth.

15.3.2.10   Pulp Stones

Pulp stones (single or multiple) occur within the pulp tissue and consist of concentric layers of mineral around dead/injured cells or collagen fibers. Irregular (linear or concentric) areas of dystrophic mineralization may also occur within the pulp tissue and are referred to as false pulp stones.

15.3.2.11   Cyst(s)

Dental cysts generally appear as discrete, membrane-lined, fluid-filled cavities within the tooth structure or alveolus.

15.3.2.12 Thrombus

Thrombosis of pulp blood vessels has been reported in incisors from rats treated with 2-butoxy ethanol (Nyska et al. 1999). Thrombi may appear granular or laminated and partly organized. They contain variable amounts of fibrin, red blood cells, and leukocytes. Thrombosis may result in coagulative necrosis of odontoblasts and/or pulp mesenchymal cells.

15.3.3 PROLIFERATIVE LESIONS OF TEETH

15.3.3.1 Odontoma

Odontomas (Brown and Hardisty 1990) (Figure 15.4) are classified as "complex" or "compound" (Dayan et al. 1994). The difference between the two is that complex odontomas show poor differentiation, whereas compound odontomas show differentiation toward normal teeth. All dental hard tissues such as enamel, dentin, and cementum as well as odontoblasts, cementoblasts, and dental pulp mesenchymal cells are present in both types of odontomas. Odontomas also have an absence of distinct areas of ameloblastic (ameloblastoma-like) epithelium unassociated with dental hard tissues.

Complex as well as compound odontomas may be malformations (hamartomas) rather than true neoplasms, although they have been shown to be chemically inducible by application of different N-nitrosourea derivatives. The odontogenic tumors described by Nozue and Kayano (1978) and by Goessner and Luz (1994) are considered to be odontomas rather than dentinomas.

Odontomas of the jaws may be diagnosed as "cementomas" when cementum-like bony substance is present. If the cementum-like structures are surrounded by fibrous tissue with cementoblasts, such tumors may be diagnosed as "cementoblastomas."

15.3.3.2 Odontoma, Ameloblastic

This variety of odontoma has proliferating ameloblastic (ameloblastoma-like) epithelium in the tumor periphery, which is unassociated with dental hard tissues. This neoplasm often shows aggressive behavior. It is usually a well-circumscribed, concentrically growing tumor (Barbolt and Bhandari 1983; Ernst and Mohr 1991; Fitzgerald 1987).

All dental tissues are found, including ameloblastic epithelium, stellate reticulum–like cells, enamel matrix, enamel, dentin, odontoblasts, cementum, cementoblasts, and pulpal tissue. The hard dental structures are usually located in the central areas of the tumor. Degenerating, keratinized, and calcified odontogenic epithelium ("ghost cells") may also be observed. Formation of reactive multinucleated giant cells within the tumor tissue in response to accumulation of keratin debris may occur. Ameloblastic odontomas tend to be locally aggressive (invasive and destructive) but do not metastasize. They have been reported to occur following administration of N-butylnitrosourea (Wang et al. 1975).

15.3.3.3 Ameloblastoma

Ameloblastomas (Ernst and Mirea 1995) do not produce dental hard tissues; this is their most distinguishing feature from odontomas. They arise from the epithelium of dentigerous cysts, remnants of the dental lamina and of the enamel organ, and the basal cell layer of the oral mucosa.

Ameloblastomas are usually large and grow concentrically. They tend to be locally invasive and destructive but do not metastasize.

They are composed of islands or nests or anastomosing strands of epithelial cells embedded in a collagenous stroma. The epithelium consists of a peripheral layer of tall columnar cells resembling the inner enamel epithelium and loosely arranged central cells similar to stellate reticulum. The epithelial islands may be solid (solid type) or may show degenerative changes in the stellate cells resulting in cyst formation (cystic type). The stroma may be focally hyalinized, but dental hard tissues (enamel, dentin, or cementum) are not produced.

Spontaneous ameloblastomas are extremely rare in rats and mice. In rats, they are chemically inducible by application of different N-nitrosourea derivatives (Berman and Rice 1980; Eisenberg et al. 1983; Pearl and Takei 1981; Smulow et al. 1983; Stoica and Koestner 1984). Ameloblastoma-like tumors (ameloblastic carcinoma, adamantoblastoma [Zegarelli 1944]) have been induced in mice by polyoma virus (Stanley et al. 1964, 1965; Gollard et al. 1992) and by local application of 3-methylcholanthrene (Greene et al. 1960).

15.3.3.4 Fibroma, Odontogenic

This is a well-circumscribed, expansible tumor, usually associated with the pulp of a continuously erupting incisor tooth (Ernst et al. 1998). They are mainly composed of cellular whorls of primitive-appearing and dental follicle-like mesenchyme separated by distinct areas of collagen.

Strands and islands of nonneoplastic, small, and mostly undifferentiated epithelial cells, representing rests of the dental epithelium, are scattered throughout the tumor.

Epithelial nests consisting of squamous cells and ghost cells are occasionally seen.

Round or irregular foci of cementum-like material can also be observed within the mesenchymal tissue. Spontaneous odontogenic fibromas have been reported in rats and mice. Odontogenic tumors with similar morphological features have been induced in Fischer rats by feeding them aflatoxins and an agar-based diet, but they were not classified as odontogenic fibromas.

15.3.3.5 Fibroma, Cementifying/Ossifying

This is a well-demarcated tumor occurring exclusively in the jaw of mice and humans (Luz et al. 1991). They often surround an incisor tooth, contain cementicles, and are considered to originate from the periodontal membrane. The appearance is suggestive of a fibroma in which bone/cementum forms by osseous metaplasia of the fibrous connective tissue component. The proliferating component consists of spindle cells resembling fibroblasts that undergo transformation to cuboidal osteoblasts/cementoblasts and form multiple, rounded, cementicle-like bodies or cementum-like trabeculae with blue-staining borders. Cell processes run perpendicular to the hard-tissue surface. Bone spicules, appearing as the letters "C" and "Y," are composed almost entirely of woven bone. The tumor is usually separated from surrounding tissue by a thin shell of newly formed cortical bone.

REFERENCES

Alaluusua, S., Lukinmaa, P.L., Pohjanvirta, R., Unkila, M., and Tuomisto, J. (1993). Exposure to 2,3,7,8-tetra-chlorodibenzo-para-dioxin leads to defective dentin formation and pulpal perforation in rat incisor tooth. *Toxicology 81*(1), 1–13.

Allen, M.J. (2003). Biochemical markers of bone metabolism in animals: uses and limitations. *Veterinary Clinical Pathology 32*, 101–113.

Baden, E.B.H. (1987). Experimental lathyrism: exostoses and aneurysmal-like bone cysts of the mandible in the rat. *Annales de Pathologie 4*, 297–303.

Barbolt, T.A. and Bhandari, J.C. (1983). Ameloblastic odontoma in a rat. *Lab Anim Sci 33*, 583–584.

Bendele, A.M. (2011). Animal models of rheumatoid arthritis. *Journal of Musculoskeletal and Neuronal Interaction 1*(4), 377–385.

Berman, J.J. and Rice, J.M. (1980). Odontogenic tumours produced in Fischer rats by a single intraportal injection of methylnitrosourea. *Arch Oral Biol 25*, 213–220.

Boss, J.H. and Misselevich, I. (2003). Osteonecrosis of the femoral head of laboratory animals: the lessons learned from a comparative study of osteonecrosis in man and experimental animals. *Veterinary Pathology Online 40*, 345–354.

Brown, A.P., Courtney, C.L., King, L.M., Groom, S.C., and Graziano, M.J. (2005). Cartilage dysplasia and tissue mineralization in the rat following administration of a FGF receptor tyrosine kinase inhibitor. *Toxicologic Pathology 33*, 449–455.

Brown, H.R. and Hardisty, J.F. (1990). Oral Cavity, Esophagus and Stomach. *In*: Pathology of the Fischer Rat, eds. Boorman, G.A., Montgomery, C.A., and MacKenzie, W.F., 1st ed., p. 16, Academic Press, Inc., San Diego, CA.

Bucher, J.R., Huff, J., Haseman, J.K., Eustis, S.L., Elwell, M.R., Davis, W.E., and Meierhenry, E.F. (1990). Toxicology and carcinogenicity studies of diuretics in F344 rats and B6C3F1 mice 1. Hydrochlorothiazide. *Journal of Applied Toxicology 10*, 359–367.

Bucher, J.R., Hejtmancik, M.R., Toft, J.D., Persing, R.L., Eustis, S.L., and Haseman, J.K. (1991). Results and conclusions of the national toxicology program's rodent carcinogenicity studies with sodium fluoride. *International Journal of Cancer 48*, 733–737.

Bullough, P.G. (2011). *Orthopaedic Pathology*. Maryland Heights, Missouri: Mosby/Elsevier.

Burkhardt, J.E., Hill, M.A., Carlton, W.W., and Kesterson, J.W. (1990). Histologic and histochemical changes in articular cartilages of immature beagle dogs dosed with difloxacin, a fluoroquinolone. *Veterinary Pathology Online 27*, 162–170.

Burkhardt, J.E., Hill, M.A., Turek, J.J., and Carlton, W.W. (1992). Ultrastructural changes in articular cartilages of immature beagle dogs dosed with difloxacin, a fluoroquinolone. *Veterinary Pathology Online 29*, 230–238.

Chamanza, R., Marxfeld, H.A., Blanco, A.I., Naylor, S.W., and Bradley, A.E. (2010). Incidences and range of spontaneous findings in control cynomolgus monkeys (*Macaca fascicularis*) used in toxicity studies. *Toxicologic Pathology 38*, 642–657.

Chang, S.C., Inui, K., Lee, W.C., Hsuan, S.L., Chien, M.S., Chen, C.H., Chang, S.J., and Liao, J.W. (2008). Spontaneous rhabdomyosarcoma in a young Sprague–Dawley rat. *Toxicologic Pathology 36*, 866–870.

Dayan, D., Waner, T., Harmelin, A., and Nyska, A. (1994). Bilateral complex odontoma in a Swiss (CD-1) male mouse. *Lab Anim 28*, 90–92.

De Souza, A.T., Cornwell, P.D., Dai, X., Caguyong, M.J., and Ulrich, R.G. (2006). Agonists of the peroxisome proliferator-activated receptor alpha induce a fiber-type-selective transcriptional response in rat skeletal muscle. *Toxicological Sciences 92*, 578–586.

Eisenberg, E., Krishna Murthy, A.S., Vawter, G.F., and Krutchkoff, D.J. (1983). Odontogenic neoplasms in Wistar rats treated with N-methylnitrosourea. *Oral Surg 55*, 481–486.

Eriksen, E. (2010). Cellular mechanisms of bone remodeling. *Reviews in Endocrine & Metabolic Disorders 11*, 219–227.

Ernst, H. and Mirea, D. (1995). Ameloblastoma in a female Wistar rat. *Exp Toxic Pathol 47*, 335–340.

Ernst, H. and Mohr, U. (1991). Ameloblastic odontoma of the mandible, rat. In: Jones, T.C., Mohr, U., and Hunt, R.D. (eds). Monographs on pathology of laboratory animals. Cardiovascular and musculoskeletal systems. Springer, Berlin Heidelberg New York Tokyo, pp. 218–224.

Ernst, H., Sander, E., Karbe, E., Nolte, T., and Mohr, U. (1992). Osteochondroma in laboratory rats: a report of 3 cases in a Fischer-344, a Sprague–Dawley, and a Wistar rat. *Toxicologic Pathology 20*, 264–267.

Ernst, H., Scampini, G., Durchfeld-Meyer, B., Brander-Weber, P., and Rittinghausen, S. (1998). Odontogenic fibroma in Sprague-Dawley rats: a report of 2 cases. *Exp Toxic Pathol 50*, 384–388.

Fitzgerald, J.E. (1987). Ameloblastic odontoma in the Wistar rat. *Toxicol Pathol 15*, 479–481.

Fletcher, A.M., Bregman, C.L., Woicke, J., Salcedo, T.W., Zidell, R.H., Janke, H.E., Fang, H., Janusz, W.J., Schlze, G.E., and Mense, M.G. (2010). Incisor degeneration in rats induced by vascular endothelial growth factor/fibroblast growth factor receptor tyrosine kinase inhibition. *Toxicol Pathol 38*, 267–279.

Frazier, K., Thomas, R., Scicchitano, M., Mirabile, R., Boyce, R., Zimmerman, D., Grygielko, E., Nold, J., DeGouville, A.C., Huet, S., Laping, N., and Gellibert, F. (2007). Inhibition of ALK5 signaling induces physeal dysplasia in rats. *Toxicologic Pathology 35*, 284–295.

Gerwin, N., Bendele, A.M., Glasson, S., and Carlson, C.S. (2010). The OARSI histopathology initiative—recommendations for histological assessments of osteoarthritis in the rat. *Osteoarthritis and Cartilage 18*[Supplement 3], S24–S34.

Gimbel, W., Schmidt, J., Brack-Werner, R., Luz, A., Strauss, P.G., Erfle, V., and Werner, T. (1996). Molecular and pathogenic characterization of the RFB osteoma virus: lack of oncogene and induction of osteoma, osteopetrosis, and lymphoma. *Virology 224*, 533–538.

Glasson, S.S., Chambers, M.G., Van Den Berg, W.B., and Little, C.B. (2010). The OARSI histopathology initiative—recommendations for histological assessments of osteoarthritis in the mouse. Osteoarthritis and Cartilage 18[Supplement 3], S17–S23.

Goessner, W. and Luz, A. (1994). Tumours of the jaws. In: Turusov, V.S. and Mohr, U. (eds). Pathology of tumours in laboratory animals. Vol 2. Tumours of the mouse, 2nd edition. IARC Scientific Publications No. 111, Lyon, pp. 141–165.

Gollard, R.P., Slavkin, H.C., and Snead, M.L. (1992). Polyoma virus-induced murine odontogenic tumors. *Oral Surg Oral Med Oral Pathol 74*, 761–767.

Greaves, P. (2000). *Histopathology of Preclinical Toxicity Studies: Interpretation and Relevance in Drug Safety Evaluation*. Amsterdam, The Netherlands: Elsevier Scientific.

Greene, G.W., Collins, D.A., and Bernier, J.L. (1960). Response of embryonal odontogenic epithelium in the lower incisor of the mouse to 3-methylcholanthrene. *Arch Oral Biol 1*, 325–332.

Gregson, R.L. and Offer, J.M. (1981). Metastasizing chondrosarcoma in laboratory rats. *Journal of Comparative Pathology 91*, 409–413.

Hall, A.P. (2005). The role of angiogenesis in cancer. *Comp Clin Path 13*, 95–99.

Hall, A.P., Westwood, F.R., and Wadsworth, P.F. (2006). Review of the effects of anti-angiogenic compounds on the epiphyseal growth plate. *Toxicologic Pathology 34*, 131–147.

Halliwell, W.H. (1997). Cationic amphiphilic drug-induced phospholipidosis. *Toxicologic Pathology 25*, 53–60.

Hansson, L.I., Menander-Sellman, K., Stenström, A., and Thorngren, K.-G. (1972). Rate of normal longitudinal bone growth in the rat. *Calcified Tissue International 10*, 238–251.

Hashimoto, K. (1984). The effect of colchicine of the pigmentation of the enamel surface in rat incisors. *Bull Tokyo Med Dent Univ 31*, 115–126.

Highman, B.R.S.G.D. (1981). Osseous changes and osteosarcomas in mice continuously fed diets containing diethylstilbesterol or 17B-estradiol. *Journal of the National Cancer Institute 67*, 653–662.

Hirano, T., Iwasaki, K., and Yamane, Y. (1988). Osteonecrosis of the femoral head of growing, spontaneously hypertensive rats. *Acta Orthopaedica Scandinavica 59*, 530–535.

Iwata, H., Yamamoto, S., Mikami, A., Yamakawa, S., Hirouchi, Y., Kobayashi, K., and Enomoto, M. (1995). A case of multiple osteochondroma in the rat. *The Journal of Veterinary Medical Science 57*(2), 339–340.

Jerome, C.P. and Peterson, P.E. (2001). Nonhuman primate models in skeletal research. *Bone 29*(1), 1–6.

Jolette, J., Wilker, C.E., Smith, S.Y., Doyle, N., Hardisty, J.F., Metcalfe, A.J., Marriott, T.B., Fox, J., and Wells, D.S. (2006). Defining a noncarcinogenic dose of recombinant human parathyroid hormone 1-84 in a 2-year study in Fischer 344 rats. *Toxicologic Pathology 34*, 929–940.

Jones, L. and Allen, M. (2011). Animal models of osteonecrosis. *Clinical Reviews in Bone and Mineral Metabolism 9*, 63–80.

Jori, F. and Cooper, J.E. (2001). Spontaneous neoplasms in captive African cane rats (*Thryonomys swinderianus* Temminck, 1827). *Veterinary Pathology Online 38*, 556–558.

Kawahara, T., Shimokawa, I., Tomita, M., Hirano, T., and Shindo, H. (2002). Effects of caloric restriction on development of the proximal growth plate and metaphysis of the caput femoris in spontaneously hypertensive rats: microscopic and computer-assisted image analyses. *Microscopy Research and Technique 59*, 306–312.

Kiebzak, G.M., Smith, R., Howe, J.C., Gundberg, C.M., and Sacktor, B. (1988). Bone status of senescent female rats: chemical, morphometric, and biomechanical analyses. *Journal of Bone and Mineral Research 3*, 439–446.

Kimura, H., Ng, J.M.Y., and Curran, T. (2008). Transient inhibition of the hedgehog pathway in young mice causes permanent defects in bone structure. *Cancer Cell 13*, 249–260.

Kronenberg, H.M. (2003). Developmental regulation of the growth plate. *Nature 423*, 332–336.

Kuijpers, M.H.M., van de Kooij, A.J., and Slootwig, P.J. (1996) The rat incisor in toxicologic pathology. *Toxicol Pathol 24*, 346–360.

Lelovas, P.P., Xanthos, T.T., Thoma, S.E., Lyritis, G.P., and Dontas, I.A. (2008a). The laboratory rat as an animal model for osteoporosis research. *Comparative Medicine 58*, 424–430.

Lindemann, G. and Nylen, M.U. (1979). Calcium fluoride containing granules produced in-vitro in rat bones. *Scand J Dent Res 87*, 381–389.

Long, P.H. and Herbert, R.A. (2002). Epithelial-induced intrapulpal denticles in B6C3F1 mice. *Toxicol Pathol 30*, 744–748.

Long, P.H., Herbert, R.A., and Nyska, A. (2004). Hexachlorobenzene-induced incisor degeneration in Sprague-Dawley rats. *Toxicol Pathol 32*, 35–40.

Long, P.H. and Leininger, J.R. (1999). Teeth. In: Maronpot, R.R., Boorman, G.A., Gaul, B.W. (eds). Pathology of the mouse. Reference and atlas. Cache River Press, Vienna, pp. 13–28.

Long, P.H., Leininger, J.R., Nold, J.B., and Lieuallen, W.G. (1993). Proliferative lesions of bone, cartilage, tooth, and synovium in rats, MST-2. In: Guides for toxicologic pathology. STP/ARP/AFIP, Washington.

Losco, P.E. (1995). Dental dysplasia in rats and mice. *Toxicol Pathol 23*(6), 677–688.

Luz, A., Goessner, W., and Murray, A.B. (1991). Ossifying fibroma, mouse. In: Jones, T.C., Mohr, U., Hunt, R.D. (eds). Monographs on pathology of laboratory animals. Cardiovascular and musculoskeletal systems. Springer, Berlin Heidelberg New York Tokyo, pp. 228–232.

Mandalunis, P.M. and Ubios, A.M. (2005). Experimental renal failure and iron overload: a histomorphometric study in rat tibia. *Toxicologic Pathology 33*, 398–403.

Marks, S.C. and Popoff, S.N. (1988). Bone cell biology: the regulation of development, structure, and function in the skeleton. *The American Journal of Anatomy 183*, 1–44.

Maurer, J.K., Cheng, M.C., Boysen, B.G., and Anderson, R.L. (1990). Two-year carcinogenicity study of sodium fluoride in rats. *J Natl Cancer Inst 82*, 1118–1126.

Movsowitz, C., Epstein, S., Fallon, M., Ismail, F., and Thomas, S. (1990). Hyperstosis induced by the bisphosphanate (2-PEBP) in the oophorectomized rat. *Calcified Tissue International 46*, 195–199.

Naito, S., Ito, M., Sekine, I., Ito, M., Hirano, T., Iwasaki, K., and Niwa, M. (2009). Femoral head necrosis and osteopenia in stroke-prone spontaneously hypertensive rats (SHRSPs). *Bone 14*, 745–753.

Nozue, T. and Kayano, T. (1978). Effects of mitomycin C in postnatal tooth development in mice with special reference to neural crest cells. *Acta Anat 100*, 85–94.

Nyska, A., Maronpot, R.R., Long, P.H., Roycroft, J.H., Hailey, J.R., Travlos, G.S., and Ghanayem, B.I. (1999). Disseminated thrombosis and bone infarction in female rats following inhalation exposure to 2-butoxyethanol. *Toxicologic Pathology 27*, 287–294.

Ominsky, M.S., Vlasseros, F., Jolette, J., Smith, S.Y., Stouch, B., Doellgast, G., Gong, J., Gao, Y., Cao, J., Graham, K., Tipton, B., Cai, J., Deshpande, R., Zhou, L., Hale, M.D., Lightwood, D.J., Henry, A.J., Popplewell, A.G., Moore, A.R., Robinson, M.K., Lacey, D.L., Simonet, W.S., and Paszty, C. (2010). Two doses of sclerostin antibody in cynomolgus monkeys increases bone formation, bone mineral density, and bone strength. *Journal of Bone and Mineral Research 25*, 948–959.

Pace, V., Persohn, E., and Heider, K. (1995). Spontaneous osteosarcoma of the meninges in an albino rat. *Veterinary Pathology Online 32*, 204–207.

Parfitt, A. (1984). The cellular basis of bone remodeling: the quantum concept reexamined in light of recent advances in the cell biology of bone. *Calcified Tissue International 36*, S37–S45.

Parfitt, A.M., Drezner, M.K., Glorieux, F.H., Kanis, J.A., Malluche, H., Meunier, P.J., Ott, S.M., and Recker, R.R. (1987). Bone histomorphometry: standardization of nomenclature, symbols, and units: report of the ASBMR histomorphometry nomenclature committee. *Journal of Bone and Mineral Research 2*, 595–610.

Pearl, G.S. and Takei, Y. (1981). Transplacental induction of ameloblastoma in rat using ethylnitrosourea (ENU). *J Oral Path 10*, 60–62.

Pritt, M.L., Hall, D.G., Recknor, J., Credille, K.M., Brown, D.D., Yumibe, N.P., Schultze, A.E., and Watson, D.E. (2008). Fabp3 as a biomarker of skeletal muscle toxicity in the rat: comparison with conventional biomarkers. *Toxicological Sciences 103*, 382–396.

Prysor-Jones, R.A. and Jenkins, J.S. (1980). Effect of excessive secretion of growth hormone on tissues of the rat, with particular reference to the heart and skeletal muscle. *Journal of Endocrinology 85*, 75–82.

Renkiewicz, R., Qiu, L., Lesch, C., Sun, X., Devalaraja, R., Cody, T., Kaldjian, E., Welgus, H., and Baragi, V. (2003). Broad-spectrum matrix metalloproteinase inhibitor marimastat-induced musculoskeletal side effects in rats. *Arthritis & Rheumatism 48*, 1742–1749.

Robinson, M., Hart, D., and Pigott (1991). The effects of diet on the incidence of periodontitis in rats. *Lab Animals 25*, 247–253.

Ryan, A.M., Eppler, D.B., Hagler, K.E., Bruner, R.H., Thomford, P.J., Hall, R.L., Shopp, G.M., and O'Neill, C.A. (1999). Preclinical Safety Evaluation of rhuMAbVEGF, an Antiangiogenic Humanized Monoclonal Antibody. *Toxicologic Pathology 27*, 78–86.

Sato, M., Vahle, J., Schmidt, A., Westmore, M., Smith, S., Rowley, E., and Ma, L.Y. (2002). Abnormal bone architecture and biomechanical properties with near-lifetime treatment of rats with PTH. *Endocrinology 143*, 3230–3242.

Schiaffino, S. and Reggiani, C. (2011). Fiber types in mammalian skeletal muscles. *Physiological Reviews 91*, 1447–1531.

Smith, S.Y., Jolette, J., and Turner, C.H. (2009). Skeletal health: primate model of postmenopausal osteoporosis. *American Journal of Primatology 71*, 752–765.

Smulow, J.B., Konstantinidis, A., and Sonnenschein, C. (1983). Age-dependent odontogenic lesions in rats after a single i.p. injection of N-nitroso-N-methylurea. *Carcinogenesis 4*, 1085–1088.

Stanley, H.R., Baer, P.N., and Kilham, L. (1965). Oral tissue alterations in mice inoculated with the Rowe substrain of polyoma virus. Periodontics *3*, 178–183.

Stanley, H.R., Dawe, C.J., and Law, L.W. (1964). Oral tumors induced by polyoma virus in mice. *Oral Surg 17*, 547–558.

Stoica, G., and Koestner, A. (1984). Diverse spectrum of tumors in male Sprague-Dawley rats following single high doses of N-ethyl-N-nitrosourea (ENU). *Am J Pathol 116*, 319–326.

Takahashi, M., Yoshida, M., Inoue, K., Morikawa, T., and Nishikawa, A. (2010). Age-related susceptibility to induction of osteochondral and vascular lesions by semicarbazide hydrochloride in rats. *Toxicologic Pathology 38*, 598–605.

Turner, C.H. and Burr, D.B. (2007). Basic biomechanical measurements of bone: a tutorial. *Bone 14*, 595–608.

Uchida, H., Kurata, Y., Hiratsuka, H., and Umemura, T. (2010). The effects of a vitamin D-deficient diet on chronic cadmium exposure in rats. *Toxicologic Pathology 38*, 730–737.

US National Toxicology Program. (1996). Toxicology and carcinogenesis studies of Sodium Fluoride (CAS NO. 7681-49-4) in F344/N Rats and B6C3F1 Mice (Drinking Water Studies) (TR No. 393), Research TrianglePark, NC, National Institute of Environmental Health Sciences.

Vahle, J.L., Sato, M., Long, G.G., Young, J.K., Francis, P.C., Engelhardt, J.A., Westmore, M.S., Linda, Y., and Nold, J.B. (2002). Skeletal changes in rats given daily subcutaneous injections of recombinant human parathyroid hormone (1-34) for 2 years and relevance to human safety. *Toxicologic Pathology 30*, 312–321.

Vassallo, J.D., Janovitz, E.B., Wescott, D.M., Chadwick, C., Lowe-Krentz, L.J., and Lehman-McKeeman, L.D. (2009). Biomarkers of drug-induced skeletal muscle injury in the rat: troponin I and myoglobin. *Toxicological Sciences 111*, 402–412.

Vonderfecht, S.L., Stone, M.L., Eversole, R.R., Yancey, M.F., Schuette, M.R., Duncan, B.A., and Ware, J.A. (2004). Myopathy related to administration of a cationic amphiphilic drug and the use of multidose drug distribution analysis to predict its occurrence. *Toxicologic Pathology 32*, 318–325.

Wadsworth, P.F. (1989). Tumours of the bone in C57BL/10J mice. *Laboratory Animals 23*, 324–327.

Wang, H., Terashi, S., and Fukunishi, R. (1975). Ameloblastic odontoma in rats induced by N-butylnitrosourea. *Gann 66*, 319–321.

Weinstock, J. (1970). Cytotoxic effects of puromycin on the golgi apparatus of pancreatic acinar cells, hepatocytes, and ameloblasts. *J Histochem Cytochem 18*, 875–876.

Westergaard, J. (1980). Structural changes induced by tetracycline in secretory ameloblasts in young rats. *Scand J Dent Res 88*, 481–495.

Westwood, F.R., Bigley, A., Randall, K., Marsden, A.M., and Scott, R.C. (2005). Statin-induced muscle necrosis in the rat: distribution, development, and fibre selectivity. *Toxicologic Pathology 33*, 246–257.

Westwood, F.R., Scott, R.C., Marsden, A.M., Bigley, A., and Randall, K. (2008). Rosuvastatin: characterization of induced myopathy in the rat. *Toxicologic Pathology 36*, 345–352.

Whittemore, L.A., Song, K., Li, X., Aghajanian, J., Davies, M., Girgenrath, S., Hill, J.J., Jalenak, M., Kelley, P., Knight, A., Maylor, R., O'Hara, D., Pearson, A., Quazi, A., Ryerson, S., Tan, X.Y., Tomkinson, K.N., Veldman, G.M., Widom, A., Wright, J.F., Wudyka, S., Zhao, L., and Wolfman, N.M. (2003). Inhibition of myostatin in adult mice increases skeletal muscle mass and strength. *Biochemical and Biophysical Research Communications 300*, 965–971.

Yabe, K., Satoh, H., Ishii, Y., Jindo, T., Sugawara, T., Furuhama, K., Goryo, M., and Okada, K. (2004). Early pathophysiologic feature of arthropathy in juvenile dogs induced by ofloxacin, a quinolone antimicrobial agent. *Veterinary Pathology Online 41*, 673–681.

Yamasaki, K. (1995). Histologic study of the femoral growth plate in beagle dogs. *Toxicologic Pathology 23*, 612–616.

Yamasaki, K. and Inui, S. (1985). Lesions of articular, sternal and growth plate cartilage in rats. *Veterinary Pathology Online 22*, 46–50.

Yarovaya, N., Kramarova, L., Borg, J., Kovalenko, S., Caragounis, A., and Linnane, A. (2002). Age-related atrophy of rat soleus muscle is accompanied by changes in fibre type composition, bioenergy decline and mtDNA rearrangements. *Biogerontology 3*, 25–27.

Yonamine, H., Ogi, N., Ishikawa, T., and Ichiki, H. (1980). Radiographic studies on skeletal growth of the pectoral limb of the beagle. *Japanese Journal of Veterinary Science 42*, 417–425.

Zegarelli, E.V. (1944). Adamantoblastomas in the Slye stock of mice. *Am J Pathol 20*, 23–87.

Zoetis, T., Tassinari, M.S., Bagi, C., Walthall, K., and Hurtt, M.E. (2003). Species comparison of postnatal bone growth and development. *Birth Defects Research Part B: Developmental and Reproductive Toxicology 68*, 86–110.

Zwicker, G.M. and Eyster, R.C. (1996). Proliferative bone lesions in rats fed a diet containing glucocorticoid for up to two years. *Toxicologic Pathology 24*, 246–250.

16 Cardiovascular System

Calvert Louden and David Brott

CONTENTS

16.1 CARDIAC

16.1.1 Introduction

The heart is the muscular pump responsible for the nutritional and functional blood supply to the pulmonary and systemic circuits and is, therefore, responsible for survival of all tissues. The effects of circulating xenobiotics can be manifested as both structural and functional changes in the heart and blood vessels in a wide variety of organs and tissues. Alterations that cause minimal effects in cardiac function can be associated with severe pathologies in another organ such as the brain or kidney because adequate blood flow is required for maintenance of normal organ function. Xenobiotics can cause functional disturbances, such as cardiac arrhythmias, that may result in severe signs, including sudden death syndrome, that are not associated with marked structural damage to the heart. Additionally, in human patients, silent, occult preexisting cardiac disease may increase the likelihood of developing cardiomyopathy from cardiotoxicity. Alterations in hepatic and renal blood flow can profoundly affect the metabolism and clearance of the xenobiotic, which can alter endothelial cell (EC) structure and function leading to severe vascular compromise. In the heart, in addition to functional disturbances, the response to xenobiotic exposure can include developmental abnormalities and structural abnormalities. The range of structural abnormalities includes hypertrophy, various types of degeneration and/or necrosis, fibrosis, subsequent repair and development of cardiomyopathy, and heart failure.

Understanding the potential mechanism of action leading to toxicity requires a thorough working knowledge of the embryology, anatomy, physiology, biochemistry, pharmacology, and molecular biology of the cardiovascular system. Evaluation of potential cardiovascular toxicity utilizes a wide spectrum of testing protocols and monitoring systems for hazard identification and selection of drug candidates early in preclinical development. These specialized procedures, such as chronic telemetry, echocardiography, magnetic resonance imaging, electrophysiology, and electrocardiography, are used in conjunction with monitoring changes such as body temperature, physical activity, and body weight (BW). However, monitoring contractile function, electrical activity, heart rate (HR), and mean arterial pressure (MAP) and assessing structural alterations in the heart and blood vessels have formed the cornerstone of cardiovascular safety evaluation in toxicological sciences.

16.1.2 Embryology Structure and Function

In reptiles, birds, and mammals, the cone-shaped muscular structure known as the heart has evolved to form a four-chambered pump with four valves (Manasek 1976). During the gastrulation process, cells of the epiblast form "fate maps" and the heart field are mapped as two separate, bilateral, and symmetric areas that migrate as a bilateral mesenchymal mesodermal sheet (Garcia-Martinez and Schoenwold 1993; Stalsberg and DeHaan 1969). The mesenchymal cells give rise to the mesothelial layer where the progenitor cells of the myocardium remain fixed to each other (Garcia-Martinez and Schoenwold, 1993). The embryonic disc, together with mesothelium of the cardiogenic plate and the endoderm, undergoes subsequent folding to form the "C"-shaped structure called the primary heart tube (De Jong et al. 1997). The central part of the cardiogenic plate will give rise to the outflow tract, embryonic ventricle, atrioventricular (AV) canal, and parts of the embryonic atrium (De Jong et al. 1997). Subsequent septation occurs and leads to the formation of the right and left atrial and ventricular chambers, while the aorta and pulmonary artery are formed from separation of the common truncus arteriosus (De Jong et al. 1997).

The heart lies within a protective fibrous sac, the pericardium, that contains a small amount of serous fluid. The pericardial sac prevents sudden cardiac dilation, assures equal end-diastolic transmural pressures throughout the ventricles, limits right ventricular stroke work, reduces friction, maintains cardiac alignment, and streamlines cardiac flow. The pericardial sac has parietal and visceral layers and is attached dorsally to the great arteries at the base of the heart, while the ventral attachment is connected to the sternum via the sternopericardial ligament except in the dog, where it is attached to the diaphragm via the phrenico pericardial ligament (Maxie and Robinson 2007). The inner layer of the pericardial sac forms an invagination that becomes the epicardium, the outer layer of the heart.

In mammals, birds, and reptiles, the four-chambered heart consists of right and left atria and right and left ventricles, and the atria and ventricles are separated by the AV valves. The cardiac muscle and valves are supported at the base of the heart by the cardiac skeleton (Robinson et al. 1983). The cardiac skeleton consists of four fibrous rings, the fibrous triangle, and the fibrous or membranous part of the ventricular septum. The fibrous triangle fills the space between the AV openings and the base of the aorta. Depending on the species, it is composed of dense fibrous connective tissue (pigs and cats), fibrocartilage (dogs), hyaline cartilage (horse), and bone (os cordis) in ruminants, and the fibrous rings can become metaplastic in older animals and form bone.

Myocardial thickness is directly related to the pressures present in each chamber, and, as such, the atria are thin and the ventricles are thick. There is variation in ventricular thickness, but in general, the left ventricular wall and the interventricular septum are—two to four times thicker than the right ventricular free wall. The higher pressures in the systemic circulation, relative to the pulmonary circuit, are primarily responsible for the marked difference in thickness between the left and right ventricles.

The valves allow blood to flow from the atria into the ventricles and prevent backflow into the atria. The valve cusps are normally thin and translucent, and the free edges overlap during closure such that fenestrations of the valve edges are usually insignificant. The valves are supported by tendinous chords (chordae tendineae) and papillary muscles, which are the site of insertion for the chordate, and these muscles project from the luminal surface of the ventricles.

The right atrium has a smooth endocardial surface, and the inflow tract opening (sinus venarum) is located between the great veins and the auricle, which has a trabeculated surface formed by pectinate muscles (Van Vleet et al. 2002). Systemic venous blood enters the right atrium from the cranial vena cava, caudal vena cava, the azygos vein, and the coronary sinus. The right ventricle has an inflow tract or sinus and an outflow tract called a conus or infundibulum. A thick muscular ridge called the supraventricular crest separates the sinus and the conus. The outflow tract is guarded by the right AV or tricuspid valve. The leaflets of the valves are anchored peripherally to the AV orifice fibrous ring, and while the atrial surface of the valve is smooth, the ventricular surface is rough and is the site of attachment for the chordae tendineae. The right ventricle is triangle-shaped, and most of the luminal surface has trabeculated muscular beams and ridges called the *trabeculae carne*. The outflow of the ventricle into the pulmonary artery is guarded by the pulmonary valve that has three semilunar shaped cusps, and this allows blood to flow into the lung. From the lungs, blood enters through the pulmonary veins and exits into the left ventricle via the left AV orifice that is guarded by the left AV valve (mitral, bicuspid). The valvular leaflets are larger and thicker than in the right AV valve, and, as in the right, they are connected to the papillary muscle by the fibrous chordae tendineae that are fewer and larger. The left ventricle has a conical shape with very thick muscular walls, and if fixed in contraction, there is marked reduction in luminal size. The left ventricular outflow tract is formed by the upper third of the ventricular septum and the ventricular surface of the septal mitral valve leaflet. The aortic opening is guarded by three semilunar cusps of the aortic valve. In comparison to the pulmonary valves, the cusps are thicker but have the comparable fibrous nodules in the center of the free edge of the cusps.

Nutritional blood supply to the heart is delivered by two major arteries: the right and left coronary arteries. These arteries arise from behind the left and right cusps of the aortic valve at the sinuses of Valsalva at the base of the aorta. The arteries tend to form a ring or crown as they encircle the base of heart in the AV or coronary groove. The left coronary artery gives rise to the left descending and left circumflex coronary arteries. The epicardial coronary arteries give rise to the intramural arteries that penetrate the myocardium. The arteries radiate over the entire heart and, in the subepicardium, give rise to perforating intramyocardial arteries that provide the nutritional blood supply to a rich capillary bed. Within the capillary bed, there are extensive anastomoses that often run parallel to the cardiac myocytes, and this is very evident on cross section where a 1:1 ratio of capillaries to cardiac myocytes can be seen (Maxie and Robinson 2007).

The conduction system of the heart is composed of a highly specialized network of conduction fibers that initiate and transmit electrical impulses throughout the organ. The sinus node (sinoatrial node; SA) or pacemaker is located subepicardially at the junction of the cranial vena cava and the right auricle. The electrical impulse from this pacemaker causes atrial depolarization and contraction, and this impulse travels through internodal bundles to the AV node that is located in the interatrial septum, cranial to the coronary sinus just beneath the septal leaflet of the tricuspid valve. The impulse is delayed in the AV node before traveling via the AV bundle (bundle of His) to the left and right bundle branches (cura) that descend on each side of the muscular ventricular septum, terminating in the Purkinje fibers, which are highly specialized, modified myocardial cells that transmit the depolarizing impulse to the ventricular myocytes. An increased concentration of Purkinje fiber–like cells has been reported in dogs as a spontaneous and incidental lesion (Ainge and Clarke 2000). This spontaneous lesion must be differentiated from histiocytoid cardiomyopathy or hamartoma, which is a developmental abnormality of the conduction system (Ainge and Clarke 2000).

The cardiac wall consists of three distinct layers: the epicardium or the outermost layer, the myocardium or the middle, thick muscular layer, and the endocardium, which is the innermost layer that is continuous with the tunica intima of the great vessels entering and leaving the heart. The epicardium, also known as visceral pericardium, is continuous with the parietal pericardium. The epicardium consists of a thin layer of mesothelium, rich with elastic fibers and connective tissue that merge with that of the myocardium. The subepicardial layer that is attached to the myocardium contains a thin layer of fibrous connective tissue and adipose tissue as well as blood vessels, nerves, and lymphatics. The cavity between the visceral and parietal pericardium contains serous fluid that lubricates the surfaces and provides frictionless cardiac motion. The myocardium is composed of cardiac myocytes that are a specialized striated muscle, embedded in a well-vascularized, connective tissue framework with nerves. These myocytes are arranged in an overlapping spiral pattern that is anchored to the cardiac skeleton. Ventricular cardiac myocytes are branching, cylindrically shaped structures that vary in size, ranging from 80 to 100 μm long and 15 to 20 μm wide (Sommer and Johnson 1979; Van Vleet et al. 2002). The individual cardiac myocytes are joined intimately at the intercalated discs, allowing them to function as a unit. The end-to-end connection by the intercalated disc creates a step-like appearance that is easily visible with scanning electron microscopy using myocyte preparations that have been separated via enzymatic digestion (Van Vleet et al. 2002). Individually, each myocyte consists of a single, centrally located nucleus, mitochondria, and contractile filaments, primarily actin and myosin (Ferrans and Thiedeman 1983). Each cardiac myocyte is limited by the sarcolemma, a structure formed by the plasma membrane or plasmalemma, and the external lamina. The plasmalemma is a trilaminar structure and is approximately 99 nm wide (Sommer and Johnson 1979). The external lamina is composed of a laminar coat, basement membrane, basal lamina, and glycocalyx (Borg et al. 1996). The external lamina contains the typical basement collagen proteins (I and IV) and glycoproteins. A network of invaginations of the sarcolemma is called the T system, and T tubules extend from the free surface throughout the cells in a transverse direction (Van Vleet et al. 2002). The sarcolemma and T tubules are required for conduction, and the sarcoplasmic reticulum stores the calcium needed for contraction. There is species variation, and myocytes can be binucleate (dogs) or multinucleate (swine). The endocardium is the inner layer of the heart that lines all four chambers and extends over the projecting structures such as the valves, chordae tendineae, and the papillary muscles.

16.1.3 EXTRACELLULAR, CELLULAR, AND SUBCELLULAR COMPONENTS

The atrial and ventricular myocardium forms a compact tissue with an interstitium that contains a wide variety of cell types that serve a unique function and purpose. The cardiac myocytes are primarily responsible for generating the force of contraction that is a measure of myocardial function. Surrounding the myocytes is the interstitium that contains a network of blood vessels, capillaries, lymphatics, and nerves that are the major components of this fibrous connective tissue matrix. Resident connective tissue cells, such as mast cells, histiocytes, fibroblasts, pericytes, and undifferentiated mesenchymal (stem) cells, are present in the interstitium (Davis et al. 2007; Robinson et al. 1983; Weber et al. 1992).

16.1.4 DISSECTION AND METHODS OF EVALUATION

A thorough external examination should be conducted; determination of BW, general body condition, and nutritional status should be recorded. Particular attention should be paid to any abnormal fluid accumulating in the abdominal and thoracic cavities and pericardial sac because this can be indicative of underlying cardiac pathology. At necropsy, the heart should be examined for any abnormality in size, shape, or color, and the circumflex and descending branches of the coronary arteries should be carefully examined. Appropriate dissection of the heart is required so that the vital anatomical structures can all be examined in the functional context of a normal-working heart. The heart is opened with an initial incision in the main pulmonary artery and extended into the right ventricle along the junction of the right ventricular free wall and the interventricular septum, down to the apex, following the septal wall and posterior border of the heart, and terminating in the right atrium. The left atrium is opened, and the endocardial surface and mitral valve are examined before the mitral annulus is incised. In dogs, a ruptured chordae tendineae is easily apparent, and abnormalities on the endocardial surface can be noted. The left ventricle is best opened by an incision between the posterior papillary muscle and the interventricular septum; this avoids cutting the chordae tendineae, continuing the incision into the aorta. In larger animals, thorough visual examination of all the valves and endocardial surface should be part of the macroscopic examination.

Because certain anatomical regions of the heart have an increased susceptibility to toxic injury that can result in unique drug-induced damage, the manner of cardiac sampling for histological examination is very important (Keenan and Vidal 2006). The patterns of macroscopic and microscopic changes in the heart chambers and coronary vessels can provide significant clues and valuable mechanistic insights. Representative sections should be examined from all four chambers, the interventricular septum, papillary muscles, and subendocardial zones. The latter is important to detect any evidence of ischemia (Greaves 2000). Several different recommendations for sectioning the heart have been proposed (Morawietz et al. 2004; Piper 1981), and recently, a standardized approach to examining key structures has been published (Keenan and Vidal 2006). In dogs, a simplified method for assessing the conduction system has been described and involves five sagittal plane sections of the sinoatrial and AV nodes (Palate et al. 1995).

TABLE 16.1

Histologic Special Stains Used in Evaluation of Cardiotoxicity

Tissue of Interest or Cellular Component	Histology Staining Procedure
Acid mucopolysaccharides	Alcian Blue, PAS
Basement membrane glycoproteins	Methenamine silver/gold (microwave)
Collagen	Gomori's, Masson, Goldner, Milligan, picric acid sirius red F3BA (Trichrome stains)
Conduction tissue (SA node, AV node, Purkinje fibers)	Trichrome stains, PAS (glycogen)
Calcium (mineralization)	Alizarin red S, von Kossa
Elastic tissue	Gomori aldehyde fuchsin, Weigert, Verhoeff-van Gieson, Orcein, May-Greu
Early myocardial damage (ischemia)	Hematoxylin-basic fuchsin-picric acid, Gomori aldehyde fuchsin, Gomori trichrome, Gomori trichrome–aniline blue, immunohistochemistry for fatty acid binding protein and troponins
Fibrin	Gram-Weigert, Mallory's phosphotungstic acid-hematoxylin, trichrome stains
Glycogen	PAS (diastase)
Lipofuscin	Ziehl-Neelsen acid fast, Kinyoun's carbol fuscin
Lipid	Oil red O (frozen sections), osmium tetroxide, Sudan black

Additional techniques to determine drug-induced cardiac structural changes include special stains (Table 16.1), morphometric analysis, immunohistochemistry, enzyme chemistry, and electron microscopy for subcellular organelles such as mitochondria. Traditional special stains for elastin and different types of collagen to determine increased fibrosis, endocardial thickening, and damaged myocardial fibers are quite useful (Bishop and Louden 1997). Detection of very early myocardial injury characterized by loss of ATPase, creatine kinase, lactate dehydrogenase, myosin, tropomyosin, and ATP, and the presence of complement C9, can be achieved using immunohistochemical stains on formalin fixed tissues (Block et al. 1983; Doran et al. 1996; Hayakawa et al. 1984; Spinale et al. 1989). Hematoxylin basic fuchsin-picric acid will stain damaged myocardial muscle fibers red, and injury can also be detected by fluorescence in hematoxylin-stained sections. In nonhuman primates, immunohistochemistry has been used to detect neural markers such as neurofilaments, glutamate receptors, and protein product of gene 9.5 (Mueller et al. 2003).

16.1.5 CARDIAC WEIGHT, DILATION, AND HYPERTROPHY

In animals and humans, heart weight (HW) varies significantly with BW and other factors such as age, sex, and body length. HW-to-BW ratio is higher in younger animals than adults. Males, in general, have a greater HW-to-BW ratio than females of the same species (Maxie and Robinson 2007). In rats, there is considerable variation in HW, depending on the strain (Tanase et al. 1982a,b). Physiologic factors such as blood pressure and genetic factors can also contribute to cardiac size and the potential for cardiac enlargement (Tanase et al. 1982a,b). HWs in rats can also be affected by dietary restriction (Kemi et al. 2000). Generally, HW-to-BW ratio is used to normalize values. However, using parameters not affected by body condition such as brain weight may be more meaningful (Sellers et al. 2007). Therefore, for the calculation of ratios, the terminal BW collected at necropsy should be used, not the weight collected the morning of necropsy. In cardiac investigative studies, to assess a potential cardiac hazard, measurement of right ventricular weight (RV), the combined left ventricular and septum weight (LV+S), and calculation of the RV- to-LV+S ratio can be of great value in pinpointing right or left side effects.

Generally, dilation and hypertrophy can be an adaptive response to mechanical, hemodynamic, hormonal, or pathological stimuli (Greaves 2007). An acute increase in volume overload of a chamber will lead to expected physiological dilation, while a chronic volume overload stimulus can result in hypertrophy (Berenji et al. 2005; Grossman 1980). Increased diastolic workload from valvular insufficiencies can also cause dilation (Hunter and Chien 1999). Dilation is a response to an increased workload in both the physiologic and pathologic states (Grossman 1980). This increased volume causes stretching of myofibers and increased contractile force of the heart, resulting in increased stroke volume and cardiac output. Chronic dilation can result in hypertrophy and change in heart shape (Dorn 2005; Grossman 1980).

A reversible increase in cardiomyocyte mass, but not myocyte number, is termed *cardiac hypertrophy*. The initiating stress factor determines the pattern of the hypertrophic (concentric or eccentric) response, and compounds that cause systemic hypertension affect the left ventricle, while pulmonary hypertension affects primarily the right ventricle. Eccentric cardiac hypertrophy occurs in a pattern similar to normal growth and is driven primarily by volume overload due to an increase in end diastolic volume and a dilated chamber (Grant et al. 1965; Grossman et al. 1975). In eccentric hypertrophy and dilation, even though there is increase in muscle mass, the walls are usually thin, and the heart tends to be globose (Grant et al. 1965; Grossman 1980; Grossman et al. 1975). Concentric hypertrophy is a disproportionate increase in ventricular wall thickness with a normal or reduced end-diastolic and chamber volume. The increased thickness of the ventricular walls will normalize the wall stress during systole because of the addition of new myofibrils (Grant et al. 1965; Grossman 1980; Grossman et al. 1975). In ventricular volume overload, there is increased wall stress during diastole, which leads to the addition of sarcomeres, fiber elongation, and chamber enlargement (Grossman 1980; Grossman et al. 1975). Chronic chamber enlargement increases systolic pressure that produces ventricular wall thickening in an attempt to normalize systolic stress. Grossly, the hypertrophic endocardium may appear opaque due to subendocardial fibrosis (Greaves 2007).

Cardiac hypertrophy develops subsequent to abnormal systolic and diastolic stresses on the cardiac myofiber. The increase in mass and size of the heart is driven by mechanical and trophic stimuli. There is recent evidence that the mechanical stresses activate growth factor–related surface receptors that induce transcription of embryonic and immediate early-response genes that influence growth and differentiation (Akazawa and Komuro 2003; Cooper 1997; Dorn 2005; Hunter and Chien 1999). Gene expression can change the phenotype of the myocyte by induction of atrial, natriuretic peptides and switching from adult to fetal forms of β myosin and skeletal α actin (Maxie and Robinson 2007). Changes in immediate early genes (C-fos, c-jun, erg-1), growth factor–related genes (TGF-β, IGF, and FGF), and vasoactive agents can play an important role in this process (Maxie and Robinson 2007). Signal transduction also plays an important role in the cardiac hypertrophy remodeling process because, in response to systemic hypertension, mice lacking gp130 cytokine receptor in myocytes do not develop cardiac hypertrophy but instead have marked increase in cardiomyocyte apoptosis, dilated cardiomyopathy, and heart failure (Hirota et al. 1999; Yamauchi-Takihara 2002). PDGFR-β upstream signaling regulates stress-induced paracrine angiogenic potential that is a critical event in the compensatory cardiac response to pressure overload-induced stress (Chintalgattu et al. 2010).

It is generally accepted that hypertrophy is an adaptive, compensatory response that diminishes wall stress and oxygen consumption (Berenji et al. 2005; Kang 2006; Pelliccia et al. 1991). In humans, ventricular hypertrophy is a marker of increased risk for development of heart failure (Berenji et al. 2005; Kang 2006). Data from some studies in humans suggest that there are clear differences between physiological and pathological hypertrophy (Pelliccia et al. 1991; Scharhag et al. 2004; Weber et al. 1992). Experimental myocardial hypertrophy has been produced as a compensatory response to exercise, hypertension, and myocardial infarction. Chronic administration of anabolic steroids, testosterone, catecholamines, thyroxine, and growth hormones can also produce a similar response (Craft-Cormney and Hansen 1980; Gilbert et al. 1985; Laks and Morady 1976; Rona 1985; Rubin et al. 1983; Sullivan et al. 1998). Although a variety of factors including endocrine, paracrine, or autocrine effects may contribute to growth in cardiac mass, it is not clear how hemodynamic stress and these interactions determine cardiac hypertrophy.

Interstitial cells also play an important role in the process of cardiac enlargement, and increased fibrosis has been reported as a contributory source of dysfunction (Weber et al. 1991). Arterial hypertension, coupled with significant increases in plasma angiotensin II and aldosterone, has been associated with increased cardiac fibroblast proliferation (Greaves 2007). Morphologically and morphometrically, fibroblast proliferation was associated with increased abnormal collagen deposition that may account for the increased stiffness of the myocardium and ultimate dysfunction (Weber et al. 1991).

16.1.6 DRUG-INDUCED CARDIAC HYPERTROPHY

Determination of HW is a routine measurement in toxicology studies, and dose-related increases in HW have been reported with cardioactive or vasoactive compounds (Greaves 2007). This includes compounds that are active pharmacologically as antiarrhythmics, sympathomimetics, calcium channel blockers, vasodilating antihypertensive drugs, α- and β-adrenergic blockers, and agents that perturb energy metabolism of cardiac myocytes such as oxfenicine (Case et al. 1984; Cruickshank et al. 1984; French et al. 1983; Gomi et al. 1985; Hoffman 1984; Sutton et al. 1986; Whitehead et al. 1979; Womble et al. 1982). This can also be seen as an off-target response as was observed with CI-959, an experimental, antiallergy/anti-inflammatory agent (Low et al. 1995). Many of these drugs have logged significant patient years and have not been reported to cause adverse cardiac effects or increase the risk of diastolic heart failure in humans (Greaves 2007). Chronic cocaine use in humans can induce pharmacologically mediated increased cardiac workload, enlarged heart, and increased HW (Brickner et al. 1991; Pozner et al. 2005). In preclinical high-dose toxicology studies, increased HW that is not associated with increased cardiac workload or morphologic changes of cellular alterations in cardiac myocytes should be considered an adaptive response and not relevant to humans (Greaves 2007). Conversely, a direct effect on the myocardial structure and/or function must also be taken into consideration, and, if necessary, special investigative studies should be conducted.

Pharmacologically, compounds that cause perturbation of cardiomyocyte energy metabolism have been reported to increase cardiac weight. In preclinical toxicology studies in rats and dogs, S-4-hydroxyphenyl glycine (oxfenicine), a cardioselective inhibitor of long chain fatty acid oxidation, caused marked increases in HW, small foci of subendocardial injury, and minimal steatosis that was indicative of lipid accumulation, but without any ultrastructural morphologic or biochemical evidence of cell damage or degeneration (Greaves et al. 1984; Higgins et al. 1985). The weight of evidence from these data suggested that exaggerated pharmacology in dogs and rats was responsible for this adaptive response (Bachmann et al. 1984; Greaves 2007). Increases in cardiac weight, myocardial discoloration, and dilated and flabby ventricles were observed in rats following administration of methyl-2-tetradecylglycidate (McNeil 3716), another selective inhibitor of long chain fatty acid oxidation (Bachmann et al. 1984). In metabolic studies to elucidate the mechanism of action (MOA), methyl-2-tetradecylglycidate was associated with progressive and dose-dependent, structural and functional damage to mitochondrial membranes (Bachmann et al. 1984). Based on these findings, it was concluded that this cardiac effect was a result of direct effect on cardiomyocyte energy metabolism (Zbinden 1986).

In the rat, intravenous, but not oral, administration of the experimental antiallergy agent CI-959 was associated with a 20% increase in cardiac weight, increased thickness of the left ventricular free wall, and cardiomyocyte hypertrophy (Greaves 2007). Light and transmission electron microscopy did not show any evidence of cell injury or damage. The effects were fully reversible after 2 weeks in the off-treatment phase (Greaves 2007). In investigational studies, the intravenous administration of CI-959 was associated with increased circulating levels of plasma catecholamine, sustained and prolonged hypotension, and inhibition of reflex tachycardia (Low et al. 1995). Administration of α and β_2 adrenoreceptor blockers did not prevent cardiac effects, but these effects were prevented when sympatholytics (nonselective β and β_1 adrenoreceptor blockers) were administered (Greaves 2007). Based on these data, it was concluded that in rats, cardiac hypertrophy was due to an off-target response via indirect stimulation of endogenous cardiac β_1 adrenoreceptors, This is because the pharmacology of CI-959 is anti-inflammatory in nature and designed to block response-coupling mechanisms that would downregulate production of inflammatory mediators and free radical generation in leukocytes (Greaves 2007; Low et al. 1995).

16.1.7 THIAZOLIDINEDIONE MECHANISM OF CARDIAC HYPERTROPHY

The thiazolidinediones, including rosiglitazone and troglitazone, are orally active antidiabetic agents that enhance hepatic glucose utilization and glycolysis through the nuclear peroxisomal proliferator-activated receptors α, γ, and δ, also referred to as PPAR β. In preclinical toxicology studies, administration of troglitazone was associated with cardiac hypertrophy in rats and mice but not monkeys (Breider et al. 1999; Oguchi et al. 2000). There was no evidence of cardiac effects with troglitazone in human clinical trials, and this may be because it was withdrawn from the market before sufficient postmarketing data became available. In contrast, the cardiac effect of rosiglitazone in humans remains controversial (Delea et al. 2003; Nikolaids and Levine 2004; Peraza et al. 2006).

Cardiac hypertrophy and peripheral edema are the two major safety concerns for this class of drug. Cardiac hypertrophy does not always require PPARγ expression in cardiomyocytes because cardiac hypertrophy was observed in both wild-type and in PPARγ null mice (Duan et al. 2005). Other models show that PPARγ ligands can inhibit cardiomyocyte hypertrophy (Asakawa et al. 2002; Yamamoto et al. 2001), and this observation is consistent with interference of NF-κB by PPARγ (Wang et al. 2002). While the specific MOA has not been elucidated for PPAR-induced cardiac effects, it is clear that PPARγ/NF-κB signaling could be involved. Because cardiac hypertrophy is a predisposing risk factor for congestive heart failure (CHF), and diabetics have an increased incidence of CHF, cardiac hypertrophy in preclinical toxicology studies requires further clarification.

In mechanistic studies, rosiglitazone and other PPARγ ligands caused increased cardiac weight, increased plasma volume, and hemodilution that were prevented with cotreatment with a diuretic agent. These preclinical observations translated into clinical edema in patients, which may or may not contribute to cardiotoxicity (Peraza et al. 2006). Receptor-mediated activity of PPARγ through PPARγ–dependent regulation of epithelial sodium channel expression may play an important role in the development of edema because deletion of PPARγ from renal collecting ducts eliminates the weight gain and fluid accumulation (Guan et al. 2005; Zhang et al. 2005). These data suggest that mechanistically, PPARγ–dependent regulation of proteins in the renal collecting duct secondarily influences fluid retention that modulates cardiac function.

In comparison to PPARγ ligands, administration of pharmacologically active PPARβ/δ ligands may be protective against cardiomyopathy (Cheng et al. 2004). Cardiomyocyte specific deletion of PPARβ/δ ligands in mice results in reduced survival because of cardiac dysfunction, progressive myocardial steatosis, cardiac hypertrophy, and CHF (Cheng et al. 2004). Mechanistically, this effect is due to the PPARβ/δ–dependent regulation of genes that control fatty acid oxidation, and as a consequence, there is decreased basal myocardial fatty acid oxidation and, ultimately, decreased functional effectiveness. In experimental studies, activation of PPARβ/δ inhibits cardiac hypertrophy by inhibiting NF-κB activation and/or signaling (Planavila et al. 2005).

16.1.8 TYROSINE KINASE–INDUCED CARDIOTOXICITY

The cardiotoxicity associated with this novel class of compounds, including some antineoplastics, covers a spectrum of adverse clinical findings that include left ventricular dysfunction (LVD), heart failure, cardiac ischemia, and myocardial infarction (Brave et al. 2008; Chen et al. 2008; Escudier et al. 2009; Llovet et al. 2008; Miller et al. 2007; Motzer et al. 2007; Seidman et al. 2002; Telli et al. 2008). Approved drugs associated with this adverse effect include sunitinib, trastuzumab, dasatinib, and sorafenib. The molecular mechanism underlying cardiotoxicity has not been elucidated, but mitochondrial perturbation and modulation of adenosine monophosphate–activated protein kinase activity have been implicated (Mellor et al. 2011). Understanding tyrosine kinase (TK) cardiotoxicity is challenging because there is a significant overlap between the signaling pathways of the therapeutic molecular target and maintenance of cardiac function and homeostasis (Mellor et al. 2011). This complex interaction and overlap makes predicting clinical cardiotoxicity from preclinical toxicology data very difficult. A summary of the preclinical and clinical effects of TK inhibitors approved for human use is summarized in Table 16.2.

16.1.9 Mechanisms of TK Cardiotoxicity

The success of targeting TKs, particularly TK inhibitors, as lifesaving cancer therapies, has prompted the need for a better understanding of the MOA associated with cardiotoxicity to significantly improve on the preclinical to clinical translation (Zhang et al. 2009). Developing a clear picture of the important signaling pathways for members of the kinome for therapeutic target selection, and secondary pharmacology screening to improve the safety profile for cardiotoxicity, is a major hurdle. Because kinases are important regulatory proteins that act through a vast, interconnected network of cellular processes, toxicity can arise from intended or unintended "bystander" targets that have no role in the desired biologic effect, for example, tumorigenesis. Determining which of these off-target kinases play a role in the maintenance of normal cardiac physiology and function will aid in selection of pharmacologically active targets and/or molecules with a low risk for cardiotoxicity. Identification of these signaling pathways will enable development and utilization of secondary pharmacology screens in preclinical toxicology studies, and this investment could reduce attrition significantly. It is clear that TK-induced cardiotoxicity is not a class effect because targeting kinase inhibitors of the epidermal growth factor receptor (EGFR) family does not seem to cause cardiotoxicity (Force et al. 2007). Therefore, potential cardiotoxicity of novel emerging targets of TK inhibition must be assessed on a case-by-case basis (Force et al. 2007).

16.1.10 Myocardial Degeneration and Necrosis, Inflammation, and Fibrosis

The myocardium can be damaged by a wide variety of insults, including infectious, ischemia, anoxia, chemical, or physical agents; however, the pattern of response to injury by cardiomyocytes is very limited. Some of these responses, such as cytoplasmic vacuolation, may be reversible, but persistence of these cytoplasmic changes will result in degeneration, necrosis, inflammation, and eventually repair by fibrous connective tissue because cardiomyocytes lack the ability to regenerate. The degree and severity of inflammation depend on the agent causing the insult, and continued contraction of myocytes plays an important role in formation of the scar tissue (Vracko et al. 1989).

In general, myocardial necrosis, myocarditis, and myocardial infarction are recognizable histologic patterns of damage that can be seen in the heart (Figure 16.1). Use of the term "necrosis" is nonspecific and is applicable to many different types of myocardial damage, while myocardial infarction implies necrosis as a result of underlying ischemia. The use of the term "myocarditis" suggests an infectious cause; however, drugs and toxins may be associated with this response, though the causation may be unclear (Feldman and McNamara 2000). In toxicology studies, spontaneous, age-related changes in the myocardium often manifest as inflammation, and this can confound interpretation in chronic toxicity studies because a clear underlying etiology is unknown.

In nonhuman primates, infiltration of inflammatory cells in the myocardium is fairly common in control animals routinely used in toxicology studies. The most common cardiac findings include inflammatory cell infiltrates, focal myocarditis, myocardial fibrosis, endocarditis, and pericarditis (Chamanza et al. 2006; Drevon-Gaillot et al. 2006; Lowenstine 2003; Qureshi 1979; Vidal et al. 2010). Noninflammatory findings that have been reported include anisokaryosis, karyomegaly, mineralization, squamous cysts, and ectopic thyroid tissue (Chamanza et al. 2006, 2010; Keenan and Vidal 2006). Spontaneous cardiomyopathy, characterized by cardiomyocyte disarray, cytoplasmic pallor, karyomegaly, vacuolization of the perimysial connective tissue, and perivascular fibrosis, has been reported (Zabka et al. 2009). The etiology of these spontaneous lesions in monkeys is not clear, and there is debate as to whether the morphologic features are comparable to chronic catecholamine-induced experimental cardiomyopathy or stress-induced cardiomyopathy (Nyska and

TABLE 16.2

Preclinical and Clinical Cardiac Effects of Targeting Tyrosinase Kinase Inhibitors

Drug/Biologic	Target	In Vitro	Safety Pharm	Preclinical Tox	Clinical	References
Bevacizumab (Avastin)	VEGF				Arterial thrombosis, hypertension	Bhargava 2009; Kilickap et al. 2003; Sica 2006
Dasatinib (Sprycel)	Bcr-Abl, Src, ckit, PBGF-β, EPHA2		QT prolongation, ↑BP	Cardiac hypertrophy, atrial and ventricular hemorrhage, myocardial necrosis, inflammation and fibrosis, valvular hemorrhage	QT prolongation and HF	Brave et al. 2008
Imatinib mesylate (Gleevec)	Bcr-Abl, PDGF-α/β, c-kit		Short ↓in BP in rats but no effects in dogs; no ECG changes	Reversible cardiac hypertrophy	Decrease in LVEF; LVD and HF	Kerkela et al. 2006
Lapatinib (Tykerb)	EFGR (Erb-1) and EFGR-2 (Erb2)		↑in systolic, diastolic and arterial BP in dogs; no effect on QT in rats and dogs	Focal fibrosis and degeneration of cardiomyocyte	Decrease in LVEF and HF and QT-prolongation	Perez et al. 2008
Nilotinib	C-kit, Bcr-Abl, PDGFR α and β		QT interval prolongation		QT interval prolongation and ventricular repolarization (?)	Weisberg et al. 2005
Sorafenib (Nexavar)	c-Raf, b-Raf, VEGFR 1-3, PDGFR α,β and c-kit	Action potential effects in isolated Purkinje fibers; hERG and ion channel effects	No ECG, BP, or HR changes	Hemorrhage and congestion, degeneration and inflammation	Infarction, ischemia, ↑BP and ECG changes	Escudier et al. 2009
Sunitinib malate (Sutent)	VEGFR 1-3, PDGFR-α and β, c-kit, FLT3, and RET kinase	↑action potential duration in canine Purkinje fibers; effects on hERG	QT interval prolongation, ↓in HR; decreased LVEF time	Pericardial inflammation, myocardial vacuolization, and increased capillary proliferation	QT interval prolongation, ↑BP, decreased LVEF, and LVD and HF	Motzer et al. 2007; Telli et al. 2008
Trastuzumab (Herceptin)	Erb2 (epidermal growth factor receptor-2)		No QT changes in rats or dogs, no effects in primates; dose-related increases in systolic, diastolic, and arterial BP	Focal myocyte degeneration and fibrosis in rats and dogs	Decreased LVEF and HF	Seidman et al. 2002

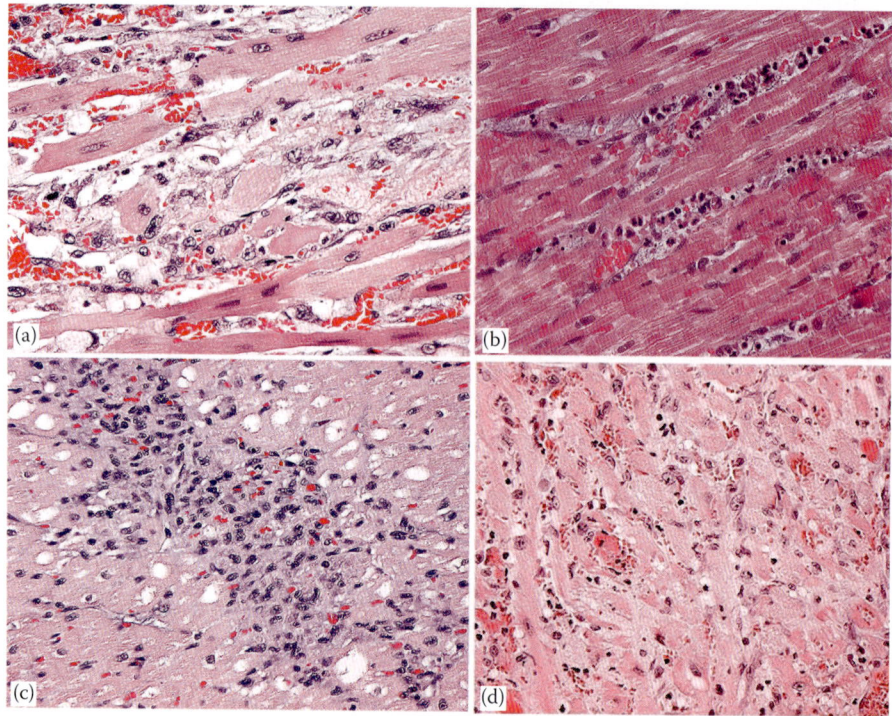

FIGURE 16.1   (a) Hematoxylin and eosin, 400×. Myocardial necrosis in the rat. (b) Hematoxylin and eosin, 400×. Acute myocardial inflammation in the dog. (c) Hematoxylin and eosin, 400×. Myocardial necrosis of myocardial cells. (d) Hematoxylin and eosin, 400×. Myocardial degeneration, necrosis and apoptosis of myocardial cells.

Gruebbel 2010; Vidal et al. 2010; Zabka et al. 2009). Biochemical measurements would be required to support the catecholamine/stress-related hypothesis.

In control, purpose-bred beagle dogs, 9–20 months of age, and using standard histologic sections of all cardiac chambers, myocardial inflammation has been reported in 2% females and 5% males (Keenan and Vidal 2006). Small foci of myocardial degeneration and necrosis, with or without inflammation and fibrous scar tissue, can be seen in routine heart sections from toxicology studies. This may or may not be associated with mineralization, and the lesion is considered to be a spontaneous incidental finding and has no specific anatomical predilection (Keenan and Vidal 2006). Focal myocardial necrosis may be due to stenosis of small intramyocardial or large branches of the coronary arteries (Luginbühl and Detweiler 1965) or due to infection with canine parvovirus, which, in older dogs, can cause cardiac inflammation and/or fibrosis (Robinson et al. 1980; Thompson et al. 1979).

In rats of most strains and with increasing age, necrotic foci, focal inflammation, and fibrosis are commonly reported as spontaneous, nontreatment-related findings (Cornwell et al. 1991; Greaves and Faccini 1992). Histologically, this lesion is characterized by variable-sized foci of dense, eosinophilic-staining myocardial fibers and pyknotic or absent nuclei with inflammatory cell infiltrates composed primarily of macrophages and fibrosis (Greaves 2007). Pigmented macrophages and mineral deposits can be seen in some older lesions. These lesions are usually subendocardial and in proximity to the papillary muscles, areas that are prone to ischemic events. While the mode of action for this common pathology in rodents is unclear, the data suggest that the lesion may be related to ischemia caused by dysfunctional myocardium (Greaves 2007). Studies in the Japanese spontaneously hypertensive rat (SHR) show that the incidence and severity of this lesion are increased in this strain when compared to normotensive rats, and particularly in rats that are older with confounding vascular pathology (Yamori and Okomoto 1976). It has been postulated that the myocardial microvasculature plays an important role in the development of these lesions because of its role in the regulation of vascular tone (Factor et al. 1984; Yamori and Okomoto 1976). Another potential mode of action may be related to metabolism and food intake because Sprague–Dawley or Wistar rats fed with a restricted or *ad libitum* diet have a decreased incidence and severity of cardiac pathology when fed with a restricted diet (Cornwell et al. 1991; Keenan et al. 1995).

Age-related myocardial degeneration, inflammation, and fibrosis can be seen in the mouse used in routine toxicology studies. In the CD-1 strain, these lesions are distributed fairly evenly throughout the myocardium (Faccini et al. 1990; Ward et al. 1979). Compared to rats, the background incidence of this lesion is less in mice, and in older mice, focal fibrosis is the prominent feature rather than necrosis and inflammation (Faccini et al. 1990; Ward et al. 1979). This spontaneous lesion commonly occurs in the ventricular myocardium below the mitral valve insertion ring and must be differentiated from viral myocarditis induced by Coxsackie or murine cytomegalovirus that induces a unique lesion characterized by prominent lymphoplasmacytic infiltrate with or without necrosis (Gang et al. 1986; Godeny and Gauntt 1987). Some mouse strains will develop inherited cardiomyopathies characterized by focal necrosis of myocardial fibers (Van Vleet and Ferrans 1986).

Of relevance to toxicology, inhibition or deficiency of vitamin K activity in mice can induce multifocal myocardial hemorrhage with secondary edema and inflammation (Allen et al. 1991). The pathology most likely reflects an effect on the coagulation pathway, and in routine toxicology studies, myocardial findings with vitamin K–mediated prolongation of prothrombin time (PT) pose an interpretative challenge for the pathologist (Allen et al. 1991).

In Hamsters, strain-specific background cardiac pathology, including myocardial necrosis, inflammation, fibrosis, and mineralization, can eventually lead to cardiomyopathy and CHF (Jasmin and Eu 1979; Karliner et al. 1981). Increased or hyperresponsiveness of myocardial cells to noradrenaline (norepinephrine), and increased activity of acid phosphatase and other lysosomal enzymes in these strains, may be an important part of the pathophysiology (Karliner et al. 1981). In addition to cardiac histopathology, lesions can also be seen in the skeletal muscle, and elevations in serum and/or plasma enzyme activity can reflect myodegeneration. This genetic disorder in the hamster is due to an autosomal recessive gene that has a mutation in the δ-sarcoglycan gene (Greaves 2007). In humans, this gene is associated with limb-girdle musculodystrophies (Nigro et al. 1997; Okazaki et al. 1996). It is important to note that when conventional hamster strains are used in routine toxicology studies, spontaneous background cardiac pathology can be seen, though the frequency and incidence are low (Greaves 2007). These lesions are characterized by focal necrosis, inflammation, and fibrosis that affect most areas of the heart, including the subendocardial zones. Atrial thrombosis can be observed with diffuse inflammation and valvular effects that include mucoid valvular degeneration, inflammation, fibrosis, and calcification. These lesions can influence the interpretation of microscopic changes in the heart in chronic toxicology studies.

Myocardial necrosis can be the result of cardiac ischemia, and the outcome of cardiac ischemic events depends not only on the intensity, size, and duration of the ischemic stimulus but also on the intrinsic defense mechanisms of the myocardium (Ravingerova 2007). The inherent protective mechanisms provide a so-called "tolerance" to myocardial ischemia/perfusion and limit the degree and magnitude of myocardial injury during ischemic events (Peart and Headrick 2008). This protective mechanism is termed "ischemic tolerance" and is induced by ischemic preconditioning, an adaptive response. Ischemic preconditioning occurs when the myocardium is exposed to brief episodes and/or cycles of ischemia/reperfusion, and this event slows myocardial ATP consumption while increasing the cardiac muscle viability when the heart is exposed to subsequent ischemic injury (Murry et al. 1986; Reimer et al. 1986).

The cardioprotective effect of ischemic preconditioning is biphasic. Classic preconditioning is the first phase and begins minutes after the "stimulus," lasting up to 2 h (Murry et al. 1986; Reimer et al. 1986). Late preconditioning, or "second window of preconditioning," is the second phase and begins 24 h post-preconditioning stimulus, lasting up to 96 h (Marber et al. 1993). Ischemic postconditioning can also occur after a period of prolonged ischemia (Zhao et al. 2003).

Cardiac ischemic tolerance reflects myocardial functional reserves that are not used when the tissue is oxygenated appropriately, and it is modulated by signal transduction pathways, transcription factors, and cellular enzymes that all converge on the main effector target, the mitochondria (Golomb et al. 2009). Therefore, drugs and/or chemicals that perturb these pathways may impair cardiac ischemic tolerance without affecting myocardial integrity or functions under normal, well-oxygenated conditions (Dzeja et al. 2007). These potential effects would not be detected during the conduct of current preclinical safety studies but could impact the outcome of ischemic events clinically in patients with cardiovascular risk (Golomb et al. 2009). This phenomenon has been described as "occult cardiotoxicity" and could be a potential source of cardiac morbidity and mortality (Golomb et al. 2009). Therefore, in preclinical safety studies, cardiovascular assessment should include an evaluation of cardiac ischemic tolerance when there is clear physiological or morphological evidence of cardiac injury particularly in longer-term, repeat-dose toxicology studies.

Ischemic preconditioning has been reproduced in many species, including some routinely used in safety testing, thus helping to establish this concept as the standard for studying mechanisms of cardioprotection (Ferdinandy et al. 2007). Classic preconditioning is mediated by modifications of existing proteins, while late preconditioning results from adaptive transcriptional regulation and protein synthesis that requires alterations in an array of genes expressed by the myocardium (Boli 2007). Some of the genes and proteins regulating this phenomenon include Bcl2, mitochondrial ATP-dependent potassium channels, connexin 43, aldehyde dehydrogenase, protein kinase C, phosphatidyl inositol 3 kinase, and mitogen-activated protein kinase (Golomb et al. 2009). Cardiac ischemic tolerance is a process that initiates and modulates signals to which cardiomyocytes are exposed, and it regulates various receptors through signal transduction pathways that ultimately send messages to intracellular end effectors, such as the mitochondria.

16.1.11 Toxicity of Cardioactive Agents

While the underlying MOA in development of cardiotoxicity is unclear, drug-induced cardiotoxicity falls into two broad categories: (1) direct cytotoxicity such as anthracyclines (Singal et al. 1987) and (2) altered function that compromises perfusion (Greaves 2000; Table 16.3).

TABLE 16.3
Cellular and Molecular Targets with Potential Biochemical and/or Cardiovascular Effects

Possible Mode of Action	Effects
Mitochondrial damage	Decreased oxidative phosphorylation and ATP levels; cytochrome c release and activation of caspase-9; mitochondrial permeability transition pore opening
Inhibition of AMP—activated protein kinase	Disruption of cellular ATP homeostasis; caspase activation
PDGFR inhibition	Effect on load and stress-induced cardiac angiogenesis, cardioprotective effects
Vasculature kinase inhibition (e.g., VEGF or VEGFR)	Inhibition of NO and prostacyclin production, hypertensive vascular change; downstream effects of PI3K
Inhibition of ion channel	hERG channels, tyrosine phosphorylation, voltage gated cardiac sodium current; volume-sensitive chloride current
Adenosine receptor inhibition	Loss of protective effects of A_1 and A_3 receptors and the downstream activation of phospholipases C and D
Functional loss of Raf-1	Cardiomyocyte apoptosis and increase in Bax/Bcl2 ratio
Functional loss of ErB2	Dilated cardiomyopathy, cardiomyocyte vacuolization, mitochondrial dysfunction

Anticancer cytotoxic drugs, such as anthracyclines, are associated with direct damage to subcellular organelles in cardiomyocytes that result in histologic changes of myocardial degeneration and necrosis. This pathology is well recognized as a "class effect," and in humans, anthracyclines at therapeutic doses are associated with adverse cardiotoxicity and are based on cumulative dose. Although the MOA is not well understood, the current evidence suggests that anthracyclines induce cardiotoxicity through generation of free radicals (Kalyanaraman et al. 1980; Singal et al. 1987; Vasquez-Vivar et al. 1997) leading to mitochondrial DNA dysfunction (Lebrecht and Walker 2007) and/or apoptosis (Arola et al. 2000; Shi et al. 2011; Wouters et al. 2005). Other potential mechanisms include decreased protein synthesis (Arena et al. 1979), decreased cardiovascular gene expression (Tong et al. 1991), and altered vasoactive amines (Bristow et al. 1980; Olson and Mushlin 1990; Tong et al. 1991).

A wide range of structurally and pharmacologically diverse agents have been reported to cause cardiotoxicity, characterized by one or all of the following: (1) necrosis of the left ventricular papillary muscles and subendocardial zones; (2) right atrial hemorrhage; and (3) medial necrosis and hemorrhage of extramural coronary arteries (Table 16.4). Some cardioactive agents, such as antihypertensives, bronchodilators, vasodilators, inotropic drugs, and catecholamines, can produce cardiac pathology that is associated with disruption of cardiac perfusion as a result of exaggerated pharmacology (Greaves 1998, 2000).

16.1.11.1   Catecholamine-Induced Cardiotoxicity

In experimental animal studies using rats, rabbits, and dogs, catecholamine-induced cardiotoxicity using model compounds, such as isoproterenol, adrenalin (epinephrine), noradrenalin (norepinephrine), salbutamol, terbutaline, and ephedrine, is well described (Boor 1987; Kline 1961; Rona et al. 1959; Simons and Downing 1985; Van Vleet and Ferrans 1986) (Figure 16.2). The characteristic, amine-induced cardiac pathology is left ventricular, subendocardial, multifocal, myocardial degeneration with involvement of the papillary muscles. Histologically, focal myocardial degeneration with contraction bands and infiltration of macrophages is seen with an absence of polymorphonuclear leukocytes (PMNs). In toxicology studies, this pattern of cardiac injury must be differentiated from the transmural, ischemic type that is seen in humans and laboratory animals when there is coronary artery occlusion (Greaves 2007). The latter is characterized primarily by PMNs. In humans, high circulating levels of endogenous catecholamines associated with pheochromocytomas and cocaine abuse are associated with contraction band necrosis (Boor 1987; Karch and Billingham 1988; Kline 1961). This finding raises the possibility that animal findings could become manifested in humans.

The MOA underlying catecholamine-induced cardiotoxicity is complex, but it is generally accepted that in laboratory animals commonly used in toxicology studies, catecholamines, administered at high doses, result in exaggerated pharmacologic and pharmacodynamic activity that causes vasoconstriction and ischemia, resulting in lower coronary artery perfusion pressure or diastolic perfusion time, increasing myocardial oxygen demand and/or intramural pressure (Dogterom et al. 1992). The pharmacology of catecholamines is diverse because of their activity on both α- and β-adrenergic receptors, and different agents may mediate cardiotoxic effects of ischemia through different mechanisms. For example, agonist effects on α receptors located on the cell surface of the vasculature mediate vasoconstriction, while the effect on vascular β_2 receptors mediates vasodilation (Dogterom et al. 1992). Data from comparative pharmacology studies show that the β_2 agonist isoprenaline induces vasodilation that is associated with more pronounced cardiotoxicity when compared to noradrenalin or adrenalin, which act primarily as α agonists but can induce both vasoconstrictor and vasodilator responses (Rona 1985). Moreover, beagle dogs continuously infused with high doses of noradrenalin had a pattern of myocardial necrosis similar to isoprenaline, though pharmacologically, noradrenalin caused tachycardia, while isoprenaline caused bradycardia (Sandusky et al. 1990). Based on this diverse and complex pharmacology, the exaggerated effects can lead to ischemia at high doses because of the "subendocardial steal hypothesis" consisting of coronary arterial spasm, hypotension, and reflex tachycardia, leading to low perfusion

TABLE 16.4

Relationship between Pharmacologic Class and Cardiotoxicity

Pharmacologic Class	Primary Target	Secondary Messenger	Compound/Drug Examples	Cardiotoxicity	Tox Species	References
Potassium channel opener	SMC K+ channels	cAMP	Minoxidil, hydralazine, nicorandil, and ZD6169	Hypotension; reflex tachycardia; atrial, subendocardial, and papillary muscle necrosis hemorrhage; medial necrosis and hemorrhage of coronary arteries (drug-induced vascular injury)	Dogs, rats	Chelly et al. 1986; Herman et al. 1989; Mesfin et al. 1987
Na, K+ ATPase pump inhibitor	Na, K+ ATPase pump	Unknown	Cardiac glycosides, digoxin, digitalis	No profound hemodynamic changes; sub-endocardial hemorrhage, papillary muscle necrosis hemorrhage; medial necrosis and hemorrhage of coronary arteries (drug-induced vascular injury)	Dogs	Bourdois et al. 1982
PDE inhibitors	PDE III, IV, and V	cAMP	SK&F 94418, SK&F 95654, SK&F 94836, milrone, theobromine, Viagra, cilomilast	Hypotension, reflex tachycardia, sub-endocardial hemorrhage, papillary muscle necrosis hemorrhage; medial necrosis and hemorrhage of coronary arteries (drug-induced vascular injury)	Dogs	Hanton et al. 1995; Joseph 2000
NOS pathway	NOS	cAMP	Sodium nitroprusside	Hypotension, reflex tachycardia, sub-endocardial hemorrhage, papillary muscle necrosis hemorrhage; medial necrosis and hemorrhage of coronary arteries (drug-induced vascular injury)	Rats	Bassil and Anand-Srivastava 2006; Brott 2006
ETRA	ETA1 or ETB1 receptors	cAMP	SB 209670; ZD1611; AZD 2574; CI-1020; bosentan	Minimal hemodynamic changes; sub-endocardial hemorrhage; medial necrosis and hemorrhage of coronary arteries (drug-induced vascular injury)	Dogs and monkeys	Albassam et al. 1999; Albassam et al. 2001; Jones et al. 2003; Louden et al. 2000; Teerlink et al. 1994
Adenosine agonists	A1 or A2 receptors	cAMP	CI-947, cyclohexyladenosine	Hypotension, tachycardia, sub-endocardial hemorrhage, papillary muscle necrosis hemorrhage; medial necrosis and hemorrhage of coronary arteries (drug-induced vascular injury)	Dogs and monkeys	Albassam et al. 1998; Metz et al. 1991
Dopamine and dopaminergic agonists	DA1 and DA2 receptors	cAMP	Fenoldopam	Hypotension, tachycardia, sub-endocardial hemorrhage, papillary muscle necrosis hemorrhage; medial necrosis and hemorrhage of coronary arteries (drug-induced vascular injury)	Rats	Bugelski et al. 1989; Hanton et al. 1995; Kerns et al. 1989b; Yuhas et al. 1985
Vitronectin receptor antagonist	αVβ3 and αVβ5	Unknown	SB-273005	Vascular SMC necrosis (aorta and renal hilar arteries), medial hypertrophy of vascular SMCs, ischemic type cardiac lesions in the heart (drug-induced vascular injury)	Rodent	Rehm et al. 2007
Histamine receptor agonist	Histamine H2 receptor	Unknown	Impromidine (SK&F 92676)	Hypotension, vasodilation, and tachycardia	Dogs and mice	Durant et al. 1978

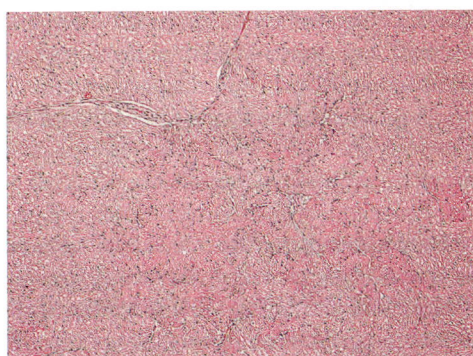

FIGURE 16.2 Hematoxylin and eosin, 200×. Myocardium after treatment with isoproterenol.

pressure, reduced diastolic perfusion time, increased myocardial oxygen demand, and perturbation in transmural blood flow (Rona et al. 1959; Simons and Downing 1985; Winsor et al. 1975).

In summary, catecholamines can induce cardiotoxic ischemia due to exaggerated vasodilation and/or excessive vasoconstriction. This hypothesis is supported by pharmacology studies that show vasoconstriction can occur in large and small coronary arteries. In large arteries, vasoconstriction is mediated largely by α_1 receptors, while in smaller resistance vessels, this response is controlled primarily by α_1 and α_2 receptors. Additionally, coronary arteries also express β receptors that can mediate vasodilation. Therefore, in high-dose toxicology studies when receptor specificity may be lost, cardiotoxicity could be the result of competing and unbalanced exaggerated pharmacology resulting in a net vasoconstriction of the coronary arteries.

16.1.11.2 Vasodilators and Positive Inotropic Agents

In dogs, structurally and pharmacologically diverse vasodilating antihypertensive and calcium channel–blocking agents produce severe hypotension, reflex tachycardia, atrial and ventricular subendocardial hemorrhage, myocyte necrosis, papillary muscle necrosis, and medial necrosis of coronary arteries (see Section 16.2). Although hemorrhage and necrosis are common features, infiltration by PMNs is not a feature as seen in myocardial infarction in humans. In toxicology studies, these lesions typically develop very early in the dosing phase, and in studies of 1-month duration or more, the lesions are generally composed of fibrous connective tissue with iron-containing, pigmented macrophages as sequela to hemorrhage. Unlike necrosis, fibrosis and subsequent repair characterize chronic lesions and are considered a response to necrosis that occurred early in the dosing phase (Herman et al. 1979).

There is extensive literature describing drug-induced cardiac pathology associated with vasodilating antihypertensive agents, cardiac glycosides, nonglycoside inotropic agents, calcium channel blockers, openers of mixed ion and potassium channels, endothelin receptor antagonists (ETRAs), and phosphodiesterase (PDE) inhibitors (Dogterom et al. 1992; Louden et al. 2000; Louden and Morgan 2001; Slim et al. 2002). Some of these drugs for human use are of varying chemical structure and pharmacologic class but are known to cause cardiac pathology without adverse clinical signs in dogs (Albassam et al. 1999; Chelly et al. 1986; Gans et al. 1980; Greaves 1998; Louden et al. 2000; Louden and Morgan 2001; Mesfin et al. 1989). In dogs, understanding cardiotoxicity pathophysiology and potential mode of action has been aided by data describing a relationship between predisposed toxicity site(s) and the distribution, density, type, and ratio of vasoactive endothelin receptors in the heart and coronary arteries (Louden et al. 2000). The composite analysis of receptor subtype profiles, mRNA expression, and regional blood flow measurements clearly supports the hypothesis that disproportionate receptor distribution is responsible for the marked functional differences in regional blood flow at the affected sites of injury (Chelly et al. 1986; Louden et al. 2000). Radioligand protein binding studies to map and quantify endothelin (ET) receptors (ET_A and ET_B) in the normal dog heart indicate a twofold greater density of ET receptors in atria when compared to the ventricles. Mapping of these same receptors indicates a marked difference between the right and left atria. This disproportionate distribution of ET receptors is responsible for a profound difference in blood flow to the right and left atria when an ETRA is administered. Collectively, these data, in conjunction with other published reports, strongly suggest that selective, site-specific cardiovascular damage in dogs is due to exaggerated pharmacology resulting in profound regional vasodilation, increased regional blood flow, and dysregulation of arterial tone (Chelly et al. 1986; Louden et al. 2000).

Some cardioactive agents produce hemodynamic effects that mediate ischemic events that result in myocardial damage. In dogs, digoxin and other cardiac glycosides produce subendocardial changes that are not associated with severe hypotension and reflex tachycardia but are more likely a reflection of localized vasoconstriction (Bourdois et al. 1982). There is also evidence that ETRAs can cause papillary muscle necrosis and left ventricle subendocardial hemorrhage without profound hypotension and reflex tachycardia (Albassam et al. 1999; Louden et al. 2000).

It is now widely accepted that hemodynamic disturbances in cardiovascular function are responsible for the unique, pathomorphological lesions in the dog heart, and data from other species support this. Minoxidil causes primarily right atrial lesions in dogs, but left atrial lesions in the miniature swine and no atrial lesion in rats or monkeys (Carson and Feenstra 1977; Herman et al. 1989). The differences in species response may be related to preferential regional anatomic distribution of the blood supply because dogs are left coronary artery dominant, making the right atrium more susceptible, while the miniature swine is the reverse, making the left atrium more susceptible (Detweiler 1989). Right atrial lesions do not develop in rats because of an extracoronary blood supply that is provided through the cardiomediastinal artery, which is a branch of the internal mammary artery (Detweiler 1989).

Subendocardial hemorrhage and papillary muscle necrosis can also be explained as alterations in hemodynamic factors. It is proposed that profound tachycardia causes shortening of diastole and reduced subendocardial perfusion time. Vasodilators compromise coronary artery autoregulation, causing reduced perfusion and exaggerated by increased HR and force of ventricular contraction (Detweiler 1989). As a consequence, hemodynamic-induced "jet lesions" on the mitral valve can be a histopathologic finding in dogs treated with positive inotropic drugs (Schneider 1991).

16.1.11.3 Cardiotoxicity Related to Exaggerated Pharmacology: Susceptibility and Relevance of Dogs

Administration of high doses of a vasoactive compound often produces biochemical disturbances and exaggerated functional responses, leading to structural damage within the cardiovascular system. The design of toxicology studies should take into consideration the pharmacologic properties of the test article, dose selection, and rationale for species of choice. This is important because when lesions develop in high-dose toxicology studies, the knowledge of the pharmacological characteristics can provide invaluable clues for understanding the mechanism of action and assessment of the relevance for potential adverse responses in humans. The cardiac pathology of right atrial and left ventricle subendocardial hemorrhage, papillary muscle necrosis, and medial hemorrhage of coronary arteries is particularly characteristic for dogs administered with high doses of potent vasodilating agents that also cause reflex tachycardia. It is now widely accepted that in most situations, this drug-induced cardiotoxicity in dogs is related to the unique sensitivity of this species to the exaggerated pharmacodynamic effects of cardioactive agents (Detweiler 1989; Dogterom et al. 1992; Louden and Morgan 2001; Louden et al. 2000; Mesfin et al. 1989).

An increase in HR is induced by reflex mechanisms due to stimulation of the sympathetic system as a result of vasodilation. This physiological response may play an important role in drug-induced cardiotoxicity because, in conscious dogs, nitroglycerin-induced reflex tachycardia is a response to the resulting systemic hypotension. In this case, the reflex tachycardia is mediated by a combination of sympathetic and parasympathetic influence because β-adrenergic and cholinergic blockades completely abolish the tachycardia without any effects on the hypotension induced by the nitroglycerin

(Vatner et al. 1974). Minoxidil also induces severe tachycardia in dogs that is mediated by parasympathetic withdrawal rather than stimulation of the sympathetic system (Mesfin et al. 1989). In contrast, in humans, minoxidil-induced tachycardia is driven primarily by sympathetic stimulation (Lowenthal and Affrime 1980). This difference in species response is primarily attributed to the high vagotonic tone in dogs, a mechanism that does not exist in humans (Lowenthal and Affrime 1980; Mesfin et al. 1989).

Complex cardiac physiological mechanisms regulate HR, MAP, and cardiac output. In normal and hypertensive individuals, direct vasodilation triggers the baroreflex counteracting forces that activate the sympathetic system and cause vasoconstriction. As a result, net hemodynamic vasodilation may be limited because of these two competing forces. There is species-specific variation in normal cardiac physiologic response. A species-specific response has been described for the peripheral vasodilator SK&F 24260 (Dogterom et al. 1992), because in dogs, the resultant tachycardia is only partly due to increased sympathetic activity compared to rats (Balazs et al. 1981; Fielden et al. 1974). In rats, the peripheral vasodilator SK&F 24210 and hydralazine-induced tachycardia are due entirely to sympathetic nervous system stimulation (Balazs et al. 1981; Fielden et al. 1974). Additionally, propranolol completely blocks hydralazine-induced tachycardia in rats, but this β blocker is only partially effective against diazoxide-induced tachycardia in dogs (Balazs et al. 1975). In hypertensive patients, diazoxide-induced alterations in HR depend on parasympathetic rather than sympathetic stimulation (Man int Veld et al. 1980).

Collectively, these data provide convincing evidence that there is no common mechanism underlying reflex tachycardia. The effects noted are a result of interacting forces because vasodilators do not have direct, stimulating effects on the heart (Rubin et. al. 1983). Reflex tachycardia, therefore, is an interplay between the autonomic nervous system, the atrial baroreflex mechanism, increased sympathetic activity, parasympathetic withdrawal (dogs), and stimulation of atrial mechanoreceptors with subsequent activation of the atrial stretch reflex.

In conclusion, the pattern of cardiotoxicity induced by vasodilators in dogs is due to a combination of the following influences: (1) shortening of the diastole period; (2) reduction of myocardial perfusion pressure due to a drop in systemic MAP; (3) stimulation of contractile force that increases the myocardial oxygen demand requirement; (4) ischemia due to insufficient oxygen delivery that can cause papillary and myocardial (focal) necrosis; and (5) subendocardial hemorrhage (Harleman et al. 1986).

16.1.11.4 Implications of Dog Cardiotoxicity and Relevance for Humans

A compound-induced lesion in the heart of dogs in a toxicology study is of concern to regulatory authorities and clinical pharmacologists. However, the emerging scientific data have provided convincing evidence that treatment-related findings in dogs generally do not signal a significant hazard for patients exposed at therapeutic doses (Sobota 1989). Structurally and pharmacologically diverse drugs such as digitalis glycosides, minoxidil, hydralazine, theobromine, milirone, nicorandil, bosentan, dopamine, and dopaminergic agonists can cause characteristic cardiac lesions in dogs, consisting of right atrial and left ventricular subendocardial hemorrhage, papillary muscle necrosis, and medial hemorrhage of coronary arteries, and in rats, mesenteric arterial lesions. These drugs have been widely used in humans, but the characteristic lesion seen in dogs has not been reported (Sobota 1989). Examination of hearts from patients with a long history of taking minoxidil is not associated with the characteristic signature cardiac pathology observed in dogs administered with this agent in toxicology studies (Sobota 1989). The lack of cardiac effects in humans cannot be explained solely by differences in systemic exposure because many of these drugs approved for use in humans have low and/or even negative preclinical to clinical safety margins (Kerns et al. 2005).

To date, there is reasonable correlation between the toxicology data in laboratory animals and prediction of adverse translatable cardiovascular effects in patients, particularly in Phase 1 clinical studies (Greaves et al. 2004). Failure to predict human cardiovascular toxicity in 1 of 10 cases was reported in a study that compared the adverse cardiotoxicity of 25 anticancer agents in humans with the findings in dog and monkey toxicology studies (Schein et al. 1970). Data from some studies suggest that monitoring of physiological parameters is highly sensitive and capable of determining potential cardiac hazards very early in preclinical safety studies (Schein et al. 1970; Zbinden 1986), and beagle dogs probably represent the most sensitive model for drug-induced electrocardiographic effects in humans. The ease of conducting electrocardiographic monitoring in dogs when compared to rats and monkeys makes dogs the model of choice for pharmacological characterization of novel cardiovascular drugs (Mitchell 2000). In one study, adverse cardiac effects derived from dog electrocardiographic monitoring predicted the outcome of cardiac toxicity in humans with all the compounds tested (Olsen et al. 2000). These data provide additional evidence supporting the use of dogs as a model for electrocardiographic cardiac hazard identification in humans.

16.1.12 CARDIOTOXICITY OF NONCARDIOACTIVE AGENTS

Pharmacologic agents that are not designed to treat cardiovascular disease may be associated with cardiotoxicity and pose a threat to human safety. The modes of action associated with cardiovascular effects of noncardiovascular drugs are common; some are poorly understood, while others are equivocal. Additionally, cardiovascular toxicity may arise indirectly from drug interactions. While progress has been made in selecting compounds with a lowered potential risk of torsades de pointes and cardiac arrhythmias, there are still significant cardiac safety hurdles that must be overcome, and many of these are unpredictable based on the preclinical toxicology data. Potential cardiotoxic effects, mode of action, and association to drug and/or drug class are shown in Table 16.5.

16.1.12.1 Cardiovascular Toxicity Induced by Inhibition of Cyclooxygenase Enzymes (COX1 and COX2)

Non-steroidal anti-inflammatory drugs (NSAIDs), including some selective inhibitors of cyclooxygenase, have been used therapeutically for years to treat chronic pain and have been linked to thrombotic events, particularly myocardial infarction and stroke. COX1 is constitutively expressed and associated with gastrointestinal toxicity, whereas COX2 is induced in the inflammatory process, making inhibition of COX2 an attractive therapeutic target unlikely to have the gastrointestinal safety risk associated with COX1 inhibition (Bombardier 2002; Grosser et al. 2006; Masferrer et al. 1992; O'Banion et al. 1992). Patients with preexisting vascular inflammatory disease could be at an increased risk for developing thrombotic adverse events when treated with COX2 inhibitors because inflammation within the vascular wall promotes localized COX2 expression that is linked to production of a potent endogenous antithrombotic, prostacyclin (Mitchell and Evans 1998). Because COX2 inhibition lowers prostacyclin production and antithrombotic activity, the net effect could be an increase in thrombotic events. This level of concern for thrombotic events was increased when it was shown that both celecoxib (McAdam et al. 1999) and rofecoxib (Catella-Lawson et al. 1999) caused significant reductions in prostacyclin metabolites but not thromboxane metabolites in the urine. Results of several studies in humans suggest that this class of agents carries an increased risk of drug-related myocardial infarction and stroke due to thrombosis (Cairns 2007; Fitzgerald 2004; Horton 2004; Topol 2004); thus, regulatory authorities have recommended a "black box" warning. ECs are the major source of prostacyclin synthase, whereas platelets are the major source of thromboxane synthase (Hamberg et al. 1975; Moncada et al. 1976). Prostacyclin is a vasodilator, inhibits platelet aggregation and adhesion, reduces cholesterol uptake and metabolism, and inhibits smooth muscle proliferation and remodeling (Mitchell and Warner 2006). In contrast, thromboxane A_2 is a potent vasoconstrictor and is prothrombotic because it promotes platelet aggregation, facilitates loading of cholesterol, and stimulates smooth muscle proliferation and vascular remodeling (Fitzgerald and Patrono 2001; Vane et al. 1998; Warner and Mitchell 2004). Cardiovascular protection is maintained in health and disease by a balance between platelet-generated thromboxane and EC-generated prostacyclin. While aspirin inhibits COX irreversibly, there is a more selective inhibition in platelets because they have no nucleus and cannot replace the inactive enzyme with newly synthesized COX enzymes, so COX inhibition in platelets is sustained for the life span of the cell (Cairns 2007; Patrono 2001). Oral doses of aspirin pass through the portal vein where platelets

TABLE 16.5

Mode of Action and Potential Cardiotoxicity of Noncardioactive Agents

Cardiotoxic Effect	Drug and/or Class	Toxicity MOA	References
Atrial fibrillation	(1) Corticosteroids/ glucocorticoids, (2) bisphosphonates, (3) ACH inhibition	(1) Efflux of cellular K+/stimulation of mineralocorticoid receptors, (2) increase in inflammatory cytokines and dysregulation of Ca++, (3) altered sympathovagal balance	(1) Fujimoto et al. 1990; Wei et al. 2004; (2) Cummings et al. 2007; (3) van der Hooft et al. 2004
Hypotension without reflex tachycardia	Phosphodiesterase V inhibition	Increased intracellular cAMP in VSMC	Cheitlin et al. 1999
Pulmonary and systemic hypertension	(1) Venlafaxine, (2) ephedra alkaloids, (3) NSAIDs, (4) fenfluramine and dexfenfluramine, (5) glycyrrhizin	(1 and 2) Increased sympathetic activity, (3) inhibit renal prostaglandins and renal perfusion that leads to sodium retention edema and hypertension, (4), pulmonary hypertension caused by agonist activity on serotonin 2B receptors, (5) inhibition of 11β-hydroxy-steroid dehydrogenase that increases cortisol, subsequent increase in mineralocorticoids and hypertension	(1 and 2) Mbaya et al. 2007; Le Corre et al. 2004; (3) Slordal and Spigset 2006; (4) Newman-Tancredi et al. 2002; Rich et al. 2000; (5) Olukoga and Donaldson 2000
Valvular heart disease	Fenfluramine, phentermine, dopamine agonists	Increase levels of serotonin	Raj et al. 2009; Zolkowska et al. 2006
Cardiomyopathy and heart failure	(1) EGFR (Trastuzumab), (2) TKI, (3) TNFα inhibitors, (4) NSAIDs, (5) Thiazolidinediones	(1) Unknown, (2) mitochondrial injury (oxidative phosphorylation) and apoptosis, (3) coagulation cascade, (4) inhibit renal prostaglandins and renal perfusion that leads to sodium retention edema and hypertension, (5) PPARγ induced stimulation of epithelial sodium channels promoting salt absorption and edema	(1) Rajagopalan et al. 2008; (2) Chu et al. 2007; (3) Raj et al. 2009; (4) Slordal and Spigset 2006; (5) Guan et al. 2005
Atherosclerosis	Protease inhibitors, e.g., ritonavir, indinavir, amprenavir	Upregulation of cholesterol uptake receptor CD36 on macrophages, impair endothelium relaxation; increase carotid intima-media thickness	Chironi et al. 2003; Dressman et al. 2003; Stein et al. 2001

are exposed to peak levels prior to hepatic metabolism (Cairns 2007; Pedersen and Fitzgerald 1984). In contrast, ECs have a nucleus, so they have the ability to synthesize COX enzymes constitutively (Patrono 2001). Therefore, regular low doses of aspirin produce a cumulative inhibition of platelet thromboxane with little or no major effect on endothelial prostacyclin, thus creating an antithrombotic environment within the vascular wall, and this is related to the vasculoprotective effects of this drug (Cairns 2007). Aspirin is unique within the NSAID family because it is the only member that is an irreversible COX inhibitor (Cairns 2007).

16.1.12.2   Mechanism of Action for Selective COX2-Induced Cardiotoxicity

The mechanistic basis for cardiotoxicity associated with some traditional NSAIDs, and the COX1-sparing but COX2-selective inhibitors, in high-risk patients, is not well understood (Cairns 2007; Vane and Warner 2000). In small vessel endothelium, during inflammation and angiogenesis, COX2 expression is stimulated by growth factors and cytokines (Crofford et al. 1994) in contrast to large vessels where laminar shear causes COX2 to be expressed constitutively, presumably to maintain homeostasis. The emerging scientific data suggest that metabolism of endocannabinoids by endothelial COX2, coupled to prostacyclin synthase, activates the nuclear hormone receptor peroxisomal proliferator-activated receptor delta (PPARδ). This activation in ECs downregulates expression of tissue factor, the primary initiator of the coagulation cascade. The selective COX2 inhibitors suppress PPARδ activity, and this suppression causes a loss of regulatory control of tissue factor expression in ECs, causing marked elevation of circulating levels of tissue factor (Ghosh et al. 2007). The net effect is that in vivo, selective COX2 inhibitors increase endothelial as well as circulating levels of tissue factor through suppression of PPARδ, thus promoting thrombosis (Ghosh et al. 2007). Furthermore, PPARδ agonists are very effective in reversing this effect and returning tissue factor levels to within normal limits (Ghosh et al. 2007). Additionally, with the reduction in prostacyclin locally and systemically, there is an imbalance of thromboxane, leading to platelet aggregation and thrombosis.

In summary, metabolism of endocannabinoids by the COX2 pathway activates PPARδ, which in turn suppresses the expression of tissue factor. Therefore, in ECs, COX2 together with prostacyclin synthase enzyme activates PPARδ, and this biological effect causes a reduction in the amount of tissue factor, an enzyme that is a critical step in the generation of thrombin and activation of the coagulation cascade. Pharmacologically, COX2 inhibitors block this cascade, causing a reduction in PPARδ activity and thus increasing tissue factor levels that can increase the risk of thrombotic events (Ghosh et al. 2007).

16.1.13 Valvular Lesions

Certain compound classes in development, as well as some marketed drugs, have been associated with serious, drug-induced valvulopathy (Elangbam 2010). Clinically, this adverse effect in humans has led to withdrawal of anorexigens and pergolide from the US market (Elangbam 2010). While the mechanism responsible for the pathogenesis of valvulopathy is not clear, the prevailing weight of evidence suggests that this response is an "off-target" effect that was not initially predicted in routine, preclinical toxicology studies. Furthermore, there are no well-established animal models or predictive screens to accurately identify this hazard in toxicology studies.

Positive inotropic agents can cause valvular lesions primarily on the mitral cusps, characterized as foci of hemorrhage, hemosiderin-laden macrophages, and/or deposits with some ground substance (Greaves 2007). These so-called "jet lesions" are the result of local blood flow changes or actual mechanical trauma to the cusps because there may be a relationship with the morphological changes and the intensity of the inotropic effect (Greaves 2007).

In preclinical toxicology studies, small molecule inhibitors of the transforming growth factor β type 1 receptor class, such as ALK5, were associated with histopathologic heart valve lesions characterized by hemorrhage, inflammation, degeneration, and proliferation of valvular interstitial cells (Anderton et al. 2011). Immunohistochemical analysis for ALK5 revealed expression on the valves but not on myocardial myocytes (Anderton et al. 2011).

In humans, appetite suppressants can be associated with drug-induced valvular disease, characterized grossly by thickness, with a shiny glistening hue and/or an opaque to off-white color. The increased thickness of the valves can lead to valvular regurgitation and has been associated with fenfluramine and phentermine (Connolly et al. 1997). Carcinoid heart disease in humans is associated with a thickened, glistening, white valvular lesion that is related to a sustained long-term increased secretion of vasoactive substances that include serotonin. Long-term serotonin administration in animal models can cause comparable morphological valve lesions (Raj et al. 2009). Furthermore, both phentermine and fenfluramine can cause an increase in circulating levels of serotonin (Zolkowska et al. 2006). Ergot-derived dopamine agonists, pergolide, and cabergoline, used to treat Parkinson's disease, can produce similar valvular lesions (Pritchett et al. 2002). Because both pergolide and cabergoline are potent agonists of serotonin 2B receptors, the cardiac valvular lesions associated with dopamine agonists and appetite suppressants may have a similar mechanism (Newman-Tancredi et al. 2002).

Based on our current knowledge, and the potential mechanistic link to 5HT-2B receptors, functional screens against this receptor, and more consistent sampling and histopathologic evaluation of the heart valves, may improve hazard identification of compounds with the potential to cause valvulopathy.

16.1.14 Neoplasia

In rat toxicology studies, primary neoplasms of the heart are rare and are generally mesenchymal in nature and poorly differentiated. Often, they appear as a diverse spectrum of spindle-shaped neoplastic cells proliferating along the endocardial surface. These tumors were widely considered as endocardial schwannomas, but the diverse expression of S100 protein within many cell types questions the validity of this marker as diagnostic for this tumor. It has been suggested that a more appropriate nomenclature would be endocardial sarcoma (Greaves 2007).

Long-term, oral administration of molecules that interact with PPARs appears to be associated with subcutaneous hemangiomas and hemangiosarcomas in 2-year rodent carcinogenicity studies (Cohen et al. 2009; Hardisty et al. 2007). The pharmacology of PPARs affects adipocytes within the subcutaneous tissues (the site of tumor development); as such, tumorigenicity may be linked to PPAR-stimulated proliferation and/or loss of differentiation of a unique stem cell population.

16.1.15 Biomarkers of Cardiovascular Effects

Cardiovascular diseases are a leading cause of death. Clinical assessment, the cornerstone of disease management, is limited to ECG, history, and physical examination as the main diagnostic tools (Chun and McGee 2004; Panju et al. 1998; Pope et al. 2000; Swap and Nagurney 2005). Additional tools, such as "biomarkers," can aid in clinical assessment and enhance diagnosis and prognosis of adverse events, both nonclinically and clinically. The overall expectation of a cardiovascular disease biomarker is that it will enhance the ability to manage patients and, optimally, patients at risk.

In toxicology studies, myocardial degeneration and necrosis, cardiac hypertrophy, and dilation are the most serious concerns. There is a need in safety testing for noninvasive, specific, and sensitive translational biomarkers for evaluating cardiac injury and remodeling. The challenge in toxicology is that such a marker, as well as analytical methods, must be applicable across multiple species, including humans (Table 16.6). Traditionally, assessment of cardiac injury focused on histopathology and functional aspects to predict human risk. However, there is an emerging interest in plasma biomarkers because, based on data from animal models, the value of such laboratory biomarkers to predict preclinical and clinical cardiotoxicity has been recognized (Vasan 2006; Walker 2006).

TABLE 16.6

Serum and or Plasma Biomarkers for Cardiac Injury and Remodeling

Myocardial Degeneration and Necrosis

Lactate dehydrogenase (LD1, LD2)

Creatine kinase (CK-1, CK-2, CK-3)

Myoglobin

Heart fatty acid binding proteins

Cardiac troponins

Myosin light chain

Cardiac Hypertrophy (Left Ventricular Remodeling)

CITP

CTP

MMPs-1,2,3,7,8,9

Osteopontin

PINP

PIIINP

TIMP-1,2,3,4

sRAGE

NT-proBNP

Scientific advancement within the field of biomarkers has enabled development of new qualified markers, and when used in conjunction with histopathology, this provides a first-tier evaluation for cardiac hazard identification (Walker 2006). Based on these data, a second tier of investigative studies can then be developed to better characterize the findings and address issues such as time of onset and relationship to systemic exposure. The combination of the first- and second-tier data can then be used to develop an appropriate clinical risk assessment and risk management strategy.

16.1.15.1 Cardiac Troponins

Measurement of cardiac troponin (cTn) concentrations in serum and/or plasma as a diagnostic biomarker for monitoring cardiac injury has been well accepted for clinical human medicine as well as in some aspects of veterinary medicine and in nonclinical toxicology studies (Collinson et al. 2001; O'Brien et al. 2006). Troponins are intracellular globular proteins, associated with myocyte contractile elements (thin filament), and differ by approximately 10–30 amino acids from the skeletal muscle isoforms (Townsend et al. 1994; Wallace et al. 2004). They are released from damaged and/or injured cardiomyocytes caused by a variety of insults, including myocardial infarction and ischemic necrosis (Feng et al. 2005; O'Brien et al. 2006). Cardiac troponins are highly conserved across species and, as such, are effective translational biomarkers of cardiotoxic injury because in humans and most laboratory animals, loss of cardiomyocyte cell membrane integrity and/or disruption causes release of this protein into the systemic circulation, where it can be easily measured in toxicology studies as well as human clinical trials (O'Brien 2008; Thygesen et al. 2007). Furthermore, the troponin (cTn T and I) assays have comparable cardiac specificity in laboratory animals and humans (Fredericks et al. 2001; O'Brien et al. 1997). However, biological validation studies will be needed to provide data in various preclinical species used for safety testing to define the diagnostic window and kinetics of circulating cTn and the correlation with histopathology and the magnitude of increases in plasma (Walker 2006). cTn is not a reliable marker of chronic myocardial injury where fibrosis, repair, and remodeling are the predominant features.

The application of cardiac troponin assays for cardiac toxicity hazard identification in nonclinical safety studies is well documented (Bertinchant et al. 2000, 2003; Bleuel et al. 1995; Cummins and Cummins 1987; Schultze et al. 2011; Walker 2006). However, differences in species cross-reactivity, precision, and dynamic range for antibodies used in cTn assays have been reported (Apple et al. 2008; Petit et al. 2007). Recently, there have been attempts to improve performance of the cTn assays that include lowering the limits of sensitivity and decreasing the sample volume to better align the nonclinical and clinical assays (Schultze et al. 2008, 2009; Todd et al. 2007; Wu et al. 2006, 2009).

For comparable types of myocardial injury, cTn T and I assays perform similarly with good translational concordance to humans (Bertinchant et al. 2000; O'Brien et al. 1997). In preclinical safety animal models of cardiotoxicity, the time to peak concentration, clearance rate, and correlation with histopathology have been studied (Bertinchant et al. 2000; O'Brien et al. 1997), and these data approximate the pattern seen in clinical patients with comparable myocardial injury. Despite the specificity of cTn, the results of cross-validation studies suggest that there is variability in cross-reactivity in dogs versus cynomolgus and rhesus monkeys as well as several automated clinical assays showed limited to no reactivity with cTn-positive serum from Han Wistar or Sprague Dawley rats (Walker 2006). Therefore, caution must be exercised when using clinical commercial assays to analyze nonhuman specimens because of unpredictable cross-reactivity and possible noncompatibility (York et al. 2007). Rodent-specific assays are now available, and progress is being made toward canine- and nonhuman primate–specific assays.

When mortality, cardiac histology, and cardiac biomarker response were compared using three outbred stocks of Sprague Dawley rats, differences in the response to a common cardiotoxic molecule were found (Schultze et al. 2011). These results suggest that in preclinical safety studies, there is a need for recognition of the potential differences in cardiotoxic response between stocks of Sprague Dawley rats and that this should be considered when selecting rats for cardiovascular safety studies, particularly if cardiovascular toxicity is suspected (Schultze et al. 2011).

16.1.15.2   Heart Fatty Acid–Binding Protein

Recently, heart fatty acid–binding protein (H-FABP) has been investigated as an early biomarker of cardiomyocyte injury and associated cell membrane disruption in humans and laboratory animals such as rats (Knowlton et al. 1989; Meng et al. 2006; Zhen et al. 2007). This low-molecular-weight protein is found abundantly in muscle (cardiac and skeletal), is released rapidly following the onset of injury, and, when used in conjunction with cTn measurements, provides strong diagnostic evidence of cardiac injury (Meng et al. 2006). However, for nonclinical safety studies, this marker lacks cardiac specificity because in rats, there is significant skeletal muscle distribution, particularly in type 1 muscle fibers such as in the soleus muscle (Zhen et al. 2007).

A major concern for pathologists and toxicologists is determining the time course between elevation of a cardiac-specific marker and the morphologic changes of myofiber necrosis. Morphologic myocardial injury with elevations in serum H-FABP and cTn, as well as loss of cTn immunoreactivity in cardiac tissue, can be detected as early as 30 min after insult; however, ultrastructural and morphologic evidence of cardiomyocyte death was not apparent until later time points (Clements et al. 2010). At later time points, there is an apparent temporal disconnect between the severity of lesion histopathology scores and the decline of cTn and H-FABP (Clements et al. 2010). While cTn and H-FABP are sensitive biomarkers of acute cardiomyocyte injury, performance of these analytes for monitoring chronic myocardial injury is questionable.

In summary, H-FABP is a good early, less sensitive, and less specific marker of cardiomyocyte injury and is released prior to necrosis (Clements et al. 2010); when used in conjunction with cTn, it provides adequate information for identification of potential cardiotoxic hazards in preclinical safety studies.

16.1.15.3   Hypertrophy and Cardiac Remodeling

There is a gap in our current understanding of the pathophysiology and biochemical events that lead to cardiac hypertrophy and remodeling in preclinical toxicology studies. In humans, it is well recognized that development of left ventricular hypertrophy is an important risk factor for the progression to diastolic heart failure, and both of these are associated with an increase in cardiovascular morbidity and mortality (Chobanian et al. 2003; Vasan et al. 2002). As some drugs can induce cardiac hypertrophy, identification of translational biomarkers would be helpful for clinical monitoring and for candidate drug selection nonclinically. Myocardial remodeling is the structural and functional response to chronic pressure overload (De Simone et al. 2008; Levy et al. 1996; Verdecchia et al. 1998). Since cardiac remodeling involves both the cardiomyocyte as well as the extracellular matrix, diagnostic biomarkers must take both elements into consideration (Levy et al. 1990; Zile et al. 2011). These specific biomarkers would constitute a profile that could be used nonclinically but could also be used to stratify potential human subjects with occult cardiac pathology (Zile et al. 2011).

Understanding the pathophysiology of cardiac structure and function remodeling is essential in identifying candidate biomarkers that are either predictors or early reporters of key events such as changes in extracellular matrix composition, particularly fibrillar collagen (Ahmed et al. 2006; Diez 2009; Gonzalez et al. 2009; Mak et al. 2009; Singh et al. 2010; Spinale 2007; Zile et al. 2011). Collagen homeostasis can be evaluated by measurements of cleaved products, rates of synthesis, processing, post-translational modification, and degradation (Ahmed et al. 2006; Diez 2009; Gonzalez et al. 2009; Singh et al. 2010; Spinale 2007). In addition to studying the extracellular matrix remodeling pathways, additional markers such as the natriuretic peptides could be included in this multipanel (Zile et al. 2011). It has been suggested that in using such an approach, a multibiomarker panel that includes changes in extracellular matrix fibrillar collagen homeostasis can be of considerable value in assessing structural remodeling (Zile et al. 2011). Data from these studies can be used to evaluate their usefulness and applicability in nonclinical models of cardiac remodeling. Such a nonclinical panel could be the basis for developing a prediction algorithm of cardiac hypertrophy and remodeling that could be used in investigative, preclinical, safety studies.

16.2 VASCULAR

16.2.1 INTRODUCTION

Structurally, the vessel wall is composed of ECs, internal and external elastic laminae, smooth muscle cells (SMCs), and perivascular adventitial collagen (type IV) containing pluripotential mesenchymal cells. The ECs, SMCs, and collagen play an important role in maintaining the integrity of the vessel wall and are also the principal targets of injury and repair. For example, a genetic defect in the mouse COL4A1 gene that plays a role in collagen assembly has been associated with increased fragility of small blood vessels (Gould et al. 2006).

ECs are the innermost lining cells of the vascular wall, and they have synthetic as well as metabolic activity and function as a physical barrier to hemodynamic forces (Gotlieb 1990). In different regions of the vascular bed, ECs have both phenotypic and functional diversity (Galley and Webster 2004) and are capable of synthesizing both anticoagulant and procoagulant molecules, as well as cytokines and growth factors (Cines et al. 1998). Sheer stress and change from laminar to turbulence flow can induce expression of genes such as tissue factor, platelet-derived growth factor (PDGF) β, and intracellular adhesion molecules (Gotlieb 1990). ECs are also responsible for regulation of vascular tone by paracrine and autocrine production and/or response to nitric oxide (NO) and endothelin-1, 2, or 3 (Arnal et al. 1999; Cines et al. 1998; Clozel et al. 1992; Teerlink et al. 1994). Expression of adhesion molecules stimulates pavementing and adherence of inflammatory cells, and this response contributes to cell migration and lipid accumulation within the vascular wall in diseases such as atherosclerosis (Ross 1999).

SMCs are primarily responsible for blood flow distribution by regulating vessel diameter, blood pressure, and vascular tone through contraction (Owens et al. 2004). They appear to have different embryonic origins including thoracic aorta-neuroectoderm, abdominal aorta-mesenchymal, and coronary artery–intracardiac mesenchyme (Ross 1999). In mature animals, these terminally differentiated cells can exhibit contractile as well as synthetic phenotypes (Miano et al. 1993) and are responsive to ion channel and surface receptor signaling. Estrogens, through binding and activation of estrogen receptors on SMCs and ECs, can have a direct vasodilatory effect but can also negatively modulate vascular response to injury (Mendelsohn and Karas 1999). In contrast, vasospasm and increased vascular reactivity are associated with anabolic steroids (Sullivan et al. 1998).

In toxicology studies, determining a potential hazard of the vascular system is accomplished primarily by physiological hemodynamic measurements (vasoconstriction/vasodilation) and morphological evaluation in rats, dogs, and monkeys. In general, toxicology studies in animals usually identify direct-acting vascular toxicants, while drugs such as the COX2 inhibitors that are associated with increased cardiovascular mortality in patients are unlikely to be detected in routine studies using normal healthy animals. Therefore, in clinical studies involving patients with a high risk of cardiovascular disease, carefully designed cardiovascular safety studies are required (Goldfine 2008).

For the cardiovascular system, evaluation of vascular toxicity in beagle dogs is particularly relevant because there is a wealth of historical nonclinical and clinical translation data that can be used to determine human relevance and risk.

Vascular injury can occur through cytotoxicity, activation of the immune system, or excessive hemodynamic activity, such as vasoconstriction and vasodilation. Preclinically, most of the treatment-related vascular pathology is caused through functional damage associated with hemodynamic effects that cause medial necrosis and hemorrhage (vascular injury). In contrast, in humans, drug-induced vasculitis (DIV) is immune-mediated. The term "vasculitis" is commonly used to describe changes that occur in the blood vessel wall and surrounding tissues, characterized by (1) lumen occlusion with or without thrombosis; (2) enlarged, hypertrophied ECs and intimal proliferation; (3) mural necrosis, hemorrhage, and inflammation; and (4) adventitial and perivascular inflammation. Because of these mechanistic and morphologic differences, the term "vasculitis" is

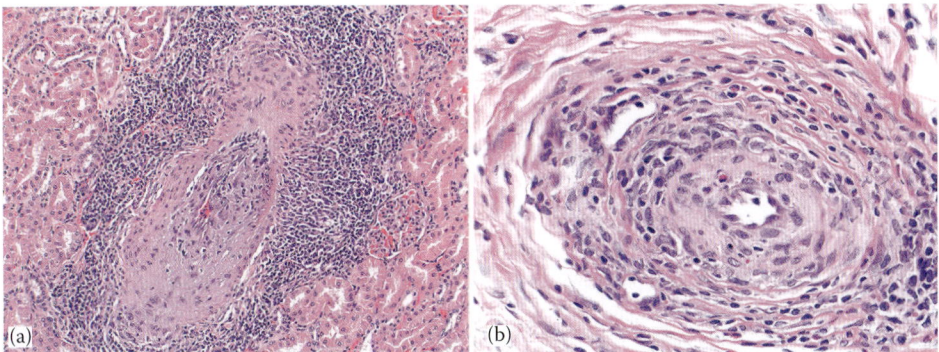

FIGURE 16.3 (a) Hematoxylin and eosin, 100×. Drug-induced vasculitis (DIV) in the dog. (b) Hematoxylin and eosin, 200×. Drug-induced vasculitis (DIV).

not preferred when documenting acute arterial lesions without prominent inflammation induced by vasoactive agents.

DIV resulting from an immune-mediated response occurs in a spectrum of vessels ranging from small cutaneous arteries to venules, in humans, monkeys, and rarely dogs (Chelly et al. 1986; Morris and Beale 1999) (Figure 16.3). It is observed macroscopically as a skin rash but may involve vessels of other organs, most commonly the kidney (Gao and Zhao 2009). In humans, DIV is complex and can involve several mechanisms (Gao and Zhao 2009), including generation of antibodies to small molecules and formation of immune complexes that can then be deposited within the vascular wall (ten Holder et al. 2002). Antibodies that react with neutrophil cytoplasm can cause release of myeloperoxidase (MPO) and hydrogen peroxide from activated neutrophils, converting the drug into a cytotoxin (Jiang et al. 1994) and ultimately leading to antineutrophil cytoplasmic antibody (ANCA) production (von Schmiedeberg et al. 1995). The possible targets for ANCA are MPO, proteinase-3, and other serine proteinases found within these granules (Jennette and Falk 1997; Saleh and Stone 2005; Savage et al. 1997). DIV in humans is of the hypersensitive, non-necrotizing type, characterized by an inflammatory infiltrate composed of mononuclear cells, eosinophils, scattered polymorphonuclear cells in the walls of arterioles, capillaries, venules, and small veins. There is no involvement of larger muscular arteries (Mullick et al. 1979). Several structural and pharmacologically diverse drugs such as the penicillins, sulfonamides, minocycline, allopurinol, thiazides, pyrazolones, retinoids, quinolones, hydantoins, propylthiouracil, hydralazine, colony-stimulating factor, and methotrexate can induce hypersensitivity vasculitis in humans (Jennette and Falk 1997; Johnson and Grimwood 1994; ten Holder et al. 2002; Table 16.7).

The most common histological and plasma marker is ANCA, and, based on immunochemistry, it is divided into cytoplasmic-stained ANCA (C-ANCA) and perinuclear stained ANCA (P-ANCA). C-ANCA is typically induced by protease-3, and P-ANCA correlates with anti-MPO, elastase, lysozyme, and lactoferrin antibodies.

16.2.2 Spontaneous Vascular Injury in Laboratory Animals

Spontaneous, stress-related, and idiopathic arterial lesions in rats and dogs add confusion and complexity to interpretation of drug-induced vascular injury and can pose a diagnostic challenge to the inexperienced pathologist. Therefore, it is important to be familiar with the differential patterns of manifestation of drug-induced versus spontaneous vascular change, especially in dogs. Blood vessels exhibit a limited and narrow spectrum of morphologic change that is characterized as medial degeneration, proliferation (intimal and adventitial), and inflammation. In dogs, degenerative and proliferative arterial diseases are often age related and generally associated with other disease

TABLE 16.7

Pharmacologically and Structurally Diverse Approved Drugs Associated with Clinical DIV in Humans

Class	Drug Examples	Reference
Analgesics	Acetaminophen, naproxen	Jahangiri et al. 1992
Antibiotics	Cephotaxime, minocycline	Feriozzi et al. 2000
Anticonvulsants	Phenytoin, carbamazepine, ethosuximide, trimethadione, primidone, valproate	Drory and Korczyn 1993
Antimicrobials	Penicillin, fluoroquinolones	Maunz et al. 2009
Antithyroid	Benzylthiouracil, carbimazole, methimazole, propylthiouracil	Pandey et al. 2008
Anti-TNFa	Adalimumab, etanercept, infliximab	Downes et al. 2011
Antituberculosis	Rifampin, pyrazinamide, isoniazid	Kim et al. 2010
Asthma	Accolate (zafirlukast), Singulair (montelukast), Azlaire (Pranlukast)	Doyle and Cuellar 2003
Cardiovascular	Hydralazine, amiodarone, atenolol	Bass 1981
CNS	Phenylpropanolamine, clozapine, thioridazine	Fallis and Fisher 1985; Penaskovic et al. 2005
Immunosuppressive	Tacrolimus (FK-506)	Nalesnik et al. 1987
Misc.	Allopurinol, D-penicillamine, levamisole, phenytoin, isotretinoin, methotrexate	Bienaime et al. 2007; Choi et al. 1998, 2000; Epstein et al. 1987; Halevy et al. 1998; Laux-End et al. 1996; ten Holder et al. 2002
Osteoporosis	Risedronate	Belhadjali et al. 2008

states (Kelly 1989). Though rare in toxicology studies, infection (bacteria, fungi, and parasites) or immune-mediated inflammatory vascular changes have been reported in dogs (Bishop 1990; Morris and Beale 1999). Spontaneous idiopathic polyarteritis of beagles, sometimes called "beagle pain syndrome," is the single most problematic issue that complicates diagnosis and interpretation of drug-induced vascular injury (Clemo et al. 2003; Louden and Morgan 2001).

16.2.2.1 Idiopathic Polyarteritis of Beagle Dogs

Idiopathic canine polyarteritis is a chronic, spontaneous, arterial disease syndrome of unknown etiology that is found primarily in laboratory beagle dogs (Kerns et al. 2001). This syndrome has a diverse clinical and histopathological manifestation and has been described as beagle pain syndrome (Hayes et al. 1989), juvenile polyarteritis syndrome (Snyder et al. 1995), necrotizing vasculitis (Stejskal et al. 1982), polyarteritis (Albassam et al. 1989; Harcourt 1978), arteritis (Hartman 1987; Morishima et al. 1990), periarteritis (Spencer and Greaves 1987), panarteritis (Kemi et al. 1990; Ruben et al. 1989), and idiopathic febrile necrotizing arteritis (Hayes et al. 1989).

Clinically, the syndrome can be presented as recurrent episodes of fever, weight loss, hunched posture, and stiff gait and neck because of cervical pain. Clinical signs are not always apparent, but in the acute febrile phase, clinical pathology findings are indicative of widespread inflammation with elevation of acute phase proteins, such as IL-6 (HogenEsch et al. 1995). The etiology of this syndrome is unknown; however, the spectra of morphologic pathology findings spanning acute, subacute, and chronic response suggest an immune-mediated injury, but this has not been confirmed with immunology-based data.

Histologically, the nature of arterial pathology is varied and depends on the number, frequency, and duration of febrile episoditic events. Idiopathic canine polyarteritis is manifested as an acute to chronic, multiorgan, polysystemic arterial disease affecting primarily small- to medium-sized arteries. While there is no organ-specific predilection, arteries in the heart, cranial mediastinum, cervical spinal meninges, and urinary bladder are frequently affected (Kerns et al. 2001; Snyder et al. 1995). Transmural neutrophilic inflammation is commonly associated with extramural, coronary arterial branches of the heart as are fibrinoid necrosis and histiocytic–lymphocytic periarterial and adventitial infiltration. Thrombosis can sometimes be seen in some acute lesions. In subacute and chronic lesions in dogs undergoing remission the arterial lesions are characterized by intimal thickening and/or hyperplasia, medial hypertrophy, ruptured and/or break in the internal elastic laminae, and perivascular mononuclear inflammatory cell infiltrates (Kerns et al. 2001; Snyder et al. 1995).

16.2.2.2 Mesenteric and Splanchnic Spontaneous Polyarteritis Syndrome in Rats

In rats, spontaneous age-related polyarteritis of medium-sized mesenteric, spermatic, and splanchnic arteries is well recognized. In older rats on longer-term studies, polyarteritis can sometimes be recognized at necropsy, with the more severely affected arteries appearing thickened and tortuous with multiple, firm, nodular formations. This lesion is sometimes referred to as "polyarteritis nodosa." The morphologic characteristics of this lesion histologically vary from acute to chronic active, or chronic inflammation, and in some instances, there is involvement of veins resulting in what is frequently referred to as polyangitis. In the acute lesion, there is infiltration of neutrophils and eosinophils, fibrinoid necrosis of the media, and disruption of the internal elastic laminae. Arterial thrombosis, fibrosis with loss of normal medial architecture, and adventitial inflammation are the characteristic features of the chronic lesion. This lesion progresses due to extensive adventitial fibroblastic proliferation, causing thickening of the arterial walls and narrowing of the lumina with eventual stenosis. In young Sprague Dawley, untreated, control rats, spontaneous medial degeneration and periarteritis of the hilar hepatic arteries have been described (Short et al. 1998). Histologically, this lesion is characterized by medial hemorrhage and vascular smooth muscle vacuolar degeneration of affected arteries. Occasionally, there is periarteritis characterized by neutrophilic or mononuclear inflammatory cell infiltrates. These hilar hepatic lesions have some common morphologic features with polyarteritis; however, it is not known if the spontaneous hilar hepatic arterial lesion is a part of the mesenteric/splanchnic polyarteritis syndrome in rats.

16.2.2.3 Other Species

Spontaneous polyarteritis has been reported in a nonhuman primate (Porter et al. 2003), and asymptomatic polyarteritis with coronary artery involvement has been reported in cynomolgus monkeys used in toxicology studies (Albassam et al. 1993; Ito et al. 1992). Spontaneous, mural, medial degeneration and/or hemorrhage of coronary arteries have also been reported in nonclinical studies (Chamanza et al. 2006; Vidal et al. 2010). Histologically, lesions are present in intramural vessels of the right or left ventricles, characterized by one or more of the following: (1) focal mural hemorrhage; (2) mural cellular debris; (3) medial SMC degeneration/regeneration; and (4) minimal perivascular mononuclear cell infiltrates (Figure 16.4). Perivasculitis/vasculitis-like lesions have been observed in renal, pulmonary, meningeal, and sciatic vessels (Chamanza et al. 2006). Spontaneous,

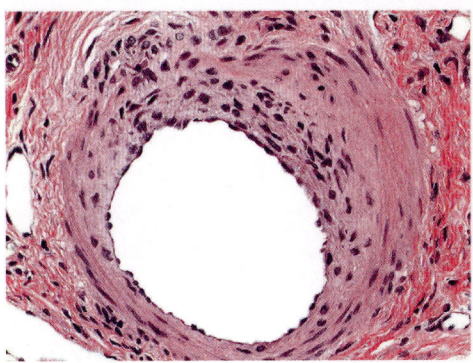

FIGURE 16.4 Hematoxylin and eosin, 200×. Spontaneous vascular lesion in the monkey.

atherosclerosis-like lesions have also been reported in monkeys (Jones and Hunt 1983). In swine, spontaneous vascular lesions are rare; however, irregular intimal thickening of the aorta, coronary arteries, and large vessels has been reported (Jones and Hunt 1983).

16.2.3 Drug-Induced Vascular Lesions

Clinical development of novel, life-saving therapies is often hindered because the nonclinical safety profiles of drug candidates are associated with silent pathological processes that are not associated with clinical signs. Moreover, noninvasive methods for the clinical monitoring of occult pathology are not currently available. In toxicology studies, drug-induced vascular injury is an example of such a situation as there are no biochemical markers for monitoring such morphological changes clinically and our understanding of the pathophysiology is limited (Figure 16.5). This type of vascular toxicity is most often associated with drug candidates that are pharmacologically active in the vascular bed (Table 16.4). Some of these are approved drugs of varying chemical structure and pharmacologic class but are known to cause occult mesenteric or coronary arterial vascular pathology without adverse clinical signs in rodents and nonrodents, respectively (Albassam et al. 1999; Chelly et al. 1986; Gans et al. 1980; Greaves 1998; Joseph 2000; Kerns et al. 1989a,b, 2000; Louden and Morgan 2001; Louden et al. 2000; Mesfin et al. 1989).

16.2.3.1 Drug-Induced Vascular Injury in Dogs

Dogs are uniquely sensitive to the development of arterial lesions that are associated with structurally and pharmacologically diverse vasoactive agents (Chelly et al. 1986; Dogterom et al. 1992;

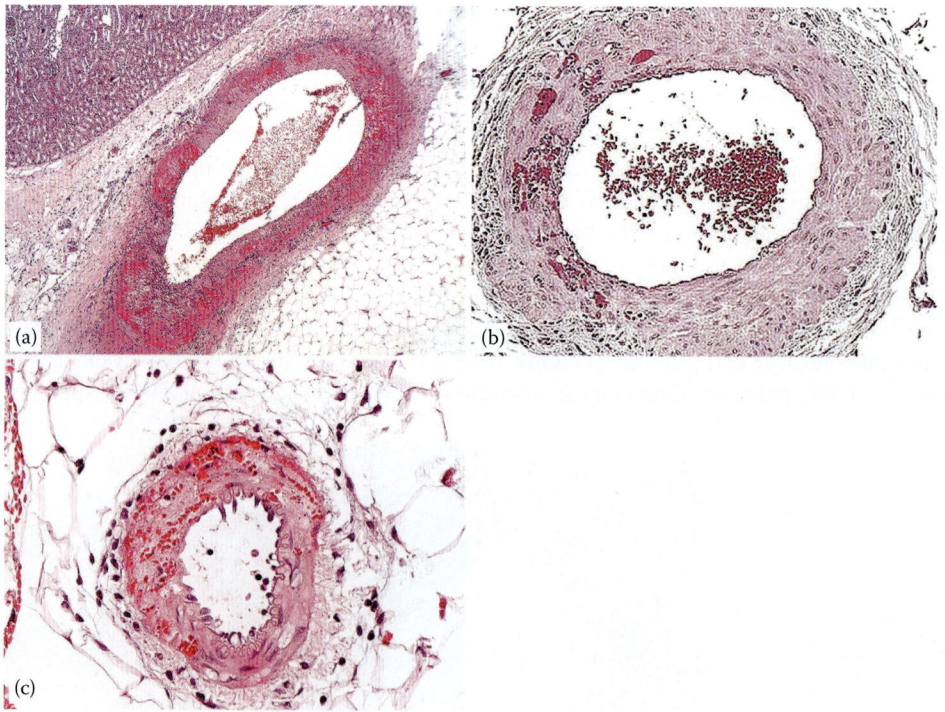

FIGURE 16.5 (a) Hematoxylin and eosin, 400×. Vascular lesion induced by an antisense oligonucleotide. (b) Hematoxylin and eosin, 400×. Canine drug-induced vascular injury (DIVI), 24 h post ETRA treatment. (c) Hematoxylin and eosin, 400×. Rat drug-induced vascular injury (DIVI), 24 h post fenoldopam (dopamine agonist) treatment.

Gans et al. 1980; Louden et al. 2000; Mesfin et al. 1989). At high doses in dogs, these agents induce a distinct morphologic coronary arterial pathology. Generally, drug-induced cardiovascular toxicity is regional with some predilection for the right side of the heart, particularly the right extramural coronary arteries. Macroscopically, hemorrhagic areas are seen in the right atrium with petechial hemorrhages or short, linear, hemorrhagic streaks overlying or adjacent to the right branches of the extramural coronary arteries. Similar small areas of hemorrhage were also seen infrequently in the left atrium. The ventricles usually remain unaffected (Louden et al. 2000; Mesfin et al. 1989).

Microscopically, vasodilators and/or positive inotropic agents such as minoxidil, hydralazine, PDE inhibitors (PDE III), or ETRA are associated with this unique coronary arterial lesion, characterized by acute, segmental changes of medial necrosis and hemorrhage that can develop as early as 12–24 h postdose following intravenous administration (Isaacs et al. 1989; Louden et al. 2000) and between 3 and 7 days with oral dosing (Mesfin et al. 1989). Medial hemorrhage can be transmural and/or circumferential, with well-preserved, extravasated red blood cells and perivascular edema. Vascular lesions are primarily seen in muscular branches of the coronary arteries, in coronary arterioles, and possibly in capillaries (Mesfin et al. 1989). Subepicardial branches of the right coronary arteries, composed of 5- to 8-cell layer thickness, are most frequently affected, while mural branches of the right and left coronary arteries are affected less frequently. Terminal arterioles and capillaries, particularly those in the outer third of the right atrial wall, are quite prominent due to enlargement because of swelling and/or activation of ECs. Chronic lesions include intimal proliferation, SMC hyperplasia with mucinous ground substance, and adventitial fibroplasia with varying degrees of mixed mononuclear inflammatory cell infiltrates.

16.2.3.2 Drug-Induced Vascular Injury in Nonhuman Primates

In nonhuman primates, segmental, medial necrosis and hemorrhage as well as inflammation and a fibroproliferative response were seen in the extramural coronary arteries following administration of an ETRA (CI-1020), an antihypertensive adenosine receptor agonist, or a PDE IV inhibitor (Albassam et al. 1998, 1999). Standard measurement of HR and/or MAP did not reveal any major hemodynamic alterations, so mechanistically, the relationship between the vascular pathology seen in nonhuman primates and altered hemodynamics is not clear.

Subchronic subcutaneous administration of a recombinant human interleukin 4 was associated with vascular pathology in a variety of tissues (Barbolt et al. 1991; Gossett et al. 1993). Vascular lesions were characterized by an obliterative/stenotic arterial and endarterial lesion with proliferation of SMCs and transmural or segmental eosinophil infiltrates in the intima and media (Barbolt et al. 1991; Gossett et al. 1993).

16.2.3.3 Drug-Induced Vascular Injury in Swine

In miniature swine, the potassium channel opener, minoxidil, is associated with left atrial and left coronary arterial lesions that are characterized microscopically by medial necrosis, hemorrhage and acute to chronic inflammation depending on duration (Herman et al. 1989). These lesions are associated with both tachycardia and hypotension (Herman et al. 1989). While the mode of action is unknown, the prevailing hypothesis is that vascular lesions are caused by overstretching of the vascular wall due to excessive and prolonged vasodilation (Herman et al. 1989).

16.2.3.4 Drug-Induced Vascular Injury in Rats

In rats, pharmacologically and structurally diverse xenobiotics of various types, such as antibiotics, immunosuppressive agents, cytotoxic anticancer drugs, cardioactive agents, and foreign proteins, can induce vascular lesions, most commonly in the splanchnic (mesenteric, pancreatic, gastric, splenic, and hepatic) beds (Kerns et al. 1989a; Yuhas et al. 1985). It is generally accepted that, in rats, drug-induced vascular lesions are induced by potent hemodynamic-altering agents. However, this is not supported by any objective data acquired through physiological or hemodynamic measurements.

Continuous intravenous infusion of fenoldopam, a dopaminergic agonist, is associated with macroscopic and microscopic vascular lesions 24 h postdosing, and lesions were seen mostly in arteries with—four to five cell layers of SMC (Joseph 2000; Joseph et al. 1997; Kerns et al. 1989a,b; Yuhas et al. 1985). Fenoldopam consistently induces a dose response in incidence and severity of lesions in rats. Regardless of dose, vascular lesions were evident only when fenoldopam was infused for 24 h. The lesion in rats is characterized by transmural, segmental, or circumferential variable-sized foci of medial SMC necrosis and hemorrhage. Focal sites will often have mostly extravasated red blood cells, some polymorphonuclear leukocytes, and a few monocytes occupying well-delineated spaces in the medial wall. Fibrin thrombi and breaks in the internal elastic lamina are uncommon findings but can be seen depending on the severity of the lesion. Ultrastructurally, there is a separation of ECs, extensive necrosis, and gaps filled with extravasated erythrocytes, leukocytes, and platelets adhered to remnants of the basal lamina (Bugelski et al. 1989; Joseph 2000). In rats, morphologically similar lesions involving the mesenteric arteries have been described following oral administration of PDE4, including the prototypic inhibitor rolipram (Larson et al. 1996; Slim et al. 2002). However, oral administration of IC542, a selective PDE4 inhibitor, was associated with a proinflammatory vascular response in rat mesenteric vessels. Coadministration of IC542 with dexamethasone completely blocked the proinflammatory vascular response in the rat mesentery (Dietsch et al. 2006). These results were in contrast to other published studies using a similar study design (Slim et al. 2002). The differences in response may be related to the selectivity of various molecules for members within the PDE family.

Vasopressor and vasoconstrictor agents can also produce medial necrosis of medium-sized arteries in rats (Greaves 2007). For example, continuous intravenous infusion or repeated injection of the potent vasoconstrictor angiotensin can induce medial necrosis in some splanchnic and renal vessels, and mechanistically, arterial damage is mediated by sustained and profound vasoconstriction (Nemes et al. 1980; Thorball and Olsen 1974). Vasoconstrictors primarily affect small caliber arteries in multiple organs, and the lesion is characterized by medial SMC fibrinoid necrosis with minimal hemorrhage (Clemo et al. 2003).

The PPAR-γ agonist GI262570X was associated with a unique but consistent vascular change in the brown adipose tissues of rats in toxicology studies (Elangbam et al. 2002) wherein round clear vacuoles were present in the tunica media of arterioles and medium-sized arteries. Occasionally, within these medial SMCs, the vacuoles were peripherally located and morphologically appeared as adipocytes (Elangbam et al. 2002). These lesions, however, did not progress to form atheroscleroticype lesions in rats following daily administration of the compound for 2 years, and the severity and incidence were reduced, suggesting that in shorter-term studies, this finding was an adaptive/compensatory response (Elangbam et al. 2002).

Neutralizing antibodies to vascular endothelial growth factor (VEGF) or inhibition/blockade of the receptor by small molecule TK inhibitors (VTK) causes hypertension, vasoconstriction, and vascular pathology (personal observation). Ergotamine and related alkaloids produce vascular arterial lesions in the tail of rats when these compounds are administered systemically. The lesion is characterized by swelling of ECs, thickening of the intima, and intimal proliferation. Thrombosis of veins, ischemia, and gangrenous necrosis of the tail develop. The lesion is mediated by intense and profound constriction of the central caudal (tail) artery and is comparable to the pathology seen when adrenalin, an endogenous vasoconstrictor, is injected locally into the tail (Lund 1951).

16.2.4 Aortic Aneurysm

In humans, genetic and familial dissecting aortic aneurysms involving primarily the thoracic aorta have been reported as disorders of Marfan's and Ehlers-Danlos type IV syndromes (Milewicz et al. 2000; Spigset 2011). Spontaneous, naturally occurring, dissecting aneurysms in the region of the ductus arteriosus have been reported in 4-day-old pups (Treumann et al. 2011), in experimental lathyrism (Boor and Langford 1997), and following administration of certain amines such as semicarbazide (Langford et al. 1999) that cause aortic aneurysm (Figure 16.6).

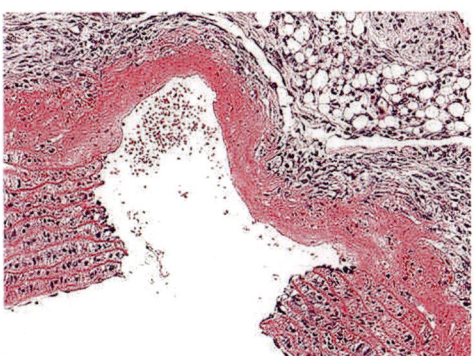

FIGURE 16.6 Hematoxylin and eosin, 200×. Aortic aneurism.

In toxicology studies, aortic necrosis, inflammation, and aneurysm formation can develop as a result of administration of xenobiotics. Although drug-induced changes to the aorta are uncommon, aortic damage and aneurysm formation (with or without necrosis and/or inflammation) have been reported with angiotensin II, catecholamines, allylamine, and beta-aminopropionitrile (Daugherty et al. 2000; Haft 1974; Haft et al. 1972; Kumar et al. 1998; Lu et al. 2008). Aortic aneurysms are characterized by focal necrosis of medial aortic SMCs, fragmentation and breaks of the elastic laminae, and breakdown in the structural integrity of the aortic wall, resulting in "outpocketing" or nodular protrusions that can lead to rupturing into the thoracic or abdominal cavities. Chronic administration of high doses of adrenalin can produce aortic calcification, reactive inflammation, and saccular aortic dilatation (Haft et al. 1972). Vascular remodeling and alteration in expression of matrix metalloproteinases have been reported as a possible mode of action for the development of aortic aneurysm (Nordon et al. 2009). In support of this hypothesis, inhibition of MMP2 and MMP9 has been associated with aortic aneurysm formation. Aortic aneurysm caused by sweet pea (*Lathyrus odoratous*) ingestion is due to inhibition of lysyl oxidase by β-aminopropionitrile. Lysyl oxidase plays an important role in cross-linking of collagen and elastin in connective tissues and, therefore, is crucial to maintaining the structural integrity of elastic arteries such as the aorta (Boor et al. 1995).

16.2.5 VASCULAR LESIONS AT OTHER SITES

Species-specific vascular SMC necrosis of the aorta and renal hilar arteries were associated with administration of a nonpeptide vitronectin receptor antagonist SB273005 in mice. Vascular lesions were characterized by necrosis, regeneration, cardiac fibrosis, and medial hypertrophy of SMCs with deposition of a PAS-positive material in the media (Rehm et al. 2007). Because there were no vascular effects in rats or monkeys, and other compounds with similar pharmacologic activity did not produce this lesion in mice, it was concluded that this lesion was not related to antagonism of vitronectin receptor (Rehm et al. 2007).

In routine toxicology studies, AN1792, a beta-amyloid immunotherapeutic agent, was not associated with adverse toxicity (Schenk et al. 1999). The compound was well tolerated in a Phase I safety and tolerability study; however, in the Phase IIa study, further development was suspended because approximately 6% of the volunteers developed symptoms of adverse inflammatory events in the brain with microhemorrhage (Orgogozo et al. 2003; Patton et al. 2006; Uro-Coste et al. 2010). In transgenic mice, this immunotherapeutic agent induced microhemorrhage with hemosiderin deposits in the brain that were Prussian blue positive, thus confirming microvascular cerebral hemorrhage (Pfeifer et al. 2002). The mechanism(s) of cerebral microvascular hemorrhage is not clear but may be related to the following: (1) NO dysfunction of the vasculature; (2) degradation of vascular extracellular matrix by metalloproteinase-9; (3) altered apolipoprotein E lipid metabolism; and/or (4) loss of mitochondrial membrane potential with decreased telomerase activity (Chiu et al. 2011; Horsburgh et al. 2000; Lee et al. 2005; Miller et al. 2010).

16.2.6 DIFFERENTIATING SPONTANEOUS FROM DRUG-INDUCED VASCULAR LESIONS

In preclinical safety studies, interpretation of drug-induced vascular changes in dogs may be confounded by sporadic and/or dose-dependent increases in the incidence of idiopathic canine polyarteritis in beagles. When making such an interpretation, it is crucial to record and document the nature and location of apparent macroscopic changes, with emphasis placed on the heart and coronary vessels. Microscopically, the histopathology profile, site predilection, and detailed characterization of the pattern and anatomical distribution should be especially noted. Arterial lesions induced by vasodilators (minoxidil, hydralazine, PDE inhibitors III–V, and ETRA) are often restricted to the extramural coronary arteries, primarily the right branches, with lower incidence normally present in the left coronary artery and left atrium. In contrast, in idiopathic polyarteritis syndrome of beagle dogs, multiple-organ, systemic involvement of medium- to small-sized arteries (in addition to the coronary arteries) is affected. The acute arterial lesion induced by vasodilators is characterized by medial hemorrhage and necrosis wherein the former may involve the endothelium, media, and adventitia. Inflammation is not a prominent feature of acute drug-induced vascular injury. The hallmark of acute idiopathic polyarteritis is prominent inflammation (periarterial and arterial) without hemorrhage. Additionally, fibrinoid necrosis and arterial thrombosis are frequently seen (Snyder et al. 1995). Idiopathic polyarteritis is not associated with secondary myocardial changes, while secondary myocardial edema due to vascular injury induced by vasodilators is observed. Intermittent-episodic fever, cervical pain, and discomfort are recognizable clinical signs of idiopathic polyarteritis, while vasodilatory vascular injury is generally silent with no clinical signs. Altered hemodynamics of hypotension, with compensatory reflex tachycardia, is an expected pharmacologic response of vasodilators, while hemodynamic changes are not a feature of idiopathic polyarteritis.

Differentiating drug-induced from spontaneous vascular changes in dogs can be problematic when vascular changes, chronic and/or chronic active, are presented simply as an increased incidence of lesions that are morphologically indistinguishable from those seen in canine idiopathic polyarteritis. Such was the case following continuous treatment with an endothelin receptor antagonist (ETRA) (Albassam et al. 2001) and minoxidil (Mesfin et al. 1989). In these situations, an association to drug treatment can be made based only on dose response and hemodynamic alterations. In addition, a non-nucleoside-reverse-transcriptase inhibitor was associated with chronic vascular lesions in dogs (Clemo et al. 2003). Because there is no human homologue for reverse transcriptase, vascular toxicity of these compounds is most likely due to an effect on subcellular organelles, and, as such, this effect must be considered as "off target." It must also be taken into consideration that compounds that are not rationally designed to be vasoactive may produce secondary "off-target" hemodynamic effects that are sufficiently profound to induce vascular lesions. Idiopathic polyarteritis in dogs may be potentiated by hemodynamic stress (Isaacs et al. 1989; Joseph et al. 1997), immunomodulating drugs (Stejskal et al. 1982), and benzodiazepines (Schlaeppi et al. 1991).

16.2.7 DRUG-INDUCED VASCULAR INJURY: MECHANISM OF ACTION(S)

Although there is considerable variation in the causes of vascular injury, the microscopic morphologic presentation is limited. Arterial injury is the end result of a series of complex interactive events that include derangements in normal vascular physiology, loss of vascular homeostatic tone, and initiation of local and systemic compensatory mechanisms. Drugs and/or chemicals cause arterial damage by directly interacting with vascular wall components or through direct or indirect interaction of drugs with the cellular and molecular pharmacological targets within the vessel wall (Figure 16.7).

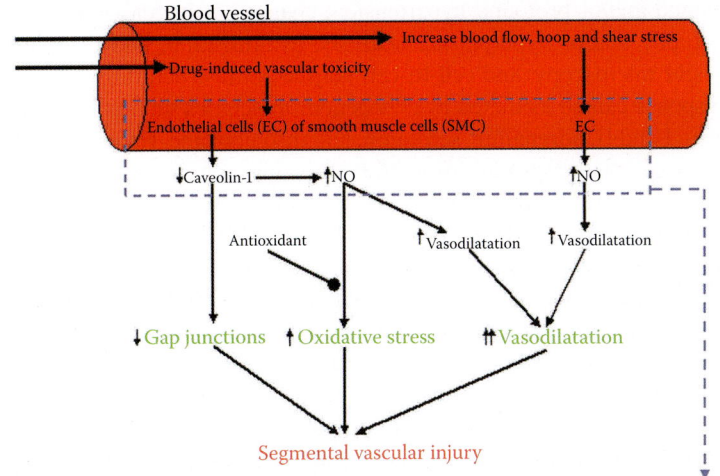

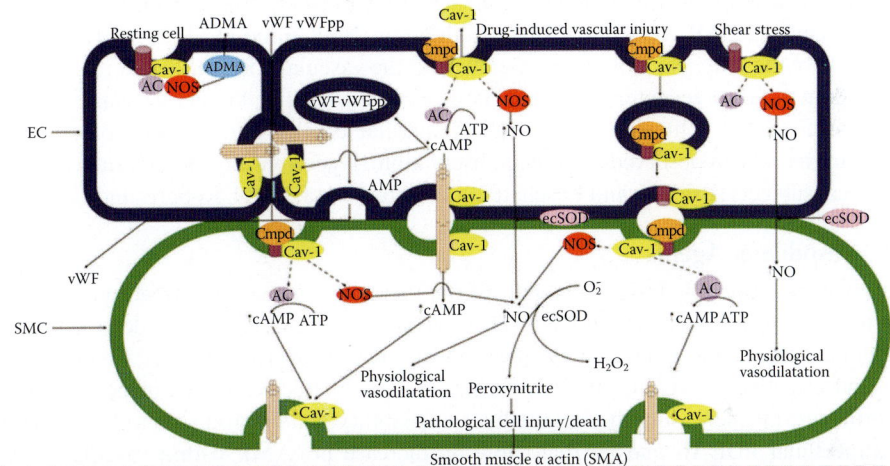

FIGURE 16.7 Potential mode of action and biomarkers for drug-induced vascular injury that involves the caveolin-1 regulated nitric oxide (NO) pathway.

16.2.7.1 Direct Acting Agents

Morphological effects of xenobiotics that directly interact with the blood vessel wall typically result in acute necrosis, thrombosis, and inflammation. The antifungal agent allylamine is a direct-acting vascular toxicant because of its effect on vascular SMCs (Boor and Hysmith 1987) but not ECs. The mechanism of toxicity may be related to the high intracellular concentration of the enzyme benzylamine oxidase within the SMC (Boor and Hysmith 1987). Inhibition of this enzyme by phenelzine prevents allylamine-induced vascular injury (Hysmith and Boor 1988). Direct-acting vascular toxicants can be detected/predicted using in vitro assays (Boor et al. 1990; Ramos et al. 1988). Other direct-acting agents cause injury through mechanisms that are not well defined and may result in lesions morphologically characterized as medial hyalinization, mineralization, and SMC hypertrophy/hyperplasia (Boor et al. 1995).

16.2.7.2 Vasoconstrictor Agents

Constriction of systemic or localized vasculature is the consequence of a physiological or chemically induced increase in vascular resistance that ultimately leads to localized or systemic hypertension.

As a response to sustained and/or profound hypertension, changes of increased medial thickness (resulting from hypertrophy and/or hyperplasia), necrosis, hyalinization, and cytoplasmic vacuolation are seen with light microscopy, and cell-to-cell hernias, ultrastructurally (Joris and Majno 1981). This vascular response can be mediated by endogenous molecules such as L-norepinephrine, endothelin-1, angiotensin I and II, adrenaline, serotonin, and thromboxane. Experimentally, arterial lesions can be induced in rats and dogs administered with endogenous vasoconstrictive agents or agonists, and the resulting physiologically induced hypertension causes a morphologically similar arterial lesion, regardless of the inciting cause (Golby and Beilin 1972; Joris and Majno 1981; Wiener and Giacomelli 1973). For example, intravenous administration of suprapharmacologic doses of endothelin-1 (ET-1), a potent ET_A agonist, causes profound vasoconstriction and the formation of medial arterial lesions that are morphologically similar to those induced by other hypertensive agents (Louden and Morgan 2001). Additionally, in anesthetized dogs, intravenous administration of low doses of ET-1 was associated with marked coronary vasoconstriction, reduction in coronary blood flow, and coronary arterial injury (Cannan et al. 1995). Another example is the pharmacologically mediated effects of VEGF. Under physiological conditions, agonist stimulation of the VEGF receptor causes intracellular, downstream activation of NO synthase (NOS) in SMCs, releasing NO that mediates SMC relaxation and vasodilation (Bouloumie et al. 1999; Bussolati et al. 2001). Because of the role in angiogenesis, members of the vascular TK family that include vascular endothelial growth factor receptor (VEGFR) have become attractive targets for cancer therapy. In nonclinical safety studies, hypertension, renal glomerular capillary injury with proteinuria, and vascular injury have been observed (personal observation). Hypertension and proteinuria have been seen in clinical subjects (Pridjian and Puschett 2002; Roberts et al. 1989; Roberts and Cooper 2001).

16.2.7.3 Vasodilator Agents

Vasodilators were rationally designed as part of the therapeutic strategy to treat hypertension and other cardiovascular diseases, such as CHF. These vasoactive agents exert their desired pharmacology by (1) direct relaxation of SMC in the arterial wall via cell surface receptors; (2) opening of K+ channels and effectively resisting the vasoconstrictive, counteractive forces of neurotransmitters and/or hormones; (3) increasing the intracellular availability and/or production of NO; (4) inhibition of intracellular PDE III and IV that cause an increase in cAMP within vascular SMC; and (5) blockade of vasoconstrictive endothelin receptors that effectively induce vasodilation. It is interesting to note that while the pharmacologic targets are quite diverse, there is often a common second intracellular messenger, hence, a common pharmacologic and toxic response (Table 16.4). Many of the compounds known to induce vascular injury have calcium and cAMP as common secondary messengers, with these molecules being regulated by the cell surface protein caveolin-1 (Park et al. 2000; Yamamoto et al. 1999).

In general, vasodilating agents significantly lower MAP, increase HR (reflex tachycardia), and increase regional coronary artery blood flow in dogs, with hemodynamic effects considered key components of the pathophysiological basis for toxicity. In fact, many approved drugs such as minoxidil, nicorandil, hydralazine, and theobromine are associated with these effects (Gans et al. 1980; Mesfin et al. 1987, 1989). However, administration of ETRA is associated with drug-induced coronary arterial lesions, but without profound hemodynamic changes in HR and MAP (Greaves 2000; Jones et al. 2003; Louden et al. 2000). In dogs, understanding ETRA-induced vascular injury, pathophysiology, and potential mode of action has been aided by data describing a relationship between sites that are prone to toxic effects, and the distribution, density, type, and ratio of vasoactive endothelin receptors in the heart and coronary arteries (Louden et al. 2000). Additionally, the composite analysis of receptor subtype profiles, mRNA expression, and regional blood flow measurements clearly support the hypothesis that this disproportionate receptor distribution is responsible for the marked functional differences in regional blood flow at the sites of injury: the right atrium and right coronary arteries (Chelly et al. 1986; Louden et al. 2000). In the dog coronary arteries, ET receptor density is five- to sixfold higher when compared to the atria and ventricles (Louden et al. 2000). ET receptor subtype characterization indicates that ET_B receptors are three times more prevalent in the right coronary arteries when compared to the left coronary arteries, and in situ hybridization studies confirm localization of these receptors to the SMC. Consequently, the composite data of expression profiles of ET receptors indicate a disproportionate distribution of ET_B receptors in the right coronary artery of dogs, thus explaining the difference in regional blood flow (Louden et al. 2000; Sumner et al. 1992; Teerlink et al. 1994). On SMCs, ET_B receptors mediate contraction, leading to a net vasodilatory effect (Louden et al. 2000; Moreland et al. 1992; Sumner et al. 1992; Teerlink et al. 1994). Collectively, these data, in conjunction with other published reports, strongly suggest that mechanistically, exaggerated pharmacology causes profound regional vasodilation, increased regional blood flow, and dysregulation of arterial tone, providing the basis for selective, site-specific, mesenteric, or coronary arterial damage in rats and dogs (Chelly et al. 1986; Joseph 2000; Louden et al. 2000).

ET receptors on the endothelium can mediate the release of NO (Chabrier 1993; Pernow and Modin 1993), which mediates the vasodilation that can be induced by antagonism of endothelin receptors and/or opening of potassium ion channels (Kuhlmann et al. 2004; Tirapelli et al. 2005; Yamaguchi et al. 2003). Fenoldopam, a dopaminergic-1 agonist, mediates renal vasodilation through the NO pathway (Venkatakrishnan et al. 2000) and preclinically induces renal and mesenteric arterial pathology (Bugelski et al. 1989; Yuhas et al. 1985). There is growing evidence that some receptors and/or ion channels act directly or indirectly through the NOS pathway to cause vascular injury as a consequence of an exaggerated pharmacological response (Brott 2006; Kerns et al. 2005; Louden and Morgan 2001). In drug-induced vascular injury, NO may mediate the prolonged and sustained vasodilation that causes dysregulation of arterial tone, leading to arterial damage (Joseph et al. 1997; Louden et al. 2000). Concomitantly, there is loss of regulation and control of key biochemical pathways in ECs and SMCs, breakdown in cell-to-cell communications, and ultimately, structural arterial wall damage (Brott 2006). Infusion of an NO donor caused mesenteric vascular pathology similar to fenoldopam, and direct interference of NO pathway by L-NAME or indirect blockade of its toxic radical nitrotyrosine by tempol attenuated this vascular pathology (Brott et al. 2007; Brott 2006).

In mice, targeted gene disruption of caveolin-1 caused impairment of NOS, NO, and calcium signaling in the cardiovascular system, causing aberrations in endothelium-dependent relaxation, contractility, and maintenance of vasculo-myogenic tone (Drab et al. 2001). Functional loss of caveolin-1 was also associated with a fivefold increase in systemic NO but no major changes in NOS expression (Drab et al. 2001; Zhao et al. 2002), suggesting that deregulation or hyperactivity of NOS was responsible for the massive increase in NO production. Caveolin-1 is expressed within the vascular wall, specifically on the phenotypically anchored primary targets of drug-induced vascular injury, endothelial and smooth muscle cells (Drab et al. 2001; Zhao et al. 2002). Within these cells, caveolin is an important mediator of many signal transduction pathways, including regulation of vascular tone (Martens et al. 2001; Yu et al. 2004). Functionally, caveolae appear to be the focal point for compartmentalizing, organizing, and modulating signal transduction activities (Linder et al. 2005; Martens et al. 2001; Yu et al. 2004) for many receptors, such as adenosine, dopaminergic-1, and endothelin, and enzymes, including PDE, NOS, and adenylyl cyclase (AC) (Table 16.8). Within ECs and/or SMCs, exaggerated pharmacologic action of these molecules or enzymes that are regulated by caveolin-1 is associated with drug-induced vascular injury. Collectively, these data suggest that caveolin-1 plays an important role in regulating NOS activity and, potentially, vascular tone. There is evidence that loss and/or reduced expression of cav-1 in SMCs and/or ECs is a critical event in drug-induced vascular injury (Brott et al. 2005a,b). In vitro studies have shown that loss of caveolin-1 is an early event that precedes SMC apoptosis. These data suggest that it is possible that drug-induced vascular injury is, in part, mediated through the NO caveolin-1 regulated pathway.

TABLE 16.8

Caveolin-1 Colocalizes with or Regulates Many Proteins and Molecules

Ion Channels

Potassium channels

Receptors

Adenosine A1

Angiotensin II

Dopaminergic

Endothelin B

Epidermal growth factor (EGF)

VEGF receptor—Flk-1

Other

Adenyl cyclase

Caspase 3

Gap junctions

Heme oxygenase-1

Nitric oxide synthase (eNOS)

Tight junctions—ZO1, occluding

16.2.8 HYPERTROPHY AND HYPERPLASIA

Hypertension is characterized histologically as a thickening of the media of muscular arteries and/or hyperplasia of SMCs. Medial hypertrophy and hyperplasia are the adaptive responses to prolonged systemic hypertension that naturally occurs in spontaneous hypertensive rats (SHRs). The disease process in this strain of rats has morphologic characteristics of the slow-developing, hypertensive vascular disease in humans and some of the rapidly evolving forms of experimentally induced hypertension in animals. Hypertensive muscular arteries have increased intramural stresses, increased wall thickness, and reduced lumina that lower arterial wall tension (Limas et al. 1980). Sustained hypertension leads to vascular remodeling, with features of EC denudation and/or injury, increased interaction and adherence of platelets and inflammatory cells, paracrine interaction with vasoactive mediators, and locally produced cytokines, as well as direct effects of catecholamine activity within the vascular wall (Coflesky et al. 1988; Fried and Reid 1985).

The SHR is a well-established model of hypertension and associated vascular remodeling, wherein there is marked variability in the morphologic characterization in different vascular beds (Ibayashi et al. 1986; Lima et al. 1985). Data from some of these studies have shown that in peripheral muscular arteries, thickening predominates, while in the aorta, both intimal and medial thickening develop (Limas et al. 980). In the aorta, there is an increased deposition of mucosubstances in the subendothelial space and thickening of interlamellar spaces by enlargement and hypertrophy of aortic SMCs without changes in the internal laminae. In contrast, in muscular arteries and arterioles, there is an increase in the number of concentric SMCs that ultrastructurally contain abundant cytoplasmic organelles that are compatible with the hyperplastic and hypertrophic phenotype. The variation in response in different vascular beds and arteries may suggest that the cellular and organelle changes are influenced by the ability of individual cells to proliferate and/or undergo hypertrophy, in response to the local humoral, toxic, and/or neurogenic factors. Additionally, the biochemical properties of the supporting structural tissues could modify the physiological (i.e., hypertension) and morphologic events that affect the outcome of vessel wall thickness (Nordborg et al. 1985).

In toxicology studies, assessment of medial changes in muscular arteries can be very difficult to evaluate histopathologically. Planimetric methodologies using nonperfusion-fixed tissues could be used for morphometric analysis of muscular arteries when vascular toxicity is suspected (Lowe 1984). However, the preferred and more accurate assessment requires a sufficient number of vessels to be studied using morphometric analysis of tissues collected using perfusion fixation at appropriate pressures (Lowe 1984).

Thickening of the medial SMC layer with reduced lumen size is the hallmark of hypertension, but novel drug candidates may also produce this effect without marked increases in systemic blood pressure, despite possible localized increases in some vascular beds. Treatment for up to 6 months with the orally active inotropic vasodilator ICI 153,110 was associated with both arterial and venous wall thickening that was a result of changes in SMC mass within the medial vessel wall. Though the morphologic changes suggest hypertension, it is also possible that marked vessel wall tension as a result of excessive vasodilation due to exaggerated pharmacology can induce an adaptive vascular response characterized by medial smooth muscle hypertrophy (Wagenaar and Wagenvoort 1978; Weibel 1958).

Within the intima of muscular arteries, particularly in humans, longitudinal smooth muscle fibers can undergo hypertrophy. This type of hypertrophy has been observed in bronchial arteries in humans but can also be seen in some systemic vessels in laboratory rats, characterized by a longitudinally arranged, nonconcentric increase in SMC size (Wagenaar and Wagenvoort 1978; Weibel 1958). These changes can also be induced in the mesenteric arteries of rats by local surgical damage and manipulation (Wagenaar and Wagenvoort 1978; Weibel 1958).

16.2.9 Pulmonary Vessels

The pulmonary tissue receives functional and nutritional blood supply from the pulmonary and bronchial circulation. Pulmonary arteries and veins are large vessels with high blood flow and low vascular resistance. Histologically, the pulmonary veins may have cardiac muscle around the walls, lack internal elastic lamina, and are located at the periphery of the acinus. A unique feature of rats is a segment of the pulmonary artery called the thick-walled, oblique muscular artery (Davies et al. 1986; Meyrick et al. 1978). This is characterized as an oblique layer of muscle that spirals around the normal muscle coat in a defined segment of the pulmonary artery (Davies et al. 1986; Meyrick et al. 1978). Muscular arteries run along the preacinar bronchi and bronchiolar airways, including the terminal bronchioles. In contrast, intra-acinar arteries may be muscular, nonmuscular, or partially muscular, and in the normal rat lung, muscular fibers are lost before the capillary bed is reached (Hislop and Reid 1978). These small, intra-acinar vessels play a very important role in pulmonary hemodynamics and response to pulmonary vascular toxicants. The pulmonary capillaries, lined by ECs, are not only important in oxygenation and gas exchange but also can be the primary target of toxicity leading to pulmonary edema.

In toxicologic investigative pathology, changes in the pulmonary vasculature should be carefully assessed, and include measurement of the right ventricular HW, because this can provide evidence of alteration in pulmonary circulatory hemodynamics. Pulmonary arterial pressure is determined by pulmonary blood flow, pressures in the left atrium and left pulmonary vein, and luminal size of the pulmonary artery.

An invasive procedure in laboratory animals is measurement of pulmonary arterial pressure. This parameter is a reliable biomarker of pulmonary hypertension that also causes changes in pulmonary vascular structure. In humans, severe pulmonary hypertension is characterized by plexiform lesions, known as plexogenic arteriopathy. Plexogenic lesions are very rarely seen in laboratory animals with confirmed pulmonary hypertension. However, in a hybrid strain of New Zealand mouse (NZB×NZW), a pulmonary vasculitis syndrome with plexiform morphologic features has been described (Harbeck et al. 1986; Staszak and Harbeck 1985). The pathogenesis of this syndrome is linked to an autoimmune-mediated process that involves both B and T cells, starting as early as 4 months of age (Harbeck et al. 1986; Staszak and Harbeck 1985). Arterioles, veins, and venules are primarily affected, with less involvement of muscular arteries. Narrowing and/or partial stenosis of vascular lumen and fragmentation of the elastic lamina with an intense lymphoid infiltrate are the key histological features (Staszak and Harbeck 1985), while necrosis is not a prominent feature.

16.2.9.1 Drug-Induced Pulmonary Vascular Changes

Administration of high doses of a human recombinant interleukin 2 (IL-2) to mice was associated with small vessel pulmonary vasculitis (Anderson and Hayes 1989). This is characterized by infiltration of lymphocytes in the interstitium as well as the walls of venules and arterioles. In rats, IL-2 administration was associated with both lymphocytic as well as an eosinophilic infiltrate (Anderson and Hayes 1989). An eosinophilic perivascular infiltrate around small vessels was associated with treatment of the immunosuppressive macrolide (FK-506, tacrolimus) (Nalesnik et al. 1987). While the explanation for the presence of eosinophils is unclear, it has been suggested that under conditions of IL-2 stimulation, lymphocytes release an eosinopoietic cytokine. There is good translation of the nonclinical toxicology findings to clinical trials, and the pulmonary vascular changes remain the dose-limiting toxicity of IL-2.

In rats, the pulmonary vascular EC is the suspected target of the mitomycin derivative, BMY-25282 (Bregman et al. 1987). The histologic features include focal EC destruction (degeneration, necrosis) and proliferation, with subintimal neutrophilic infiltrate, mononuclear cells, and fibrin deposition. Adventitial fibrosis with mononuclear cells can also be seen (Bregman et al. 1987).

Intravenous administration of large volumes, an increased infusion rate of saline, or large-molecular-weight substances such as polysaccharides can cause pulmonary vasculitis (Johnson et al. 1984; Morton et al. 1997). Frequently, fragments of skin, hair, or keratin punched out during the injection procedure can be seen in pulmonary vessels of laboratory animals in toxicology studies (Morton et al. 1997; Tekeli 1974).

16.2.9.2 Pulmonary Hypertension

Pulmonary hypertension can be the result of a variety of causes that include idiopathic pulmonary venous hypertension (associated with pulmonary disorders and hypoxemia), thrombolic and embolic hypertension, and hypertension due to pulmonary vessel damage from mechanical obstruction and inflammation (Kumar and Holden 1986; Simonneau et al. 2004). In toxicology studies, histopathological changes in the pulmonary vasculature can be assessed by measuring the ratio of the right ventricle weight to the weight of the left ventricle plus septum. Pulmonary hypertension is associated with right ventricular hypertrophy and remodeling of the vasculature, characterized by medial hypertrophy. There is typically a proportional increase in muscular arteries around bronchioles and alveolar ducts and walls (Louden et al. 1998; Meyrick and Reid 1981). Hypoxia and vasoconstriction play an important role in the development of pulmonary hypertension (Coflesky et al. 1988; Fried and Reid 1985). Hyperoxia can also induce right ventricular hypertrophy and medial hypertrophy of the pulmonary vasculature, including muscularization of small veins in the alveolar region (Coflesky et al. 1988; Hu and Jones 1989).

In humans, the appetite suppressants aminorex, phentermine, chlorpheniramine, fenfluramine, and dexfenfluramine are associated with pulmonary hypertension (Greaves 2007). In dogs, amphetamines and aminorex can induce transient increases in pulmonary arterial pressures (Will and Bisgard 1972). Although pulmonary hypertension can be induced in the rat with a single intravenous dose of monocrotaline pyrrole, the histologic changes are not comparable to the well-characterized plexiform lesion seen in humans, and, as such, there are no relevant animal models for human pulmonary hypertension. Monocrotaline-induced pulmonary hypertension in rats may be mediated, in part, by the potent endogenous vasoconstrictor endothelin-1 (Miyauchi et al. 1993). Other studies have suggested that remodeling proteins, such as osteopontin, play a significant role in monocrotaline-induced pulmonary hypertension (Louden et al. 1998).

16.2.10 BIOMARKERS OF VASCULAR TOXICITY

A finding of drug-induced vascular injury in toxicology studies can result in regulatory pressure to provide data to confirm that a drug candidate is reasonably safe for administration to humans, especially when the safety margins are low or negative. This is in light of the fact that several approved drugs are known to cause vascular injury in rodents and nonrodents in nonclinical safety studies yet have no effects in humans (Sobota 1989).

Endothelial and SMCs play an important role in the regulation of vascular tone, and these cells are the primary targets of toxic injury. Therefore, both physiological and biochemical markers of endothelial and SMCs should be evaluated to identify and develop translational markers (Table 16.9).

16.2.10.1 Physiological Biomarkers of Vascular Toxicity

16.2.10.1.1 HR and MAP

In nonclinical safety studies, vascular toxicity is associated with structurally and pharmacologically diverse agents. In dogs, vascular toxicity is often associated with profound cardiovascular hemodynamic changes in MAP and HR. These parameters have been used as biomarkers to monitor potential vascular toxicity in humans at therapeutic doses (Dogterom et al. 1992). In nonclinical studies in dogs, minoxidil, a potent antihypertensive agent, causes profound decreases in MAP, with compensatory increases in HR as well as vascular lesions (Mesfin et al. 1989). Similar findings have been reported following hydralazine administration (Mesfin et al. 1987). However, recent experiences with ETRAs, a novel class of vasoactive agents, suggest that in comparison to minoxidil, profound hemodynamics changes (MAP and HR) are not a prerequisite for development of coronary artery lesions in dogs (Albassam et al. 2001; Louden et al. 2000). For ETRAs, the lack of concordance with HR and MAP suggests that extrapolation of the potential risk to the human population can be made only on the basis that the dog is a very sensitive species (Albassam et al. 2001; Dogterom et al. 1992; Louden et al. 2000). This species sensitivity response is supported by data in monkeys administered the ETRA CI-1020 that required higher systemic exposure and longer duration of treatment to develop less severe coronary artery lesions (Albassam et al. 1999).

16.2.10.1.2 Regional Blood Flow

In dogs, drug-induced vascular injury is associated with vasodilation and increased blood flow, changes that precede arterial damage. Increases in regional coronary artery blood flow have been reported with minoxidil (Humphrey and Zins 1984; Mesfin et al. 1989), hydralazine (Chelly et al. 1986; Mesfin et al. 1987), SB209670 (Louden et al. 2000), and adenosine agonists (Albassam et al. 1998; Metz et al. 1991). In rats, mesenteric arterial damage and increases in mesenteric arterial blood flow were associated with administration of minoxidil, fenoldopam, and SKF 95654 (Joseph 2000). In dogs and humans, exercise can cause an increase in coronary artery blood flow, suggesting that physiological regulation plays a critical role in maintaining vascular integrity. In humans, because of the relationship between vasodilation and blood flow, flow-mediated dilatation can be used to determine and measure regional blood flow and drug-related effects.

16.2.10.2 Biochemical Biomarkers of Vascular Toxicity

16.2.10.2.1 EC Biomarkers

Damage and/or injury to ECs can cause a release of several molecules and/or proteins that could serve as biomarkers of vascular injury. These include von Willebrand factor (vWF), vWF propeptide (vWFpp), vascular endothelial growth factor (VEGF), endothelin (ET), asymmetric dimethylarginine (ADMA), NO, and caveolin-1. It has also been suggested that, as a consequence of arterial damage, ECs and/or microparticles are released from the site of injury and can be measured as a biomarker of vascular injury (McFarland et al. 2004; Scicchitano et al. 2003).

TABLE 16.9

Potential Biomarkers of the Vascular System

Biomarker (Type and Source)	Assay Availability (R: rat, D: dog, H: human)	Biomarker (Reference)
Functional	R, D, H	Blood flow (Louden et al. 2000); blood pressure (systolic, diastolic, pulse) (Dogterom et al. 1992); erythrocyte sedimentation rate (Finke et al. 2011); HR (Dogterom et al. 1992)
Biochemical		
Endothelial cell	R, D, H	Caveolin-1 (Brott et al. 2005b); eotaxin (Øynebråten et al. 2004); e-selectin (Zhang et al. 2010); PDGF (Paulus et al. 2011); platelet endothelial cell adhesion molecule-1 (PECAM-1) (Zhang et al. 2010); P-selectin (Zhang et al. 2010); prostacyclin (PGI2) (Blank et al. 2002); serum nitrite (Sheth et al. 2011); soluble intercellular adhesion molecule (sICAM-1) (Tesfamariam and DeFelice 2007); soluble thrombomodulin (sTM) (Blank et al. 2002; Kerns et al. 2005; Tesfamariam and DeFelice 2007); soluble vascular cell adhesion protein-1 (sVCAM-1) (Tesfamariam and DeFelice 2007); thrombospondin 1 (Moxon et al. 2011); tissue plasminogen activator (tPA) (Tesfamariam and DeFelice 2007); urokinase plasminogen activator (uPA) (Paulus et al. 2011); vascular cell adhesion molecule 1 (VCAM-1) (Zhang et al. 2011b); VEGF (Tesfamariam and DeFelice 2007); VWF (Brott 2005b; Newsholme et al. 2000)
	R, H	Endocan (ESM-1) (Paulus et al. 2011); endothelial microparticles (Kerns et al. 2005); junctional adhesion molecule A (JAM-A; CD321) (Zhang et al. 2010); platelet activating factor (PAF) (Zhang et al. 2011b); sE-Selectin (Kerns et al. 2005); sVEGF-receptor-1 (sFlt-1) (Paulus et al. 2011)
	D, H	VWFpp (Katein et al. 2008; van Mourik et al. 1999)
	H	α1,3-Fucosyltransferase VI (Schnyder-Candrian et al. 2000)
Smooth muscle cell	R, D, H	Asymmetric dimethylarginine (ADMA) (Zhang et al. 2010); Caveolin-1 (Brott et al. 2005b); Smooth muscle alpha actin (Brott et al. 2005b)
	R, H	H-Caldesmon (Smolock et al. 2009); smoothelin (Van Eys et al. 2007); SM22/transgelin (Li et al. 1996)
	H	H1-Calponin (Qu et al. 2008)

Category		Details
Inflammation or cytokine	R, D, H	Acute phase proteins (Watterson et al. 2009); CCL2/MCP-1 (Lee et al. 2011); CCL3/MIP1 (Labonte et al. 2009); CCL19 (Yang et al. 2007); C-reactive protein (Brott et al. 2005a); haptoglobin (Brott 2006a); IL-1a (Zhang et al. 2011a); IL-1b (Zhang et al. 2011a); IL6 (Blank et al. 2002); IL-8 (Zhang et al. 2010); MCP1 (Aplin et al. 2010); MIP-1 (Ozer et al. 2005); TNFα (Tesfamariam and DeFelice 2007)
	R, H	Tenascin-C (Suzuki et al. 2011)
	D, H	Serum amyloid A (Kerns et al. 2005)
Coagulation or platelets	R, D, H	APTT or PTT (Brott et al. 2005a); CD61 (Galindo et al. 2009); D-dimers (Paulus et al. 2011); fibrinogen (Brott 2006); homocysteine (Yan et al. 2010); prothrombin time (PT) (Brott 2006); thromboxane A2 (TXA2) (Blank et al. 2002); tissue factor (Kerns et al. 2005); tissue-type plasminogen activator (tPA) (Huber et al. 2002)
	R, H	CD63 (Doi et al. 2001); plasminogen activator inhibitor-1 (PAI-1) (Tesfamariam and DeFelice 2007); sCD40L (Tesfamariam and DeFelice 2007)
	R	α2-macroglobulin (Zhang et al. 2006)
	H	Factor XIIIa (Schaumburg-Lever et al. 1994)
Extracellular matrix	R, D, H	MMP9 (Ramos-Fernandez et al. 2011); sCD44 (hyaluronic acid) (Kerns et al. 2005); tissue inhibitor of metalloproteinases-1 (TIMP-1) (De la Sierra and Larrousse 2010)
	R, H	MMP8 (matrix metalloproteinase) (Pradhan-Palikhe et al. 2010)
Circulation	R, D, H	ANCA (Kerns et al. 2005); calcitonin gene-related protein (CGRP) (Zheng et al. 2010); circulating endothelial cells (Kerns et al. 2005); endothelial progenitors (Kerns et al. 2005); FasL (CD95L) (Kerns et al. 2005); histamine (Kerns et al. 2005); neutrophil count (Kerns et al. 2005); neutrophil gelatinase-associated lipocalin (NGAL) (Chen et al. 2009); NO (Zhang et al. 2011); placental growth factor (PLGF) (van Steenkiste et al. 2009)
	R, H	Angiotensin II converting enzyme (ACE 1) (Prosser et al. 2010); osteoprotegerin (Zannettino et al. 2005)
	D, H	Anti-elastase antibody (Savige et al. 1991); anti-lysosome antibody (Savige et al. 1991); anti-myeloperoxidase antibody (Kerns et al. 2005); anti-proteinase 3 antibody (Kerns et al. 2005)
Immunohistochemistry	R, D, H	Annexin V (Kerns et al. 2005); caspase 3 (Chiu et al. 2011); claudin (Brott 2006); clusterin (Moxon et al. 2011); collagen stain (Cho et al. 2010); nitrotyrosine (Zhang et al. 2011); trichrome stain (Cho et al. 2010); TUNEL (Kerns et al. 2005)

vWF and its propeptide (vWFpp) have been studied as potential markers of EC perturbation (van Mourik et al. 1999) and drug-induced vascular injury (Louden et al. 2006) due to vWF and vWFpp release into the circulation being controlled by well-defined constitutive and regulated pathways, as well as biochemical processes. However, vWFpp levels are lower in plasma because of its shorter half-life than VWF (van Mourik et al. 1999). The plasma levels and vWF/vWFpp ratio can be used to distinguish between acute and chronic EC perturbation (van Mourik et al. 1999).

In models of drug-induced vascular injury, plasma vWF was evaluated to assess its utility as a potential marker of vascular injury in rats and dogs (Brott et al. 2005a; Newsholme et al. 2000). Minor increases in plasma vWF were observed following administration of a potassium channel opener (Brott et al. 2005a) and fenoldopam (Newsholme et al. 2000). This observation, in conjunction with other reports, raises the possibility that the transient, 2- to 6-h increase in circulating plasma vWF could be an indicator of EC activation/perturbation prior to morphologic evidence of vascular damage (Brott et al. 2005a; Newsholme et al. 2000) because levels returned to baseline prior to vascular injury being confirmed histologically (Brott et al. 2005b). Additional studies in dogs indicated that minimal lesions induced by a potassium channel opener did not result in increased vWF levels (Katein et al. 2008); thus, vWF does not seem to be a suitable marker for use in toxicology studies to monitor progressive vascular damage. It has been suggested that analyzing the vWF/vWFpp ratio in humans, dogs, and baboons allows discrimination between chronic and acute phases of EC perturbation, activation, and injury (Brott et al. 2005b; Louden et al. 2006; van Mourik et al. 1999).

VEGF and ADMA are secretory products from EC as well as other cells in the body that affect endothelial and SMC function and therefore could have utility as diagnostic markers of vascular injury. The biochemical pharmacology implicates VEGF activation of vascular TK receptors to be the cause of vasodilation and, consequently, hypotension through the NO pathway (Bussolati et al. 2001; Hennequin et al. 1999).

ADMA generated considerable interest when it was shown to inhibit all three forms of NOS and when clinically, ADMA levels were elevated in patients with pulmonary hypertension (Gorenflo et al. 2001; Saitoh et al. 2003). Therefore, compounds that inhibit the NOS, VEGF, and/or VEGF vascular TK receptors are likely to cause drug-induced vascular lesions that are mechanistically related to hypertension, making ADMA a good biochemical biomarker because it can be measured easily in plasma.

Activation of ECs also plays a critically important role in the evolution of drug-induced vascular injury. In response to this stimulation and activation, ECs can release endothelial-specific substances that may serve as biomarkers of injury. These potential biomarkers include adhesion molecules, cytokines, chemokines, procoagulant and anticoagulant molecules, NO-derived products, and acute phase reactants (Zhang et al. 2010). A robust strategy using a pathologic basis for identification of biomarkers of EC activation has been proposed. This includes recommended surrogate markers for activation, markers that are potentially useful but not yet qualified or validated, and emerging markers (Zhang et al. 2010).

16.2.11 INVESTIGATIONAL *IN VIVO* STUDIES

16.2.11.1 MicroRNAs (miRNAs)

Because there is a strong interest in developing novel approaches to monitor organ toxicity, the discovery of small, noncoding RNAs (called miRNAs) that regulate gene expression have drawn considerable interest because they could potentially serve as biomarkers. Hartmann and Thum (2011) determined that changes in miRNAs could be a reflection of vascular function (and dysfunction). Thomas et al. (2011) explored the utility of miRNAs as an emerging diagnostic marker for vascular injury induced by fenoldopam and dopamine. More studies will be required to further qualify and validate these markers in drug-induced vascular toxicities so as to determine their nonclinical usefulness to predict human safety.

16.2.12 Drug-Induced Vascular Lesions: Implications for Humans

Quantitative and/or qualitative characterization of the potentially adverse effects of a drug substance on a specific cell population is a key element in determining the approach to risk assessment that will be used to assess risk. Adequate assessment of human risk is best accomplished when all relevant scientific data summarizing hazard identification, dose response of the identified hazard, comparative systemic exposure, and risk characterization can be analyzed both quantitatively and qualitatively. The species-specific metabolite profile; differences in distribution, sensitivity, and functionality of the molecular target; and the therapeutic index are all important factors that must be considered when assessing the potential of a drug in laboratory animals to cause adverse effects in humans. It is also important to note that adverse cardiovascular toxicology findings at high doses in animal studies may have no relevance to humans at therapeutic doses. Despite the higher exposure of minoxidil in humans through topical administration for the treatment for hypertension, the signature cardiovascular findings have not been observed in humans. The physiological and toxicologic response to minoxidil varies between species, and presumably, the biochemical mechanisms and controlling forces that regulate vascular tone and vasodilation are different in dogs compared to humans.

Clinical experience and epidemiology are other factors that should be considered with the aim of establishing a correlation between arterial toxicity in laboratory animals and humans. Based on current clinical data, drugs such as digoxin, hydralazine, fenoldopam, theobromine, and minoxidil are all associated with vascular lesions in laboratory animals, yet these drugs have been safely administered to humans for many years. Regarding the ETRAs, it is noteworthy that there are species differences in the distribution and function of endothelin receptors in dogs and humans, so a variation in vascular response to these drugs could be predicted (Louden et al. 2000). The experience and knowledge of the unique, specie-specific pattern of cardiovascular toxicity in dogs have formed the basis for challenging the validity of conducting chronic toxicity studies in this species at doses associated with arterial toxicity, as this has no relevance to humans; thus, these data contribute little to the overall assessment of human risk for the compound being evaluated.

Arterial lesions in toxicology studies pose an exceptional clinical challenge because there are no unequivocal biochemical diagnostic markers for monitoring and/or confirming in humans. Thus, estimation of human risk for therapeutic agents that are associated with adverse cardiotoxicity in dogs must take into consideration (1) species-specific response; (2) comparative systemic exposure; (3) interspecies scaling; (4) no-effect doses in relevant toxicology species; (5) therapeutic margins; and (6) risk–benefit ratio. Assessment of this risk can be greatly improved if data from investigative studies in animals show that the mechanism of injury may not be applicable to humans. The cumulative toxicology data linked to the clinical experience suggest that coronary arterial lesions in dogs can lead to an erroneous and irrelevant extrapolation to humans.

REFERENCES

Ahmed, S. H., Clark, L. L., Pennington, W. R., Webb, C. S., Bonnema, D. D., Leonardi, A.H., McClure, C. D., Spinale, F. G., Zile, M.R. 2006. Matrix metalloproteinases/tissues inhibitors of matalloproteinases: relationship between changes in proteolytic determinants of matrix composition and structural, functional and clinical manifestations of hypertensive heart disease. *Circulation* 113:2089–2096.

Ainge, G. and Clarke, C. J. 2000. Spontaneous myocardial concentration of Purkinje fiber-like cells in a beagle dog. *Toxicol Pathol* 28:827–828.

Akazawa, H. and Komuro, I. 2003. Roles of cardiac transcription factors in cardiac hypertrophy. *Circ Res* 92:1079–1088.

Albassam, M. A., Metz, A. L., Potoczak, R. E., Gallagher, K. P., Haleen, S., Hallak, H., McGuire, E. J. 2001. Studies on coronary arteriopathy in dogs following administration of CI-1020, an endothelin A receptor antagonist. *Toxicol Pathol* 29:277–284.

Albassam, M. A., Metz, A. L., Gragtmans, N. J., King, L. M., Macallum, G. E., Hallak, H., McGuire, E. J. 1999. Coronary arteriopathy in monkeys following administration of CI-1020, an endothelin A receptor antagonist. *Toxicol Pathol* 27:156–164.

Albassam, M. A., Smith, G. S., Macallum, G. E. 1998. Arteriopathy induced by adenosine agonist-antihypertensive in monkeys. *Toxicol Pathol* 26:375–380.

Albassam, M. A., Lillie, L. E., Smith, G. S. 1993. Asymptomatic polyarteritis in a cynomolgus monkey. *Lab Anim* Sci 43:628–629.

Albassam, M. A., Houston, B. J., Greaves, P., Barsoum, N. 1989. Polyarteritis in a beagle. *J Am Vet Med Assoc* 194:1595–1597.

Allen, A. M., Hansen, C. T., Moore, T. D., Knapka, J., Ediger, R. D., Long, P. H. 1991. Hemorrhagic cardiomyopathy and hemothorax in vit K deficient mice. *Toxicol Pathol* 19:589–596.

Anderson, T. D. and Hayes, T. J. 1989. The toxicity of human recombinant interleukin-2 in rats. Pathologic changes are characterized by marked lymphocytic and eosinophilic proliferation and multisystem involvement. *Lab Invest* 60:331–346.

Anderton, M. J., Mellor, H. R., Bell, A., Sadler, C., Pass, M., Powell, S., Steele, S. J., Roberts, R. A., Heier, A. 2011. Induction of heart valve lesions by small molecule ALK5 inhibitors. *Toxicol Pathol* 39:916–924.

Aplin, A. C., Fogel, E., Nicosia, R. F. 2010. MCP-1 promotes mural cell recruitment during angiogenesis in the aortic ring model. *Angiogenesis* 13:219–226.

Apple, F. S., Murakami, M. M., Ler, R., Walker, D., York, M. 2008. HESI Technical Committee of Biomarkers Working Group on Cardiac Troponins. Analytical characteristics of commercial cardiac troponin I and T immunoassays in serum of rats, dogs and monkeys with induced myocardial injury. *Clin Chem* 54:1982–1989.

Arena, E., D'Alessandro, N., Dusonchet, L., Geraci, M., Rausa, L., Sanguedolce, R. 1979. Repair kinetics of DNA, RNA and proteins in the tissues of mice treated with doxorubicin. *Arzneimittelforschung* 29:901–902.

Arnal, J. F., Dinh-Xuan, A. T., Pueyo, M., Darblade, B., Rami, J. 1999. Endothelium-derived nitric oxide and vascular physiology and pathology. *Cell Mol Life Sci* 55:1078–1087.

Arola, Q. J., Saraste, A., Pulkki, K., Kallajoki, M., Parvinen, M., Voipio-Pulkki, L. M. 2000. Acute doxorubicin cardiotoxicity involved cardiomyocyte apoptosis. *Cancer Res* 60:1789–1792.

Asakawa, M., Takano, H., Nagai, T., Uozumi, H., Hasegawa, H., Kubota, N., Saito, T., Masuda, Y., Kadowaki, T., Komuro, I. 2002. Peroxisome proliferator-activated receptor gamma plays a critical role in inhibition of cardiac hypertrophy in vitro and in vivo. *Circulation* 105:1240–1246.

Bachmann, E., Weber, E., Zbinden, G. 1984. The effect of methyl-2-tetradecylglycidate (McNeil 3716) on heart mitochondrial metabolism in rats. *Biochem Pharmacol* 33:1947–1950.

Balazs, T., Ferrans, V. J., El-Hage, A., Ehrreich, S. J., Johnson, G. L., Herman, E. H., Atkinson, J. C., West, W. L. 1981. Study of the mechanism of hydralazine-induced myocardial necrosis in the rat. *Toxicol Appl Pharmacol* 59:524–534.

Balazs, T., Herman, H. E., Earl, F. L., Wolff, F. W. 1975. Cardiotoxicity studies with diazoxide, reserpine, guanethidine, and combinations of diazoxide and propranolol in dogs. *Toxicol Appl Pharmacol* 33:498–503.

Barbolt, T. A., Gossett, K. A., Cornacoff, J. B. 1991. Histomorphologic observations for cynomolgus monkeys after subchronic subcutaneous injection of a recombinant human interleukin-4. *Toxicol Pathol* 21:251–257.

Bass, B. H. 1981. Hydralazine lung. *Thorax* 36:695–696.

Bassil, M., Anand-Srivastava, M. B. 2006. Nitric oxide modulated Gi-protein expression and adenylyl cyclase signaling in vascular smooth muscle cells. *Free Radic Biol Med* 41:1162–1173.

Belhadjali, H., Slim, R., Aouam, K., Youssef, M., Zili, J. 2008. Cutaneous vasculitis induced by risedronate. *Allergy* 63:1405.

Berenji, K., Drazner, M. H., Rothermel, B. A., Hill, J. A. 2005. Does load-induced ventricular hypertrophy progress to systolic heart failure *Am J Physiol-Heart and Circ Phys* 289:H8–H16.

Bertinchant, J. P., Polge, A., Juan, J. M., Oliva-Laurarie, M. C., Giuliani, I., Marty-Double, I., Marty-Double, C., Burdy, J. Y., Fabbro-Peray, P., Laprade, M., Bali, J. P., Granier, C., de la Coussaye, J. E., Dauzat, M. 2003. Evaluation of cardiac troponin I and T levels as markers of myocardial damage in doxorubicin-induced cardiomyopathy rats, and their relationship with echocardiographic and histological findings. *Clin Chem Acta* 329:39–51.

Bertinchant, J. P., Robert, E., Polge, A., Marty-Double, I., Fabbro-Peray, P., Poirey, S., Aya, G., Juan, J. M., Ledermann, B., de la Coussaye, J. E., Dauzat, M. 2000. Comparison of the diagnostic value of cardiac troponin I and T determinations for detecting early myocardial damage and the relationship with histological findings after isoprenaline-induced cardiac injury in rats. *Clin Chem Acta* 298:13–28.

Bhargava, P. 2009. VEGF kinase inhibitors: How do they cause hypertension? *Am J Physiol Regul Integr Comp Physiol* 297:R1–R5.

Bienaime, F., Clerbaux, G., Plaisier, E., Mougenot, B., Ronco, P., Rougier, J. P. 2007. D-penicillamine-induced ANCA-associated crescentic glomerulonephritis in Wilson disease. *Am J Kidney Dis* 50:821–825.

Bishop, S. P., Louden, C. 1997. Morphologic evaluation of the heart and blood vessels. In *Comprehensive Toxicology* (eds. Bishop, S. P. and Kerns, W. D.), vol. 6, pp. 5–26. Elsevier Science, New York.

Bishop, S. P. 1990. Animal models of vasculitis. *Toxicol Pathol* 17:109–117.

Blank, M., Shoenfeld, Y., Tavor, S., Praprotnik, S., Boffa, M. C., Weksler, B., Walenga, M. J., Amiral, J., Eldor, A. 2002. Anti-platelet factor 4/heparin antibodies from patients with heparin induced thrombocytopenia provoke direct activation of microvascular endothelial cells. *Int Immunol* 14:121–129.

Bleuel, H., Deschl, U., Bertsch, T., Bolz, G., Rebel, W. 1995. Diagnostic efficiency of troponin T measurements in rats with experimental myocardial cell damage. *Exp Toxicol Pathol* 47:121–127.

Block, M. I., Said, J. W., Siegel, R. J., Fishbein, M. C. 1983. Myocardial myoglobin following coronary artery occlusion. An immunohistochemistry study. *Am J Pathol* 111:374–379.

Boli, R. 2007. Preconditioning: A paradigm shift in the biology of myocardial ischemia. *Am J Physiol* 292:H19–H27.

Bombardier, C. 2002. An evidence-based evaluation of the gastrointestinal safety of coxibs. *Am J Cardiol* 89:3D–9D.

Boor, P. J., Langford, S. D. 1997. Pathogenesis of medial lesions caused by chemical agents. In *Comprehensive Toxicology* (eds. Snipes, G., McQueen, C., and Gandolfi, J.), pp. 309–332. Elsevier Science, New York, NY.

Boor, P. J., Gotlieb, A. I., Joseph, E. C., Kerns, W. D., Roth, R. A., Tomaszewski, K. R. 1995. Chemical-induced vasculature injury. *Toxicol Appl Pharmacol* 132:177–195.

Boor, P. J., Hysmith, R. M., Sanduja, R. 1990. A role for a new vascular enzyme in the metabolism of xenobiotic amines. *Circ Res* 66:249–252.

Boor, P. J., Hysmith, R. M. 1987. Allylamine cardiovascular toxicity. *Toxicology* 44:129–145.

Boor, P. J. 1987. Amines and the heart. *Arch Pathol Lab Med* 111:930–932.

Borg, T. K., Rubin, K., Carver, W., Samarel, A., Terracio, L. 1996. The cell biology of the cardiac interstitium. *Trends Cardiovasc Med* 6:65–70.

Bouloumie, A., Schini-Kerth, V. B., Busse, R. 1999. Vascular endothelial growth factor up-regulates nitric oxide synthase expression in endothelial cells. *Cardiovasc Res* 41:773–780.

Bourdois, P. S., Dancla, J. L., Faccini, J. M., Nachbaur, J., Monro, A. M. 1982. The subacute toxicology of digoxin in dogs: clinical chemistry and histopathology of heart and kidneys. *Arch Toxicol* 51:273–283.

Brave, M., Goodman, V., Kaminskas, E., Farrell, A., Timmer, W., Pope, S., Harapanhall, R., Saber, H., Morse, D., Bullock, J., Men, A., Noory, C., Ramchandani, R., Kenna, L., Gobburu, J., Jiang, X., Sridhara, R., Justice, R., Pazdur, R. 2008. Sprycel for chronic myeloid leukemia and Philadelphia chromosome-positive acute lymphoblastic leukemia resistant to or intolerant of imatinib mesylate. *Clin Cancer Res* 14:352–359.

Bregman, C. L., Comereski, C. R., Buroker, R. A., Hirt, R. S., Madissoo, H., Holtendorf, G. H. 1987. Single-dose and multiple-dose intravenous toxicity studies of BMY-25282 in rats. *Fundam Appl Toxicol* 9:90–109.

Breider, M. A., Gough, A. W., Haskins, J. R., Sobocinski G., de la Iglesia, F. A. 1999. Troglitazone-induced heart and adipose tissue cell proliferation in mice. *Toxicol Pathol* 27:545–552.

Brickner, M. E., Willard, J. E., Eichorn, E. J., Black, J., Grayburn, P. A. 1991. Left ventricular hypertrophy associated with chronic cocaine abuse. *Circulation* 84:1130–1135.

Bristow, M. R., Sageman, W. S., Scott, R. H., Billingham, M. E., Bowden, R. E., Kernoff, R. S., Snidow, G. G., Daniels, J. R. 1980. Acute and chronic cardiovascular effects of doxorubicin in the dog: the cardiovascular pharmacology of drug-induced histamine release. *J Cardiovasc Pharmacol* 2:487–515.

Brott, D., Foster-Brown, L., Richardson, R. J., Louden, C. 2007. The role of nitric oxide pathway in fenoldopam-induced vascular injury. *Toxicologist*, 2110A.

Brott, D. A. 2006. Mechanistic studies and potential diagnostic markers of drug-induced vascular injury. PhD Dissertation, The University of Michigan.

Brott, D. A., Jones, H. B., Gould, S., Valentin, J. P., Evans, G., Richardson, R. J., Louden, C. 2005a. Current status and future directions for diagnostic markers of drug-induced vascular injury. *Cancer Biomark* 1:15–28.

Brott, D., Gould, S., Jones, H., Schofield, J., Prior, H., Valentin, J. P., Bjurstrom, S., Kenne, K., Schuppe-Koistinen, I., Katein, A., Foster-Brown, L., Betton, G., Richardson, R., Evans, G., Louden, C. 2005b. Biomarkers of drug-induced vascular injury. *Toxicol Appl Pharmacol* 207:S441–S445.

Bugelski, P. J., Vockley, C. M., Sowinski, J. M., Arena, E., Berkowitz, B. A., Morgan, D. G. 1989. Ultrastructure of an arterial lesion induced in rats by fenoldopam mesylate, a dopaminergic vasodilator. *Br J Exp Pathol* 70:153–165.

Bussolati, B., Dunk, C., Grohman, M., Kontos, C. D., Mason, J., Ahmed, A. 2001. Vascular endothelial growth factor receptor-1 modulates vascular endothelial growth factor-mediated angiogenesis via nitric oxide. *Am J Pathol* 159:993–1008.

Cairns, J. A. 2007. The coxibs and traditional nonsteroidal anti-inflammatory drugs: A current perspective on cardiovascular risks. *Can J Cardiol* 23:125–131.

Cannan, C. R., Burnett, J. C. Jr., Brandt, R. R., Lerman, A. 1995. Endothelin at pathophysiological concentrations mediates coronary vasoconstriction via the endothelin-A receptor. *Circulation* 92:3312–3317.

Carson, R. G., Feenstra, E. S. 1977. Toxicologic studies with the hypotensive agent minoxidil. *Toxicol Appl Pharmacol* 39:1–5.

Case, M. T., Sibiniski, L. J., Steffen, G. R. 1984. Chronic oral toxicity and oncogenicity studies of flecainide an antiarrhythmic, in rats and mice. *Toxicol Appl Pharmacol* 73:232–242.

Catella-Lawson, F., McAdam, B., Morrison, B. W., Kapoor, S., Kujubu, D., Antes, L., Lasseter, K. C., Quan, H., Gertz, B. J., FitzGerald, G. A. 1999. Effects of specific inhibition of cyclooxygenase-2 on sodium balance, hemodynamics, and vasoactive eicosanoids. *J Pharmacol Exp Ther* 289:735–741.

Chabrier, P. E. 1993. The role of endothelin in the vessel wall. *Bailleres Clin Hematol* 6:577–563.

Chamanza, R., Marxfeld, H. A., Blanco, A. I., Naylor, S. W., Bradley, A. E. 2010. Incidences and range of spontaneous findings in control cynomolgus monkeys (*Macaca fascicularis*) used in toxicity studies. *Toxicol Pathol* 38:642–657.

Chamanza, R., Parry, N. M., Rogerson, P., Nicol, J. R., Bradley, A. E. 2006. Spontaneous lesions of the cardiovascular system in purpose-bred laboratory nonhuman primates. *Toxicol Pathol* 34:357–363.

Cheitlin, M. D., Hutter, A. M. Jr., Brindis, R. G., Ganz, P., Kaul, S., Russell, R. O. Jr., Zusman, R. M. 1999. ACC/AHA expert consensus document: use of sildenafil (Viagra) in patients with cardiovascular disease: American College of Cardiology/American Heart Association. *J Am Coll Cardiol* 33:273–282.

Chelly, J. E., Doursout, M. F., Begaud, B., Tsao, C. C., Hartley, C. J. 1986. Effects of hydralazine on regional blood flow in conscious dogs. *J Pharmacol Exp Ther* 238:665–669.

Chen, M., Wang, F., Zhao, M. H. 2009. Circulating neutrophil gelatinase-associated lipocalin: A useful biomarker for assessing disease activity of ANCA-associated vasculitis. *Rheumatology (Oxford)* 48:344–348.

Chen, M. H., Kerkela, R., Force, T. 2008. Mechanism of cardiac dysfunction associated with tyrosine kinase inhibitor cancer therapeutics. *Circulation* 118:84–95.

Cheng, L., Ding, G., Qin, Q., Huang, Y., Lewis, W., He, N., Evans, R. M., Schneider, M. D., Brako, F. A., Xiao, Y., Chen, Y. E., Yang, Q. 2004. Cardiomyocyte restricted peroxisome proliferator-activated receptor-delta deletion perturbs myocardial fatty acid oxidation and leads to cardiomyopathy. *Nat Med* 10:1245–1250.

Chintalgattu, V., Ai, D., Langley, R. R., Zhang, J., Bankson, J. A., Shih, T. L., Reddy, A. K., Coombes, K. R., Daher, I. N., Pati, S., Patel, S. S., Pocius, J. S., Taffet, G. E., Buja, L. M., Entman, M. L., Khakoo, A. Y. 2010. Cardiomyocyte PDGFR-beta signaling is an essential component of the mouse cardiac response to load-induced stress. *J Clin Invest* 120:472–484.

Chironi, G., Escaut, L., Gariepy, J., Cogny, A., Teicher, E., Monsuez, J. J., Levenson, J., Simon, A., Vittecoq, D. 2003. Brief report: carotid-intima media thickness in heavily pretreated HIV-infected patients. *J Acquir Immune Defic Syndr* 32:490–493.

Chiu, W. T., Shen, S. C., Yang, L. Y., Chow, J. M., Wu, C. Y., Chen, Y. C. 2011. Inhibition of HSP90-dependent telomerase activity in amyloid b-induced apoptosis of cerebral endothelial cells. *J Cell Physiol* 226:2041–2051.

Cho, G. S., Roelofs, K. J., Ford, J. W., Henke, P. K., Upchurch, G. R. Jr. 2010. Decreased collagen and increased matrix metalloproteinase-13 in experimental abdominal aortic aneurysms in males compared with females. *Surgery* 147:258–267.

Chobanian, A. V., Bakris, G. L., Black, H. R., Cushman, W. C., Green, L. A., Izzo, J. L. Jr., Jones, D. W., Materson, B. J., Opaaril, S., Wright, J. T. Jr., Roccella, E. J. 2003. National Heart, Lung and Blood Institute Joint National Committee on Prevention, Detection, Evaluation and Treatment of High Blood Pressure; National High Blood Pressure Education Program Coordinating Committee. The seventh Report of the Joint National Committee on Prevention, Detection, Evaluation, and Treatment of High Blood Pressure: the JNC 7 report. *JAMA* 289:2560–2572.

Choi, H. K., Merkel, P. A., Walker, A. M., Niles, J. L. 2000. Drug-associated antineutrophil cytoplasmic antibody-positive vasculitis: prevalence among patients with high titers of antimyeloperoxidase antibodies. *Arthritis Rheum* 43:405–413.

Choi, H. K., Merkel, P. A., Niles, J. L. 1998. ANCA-positive vasculitis associated with allopurinol therapy. *Clin Exp Rheumatol* 16:743–744.

Chu, T. F., Rupnick, M. A., Kerkela, R., Dallabrida, S. M., Zurakowski, D., Nguyen, L., Woulfe, K., Pravda, E., Cassiola, F., Desai, J. 2007. Cardiotoxicity associated with tyrosine kinase inhibitor sunitinib. *Lancet* 370:2011–2019.

Chun, A. A., McGee, S. R. 2004. Bedside diagnosis of coronary artery disease: a systematic review. *Am J Med* 117:334–343.

Cines, D. B., Pollak, E. S., Buck, C. A, Loscalzo, J., Zimmerman, G. A., McEver, R. P., Pober, J. S., Wick, T. M., Konle, B. A., Scwartz, B. S., Barnathan, E. S., Mcrae, K. R., Hug, B. A., Schmidts, A. M., Stern, D. M. 1998. Endothelial cells in physiology and in the pathophysiology of vascular disorders. *Blood* 91:3527–3561.

Clements, P., Brady, S., York, M., Berridge, B., Mikaelian, I., Nicklaus, R., Gandhi, M., Roman, I., Stamp, C., Davies, D., McGill, P., Williams, T., Pettit, S., Walker, D., ILSI HESI Cardiac Troponins Working Group Turton J. 2010. Time course characterization of serum cardiac troponins, heart fatty acid-binding protein, and morphologic findings with isoproterenol-induced myocardial injury in the rat. *Toxicol Pathol* 38:703–714.

Clemo, F. S., Evering, W. E., Snyder, P. W., Albassam, M. A. 2003. Differentiating spontaneous from drug-induced vascular injury in the dog. *Toxicol Pathol* 31S:25–31.

Clozel, M., Gray, G. A., Breu, V., Loffler, B. M., Osterwalder, R. 1992. The endothelin B receptor mediates both vasodilation and vasoconstriction in vivo. *Biochem Biophys Res Commun* 186:867–873.

Coflesky, J. T., Adler, K. B., Woodcock-Mitchell, J., Mitchell, J., Evans, J. N. 1988. Proliferative changes in the pulmonary arterial wall during short-term hyperoxic injury to the lung. *Am J Pathol* 132:563–573.

Cohen, S. M., Storer, R. D., Criswell, K. A., Doerrer, N. G., Dellarco, V. L., Pegg, D. G., Wojcinski, Z. W., Malarkey, D. E., Jacobs, A. C., Klaunig, J. E., Swenberg, J. A., Cook, J. C. 2009. Hemangiosarcoma in rodents: Mode-of-action evaluation and human relevance. *Toxicol Sci* 111(1):4–18.

Collinson, P. O., Boa, F. G., Gaze, D. E. 2001. Measurement of cardiac troponins. *Ann Clin Biochem* 38:423–449.

Connolly, H. M., Crary, J. L., McGoon, M. D., Hensrud, D. D., Edwards, B. S., Edwards, W. D., Schaff, H. V. 1997. Valvular heart disease associated with fenfluramine-phentermine. *N Engl J Med* 337:581–588.

Cooper, G. 1997. Basic determinants of myocardial hypertrophy: a review of molecular mechanisms. *Annu Rev Med* 48:13–23.

Cornwell, G. G., Thomas, B. P., Snyder, D. L. 1991. Myocardial fibrosis in aging germ-free and conventional Lobund-Wistar rats: the protective effects of diet restriction. *J Gerentol* 46:B167–B169.

Craft-Cormney, C., Hansen, J. T. 1980. Early ultrastructural changes in the myocardium following thyroxine-induced hypertrophy. *Virchows Arch B Cell Pathol Incl Mol Pathol* 33:267–273.

Crofford, L. J., Wilder, R. L., Ristimaki, A. P., Sano, H., Remmers, E. F., Epps, H. R., Hla, T. 1994. Cyclooxygenase-1 and -2 expression in rheumatoid synovial tissues. Effects of interleukin-1 beta, phorbol ester, and corticosteroids. *J Clin Invest* 93:1095–1101.

Cruickshank, J. M., Fitzgerald, J. D., Tucker, M., Love, S. 1984. Beta-adrenoreceptor blocking drugs: pronethalol, propanol and practolol. In *Safety Testing of New Drugs, Laboratory Predictions and Clinical Performance* (eds. Lawerence, D. R., McLean, A. E. M., and Weatheral, M.), pp. 93–123. Academic Press, London.

Cummings, S. R., Schwartz, A. V., Black, D. M. 2007. Alendronate and atrial fibrillation. *N Engl J Med* 356:1895–1896.

Cummins, B., and Cummins, P. 1987. Cardiac specific troponin-I release in canine experimental myocardial infarction: development of a sensitive enzyme-linked immunoassay. *J Mol Cell Cardiol* 19:999–1010.

Daugherty, A., Manning, M. W., Cassis, L. A. 2000. Angiotensin II promotes atherosclerotic lesions and aneurysms in apolipoprotein E-deficient mice. *J Clin Invest* 105:1605–1612.

Davies, P., Burke, G., Reid, L. 1986. The structure of the wall of the rat intraacinar pulmonary artery: an electron microscopic study of microdissected preparations. *Microvasc Res* 32:50–63.

Davis, D. R., Wilson, K., Sam, M. J., Kennedy, S. E., Mackman, N., Charlesworth, J. A., Erlich, J. H. 2007. The development of cardiac fibrosis in low tissue factor mice is gender-dependent and is associated with differential regulation of urokinase plasminogen activator. *J Mol Cell Cardiol* 42:559–571.

De Jong, F., Moorman, A. F. M., Viragh, S. 1997. Cardiac development: Prospects for a morphologically integrated molecular approach. In *Comprehensive Toxicology* (eds. Bishop, S. P. and Kerns, W. D.), vol. 6, pp. 5–26. Elsevier Science, New York.

De la Sierra, A., Larrousse, M. 2010. Endothelial dysfunction is associated with increased levels of biomarkers in essential hypertension. *J Hum Hypertens* 24:373–379.

De Simone, G., Gottdiener, J. S., Chinali, M., Maurer, M. S. 2008. Left ventricular mass predicts heart failure not related to previous myocardial infarction: The Cardiovascular Health Study. *Eur Heart J* 29:741–747.

Delea, T. E., Edelsberg, J. S., Hagiwara, M., Oster, G., Phillips, L. S. 2003. Use of thiazolidinediones and risk of heart failure in people with type 2 diabetes: a retrospective cohort study. Diabetes Care 26:2983–2989.

Detweiler, D. K. 1989. Spontaneous and induced arterial disease in the dog: pathology and pathogenesis. *Toxicol Pathol* 17:94–108.

Dietsch, G. N., Diplma, C. R., Eyre, R. J., Pham, T. Q., Poole, K. M., Pefaur, N. B., Welch, W. D., Trueblood, E., Kerns, W. D., Kanaly, S. T. 2006. Characterization of the inflammatory response to a highly selective PDE4 inhibitor in the rat and the identification of biomarkers that correlate with toxicity. *Toxicol Pathol* 34:39–51.

Diez, J. 2009. Towards a new paradigm about hypertensive heart disease. *Med Clin North Am* 93:637–645.

Dogterom, P., Zbinden, G., Rezik, G. K. 1992. Cardiotoxicity of vasodilators and positive inotropic/vasodilating drugs in dogs: An overview. *Crit Rev Toxicol* 22:203–241.

Doi, Y., Kudo, H., Nishino, T., Kayashima, K., Kiyonaga, H., Nagata, T., Nara, S., Morita, M., Fujimoto, S. 2001. Synthesis of calcitonin gene-related peptide (CGRP) by rat arterial endothelial cells. *Histol Histopathol* 16:1073–1079.

Doran, J. P., Howie, A. J., Townend, J. N., Bonser, R. S. 1996. Detection of myocardial infarction by immunohistochemical staining for C9 on formalin fixed paraffin wax embedded sections. *J Clin Pathol* 49:34–37.

Dorn, G. W. 2005. Physiological growth and pathological genes in cardiac development and cardiomyopathy. *Trends Cardiovasc Med* 15:185–189.

Downes, M. R., Prendiville, S., Kiely, C., Lenane, P., Mulligan, N. 2011. Cutaneous reactions to adalimumab administration. *Ir Med J* 104:122–123.

Doyle, M. K., Cuellar, M. L. 2003. Drug-induced vasculitis. *Expert Opin Drug Saf* 2:401–409.

Drab, M., Verkade, P., Elger, M., Kasper, M., Lohn, M., Lauterbach, B., Menne, J., Lindschau, C., Mende, F., Luft, F. C., Schedl, A., Haller, H., Kurzchalia, T. V. 2001. Loss of caveolae, vascular dysfunction, and pulmonary defects in Caveolin-1 gene-disrupted mice. *Science* 293:2449–2452.

Dressman, J., Kincer, J., Matveev, S. V., Guo, L., Greenberg, R. N., Guerin, T., Meade, T., Li, X. A., Zhu, W., Uittienbogaard, A., Wilson, M. E., Smart, E. J. 2003. HIV protease inhibitors promote atherosclerotic lesion formation independent of dyslipidemia by increasing CD36-dependent cholesteryl ester accumulation in macrophages. *J Clin Invest* 111:389–397.

Drevon-Gaillot, E., Perron-Lepage, M. R., Clement, C., Burnett, R. 2006. A review of background findings in cynomolgus monkeys (*Macaca fascicularis*) from three different geographical origins. *Exp Toxicol Pathol* 58:77–88.

Drory, V. E., Korczyn, A. D. 1993. Hypersensitivity vasculitis and systemic lupus erythematosus induced by anticonvulsants. *Clin Neuropharmacol* 16:19–29.

Duan, S. Z., Ivashchenko, C. Y., Russell, M. W., Milstone, D. S., Mortensen, R. M. 2005. Cardiomyocyte-specific knockout and agonist of peroxisome proliferator-activated receptor-gamma both induce cardiac hypertrophy in mice. *Cir Res* 97:372–379.

Durant, G. J., Duncan, W. A., Ganellin, C. R., Parsons, M. E., Blakemore, R. C., Rasmussen, A. C. 1978. Impromidine (SK&F 92676) is a very potent and specific agonist for histamine H2 receptors. *Nature* 276:403–404.

Dzeja, P. P., Bast, P., Pucar, D., Wieringa, B., Terzic, A. 2007. Defective metabolic signaling in adenylate kinase AKI gene knock-out hears compromises post-ischemic coronary reflow. *J Biol Chem* 282:31366–31372.

Elangbam, C. S. 2010. Drug-induced valvulopathy: An update. *Toxicol Pathol* 38:837–848.

Elangbam, C. S., Brodie, T. A., Brown, H. R., Nold, J. B., Raczniak, T. J., Tyler, R. D., Lightfoot, R. M., Wall, H. G. 2002. Vascular effects of GI262570X (PPAR-γ agonist) in brown adipose tissue of Han Wistar Rats: A review of 1-month, 13 week, 27 week and 2-year oral toxicity studies. *Toxicol Pathol* 30:420–426.

Epstein, E. H. Jr., McNutt, N. S., Beallo, R., Thyberg, W., Brody, R., Hirsch, A., LaBraico, J. M. 1987. Severe vasculitis during isotretinoin therapy. *Arch Dermatol* 123:1123–1125.

Escudier, B., Eisen, T., Stadler, W. M., Szczylik, C., Oudard, S., Siebels, M., Negrier, S., Chevreau, C., Solska, E., Desai, A. A., Rolland, F., Demkow, T., Hutson, T. E., Gore, M., Freeman, S., Schwartz, B., Shan, M., Simantov, R., Bukowski, R. M.; TARGET Study Group. 2009. Sorafenib in advanced clear-cell renal-cell carcinoma. *N Engl J Med* 356:125–134.

Faccini, J. M., Abott, D. P., Paulus, G. J. 1990. Cardiovascular System. In *Mouse Histopathology. A Glossary for Use in Toxicity and Carcinogenicity Studies*, pp. 64–65. Elsevier, Amsterdam.

Factor, S. M., Minase, T., Cho, S., Fein, F., Capasso, J. M., Sonnenblick, E. H. 1984. Coronary microvascular abnormalities in the hypertensive-diabetic rats. A primary cause of cardiomyopathy? *Am J Pathol* 116:9–20.

Fallis, R. J., Fisher, M. 1985. Cerebral vasculitis and hemorrhage associated with phenylpropanolamine. *Neurology* 35:405–407.

Feldman, A. M., McNamara, D. 2000. Myocarditis. *N Engl J Med* 343:1388–1398.

Feng, X., Taggart, P., Hall, L., Bryant, S., Sansone, J., Kemmerer, M., Herlich, J., Lord, P. 2005. Limited additional release of cardiac troponin I and T in isoproterenol-treated beagle dogs with cardiac injury. *Clin Chem* 51:1305–1307.

Ferdinandy, P., Schulz, R., Baxter, G. F. 2007. Interaction of cardiovascular risk factors with myocardial ischemia/reperfusion injury, preconditioning, and postconditioning. *Pharmacol Rev* 59:418–458.

Feriozzi, S., Muda, A. O., Gomes, V., Montanaro, M., Faraggiana, T., Ancarani, E. 2000. Cephotaxime-associated allergic interstitial nephritis and MPO-ANCA positive vasculitis. *Ren Fail* 22:245–251.

Ferrans, V. J., Thiedeman, K. U. 1983. Ultrastructure of the normal heart. In *Cardiovascular Pathology* (eds. Silver, M. D.), vol. I, pp. 31–86. Churchill Livingstone, New York.

Fielden, R., Owen, D. A., Taylor, E. M. 1974. Hypotensive and vasodilator actions of SK&F 24260, a new dihydropyridine derivative. *Br J Pharmacol* 52:323–332.

Finke, C., Schroeter, J., Kalus, U., Ploner, C. J. 2011. Plasma viscosity in giant cell arteritis. *Eur Neurol* 66:159–164.

Fitzgerald, G. A. 2004. Coxibs and cardiovascular disease. *N Engl J Med* 351:1709–1711.

Fitzgerald, G. A., Patrono, C. 2001. The coxibs, selective inhibitors of cyclooxygenase-2. *N Engl J Med* 345:443–442.

Force, T., Krause, D. S., Van Etten, R. A. 2007. Molecular mechanisms of cardiotoxicity of tyrosine kinase inhibition. *Nat Rev Cancer* 7:332–344.

Fredericks, S., Merton, G. K., Lerena, M. J., Heining, P., Carter, N. D., Holt, D. W. 2001. Cardiac troponins and creatine kinase content of striated muscle in common laboratory animals. *Clin Chem Acta* 304:65–74.

French, W. J., Adomian, G. E., Averill, W. K. 1983. Chronic infusion of verapamil produces increased heart weight in conscious dogs. *Clin Res* 31:184A.

Fried, R., Reid, L. M. 1985. The effects of isoproterenol on the development and recovery of hypoxic pulmonary hypertension. A structural and haemodynamic study. *Am J Pathol* 121:102–111.

Fujimoto, S., Kondoh, H., Yamamoto, Y., Hisanaga, S., Tanaka, K. 1990. Holter electrocardiogram monitoring in nephritic patients during methylprednisolone pulse therapy. *Am J Nephrol* 10:231–236.

Galindo, M., Gonzalo, E., Martinez-Vidal, M. P., Montes, S., Redondo, N., Santiago, B., Loza, E., Pablos, J. L. 2009. Immunohistochemical detection of intravascular platelet microthrombi in patients with lupus nephritis and anti-phospholipid antibodies. *Rheumatology* 48:1003–1007.

Galley, H. F., Webster, N. R. 2004. The physiology of the endothelium. *Br J Anaes* 93:105–113.

Gang, D. L., Barrett, L. V., Wilson, E. J., Rubin, R. H., Medearis, D. N. 1986. Myopericarditis and enhanced dystrophic cardiac calcification in in murine cytomegalovirus infection. *Am J Pathol* 124:207–215.

Gans, J. H., Korson, R., Cater, M. R., Ackerly, C. C. 1980. Effects of short-term and long-term theobromine administration to male dogs. *Toxicol Appl Pharmacol* 53:481–496.

Gao, Y., Zhao, M. H. 2009. Review article: drug-induced anti-neutrophil cytoplasmic antibodies associated vasculitis. *Nephrology (Carlton)* 14:33–41.

Garcia-Martinez, V., Schoenwolf, G. C. 1993. Primitive-streak origin of the cardiovascular system in avian embryos. *Dev Biol* 19:128–159.

Ghosh, M., Wang, H., Ai, Y., Romeo, E., Luyendyk, J. P., Peters, J. M., Mackman, N., Dey, S. K., Hla, T. 2007. COX-2 suppresses tissue factor expression via endocannabinoid-directed PPARδ activation. *J Exp Med* 204:2053–2061.

Gilbert, P. L., Siegel, R. J., Melmed, S., Sherman, C. T., Fishbein, M. C. 1985. Cardiac morphology in rat with growth hormone-producing tumors. *J Mol Cell Cardiol* 17:805–811.

Godeny, E. K., Gauntt, C. J. 1987. In situ immune autoradiographic identification of cells in heart tissues of mice with coxsackievirus B3-induced myocarditis. *Am J Pathol* 129:267–276.

Golby, F. S., Beilin, L. J. 1972. New thoughts on essential hypertension. *Br Med J* 2:594–595.

Goldfine, A. B. 2008. Assessing the cardiovascular safety of diabetes therapies. *N Engl J Med* 359:1092–1095.

Golomb, E., Nyska, A., Schwalb, H. 2009. Occult cardiotoxicity— toxic effects on cardiac ischemic tolerance. *Toxicol Pathol* 37:572–593.

Gomi, T., Yamamoto, H., Ozeki, M., Fujikura, M., Hirao, A., Kobayashi, M., Tateishi, T., Yumoto, S., Okumura, M., Aikawa, K. 1985. Acute and subacute toxicity of 2,6-dimethyl-3,5-dimethoxycarbonyl-4-(o-difluoromethoxyphenyl)-1, 4-dihydropyridine (PP-1466). *Arzneimittel-Forschung* 35:915–922.

Gonzalez, A., Lopez, B., Ravassa, S., Beaumont, J., Arias, T., Hermida, N., Zudaire, A., Diez, J. 2009. Biochemical markers of myocardial remodeling in hypertensive disease. *Cardiovasc Res* 81:509–518.

Gorenflo, M., Zheng, C., Werle, E., Fiehn, W., Ulmer, H. E. 2001. Plasma levels of asymmetrical dimethyl-L-arginine in patients with congenital heart disease and pulmonary hypertension. *J Cardiovasc Pharmacol* 37:489–492.

Gossett, K. A., Barbolt, T. A., Carnnacoff, J. B., Zelinger, D. J., Dean, J. H. 1993. Clinical–pathologic alterations associated with subcutaneous administration of recombinant interleukin-4 to cynomolgus monkeys. *Toxicol Pathol* 21:46–53.

Gotlieb, A. I. 1990. The endothelial cytoskeleton: organization in normal and regenerating endothelium. *Toxicol Pathol* 18:603–617.

Gould, D. B., Phalan, F. C., van Mil, S. E., Sundberg, J. P., Vahedi, K., Massin, P., Bousser M. G., Heutink, P., Miner, J. H., Tournier-Lasserve, E., John, S. W. 2006. Role of COL4A1 in small-vessel disease and hemorrhage and stroke. *N Engl J Med* 354:1489–1496.

Grant, C., Greene, D. G., Bunnell, I. L. 1965. Left ventricular enlargement and hypertrophy. A clinical and angiocardiographic study. *Am J Med* 39:895–904.

Greaves, P. 2007. *Histopathology of Preclinical Toxicity Studies*. Elsevier Academic Press, Amsterdam.

Greaves, P., Williams, A., Eve, M. 2004. First dose of potential new medicines to humans: How animals help. *Nat Rev Drug Disc* 3:226–236.

Greaves, P. 2000. Patterns of cardiovascular pathology induced by diverse cardioactive drugs. *Toxicol Lett* 112–113:547–552.

Greaves, P. 1998. Patterns of drug-induced cardiovascular pathology in the beagle dog: relevance for humans. Exp *Toxicol Pathol* 40:283–293.

Greaves, P. and Faccini, J. M., Cardiovascular System. 1992. *A Glossary for Use in Toxicity and Carcinogenicity Studies*, pp. 91–104. Elsevier, Amsterdam.

Greaves, P., Martin, J., Mitchell, M. C. 1984. Cardiac hypertrophy in the dog and rat induced by oxfenicine, an agent which modifies muscle metabolism. *Arch Toxicol Suppl* 7:488–493.

Grosser, T., Fries, S., FitzGerald, G. A. 2006. Biological basis for the cardiovascular consequences of COX-2 inhibition: Therapeutic challenges and opportunities. *J Clin Invest* 116:4–15.

Grossman, W. 1980. Cardiac hypertrophy: useful adaption or pathological process? *Am J Med* 69:576–584.

Grossman, W., Jones, D., McLaurin, L. P. 1975. Wall stress and patterns of hypertrophy. *J Clin Invest* 56:56–64.

Guan, Y., Cha, C., Rao, R., Lu, W., Kohan, D. E., Magnuson, M. A., Redha, R., Zhang, Y., Breyer, M. D. 2005. Thiazolidinediones expand body fluid volume through PPAR gamma stimulation of ENaC-mediated renal salt absorption. *Nat Med* 11:861–866.

Haft, J. I. 1974. Cardiovascular injury induced by sympathetic catecholamines. *Prog Cardiovasc Dis* 17:73–86.

Haft, J. I., Kranz, P. D., Albert, F. J., Fani, K.L. 1972. Intravascular platelet aggregation in the heart induced by norepinephrine. *Circulation* 46:698–708.

Halevy, S., Giryes, H., Avinoach, I., Livni, E., Sukenik, S. 1998. Leukocytoclastic vasculitis induced by low-dose methotrexate: in vitro evidence for an immunologic mechanism. *J Eur Acad Dermatol Venereol* 10:81–85.

Hamberg, M., Svensson, J., Samuelsson, B. 1975. Thromboxanes: a new group of biologically active compounds derived from prostaglandin endoperoxides. *Proc Natl Acad Sci USA* 72:2994–2998.

Hanton, G., Le Net, J. L., Ruty, B., Leblanc, B. 1995. Characterization of the arteritis induced by infusion of rats with UK-61,260, an inodilator, for 24 h. A comparison with the arteritis induced by fenoldopam mesylate. *Arch Toxicol* 69:698–704.

Harbeck, R. J., Launder, T. and Staszak, C. 1986. Mononuclear cell pulmonary vasculitis in NZB/W mice. Immunohistochemical characterization of infiltrating cells. *Am J Pathol* 123:204–211.

Harcourt, R. A. 1978. Polyarteritis in a colony of beagles. *Vet Rec* 102:519–522.

Hardisty, J. F., Elwell, M. R., Ernst, H., Greaves, P., Kolenda-Roberts, H., Malarkey, D. E., Mann, P. C., Tellier, P. A. 2007 Histopathology of hemangiosarcomas in mice hamsters and liposarcomas/fibrosarcomas in rats associated with PPAR agonists. *Toxicol Pathol* 35:928–941.

Harleman, J. H., Joseph, E. C., Eden, R. J., Walker, T. F., Major, I. R., Lamb, M. S. 1986. Cardiotoxicity of a new inotrope/vasodilator drug (SK&F 94120) in the dog. *Arch Toxicol* 59:51–55.

Hartman, H. A. 1987. Idiopathic extramural coronary arteritis in beagle and mongrel dogs. *Vet Pathol* 24:537–544.

Hartmann, D., Thum, T. 2011. MirocRNAs and vascular (dys)function. *Vascul Pharmacol* 55:92–105.

Hayakawa, B. N., Jorgensen, A. O., Gotlieb, A. I., Zhao, M. S., Liew, C. C. 1984. Immunofluorescent microscopy for identification of human necrotic myocardium. *Arch Pathol Lab Med* 198:284–286.

Hayes, T. J., Roberts, G. K., Halliwell, W. H. 1989. An idiopathic febrile necrotizing arteritis syndrome in the dog: beagle pain syndrome. *Toxicol Pathol* 17:129–137.

Hennequin, L. F., Thomas, A. P., Johnstone, C., Stokes, E. S., Ple, P. A., Lohman, J. J., Ogilvie, D. J., Wedge, S. R., Curwen, J. O., Kendrew, J., Lambert-van der Brempt, C. 1999. Design and structure-activity relationship of a new class of potent VEGF receptor tyrosine inhibitors. *J Med Chem* 42:5369–5389.

Herman, E. H., Ferrans, V. J., Young, R. S., Balazs, T. 1989. A comparative study of minoxidil-induced myocardial lesions in beagle dogs and miniature swine. *Toxicol Pathol* 17(1):182–192.

Herman, E. H., Balazs, T., Young, R., Earl, F. L., Krop, S., Ferrans, V. J. 1979. Acute cardiomyopathy induced by the vasodilating antihypertensive agent minoxidil. *Toxicol Appl Pharmacol* 47:493–503.

Higgins, A. J., Faccini, J. M., Greaves, P. 1985. Coronary hyperemia and cardiac hypertrophy following inhibition of fatty acid oxidation. Evidence of a regulatory role for cytosolic phosphorylation potential. In *Advances in Myocardiology* (eds. Dhalla, N. S., Hearse, D. J.), pp. 329–338, Plenum Press, New York.

Hirota, H., Chen, J., Betz, U. A., Rajewsky, K, Gu, Y., Ross, J. Jr., Müller, W., Chien, K. R. 1999. Loss of a gp130 cardiac muscle cell survival pathway is a critical event in the onset of heart failure during biochemical stress. *Cell* 97:189–198.

Hislop, A., Reid, L. 1978. Normal structure and dimensions of the pulmonary arteries in the rat. *J Anat* 125:209–221.

Hoffman, K. 1984. Toxicological studies with nitrendipine. In *Nitrendipine* (eds. Scriabine, A., Vanov, S., Deck, K.), pp. 25–31, Urban Schwarzenberg, Baltimore, MD.

HogenEsch, H., Snyder, P. W., Scott-Moncrief, C. R., Glickman, L. T., Felsburg, P. J. 1995. Interleukin -6 activity in dogs with juvenile polyarteritis syndrome: Effect of corticosteroids. *Clin Immunol Immunopathol* 77:107–110.

Horsburgh, K., McCarron, M. O., White, F., Nicoll, J. A. 2000. The role of apolipoprotein E in Alzheimer's disease, acute brain injury and cerebrovascular disease: evidence of common mechanisms and utility of animal models. *Neurobiol Aging* 21:245–255.

Horton, R. 2004. Vioxx, the implosion of Merck, and aftershocks at the FDA. *Lancet* 364:1995–1996.

Hu, L. M. and Jones, R. 1989. Injury and remodeling of pulmonary veins by high oxygen. A morphometric study. *Am J Pathol* 134:253–462.

Huber, D., Cramer, E. M., Kaufmann, J. E., Meda, P., Massé, J. M., Kruithof, E. K., Vischer, U. M. 2002. Tissue-type plasminogen activator (t-PA) is stored in Weibel-Palade bodies in human endothelial cells both in vitro and in vivo. *Blood* 99:3637–3645.

Humphrey, S. J., Zins, G. R. 1984. Whole body and regional hemodynamic effects of minoxidil in the conscious dogs. *J Cardiovasc Pharmacol* 6:979–988.

Hunter, J. J., Chien, K. R. 1999. Mechanisms of disease-signalling pathways for cardiac hypertrophy and failure. *N Engl J Med* 341:1276–1283.

Hysmith, R. M., Boor, P. J. 1988. Role of benzylamine oxidase in the cytotoxicity of allylamine toward aortic smooth muscle cells. *Toxicology* 51:133–145.

Ibayashi, S., Ogata, J., Sadoshima, S., Fujii, K., Yao, H., Fujishima, M. 1986. The effect of long-term antihypertensive treatment on medial hypertrophy of cerebral arteries in spontaneously hypertensive rats. *Stroke* 17:515–519.

Isaacs, K. R., Joseph, E. C., Betton, G. R. 1989. Coronary vascular lesions in dogs treated with phosphodiesterase III inhibitors. *Toxicol Pathol* 17:153–163.

Ito, T., Chatani, F., Sasaki, S., Ando, T., Miyajima, H. 1992. Spontaneous lesion in cynomolgus monkeys used in toxicity studies. *Exp Anim* 41:455–469.

Jahangiri, M., Jayatunga, A. P., Bradley, J. W., Goodwin, T. J. 1992. Naproxen-associated vasculitis. *Postgrad Med J* 68(803):766–767.

Jasmin, G., Eu, H. Y. 1979. Cardiomyopathy of hamster dystrophy. *Ann NY Acad Sci* 317:46–58.

Jennette, J. C., Falk, R. J. 1997. Small-vessel vasculitis. *N Engl J Med* 337:1512–1523.

Jiang, X., Khursigara, G., Rubin, R. L. 1994. Transformation of lupus-inducing drugs to cytotoxic products by activated neutrophils. *Science* 266:810–813.

Johnson, K. J., Glovsky, M. and Schrier, D. 1984. Pulmonary granulomatosis vasculitis induced in rats by treatment with glucan. *Am J Pathol* 114:515–516.

Johnson, M. L., Grimwood, R. E. 1994. Leukocyte colony stimulating factors. A review of associated neutrophilic dermatoses and vasculitides. *Arch Derm* 130:77–81.

Jones, H. B., Macpherson, A., Betton, G. R., David, A. S., Siddall, R., Greaves, P. 2003. Endothelin antagonist-induced coronary and systemic arteritis in the beagle dog. *Toxicol Pathol* 31(3):263–272.

Jones, T. C., Hunt, R. D. 1983. *Veterinary Pathology* 5th ed. Lea & Febiger, Philadelphia.

Joris, I., Majno, G. 1981. Medial changes in arterial spasm induced by L-norepinephrine. *Am J Pathol* 105:212–222.

Joseph, E. C. 2000. Arterial lesions induced by phosphodiesterase II (PDE III) inhibitors and DA1 agonist. *Toxicol Lett* 112–113:537–546.

Joseph, E. C., Mesfin, G., Kerns, W. D. 1997. Pathogenesis of arterial lesions caused by vasoactive compounds in laboratory animals. In *Cardiovascular Toxicology* (eds. Bishop, S. P., Kerns, W. D.), pp. 279–307. Pergamon, New York.

Kalyanaraman, B., Perez-Reyes, E., Mason, R. P. 1980. Spin-trapping and direct electron spin resonance investigations of the redox metabolism of quinine anticancer drugs. *Biochim Biophys Acta* 630:119–130.

Kang, Y. J. 2006. Cardiac hypertrophy: a risk factor for QT-prolongation and cardiac sudden death. *Toxicol Pathol* 34:58–66.

Karch, S. B., Billingham, M. E. 1988. The pathology and etiology of cocaine-induced heart disease. *Arch Pathol Lab Med* 112:225–230.

Karliner, J. S., Alabaster, C., Stephens, H., Barnes, P., Dollery, C. 1981. Enhanced noradrenaline response in cardiomyopathic hamsters: A possible relation to changes in adrenoreceptors studied by radioligand binding. *Cardiol Vasc Res* 15:296–304.

Katein, A., Brott, D., Richardson, R. J., Louden, C. 2008. Plasma von Willebrand factor (VWF) as a potential preclinical drug-induced vascular injury (DIVI) biomarker. *Toxicologist* 388A.

Keenan, C. M., Vidal, J. D. 2006. Standard morphologic evaluation of the heart in the laboratory dog and monkey. *Toxicol Pathol* 34:67–74.

Keenan, K. P., Soper, K. A., Hertzog, P. R., Gumprecht, L. A., Smith, P. F., Mattson, B. A., Ballam, G. C., Clark, R. L. 1995. Diet, overfeeding, and moderate dietary restriction in control Sprague–Dawley rats: II. Effects on age-related proliferation and degenerative lesions. *Toxicol Pathol* 23:287–302.

Kelly, D. F. 1989. Classification of naturally occurring arterial disease in the dog. *Toxicol Pathol* 17:77–93.

Kemi, M., Keenan, K. P., McCoy, C. Hoe, C. M., Soper, K. A., Ballam, G. C., van Zwieten, M. J. 2000. The relative protective effects of moderate dietary restriction versus dietary modification on spontaneous cardiomyopathy in male Sprague–Dawley rats. *Toxicol Pathol* 28:285–296.

Kemi, M., Usui, T., Narama, I., Takahashi, R. 1990. Histopathology of spontaneous panarteritis in beagle dogs. *Jpn J Vet Sci* 52:55–61.

Kerkela, R., Grazette, L., Yacobi, R., Iliescu, C., Patten, R., Beahm, C., Waalters, B., Shevtsov, S., Pesant, S., Clubb, F. J., Rosenzweig, A., Salomon, R. N., Van Etten, R. A., Alroy, J., Curande, J. B., Force, T. 2006. Cardiotoxicity of the cancer therapeutic agent imatinib mesylate. *Nat Med* 12:908–916.

Kerns, W., Schwartz, L., Blanchard, K., Burchiel, S., Essayan, D., Fung, E., Johnson, R., Lawton, M., Louden, C., MacGregor, J., Miller, F., Nagarkatti, P., Robertson, D., Snyder, P., Thomas, H., Wagner, B., Ward, A., Zhang, J. Expert Working Group on Drug-Induced Vascular Injury. 2005. Drug-induced vascular injury—a quest for biomarker. *Toxicol Appl Pharmacol* 203:62–87.

Kerns, W. D., Roth, L., Hosokawa, S. 2001. Idiopathic canine polyarteritis. In *Pathology of the Ageing Dog* (eds. Mohr, U., Carlton, W. W., Dungworth, D. L., Benjamin, S. A., Capen, C. C., Hahn, F. F.), vol. 2, pp. 118–126. Iowa State University Press, Ames, IA.

Kerns, W. D., Arena, E., Macia, R. A., Bugelski, P. J., Matthews, W. D., Morgan, D. G. 1989a. Pathogenesis of arterial lesions induced by dopaminergic compounds in the rat. *Toxicol Pathol* 17:203–213.

Kerns, W. D., Arena, E., Morgan, D. G. 1989b. Role of dopaminergic and adrenergic receptors in the pathogenesis of arterial lesions induced by fenoldopam mesylate and dopamine in the rat. *Am J Pathol* 135:339–349.

Kilickap, S., Abali, H., Celik, I. 2003. Bevacizumab, bleeding, thrombosis and warfarin. *J Clin Oncol* 21:3542.

Kim, J. H., Moon, J. L., Kim, J. E., Choi, G. S., Park, H. S., Ye, Y. M., Yim, H. 2010. Cutaneous leukocytoclastic vasculitis due to anti-tuberculosis medications, rifampin and pyrazinamide. *Allergy Asthma Immunol Res* 2:44–48.

Kline, I. K. 1961. Myocardial alterations associated with pheochromocytomas. *Am J Pathol* 38:539–551.

Knowlton, A. A., Apstein, C. S., Saouf, R., Brecher, P. 1989. Leakage of heart fatty acid-binding protein with ischemia and reperfusion in the rat. *J Moll Cell Cardiol* 21:577–583.

Kuhlmann, C. R., Trumper, J. R., Abdallah, Y., Wiebke, L. D., Schaefer, C. A., Most, A. K., Backenkohler, U., Neumann, T., Walther, S., Piper, H. M., Tillmanns, H., Erdogan, A. 2004. The K+ channel opener NS1619 increases endothelial NO-synthesis involving p42/p44 MAP-kinase. *Thromb Haemost* 92:1099–1107.

Kumar, D., Trent, M. B., Boor, P. J. 1998. Allylamine and beta-aminopropionitrile induced aortic medial necrosis: mechanisms of synergism. *Toxicology* 125:107–115.

Kumar, D., Holden, W. E. 1986. Drug-induced pulmonary vascular disease—mechanisms and clinical patterns. *West J Med* 145:343–349.

Labonte, L., Li, Y., Yang, L., Gillingham, A., Halpenny, M., Giulivi, A., Sills, T., Evans, K., Zanke, B., Allan, D. S. 2009. Increased plasma EPO and MIP-1 alpha are associated with recruitment of vascular progenitors but not CD34(+) cells in autologous peripheral blood stem cell grafts. *Exp Hematol* 37:673–678.

Laks, M. M., Morady, F. 1976. Norepinephrine-the myocardial hypertrophy hormone? *Am Heart J* 91:674–675.

Langford, S. D., Trent, M. B., Balakumaran, A., Boor, P. J. 1999. Developmental vasculotoxicity associated with inhibition of semicarbazide-sensitive amine oxidase. *Toxicol Appl Pharmacol* 155:237–244.

Larson, J. L., Pino, M. V., Geiger, L. E., Simeone, C. R. 1996. The toxicity of repeated exposures to rolipram, a type IV phosphodiesterase inhibitor, in rats. *Pharmacol Toxicol* 78:44–49.

Laux-End, R., Inaebnit, D., Gerber, H. A., Bianchetti, M. G. 1996. Vasculitis associated with levamisole and circulating autoantibodies. *Arch Dis Child* 75:355–356.

Le Corre, P., Parmer, R. J., Kailsman, M. T., Kennedy, B. P., Skaar, T. P., Ho, H., Leverage, R., Smith, D. W., Ziegler, M. G., Insel, P. A., Schork, N. J., Flockhart, D. A., O'Connor, D. T. 2004. Human sympathetic activation by alpha2-adrenergic blockade with yohimbine: bimodal, epistatic influence of cytochrome P450-mediated drug metabolism. *Clin Pharmacol Ther* 76:139–153.

Lebrecht, D., Walker, U. A. 2007. Role of mtDNA lesions in anthracycline cardiotoxicity. *Cardiovasc Toxicol* 7(2):108–113.

Lee, H. Y., Lee, S. Y., Kim, S. D., Shim, J. W., Kim, H. J., Jung, Y. S., Kwon, J. Y., Baek, S. H., Chung, J., Bae, Y. S. 2011. Sphingosylphosphorylcholine stimulates CCL2 production from human umbilical vein endothelial cells. *J Immunol* 186:4347–4353.

Lee, J. M., Yin, K., Hsin, I., Chen, S., Fryer, J. D., Holtzman, D. M., Hsu, C. Y., Xu, J. 2005. Matrix metalloproteinase-9 in cerebral-amyloid-angiopathy-related hemorrhage. *J Neurol Sci* 229–230:249–254.

Levy, D., Larson, M. G., Vasan, R. S., Kannel, W. B., Ho, K. K. 1996. The progression from hypertension to congestive heart failure. *JAMA* 275:1557–1562.

Levy, D., Labib, S. B., Anderson, K. M., Christiansen, J. C., Kannel, W. B., Castetelli, W. P. 1990. Determinants of sensitivity and specificity of electrocardiographic criteria for left ventricular hypertrophy. *Circulation* 81:1144–1146.

Li, L., Miano, J. M., Cseriesi, P., Olson, E. N. 1996. SM22 alpha, a marker of adult smooth muscle, is expressed in multiple myogenic lineages during embryogenesis. *Circ Res* 78:188–195.

Lima, J. A., Becker, L. C., Melin, J. A., Lima, S., Kallman, C. A., Weisfeldt, M. L., Weiss, J. L. 1985. Impaired thickening of nonischemic myocardium during acute regional ischemia in the dog. *Circulation* 71:1048–1059.

Limas, C., Westrum, B., Limas, C. J. 1980. The evolution of vascular changes in the spontaneously hypertensive rat. *Am J Pathol* 98:357–384.

Linder, A. E., McCluskey, L. P., Cole, K. R. 3rd, Lanning, K. M., Webb, R. C. 2005. Dynamic association of nitric oxide downstream signaling molecules with endothelial caveolin-1 in rat aorta. *J Pharmacol Exp Ther* 314:9–15.

Llovet, J. M., Ricci, S., Mazzafero, V., Hilgard, P., Gane, E., Blanc, J. F., de Oliveria, A. C., Santaro, A., Raoul, J. L., Forner, A. 2008. Sorafenib in advanced hepatocellular carcinoma. *N Engl J Med* 359:378–390.

Louden, C., Brott, D., Katein, A., Kelly, T., Gould, S., Jones, H., Betton, G., Valentin, J. P., Richardson, R. J. 2006. Biomarkers and mechanisms of drug-induced vascular injury in non-rodents. *Toxicol Pathol* 34:19–26.

Louden, C., Morgan, D. G. 2001. Pathology and pathophysiology of drug-induced arterial injury in laboratory animals and its implications on the evaluation of novel chemical entities for human clinical trials. *Pharmacol Toxicol* 89:158–170.

Louden, C. S., Nambi, P., Pullen, M. A., Thomas, R. A., Tierney, L. A., Solleveld, H. A., Schwartz, L. W. 2000. Endothelin receptor subtype distribution predisposes coronary arteries to damage. *Am J Pathol* 157:123–134.

Louden, C., Murphy, D., Thomas, H., Ellison, J., Wang, X., Gossett, K., Solleveld, H. 1998. Temporal and spatial expression of osteopontin following experimental pulmonary hypertension in the rat. *Cardiovasc Pathobiol* 2:135–148.

Low, J. E., Metz, A. L., Mertz, T. E., Henry, S. P., Knowlton, P., Lowen, G., Sommers C. S., Robertson, D. G., Olszewski, B. J., Schroeder, R. L., 1995. Cardiac hypertrophy in rats after intravenous administration of CI-959, a novel anti inflammatory compound, morphologic features and pharmacokinetic and pharmacodynamic mechanisms. *J Cardiovasc Pharm* 25:930–939.

Lowe, J. 1984. Method for morphometric analysis of arterial structure. *J Clin Pathol* 37:1413–1415.

Lowenstine, L. J. 2003. A primer of primate pathology: lesions and nonlesions. *Toxicol Pathol* 31 Suppl:92–102.

Lowenthal, D. T., Affrime, M. B. 1980. Pharmacology and pharmacokinetics of minoxidil. *J Cardiovasc Pharmacol* 2(Suppl 2):S93–S106.

Lu, H., Rateri, D. L., Cassis, L. A., Daugherty, A. 2008. The role of the renin–angiotensin system in aortic aneurysmal diseases. *Curr Hypertens Rep* 10:99–106.

Luginbühl, H., Detweiler, D. K. 1965. Cardiovascular lesions in dogs. *Ann NY Acad Sci* 127:517–540.

Lund, F. 1951. Vasodilator drugs against experimental peripheral gangrene. A method of testing the effect of vasodilator drugs on constricted peripheral vessels. *Acta Physiol Scand* 2 (Suppl 82):4–79.

Mak, G. J., Ledwidge, M. T., Watson, C. J., Phelan, D. M., Dawkins, I. R., Murphy, N. F., Patle, A. K., Baugh, J. A., McDonald, K. M. 2009. Natural history of markers of collagen turnover in patients with early diastolic dysfunction and impact of eplerenone. *J Am Coll Cardiol* 54:1674–1682.

Man int Veld, A. J., Wenting, G. J., Boomsma, M. A., Verhoeven, R. P., Schalekamp, M. P. 1980. Sympathetic and parasympathetic components of reflex cardiostimulation during vasodilator treatment of hypertension. *Br J Clin Pharmacol* 9:547–551.

Manasek, F. J. 1976. In *The Cell surface in Animal Embryogenesis and Development* (eds. Poste, G., Nicolson, G. L.), pp. 546–596. Elsevier Biomedical, Amsterdam.

Marber, M. S., Latchman, D. S., Walker, J. M., Yellon, D. M. 1993. Cardiac stress protein elevation 24 hours after brief ischemia or heat stress is associated with resistance to myocardial infarction. *Circulation* 88:1264–1272.

Martens, J. R., Sakamoto, N., Sullivan, S. A., Grobaski, T. D., Tamkun, M. M. 2001. Isoform-specific localization of voltage-gated K+ channels to distinct lipid raft populations. Targeting of Kv1.5 to caveolae. *J Biol Chem* 276:8409–8414.

Masferrer, J. L., Seibert, K., Zweifel, B., Needleman, P. 1992. Endogenous glucocorticoids regulate an inducible cyclooxygenase enzyme. *Proc Natl Acad Sci USA* 89:3917–3921.

Maunz, G., Conzett, T., Zimmerli, W. 2009. Cutaneous vasculitis associated with fluoroquinolones. *Infection* 37:466–468.

Maxie, M. G., Robinson, W. F. 2007. The cardiovascular system. In *Maxie, Jubb, Kennedy and Palmer's Pathology of Domestic Animals* (eds. Maxie, M. G., Jubb, K. V., Kennedy, P. C., Palmer, N. C.), pp. 1–10. Elsevier, Saunders.

Mbaya, P., Alam, F., Ashim, S., Bennett, D. 2007. Cardiovascular effects of high dose venlafaxine XL in patients with major depressive disorder. *Hum Psychopharmacol* 22:129–133.

McAdam, B. F., Catella-Lawson, F., Mardini, I. A., Kapoor, S., Lawson, J. A., FitzGerald, G. A. 1999. Systemic biosynthesis of prostacyclin by cyclooxygenase (COX)-2: the human pharmacology of a selective inhibitor of COX-2. *Proc Natl Acad Sci USA* 96:272–277.

McFarland, D. C., Scicchitano, M. S., Thomas, R. A., Narayanan, P. K., Schwartz, L. W., Thomas, H. C. 2004. 6-color flow-sorting of rat circulating endothelial cells and Taqman real-time PCR analysis. *Cytometry* 59A:65.

Mellor, H. R., Bell, A. R., Valentin, J. P., Roberts, R. A. 2011. Cardiotoxicity associated with targeted kinase pathways in cancer. *Toxicol Sci* 120:14–32.

Mendelsohn, M. E., Karas, R. H. 1999. The protective effects of estrogen on the cardiovascular system. *N Engl J Med* 340:1801–1811.

Meng, X., Ming, M., Wang, E. 2006. Heart fatty acid binding protein as a marker for postmortem detection of early myocardial damage. *Forensic Sci Int* 150:11–16.

Mesfin, G. M., Piper, R. C., DuCharme, D. W., Carlson, R. G., Humphrey, S. J., Zins, G. R. 1989. Pathogenesis of cardiovascular alterations in dogs treatment with minoxidil. *Toxicol Pathol* 17:164–181.

Mesfin, G. M., Shawaryn, G. G., Higgins, M. J. 1987. Cardiovascular alterations in dogs treated with hydralazine. *Toxicol Pathol* 15:409–416.

Metz, A. L., Dominick, M. A., Suchanek, G., Gough, A. W. 1991. Acute cardiovascular toxicity induced by an adenosine agonist-antihypertensive in beagles. *Toxicol Pathol* 19:98–107.

Meyrick, B., Reid, L. 1981. The effect of chronic hypoxia on pulmonary arteries in young rats. *Exp Lung Res* 2:257–271.

Meyrick, B., Hislop, A., Reid, L. 1978. Pulmonary arteries of normal rats: the thick walled oblique muscular segment. *J Anat* 12:209–221.

Miano, J. M., Vlasic, N., Tota, R. R., Stemerman, M. B. 1993. Smooth muscle cell immediate-early gene and growth factor activation follows vascular injury. A putative in vivo mechanism for autocrine growth. *Arterioscler Thromb* 13:211–219.

Milewicz, D. M., Urban, Z., Boyd, C. 2000. Genetic disorders of the elastic fiber system. *Matrix Biol* 19:471–480.

Miller, A. A., Budzyn, K., Sobey, C. G. 2010. Vascular dysfunction in cerebrovascular disease: mechanisms and therapeutic intervention. *Clin Sci (Lond)* 119:1–17.

Miller, K., Wang, M., Gralow, J., Dickler, M., Cobleigh, M., Perez, E. A., Shenkier, T., Cella, D., Davidson, N. E. 2007. Paclitaxel plus bevacizumab versus paclitaxel alone for metastatic breast cancer. *N Engl J Med* 357:2666–2676.

Mitchell, A. R. 2000. Hypertension in dogs: the value of comparative medicine. *J Royal Soc Med* 93:451–452.

Mitchell, J. A., Evans, T. W. 1998. Cyclooxygenase-2 as a therapeutic target. *Inflamm Res* 47(Suppl 2):S88–S92.

Mitchell, J. A., Warner, T. D. 2006. COX isoforms in the cardiovascular system: Understanding the activities of non-steroidal anti-inflammatory drugs. *Nat Rev Drug Discov* 5:75–86.

Miyauchi, T., Yorikane, R., Sakai, S., Sakurai, T., Okada, M., Nishikibe, M., Yano, M., Yamaguchi, I., Sugisshita, Y., Goto, K. 1993. Contribution of endogenous endothelin-1 to the progression of cardiopulmonary alterations in rats with monocrotaline-induced pulmonary hypertension. *Circ Res* 73:887–897.

Moncada, S., Gryglewski, R., Bunting, S., Vane, J. R. 1976. An enzyme isolated from arteries transforms prostaglandins endoperoxides to an unstable substance that inhibits platelet aggregation. *Nature* 263:663–665.

Morawietz, G., Ruel-Fehlert, C., Kitteel, B., Bube, A., Keane, K., Halm, S., Heuser, A., Hellmann, J. 2004. Revised guides for organ sampling and trimming in rats and mice. Part 3: A joint publication of the RITA and NACAD groups. *Exp Toxicol Pathol* 55:433–449.

Moreland, S., McCullen, D. M., Delaney, C. L., Lee, V. G., Hunt, J. T. 1992. Venous smooth muscle cell contains vasoconstrictor like ETB like receptors. *Biochem Biophys Res Commun* 184:100–106.

Morishima, H., Nonoyama, T., Sasaki, S., Miyajima, H. 1990. Spontaneous lesions in beagle dogs used in toxicity studies. *Exp Anim* 39:239–248.

Morris, D. O., Beale, K. M. 1999. Cutaneous vasculitis and vasculopathy. *Vet Clin North Am Small Anim Pract* 29:1325–1335.

Morton, D., Safron, J. A., Glosson, J., Rice, D. W., Wilson, D. M., White, R. D. 1997. Histologic lesions associated with intravenous infusions of large volumes of isotonic saline in rats for 30 days. *Toxicol Pathol* 25:390–394.

Motzer, R. J., Hutson, T. E., Tomczak, P., Michaelson, M. D., Bukowski, R. M., Rixe, O., Oudard, S., Negrier, S., Szcylik, C., Kim, S. T., Chen, I., Bycott, P. W., Baum, C. M., Figlin, R. A. 2007. Sunitinib versus interferon alfa in metastatic renal-cell carcinoma. *N Engl J Med* 356:115–124.

Moxon, J. V., Padula, M. P., Clancy, P., Emeto, T. I., Herbert, B. R., Norman, P. E., Golledge, J. 2011. Proteomic analysis of intra-arterial thrombus secretions reveals a negative association of clusterin and thrombospondin-1 with abdominal aortic aneurysm. *Atherosclerosis* 219:432–439.

Mueller, R. W., Gill, S. S., Pulido, O. M. 2003. The monkey heart (Macaca fascicularis) neural structures and conducting system: an immunochemical study of selected neural biomarkers and glutamate receptors. *Toxicol Pathol* 31:227–234.

Mullick, F. G., McAllister, H. A., Wagner, B. M., Fenoglio, J. J. Jr. 1979. Drug-related vasculitis: clinicopathological correlations in 30 patients. *Hum Pathol* 10:313–325.

Murry, C. E., Jennings, R. B., Reimer, K. A. 1986. Preconditioning with ischemia: a delay of lethal cell injury in ischemic myocardium. *Circulation* 74:1124–1136.

Nalesnik, M. A., Todo, S., Murase, N., Gryzan, S., Lee, P. H., Makowka, L., Starzl, T. E. 1987. Toxicology of FK-506 in Lewis rat. *Transplant Proc* 5(Suppl 6):89–92.

Nemes, Z., Dietz, R., Mann, J. F., Luth, J. B., Gross, F. 1980. Vasoconstriction and increased blood pressure in the development of accelerated vascular disease. *Virchow Arch A Pathol Anat Histol* 386:161–173.

Newman-Tancredi, A., Cussac, D., Quenteric, Y., Touzard, M., Verrile, L., Carpenter, N., Millan, M. J. 2002. Differential action of anti Parkinson agents at multiple classes of monaminergic receptor III: Agonists and antagonist properties of serotonin, 5-HT(1) and 5-HT(2), receptor subtypes. *J Phamacol Exp Ther* 303:815–822.

Newsholme, S. J., Thudium, D. T., Gossett, K. A., Watson, E. S., Schwartz, L. W. 2000. Evaluation of plasma von Willebrand factor as a biomarker for acute arterial damage in rats. *Toxicol Pathol* 28:688–693.

Nigro, V., Okazaki, Y., Belsito, A., Piluso, G., Matsuda, Y., Politano, L., Nigro, G., Ventura, C., Abbondanza, C., Molinari, A. M., Acampora, D., Nishimura, M., Hayashizaki, Y., Puca, G. A. 1997. Identification of the Syrian hamster cardiomyopathy gene. *Hum Mol Gen* 6:601–607.

Nikolaids, L. A., Levine, T. B. 2004. Peroxisome proliferator activator receptor (PPAR), insulin, and cardiomyopathy: friends or foes for the diabetic patient with heart failure? *Cardiol Rev* 12:158–170.

Nordborg, C., Fredriksson, K., Johansson, B. B. 1985. Internal carotid and vertebral arteries of spontaneously hypertensive and normotensive rats. A morphometric study on extracranial, intraosseous, and intracranial arterial segments. *Acta Pathol Microb Immunol Scan A* 93:153–158.

Nordon, I. M., Hinchliffe, R. J., Holt, P. J., Loftus, I. M., Thompson, M. M. 2009. Review of current theories for abdominal aortic aneurysm pathogenesis. *Vascular* 17:253–263.

Nyska, A., Gruebbel, M. M. 2010. Letter to the editor. *Toxicol Pathol* 38:511.

O'Banion, M. K., Winn, V. D., Young, D. A. 1992. cDNA cloning and functional activity of a glucocorticoid-regulated inflammatory cyclooxygenase. *Proc Natl Acad Sci USA* 89:4888–4892.

O'Brien, P. J. 2008. Cardiac troponin is the most effective translational safety biomarker for myocardial injury in cardiotoxicity. *Toxicology* 245:206–218.

O'Brien, P. J., Smith, D. E., Knechtel, T. J., Marchak, M. A., Pruimboom-Brees, I., Brees, D. J., Spratt, D. P., Archer, F. J., Butler, P., Potter, A. N., Provost, J. P., Richard, J., Synder, P. A., Regan, W. J. 2006. Cardiac troponin I, is a sensitive, specific biomarker of cardiac injury in laboratory animals. *Lab Anim* 40:153–171.

O'Brien, P. J., Dameron, G. W., Beck, M. L., Kang, Y. J., Erickson, B. K., Di Battista, T. H., Miller, K. E., Jackson, K. N., Mittelstadt, S. 1997. Cardiac troponin T, is a sensitive, specific biomarker of cardiac injury in laboratory animals. *Lab Anim Sci* 47:486–495.

Oguchi, M., Wada, K., Homna, H., Tanka, A., Kaneko, T., Sakakibara, S., Ohsumi, J., Serizawa, N., Fujiwara, T., Horikoshi, H. 2000. Molecular design, synthesis and hypoglycemic activity of a series of thiazolidine-2-4-diones. *J Med Chem* 43:3052–3066.

Okazaki, Y., Okuizumi, H., Ohsumi, T., Nomura, O., Takada, S., Kamiya, M., Sasaki, N., Matsuda, Y., Nishimura, M., Tagaya, O., Muramatsu, M., Hayashizaki, Y. 1996. A genetic linkage map of the Syrian hamster and localization of cardiomyopathy locus on chromosome 9qa2.1-bl using RLGS spot mapping. *Nat Gen* 13:87–90.

Olsen, H., Betton, G., Robinson, D., Thomas, K., Monro, A., Kolaja, G., Lilly, P., Sanders, J., Sipes, G., Bracken, W., Dorato, M., Van Deun, K., Smith, P., Berger, B., Heller, A. 2000. Concordance of toxicity of pharmaceuticals in humans and in animals. *Reg Toxicol Pharm* 32:56–67.

Olson, R. Mushlin, P. 1990. Doxorubicin cardiotoxicity: analysis of prevailing hypothesis. *FASEB J* 4:3076–3086.

Olukoga, A,. Donaldson, D. 2000. Liquorice and its health implications. *J R Soc Health* 120:83–89.

Orgogozo, J. M., Gilman, S., Dartigues, J. M., Laurent, B., Puel, M., Kirby, L. C., Jouanny, P., Dubois, B., Eisner, L., Flitman, S., Michel, B. F., Boada, M., Frank, A., Hock, C. 2003. Subacute meningoencephalitis in a subset of patients with AD after Abeta42 immunization. *Neurology* 61:46–54.

Owens, G. K., Kumar, M. S., Wamhoff, B. R. 2004. Molecular regulation of vascular smooth muscle cell differentiation in development and disease. *Physiol Rev* 84:767–801.

Øynebråten, I., Bakke, O., Brandtzaeg, P., Johansen, F. E., Haraldsen, G. 2004. Rapid chemokine secretion from endothelial cells originates from 2 distinct compartments. *Blood* 104:314–320.

Ozer, H. T., Erken, E., Gunesacar, R., Kara, O. 2005. Serum RANTES, MIP-1alpha, and MCP-1 levels in Behcet's disease. *Rheumatol Int* 25:487–488.

Palate, B. M., Denoël, S. R., Roba, J. L. 1995. A simple method for performing routine histopathological examination of the cardiac conduction tissue in the dog. *Toxicol Pathol* 23:56–62.

Pandey, S., Kushwaha, R. S., Mehndiratta, P., Mehndiratta, M. M. 2008. Carbimazole induced ANCA positive vasculitis. *J Assoc Phys India* 56:801–803.

Panju, A. A., Hemmelgarn, B. R., Guyatt, G. H., Simel, D. L. 1998. A rational clinical examination. Is this patient having a myocardial infarction? *JAMA* 280:1256–1263.

Park, H., Go, Y. M., Darji, R., Choi, J. W., Lisanti, M. P., Maland, M. C., Jo, H. 2000. Caveolin-1 regulates shear stress-dependent activation of extracellular signal-regulated kinase. *Am J Physiol Heart Circ Physiol* 278:H1285–H1293.

Patrono, C. 2001. Aspirin: new cardiovascular uses for an old drug. *Am J Med* 110:62S–65S.

Patton, R. L., Kalback, W. M., Esh, C. L., Kokjohn, T. A., Van Vickle, G. D., Luehrs, D. C., Kuo, Y. M., Lopez, J., Burne, D., Ferrer, I., Masliah, E., Newel, A. J., Beach, T. G., Castano, E. M., Roher, A. E. 2006. Amyloid-beta peptide remnants in AN-1792-immunized Alzheimer's disease patients: a biochemical analysis. *Am J Pathol* 169:1048–1063.

Paulus, P., Jennewein, C., Zacharowski, K. 2011. Biomarkers of endothelial dysfunction: can they help us deciphering systemic inflammation and sepsis? *Biomarkers* 16:4311–521.

Peart, J. N., Headrick, J. P. 2008. Sustained cardioprotection: exploring unconventional modalities. *Vascul Pharmacol* 49:63–70.

Pedersen, A. K., FitzGerald, G. A. 1984. Dose-related kinetics of aspirin. Presystemic acetylation of platelet cyclooxygenase. *N Engl J Med* 311:1206–1211.

Pelliccia, A., Maron, B. J., Spataro, A., Proschan, M. A., Spirito, P. 1991. The upper limit of physiologic cardiac hypertrophy in highly trained elite athletes. *N Engl J Med* 324:295–301.

Penaskovic, K. M., Annamraju, S., Kraus, J. E. 2005. Clozapine-induced allergic vasculitis. *Am J Psych* 162:1543.

Peraza, M. A., Burdick, A. D., Marin, H. E., Gonzalez, F. J., Peters, J. M. 2006. The toxicology of ligands for peroxisome proliferator-activated receptors (PPAR). *Toxicol Sci* 90:269–295.

Perez, E. A., Koehler, M., Byrne, J., Preston, A. J., Rappold, E., Ewer, M. S. 2008. Cardiac safety of lapatinib: pooled analysis of 3689 patients enrolled in clinical trials. *Mayo Clin Proc* 83:679–686.

Pernow, J., Modin, A. 1993. Endothelin regulation of coronary vascular tone in vitro: contribution of endothelin receptor subtypes and nitric oxide. *Eur J Pharmacol* 243:281–286.

Petit, S., York, M., Walker, D., Apple, F., Herman, E., Brady, S., Turton, J., Berridge, B., Nicklaus, R., Clements, P., Mikaelian, I., and HESI Biomarker Committee, Cardiac Troponin Expert Working Group. 2007. Comparison of commercial cardiac troponin (cTn) assays for evaluation of myocardial injury in the laboratory rat and dog and cynomolgus and rhesus monkey, and kinetics properties of serum cTn in rats with acute cardiotoxicity. *Toxicologist* [CD ROM]:48.

Pfeifer, M., Boncristiano, S., Bondolfi, L., Stalder, A., Deller, T., Staufenbiel, M., Mathews, P. M., Jucker, M. 2002. Cerebral hemorrhage after passive anti-Abeta immunotherapy. *Science* 298:1379.

Piper, R. C. 1981. Morphologic evaluation of the heart in toxicology studies. In *Cardiac Toxicology* (ed. Balazs, T.), vol. 3, pp. 111–136. CRC Press, Boca Raton.

Planavila, A., Laguna, J. C., Vazques-Carrera, M. 2005. Atorvastatin improves peroxisome proliferator-activated receptor signaling in cardiac hypertrophy by preventing nuclear factor-kappa B activation. *Biochim Biophys Acta* 1687:76–83.

Pope, J. H., Aufderheide, T. P., Ruthazer, R., Woolard, R. H., Feldman, J. A., Beshansky, J. R., Griffith, J. L., Selker, H. P. 2000. Missed diagnoses of acute cardiac ischemia in the emergency department. *N Engl J Med* 342:1163–1170.

Porter, B. F., Frost, P., Hubbard, G. B. 2003. Polyarteritis nodosa in a cynomolgus macaque (*Macaca fascicularis*). *Vet Pathol* 40:570–573.

Pozner, C. N., Levine, M., Zane, R. 2005. The cardiovascular effects of cocaine. *J Emerg Med* 29:173–178.

Pradhan-Palikhe, P., Vikatmaa, P., Lajunen, T., Palikhe, A., Lepantalo, M., Tervahartiala, T., Salo, T., Saikhu, P., Leinonen, M., Pussinen, P. J., Sorsa, T. 2010. Elevated MMP-8 and decreased myeloperoxidase concentrations associate significantly with the risk for peripheral atherosclerosis disease and abdominal aortic aneurysm. *Scand J Immunol* 72:150–157.

Pridjian, G., Puschett, J. B. 2002. Preeclampsia Part 1: clinical and pathophysiologic considerations. *Obstet Gynecol Surv* 57:598–618.

Pritchett, A. M., Morrison, J. F., Edwards, W. D., Schaff, H. V., Connolly, H. M., Espinosa, R. E. 2002. Valvular heart disease in patients taking pergolide. *Mayo Clin Proc* 77:1280–1286.

Prosser, H. C., Richards, A. M., Forster, M. E., Pemberton, C. J. 2010. Regional vascular response to proangiotensin-12 (PA12) through the rat arterial system. *Peptides* 31:1540–1545.

Qu, M. J., Liu, B., Qi, Y. X., Jiang, Z. L. 2008. Role of rac and rho-gdi alpha in the frequency-dependent expression of h1-calponin in vascular smooth muscle cells under cyclic mechanical strain. *Ann Biomed Eng* 36:1481–1488.

Qureshi, S. R. 1979. Chronic interstitial myocarditis in primates. *Vet Pathol* 16:486–487.

Raj, S. R., Stein, M., Saavedra, P. J., Roden, D. M. 2009. Cardiovascular effects of non-cardiovascular drugs. *Circulation* 120:1123–1132.

Rajagopalan, V., Zucker, I. H., Jones, J. A., Carlson, M., Ma, Y. J. 2008. Cardiac ErbB1/ErbB2 mutant expression in young adult mice leads to cardiac dysfunction. *Am J Physiol Heart Circ Physiol* 295:H543–H554.

Ramos, K., Grossman, S. L. Cox, L. R. 1988. Allylamine-induced vascular toxicity in vitro: prevention by semicarbazide-sensitive amine oxidase inhibitors. *Toxicol Appl Pharmacol* 95:61–71.

Ramos-Fernandez, M., Bellolio, M. F., Stead, L. G. 2011. Matrix metalloproteinase-9 as a marker for acute ischemic stroke: a systematic review. *J Stroke Cerebrovasc Dis* 20:47–54.

Ravingerova, T. 2007. Intrinsic defensive mechanisms in the heart: a potential novel approach to cardiac protection against ischemic injury. *Gen Physiol Biophys* 26:3–13.

Rehm, S., Thomas, R. A., Smith, K. S., Mirabile, R. C., Gales, T. L., Eustis, S. L., Boyce, R. W. 2007. Novel vascular lesions in mice given a non-peptide vitronectin receptor antagonist. *Toxicol Pathol* 35:958–971.

Reimer, K. A., Murry, C. E., Yamasawa, I., Hill, M. L., Jennings, R. B. 1986. Four brief periods of myocardial ischemia cause no cumulative ATP loss or necrosis. *Am J Physiol* 251:H1306–H1315.

Rich, S., Rubin, L., Walker, A. M., Schneeweiss, S., Abenhaim, L. 2000. Anorexigens and pulmonary hypertension in the United States: results from the surveillance of North American pulmonary hypertension. *Chest* 117:870–874.

Roberts, J. M., Cooper, D. W. 2001. Pathogenesis and genetics of pre-eclampsia. *Lancet* 357:53–56.

Roberts, J. M., Taylor, R. N., Musci, T. J., Rodgers, G. M., Hubel, C. A., McLaughlin, M. K. 1989. Preeclampsia: an endothelial cell disorder. *Am J Obstet Gynecol* 161:1200–1204.

Robinson, T. F., Cohen-Gould, L., Factor, S. M. 1983. Skeletal framework of mammalian heart muscle. Arrangement of inter- and pericellular connective tissue structures. *Lab Invest* 49:482–498.

Robinson, W. F., Huxtable, C. R., Pass, D. A. 1980. Canine parvovirus myocarditis. A morphologic description of the natural disease. *Vet Pathol* 17:282–293.

Rona, G. 1985. Catecholamine cardiotoxicity. *J Mol Cell Cardiol* 17:291–306.

Rona, G., Chappel, C. I., Balazs, T., Gaudry, R. 1959. An infarct like myocardial lesion and other toxic manifestations produced by isoproterenol in the rat. *Arch Pathol* 67:443–459.

Ross, R. 1999. Atherosclerosis—an inflammatory disease. *N Engl J Med* 340:115–126.

Ruben, Z., Deslex, P., Nash, G., Redmond, N. I., Poncet, M., Dodd, D. C. 1989. Spontaneous disseminated panarteritis in laboratory beagle dogs in a toxicity study: possible genetic predilection. *Toxicol Pathol* 17:145–152.

Rubin, S. A., Fishbein, M. C., Swan, H. J. 1983. Compensatory hypertrophy in the heart after myocardial infarction in the rat. *J Am Coll Cardiol* 1:1435–1441.

Saitoh, M., Osanai, T., Kamada, T., Matsunaga, T., Ishizaka, H., Hanada, H., Okumura, K. 2003. High plasma level of asymmetric dimethylarginine in patients with acute exacerbated congestive heart failure: role in reduction of plasma nitric oxide level. *Heart Vessels* 18:177–182.

Saleh, A., Stone, J. H. 2005. Classification and diagnostic criteria in systemic vasculitis. *Best Pract Res Clin Rheumatol* 19:209–221.

Sandusky, G. E., Means, J. R., Todd, G. C. 1990. Comparative cardiovascular toxicity in dogs given inotropic agents by continuous intravenous. *Toxicol Pathol* 18:268–278.

Savage, C. O., Harper, L., Adu, D. 1997. Primary systemic vasculitis. *Lancet* 349:553–558.

Savige, J. A., Gallicchio, M., Chang, L., Parkin, J. D. 1991. Autoantibodies in systemic vasculitis. *Aust N Z J Med* 21:433–437.

Scharhag, J., Urhausen, A., Kindermann, W. 2004. Suggested new upper limit of physiologic cardiac hypertrophy determined in Japanese ultramarathon runners must be interpreted cautiously. *J Am Coll Cardiol* 44:470–471.

Schaumburg-Lever, G., Gehring, B., Kaiserling, E. 1994. Ultrastructural localization of factor XIIIa. *J Cutan Pathol* 21:129–134.

Schein, P. S., Davis, R. D., Carter, R. S., Newman, J., Schein, D. R., Rall, D. P. 1970. The evaluation of anti-cancer drugs in dogs and monkeys for the prediction of qualitative toxicities in man. *Clin Pharmacol Ther* 11:3–40.

Schenk, D., Barbour, R., Cunn, W., Gordon, G., Grajeda, H., Guido, T., Hu, K., Huang, J., Johnson-Wood, K., Khan, K., Kholodenko, D., Lee, M., Liao, Z., Lieberburg, I., Motter, R., Mutter, L., Soriano, F., Shopp, G., Vasquez, N., Vandevert, C., Walker, S., Woqulis, M., Yednock, T., Games, D., Seubert, P. 1999. Immunization with amyloid-beta attenuates Alzheimer-disease-like pathology in the PDAPP mouse. *Nature* 400:173–177.

Schlaeppi, B., Roncari, G., Zahm, P. 1991. Vascular toxicity in dogs associated with overdose of a novel benzodiazepine receptor partial agonist. *Arc Toxicol* 65:73–80.

Schneider, P. 1991. Hemodynamically induced heart lesions in the dog after administration of cardioactive substances. *Exp Pathol* 40:155–159.

Schnyder-Candrian, S., Borsig, L., Moser, R., Berger, E. G. 2000. Localization of alpha 1,3-fucosyltransferase VI in Weibel-Palade bodies of human endothelial cells. *Proc Natl Acad Sci USA* 97:8369–8374.

Schultze, A. E., Bradley, W., Main, D., Hall, D. G., Wherly, P., Hoffman, H. Y., Lee, C., Ackerman, B. L., Pritt, M. L., Smith, H. W. 2011. A comparison of mortality and cardiac biomarker response between three outbred stocks of Sprague Dawley rats treated with isoproterenol. *Toxicol Pathol* 39:576–588.

Schultze, A. E., Carpenter, K. H., Wians, F. H., Agee, S. J., Minyard, J., Lu, Q. A., Todd, J., Konrad, R. J. 2009. Longitudinal studies of cardiac troponin-I concentrations in serum from male Sprague-Dawley rats: Baseline reference ranges and effects of handling and placebo dosing on biological variability. *Toxicol Pathol* 37:754–760.

Schultze, A. E., Konrad, R. J., Credille, K. M., Lu, Q. A., Todd, J. 2008. Ultra sensitive cross-species measurement of cardiac troponin-I using the Erenna immunoassay system. *Toxicol Pathol* 36:777–782.

Scicchitano, M., Thomas, R., McFarland, D., Narayanan, P., Thomas, H., Tierney, L., Schwartz, L. 2003. Transcriptional phenotyping of circulating endothelial cells from sorted rat whole blood. *Vet Pathol* 40:626a.

Seidman, A., Hudis, C., Pierri, M. K., Shak, S., Paton, V., Ashby, M., Murphy, M., Stewart, S. J., Keefe, D. 2002. Cardiac dysfunction in the trastuzumab clinical trials experience. *J Clin Oncol* 20:1215–1221.

Sellers, R. S., Morton, D., Michael, B., Roome, N., Johnson, J. K., Yano, B. L., Perry, R., Schafer, K. 2007. Society of Toxicologic Pathology position paper: organ weight recommendations for toxicology studies. *Toxicol Pathol* 35:751–755.

Sheth, C. M., Enerson, B. E., Peters, D., Lawton, M. P., Weaver, J. L. 2011. Effects of modulating in vivo nitric oxide production on the incidence and severity of PDE4 inhibitor-induced vascular injury in Sprague-Dawley rats. *Toxicol Sci* 122:7–15.

Shi, J., Abdelwahid, E., Wei, L. 2011. Apoptosis in anthracycline cardiomyopathy. *Curr Pediatr Rev* 7(4):329–336.

Short, B., Louden, C., Schwartz, L. S., Solleveld, H. 1998. Degeneration and periarteritis of hepatic arteries in young Sprague–Dawley rats. *Toxicol Pathol* 26:483(abstract).

Sica, D. A. 2006. Angiogenesis inhibitors and hypertension: an emerging issue. *J Clin Oncol* 24:1329–1331.

Simonneau, G., Galie, N., Rubin, L. J., Langleben, D., Seeger, W., Domenighetti, G., Gibbs, S., Lebrec, D., Speich, R., Beghetti, M., Rich, S., Fishman, A. 2004. Clinical classification of pulmonary hypertension. *J Am Coll Cardiol* 43:5S–12S.

Simons, M., Downing, S. E. 1985. Coronary vasoconstriction and catecholamine cardiomyopathy. *Am Heart J* 109:297–304.

Singal, P. K., Deally, C. M., Weinberg, L. E. 1987. Subcellular effects of adriamycin in the heart: A concise review. *J Mol Cell Cardiol* 19:817–828.

Singh, M., Foster, C. R., Dalal, S., Singh, K. 2010. Osteopontin role in extracellular matrix deposition and myocardial remodeling post-MI. *J Mol Cell Cardiol* 48:538–543.

Slim, R. M., Robertson, D. G., Albassam, M., Reily, M. D., Robosky, L., Dethloff, L. A. 2002. Effect of dexamethasone on the metabonomics profile associated with phosphodiesterase inhibitor-induced vascular lesions in rats. *Toxicol Appl Pharmacol* 183:108–116.

Slordal, L., Spigset, O. 2006. Heart failure induced by non-cardiac drugs. *Drug Saf* 29:567–586.

Smolock, E. M., Trappanese, D. M., Chang, S., Wang, T., Titchenell, P., Moreland, R. S. 2009. siRNA-mediated knockdown of h-caldesmon in vascular smooth muscle. *Am J Physiol Heart Circ Physiol* 297:H1930–H1939.

Snyder, P. W., Kazacos, E. A., Scott-Moncrieff, J. C., HogenEsch, H., Carlton, W. W., Glickman, L. T., Felsburg, P. J. 1995. Pathologic features of naturally occurring juvenile polyarteritis in Beagle dogs. *Vet Pathol* 32:337–345.

Sobota, J. T. 1989. Review of cardiovascular findings in humans treated with minoxidil. *Toxicol Pathol* 17:193–202.

Sommer, J. R., Johnson, E. A. 1979 Ultrastructure of cardiac muscle. In *Hand of Physiology* (eds. Berne, R. M., Sperelakis, N., Geiger, S. R.), vol. I, pp. 113–118. The American Physiology Society, Bethesda, MD.

Spencer, A., Greaves, P. 1987. Periarteritis in a beagle colony. *J Comp Pathol* 97:121–128.

Spigset, O. 2011. Drug-induced aortic aneurysms, ruptures and dissections. In *Etiology, Pathogenesis and Pathophysiology of Aortic Aneurysms and Aneurysm Rupture* (ed. Grundmann, R.), pp. 159–174. InTech Open Access Publisher. ISGM: 978-953-307-523-5.

Spinale, F. D., Schulte, B. A., Crawford, F. A. 1989. Demonstration of early ischemic injury in porcine right ventricular myocardium. *Am J Pathol* 134:693–704.

Spinale, F. G. 2007. Myocardial matrix remodeling and the matrix metalloproteinases: influence on cardiac form and function. *Physiol Rev* 87:1285–1342.

Stalsberg, H., DeHaan, R. L. 1969. The precardiac areas and formation of the tubular heart in the chick embryo. *Dev Biol* 19:128–159.

Staszak, C., Harbeck, R. J. 1985. Mononuclear-cell pulmonary vasculitis in NZB/W mice. Histopathologic evaluation of spontaneously occurring pulmonary infiltrates. *Am J Pathol* 120:99–105.

Stein, J. H., Klein, M. A., Bellehumeur, J. L., McBride, P. E., Wiebe, D. A., Otvos, J. D., Sosman, J. M. 2001. Use of human immunodeficiency virus-1 protease inhibitors is associated with atherogenic lipoproteins changes and endothelial dysfunction. *Circulation* 104:257–262.

Stejskal, V., Havu, N., Malmfors, T. 1982. Necrotizing vasculitis as an immunological complication in toxicity study. *Arch Toxicol Suppl* 5:283–286.

Sullivan, M. L., Martinez, C. M., Gennis, P., Gallagher, E. J. 1998. The cardiotoxicity of anabolic steroids. *Prog Cardiovasc Dis* 41:1–15.

Sumner, M. J., Cannon, T. R., Mundin, J. W., White, D. G., Watts, I. S. 1992. Endothelin ETA and ETB receptors mediate vascular smooth muscle contraction. *Br J Pharmacol* 107:858–860.

Sutton, T. J., Darby, A. J., Johnson, P., Leslie, G. B., Walker, T. F. 1986. Dyspnoea and thoracic spinal deformation in rats after prizidilol (SK&F 92657). *Hum Toxicol* 5:183–187.

Suzuki, H., Kanamaru, K., Shiba, M., Fujimoto, M., Imanaka-Yoshida, K., Yoshida, T., Taki, W. 2011. Cerebrospinal fluid tenascin-c in cerebral vasospasm after aneurismal subarachnoid hemorrhage. *J Neurosurg Anesthesiol* 23:310–317.

Swap, C. J., Nagurney, J. T. 2005. Value and limitations of chest pain history in the evaluation of patients with suspected acute coronary syndromes. *JAMA* 294:2623–2629.

Tanase, H., Yamori, Y., Hansen, C. T., Lovenberg, W. 1982a. Heart size in inbred strains of rats. Part 1: Genetic determination of the development of cardiovascular enlargement in rats. *Hypertension* 4:864–872.

Tanase, H., Yamori, Y., Hansen, C. T., Lovenberg, W. 1982b. Heart size in inbred strains of rats. Part 2: Cardiovascular DNA and RNA contents during the development of cardiac enlargement in rats. *Hypertension* 4:872–880.

Teerlink, J. R., Breu, V., Sprecher, U., Clozel, M., Clozel, J. P. 1994. Potent vasoconstriction mediated by endothelin ETB receptors in canine coronary arteries. *Circ Res* 74:105–114.

Tekeli, S. 1974. Occurrence of hair fragment emboli in the pulmonary vascular system of rats. *Vet Pathol* 11:482–485.

Telli, M. L., Witteles, R. M., Fisher, G. A., Srinivas, S. 2008. Cardiotoxicity associated with cancer therapeutic agent sunitinib malate. *Ann Oncol* 19:1613–1618.

ten Holder, S. M., Joy, M. S., Falk, R. J. 2002. Cutaneous and systemic manifestations of drug-induced vasculitis. *Ann Pharmacother* 36:130–147.

Tesfamariam, B., DeFelice, A. F. 2007. Endothelial injury in the initiation and progression of vascular disorders. *Vasc Pharmacol* 46:229–237.

Thomas, R. A., Frazier, K. S., Thomas, H. C., Scicchitano, M. S. 2011. microRNA changes in rat mesentery and plasma associated with drug-induced vascular injury. *Toxicologist CD*, 120:2725A (late-breaking).

Thompson, H., McCandlish, I. A., Cornwell, H. I., Wright, N. G., Rogerson, P. 1979. Myocarditis in puppies. *Vet Record* 104:107–108.

Thorball, N., Olsen, F. 1974. Ultrastructural pathological changes in intestinal submucosal arterioles in angiotensin induced acute hypertension in rats. *Acta Pathol Microbiol Immunol Scand A* 82:703–714.

Thygesen, K., Alpert, J. S., White, H. D., Joint ESC/ACCF/AHA/WHF Task Force for the Redefinition of Myocardial Infarction. 2007. Universal definition of myocardial infarction. *Circulation* 116:2634–2653.

Tirapelli, C. R., Casolari, D. A., Yogi, A., Montezano, A. C., Tostes, R. C., Legros, E., D'Orleans-Juste, P., de Oliveira, A. M. 2005. Functional characterization and expression of endothelin receptors in rat carotid artery: involvement of nitric oxide, a vasodilator prostanoid and the opening of K+ channels in ETB-induced relaxation. *Br J Pharmacol* 146:903–912.

Todd, J., Freese, B., Lu, A., Held, D., Morey, J., Livingston, R., Goix, P. 2007. Ultra-sensitive femtogram level flow-based immunoassays using single molecule counting clinical chemistry. *Clin Chem* 53:1990–1995.

Tong, J., Ganguly, P. K., Singal, P. K. 1991. Myocardial adrenergic changes at two stages of heart failure due to adriamycin treatment in rats. *Am J Physiol Heart Circ Physiol* 260:H909–H916.

Topol, E. J. 2004. Failing the public-rofecoxib, Merck and the FDA. *N Eng J Med* 351:1707–1709.

Townsend, P. J., Farza, H., MacGeoch, C., Spurr, N. K., Wade, R., Gahlmann, R., Yacoub, M. H., Barton, P. J. 1994. Human cardiac troponin T: identification of fetal isoforms and assignment of the TNNT2 locus to chromosome 1q. *Genomics* 21:311–316.

Treumann, S., Schneider, S., Gröters, S., Moore, N. P., Boor, P. J. 2011. Spontaneous occurrence of dissecting aneurysms in the region of the ductus arteriosus in four-day-old Wistar rat pups. *Toxicol Pathol* 39:969–974.

Uro-Coste, E., Russano de Paiva, G., Guibeau-Frugier, C., Sastre, N., Ousset, P. J., da Silva, N. A., Lavialle-Guilotreau, V., Vellas, B., Delisle, M. B. 2010. Cerebral amyloid angiopathy and microhemorrhages after amyloid beta vaccination: case report and brief review. *Clin Neuropathol* 29:209–216.

van der Hooft, C. S., Heeringa, J., van Herpen, G., Kors, J. A., Kingma, J. H., Stricker, B. H. 2004. Drug-induced atrial fibrillation. *J Am Coll Cardiol* 44:2117–2124.

Van Eys, G. J., Niessen, P. M., Rensen, S. S. 2007. Smoothelin in vascular smooth muscle cells. *Trends Cardiovasc Med* 17:26–30.

van Mourik, J. A., Boertjes, R., Huisveld, I. A., Fijnvandraat, K., Paikrt, D., van Genderen, P. J., Fijnheer, R. 1999. Von Willebrand factor propeptide in vascular disorders: a tool to distinguish between acute and chromic endothelial cell perturbation. *Blood* 94:179–185.

van Steenkiste, C., Geerts, A., Vanheule, E., Van Vlierberghe, H., De Vos, F., Olievier, K., Cateleyn, C., Laukens, D., De Vos, M., Stassen, J. M., Carmeliet, P., Colle, I. 2009. Role of placental growth factor in mesenteric neoangiogenesis in a mouse model of portal hypertension. *Gastroenterology* 137:2112–2124.

Van Vleet, J. F., Ferrans, V. J., Herman, E. 2002. Cardiovascular and skeletal systems. In *Handbook of Toxicologic Pathology*, 2nd ed. (eds. Haschek, W., Rousseaux, C. G., Wallig, M. A.), pp. 363–455. Academic Press, San Diego CA.

Van Vleet, J. F., Ferrans, V. J. 1986. Myocardial diseases of animals. *Am J Pathol* 124:98–178.

Vane, J. R., Warner, T. D. 2000. Nomenclature for COX-2 inhibitors. *Lancet* 356:1373–1374.

Vane, J. R., Bakhle, Y. S., Botting, R. M. 1998. Cyclooxygenase 1 and 2. *Annu Rev Phamacol Toxicol* 38:97–120.

Vasan, R. S. 2006. Biomarkers of cardiovascular disease. Molecular basis and practical considerations. *Circulation* 113:2335–2362.

Vasan, R. S., Beiser, A., Seshadri, S., Larson, M. G., Kannel, W. B., D'Agostino, R. B., Levy, D. 2002. Residual lifetime risk for developing hypertension in middle-aged women and men: the Framingham Heart Study. *JAMA* 287:1003–1010.

Vasquez-Vivar, J., Martasek, P., Hogg, N., Masters, B. S., Pritchard, K. A. Jr., Kalyanaraman, B. 1997. Endothelial nitric oxide synthase-dependent superoxide generation from adriamycin. *Biochemistry* 36:11293–11297.

Vatner, S. F., McRitchie, R. J, Maroko, P. R., Patrick, T. A., Braunwald, E. 1974. Effects of catecholamines, exercise, and nitroglycerin on the normal and ischemic myocardium in conscious dogs. *J Clin Invest* 54:563–575.

Venkatakrishnan, U., Chen, C., Lokhandwala, M. F. 2000. The role of intrarenal nitric oxide in the natriuretic response to dopamine-receptor activation. *Clin Exp Hypertens* 22:309–324.

Verdecchia, P., Schillaci, G., Borgioni, C., Ciucci, A., Gattobigio, R., Zampi, I., Porcellati, C. 1998. Prognostic value of new electrocardiographic method for diagnosis of left ventricular hypertrophy in essential hypertension. *J Am Coll Cardiol* 31:383–390.

Vidal, J. D., Drobatz, L. S., Holliday, D. F., Geiger, L. E., Thomas, H. C. 2010. Spontaneous findings in the heart of Mauritian-origin cynomolgus macaques (Macaca fascicularis). *Toxicol Pathol* 38:297–302.

Von Schmiedeberg, S., Goebel, C., Gleichmann, E., Uetrecht, J. 1995. Neutrophils and drug metabolism. *Science* 268:585–586.

Vracko, R., Thorning, D., Frederickson, R. G. 1989. Connective tissue cells in healing rat myocardium. A study of cell reactions in rhythmically contracting environment. *Am J Pathol* 134:99–106.

Wagenaar, S. S., Wagenvoort, C. A. 1978. Experimental production of longitudinal smooth muscle cells in the intima of muscular arteries. *Lab Invest* 39:37–374.

Walker, D. 2006. Serum chemical biomarkers of cardiac injury for nonclinical safety testing. *Toxicol Pathol* 34:94–104.

Wallace, K. B., Hausner, E., Herman, E., Holt, G. D., Macgregor, J. T., Metz, A. L., Murphy, E., Rosenblum, I. Y., Sistare, F. D., York, M. J. 2004. Serum troponins as biomarkers of drug-induced cardiac toxicity. *Toxicol Pathol* 32:106–121.

Wang, N., Verna, L., Chen, N. G., Chen, J., Li, H., Forman, B. M., Stemerman, M. B. 2002. Constitutive activation of peroxisome proliferator-activated receptor-gamma suppresses pro-inflammatory adhesion molecules in human vascular endothelial cells. *J Biol Chem* 277:34176–34181.

Ward, J. M., Goodman, D. G., Squire, R. A., Chu, K. C., Linhart, M. S. 1979. Neoplastic and non-neoplastic lesions in ageing (C57B/6NX C3H/HeN) F1 (B6C3F1) mice. *J Natl Cancer Inst* 63:849–854.

Warner, T. D., Mitchell, J. A. 2004. Cyclooxygenase: New forms, new inhibitors and lessons from the clinic. *FASEB J* 18:790–804.

Watterson, C., Lanevschi, A., Horner, J., Louden, C. 2009. A comparative analysis of acute-phase proteins as inflammatory biomarkers in preclinical toxicology studies: implications for preclinical to clinical translation. *Toxicol Pathol* 37:28–33.

Weber, K. T., Brilla, C. G., Campbell, S. E., Zhou, G., Matsubara, L., Guarda, E. 1992. Pathologic hypertrophy with fibrosis: structural basis for myocardial failure. *Blood Pressure* 1:75–85.

Weber, K. T., Brilla, C. G., Janicki, J. S. 1991. Signals for the remodeling of the cardiac interstitium in systemic hypertension. *J Cardiovasc Pharmacol* 17(Suppl 2):S14–S19.

Wei, L., MacDonald, T. M., Walker, B. R. 2004. Taking glucocorticoids by prescription is associated with subsequent cardiovascular disease. *Ann Intern Med* 141:764–770.

Weibel, E. 1958. Entstehung der Längsmuskulatur in den Ästen der A. Bronchialis. *Zschr Zellforsch* 47: 440–468.

Weisberg, E., Manley, P. W., Breitenstein, W., Bruggen, J., Cowan-Jacob, S. W., Raay, A., Huntlt, B., Fabbro, D., Fendrich, G., Hall-Myeres, E., Kung, A. L., Mestan, J., Daley, G. Q., Callahan, L., Catley, L., Cavazza, C., Azam, M., Neuberg, D., Wright, R. D., Gillilan, D. G., Griffin, J. D. 2005. Characterization of AMN107 a selective inhibitor of native and mutant Bcr-Abl. *Cancer Cell* 7:129–141.

Whitehead, P. N., Chesterman, H., Street, A. E. 1979. Toxicity of nicardipine hydrochloride, a new vasodilator, in the beagle dog. *Toxicol Lett* 4:57–59.

Wiener, J., Giacomelli, F. 1973. The cellular pathology of experimental hypertension, VII. Structure and permeability of the mesenteric vasculature in angiotensin-induced hypertension. *Am I Path* 72:221–240.

Will, J. A., Bisgard, G. E. 1972. Haemodynamic effects of oral aminorex and amphetamine in unanaesthetized beagle dogs. *Thorax* 27:120–126.

Winsor, T., Mills, B., Winbury, M. M., Howe, B. B., Berger, H. J. 1975. Intramyocardial diversion of coronary blood flow: effects of isoproterenol-induced subendocardial ischaemia. *Micro Vasc Res* 9:261–278.

Womble, J. R., Larson, D. F., Copeland, J. G. 1982. Low-dose oral terbutaline therapy rapidly induces significant cardiac hypertrophy. *Clin Pharmacol Ther* 31:283–284.

Wouters, K. A., Kremer, L. C. Miller, T. L., Herman, E. H., Lipshultz, S. E. 2005. Protecting against anthracyclin-induced myocardial damage: a review of the most promising strategies. *Br J Haematol* 131(5):561–578.

Wu, A. H., Lu, Q. A., Todd, J., Moecks, J., Wians, F. 2009. Short and long-term biological variation in cardiac troponin I with a high sensitivity assay: Implication for clinical practice. *Clin Chem* 55:52–58.

Wu, A. H., Fukushima, N., Puskas, R., Todd, J., Goix, P. 2006. Development and preliminary clinical validation of a high sensitivity assay for cardiac troponin using a capillary flow (single molecule) fluorescence detector. *Clin Chem* 52:2157–2159.

Yamaguchi, T., Murata, Y., Fujiyoshi, Y., Doi, T. 2003. Regulated interaction of endothelin B receptor with caveolin-1. *Eur J Biochem* 270:1816–1827.

Yamamoto, K., Ohki, R., Lee, R. T., Ikeda, U., Shimada, K. 2001. Peroxisome proliferator-activated receptor gamma activators inhibit cardiac hypertrophy in cardiac myocytes. *Circulation* 104:1670–1675.

Yamamoto, M., Okamura, S., Oka, N., Schwencke, C., Ishikawa, Y. 1999. Downregulation of caveolin expression by cAMP signal. *Life Sci* 64:1349–1357.

Yamauchi-Takihara, K. 2002. Gp-130 mediated pathway and left ventricular remodeling. *J Cardiac Failure* 8:S374–S378.

Yamori, Y., Okomoto, K. 1976. The Japanese spontaneously hypertensive rat (SHR). *Clin Exp Pharmacol Physiol Suppl* 3:1–4.

Yan, T. T., Li, Q., Zhang, X. H., Wu, W. K., Sun, J., Li, L., Zhang, Q., Tan, H. M. 2010. Homocysteine impaired endothelial function through compromised vascular endothelial growth factor/Akt/endothelial nitric oxide synthase signaling. *Clin Exp Pharmacol Physiol* 37:1071–1077.

Yu, P., Yang, Z., Jones, J. E., Wang, Z., Owens, S. A., Mueller, S. C., Felder, R. A., Jose, P. A. 2004. D1 dopamine receptor signaling involves caveolin-2 in HEK-293 cells. *Kidney Int* 66:2167–2180.

Yang, B. G., Tanaka, T., Jang, M. H., Bai, Z., Hayasaka, H., Miyasaka, M. 2007. Binding of lymphoid chemokines to collagen IV that accumulates in the basal lamina of high endothelial venules: its implications in lymphocyte trafficking. *J Immunol* 179:4376–4382.

York, M., Scudamore, C., Brady, S., Chen, C., Wilson, S., Curtis, M., Evans, G., Griffiths, W., Whayman, M., Williams, T., Turton J. 2007. Characterization of troponin responses in isoproterenol-induced cardiac injury in the Hanover Wistar rat. *Toxicol Pathol* 35(4):606–617.

Yuhas, E. M., Morgan, D. G., Arena, E., Kupp, R. P., Saunders, L. Z., Lewis, H. B. 1985. Arterial medial necrosis and hemorrhage induced in rats by intravenous infusion of fenoldopam mesylate, a dopaminergic vasodilator. *Am J Pathol* 119:83–91.

Zabka, T. S., Irwin, M., Albassam, M. A. 2009. Spontaneous cardiomyopathy in cynomolgus monkeys (Macaca fascicularis). *Toxicol Pathol* 37:814–818.

Zannettino, A. C., Holding, C. A., Diamond, P., Atkins, G. J., Kostakis, P., Farrugia, A., Gamble, J., To, L. B., Findlay, D. M., Haynes, D. R. 2005. Osteoprotegerin(OPG) is localized to the Weibel-Palade bodies of human vascular endothelial cells and is physically associated with von Willebrand factor. *J Cell Physiol* 204:714–723.

Zbinden, G. 1986. Detection of cardiotoxic hazards. *Arch Toxicol Suppl* 9:178–187.

Zhang, H., Zhang, A., Kohan, D. E., Nelson, R. D., Gonzalez, F. J., Yang, T. 2005. Collecting-duct specific deletion of peroxisome proliferator-activated receptor gamma blocks thiazolidinedione-induced fluid retention. *Proc Natl Acad Sci USA* 102:9406–9411.

Zhang, J., Defelice, A. F., Hanig, J. P., Colatsky, T. 2010. Biomarkers of endothelial cell activation serve as potential surrogate markers for drug-induced vascular injury. *Toxicol Pathol* 38:865–871.

Zhang, J., Yang, P. L., Gray, N. S. 2009. Targeting cancer with small molecule kinase inhibitors. *Nat Rev Cancer* 9:28–39.

Zhang, L., Li, H. Y., Li, H., Zhao, J., Su, L., Zhang, Y., Zhang, S. L., Miao, J. Y. 2011a. Lipopolysaccharide activated phosphatidylcholine-specific phospholipase C and induced IL-8 and MCP-1 production in vascular endothelial cells. *J Cell Physiol* 226:1694–1701.

Zhang, Y., Ge, G., Greenspan, D. S. 2006. Inhibition of bone morphogenetic protein 1 by native and altered forms of alpha2-macroglobulin. *J Biol Chem* 281:39096–39104.

Zhang, Z., Chu, G., Wu, H. X., Zou, N., Sun, B. G., Dai, Q. Y. 2011b. IL-8 reduces VCAM-1 secretion of smooth muscle cells by increasing p-ERK expression when 3-D co-cultured with vascular endothelial cells. *Clin Invest Med* 34:E138–E146.

Zhao, Y. Y., Liu, Y., Stan, R. V., Fan, L., Gu, Y., Dalton, N., Chu, P. H., Peterson, K., Ross, J. Jr., Chien, K. R. 2002. Defects in caveolin-1 cause dilated cardiomyopathy and pulmonary hypertension in knockout mice. *Proc Natl Acad Sci USA* 99:11375–11380.

Zhao, Z. Q., Corvera, J. S., Halkos, M. E., Kerendi, F., Wang, N. P., Guyton, R. A., Vinten-Johansen, J. 2003. Inhibition of myocardial injury by ischemic postconditioning during reperfusion: comparison with ischemic preconditioning. *Am J Physiol Heart Circ Physiol* 285:H579–H588.

Zhen, E. Y., Berna, M. J., Jin, Z., Pritt, M. L., Watson, D. E., Ackermann, B. L., Hale, J. E. 2007. Quantification of heart fatty acid-binding protein as a biomarker for drug-induced cardiac and musculoskeletal necroses. *Proteomics* 1:661–671.

Zheng, S., Li, W., Xu, M., Bai, X., Zhou, Z., Han, J., Shyy, J. Y., Wang, X. 2010. Calcitonin gene related peptide promotes angiogenesis via AMP-activated protein kinase. *Am J Physiol Cell Physiol* 299:C1485–C1492.

Zile, M. R., Desantis, S. M., Baicu, C. F., Stroud, R. E., Thompson, S. B., McClure, C. D., Mehurg, S. M., Spinale, F. G. 2011. Plasma biomarkers that reflect determinants of matrix composition identify the presence of left ventricular hypertrophy and diastolic heart failure. *Circ Heart Fail* 4:246–256.

Zolkowska, D., Rothman, R. B., Baumann, M. H. 2006. Amphetamine analogs increase plasma serotonin: implications for cardiac and pulmonary disease. *J Pharmacol Exp Ther* 318:604–610.

17 Endocrine Glands

Sundeep Chandra, Mark J. Hoenerhoff, and Richard Peterson

CONTENTS

17.1   INTRODUCTION

The endocrine system is one of the body's major homeostatic control systems whose aim is to maintain normal function and development in the face of a constantly changing environment. Working in tandem with the nervous system, which is mainly responsible for rapid and immediate responses, the endocrine system tends to act in a slower and more sustained manner to regulate a diverse set of processes. Multiple endocrine glands also work in concert with one another to form complex feedback loops, which tightly regulate critical physiological processes. Like all homeostatic control systems, the capacity to maintain physiological parameters within normal bounds is finite, and when this capacity is exceeded by chemical or drug exposure, or environmental stressors, adverse consequences can ensue. Chemicals can cause endocrine abnormalities via different mechanisms, including direct alteration of hormone production, changes in the regulation of the hormonal axis, effects on hormonal transport, binding and signaling, as well as similar changes to counterregulatory hormone systems. The objective of this chapter is to provide a broad overview of common spontaneous morphological changes in endocrine organs (pituitary gland, adrenal glands, thyroid gland, parathyroid gland, and the pancreatic islets), with examples of xenobiotic-induced changes, predominantly in rodents.

17.2   PITUITARY GLAND

17.2.1   NORMAL STRUCTURE AND FUNCTION

The pituitary gland or hypophysis is situated within the sella turcica and, together with the hypothalamus, coordinates the structural integrity and functions of other endocrine glands. The pituitary stalk serves as an anatomic and functional connection to the hypothalamus (Figure 17.1a). The

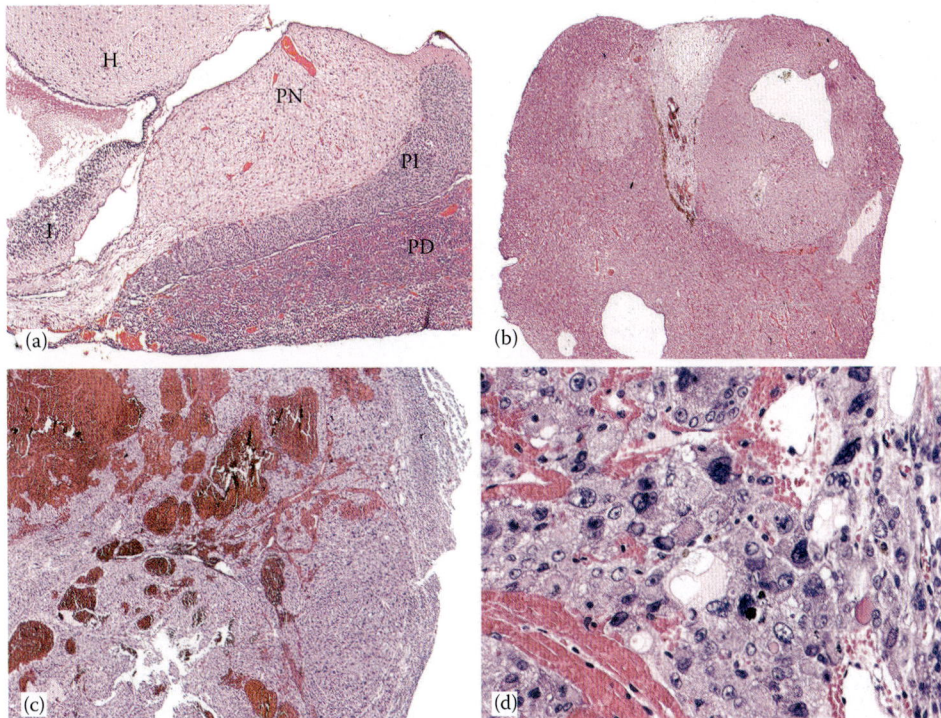

FIGURE 17.1 (a) Sagittal section of the pituitary and hypothalamus (H) showing infundibulum (I), pars nervosa (PN), pars intermedia (PI), and pars distalis (PD). (b) Pituitary gland from an aged rat showing a focus of hyperplasia (left) and an adenoma of the pars distalis on the right. (c and d) Low- and high-magnification images of pituitary carcinoma originating in the pars distalis in a rat.

hypothalamus contains nerve cell bodies that synthesize hypophysiotropic-releasing and -inhibiting hormones, as well as the neurohypophyseal hormones of the posterior pituitary (arginine vasopressin [AVP] or antidiuretic hormone and oxytocin [OT]).

The pituitary gland is divided into the anterior and posterior pituitary, two regions distinctive in their embryology, anatomy, and function. The anterior lobe (or adenohypophysis) is embryonically derived from an ectodermal evagination, the hypophyseal recess, or Rathke's pouch, while the posterior lobe (or neurohypophysis) is derived from the diencephalic neuroectoderm. The anterior lobe is composed of an anterior portion (or pars distalis) and an intermediate lobe (or pars intermedia), and the pars tuberalis, which represents a dorsal projection or sleeve of cells, is situated around or along the infundibular stalk (Figure 17.1a). The median eminence of the tuber cinereum, the infundibular stalk, and the infundibular processes together make up the neurohypophysis or posterior lobe. Blood supply to the gland is from several sources.

The anterior pituitary is a heterogeneous gland with multiple cell types that secrete hormones with unique functions. It consists of five major cell types that produce six traditionally recognized hormones: (1) corticotrophs that secrete adrenocorticotropic hormone (ACTH); (2) thyrotrophs that secrete thyroid-stimulating hormone (TSH); (3) gonadotrophs that secrete luteinizing hormone (LH) and follicle-stimulating hormone (FSH); (4) somatotrophs that secrete growth hormone (GH); and (5) lactotrophs that secrete prolactin (PRL). These hormone cells have been traditionally divided into acidophils, basophils, and chromophobes on the basis of their staining characteristics using hematoxylin and eosin and other techniques; however, the staining characteristics do not accurately reflect the type of hormones that are synthesized by these cells. An overview of each pituitary cell type, secretory profiles, and regulation of the hormone products and biological actions is listed in Table 17.1.

TABLE 17.1

Pituitary Cell Types, Secretory Profiles, Regulation of Hormonal Products, and Biological Actions

	Gonadotrophs	Thyrotrophs	Lactotrophs	Somatotrophs	Corticotrophs
Primary Hormone	FSH, LH	TSH	PRL	GH	ACTH
Secretory product	Glycoprotein αβ subunits	Glycoprotein αβ subunits	Polypeptide	Polypeptide	Polypeptide
Cellular features					
Staining population	Basophilic, 10%–15%	Basophilic, 10%	Basophilic, 15%–20%	Acidophilic, 30%–50%	Basophilic, 15%–20%
Target tissue	Ovary, testis	Thyroid gland	Mammary gland	Liver, bone, muscle	Adrenal glands
Primary inhibitors of secretion (negative feedback)	Estrogen, progesterone, testosterone, inhibin	T3, T4	Dopamine	Somatostatin	Glucocorticoids
Stimulators	GnRH, estrogen	TRH	Estrogen, TRH	GHRH, GHS	CRH, VP

Note: GHS = growth hormone secretagogues.

The posterior pituitary (neurohypophysis) does not contain neuroendocrine cells. Instead, it consists of the axonal terminals of two groups of hypothalamic neurons that secrete AVP and OT. The neurohypophysis contains an intrinsic population of cells, the pituicytes, and the terminal parts of the axons of secretory neurons, the bodies of which are located in the supraoptic and paraventricular nuclei in the hypothalamus. The fibers from these cells converge upon the median eminence and run down the infundibular stem into the infundibular process where they end intimately related to the capillary vasculature. Spherical bodies of variable size known as Herring bodies are also present in the fibers and represent secretory material. Pituicytes, as specialized astrocytes, are the main glial cells of the neural lobe. They are in intimate contact with the perivascular space of the sinusoidal vessels. Pituicytes are characterized by the expression of specific membrane-bound receptors for opioids, vasopressin, and b-adrenoceptors (Wittkowski 1988). Mitotic activity in the pituicytes can be greatly increased when isotonic lithium is administered after water deprivation and rehydration. The mitotic activity in these conditions is related to a physiological attempt to maintain homeostasis rather than a response to injury or the development of neoplasia (Levine et al. 2000, 2002). The neurohypophysis is joined to the hypothalamus via the infundibular stalk. Both AVP and OT are synthesized as preprohormones. As the biosynthetic precursor molecules travel along the axons in secretion granules from the neurosecretory neurons, the precursors are cleaved into the active hormones. With removal of the signal peptide and glycosylation of the polypeptide in the endoplasmic reticulum, the respective prohormones are produced and packaged into neurosecretory granules. Plasma osmolality is the principal stimulus for the release of AVP from SON and PVN through osmoreceptors located in these areas. Estrogen is known to modulate OT gene expression in various species. Like other hypothalamic neurons, AVP and OT secretion are under a myriad of neural and endocrine controls (Cheung and Lustig 2007; Sam and Frohman 2008).

17.2.2 Nonproliferative Lesions

Spontaneous nonproliferative background lesions are uncommon except for pituitary cysts in the adenohypophysis or neurohypophysis. These cysts are common spontaneous findings in laboratory rats and beagle dogs. They are lined by ciliated cuboidal to columnar or squamous epithelium. Portions of Rathke's pouch, the embryologic structure that ultimately gives rise to the pituitary, may persist in the pituitary of adult rats. Remnants of Rathke's pouch are often closely associated with Rathke's cleft, which separates the pars distalis from the pars intermedia. Rathke's pouch remnants appear as variably sized tubular or glandular structures lined by ciliated or squamous epithelium.

17.2.2.1 Atrophy

Loss of anterior pituitary cell mass can occur under circumstances of reduced demand, and this loss may be associated with reduced weight. Aging in rats is associated with a reduction in the hypothalamic content of releasing hormones and the capacity of the pituitary to synthesize or release FSH, LH, and TSH; these differences may be partly due to differences in pituitary tumor incidence and their space occupying effects (Bedrak et al. 1983; Chen 1984). Physiological alterations that result in increased activity of the hypothalamus, such as water deprivation or lactation, may result in involution of the pars intermedia. Rats administered bromocriptine, a dopamine receptor agonist, decreased the cell number and thickness of the pars intermedia in association with reduction in synthesis of pro-opiomelanocortin–derived peptides and mRNA (Chronwall et al. 1987).

17.2.2.2 Hypertrophy

Direct, drug-induced, nonproliferative lesions primarily affecting the pituitary are uncommon. Morphological changes observed in this gland are secondary to the pharmacology of the drug and/or reflect alterations in gonadal or endocrine tissues that are linked to the pituitary by a feedback mechanism.

The pituitary is composed of several cell types as described earlier, each responsible for the production of specific hormones. In the past, it was thought that one cell could make only one hormone; the concept of plurihormonality was poorly understood. However, the molecular factors that determine hormone production have now been deciphered and transcription factors that target specific hormone genes identified. These factors have clarified three main pathways of cell differentiation. ACTH-producing corticotrophs are determined by corticotropin upstream transcription-binding element (CUTE) proteins including neuroD1/beta 2. Bihormonal gonadotrophs require expression of steroidogenic factor-1 (SF-1). The complex family of Pit-1-expressing cells can mature into somatotrophs, mammosomatotrophs, lactotrophs, or thyrotrophs with the additional expression of estrogen receptor (ER) alpha, which enhances PRL secretion, or thyrotroph embryonic factor (TEF), which stimulates TSH-beta production. The recognition of these molecular determinants of adenohypophyseal cytodifferentiation has clarified the patterns of plurihormonality (Asa and Ezzat et al. 1999).

Adenohypophyseal cells are not irreversibly committed to the production of one single hormone, and cell phenotype can change in response to functional demand. Morphologic changes in the pituitary can be observed secondary to changes in the dependent tissues. In patients with protracted primary hypothyroidism, the pituitary is enlarged due to the lack of feedback inhibition by thyroid hormone, and there is thyrotroph hyperplasia and the formation of "thyroidectomy" or "thyroid deficiency" cells. Pituitary thyrotroph hyperplasia resulting from prolonged primary hypothyroidism has been reported in humans, mice, and rats. For example, depletion of thyroid hormones, such as after thyroidectomy, or increased clearance of thyroid hormone, secondary to hepatocellular microsomal enzyme induction, can lead to hypertrophy of thyrotrophs and a decrease in staining intensity for TSH in the pituitary (Zabka et al. 2011; Ozawa 1991). A number of thyroidectomy cells are also immunoreactive for GH, revealing the presence of bihormonal cells containing both GH and TSH indicating that somatotrophs may transform to thyrotrophs. Thus, in addition to multiplication of thyrotrophs, transdifferentiation of GH cells to thyrotrophs contributes to the increase of TSH-producing cells, and these bihormonal cells are termed "thyrosomatotrophs." Further, in hypothyroidism, there is transdifferentiation of somatotrophs into thyrotrophs through bihormonal intermediate thyrosomatotrophs during thyrotroph hyperplasia in both rodent and human pituitaries. There is a shift in the relative populations of somatotrophs toward thyrotrophs (Nolan et al. 2004; Vidal et al. 2001).

Lactotroph hyperplasia is a prominent finding in the adenohypophysis of pregnant women with concurrent increases in the amount of prolactin (PRL) mRNA and mitoses in PRL-immunoreactive cells. In pregnancy, somatotrophs are recruited to produce PRL, express PRL mRNA, and transform to bihormonal mammosomatotrophs and possibly later to lactotrophs, contributing to PRL production (Stefaneanu et al. 1992). Similar to transdifferentiation of somatotrophs to thyrotrophs in hypothyroidism, there is transdifferentiation of somatotrophs into bihormonal mammosomatotrophs in gestational lactotroph hyperplasia during pregnancy.

The effect of gonadectomy on the gonadotrophs of the pituitary has been widely investigated. Hypertrophy of the gonadotrophs is observed after ovariectomy (OVX) or castration, and release of gonadotrophins increases as a function of time after OVX. Ultrastructural and immunohistochemical studies have shown that affected gonadotrophs contain decreased numbers of secretory granules and vacuolated rough endoplasmic reticulum, both containing FSH and LH (Tixier-Vidal et al. 1975). Some of the dilated residues of endoplasmic reticulum fuse to form the large vacuoles typical of the signet ring appearance of "castration cells." Treatment of rats with the antiandrogen flutamide produced a hypertrophy–hyperplasia of the FSH cells and hypertrophy of LH-secreting cells, with marked alterations at the ultrastructural level suggesting a hyperstimulation stage (Cónsole et al. 2001). A similar morphologic change (hydropic degeneration) was observed in the anterior pituitary of rats secondary to hyponatremia and (or?) uremia (Levine and Saltzman 2004).

Estrogen treatment reverses the effects of OVX on gonadotroph size and morphology and secretion of gonadotrophins (Sánchez-Criado et al. 2006). Estrogens stimulate proliferation of the prolactin (PRL)-producing lactotroph and enhance lactotroph survival (Spady et al. 1999). Morphological and immunohistochemical studies of the pituitary gland of rats treated with diethylstilboestrol or estradiol for periods of up to 16 weeks revealed enlarged congested glands containing large prolactin-positive pituitary cells with large nuclei and numerous mitotic figures (Lloyd 1983; Lloyd and Mailloux 1987; Niwa et al. 1987).

The degree of prolactin cell hyperplasia appears to be time dependent. Serum prolactin levels in rats treated with estrogen increase in parallel with pituitary hyperplasia (Lyle et al. 1984). Rat strains vary in their sensitivity to the effects of estrogens on the pituitary gland. In addition, estrogens also modulate pituitary angiogenesis and enhance the expression of proangiogenic factors (Lombardero et al. 2009). Through these actions on lactotroph proliferation and survival, estrogens induce or contribute to the development of PRL-producing pituitary tumors in several rat strains. Experimentally, estrogen-induced pituitary tumors can be observed fairly early in life. Female Fischer 344 rats treated subcutaneously with 5 mg/animal of estradiol dipropionate (ED) once every 2 weeks for 13 weeks developed an adenoma as early as week 5, and a carcinoma was noted at week 7 posttreatment (Satoh et al. 1997). Estrogens have a biphasic effect on pituitary cell proliferation in vitro, with higher concentrations of estradiol having an inhibitory effect on cell growth, while lower concentrations stimulate PRL secretion (Lloyd et al. 1991).

17.2.3 PROLIFERATIVE LESIONS

17.2.3.1 Hyperplasia

Focal and diffuse hyperplasia. Proliferative lesions in the intermedia and nervosa are rare. Although pituitary adenoma is a common proliferative lesion, focal and diffuse hyperplasias represent a continuum of proliferative lesions with overlapping histopathological features (Figure 17.1b). Diffuse hyperplasia affects one or more of the pituitary cell populations, and altered cells are typically interspersed with unaffected cells, while focal hyperplasia is characterized by foci of pituitary cells that show altered tinctorial properties, with little or no compression of the surrounding normal tissue. Diffuse hyperplasia occurs spontaneously in aging rats and in response to lactation, surgical resection of endocrine tissues, administration of sex hormones, oral contraceptives, trophic factors, and other agents that induce prolonged changes to the endocrine system (Furth et al. 1973).

Dogs with primary hypothyroidism have enlarged pituitary glands with thyrotroph hyperplasia (Diaz-Espiñeira et al. 2008). Large, vacuolated thyroid deficiency cells and decreased numbers of mammotrophs were observed microscopically, and some cells stained for both GH and TSH, indicating transdifferentiation. Thyrotroph hyperplasia can be observed with concurrent corticotroph adenoma (Teshima et al. 2009). Treatment of ovariectomized beagles with high doses of cyproterone acetate (synthetic progesterone) produced hyperplasia and hypertrophy of GH-producing cells, leaving prolactin-containing cells generally unchanged (El Etreby 1978b). On the contrary, administration of porcine GH to dogs produced increased pituitary weight and histologically enlarged vacuolated cells that stained for GH (Laroque et al. 1998). Female beagles treated with estrogen had hypertrophy and hyperplasia of prolactin-containing cells (El Etreby 1978a). Aging dogs have diffuse hypertrophy and hyperplasia of GH-containing cells with proliferative changes in the mammary gland.

17.2.3.2 Neoplasia

Spontaneous pituitary adenomas are common in certain strains of laboratory rat, with females being more commonly affected. Adenoma of the pars distalis (Figure 17.1b) is a fairly common proliferative lesion in rats, with a high incidence of up to 70% in the Sprague–Dawley rats. In the latter strain, pituitary adenoma is also the most common cause of death, especially in female rats during the conduct of carcinogenicity studies (Son and Gopinath 2004a, 2004b). Pituitary tumors can be observed in young adult Sprague–Dawley rats as early as 19 weeks of age (Ikezaki et al. 2011), and in a carcinogenicity study, adenomas of the pars distalis were observed by the 33rd week, with an incidence of almost 35% in female Sprague–Dawley rats by week 50 (Son and Gopinath 2004b). While the most common early tumor in the Sprague–Dawley rat occurs in the pituitary gland of females, the most common early tumor in the Han Wistar strain was malignant lymphoma in both sexes (Son et al. 2010), indicating strain differences in tumor onset. Pituitary adenoma is also common in the Han rat, with a 33.9% incidence in males and 54.6% incidence in females (Carlus et al. 2011).

Most pituitary neoplasms in rats have been considered chromophobe adenomas of the pars distalis, with variable histological appearance (Helminski et al. 1989). In aging male Wistar rats, the spontaneous pituitary adenomas may originate from undifferentiated cells, PRL-, GH- and TSH-secreting cells, in diminishing order of frequency (Fong et al. 1982). Although most spontaneous pituitary tumors in Sprague–Dawley and Fischer 344 rats are immunoreactive for prolactin (PRL), immunoreactivity as well as lack of any specific immunoreactivity have also been reported (Sandusky et al. 1988; McComb et al. 1984, 1985). The development of tumors and hyperplasia of prolactin-secreting cells is accompanied by increasing serum levels of prolactin. Elevated serum prolactin resulting in mammary tumors is commonly observed in rats. Rodent mammary tumors resulting from elevated prolactin were assumed to be a rodent- specific phenomenon and not necessarily relevant to humans (Sistare et al. 2011). However, recent reports contradict the previous assumptions and suggest that drugs and chemicals causing rodent prolactin-induced mammary carcinogenesis may pose a risk to humans via the same mechanism if exposures also increase prolactin secretion in humans (Harvey 2005, 2012).

Since the majority of these tumors contain prolactin cells, it has been suggested that decreased hypothalamic content of dopamine observed in older rats may be an important factor as dopamine is the main inhibitory factor for prolactin (Prysor-Jones et al. 1983). The higher incidence of pituitary adenomas in females suggests that estrogen is involved, either by a direct effect on the pituitary cells or through inhibition of dopamine. A small number of spontaneous adenomas also develop from cells of the intermediate lobe in rats and show immunohistochemical staining for ACTH (McComb et al. 1984, 1985).

Multiple studies have shown the influence of dietary factors on both the incidence and onset of pituitary tumors in rats (Keenan et al. 1995a,b; Duffy et al. 2008). A lower incidence of pituitary tumors in rats fed with a restricted diet was associated with decreased circulating levels of prolactin, estradiol, LH, and IGF-1; reduced volume of GH and prolactin-containing cells; and a lower proliferation index in the pituitary gland (Molon-Noblot et al. 2003).

Pituitary carcinomas cannot be readily distinguished from adenomas based on the nature of the cells and the architectural pattern of the neoplasm (Figure 17.1c and d). Differentiating factors between adenomas and carcinomas include the presence of distant metastasis or aggressive local invasion of the adjacent brain or the sphenoid bone, the latter representing the most common evidence of malignancy. Local invasion must be differentiated from expansive growth commonly seen with adenomas (Majka et al. 1990).

Other proliferative lesions, including craniopharyngioma (Pace et al. 1997; Heider 1986) and pituicytoma (Satoh et al. 2000), are rare neoplasms, and isolated cases have been described. Adenomas of the pars intermedia are uncommon in rats. Spontaneous pituitary neoplasms are less common in mice. The FVB/N mouse strain has a high prevalence of prolactin-secreting pituitary proliferative lesions (hyperplasia and adenoma), with secondary effects on the mammary gland (Wakefield et al. 2003). Similar to rats, dietary restriction reduced the incidence of pituitary and other tumors in diet-restricted B6C3F1 mice compared with ad libitum–fed controls. Pituitary adenomas have been reported in beagle dogs. The neoplasms in dogs appeared as small nodules (2–3.5 mm in diameter), and histologically, the tumors were composed of ACTH, immature or intermediate zone, cells (Attia 1980). In a retrospective study, spontaneous pituitary adenomas that caused either gross enlargement of the gland or microadenomas that were identified on histologic examination were observed in 14 of 491 cynomolgus macaques (*Macaca fascicularis*). Pituitary weight was increased due to these tumors. A total of 35 adenomas were identified, with mixed histologic appearance and hormone expression, although a majority of the tumors stained immunohistochemically for prolactin (Remick et al. 2006).

17.3 THYROID GLAND

17.3.1 NORMAL STRUCTURE AND FUNCTION

The thyroid gland plays an important role in the regulation of numerous physiological processes in the body, including normal growth and development and basic metabolic processes. The thyroid is the largest organ that functions exclusively as an endocrine gland (Capen et al. 2002). In mammals, it is composed of two endocrine cell populations that are responsible for the synthesis of two distinct hormones. The first cell population is the follicular epithelial cells, which synthesize and secrete the thyroid hormones, including triiodothyronine (T3) and thyroxine (T4). Follicular morphology may vary depending on several factors, including nutritional or endocrine status, environment, age, sex, and species, among others. For example, in male rats, the thyroid tends to be larger as a whole, and the volume of the follicular epithelial cells tends to be greater compared with that of females, while follicles in females tend to contain a greater volume of colloid (Hardisty and Boorman 1990). With increasing age, follicles become more variable and larger in size, the amount of stroma increases, colloid tincture becomes more eosinophilic (Hardisty and Boorman 1999), and many inactive follicles with flattened epithelium are interspersed among active follicles.

The second cell population within the thyroid gland is made up of C-cells, which are so named because they produce calcitonin, a hormone critical in the regulation of calcium and phosphorous homeostasis, as well as normal bone metabolism (Hardisty and Boorman 1990, 1999; Capen et al. 2002). C-cell numbers comprise approximately 10% of follicular cells and occur singly or in clusters between the basal region of the follicular epithelium and the follicular basement membrane. C-cells are polygonal to round, with large, round, central nuclei and moderately pale cytoplasm with numerous secretory granules containing calcitonin and catecholamines. These granules are inconspicuous and poorly visualized with hematoxylin and eosin but may be demonstrated with various silver stains (Grimelius) due to their catecholamine content, or by immunolabeling with antibodies for calcitonin (Hardisty and Boorman 1999), and are electron dense by transmission electron microscopy (TEM).

17.3.2 Thyroid Hormones

The thyroid gland is unique among all other organs in the body in that it can accumulate iodine in large quantities and incorporate it into hormones (Capen and Martin 1989a). Furthermore, it is unique among endocrine glands in that the synthesis of the final hormone product(s) occurs extracellularly within the glandular lumen in the form of colloid, rather than intracellularly (Capen and Martin 1989a; McClain 1992). While this extracellular location is a very unusual storage location for hormones produced by an endocrine gland, the ability to store a large reserve of hormone in the follicular lumen allows for a large, available reserve of this important metabolic hormone and enables mammals to withstand long periods of iodine deprivation (Greco and Stabenfeldt 2007).

A majority (>99%) of thyroid hormones are bound to plasma proteins. In rats, thyroid hormones are primarily bound to transthyretin and albumin, while in humans, dogs, and nonhuman primates (NHPs), they are transported bound to an additional protein, thyroxine binding globulin (TBG), which represents a significant species difference in thyroid hormone function and accounts for significant species differences in proliferative lesions due to chronic TSH stimulation (discussed later). Only those hormones not bound to protein are able to bind to cell receptors and be hormonally active. Free thyroid hormones are the primary mediators in the control of metabolism and, following their release, exert effects on several different target tissues within the organism. Thyroid hormones increase carbohydrate, protein, and lipid metabolism, glycolysis, gluconeogenesis and intestinal glucose absorption, oxygen consumption, and heat production (Capen and Martin 1989a; Greco and Stabenfeldt 2007). They are essential for normal growth and development of the central nervous system (CNS), as well as normal neural function in the adult animal. In the cardiovascular system, thyroid hormones increase the heart rate, cardiac output, and blood pressure and are necessary for normal contractility of cardiac muscle (Capen and Martin 1989a). An increase in unbound thyroid hormones also results in a decrease in circulating TSH, through the negative feedback mechanism with the pituitary and hypothalamus, and conversely, a decrease in free hormones results in increased TSH production.

17.3.3 Nonproliferative Lesions

17.3.3.1 Congenital Lesions

Because of its close proximity to the aortic sac during development, accessory thyroid tissue may be observed within the ventral neck along the midline or in the mediastinum (Capen and Martin 1989b). These embryonic rests are composed of normal-appearing follicles that retain hormonal function but are devoid of C-cells. In dogs, presence of this accessory tissue is quite common, and up to 50% of dogs have ectopic thyroid remnants, which have been associated with neoplastic transformation in this species. Ectopic thymus, composed of clusters of normal lymphoid tissue with typical cortical and medullary regions, may also be observed within or in close proximity to the thyroid gland (Hardisty and Boorman 1990).

Thyroid cysts may occur in all species, most commonly in rats and dogs, and may be lined by either keratinizing or nonkeratinizing squamous epithelium (ultimobranchial) or cuboidal to columnar and occasionally ciliated epithelial cells (thyroglossal duct) (Capen et al. 2002). Cysts arising from the ultimobranchial bodies (ultimobranchial cysts) are located centrally within the thyroid, are lined by attenuated squamous epithelium, and contain cellular debris. The less common thyroglossal duct cyst occurs in the cranioventral neck along the ventral midline, as a result of persistence of a segment of the thyroglossal duct that is retained during development. Thyroglossal duct cysts may give rise to papillary carcinomas in dogs (Capen and Martin 1989a).

17.3.3.2 Atrophy/Degeneration

Atrophy of the thyroid gland may result from direct damage due to chronic inflammation, disruption of thyroid hormone synthesis, or decreased stimulation due to a lack of TSH. For example, chronic lymphocytic thyroiditis will result in atrophy of the follicular epithelium as a result of chronic damage and degeneration due to inflammation. Atrophy due to a lack of stimulation by TSH is a primary atrophy of follicular epithelial cells. A functional follicular thyroid tumor may result in significant atrophy of the contralateral gland due to excessive thyroid hormone production, with a compensatory decrease in circulating TSH levels. Alternatively, a hypothalamic or pituitary lesion that results in loss of TRH or TSH production, respectively, can lead to diffuse thyroid atrophy and hypothyroidism (Capen et al. 2002). Drugs, chemicals, or dietary imbalances that alter thyroid

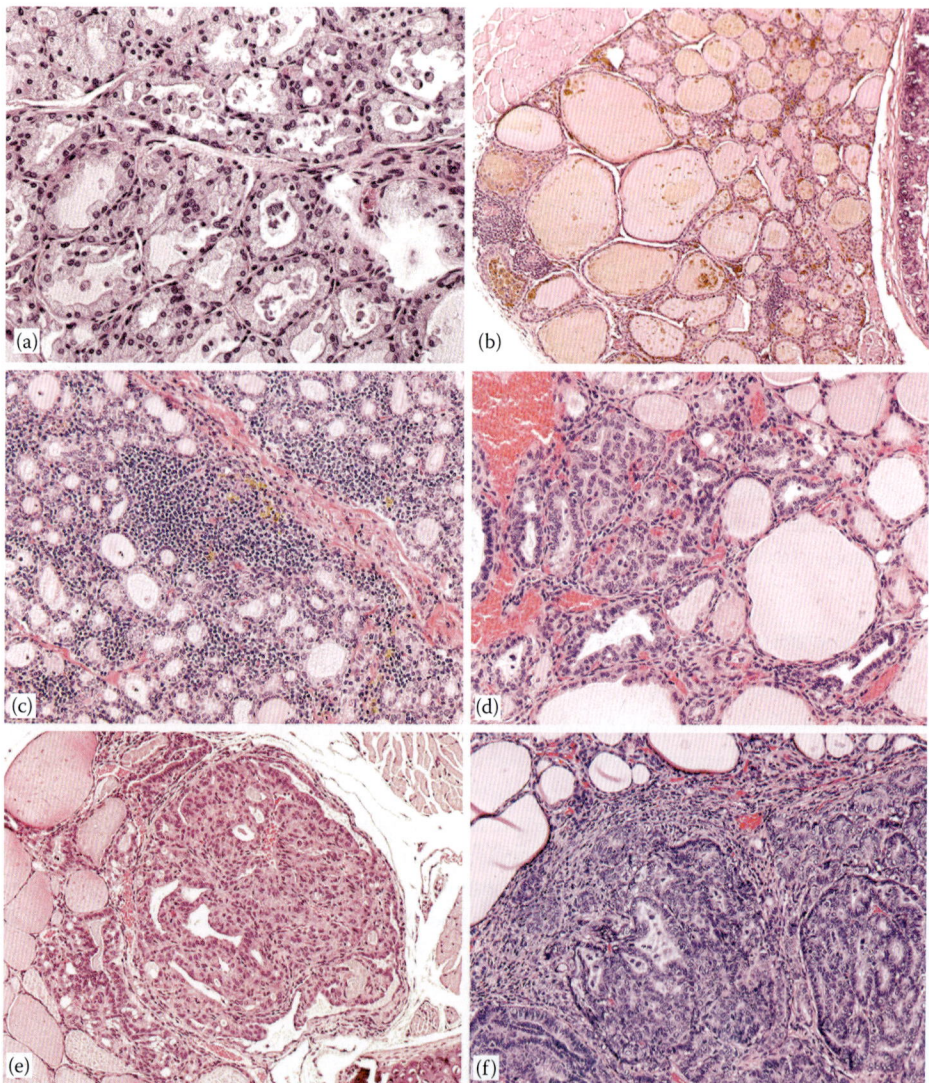

FIGURE 17.2   (a) Diffuse follicular atrophy and degeneration in a rat; epithelial cells are irregular, with pyknotic nuclei, loss of cell–cell contact, and exfoliation into follicular lumens. (b) Diffuse follicular pigmentation and alteration of colloid tincture and multifocal granularity in a mouse. (c) Moderate to severe thyroiditis in a rat characterized by multifocal to coalescing infiltrates of lymphocytes and plasma cells. (d) Focal follicular hyperplasia in a mouse; note the small, irregular follicles composed of crowded epithelial cells containing large hyperchromatic nuclei without compression of adjacent parenchyma. (e) Thyroid follicular adenoma in a mouse; note well demarcated expansile proliferation of fairly well-differentiated follicular epithelial cells. (f) Thyroid carcinoma in a mouse; note the infiltrative nests and tubules of poorly differentiated follicular epithelial cells with large pleomorphic nuclei.

function and lead to low thyroid hormone levels can lead to atrophy. Atrophic changes may include low cuboidal to flattened follicular epithelial cells with loss of characteristic endocytosis of colloid. Follicular epithelial cells may be degenerate, with the presence of pyknotic or karyorrhectic cellular debris, or exfoliated cells within follicular lumens (Figure 17.2a). Idiopathic follicular atrophy occurs in several dog breeds and is characterized by loss of thyroid follicles with replacement by adipose tissue and minimal inflammation, without involvement of thyroid C-cells. Exposure to a variety of drugs, chemicals, and nutritional imbalances affects thyroid hormone synthesis and function and may result in atrophy of the thyroid gland. Injection of male rats with gossypol, a natural phenolic aldehyde produced by the cotton plant (*Gossypium*), results in a significant reduction of thyroid hormones and dose-related degeneration and atrophy of the thyroid gland (Rikihisa and Lin 1989).

17.3.3.3 Pigmentation and Accumulations

Pigmentation of the thyroid gland occurs with treatment by various drugs and chemicals (Figure 17.2b). Black pigmentation of the thyroid gland has been reported in rats, mice, dogs, monkeys, and humans treated with minocycline, commonly used for the treatment of acne in adolescents (Benitz et al. 1967; Enochs et al. 1993; Medeiros et al. 1984; Sanchez et al. 2004), and other tetracycline derivatives (Deichmann et al. 1964; Moller and Rausing 1980). Minocycline has been associated with altered thyroid function, and the brownish pigment that accumulates in follicles is thought to be an oxidation product of minocycline by thyroid peroxidases (Taurog et al. 1996). In rats, chronic administration of minocycline leads to thyroid dysfunction and development of follicular hyperplasia/goiter (Capen 1997). It stains with Masson–Fontana histochemical stain and is sensitive to bleaching by potassium permanganate, properties that are characteristic of melanin (Reid 1983; Tajima et al. 1985). Rats treated with clozapine, an antipsychotic medication, show a brown discoloration of the thyroid gland as a result of lipofuscin accumulation. Dark brown to black discoloration and enlargement of the thyroid in Gunn rats have been attributed to follicular epithelial accumulation of altered colloid protein, resulting from an enzymatic defect in the thyroid gland leading to abnormal colloid proteolysis (Gomba et al. 1976). Lipofuscin accumulation occurs spontaneously in older dogs, monkeys, and guinea pigs (Gordon et al. 1984), as well as in humans (Dempsey 1949; Heimann 1966). As mentioned above, lipofuscin accumulation also occurs in rats treated with clozapine and other antipsychotic agents (Sayers and Amsler 1977) and certain aniline analgesics (Pataki et al. 1975). Melanosis occurs in 60% of aging B6;129 mice, most often affecting the parathyroid gland (Haines et al. 2001).

Amyloidosis is commonly observed in the CD1 mice (and less frequently in other mouse strains as well as in hamsters) in 2-year carcinogenicity studies and is a major cause of death in this strain due to glomerular amyloid accumulation and chronic renal disease (CRD) (Frith and Chandra 1991; Majeed 1993). In severe cases, it accumulates in the thyroid and parathyroid glands, among other organs, and is characterized by a diffuse expansion of the interstitial tissues with faintly eosinophilic, amorphous material, with separation and possible atrophy and loss of thyroid follicles and/or parathyroid chief cells. Amyloid is occasionally seen in thyroid C-cell adenomas in rats (Hardisty and Boorman 1990). As a cause of CRD, amyloidosis can contribute indirectly to parathyroid hyperplasia as a result of calcium loss through the kidneys.

17.3.3.4 Inflammatory Lesions

Inflammatory lesions of the thyroid are generally uncommon in untreated laboratory animals. Mild lesions consisting of focal inflammatory foci (Figure 17.2c) may be observed sporadically in the thyroid gland of rodents, dogs, and primates, but are typically of minimal significance (La Perle and Capen 2007). They may represent extension of inflammation from adjacent tissues or are part of systemic disease, or they may occur in association with occasional follicles exhibiting cystic or degenerative changes. In rats, inflammatory lesions of the tunica media and adventitia may be seen with polyarteritis nodosa (Hardisty and Boorman 1990). A similar incidence and character of inflammatory lesions are typical for the parathyroid as well. Although most inflammatory lesions of the thyroid are mild and sporadic, an autoimmune lymphocytic thyroiditis has been recognized in dogs, some rat strains, obese strains of chickens, and marmosets, which results in hypothyroidism and morphologically resembles Hashimoto's disease in humans (Capen 2001; Conaway et al. 1985; Gosselin et al. 1981; Guzman and Radi 2007; Levy et al. 1972; Tucker 1962). The disease is characterized by the presence of circulating antithyroid autoantibodies and a diffuse or multifocal infiltrate of lymphocytes, plasma cells, and macrophages with the formation of prominent germinal centers in the thyroid gland. There is significant loss of follicular epithelial cells and colloid and the presence of enlarged follicular epithelial cells and multinucleate giant cells (Fritz et al. 1970). Squamous metaplasia may occur secondary to chronic thyroiditis in beagles (Zayed et al. 1998). In rats, the Buffalo and BioBreeding/Worchester (BB/W) strains are prone to developing lymphocytic thyroiditis spontaneously or in response to treatment with carcinogenic or immunomodulatory agents (Silverman and Rose 1974, 1975; Yanagisawa et al. 1986). Susceptibility to developing autoimmune thyroiditis varies considerably between rodent species or strains (Rose 1985). Most rat strains, including the Fischer 344 (Hardisty and Boorman 1990) and Wistar (La Perle and Capen 2007) strains, do not develop the disease; however, some resistant strains can develop the disease following whole-body radiation or other means of immunosuppression (Kitchen et al. 1979; Penhale et al. 1973). In dogs, the condition is most common in the beagle and may be familial as in humans (Capen 2001; Musser and Graham 1968). Minimal to mild amounts of lymphocytic inflammation in the thyroid and parathyroid have been reported in a few cynomolgus macaques from a large cohort of control animals, with histologic features of lymphoid follicle formation and loss of thyroid follicles resulting in a few remaining follicles lined by hypertrophied epithelium (Chamanza et al. 2010). One report characterizes inflammatory lesions in the thyroid of a cynomolgus macaque morphologically resembling Hashimotos' disease (Guzman and Radi 2007).

17.3.4 PROLIFERATIVE LESIONS

17.3.4.1 Thyroid Follicular Epithelium

Spontaneous thyroid follicular tumors are rare in rats and mice, and the majority are benign (Thomas and Williams 1999). The overall frequency in all mouse strains is approximately 1% (Thomas and Williams 1996). According to the NTP historical database (May 2011, all routes, all vehicles), in the B6C3F1 mouse strain, the incidence of follicular adenomas in males is 7/1143 (0.61%) and in females is 5/1187 (0.42%). Likewise, the incidence of follicular carcinomas is very low: 4/1143 (0.96%) in males and 6/1187 (0.51%) in females. Proliferative thyroid follicular lesions are more common in rats than in mice, and males are more prone to developing such lesions than females in response to chronic TSH stimulation (Capen 1994). The overall incidence in rats is less than 3% (Thomas and Williams 1994), and according to the NTP historical database, the incidence of thyroid follicular adenomas in the F344 rat strain is 13/1239 (1.05%) in males and 8/1186 (0.67%) in females. The incidence of follicular carcinomas in the F344 rat is 10/1239 (0.81%) in males and 5/1186 (0.42%) in females. In a study of 930 control Wistar rats, there was an incidence of thyroid follicular adenomas of 3.9% in males and 2.8% in females (Poteracki and Walsh 1998).

Follicular cell hyperplasia may be focal, multifocal/nodular, or diffuse in nature. Glands affected by diffuse hyperplasia are typically enlarged bilaterally and may be dark red to reddish-brown in color. Small focal hyperplasias may not be grossly visible. Focal or multifocal hyperplasia may arise in preexisting diffuse hyperplasia and, in a histologically normal gland, may blend imperceptibly with adjacent tissue (Figure 17.2d). Follicles may be variable in size, with maintenance of normal follicular architecture. In rodents, progression from focal or diffuse hyperplasia to adenoma is common (Capen et al. 2002). Diffuse hyperplasia is characterized by an increase in the number of follicular epithelial cells throughout both glands, often in a microfollicular pattern composed of glands lined by cuboidal epithelial cells that may show papillary infoldings or piling into glandular lumens.

Atypia is not present. Hypertrophy is characterized by increased height of follicular epithelial cells and is often associated with hyperplasia associated with chronic TSH stimulation. The height/size of the follicular epithelium reflects the hormonal activity of the thyroid gland, with more active glands containing tall columnar epithelium and inactive follicles lined by flattened or low cuboidal epithelial cells.

Follicular adenomas are reddish-brown to yellow gray in color and soft. Histologically, they are expansile, well-demarcated, unencapsulated proliferations of well-differentiated thyroid follicular epithelial cells arranged in complex branching papillary projections, dilated cystic proliferations, or solid sheets of variably sized follicles lined by one or multiple layers of well-differentiated epithelium, which compresses the adjacent normal thyroid tissue (Figure 17.2e). Compression of adjacent tissue may form a pseudocapsule. Follicular or solid patterns composed of small follicles with scant cytoplasm are termed "microfollicular," whereas those with large or irregular follicles are "macrofollicular" (Botts et al. 1991). Cells are cuboidal to columnar, with large hyperchromatic nuclei and an increased nuclear-to-cytoplasmic ratio. Mitoses are rare. Adenomas may be solitary, multiple, unilateral, or bilateral. Lesions that arise as a result of chronic TSH stimulation may progress to hormone independence, usually corresponding to progression to a more aggressive phenotype. Removal of the TSH stimulus may cause regression in hormone-dependent tumors (Capen et al. 2002). Follicular adenomas that secrete thyroid hormones may induce involution of adjacent follicles due to inhibition of TSH secretion.

Thyroid follicular carcinomas (Figure 17.2f) are very vascular, typically reddish-brown in color, and soft. Histologically, they may exhibit similar morphologic patterns as adenomas and may be well differentiated and difficult to differentiate from adenoma. Solid carcinomas may be difficult to differentiate from C-cell neoplasm but tend to have a denser cytoplasm and better-defined cell borders with a coarser chromatin pattern (Capen et al. 2002). Carcinomas tend to have a more variable or heterogeneous cellular growth pattern and may show evidence of cellular atypia and invasion of vascular, lymphatic, or adjacent thyroid gland and associated tissues. Highly malignant variants may not have recognizable follicular structures and may be associated with a scirrhous response. Carcinomas may be encapsulated and show evidence of capsular invasion. These neoplasms tend to be highly vascularized, and necrosis is common. The mitotic rate is variable but can be quite high, and distant metastases, predominantly to regional lymph nodes and lung, are uncommon. The incidence of benign and malignant tumors markedly increases when animals are fed with a low-iodine diet or are exposed to chemicals that alter thyroid hormone homeostasis. Goitrogens can increase incidence of tumors even further following administration of a mutagen.

17.3.4.2 Thyroid C-Cells

Focal and diffuse C-cell hyperplasia and adenomas are fairly common lesions in aged rats (Botts et al. 1991; Hardisty and Boorman 1990). Conversely, C-cell proliferative lesions are uncommon in the mouse. C-cell hyperplasia may be focal, multifocal, or diffuse. Focal hyperplastic lesions may be difficult to differentiate from small C-cell adenomas and are composed of clusters of well-differentiated polygonal to round cells with abundant pale cytoplasm and central round nuclei (Figure 17.3a). Hyperplastic foci may be variably compressive, making differentiation even more difficult. Diffuse C-cell hyperplasia is characterized by an increase in histologically normal C-cells distributed relatively uniformly between follicles (Figure 17.3b). Atypia is generally not present in hyperplasia but may be observed in adenomas. In humans, C-cell hyperplasia may be associated with multiple endocrine neoplasia (MEN) and the development of C-cell medullary carcinoma (La Perle and Capen 2007). When associated with hypercalcemia or hyperparathyroidism, C-cell hyperplasia is typically diffuse in nature. In humans and rats, when associated with the development of neoplasia, hyperplasia tends to be diffuse and nodular and associated with increased serum calcitonin levels. A vitamin D–deficient diet is associated with a decreased incidence of C-cell tumors, whereas an increase in proliferative C-cell lesions is seen in animals on a high-protein diet.

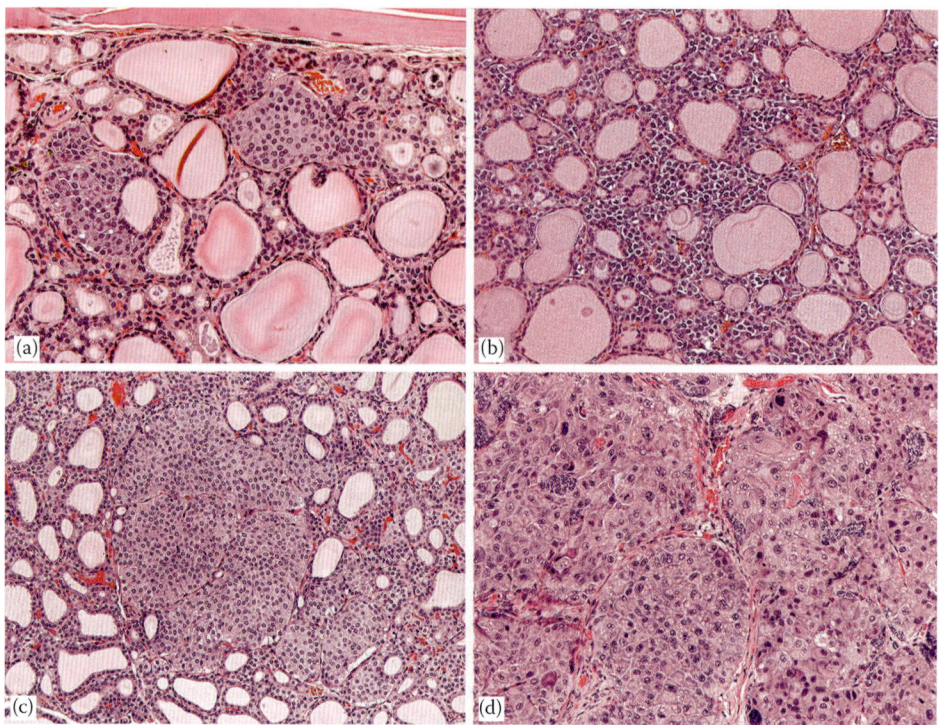

FIGURE 17.3 (a) Focal C-cell hyperplasia in a rat; note multiple discrete foci of morphologically normal C-cells expanding the interstitium. (b) Diffuse C-cell hyperplasia in a rat; the interstitium is expanded diffusely by increased numbers of well-differentiated C-cells. (c) Cell adenoma in a rat composed of sheets and lobules of well-differentiated C-cells, mildly compressing the adjacent parenchyma. (d) C-cell carcinoma characterized by infiltrative lobules of poorly differentiated C-cells exhibiting marked anitocytosis and aniso-karyosis, multinucleated cells, and occasional mitoses.

C-cell adenomas are very common in aged F344 rats and occur more frequently in males than in females (Capen et al. 2002; Hardisty and Boorman 1990). The NTP historical database indicates that spontaneous C-cell adenomas occur at an incidence of 191/1239 (15.42%) in males and 144/1186 (12.14%) in females. C-cell adenomas have not been reported in the B6C3F1 mouse (NTP historical controls, May 2011). In a study of 930 control Wistar rats, the incidence of thyroid C-cell adenoma was 5.8% in males and 8.4% in females (Poteracki and Walsh 1998). Grossly, these tumors are typically white to whitish yellow in color with a firm consistency. As with follicular adenomas, C-cell adenomas can be single, multiple, unilateral, or bilateral and are often expansile, causing compression of adjacent parenchyma, but do not invade (Figure 17.3c). Neoplastic cells are arranged in clusters or sheets, with scant stroma, and are typically very well differentiated and unencapsulated. Historically, the distinction between focal hyperplasia and adenoma has been designated by size; those lesions less than five follicles in diameter are considered hyperplasias, whereas larger lesions are considered adenomas. However, features of compression, atypia, and other features of neoplasia should be taken into consideration when differentiating large focal hyperplasias from smaller adenomas. The presence of amyloid, diagnostic in human tumors, is very infrequent in rodents (Capen et al. 2002).

Spontaneous C-cell (medullary) carcinomas are reported in the F344 rat at a low incidence: 28/1239 (2.26%) in males and 14/1186 (1.18%) in females. These tumors are exceedingly rare in B6C3F1 mice, as only one (in a male mouse) has been reported in the NTP database. C-cell carcinomas are firm in consistency, whitish-yellow to pale tan, and poorly vascularized. Similar to adenomas, C-cell carcinomas may be unilateral or bilateral. Cells are arranged in sheets, cords, and lobules separated by a fine fibrovascular stroma and may appear well differentiated and indistinguishable from adenomas, or pleomorphic with frequent mitoses (Figure 17.3d). Poorly differentiated tumors may have a spindyloid appearance and exhibit weak immunoreactivity for calcitonin (DeLellis et al. 1979, 1987). Evidence of local invasion or distant metastases to regional lymph nodes and lung may be observed. Proliferative lesions of C-cells have been described in multiple species, including dogs, bulls, cats, rats, mice, and hamsters (Capen and Black 1974; DeLellis et al. 1979; Leav et al. 1976; Van Zwieten et al. 1983). In rats, the Long–Evans strain develops C-cell hyperplasia that progresses to neoplasia in a similar fashion as the familial disease in humans that is part of the MEN syndrome, as a result of mutation of the Ret proto-oncogene (Wilhelm and Prinz 2004). Chemically induced C-cell tumors are very rare and have been associated with a number of NTP chemicals in F344 rats, including 2,4-diaminoanisole sulfate, 4,4′-methylenedianiline dihydrochloride, 1,5-naphthalenediamine, phosphamidon, stannous chloride, tetrachlorvinphos, and ziram.

17.3.4.3 Mechanisms of Chemically Induced Thyroid Follicular Hyperplasia and Neoplasia

There are numerous drugs, chemicals, and physiologic alterations that increase tumor development in rodents. When extrapolating data from carcinogenicity studies in rats and mice to humans, one must remember that there are significant species differences in thyroid hormone synthesis, transport, and metabolism in rodents compared to humans that influence tumor development in rodent species (Capen 1994; Capen and Martin 1989a; McClain 1995; Thomas and Williams 1999). In general, rats are more sensitive to developing proliferative lesions of the thyroid gland than mice and markedly more sensitive than humans in response to exposure to drugs and other compounds. Furthermore, male rats are more sensitive than females due to higher circulating levels of TSH. The increased incidence of proliferative thyroid lesions in rodents is related, in part, to their increased sensitivity to TSH stimulation due to species-specific differences in thyroid hormone half-life and serum protein binding and transport. In addition, differences in thyroid hormone metabolism play a role in thyroid proliferation in rodents compared to humans.

The plasma half-life of T4 is significantly shorter in rats (12–24 h) than in humans (5–9 days). This results in increased turnover of thyroid hormones in rodents, with serum TSH being 25-fold higher in rodents than in humans, with subsequent increased stimulation of thyroid follicular epithelial cells (McClain 1995). There are significant differences between rodents and humans in serum protein transport of thyroid hormones. Rodents (as well as birds, amphibians, and fish) lack thyroxine-binding globulin (TBG), which in dogs, humans, and NHPs is a high-affinity binding protein for T4 (and to a lesser extent T3). While a majority of thyroid hormones in rodents are bound to albumin, TBG is the main binding protein for T4 in primates. The binding affinity of TBG for T4 is markedly higher than that of albumin or prealbumin (1000-fold greater), the major transport proteins in rodents (Capen 1994). T3 is transported bound to TBG and albumin in dogs, NHPs, and humans and to albumin only in rats and mice (Capen 1994). This results in more rapid turnover of thyroid hormones in rodents, with increased TSH stimulation on follicular epithelial cells (Alison et al. 1994; Capen 1997; McClain 1995; Thomas and Williams 1999). This higher activity in rodents is also reflected in the histologic appearance of the thyroid gland, that is, small follicles with relatively small amounts of colloid and cuboidal epithelium, with larger follicles containing more colloids located more peripherally, in contrast to primate thyroid glands in which the entire structure is composed of large, distended follicles containing abundant colloid, lined by flattened follicular epithelium (McClain 1992).

Chronic TSH stimulation of the rodent thyroid gland is a major mechanism of thyroid follicular hyperplasia and neoplasia in rodents. While excessive TSH stimulation alone is enough to induce high incidences of thyroid tumors in rodents (Capen 1997), differences in xenobiotic metabolism significantly affect the proliferative response of the thyroid gland to various drugs and chemicals in rodents compared to humans. While there are few direct-acting thyroid carcinogens in laboratory animals, several nongenotoxic compounds, including natural goitrogens, drugs, environmental chemicals, and other agents, significantly influence the development of proliferative lesions in rodent thyroid. The common mechanism of increased thyroid hyperplasia, hypertrophy, and tumorigenesis is chronic stimulation of the thyroid by TSH due to alterations in the balance of thyroid hormones and disruption of the negative feedback system of the thyroid. Virtually all compounds that induce thyroid follicular tumors in rodents have been shown to interfere with this negative feedback system (Thomas and Williams 1999). Any compound that interferes with thyroid hormone synthesis, secretion, or metabolism will significantly impair the hypothalamic–pituitary–thyroid hormone axis and potentially result in thyroid follicular hyperplasia and tumorigenesis.

17.3.4.4 Interference with Thyroid Function by Goitrogenic Compounds

Thyroid follicular hyperplasia (goiter) may occur in all species and results from iodine-deficient diets, iodide excess, or goitrogenic compounds that interfere with thyroid hormone synthesis. Goitrogenic compounds elicit their effects through interference with thyroid hormone synthesis, secretion, excretion, or peripheral metabolism of thyroid hormones (Capen 1994), leading to decreased T3 and T4 levels in the circulation, with a compensatory increase in TSH secretion and stimulation of thyroid follicular epithelial cells. Iodine-deficient diets lead to chronic low levels of circulating thyroxine, which induces the feedback mechanism of the hypothalamic–pituitary–thyroid axis, resulting in secretion of TSH (Axelrad and Leblond 1955). Xenobiotic compounds that alter any step in the synthesis, secretion, or metabolism of thyroid hormones can lead to goiter or neoplasia in susceptible species.

17.3.4.4.1 Inhibition of Thyroid Hormone Synthesis

Inhibition of synthesis of thyroid hormones occurs in rodents exposed to compounds that interfere with either iodine uptake (trapping) by the thyroid gland, which is the first step in thyroid hormone synthesis, or inhibition of thyroid peroxidase (organification), the second step in thyroid hormone synthesis (Alison et al. 1994; Capen 1997). Interference with uptake of iodine by the thyroid gland occurs in rodents exposed to anions that act as competitive inhibitors of iodide transport, including perchlorate, thiocyanate, and pertechnetate (Capen 1994; Crofton 2008). Perchlorate competes with iodine for uptake by the thyroid gland, which results in the decreased availability of iodine for the thyroid gland, which in turn results in hypothyroidism (Yu et al. 2002). The kinetics of inhibition of iodine uptake by perchlorate in humans and rodents is very similar; however, species differences in thyroid hormone biology prevent extrapolation between rodents and humans in terms of downstream adverse effects in humans (Miller et al. 2009).

Interference with thyroid peroxidase is caused by various thionamides (thiouracil, thiourea, propylthiouracil, methimazole, aminotriazole, carbimazole), aniline derivatives (sulfonamides, para-aminobenzoic acid, para-aminosalicylic acid, amphenone), and phenols (resorcinol, phloroglucinol, 2,4-dihydroxybenzoic acid) (Capen 1994; Heath and Littlefield 1984; Takayama et al. 1986; Todd 1986). Interference with organification by inhibition of thyroid peroxidase prevents the oxidation of iodide to iodine, as well as the formation of T3 and T4 by monoiodotyrosine (MIT) and diiodotyrosine (DIT) molecules (Capen 1998). Rats, mice, hamsters, pigs, and dogs are sensitive species to sulfonamide-induced thyroid hormone dysfunction, whereas guinea pigs, NHPs, and humans are resistant, making the thyroid gland in rats and mice more susceptible to proliferative lesions through this mechanism (Alison et al. 1994; Capen 1994; McClain 1995). However, thiocarbamide drugs (methimazole, propylthiouracil, carbimazole) are used to block thyroid hormone synthesis in hyperthyroid patients, and occupational exposure to workers exposed to chemicals with similar chemical structure (aminotriazole herbicide, thiourea) can cause hypothyroidism (Baccarelli et al. 2000; Hood et al. 1999).

17.3.4.4.2 Inhibition of Thyroid Hormone Secretion

Relatively few chemicals interfere with the secretion of thyroid hormones. Excess dietary iodide is known to cause inhibition of thyroid hormone synthesis in animals and humans, leading to decreased thyroid hormone levels, goiter, and hypothyroidism (Capen 1994). Iodide excess interferes with uptake of iodine by the thyroid gland and with normal colloid proteolysis by decreasing lysosomal protease activity, thereby blocking the release of T3 and T4 from thyroglobulin. Excess iodide also disrupts the peroxidation of iodide to iodine and formation of DIT from MIT (Capen and Martin 1989a). Similarly, lithium interferes with thyroid hormone release in humans and animals through inhibition of cAMP release necessary for colloid droplet formation, leading to hypothyroidism and goiter. As previously discussed, various pigments resulting from metabolism of compounds such as minocycline, other tetracycline derivatives, or the antipsychotic clozapine accumulate in the thyroid gland and alter thyroid function. Inhibition of thyroid hormone secretion due to abnormal colloid proteolysis in Gunn rats leads to altered thyroid function (Gomba et al. 1976).

17.3.4.4.3 Alterations in Thyroid Hormone Metabolism and Clearance

Xenobiotic compounds that increase the rate of peripheral metabolism of thyroid hormones include inhibitors of 5′-deiodinase and hepatic microsomal enzyme inducers. Inhibition of 5′-deiodinase, the major enzyme responsible for conversion of T4 to active T3, leads initially to increases in serum T4. This is followed by conversion of T4 by the same enzyme, 5-deiodinase, leading to marked increases in the inactive form of T3, reverse T3 (rT3). Furthermore, there is accumulation of rT3 resulting from inhibition of 5′-deiodinase due to an inability to further degrade rT3 to DIT (Alison et al. 1994; Capen and Martin 1989a). Low circulating levels of active T3 results in stimulation of the pituitary to secrete TSH, resulting in chronic stimulation of the thyroid follicular epithelium, hyperplasias, and tumorigenesis. Feeding of the nongenotoxic food color additive FD&C Red No. 3 (erythrosine), a well-known inhibitor of 5′-deiodinase and rat thyroid carcinogen, is associated with follicular epithelial hyperplasia and benign adenomas in male rats, but not mice or gerbils (Alison et al. 1994; Borzelleca et al. 1987; Capen and Martin 1989a). Several iodinated compounds (tetraiodofluoresceine, amiodarone, iodinated contrast media), UV inhibitors (octyl-methoxycinnamate), propylthiouracil, and a selenium-deficient diet have also been shown to inhibit 5′-deiodinase activity (Crofton 2008; McClain 1995).

Induction of hepatic microsomal enzymes by xenobiotics is a well-known phenomenon in rodents that occurs due to species-specific differences in the metabolism of thyroid hormones. Chemical induction of microsomal hepatic enzymes causes increased metabolism and excretion of thyroid hormones. Chronic administration of these compounds leads to persistent decreases in serum thyroid hormones, with stimulation of the hypothalamic–pituitary–thyroid axis, and subsequent TSH stimulation of the thyroid gland and increased incidence of proliferative lesions (Alison et al. 1994; Capen 1997; Hood et al. 1999; Richardson and Klaassen 2010a,b; Yoshizawa et al. 2007). Compounds associated with induction of thyroid hormone metabolism by hepatic microsomal enzymes in rats include CNS drugs (phenobarbital, benzodiazepines), calcium channel blockers (nicardipine, bepridil), steroids (spironolactone), retinoids, chlorinated hydrocarbons (chlordane, dichlorodiphenyltrichloroethane (DDT), 2,3,7,8-tetrachlorodibenzodioxin (TCDD)), and polyhalogenated biphenyls (PCBs) (Capen 1994). An increased turnover of thyroid hormones leading to sustained TSH increase through this mechanism occurs predominantly in rodents because UDP-glucuronyltransferases, the enzymes responsible for T3 and T4 glucuronidation and biliary excretion, are easily induced in rodent species (Capen 1997; Hood et al. 1999, 1999; McClain 1989; Richardson and Klaassen 2010b). Chronic exposure to TCDD induces a dose-related increase in thyroid follicular adenomas in male Osborne–Mendel rats and B6C3F1 mice and follicular cell hypertrophy in F344 rats (Yoshizawa et al. 2007, 2010). Furthermore, the high turnover of thyroid hormones in rodent species due to differences in half-life and serum protein binding and transport make the rodent thyroid gland markedly more sensitive to development of proliferative lesions due to chronic TSH stimulation.

Compounds inducing hepatic microsomal enzymes in the liver, such as phenobarbital, PCBs, and pregnenolone-16a-carbonitrile (PCN), also lead to increased metabolism and excretion of thyroid hormones (Hood et al. 1999; Vansell et al. 2004). Phenobarbital induces follicular cell hypertrophy and hyperplasia and increases thyroid weight in rodents through increased hepatic clearance of T4 due to glucuronidation. PCBs increase metabolism and excretion of thyroid hormones to a greater extent than phenobarbital and also interfere with normal colloid proteolysis and secretion of thyroid hormones, making them more potent inducers of thyroid proliferative lesions (Alison et al. 1994; McClain 1989). PCN and phenobarbital increase T4 glucuronidation and also increase serum levels of TSH, resulting in thyroid follicular proliferation (Vansell et al. 2004). Similar effects on the NHP thyroid gland are not observed with inducers of hepatic microsomal enzymes (Waechter et al. 1999), and although studies in humans exposed to hepatic enzyme inducers show conflicting evidence of alterations in thyroid function (Baccarelli et al. 2000), overall epidemiologic studies have failed to show a connection between exposure to hepatic microsomal inducers and an increased risk of thyroid tumorigenesis (Curran and DeGroot 1991; Olsen et al. 1989; Shirts et al. 1986; Yoshizawa et al. 2007).

The development of thyroid follicular hypertrophy, hyperplasia, and subsequently adenomas or carcinomas through chronic TSH stimulation due to interference with one or more steps of thyroid hormone synthesis, secretion, or metabolism is typically associated with nongenotoxic compounds. Furthermore, a no observable adverse effect level (NOAEL) can be established in rodents exposed to such compounds, indicating that there is a threshold effect on the pituitary–thyroid axis, below which the risk for thyroid neoplasia is minimal (Paynter et al. 1988). The rodent thyroid is markedly more sensitive to the tumorigenic effects of chronic TSH stimulation, due to differences in thyroid hormone binding and metabolism, than the NHP or human thyroid gland. Even in areas where there is severe iodine deficiency and endemic goiter reported in human subjects, there is no evidence of increased risk for thyroid neoplasia. These data indicate that compounds that cause thyroid hormone axis imbalance leading to chronic TSH stimulation appear to have little bearing on human thyroid carcinogenesis (Alison et al. 1994; Capen 1997). It has been suggested that TSH stimulation of the thyroid would likely result in thyroid tumorigenesis only if combined with other metabolic or immunologic abnormalities. Furthermore, such compounds would likely have a significant toxicologic effect in humans before exposure would increase risk for thyroid tumorigenesis (McClain 1995).

17.3.4.5 Direct Acting Thyroid Mutagens

A majority of chemicals inducing thyroid tumorigenesis in rodents are nongenotoxic and function through the above mechanisms, while tumorigenesis induced by genotoxic compounds is uncommon. However, there are a number of mutagens that have been used to induce thyroid tumors in laboratory animals. Aromatic amines, polycyclic hydrocarbons, azo dyes, dichlorobenzene, 2-acetylaminofluorene, nitrosamines, and nitrosoureas have all been used to induce thyroid tumors in rodents (McClain 1989; Thomas and Williams 1999). A significant mutagenic inducer of thyroid neoplasms in humans and laboratory animals is irradiation (x-ray or iodine radioisotopes). Studies have indicated an increased incidence of thyroid neoplasia in children in areas of nuclear accidents and who are exposed to a high degree of irradiation, such as at the Chernobyl nuclear power plant (Jargin 2011), the Marshall islands (Land et al. 2010), and Hiroshima/Nagasaki (Nakachi et al. 2008). Irradiation has a mutagenic effect on thyroid follicular epithelium as well as growth-promoting effects due to TSH release from the pituitary. Follicular carcinomas induced by irradiation occur at a higher rate in males than females, whereas castration reduces the incidence in irradiated males versus females (Capen 1994). Goitrogens, including dietary deficiency or excess of iodine, are powerful promoters of thyroid carcinogenesis and have been used to significantly increase the induction of thyroid neoplasia (Kanno et al. 1992; McClain 1995; Ohshima and Ward 1986; Thomas and Williams 1999).

17.4 PARATHYROID GLAND

17.4.1 Normal Structure and Function

The parathyroid gland is the major organ regulating calcium and phosphorous homeostasis in the body. Working in concert with thyroid C-cells, the parathyroid is responsible for maintaining physiologic levels of calcium and phosphorous necessary for adequate bone integrity and basic metabolic processes. Diseases or compounds that cause alterations in calcium homeostasis can alter the response of the parathyroid, resulting in proliferative lesions including tumorigenesis.

The functional unit of the parathyroid gland is the chief cell. These cells are responsible for the production of parathyroid hormone (PTH), which is a critical hormone responsible for maintaining calcium homeostasis, acting in concert with calcitonin produced by C-cells of the thyroid gland. By TEM, chief cells contain numerous electron-dense, ovoid secretory granules, 100–300 nm in diameter, surrounded by a limiting membrane (Hardisty and Boorman 1999). These granules contain small amounts of preformed PTH that may be immediately released, but the parathyroid can synthesize and secrete large amounts of hormone on demand. Rats have relatively few of these secretory granules, while they are numerous in the mouse (Capen and Rosol 1989). Active chief cells have increased numbers of organelles and secretory granules, resulting in increased cytoplasmic electron density. In some species such as dogs and rats, multinucleate cells have also been observed in active glands (Capen 1983; Meuten et al. 1984; Oksanen 1980) (Figure 17.4a). Quiescent chief cells, also called "clear cells," occur in small clusters or are singly interspersed among chief cells and are larger with more abundant pale cytoplasm and large hyperchromatic nuclei (Hardisty and Boorman 1999). These cells, also termed "oxyphil cells" in humans and other species, including the bovine and horse (Greco and Stabenfeldt 2007; La Perle and Capen 2007), tend to increase in number with age, by TEM exhibit poorly developed organelles and few secretory granules but numerous large mitochondria compared to chief cells, are not responsive to changes in serum calcium, and are thought to possibly reflect age-related changes of normal chief cells (Capen and Rosol 1989).

17.4.2 CALCITONIN AND PARATHYROID HORMONE

Calcium and phosphorous homeostasis is regulated by key hormones from the thyroid and parathyroid, calcitonin and parathyroid hormone, respectively. Parathyroid hormone (parathormone/PTH), an 84-amino acid polypeptide, is the primary hormone responsible for calcium homeostasis. It is rapidly secreted from secretory granules in parathyroid chief cells in response to relatively small decreases in serum calcium (Capen and Rosol 1989). PTH has a short half-life (2–5 min) and acts rapidly on target cells in the bone and kidney, and also indirectly on the intestine, to increase levels of calcium and decrease phosphorous in extracellular fluids (Greco and Stabenfeldt 2007). PTH acts on bone to promote bone resorption through effects on osteoclast and osteoblast function, and on the distal tubules and loop of Henle of the kidney to increase renal calcium and magnesium reabsorption. Chronic secretion of PTH results in increased numbers of osteoclasts and osteoblasts in bone and ongoing bone remodeling with increased bone resorption as well as formation. In addition, PTH also decreases renal phosphorous, sodium, and bicarbonate reabsorption in proximal tubules by inhibiting sodium-dependent phosphate cotransport in the brush border, leading to increased excretion in the urine (Capen 1983). PTH mediates activation of vitamin D3 in the kidney through increasing activity of alpha-1 hydroxylase, the enzyme responsible for hydroxylating (activating) inactive vitamin D (25-hydroxyvitamin D, calcitriol) in the proximal tubules. Increased activation of vitamin D by the actions of PTH increases absorption of calcium from the intestinal tract. In response to normalization of serum calcium, there is a negative feedback on the parathyroid gland through activation of the calcium sensing receptor (CaSR) on parathyroid chief cells that inhibits PTH secretion, gene expression, and chief cell proliferation and promotes calcitonin secretion from thyroid C-cells (Kantham et al. 2009).

Calcitonin, a 32-amino acid peptide, has the opposite effect on blood calcium. It is present within secretory granules of C-cells of the thyroid gland, is released in response to increased levels of calcium in extracellular tissues, and plays a compensatory role acting as a counterbalance to PTH. Calcitonin decreases serum calcium and promotes movement into cells, primarily through effects on bone; it decreases bone resorption by inhibition of osteoclast function and increases phosphate mobilization to bone. Additionally, it blocks renal reabsorption of calcium and phosphorous and increases their excretion, and it decreases intestinal absorption by inhibiting gastrin and gastric acid secretion (Greco and Stabenfeldt 2007). Physiologic release of calcitonin regularly occurs as a result of stimulation by gastrointestinal hormones (gastrin, pancreozymin, glucagon) following meals to prevent postprandial hypercalcemia and protects the maternal skeleton during pregnancy against excessive calcium and phosphorous loss (Capen and Martin 1989a). Although evidence is lacking that xenobiotics affect the functions of calcitonin, C-cell function may be altered by any compound interfering with calcium homeostasis.

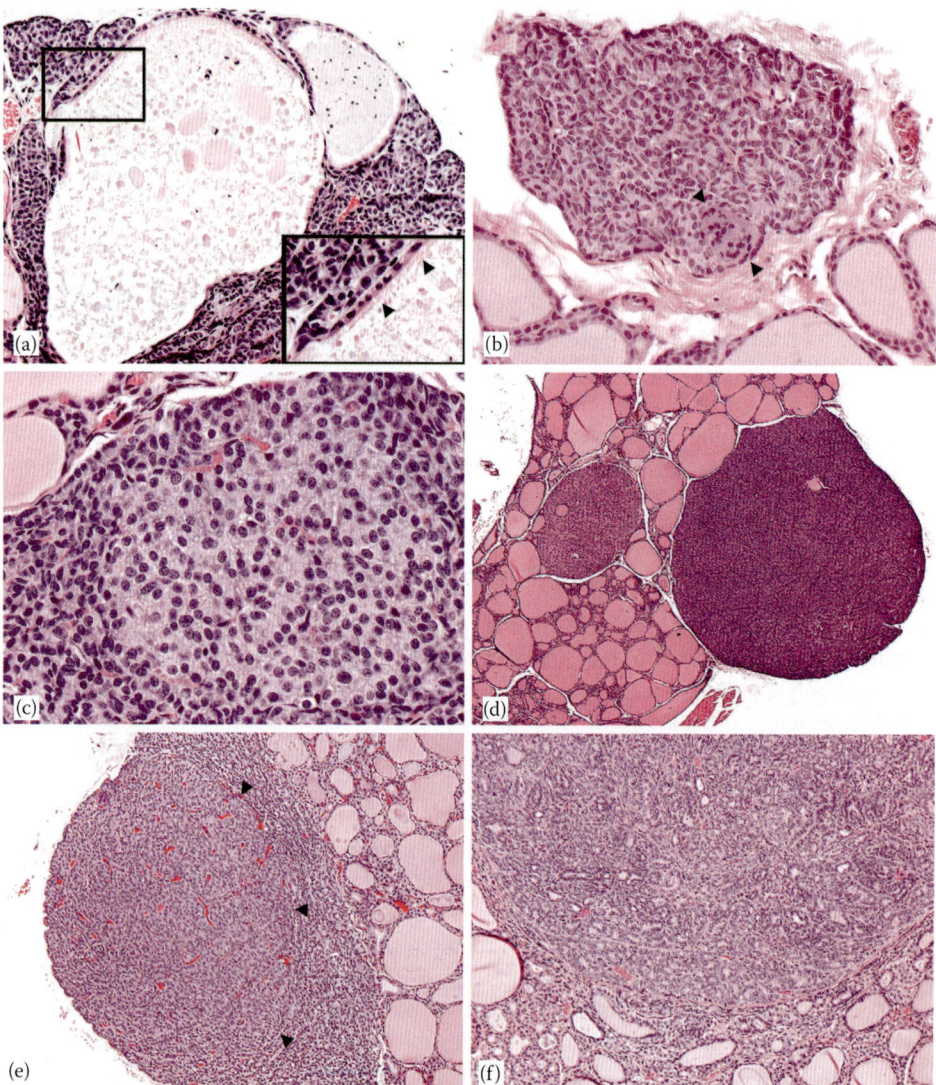

FIGURE 17.4   (a) Parathyroid cyst lined by ciliated epithelium in a rat (inset, arrowheads). (b) Multinucleate syncytial cell in a rat (arrowheads) characterized by fusion of multiple parathyroid chief cells. (c) Focal chief cell hypertrophy in a rat; note enlarged cells with increased lightly basophilic cytoplasm and well-differentiated nuclei, without compression of the adjacent parenchyma. (d) Diffuse hyperplasia of parathyroid in a rat causing marked expansion of the gland above the thyroid surface; note adjacent thyroid C-cell adenoma on the left. (e) Parathyroid adenoma in a rat composed of expansile clusters of well-differentiated chief cells causing compression of adjacent parathyroid parenchyma (arrowheads). (f) Parathyroid carcinoma in a rat composed of palisading rows, tubules, and rosettes of poorly differentiated chief cells.

17.4.3   VITAMIN D_3

The third primary hormone responsible for maintenance of calcium in the body is vitamin D_3 (1,25-dihydroxyvitamin D) or cholecalciferol. Vitamin D_3 is required for calcium absorption from the proximal small intestine and phosphorous absorption from the distal small intestine. This hormone is produced entirely in the skin through conversion of a provitamin, 7-dehydrocholesterol, to inactive vitamin D3 (25-hydroxyvitamin D) by cleavage via exposure to ultraviolet light in the epidermis. Inactive vitamin D3 is hydrolyzed in the liver and then in the kidney to the active molecule, 1,25-dihydroxyvitamin D. As low levels of calcium in the blood stimulate PTH secretion, this increases synthesis of vitamin D3 and, subsequently, intestinal absorption of calcium from the intestine. While PTH increases vitamin D3 synthesis, calcitonin inhibits its activation in the kidney. Decreased production of vitamin D3 due to CRD leads to decreased absorption of calcium from the intestinal tract. Alterations in vitamin D3 levels can have a significant impact on calcium homeostasis.

17.4.4 Nonproliferative Lesions

17.4.4.1 Congenital Lesions

Ectopic parathyroid tissue may be observed in all species in the anterior neck or, because of its close proximity during development, within the thymus. Conversely, ectopic thymus may also be present within or adjacent to the parathyroid glands. Parathyroid tumors that arise within the precardiac mediastinum are derived from ectopic parathyroid tissue (Rosol and Capen 1989). Parathyroid cysts have been reported as spontaneous lesions in dogs and rats and occasionally other species. These occur as a result of persistence of the duct connecting the parathyroid to the thymic primordium during development. Cysts are lined by cuboidal to columnar epithelial cells that may be ciliated (Capen and Rosol 1989) (Figure 17.4b). Parathyroid cysts have been reported in carcinogenicity studies in rats exposed to dihydrotachysterol and calcium acetate secondary to necrosis of chief cells and subsequent retention of necrosis cellular debris and secretory material (Hardisty and Boorman 1999). Chamanza et al. (2010) showed that cysts of the parathyroid and thyroid glands as well as ectopic thymus within the parathyroid or thyroid glands were among the most common spontaneous lesions in a series of 570 control cynomolgus macaques used in toxicology studies (Chamanza et al. 2010). Congenital thyroid cysts and dilated cystic follicles were twice as common in males as in females.

17.4.4.2 Inflammatory Lesions

Mild lymphocytic infiltrates have been reported in the parathyroid (and thyroid) gland in cynomolgus macaques (Chamanza et al. 2010). Similar to the thyroid, diffuse lymphocytic parathyroiditis is associated with infiltrates of lymphocytes, plasma cells, and macrophages, and in severe cases, parathyroid tissue is eventually replaced by lymphocytes and fibrosis.

17.4.4.3 Atrophy/Degeneration

Atrophy of the parathyroid gland may occur secondary to direct injury (such as lymphocytic parathyroiditis) (Lupulescu et al. 1968) or neoplasia (including parathyroid tumors), or by hormonal factors such as chronic hypercalcemia (Goedegebuure and Hazewinkel 1986). While the parathyroid gland is an uncommon target for direct injury by chemicals, any compound that alters calcium homeostasis may result in changes in this organ. Animals with diffuse lymphocytic parathyroiditis may have significant degeneration and subsequent atrophy of the parathyroids, leading to loss of chief cells and replacement by fibrosis (Lupulescu et al. 1968). Functional parathyroid tumors, usually adenomas, may secrete large amounts of PTH. The presence of such a tumor in one parathyroid gland can lead to diffuse atrophy of the adjacent and contralateral parathyroids as a result of negative feedback on the chief cells (Rosol and Capen 1989). Finally, cancer-associated hypercalcemia may be associated with hypercalcemic states and atrophy of the parathyroids. Primary hematologic malignancies cause local bone destruction and resorption leading to increased serum calcium levels. Similarly, solid tumors that metastasize to bone may contribute to significant hypercalcemia through bony remodeling (Komatsu et al. 2005). Lastly, humoral hypercalcemia of malignancy (HHM) is associated with certain tumors that secrete a parathyroid hormone-related peptide (PTH-rP) that promotes hypercalcemia through actions on bone, kidney, and the intestine (Rosol and Capen 1989). All of these conditions result in atrophic changes that include loss of cytoplasm, reduction in organelles and secretory granules, and increased lipid and lipofuscin deposition in the cytoplasm (La Perle and Capen 2007). With marked atrophy, parathyroid glands may be undetectable or reduced such that only a small number of inactive chief cells remain interspersed in the connective tissue stroma and abundant adipose tissue. Vacuolar changes in parathyroid chief cells have been observed in rats following acute, subchronic, and chronic exposures to 2,2′-methylenebis (4-ethyl-6-tert-butylphenol), a synthetic antioxidant (Takagi et al. 1992, 1996).

17.4.5 Proliferative Lesions

17.4.5.1 Chief Cell Hyperplasia

Parathyroid hyperplasia is usually due to disorders of calcium regulation (Botts et al. 1991). Hyperplasia is common with increasing age in F344 rats, usually as a result of chronic progressive nephropathy (CPN), particularly in males (Hardisty and Boorman 1990). Focal hyperplasia, less common than diffuse, may be unilateral or bilateral and may arise within preexisting diffuse hyperplasia. Focal hyperplastic lesions may be slightly compressive or merge imperceptibly with surrounding normal tissue (Figure 17.4c). Large focal hyperplastic lesions may be difficult to differentiate from small adenomas, and the only discriminating factor to separate the lesions may be the lack of compression by hyperplasias (Botts et al. 1991). Focal hyperplasia is uncommon in laboratory species and usually nonfunctional (Rosol and Capen 1989). Conversely, bilateral, diffuse chief cell hyperplasia and hypertrophy, secondary to nephropathy, are the most common parathyroid lesions in the F344 rat and very common in hamsters and some strains of mice, where they are most often associated with renal amyloidosis (Frith and Chandra 1991; Hardisty and Boorman 1999; Pour 1983). Parathyroid glands are rarely targets of toxicity by chemicals, but administration of compounds that interfere with calcium homeostasis or a chronic low-calcium diet can result in chronic stimulation of chief cells and diffuse hyperplasia. Hyperplasia due to dysregulation of calcium homeostasis or renal disease is bilateral and diffuse and is not associated with progression to neoplasia (Rosol and Capen 1989). With diffuse hyperplasia, there is global enlargement of the gland, with extension beyond the surface of the thyroid gland histologically (Figure 17.4d). Chief cells are polygonal, with increased amounts of lightly eosinophilic to pale vacuolated cytoplasm and round to fusiform nuclei. Cells may appear deeply basophilic to eosinophilic to clear in tincture depending on their hormonal activity. Aside from chronic kidney disease, chief cell hyperplasia has been associated with irradiation, various chemicals and hormones (deoxycorticosterone acetate, alloxan, calcitonin), and other physiologic alterations (adrenalectomy, nephrectomy) (Hardisty and Boorman 1990).

17.4.5.2 Chief Cell Neoplasms

Parathyroid gland tumors are uncommon in all species but occur with low incidence in dogs, rats, mice, and Syrian hamsters (Rosol and Capen 1989). There are little data on the neoplastic response of the parathyroid gland to chemical exposure. In fact, there have been no studies in the NTP that have confirmed a carcinogenic response in the parathyroid gland in response to chemical exposure in rats or mice (Hardisty and Boorman 1990, 1999; Huff et al. 1991). Similar to chief cell hyperplasia, adenomas are occasionally seen in rats as a result of chronic calcium loss due to nephropathy. In terms of spontaneous chief cell adenomas, according to the NTP historical control database, F344 rats have an incidence of 5/1186 (0.42%) in males and 5/1123 (0.45%) in females. In a study of 930 control Wistar rats, parathyroid adenomas were only seen in males (1.9%) (Poteracki and Walsh 1998). Spontaneous parathyroid adenomas have not been reported in B6C3F1 mice at the NTP. Adenomas in rats are reddish-brown to whitish-gray in color, encapsulated, and solitary, causing enlargement of a single lobe. Histologically, they are typically expansile and compressive, composed of sheets and packets of densely arranged, well-differentiated chief cells separated by a fine fibrovascular stroma (Figure 17.4e). The cytologic appearance of chief cells may be similar to hyperplasias and depends on the functional state of the tumor. Nonfunctional tumors tend to be composed of sheets, lobules, or acini of cuboidal to polygonal cells, whereas cells of functional tumors are more densely packed into clusters, are lightly eosinophilic, and may have increased cytoplasmic volume (Rosol and Capen 1989). The cellular pattern may also be very similar to hyperplastic lesions or may be organized in a papillary, cystic, or acinar fashion. Pleomorphism and mitotic rate are generally low but may be variable. Multiple white, pinpoint foci may be observed in thyroid glands in animals with functional parathyroid adenomas; these are areas of C-cell hyperplasia responding to chronic hypercalcemia (Botts et al. 1991; Rosol and Capen 1989).

Parathyroid carcinomas are extremely rare in laboratory and domestic species. In fact, these tumors are so rare that none have been reported in the NTP rodent bioassay database. One case of parathyroid carcinoma was reported in an OFA rat (Pour et al. 1983), and a second in a Wistar rat (Pace et al. 2003), characterized by sheets and nodules of poorly differentiated and pleomorphic cells with local invasion of the capsule (Figure 17.4f).

17.4.5.3 Alterations of Calcium Homeostasis and Parathyroid Function

17.4.5.3.1 Primary Hyperparathyroidism

Primary chief cell tumors may be functional PTH-secreting lesions in humans, dogs, and cats but are usually nonfunctional in rats (Capen et al. 2002; Rosol and Capen 1989). Excessive PTH secretion from functional parathyroid tumors is independent of circulating calcium levels and results in persistent hypercalcemia, excessive renal calcium and phosphorous excretion, and excessive bony resorption. Excessive calcium excretion in the kidneys may lead to the formation of calculi, and bone resorption leads to generalized weakening and fractures of long bones or vertebrae (Capen and Rosol 1989).

Common treatments for osteoporosis in humans include hormones and drugs that inhibit osteoclast resorption and osteoblast function in the bone, including estrogens, calcitonin, and bisphosphonates (Sato et al. 2002). Treatment with recombinant PTH has been shown to reduce fractures in osteoporotic women, and recombinant PTH is the only compound that has been shown to increase bone volume and rate of bone formation and reduce fracture rate in humans (Neer et al. 2001; Sato et al. 2002). Treatment of rats with human recombinant PTH has been shown to increase bone mass and strength in the femur and vertebrae but decrease strength in the midshaft femur. However, the effects on cortical bone by PTH are species dependent. The degree of PTH effects on bone is substantially greater in rats than in humans (Vahle et al. 2002, 2008). In humans and NHPs, PTH stimulates intracortical remodeling without a significant increase in cortical bone mass. Treatment with PTH results in intracortical remodeling and increased porosity toward the endocortical surface, retaining biomechanical strength (Lotinun et al. 2004). In rats, which lack Haversian canals, bony remodeling cannot occur in cortical bone due to a lack of cortical porosity. This results in appositional formation of bone along existing endocortical and periosteal surfaces without cortical remodeling, increased bone mass, decreased marrow space, altered bone structure, and subsequent loss of strength (Lotinun et al. 2004; Vahle et al. 2002). In addition, growth plates and longitudinal skeletal growth persist throughout life in rats, as opposed to NHPs, in which by 18–30 years, growth plates close and longitudinal skeletal growth ceases (Vahle et al. 2002). Osteosarcomas and other proliferative bone lesions have been observed in rodents in long-term studies using PTH (Jolette et al. 2006; Vahle et al. 2004), whereas in NHPs, proliferative bone lesions have not been observed (Vahle 2008). The effects of PTH on bone in humans are very similar to those in NHPs, and bone lesions in rodents are thought to arise from chronic hormone receptor-mediated stimulation leading to increases in bone mass that, due to significant species differences, would not be observed in humans exposed to PTH (Vahle et al. 2002). Furthermore, the effects of PTH exposure are dose related and depend on treatment duration; exposure to PTH in humans is short term and typically well after skeletal maturity. In rodents, near lifetime exposures during skeletal maturity to high levels of PTH are not representative of human exposures (Vahle et al. 2004, 2007). The significant differences in physiology between the rodent and primate skeleton, lack of neoplastic lesions in primates, and differences in treatment duration and dose suggest that exposure of humans to PTH and PTH-like compounds for the treatment of osteoporosis holds little concern for risk of neoplasia (Hodsman et al. 2005; Vahle et al. 2007).

17.4.5.3.2   Secondary Hyperparathyroidism

Long-term dietary imbalances or CRD is a cause of diffuse parathyroid hyperplasia and secondary hyperparathyroidism (Rosol and Capen 1989). Nutritional hyperparathyroidism occurs in NHPs, dogs, cats, and laboratory rodents fed with diets that are improperly formulated. Long-term feeding of diets low in calcium or high in phosphorous or feeding New World primates housed indoors (without exposure to UV light) with diets low in vitamin D3 contributes to hypocalcemia, hyperplasia of parathyroid glands, and excessive secretion of PTH in an attempt to increase serum calcium levels, leading to secondary hyperparathyroidism (Capen 2001). Diets low in calcium obviously limit the intake of calcium ions, contributing to hypocalcemia and stimulation of the parathyroid to secrete PTH. The most common cause of secondary hyperparathyroidism is the feeding of diets high in phosphorous (La Perle and Capen 2007). Phosphorus indirectly stimulates the parathyroid gland by decreasing blood calcium levels. New World primates exhibit target organ resistance to vitamin D compared to Old World primates and humans due to a vitamin D response element-binding protein that inhibits DNA binding and downstream function of vitamin D signaling (Angelo et al. 2002; Chen et al. 2000). Therefore, these animals require extremely high amounts of vitamin D and exposure to UV light for adequate calcium absorption in order to prevent bone resorption and osteomalacia. Long-term feeding of diets high in phosphorus decreases serum calcium, leading to PTH stimulation and bone resorption. In New World primates, a diet high in phosphorus and low in calcium is associated with osteomalacia and a disease syndrome called "simian bone disease" (Liu 2002). Animals with this disorder have kyphosis, an increased incidence of fractures of long bones, and thickening of maxillary and mandibular bones with displacement of teeth.

In CRD, glomerular filtration rate (GFR) decreases as a result of loss of functional nephron mass. Decreased GFR leads to retention of phosphorus and decreased calcium reabsorption through renal tubular loss, resulting in effects due to high serum phosphorus. CRD also impairs activation of vitamin D in the kidney and, subsequently, decreases intestinal absorption of calcium. Loss of functional vitamin D and retention of phosphorus lead to hypocalcemia and chronic stimulation of the parathyroid gland, excessive PTH secretion, and mobilization of calcium from the skeleton. In dogs, this results in bone resorption with osteoblastic proliferation and deposition of poorly mineralized osteoid and fibrous connective tissue, predominantly in zones of increased bone turnover such as the facial bones, maxillae, and mandibles, resulting in loosening of teeth and the syndrome of fibrous osteodystrophy (Capen and Rosol 1989). In rats, parathyroid gland hyperplasia resulting from exacerbation of CPN by various compounds can lead to metastatic calcification of various organs, including heart, aorta, and other soft tissues (Bucher et al. 1990; Hooth et al. 2004). Several compounds evaluated by the NTP were shown to induce parathyroid chief cell hyperplasia by exacerbation of CPN in rats (secondary renal hyperparathyroidism), including dipropylene glycol, furosemide, hydrochlorothiazide, acetaminophen, quercetin, mercuric chloride, C.I. pigment red, C.I. acid orange 3, primidone, phenolphthalein, o-benzyl-p-chlorophenol, nitrofurantoin, and coumarin.

17.4.5.3.3   Pseudohyperparathyroidism (Humoral Hypercalcemia of Malignancy)

Various malignancies in humans and animals have systemic effects that mimic excess PTH secretion due to the production of a PTH-rP that acts on PTH receptors to promote hypercalcemia through bone resorption, retention of calcium and excretion of phosphorous by the kidney, increased activation of vitamin D, and increased absorption of calcium from the intestinal tract, leading to the syndrome of HHM (Rosol and Capen 1989). HHM is a well-recognized syndrome in animals (particularly dogs) and humans and is characterized by hypercalcemia, hypophosphatemia, and increased bone resorption due to secretion of PTH-rP from tumor cells (Capen 2001). Elevated PTH-rP levels are found in up to 88% of cancer patients with hypercalcemia (Komatsu et al. 2005), and HHM is the most common cause of hypercalcemia in animals (La Perle and Capen 2007). Other proteins may act synergistically with PTH-rP to promote hypercalcemia, such as TGFa, TGFb, IL1, TNFa, 1,25 dihydroxyvitamin D, and prostaglandins (Grone et al. 1992; Rosol and Capen 1989). Tumors most commonly associated with HHM in humans include squamous cell carcinoma, renal cell carcinoma, and lymphosarcoma; in dogs, it is associated with lymphosarcoma, apocrine gland adenocarcinoma of the anal sac, and other solid carcinomas (Capen et al. 2002; Rosol and Capen 1989). In vitro and rodent models have been developed to study this syndrome with clinicopathologic features similar to the disease in humans, including a rat Leydig cell tumor line, rat Walker mammary carcinosarcoma, nude mouse canine apocrine anal sac adenocarcinoma xenograft model (Grone et al. 1992; Rosol et al. 1986), and rat pulmonary adenocarcinoma xenograft models (Gittes and Radde 1966; Komatsu et al. 2005). Other rodent models developed to study HHM and primary hyperparathyroidism in humans involve infusion of PTH or PTH-rP (Doppelt et al. 1981; Endo et al. 2000; Grone et al. 1992; Jaeger et al. 1987; Komatsu et al. 2005) or implantation of parathyroid fragments (Gittes and Radde 1966). The osteoclastic effects of PTH-rP are not restricted to bone; incisor fractures have been reported in nude rats implanted with PTH-rP expressing human large-cell lung cancer cell line, characterized by hypercalcification and thinning of dentin, caused by PTH-rP effects on odontoblasts (Kato et al. 2003, 2005).

17.4.5.4 Irradiation, Xenobiotics, Heavy Metals, and Alterations in Parathyroid Function

Relatively few xenobiotics have been associated with the induction of parathyroid gland tumors in chronic rodent bioassays. Exposure to the pesticide rotenone has been associated with the development of parathyroid adenomas in high-dose groups of male rats, although it is uncertain whether this increased incidence was an effect of exposure or increased survival in the high-dose groups, particularly in the absence of hyperplastic lesions in that study (Capen and Rosol 1989). Parathyroid adenomas have been induced by exposure to radioactive iodine or X-irradiation in the rat (Capen 2001; Capen and Rosol 1989; Greaves 2007; Hardisty and Boorman 1990) and can be enhanced by feeding a diet low in calcium or vitamin D (Wynford-Thomas et al. 1983). Impairment of parathyroid function with disruption of calcium homeostasis may occur with exposure to several metals (Baccarelli et al. 2000). Cadmium, a reported environmental risk factor for osteoporosis, interferes with renal activation of vitamin D and inhibits the renal reabsorption, intestinal absorption, and bone incorporation of calcium, leading to increased long bone fracture and osteopenia in rats (Brzoska and Moniuszko-Jakoniuk 2005). Iron lactate administered intravenously to rats causes rapid degranulation of secretory granules and elaboration of PTH, leading to transiently increased osteoclastic activity and bone resorption (Matsushima et al. 2005). Aluminum inhibits PTH release from porcine chief cells (Bourdeau et al. 1987) and is associated with inhibition of osteoclast and osteoblast activity, leading to osteomalacia (Jeffery 1996; Baccarelli et al. 2000). Exposure to lead is associated with direct bone toxicity, vitamin D deficiency, and secondary hyperparathyroidism (Rosen et al. 1980).

17.5 ADRENAL GLANDS

17.5.1 Normal Structure and Function

The adrenal gland is reported to be the most common endocrine organ associated with chemically induced lesions (Ribelin 1984). In surveys based on chemically induced endocrine lesions seen in in vivo toxicology studies, the order of endocrine organ toxicity by frequency of reported effects was as follows: adrenal > testes > thyroid > ovary > pancreas > pituitary > parathyroid (Ribelin 1984; Colby and Longhurst 1992) with the adrenal cortex, rather than the medulla, being the most frequent site of toxicity.

The adrenal gland contains two distinct endocrine regions, the medulla and the cortex. The adrenal cortex is required for life, particularly the secretion of aldosterone, but the functions of the medulla are not essential for life (Rosol et al. 2001). In mammals, the adrenal cortex and medulla are formed during embryogenesis by two distinct cell populations deriving from mesodermal and neuroectodermal origins (Hammer et al. 2005). The adrenal cortex derives from the mesenchymal cells attached to the coelomic cavity adjacent to the urogenital ridge. Embryonically, the adrenal medulla is derived from the ectodermal tissue of the neural crest and initially develops quite separately from the cortex. Eventually, the group of developing cortical cells is invaded by the precursor medullary cells, which they surround, forming the embryonic adrenal, which then migrates and relocates near the kidney. The medulla constitutes 10%–20% of the gland and secretes the catecholamine hormones adrenalin and noradrenaline.

17.5.2 Adrenal Cortex

The adrenal cortex is characterized by three layers, the zona glomerulosa (ZG), zona fasciculata, and zona reticularis, although there are species differences in the organization of these zones. The zona fasciculata constitutes the bulk of the cortex in laboratory animals. The zona reticularis is prominent in humans, but it is not clearly distinguishable in some rodents, particularly in the mouse. Adrenocorticotropic hormone (ACTH, corticotropin) is the primary regulator for fetal adrenal development and adult adrenal functions. ACTH exerts its effects mainly through a guanine nucleotide-binding protein (G protein)–coupled receptor, the ACTH receptor (ACTHR), present in the plasma membrane of adrenocortical cells. ACTHR expression has been demonstrated in all three zones of the cortex in humans and rodents, although the expression level in each zone appears to vary among species (Xia and Wikberg 1996; Reincke et al. 1998; Müller et al. 2001).

ACTH stimulates the synthesis and secretion of glucocorticoids, mineralocorticoids, and adrenal androgen via ACTHR (Kater et al. 1989); it also induces the proliferation of adrenocortical cells (Imai et al. 1990). The primary site for mitogenic action of ACTH is the ZG. Chronic hypersecretion of ACTH induces bilateral, diffuse hyperplasia of the adrenals (Bland et al. 2003); thus, ACTH has been considered a mitogenic hormone for adrenals. The outer fasciculata is the primary adrenal zone responsible for compensatory growth, though proliferating cells can be observed in the ZG in the early stages (Engeland et al. 2005). In aged animals, adrenocortical cells are less susceptible to the lack of ACTH, possibly as a result of their decreased functional ability (Almeida et al. 2006).

17.5.2.1 Steroidogenesis in Cortex

The adrenal gland is the most important steroidogenic organ, and steroidogenic processes take place in the adrenal cortex, which is histologically and functionally divided into three concentric zones: the outer ZG, the intermediate zona fasciculata, and the inner zona reticularis. A simplified view of adrenal steroidogenesis is depicted below.

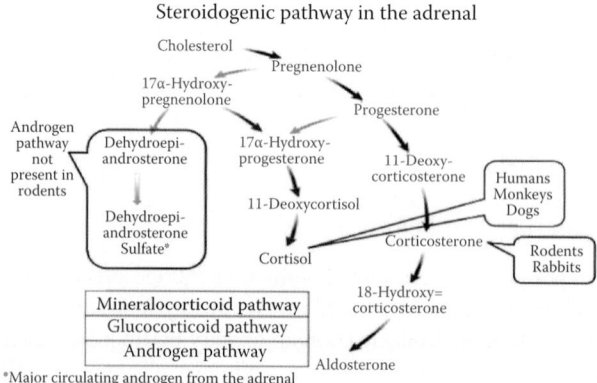

Steroidogenic pathway in the adrenal

Adrenal corticosteroids are essential for life. Three main types of hormones are produced by the adrenal cortex: glucocorticoids (cortisol, corticosterone), mineralocorticoids (aldosterone, deoxycorticosterone), and the sex steroids (mainly the androgen precursors dehydroepiandrosterone [DHEA] and androstenedione). Mineralocorticoids are essential for survival as they tightly regulate the Na+/

K+ balance in extracellular fluids and blood pressure homeostasis. Glucocorticoids are important in glucose homeostasis and the response of the organism to stressors and are also important in fetal lung development, immune modulation, and maintenance of normal function of a variety of tissues.

Steroid production is regulated by specific external stimuli, such as ACTH, which increases mainly glucocorticoid and, to a lesser extent, induces androgen production via the cAMP-mediated protein kinase A (PKA) pathway (Rainey 1999) and activates factors such as steroidogenic acute regulatory (StAR) protein (Stocco 2001) and steroidogenic factor-1 (SF-1) (Morohashi and Omura 1996; Morohashi et al. 1992). Angiotensin II and potassium selectively increase mineralocorticoid synthesis (Schimmer and Parke 1996) via the inositol triphosphate/diacylglycerol-mediated protein kinase C (PKC) pathway (Rainey 1999).

Cholesterol is the precursor for all adrenal steroidogenesis. The principal source of this cholesterol is provided from the circulation in the form of low-density lipoprotein (LDL) cholesterol. Uptake is by specific cell surface LDL receptors present on adrenal tissue; LDL is then internalized by means of receptor-mediated endocytosis. The resulting vesicles fuse with lysozymes, and free cholesterol is produced following hydrolysis. Cholesterol can also be generated de novo within the adrenal cortex from acetyl coenzyme A. The initial hormone-dependent rate-limiting step is the transport of intracellular cholesterol from the outer to inner mitochondrial membrane for conversion to pregnenolone by cytochrome P450scc. The movement of cholesterol into the mitochondria is mediated by the StAR protein. StAR is induced by an increase in intracellular cAMP following binding of corticotropin (ACTH) to its cognate receptor, providing the first important rate-limiting step in adrenal steroidogenesis.

After uptake of cholesterol to the mitochondrion, cholesterol is cleaved by the P450 cholesterol side chain cleavage enzyme (P450scc or CYP11A) to form pregnenolone. As mentioned earlier, this is the single most important rate-limiting step of steroid hormone biosynthesis. In the cytoplasm, pregnenolone is converted to progesterone by the type II isozyme 3β-hydroxysteroid dehydrogenase (3β-HSD). Progesterone is hydroxylated to 17OH-progesterone through the activity of P450c17. 17-Hydroxylation is an essential prerequisite for glucocorticoid synthesis (ZG does not express P450c17). P450c17 also possesses 17, 20-lyase activity, which results in the production of the C19 adrenal androgen precursors, DHEA and androstenedione. Adrenal androstenedione secretion is dependent upon the conversion of DHEA to androstenedione by 3β-HSD. The 17, 20-lyase activity of CYP17 is low in the adult adrenal cortex and is exclusive to the zona reticularis, where it converts the two 17α-hydroxylated steroids to the weak androgens, DHEA and androstenedione.

21-Hydroxylation of either progesterone (ZG) or 17-OH-progesterone (zona fasciculata) is performed by the product of the CYP21A2 gene, P450c21 (CYP21), which exerts 21-hydroxylase activity to yield deoxycorticosterone or 11-deoxycortisol, respectively. CYP21, an enzyme unique to the adrenal cortex, is essential for the biosynthesis of both mineralocorticoids and glucocorticoids. It is expressed in the smooth endoplasmic reticulum of all three adrenocortical zones and is responsible for the conversion of progesterone and 17α-hydroxyprogesterone to 11-deoxycorticosterone (mineralocorticoid pathway) and 11-deoxycortisol (glucocorticoid pathway), respectively (Sasano et al. 1988). These precursors, in turn, are converted in the mitochondria to the biologically active hormones, aldosterone and cortisol, by aldosterone synthetase (CYP11B2) and steroid 11β-hydroxylase (CYP11B1), respectively. These two mitochondrial enzymes are also unique to the adrenal cortex. CYP11B1, which is expressed in the zonae fasciculata and reticularis (Erdmann et al. 1995), has strictly 11β-hydroxylase activity, whereas CYP11B2, which is expressed only in the ZG (Pascoe et al. 1995), has additional 18-hydroxylase/aldosterone synthetase activity, explaining the zone selectivity of adrenocortical steroid biosynthesis. The weak adrenal androgens are formed by CYP17, a single enzyme with both 17α-hydroxylase and 17, 20-lyase activities. CYP17 hydroxylates pregnenolone and progesterone to form the respective 17α-hydroxysteroids, a process that occurs in the zonae reticularis and fasciculata but not in the ZG (Reincke et al. 1998). The rat adrenal gland has negligible expression of CYP17 and, therefore, secretes corticosterone instead of cortisol and has no significant androgen secretion (Hinson and Raven 2006).

Aldosterone formation occurs in the ZG. The circulating renin–angiotensin system (RAS) is a major regulator of aldosterone secretion. The RAS–aldosterone system is important in the control of salt and water balance and of blood pressure. The activity of RAS is determined predominantly by control of renin secretion from the kidney in addition to a local RAS in the ZG (Mulrow et al. 1988). The complete RAS is present in the adrenal cortex: prorenin, renin, angiotensinogen, angiotensin I and II, and converting enzyme. In the rat, renin production is under physiological control and can be influenced by ACTH, changes in electrolyte balance, and the genetic background of the animal (Mulrow 1998). There is a close correlation between adrenal renin and aldosterone production. Angiotensin can bind to two types of G protein coupled receptors, the AT1 and AT2 receptors. Both receptors are found on cells from the ZG, the site of aldosterone synthesis. Angiotensin II, acting via the AT1 receptor, stimulates the synthesis of aldosterone at early and late steps in the pathway. Its effect on aldosterone is influenced by a number of other factors such as plasma potassium levels, sodium status, other peptides such as ANP, and adrenomedullin and proadrenomedullin N-terminal peptide (Mulrow 1999). A low-sodium diet or a high-potassium diet, or nephrectomy, markedly increases the adrenal renin concentration in the ZG cells without any effect on the fasciculata–medullary cells. Angiotensin II, besides being one of the main agonists for the secretion of aldosterone, also stimulates proliferation of ZG cells, a process mediated by mitogen-activated protein kinases (MAPKs). Aldosterone controls sodium transport across epithelial cells, but recently, novel effects on the heart have been described (Lumbers 1999).

17.5.2.2 Xenobiotics Acting on Hypothalamic–Pituitary–Adrenal Axis

The hypothalamic–pituitary–adrenal (HPA) axis regulates the body's response to stress, which is mediated through the interaction of the hypothalamus, the pituitary, and the adrenal glands via several hormones in a negative-feedback fashion. Corticotropin-releasing hormone (CRH) is produced by the hypothalamus in response to a brain-derived stimulus, which in turn stimulates the production of ACTH from the pituitary. ACTH then stimulates the release of cortisol/corticosterone from the adrenal glands. Cortisol/corticosterone binds to receptors on the hypothalamus, further suppressing release of CRH and ACTH, thus inhibiting further cortisol/corticosterone production. Exogenous corticosteroids in the bloodstream decrease endogenous cortisol/corticosterone production, thereby disrupting the normal function of the HPA axis. As well as directly operating on the adrenal cortex, certain drugs can suppress adrenocortical function by inhibition of hormones higher in the endocrine axis at the level of the hypothalamus or pituitary, but the end result of deficits in glucocorticoid secretion is the same as that of a direct-acting adrenocortical enzyme inhibitor. For example, valproic acid, bromocriptine, cyproheptadine, ketanserin, ritanserin, somatostatin analogs, and glucocorticoids can suppress pituitary ACTH secretion and, in turn, adrenal glucocorticosteroid secretion as the endpoint, in both humans and rats; valproic acid also suppresses hypothalamic corticotropin-releasing hormone (Mercado-Asis et al. 1997; Kasperlik-Załuska et al. 2005; Sonino et al. 2005). The importance of this is that these compounds suppress the adrenal gland by a mechanism likely to be detected only by in vivo studies, with intact HPA axis function, which, in turn, affects any proposed assessment strategy for adrenal function.

17.5.2.3 Why Is the Adrenal Gland a Target of Toxicity?

The adrenal gland expresses numerous xenobiotic metabolizing enzymes and is rich in lipids with the potential to accumulate lipophilic compounds; it is therefore vulnerable to chemical toxicity. Identified factors predisposing the adrenal gland to toxic insult in vivo include the large number of potential toxicological targets such as receptors, enzymes, and peripheral hormone carrier molecules; high vascularization and disproportionately large blood volume received per unit mass; the high content of unsaturated fatty acids in adrenocortical cell membranes susceptible to lipid peroxidation; lipophilicity due to rich cholesterol and steroid content; and the high content of cytochrome P450 (CYP) enzymes present in the adrenal cortex, which normally catalyze steroidogenesis but which can also produce reactive metabolites of toxicants and hydroxylation reactions that may generate free radicals (Hinson and Raven 2006). Effects of altered glucocorticoid levels have been well documented clinically in patients with adrenal insufficiency (Addison's disease) or Cushing's syndrome (a generic term for manifestations of GC excess by any cause) as well as Cushing's disease (hypercortisolism, specifically due to pituitary ACTH hypersecretion).

17.5.2.4 Species Differences

In contrast to other mammals, mice and rats do not have a functionally distinct zona reticularis and lack expression of 17α-hydroxylase expression. Therefore, adrenals from mice and other rodents are devoid of the secretion of adrenal androgens. A specific feature of the mouse (and rabbit) adrenal cortex is the so-called X-zone, a putative postpartal remnant of the fetal adrenal zone located at the junction of the cortex and medulla. In males, this zone disappears rapidly with the approach of puberty (5 weeks), whereas in females, it continues to increase in size to reach a maximum at about 9 weeks and gradually regresses once they reach sexual maturity (Figure 17.5a). There is delayed disappearance of the adrenal X-zone in obese hyperglycemic mice, probably related to hypogonadism (Naeser 1975). In mice, growth and function of the adrenal glands are markedly influenced by gender and age. Female mice have heavier adrenal glands, with a higher volume of the zona fasciculata, and the total circulating corticosterone is higher in females between weeks 5 and 11 compared to male mice (Bielohuby et al. 2007). Likewise, homogenates of adrenals from female rats produced more corticosterone than homogenates from males of corresponding age, and similar to mice, adrenal weights are higher in females than in males. In contrast to mice and rats, adrenal glands of adult male hamsters are larger and secrete more cortisol than those of females, and adrenal weights are higher in males (Malendowicz and Nussdorfer 1984). Calcified (mineralization) foci at the junction between adrenal cortex and medulla are commonly observed in different NHPs used in drug safety studies and are considered to be remnants of the fetal zone (Majeed and Gopinath 1980; Kast et al. 1994).

17.5.3 NONPROLIFERATIVE LESIONS

Common spontaneous lesions of the adrenal cortex encountered in routine toxicity studies are discussed below.

Accessory cortical tissue. This denotes the presence of concomitant adrenocortical tissue outside the adrenal capsule or in the periadrenal tissue. It is composed of normal cortex, either detached from the adrenal gland or attached to the gland but separated from it by a complete fibrous capsule (Figure 17.5b). These nodules generally lack the distinct zonal arrangement of the adrenal cortex and are devoid of medullary tissue.

Angiectasis/telangiectasis (Figure 17.5c). Both aged rats and mice develop telangiectasis in the adrenal cortex because of marked dilatation of cortical capillaries after loss of parenchymal cells. This is a common lesion in aging female rats, whereas it is rarely found in mice (Frith et al. 2000).

Extramedullary hematopoiesis. Extramedullary hematopoiesis is occasionally observed in the adrenal cortex in rodents and may contain erythrocytic and/or granulocytic cells. This change must be differentiated from inflammation. When it is found in the adrenal gland, usually, prominent extramedullary hematopoiesis is also present in the spleen (Frith et al. 2000).

Amyloidosis. In aging mice of several strains, adrenal amyloidosis is common. It occurs most frequently in mice of the A, L, C3H, C57, and CBA strains. In contrast, adrenal amyloidosis is rarely seen in rats. In F344 rats, it has been reported in the absence of general amyloidosis. The deposits usually start in the zona reticularis and, in severe cases, may largely replace this zone (Nyska and Maronpot 1999).

Lipofuscin deposition. Aged mice and rats may develop lipofuscin deposition ("brown degeneration") in adrenal cortical cells and macrophages in the zona reticularis (Rosol et al. 2001). However, its presence in young rats may be indicative of excessive cellular organelle

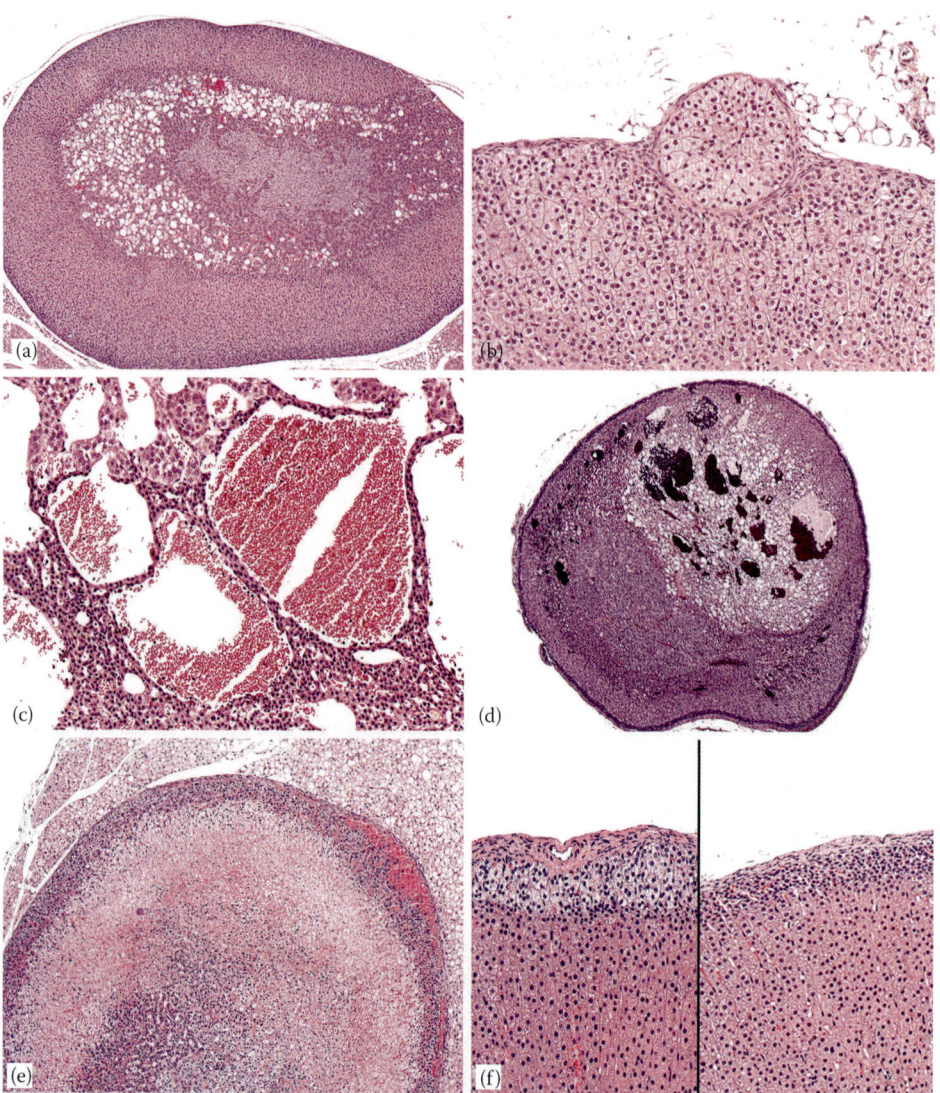

FIGURE 17.5 (a) Adrenal gland from a young female mouse showing vacuolation of the X-zone. (b) Accessory adrenocortical nodule in a mouse. The nodule is surrounded by a thin capsule. (c) Angiectasis (peliosis) in an aging female rat. (d) Cystic degeneration in an aged rat. (e) Diffuse necrosis of the zona fasciculata in a mouse secondary to xenobiotic administration. (f) On the left, increased vacuolation and hypertrophy of the ZG in a female rat, a microscopic finding that can be observed due to perturbation in the renin–angiotensin system. Unaffected ZG is shown on the right.

turnover or defective cell metabolism. Lipofuscin pigmentation may be associated with severe hormone-induced atrophy, and the severity can be enhanced by the administration of estrogens and adrenocorticosteroids. In mice, the accumulation of ceroid pigment is prominent in the degenerating X-zone at the corticomedullary interface, and in some strains, especially BALB/c, it is a relatively common finding. In aged hamsters, dense aggregates of ceroid pigment may also accumulate at the corticomedullary junction (Nickerson 1979).

Focal cortical vacuolation (focal fatty change) and cystic degeneration. Focal cortical vacuolar change is a spontaneous finding, especially in aged rats, in contrast to diffuse cortical vacuolation that may be secondary to xenobiotic treatment or due to stress. The histologic appearance of focal cortical vacuolation varies from multiple small vacuoles to single large, clear cytoplasmic vacuoles (Frith et al. 2000). Cystic degeneration is considered to be a continuum of focal cortical vacuolation, particularly severe forms in which there is cell loss with the resultant formation of cystic and/or blood-filled spaces. Cystic degeneration (Figure 17.5d) is predominantly observed in aging female Sprague–Dawley rats. This lesion can mimic vacuolar degeneration due to chemically induced toxicity. If the vacuolar degeneration is severe, there will be loss of cortical cells, possibly mineralization, and vascular ectasia (Hamlin and Banas 1990).

17.5.3.1 Hypertrophy

17.5.3.1.1 Zona Fasciculata Hypertrophy

Adrenocortical hypertrophy (increase in size; usually increased thickness involving the zona fasciculata with increased cell size and/or number) is a common finding in toxicology studies. Adrenocortical hypertrophy is readily induced in the rat by ACTH treatment and reverses upon removal of ACTH stimulation (Akana et al. 1983). Adrenocortical hypertrophy is seen grossly as an increase in gland size and weight due to an increase in the width of the cortex (Rosol et al. 2001; Harvey and Sutcliffe 2010; Harvey et al. 2007). Adrenal weights can be relatively insensitive depending on study design, and the organ-to-brain weight ratio appears to be most predictive for adrenal weights (Bailey et al. 2004). The zona fasciculata is most often affected in cortical hypertrophy. Adrenocortical hypertrophy is usually the result of ACTH overstimulation and can arise as a result of the stress response, but it may also occur due to deficient glucocorticoid feedback regulation of ACTH due to toxicity to the adrenal cortex. Histologically, the cells of the zona fasciculata have larger vesicular nuclei, prominent nucleoli, and dense eosinophilic cytoplasm with a reduction in cytoplasmic lipid vacuoles. Following cessation of stress or withdrawal of ACTH administration, repletion of lipid occurs in an outward fashion starting at the junction of the zona fasciculata and zona reticularis. Chronic variable stress induces hyperplasia in the outer zona fasciculata, hypertrophy in the inner zona fasciculata and medulla, and reduced cell size in the ZG (Ulrich-Lai et al. 2006).

Differentiation of stress-induced adrenocortical hypertrophy compared with adrenocortical hypertrophy resulting from direct toxicity and inhibition of glucocorticoid steroidogenesis is vital. In stress, activation of the HPA axis will result in increased glucocorticoid secretion (corticosterone in rats and mice and cortisol in dogs, NHPs, and humans), which usually produces detectable effects elsewhere, indicating functional competency of the gland. Increased glucocorticoid production should have observable effects in other tissues such as the lymphoid system. Typically, this is seen as lymphocytolysis in the thymus resulting in thymic atrophy. Experimentally, thymic atrophy is a well-known consequence of stress (Buckingham 2008) and has been shown in rats following repeated administration of corticosterone (Harvey et al. 1992). Experimentally, rats administered corticosterone mimicking physiologically relevant blood concentrations approximating stress values had reduced body weight gain, coupled with lower thymus, prostate, and seminal vesicle weights. The findings were attributed to both the direct effects of corticosterone (body weight and thymus weight) and the inhibition by corticosterone of LH and testosterone (Harvey et al. 1992; Kamel and Kubajak 1987; Sankar et al. 2000). This combination of findings, including reduced body weights and lower thymus, prostate, and seminal vesicle weights indicative of the effects of corticosterone, in combination with enlarged adrenal gland, indicative of ACTH stimulation, may prove to be useful markers of adrenocortical steroid production and, therefore, adrenocortical competency, in the absence of direct data such as blood corticosterone concentration. In addition to cortical hypertrophy, genuine stress can also produce adrenomedullary hypertrophy (Ulrich-Lai et al. 2006).

Urine corticosterone and its metabolites may be potential biomarkers of stress in rats. The combined findings of increased urinary corticosterone and changes in blood lymphocyte and neutrophil differential counts, with decreased thymus weight or cellularity, aid in recognizing drug-induced stress response (Pruett et al. 2008).

Adrenocortical hypertrophy may occur in the absence of other adrenocortical lesions such that a toxicopathological mechanism is not obvious, for example, pharmacological inhibition of steroidogenesis at the biochemical level. Adrenocortical toxicity is indicated in cases of increases in blood ACTH and/or with adrenocortical hypertrophy, but without supplementary evidence such as atrophy of the thymus. Even a normal range of glucocorticoid blood levels in this situation may be indicative of adrenocortical steroidogenic impairment since it may be the case that much higher levels of endogenous ACTH are required to maintain failing adrenocortical steroidogenesis (Harvey and Sutcliffe 2010).

Stress increases ACTH secretion (Buckingham 2008) as does a direct-acting adrenocortical toxicant that inhibits steroidogenesis, for example, aminoglutethimide (Akana et al. 1983), resulting in increased ACTH due to loss of feedback regulation. Stress is endocrinologically characterized by increased ACTH and increased glucocorticoid (Buckingham 2008). Therefore, if both increased ACTH and glucocorticoids are seen in the blood, a stress etiology can be considered, but it is important to recognize that certain drugs can increase ACTH secretion via pharmacological mechanisms (Kumari et al. 1997) at the level of the hypothalamus (Colagiovanni et al. 2006; Colagiovanni and Meyer 2008; Kumari et al. 1997).

17.5.3.1.2 ZG Hypertrophy

Angiotensin II (Ang II) is one of the most important stimuli of rat adrenal glomerulosa cells that promote cellular hypertrophy but not proliferation (Otis et al. 2005). In the absence of other trophic factors, ACTH also stimulates the growth of the ZG, although it is a trophic factor for the fasciculata. Administration of renin or angiotensin II increases aldosterone secretion and the thickness (hypertrophy) of the ZG (Figure 17.5e). Likewise, salt depletion, potassium loading, ischemia, renovascular hypertension, and administration of ACTH all lead to cell enlargement and widening of the ZG (Nussdorfer 1986; McEwan et al. 1996). Epithelial cells of the zona reticularis also respond to Ang II and sodium restriction (McEwan et al. 1996).

17.5.3.1.3 Atrophy

Bilateral atrophy usually results from deficiency of ACTH due to destructive lesions in the pituitary gland. Atrophy of the zona fasciculata in toxicity studies is usually due to endogenous corticosteroids from a steroid-producing neoplasm or from exogenous administration of corticosteroids. Unilateral atrophy may occur in the presence of a corticosteroid-secreting neoplastic lesion in the contralateral adrenal cortex. Chronic adrenal cortical atrophy is accompanied by thickening of the fibrous tissue of the capsule. Rats treated with exemestane, an inhibitor of the cytochrome-P450 aromatase (P450$_{arom}$), had decreased adrenal weights and decreased cell size in both the zona fasciculata and pituitary pars distalis (Mirsky et al. 2011). Similarly, rats administered PD 138142-15, a substituted urea hypolipidemic and potential anti-atherosclerotic agent, had decreased ACTH-stimulated cortisol levels with concurrent atrophy, principally of the zona fasciculata and zona reticularis (Wolfgang et al. 1995).

Atrophy of the zona reticularis with decreased adrenal weight is observed in female rats administered with 1-alpha-methyltestosterone (Okazaki et al. 2002). Perturbation of the RAS is associated with atrophy of the ZG. Rats treated with atrial natriuretic peptide exhibit atrophy of the ZG (Mazzocchi et al. 1987). Likewise, rats treated with an inhibitor of angiotensin-converting enzyme captopril have a decrease in the volume of glomerulosa cells associated with smaller nuclear and mitochondrial volumes and reduced surface areas of mitochondrial cristae and membranes of the endoplasmic reticulum (Mazzocchi and Nussdorfer 1984; McEwan et al. 1996). These effects were completely abolished by concomitant administration of angiotensin II. Prolonged infusion of rats with atrial natriuretic factor induced atrophy of the ZG and a lowering of plasma concentrations of aldosterone, with changes in plasma renin activity (Nussdorfer et al. 1988).

17.5.3.1.4   Necrosis

Spontaneous adrenal cortical necrosis is uncommon in rats and mice, and it is beyond the scope of this chapter to list xenobiotic-associated cortical necrosis (Figure 17.5f). Examples of compounds causing adrenocortical toxicity and their molecular targets are listed in several publications (Ullerås et al. 2008; Harvey and Everett 2003; Harvey et al. 2007; Nishizato et al. 2010; Szabo and Lippe 1989). In addition to xenobiotics like the DDT derivative o,p′-DDD, pharmaceutical compounds such acyl-coenzyme A:cholesterol acyltransferase (ACAT) and tyrosine kinase inhibitors cause necrosis due to direct toxicity to adrenocortical cells (Patyna et al. 2008; Dominick et al. 1993). Cortical necrosis with ACAT inhibitors was observed in multiple species, including dogs, rabbits, monkeys, and guinea pigs (Dominick et al. 1993; Reindel et al. 1994). Further, in healthy rats, exogenous ACTH can cause adrenal degeneration in a dose-dependent manner (Burkhardt et al. 2011).

17.5.3.1.5   Vacuolation

The three zones of the adrenal cortex normally have some degree of vacuolation, with the extent of the vacuolar appearance varying between zones reflecting a state of cellular activity. In the normal rat, the zona fasciculata contains the most prominent vacuoles. These vacuoles contain neutral lipid and cholesterol and can become larger or more prominent in some species with advancing age (Hamlin and Banas 1990; Ribelin et al. 1984). Increased cortical vacuolation is a common morphologic lesion (Figure 17.6a) that can be due to inhibition of cholesterol biosynthesis or metabolism and to disruption of cytochrome P450 enzymes leading to accumulation of cholesterol and steroid precursors. Compounds that inhibit enzymes involved in the synthesis of corticosteroids increase storage of nonutilized steroid precursors and induce adrenocortical hyperplasia by a negative-feedback mechanism that stimulates ACTH secretion. This hyperplastic process can be accompanied by an accumulation of cholesterol and steroid precursors in the cytoplasm of adrenocortical cells giving rise to collections of clear cells with a foamy appearance, sometimes with cholesterol cleft formation.

Triaryl phosphates are an example of a group of organophosphates that result in impaired cholesterol metabolism and increased cytoplasmic lipid vacuolation (Latendresse et al. 1994). DMNM (-[1,4-dioxido-3-methylquinoxalin-2-yl]-N-methylnitrone) is an antibiotic that causes impaired steroidogenesis likely by blocking the conversion of cholesterol to pregnenolone. After acute exposure, it results in cytoplasmic vacuolation of the zonae fasciculata and reticularis (Yarrington et al. 1981, 1985). Increased lipid droplets were observed in the zonae fasciculata and reticularis treated with ketoconazole and another antimycotic drug clotrimazole in rats and dogs. These antimycotic drugs inhibit a number of cytochrome P450–dependent steroidogenic enzymes in the cortex (Pont et al. 1982; Mason et al. 1985; Houston et al. 1988). Aminoglutethimide, an amino acid derivative of the hypnotic glutethimide, inhibits several P450-mediated hydroxylation steps in the adrenal cortex, leading to increased width of the zona fasciculata composed of cells containing cytoplasmic lipid droplets (Zak et al. 1985). Similar findings are observed in rats administered with the steroidogenic inhibitor U-8113 (an analog of amphenone B), with increased adrenal gland weight with hypertrophy and vacuolation of the zonae fasciculata and reticularis (Sharawy et al. 1978).

In addition, vacuolation of the zonae fasciculata and reticularis can also be observed with cationic amphiphilic compounds that cause generalized phospholipidosis, though the biochemical mechanism is different. Vacuolation of adrenocortical cells due to phospholipidosis was observed in rats administered with PNU-177864, a dopamine D3 receptor antagonist (Rudmann et al. 2004). Ultrastructural evaluation of the adrenal cortex can often provide important mechanistic clues beyond that which can be observed by light microscopy. For example, cytoplasmic lamellar lysosomal bodies (myelin figures) are diagnostic for phospholipidosis, and for chemicals that impair the activity of cytochrome P450 enzymes, changes are seen in the smooth endoplasmic reticulum or mitochondria. Long duration of treatment with compounds that cause marked vacuolar degeneration may lead to cell death, accumulation of cholesterol, fibrosis, and lipid droplets in macrophages.

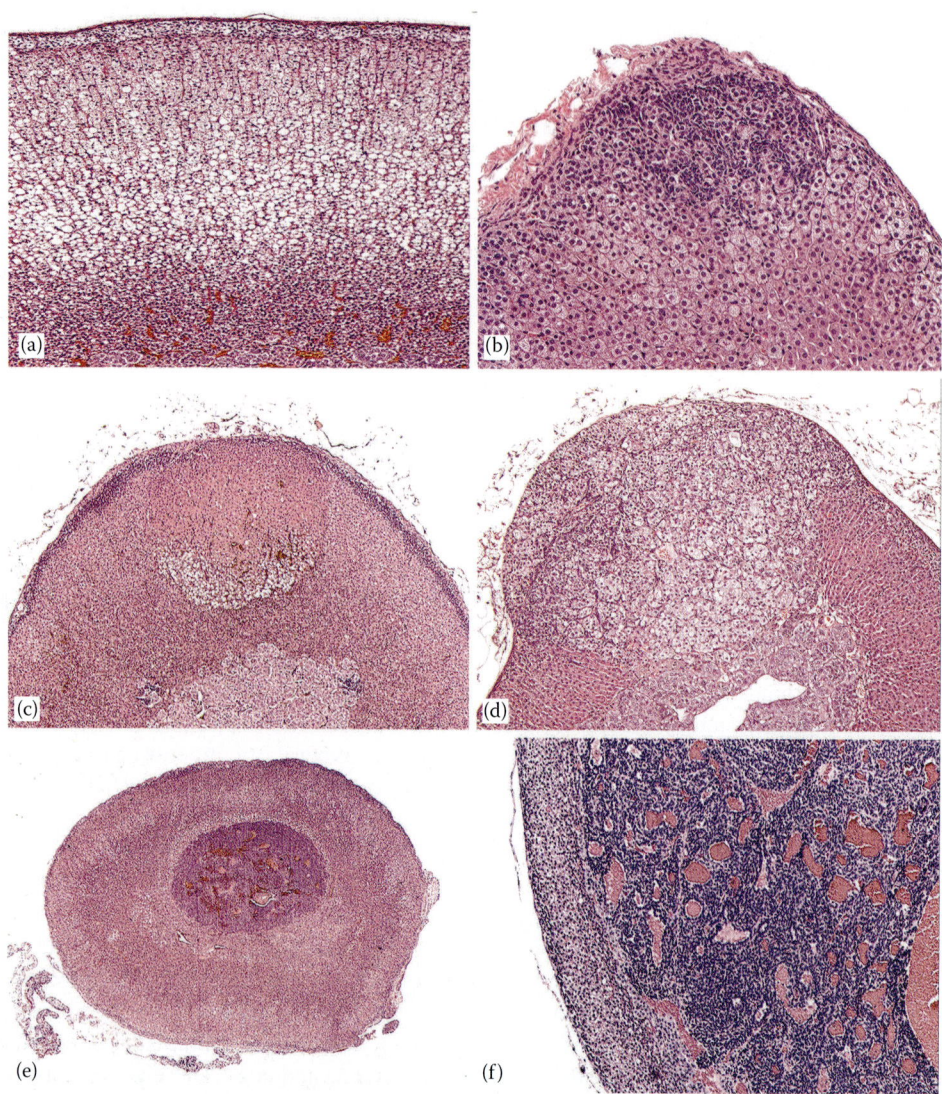

FIGURE 17.6 (a) Increased vacuolation of the zona fasciculata in a rat. (b) Subcapsular cell hyperplasia in a mouse. (c) Focal cortical hyperplasia in a rat. Similar focal lesions have also been diagnosed as focal cortical hypertrophy and focus of cellular alteration. (d) Subcapsular cell adenoma from a mouse composed of type A (spindle cells) and type B (polygonal cells). (e and f) Low- and high-magnification images of benign pheochromocytoma in a rat.

17.5.4 PROLIFERATIVE LESIONS

17.5.4.1 Subcapsular Cell Hyperplasia

Subcapsular cell hyperplasia (spindle cell hyperplasia) is a common, age-related change in mice and is enhanced after gonadectomy. The function of these spindle cells is unknown. Subcapsular hyperplasia (Figure 17.6b) can be focal or diffuse, and these hyperplastic foci are composed of spindle cells (type A) or polygonal cells (type B), or both. This can appear as a fairly uniform thickening of the capsule; develop as localized, wedge-shaped proliferations beneath the capsule; or become an extensive mass replacing much of the cortex. Subcapsular adenomas are derived from the same cell population in varying combinations (Nyska and Maronpot 1999).

17.5.4.2   Focal Hyperplasia, Focal Hypertrophy, and Foci of Cellular Alteration

Diffuse hyperplasia of the adrenal cortex is a relatively uncommon manifestation of chemically induced lesions (Rosol et al. 2001). Focal, small-to-large aggregates of small or hypertrophied cells that differ cytologically from the surrounding normal parenchyma are commonly observed in the zona fasciculata of rats and mice, as well as in dogs and NHPs. These foci may show a variety of cytoplasmic alterations (basophilic, eosinophilic, or vacuolated) with minimal compression of the adjacent parenchyma, unlike an adenoma (Figure 17.6c). The morphological features of focal hyperplasia and focal hypertrophy often overlap, and it is not known if these focal lesions represent true foci of hyperplasia, or collections of cells with altered functional state, or both. Their classification has been the source of dispute. Focal hyperplasia must be distinguished from adenoma.

17.5.4.3   Adenoma and Carcinoma

Spontaneous cortical adenomas and carcinomas are uncommon in both rats and mice. Subcapsular cell adenomas (Figure 17.6d) are observed in old mice, and these adenomas are composed of type A (spindle) and type B (polygonal) cells similar to the subcapsular cell hyperplasia. Morphological features of focal (nodular) hyperplasia and adenoma often overlap such that compression of the surrounding gland is used as a diagnostic feature of adenoma. Carcinomas of the cortex are large lesions that compress the surrounding parenchyma and are composed of large, polyhedral, or pleomorphic cells with an eosinophilic or vacuolated cytoplasm. Blood-filled spaces and localized areas of necrosis are common. Atrophy of the contralateral adrenal cortex may occur if the carcinoma is functional and secretes corticosteroids. Although the adrenal gland, and especially the cortex, is reported to be the most common endocrine organ associated with chemically induced lesions, a review of the NTP database reveals very few chemicals associated with site-specific induction of tumors in the cortex. Chemically induced tumors were mostly adenomas and predominantly seen in rats. Chemicals associated with tumor induction in the adrenal cortex include 2-dibromo-3-chloropropane, parathion tetrachlorvinphos, 3,3′,4,4′-tetrachloroazobenzene, 3,3′,4,4′,5-pentachlorobiphenyl, and 4-vinylcyclohexene.

17.5.4.4   In Vitro Methods to Identify Mechanisms of Toxicity

Once direct adrenocortical toxicity has been identified, the use of in vitro systems will be useful to investigate the precise mechanisms. The human adrenocortical carcinoma-derived cell line H295R has been widely used to study adrenocortical function, regulation of steroidogenesis, and screening of enzymatic inhibitors (Johansson et al. 2002; Sanderson et al. 2002; Müller-Vieira et al. 2005). This cell line expresses all the key enzymes necessary for steroidogenesis and the production of all the major steroids such as progesterone, androgens, estrogens, glucocorticoids, and the mineralocorticoid aldosterone (Zhang et al. 2005). In contrast to the human adrenal cortex in vivo, the H295R cells express aromatase and produce sex hormones such as testosterone and estradiol (Rainey et al. 1994). In the context of adrenal gland toxicology, though the priority is to identify compounds causing functional suppression of the adrenal gland, this in vitro cell line is used to detect up-regulation as well as down-regulation of steroidogenesis. Given that a number of the tested chemicals have been characterized as more or less specific inhibitors of the steroidogenic cytochrome P450 enzymes, it is not surprising that the general effect is toward inhibition of steroidogenesis and hormone secretion. The H295R in vitro system has a potential for high-throughput screening not only to characterize the effects of chemicals on endocrine systems but also to prioritize chemicals for additional testing. The in vitro assay is generally useful for detecting direct effects on adrenal cells. A limitation of this model is that substances requiring metabolic activation or indirect effects on the adrenal gland due to disruption of the HPA axis cannot be adequately identified. In addition to H295R, a primary culture system of adrenocortical cells from dogs has been used. An added advantage of the canine system is a direct correlation to in vivo toxicology study data (Morishita et al. 2001).

17.6 ADRENAL MEDULLA

17.6.1 NORMAL STRUCTURE AND FUNCTION

The medulla comprises about 10%–20% of the volume of the adrenal gland. It derives from the neural crest and consists of three types of cells: chromaffin, neuronal (ganglion-like), and sustentacular cells (Carney 1992; Cormack, 1989). Chromaffin and ganglion-like cells are descendent from a common sympathoadrenal neuroblastic precursor (Tischler et al. 1977), express neuronal cytoskeletal proteins, and exhibit catecholaminergic properties. Sustentacular cells are stromal or supportive cells and possess morphologic, functional, and antigenic properties similar to those of Schwann and satellite cells. The chromaffin cells are the sites of synthesis and storage of catecholamines. In rats, there are three types of chromaffin cells: epinephrine (E) cells (the majority), norepinephrine (NE) cells, and small granule-containing cells (Pace et al. 2002; Rosol et al. 2001). The ratios of E/NE-type cells and of stored E/NE in young adult rats are each about 4/1 (Tischler 1989).

The most important hormones of the medulla are the catecholamines adrenaline, noradrenaline, and dopamine. Their biosynthesis begins with tyrosine, which is metabolized by tyrosine hydroxylase (TH) as the rate-limiting step, to form 3,4-dihydroxyphenylalanine (dopa). A decarboxylase converts dopa into dopamine, which is hydroxylated to produce noradrenaline. Noradrenaline is methylated to adrenaline by phenylethanolamine N-methyltransferase (PNMT) in the medulla. High concentrations of adrenaline and noradrenaline are stored in the cells of the adrenal medulla and the peripheral nerves in membrane-bound secretory vesicles. The vesicles in the medulla release mainly adrenaline into the blood. The catecholamines that are released into the blood react with receptors in the organs and blood vessels, which in turn activate intracellular signal chains via membrane-bound G proteins. Stimulation of the receptors produces a rise in glucose and free fatty acids in the blood and increases basal metabolic rate, muscular perfusion contractility of the heart muscle, heart rate, and blood pressure.

The secretion of catecholamines is controlled by sympathetic innervation. Production and secretion of catecholamines are triggered by acute events such as stress, trauma, and shock, as well as by fasting, hypoxia, hypoglycemia, or pharmacologically active substances such as nicotine, reserpine, or retinoic acid. The cardinal symptom of acute and chronic release of catecholamines is increased blood pressure.

In addition to catecholamines, adrenal chromaffin cells produce a variety of neuropeptides, which are stored in the same secretory granules. Neurotensin and neuropeptide-Y (NPY), for example, are present in NE-type cells, while enkephalins are present in cells of both types. Serotonin and histamine may also be present (Tischler 1989).

17.6.2 NONPROLIFERATIVE LESIONS

The adrenal medulla is a less common site of chemically induced nonproliferative lesions, though proliferative lesions of the medulla are common in rodents, especially rats. Scientific literature on acute toxicity and/or nonproliferative lesions of the adrenal medulla is rather limited. Medullary chromaffin cells in rats are susceptible to acute necrosis and cytolysis by salinomycin, followed by regeneration in as little as 24 h (Chen-Pan et al. 1999). Degeneration of the adrenal medulla has been reported in mice administered with ciguatoxin or ciguatoxin-4c (Terao et al. 1991).

17.6.3 PROLIFERATIVE LESIONS

Spontaneous proliferative lesions of the adrenal medulla are common in aging rats, while both spontaneous and chemically induced pheochromocytomas (tumors originating from chromaffin cells) are rare in mice. These lesions, which include focal (nodular) hyperplasia, diffuse hyperplasia, and pheochromocytoma, occur most frequently in male rats, with a reported frequency of over 80% in the Wistar strain and over 30% in the Fischer 344 and Sprague–Dawley strains (Strandberg

1996). The adrenal medulla in many strains of rats develops diffuse and nodular hyperplasia and, in some instances, neoplasia, either spontaneously with aging or after prolonged exposure to a variety of hormones, drugs, and other agents. These agents include hormones or drugs, which affect the hypothalamic–endocrine axis or the autonomic nervous system, dietary factors, miscellaneous drugs and toxins, and radiation. Their diversity suggests that they might, in some instances, affect the adrenal medulla indirectly by acting as systemic stressors. Within any given strain of rat, adrenal medullary hyperplasia and neoplasia occur most frequently in older animals and in males. The evolution of adrenal medullary proliferative changes from diffuse hyperplasia through diffuse and nodular hyperplasia and neoplasia is accompanied by increased production of NE and decreased E/NE ratios (Tischler 1989). In rodents, the principle diagnostic difficulty in the medulla is that hyperplasia forms a continuous histological spectrum with neoplastic growth (pheochromocytomas). This difficulty has given rise to controversy among regulatory authorities about the safety of xenobiotics that produce medullary hyperplasia in rats. Diffuse hyperplasia is characterized by an expansion of the medullary volume by increased numbers of chromaffin cells without the formation of nodules, whereas focal hyperplasia is recognized by the presence of localized aggregates of medullary cells, cytologically distinct from normal surrounding parenchyma. In rodents, cells in these foci usually possess scanty basophilic cytoplasm and enlarged nuclei.

Pheochromocytoma (Figure 17.6e and f) is the most common adrenal medullary tumor in rodents, and these tumors are often found in a background of diffuse adrenomedullary hyperplasia (Tischler et al. 1985). The incidence of pheochromocytoma is highly strain dependent, with an incidence ranging from 0% to 86%. Some strains (e.g., F344, Sprague–Dawley) are particularly liable to develop focal hyperplasia and neoplasia of the medulla, both spontaneously with advancing age and following administration of xenobiotics. Morphologically, benign pheochromocytomas are characterized by monomorphic, small, basophilic cells with few, if any, mitoses, whereas malignant pheochromocytomas exhibit pleomorphism, a higher rate of mitoses, multinucleated giant cells, necrosis, infiltrative growth, and, in rare cases, metastasis to the lungs, lymph nodes, or bone marrow. These tumors are highly vascular with concurrent hemorrhage and necrosis. Cells are large and rich in cytoplasm (so-called "secretory" cells) or small, poor in cytoplasm, and basophilic. All pheochromocytomas are strongly immunoreactive for TH, the rate-limiting enzyme in catecholamine synthesis. Subpopulations of chromaffin cells express chromogranin A (CGA) positivity (Pace et al. 2002).

Chronic treatment with xenobiotics, such as the antihypertensive drug reserpine and vitamin D3, stimulates chromaffin cell proliferation and induces pheochromocytomas in rats (Rosol et al. 2001). Pheochromocytomas occur with a relatively higher frequency in male rats, especially when the following conditions are involved: hypoxia (impaired respiration or pulmonary toxicity); uncoupling of oxidative phosphorylation; disturbance in calcium homeostasis (e.g., in the case of kidney damage); disturbance of the hypothalamic endocrine axis; and acute stress and overfeeding. Altered calcium homeostasis is indirectly involved in the pathogenesis of pheochromocytomas. High doses of slowly or poorly absorbed sugars such as lactose or sugar alcohols such as mannitol, sorbitol, xylitol, and lactitol increase the absorption of calcium from the small intestine in rats. Though the mechanism is not completely understood, a role for calcium has been postulated. Ca2+ up-regulates TH and, thus, the synthesis of catecholamines. The underlying biochemical mechanisms suggest that other substances that interfere with these biochemical endpoints also produce pheochromocytomas (Greim et al. 2009). In rats, a series of nongenotoxic mechanisms result in proliferation of chromaffin cells. An association between chronic pulmonary lesions, fibrosis, inflammation, and hypoxemia in the induction of pheochromocytoma has been observed in F344 male rats (Ozaki et al. 2002). In addition, genetic background, chronic high levels of GH, or prolactin associated with pituitary tumors, dietary factors, and stimulation of the autonomic nervous system also play a role in the induction of medullary tumors.

Rat tumors have a greater phenotypic diversity than human tumors and are not limited to the noradrenergic phenotype (Powers et al. 2008). Gene expression profiling of rat pheochromocytoma has revealed both generic and specific parallels between rat and human tumors (Elkahloun et al. 2006), though pheochromocytomas are rare in humans. According to one report, the relevance of rat pheochromocytomas as a model for their human counterparts is uncertain. There is no indication that pheochromocytomas in animals are induced by chemical substances via genotoxic mechanisms (Ozaki et al. 2002). Their occurrence following administration of a toxic agent in animal experiments should be assessed as a secondary effect with little relevance for human risk (Greim et al. 2009).

Pheochromocytoma-induced cardiomyopathy (Kassim et al. 2008) primarily from release of catecholamines from the tumor, is a well-recognized entity in humans and has been experimentally induced in rats. Catecholamines and their oxidation products cause a direct toxic effect on the myocardium. The findings are characterized by increased heart weights, increased systolic blood pressure with multifocal lesions of enhanced interstitial and replacement fibrosis, granularity of the cytoplasm and contraction band necrosis, and mixed inflammatory infiltrates (Mobine et al. 2009; Rosenbaum et al. 1988; Hoffman 1987). In addition to cardiac lesions, hepatic necrosis and nephrosclerosis have been associated with pheochromocytomas (Cheng 1980). Urinary or plasma fractionated catecholamines, metanephrines, and serum chromogranin-A levels have been used as serum biomarkers of pheochromocytomas in humans. The presence of serum markers is also common in cases of medullary hyperplasia (van der Harst et al. 2002).

Spontaneous and chemically induced pheochromocytomas are rare in mice. Similar to rats, most tumors express immunoreactivity for TH, and, in addition, the tumors are variably positive for PNMT and CGA (Tischler et al. 1996; Hill et al. 2003). It has been suggested that, based on frequency, morphology, and immunophenotype, mice may be a more appropriate model (versus rats) for human adrenal medullary pathology (Tischler et al. 1996).

Other proliferative lesions of the medulla, including ganglioneuroma and neuroblastoma, are rare in rodents. Ganglioneuromas are composed of well-differentiated ganglion cells mixed with satellite cells, Schwann cells, and neurites within an eosinophilic neurofibrillar matrix. They are often found together with pheochromocytomas. The incidence of ganglioneuroma is extremely low and must be differentiated from the more common complex pheochromocytomas, which consist of fewer neural components (<80% of the mass) (Reznik et al. 1980; Goelz et al. 1998; Pace et al. 2002). Ganglion cells exhibit peripherin and beta-tubulin immunoreactivity. Neuroblastomas are composed of small cells with round to ovoid hyperchromatic nuclei and scant cytoplasm. Neuroblastomas are very rare tumors in laboratory rats (Reznik and Germann 1996). Distant metastasis has not been reported in spontaneous tumors. Spontaneous neuroblastoma is rare in mice (Maita et al. 1988). Aguzzi et al. (1990) reported that transgenic mice carrying a cDNA to the polyoma virus middle T antigen linked to the thymidine kinase promoter developed neuroblastoma in multiple organs, including the adrenal glands, by 2–3 months of age. These tumors expressed the N-myc oncogene and metastasized.

17.7 PANCREATIC ISLETS

17.7.1 NORMAL STRUCTURE AND FUNCTION

The multiple cell types of the pancreatic islets of Langerhans (pancreatic islets) are incorporated into a "sea" of exocrine pancreatic tissue. In mammals, the endocrine tissue (islets) comprise <5% and the exocrine tissue comprises the remaining >95% of the pancreas. In all mammals, the pancreas is located on the left side of the peritoneal cavity, between the spleen and the pyloric region of the stomach. The pancreas runs along the duodenum and terminates within the mesentery/omentum. The pancreas generally consists of poorly demarcated areas referred to as the body and tail, but there is substantial interspecies variation, and the anatomic terminology varies as well. The distribution and number of islets differ between the areas of the pancreas and between species.

During embryonal development, the pancreas arises from the duodenal endoderm (develops into the dorsal pancreas) and the hepatic diverticulum endoderm (develops into the ventral pancreas), which then fuse to form the developing pancreas. The mature pancreas consists primarily of the acinar tissue, which is discussed elsewhere in this book, and the pancreatic islets (Islets of

Langerhans), which arise multifocally by budding off of the developing acini and undergo a genetic switch to synthesizing certain protein hormones such as insulin, glucagon, pancreatic polypeptide, ghrelin, and somatostatin (Carlson 1988). The pancreatic islet cells develop through a series of differentiation steps, from primary multipotential progenitor cells that divide to form secondary multipotential precursor cells, which can then differentiate into acinar and bipotential progenitor cells. The bipotential progenitor cells differentiate into ductular cells and endocrine precursor cells. The endocrine precursor cells then undergo a series of cellular divisions and differentiation steps to an endocrine precursor cell, which, depending on the presence of certain transcription factors, will differentiate into α-, δ-, ε-, pancreatic peptide (PP)-, or immature β-cells. Immature β-cells will then differentiate into mature β-cells in the presence of the following transcription factors: Pdx1^{HI}, Mnx1, Nkx6.1, NeuroD, Nkx2.2, MafA, Pax4, Foxa1, and Foxa2 (Pan and Wright 2011).

Pancreatic islets are well-organized groups of endocrine cells that are distributed throughout the exocrine pancreas. The majority of the endocrine cells are located within the islets, but individualized or small clusters of pancreatic islet hormone immunoreactive cells (primarily insulin expressing) are seen scattered throughout the exocrine pancreas, especially near the acinar ducts (Figure 17.7a). There are several cell types that synthesize and secrete particular peptide hormones

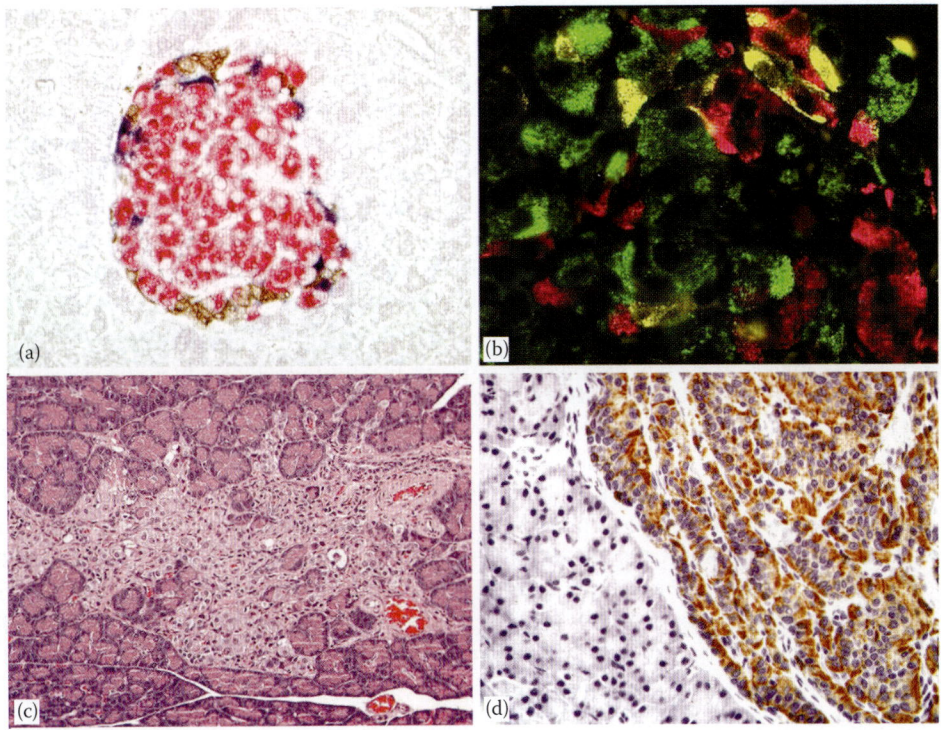

FIGURE 17.7 (a) Sprague-Dawley rat, pancreatic islet, triple immunohistochemistry for insulin (red), glucagon (brown), and somatostatin (blue). Streptavidin–biotin complex labeling. (b) C57BL/6 mouse, pancreatic islet (peripheral), triple immunofluorescence for insulin (green), glucagon (red), and somatostatin (yellow). Note the characteristic cytoplasmic secretory granules in the three islet cell types and the interactions of the three cell types at the periphery of the rodent pancreatic islet. (c) ZDF *fa/fa* rat, 17 weeks of age, pancreatic islet, H&E. Note the disorganization of the islet, the presence of fibrosis and decrease in the number of β-cells. Beta cells that are present are vacuolated and there is evidence of β-cell apoptosis. (d) Ferret (*Mustela putorius furo*), islet cell adenoma (insulinoma), insulin immunohistochemistry, streptavidin–biotin complex method. Note the presence of well-differentiated neoplastic islet cells (β-cells) arranged in "packets." The mass is encapsulated and lacks cellular atypia and invasiveness.

including α-cells (glucagon), β-cells (insulin), δ-cells (somatostatin), ε-cells (ghrelin), and PP-cells (pancreatic polypeptide) (Figure 17.7b).

Pancreatic islets in all species are characterized by a prominent microcirculation consisting of a network of capillaries, which is important in the rapid distribution of islet hormones systemically (i.e., endocrine). Capillaries that invest an islet come into intimate contact with all cell types (α-, β-, δ-, ε-, and PP-cells) and also allow paracrine interactions within the islet, thus tightly regulating homeostatic control of blood glucose levels (Kanno et al. 2002). There are certainly interspecies differences in how the capillaries invest pancreatic islets.

Islets contain a minor stromal component that can become more prominent when there is damage to the islets (i.e., fibrosis/fibroplasia). Depending upon the species, the islets can also have a fibrous capsule separating them from the surrounding exocrine tissue.

Ultrastructurally, pancreatic islet cells are rather homogeneous in appearance. They are polyhedral in shape with abundant cytoplasm and many neuroendocrine granules. The neuroendocrine granule content differs ultrastructurally based on the cell type: α-cells have electron-dense core granules with a clear halo; β-cells contain an electron-dense crystalline core; and δ-cells have variably sized granules that can range from dense to flocculent. The rough endoplasmic reticulum is modest, there are occasional mitochondria, and a Golgi complex is present. The migration of granules to the cell membrane for release can be appreciated ultrastructurally (Ghadially 1997).

Cell-to-cell interactions in the pancreatic islet are fairly complex and integral in regulating blood glucose levels (i.e., glycemia) (Jain and Lammert 2009). Beta-cells are associated with each other by gap junctions (six connexins form a tubular structure called a connexon, and connexons from adjacent cells form channels). Ions and metabolites can pass between cells, leading to synchronized responses, and are also important in controlling β-cell synthesis, storage, and secretion of insulin (Charollais et al. 2000). Connexin 36 (Cx36) appears to be critical in this regard based upon knockout mouse studies (Ravier et al. 2005). Another set of molecules that have been shown to be important in islet cell communication/interactions in the mouse and human are the Ephs, a family of receptor tyrosine kinases, types EphA and EphB, and their respective ligands, the ephrins (ephrin A and ephrin B). This allows bidirectional signaling between β-cells controlling insulin secretion (Konstantinova et al. 2007; Pasquale 2008). Mice deficient in ephrin-A5 are glucose intolerant, and their β-cells are unable to secrete appropriate levels of insulin in response to a glucose challenge (Konstantinova et al. 2007; Pasquale 2008). Alpha-cells interact via neural cell adhesion molecule (NCAM), which is supported by studies in NCAM knockout mice, where α-cells are intermingled with β-cells throughout the islet, versus wild-type mice, where α-cells are preferentially located at the periphery of the islet (Esni et al. 1999). Beta-cells and α-cells are also able to communicate/interact with each other. Beta-cells secrete Zn^{2+}, γ-aminobutyric acid (GABA), and insulin, which are all inhibitory on α-cells (Franklin et al. 2005). Alpha-cells express insulin receptors, where insulin acts as paracrine α-cell inhibitor (Kawamori et al. 2009). Somatostatin, secreted from δ-cells, is a paracrine inhibitor of α-cells and β-cells via somatostatin receptors (Cejvan et al. 2003). Ghrelin, secreted by ε-cells, also acts as a paracrine inhibitor of insulin secretion from β-cells in mice, rats, and humans (Dezaki et al. 2007).

17.7.2 Species Differences

Rats and mice have similar pancreatic anatomy and islet morphology (Table 17.2). Rodent pancreatic islets have a zonal distribution of cell types. Beta-cells are the predominant cell type and are located centrally within the islet, whereas α-, δ-, and PP-cells are present in lower numbers and are located at the periphery. Delta-cells associate intimately with α- and β-cells in the peripheral area of the islets. PP-cells are variable in number, and δ-cells can increase in number and become more centrally located during development of diabetes mellitus in susceptible strains/models (Adeghate and Ponery 2002). Rabbits are similar to rodents in regards to pancreatic islet morphology.

TABLE 17.2
Species Differences in Pancreatic and Islet Morphology

Species	Strain	Pancreas Morphology	Islet Endocrine Cell Distribution
Rat	Wistar	Body (dorsal) Left lobe (dorsal) Right lobe (dorsal, ventral)	β-cells central, α-cells at periphery forming a mantle, rare δ- and PP cells at periphery.
Mouse	Balb/c-nu/nu SKH-1	Splenic lobe Duodenal lobe	β-cells central, α-cells at periphery forming a mantle, rare δ- and PP cells at periphery.
Dog	Beagle Other breeds	Left lobe (splenic) Right lobe (duodenal) Body	Left lobe and body: α- and β-cells central and/or peripheral, few δ- and PP-cells (10%). Right lobe: single or small groups of β-cells, single α-cells, rare δ-cells, frequent PP-cells (90%).
Minipig	Göttingen	Right or head (duodenal portion) Left or tail (splenic portion)	Small islets with few β-cells, large islets with central β-cells. Large islets with peripheral β-cells. α-cells are rare in the right lobe and more frequent in the left lobe. δ-cells are rare and peripheral in islets. PP-cells are located in the right lobe as single cells, small groups, or peripheral in islets.
NHP	*Macaca fascicularis*	Head Body Tail	β-cells (70%–80% of total islet area) peripheral in islets and located as single or small groups in the exocrine pancreas. α-cells (7% of total islet area) are located centrally in islets or scattered individually in the exocrine pancreas. Scattered δ-cells (5% of total islet area) within the islets. PP-cells (4%–5% of total islet area) are located peripheral in islets or scattered within the exocrine pancreas.
Human	*Homo sapiens*	Head Body Tail	Highly variable composition, complex arrangements of islet cells. Beta cell volume is in the range of 52%–75% in nondiabetics. Islets from the uncinate process of the pancreas are PP-rich with a minority of β-cells.

Morphologically, the canine pancreas consists of three regions: left or splenic lobe, the right or duodenal lobe, and the intervening body. By using immunohistochemistry for insulin, as a marker for β-cells, and quantification using computer-assisted morphometry, Govendir et al. (1999) have shown that β-cell volume across the three areas of the pancreas differed with a significantly higher β-cell volume in the body and left lobes, 0.98 ± 0.05 and 0.97 ± 0.08 mm^3, respectively, when compared with the right lobe (0.67 ± 0.06 mm^3). This group also showed the potential pitfalls in determining β-cell volume. Their results depended on the orientation of sectioning of the pancreas (Govendir et al. 1999; Wieczorek et al. 1998).

In the canine, large compact islets were present primarily in the left lobe, and smaller islets and single endocrine cells were primarily located in the right lobe (Wieczorek et al. 1998). This is consistent with the findings of decreased β-cell volume in the right lobe (Govendir et al. 1999). In the right lobe, there is a preponderance of PP cells with scattered small groups of β-cells and rare α- and δ-cells (Wieczorek et al. 1998). Beta- (>60% of islet cells) and α-cells were located primarily within the islets in the left lobe, either centrally located or at the periphery, whereas δ- and PP-cells are also present within the islets at a lower frequency and also scattered in the exocrine pancreas.

The porcine (Göttingen minipig) pancreas is composed of two lobes, the right or head (duodenal portion) and the left or tail (splenic portion). Islets in the pig are more variable in size and have a looser structure when compared with other species. Porcine pancreatic islets also lack a complete capsule separating endocrine from exocrine pancreatic cells. Beta-cells are the most prevalent cell type, and they are found in three different patterns: small islets with few β-cells, large islets that have frequent β-cells located centrally (similar to rodents), and large islets with the reverse pattern (β-cells located peripherally with non-β-cells located centrally) (Wieczorek et al. 1998).

The pancreas in NHPs consists of a head, body, and tail, and the islets are arranged differently than those of rodents, minipigs, and dogs. The β-cells are located peripherally, and the α-cells are located centrally within the islets with scattered δ-cells and rare peripheral PP cells. There are some similarities to islets in humans (see below). In the head of the NHP pancreas, islets tend to have more PP-cells when compared with the body and tail. Islets in NHP can be characterized as either PP-cell rich or β-cell rich, where the PP-cell-rich islets are located in the posterior pancreatic head, whereas β-cell-rich islets are distributed throughout the rest of the pancreas (Wieczorek et al. 1998). In NHP, amyloid accumulation within islets is considered to be a marker of developing type 2 diabetes mellitus, which has also been reported in human diabetics (Schneider et al. 1980) and diabetic cats. There is conflicting evidence whether the accumulation of amyloid (likely derived from islet-associated polypeptide [IAPP] co-secreted with insulin by β-cells) within islets is the cause of or an effect of the β-cell dysfunction characteristic of type 2 diabetes (De Koning et al. 1993).

Human pancreatic islets lack the more regimented cellular organization that exists in other mammals. Beta-cells are intermingled with α- and δ-cells and are associated with the microvasculature within the islets in a random fashion. Beta-cells are not arranged in clusters as is common in other mammals. Although the majority of islet cells in humans are β-cells, they are intimately associated with the other cell types (e.g., α- and δ-cells), suggesting complex paracrine interactions between islet cells in humans. The fact that the arrangement of islet cell types with the microvasculature is random suggests that the paracrine effects are not based upon a defined distance from or proximity to islet capillaries. In comparison with rodents and other mammals, humans have a lower proportion of β-cells, a higher proportion of α-cells, and a less well-coordinated oscillatory activity as experimentally observed in isolated human islets. Pancreatic islets in diabetic patients do not appear morphologically different from nondiabetics except for the presence of amyloid. In conclusion, the differences between human islets and the islets of other mammals suggest major functional differences that make the appropriate translational animal model for diabetes mellitus difficult to identify (Bonner-Weir and O'Brien 2008; Cabrera et al. 2006).

17.7.3 CLINICAL CHEMISTRY PARAMETERS

The most commonly evaluated pancreatic islet function serum endpoints in laboratory animal models are serum glucose and insulin. Levels of glycosylated hemoglobin (HbA1c) can also be

TABLE 17.3

Reference Range Values for Serum Glucose and Insulin Levels from the Literature

Species	Strain	Insulin Reference Range	Glucose Reference Range	Reference
Rat	Wistar	12 ± 1 μU/mL		Giridharan et al. 1997
	ZDF, Lean, *Fa/Fa*	51.2 ± 4.7 μU/mL		Blonz et al. 1985
	ZDF, Obese, *fa/fa*	177.1 ± 32.0 μU/mL		Blonz et al. 1985
	GK			
Dog	Various Breeds	5–25 μIU/mL	60–120 mg/dL	Reimers 1998
	Beagle	N/A	97.3 ± 9.1 mg/dL	Marshall Bio.
	Mongrel	N/A	104.1 ± 9.2 mg/dL	Marshall Bio.
Ferret		10–40 μIU/mL	115.2 ± 24.2 mg/dL	Reimers 1998
				Marshall Bio.
Minipig	Göttingen	1.0–11.0 μg/100 mL	94.6 ± 12.8 mg/dL	Hannon et al. 1990
				Marshall Bio.
NHP	*Macaca fascicularis*	459 ± 409 pmol/L		Wagner et al. 1996

measured in animal models of diabetes mellitus. Insulin is measured by immunoassays (routinely used) or bioassays (complex with inconsistent results). Less common techniques include high-performance liquid chromatography (HPLC) and stable isotope dilution mass spectrometry assays (Chevenne et al. 1999). Glucose levels are normally kept within a fairly narrow range. With development of diabetes mellitus, animals become hyperglycemic, and glucosuria becomes detectable when serum glucose levels pass a threshold and is then excreted through the kidneys. Reference ranges for serum insulin in common laboratory animals are shown in Table 17.3. Due to a variety of sources, the reference ranges are in different units (Blonz et al. 1985; Reimers 1998; Giridharan et al. 1997; Wagner et al. 1996; Hannon et al. 1990; Marshall BioResources 2006).

17.7.4 NONPROLIFERATIVE LESIONS

Pancreatic islet inflammation (synonyms: islitis, insulitis, inflammatory cell infiltrate): Inflammatory cells (mostly mononuclear) can sometimes be seen within normal pancreatic islets, although they are more commonly seen in disease models during development of type 1 diabetes mellitus, resulting in β-cell destruction and loss. The inflammatory infiltrates most commonly seen are lymphocytes and/or macrophages (Anderson 1970; Marliss et al. 1982; Yale and Marliss 1984; Stokes 1986; Wagner et al. 2001).

Damage secondary to acute pancreatitis: Pancreatic islets can be affected (bystander effect) negatively during acute pancreatitis, and this most commonly occurs in dogs. Acute pancreatitis can be associated with edema, a mixed inflammatory cell infiltrate, fat saponification, and islet as well as exocrine tissue necrosis. Severe acute pancreatitis can lead to type 1 diabetes mellitus.

Spontaneous pancreatic islet fibrosis/hemorrhage: In Sprague–Dawley (CD(SD)IGS) rats, pancreatic islet hemorrhage and fibrosis have been shown to occur spontaneously, in males more often than in females and increasing in incidence with age. Spontaneous hemorrhage occurs and is associated with hemosiderin-laden macrophages and an inflammatory cell infiltrate of variable severity. Fibrous connective tissue eventually ensues separating the islet cells (Imaoka et al. 2007). Based upon the apparent sex bias of the lesion, Imaoka et al. investigated the effect of estradiol therapy and ovariectomy. They showed that estrogen treatment in males/ovariectomy in females did not abrogate development of spontaneous islet hemorrhage but did inhibit inflammation and development of islet fibrosis. In males treated with estradiol, there was no change in incidence of islet hemorrhage, although ovariectomy in female rats did cause an increase in incidence of the lesion (Imaoka et al. 2009).

Islet cell vacuolation: Vacuolation of the islet cells is not a specific finding and can represent an accumulation of glycogen, hydropic degeneration that can be seen spontaneously during diabetogenesis in several of the rodent models, following treatment with alloxan and streptozotocin in several species (Lenzen 2008; Kim and Steinberg 1984), and can even represent fixation artifact.

Amyloidosis: Islet amyloid polypeptide (IAPP; synonym: amylin) is co-secreted with insulin by β-cells and can accumulate and polymerize in pancreatic islets in cats, NHPs, and humans (Butler et al. 1990; Westermark et al. 1987; Palotay and Howard 1982). IAPP fibrils have been shown to induce apoptosis of β-cells in culture (Lorenzo et al. 1994). Pancreatic islet amyloid accumulation is commonly seen in mice on chronic toxicity studies, where it is associated with multisystemic amyloidosis, and not related to IAPP accumulation/polymerization (Williams 1964).

Several viruses have been shown to have a predilection for infection and cytolysis of β-cells in laboratory animal species and humans, ultimately leading to type 1 diabetes mellitus (Jun and Yoon 2003). These viruses include Coxsackie B virus in mice, NHPs, and humans (Hou et al. 1993; Yoon et al. 1978) and encephalomyocarditis virus in mice and hamsters (Yoon et al. 1980; Craighead and McLane 1968). Reovirus in mice (Onodera et al. 1978) and Kilham rat virus in rats (Guberski et al. 1991) have not been shown to directly infect rodent β-cells and are likely inducers of anti-β-cell autoimmunity.

17.7.4.1 Manifestations of Toxicity

17.7.4.1.1 Agents that Cause Islet Cell Degeneration/Necrosis

Alloxan (multiple species): Alloxan is a pyrimidine derivative that has also been shown to be toxic to pancreatic islet cells. Alloxan elicits β-cell necrosis by inhibiting glucokinase leading to inhibition of glucose-induced insulin secretion and by inducing reactive oxygen species formation in β-cells leading to oxidative stress and necrosis (Lenzen 2008). Following treatment with alloxan, β-cells become vacuolated/swollen and then undergo necrosis (Deeds et al. 2011; Patent and Alfert 1967; Dunn et al. 1943).

Streptozotocin (multiple species): Streptozotocin (STZ) is a broad-spectrum, glucosamine–nitrosourea antibiotic that is toxic to β-cells (males > females and C57BL/6 and CD-1 mice being sensitive). STZ has structural similarities to glucose and is preferentially transported into the β-cell via the GLUT2 glucose transporter, where it causes DNA and protein alkylation and NO production, ultimately leading to β-cell necrosis (Deeds et al. 2011; Bugger and Abel 2009; Lenzen 2008; Kim and Steinberg 1984). Following treatment with STZ, β-cells become vacuolated/swollen and then undergo necrosis (Deeds et al. 2011; Patent and Alfert 1967; Dunn et al. 1943).

Cyclosporin A (mice, rats, and humans): Treatment of rats with cyclosporin A for 7 days resulted in severe β-cell vacuolization and degranulation with ultrastructural evidence of endoplasmic reticulum dilation, markedly decreased serum and pancreatic insulin levels, and significantly increased serum glucose (Helmchen et al. 1984; Bani-Sacchi et al. 1990). A prostaglandin E_1 analog has been shown to prevent these changes (i.e., β-cell morphologic changes and, subsequently, the changes seen in insulin and glucose), perhaps via membrane stabilizing effects involving lysosomes and/or the cell as a whole (Löhr et al. 1989).

Zinc chelators: Zinc chelators such as dithizone and 8-hydroxy-quinoline are capable of inducing diabetes in rodents and rabbits. This is likely through an oxidant effect on β-cells. Zn is co-released from β-cell secretory granules with insulin. Chelating Zn could predispose β-cells to oxidative damage (Thompson 2008; Taylor 2005).

17.7.5 PROLIFERATIVE LESIONS

Nesidioblastosis is defined as a hyperfunctional change in islets that might be enlarged or normal sized. The characteristic changes are β-cell hypertrophy and proliferation of pancreatic ductular cells (Capen 2002).

Islet/islet cell hyperplasia: An increase in the number of islets or in the number/mass of islet cells and/or increased mitotic figures can be seen in regenerative responses in the islet (Capen 2002).

Islet cell adenoma: An islet cell adenoma (synonyms: insulinoma, glucagonoma, somatostatinoma, etc.) is defined as a benign neoplasm of pancreatic islet cells that is well demarcated from the surrounding pancreatic exocrine tissue by a fibrous capsule (Figure 17.7c). These neoplasms are generally solitary and less than 2 cm in diameter. The neoplastic cells are separated into small packets/lobules or trabeculae by a fine fibrovascular stroma. Neoplastic cells are well differentiated with rare mitotic figures (Capen 2002). Multiple islet cell adenomas are rare but have been seen in some species in combination with adrenal pheochromocytoma and likely represent a multiple endocrine neoplasm (MEN) syndrome (Capen 2002). Islet cell adenomas are usually composed of one type of endocrine cell that produces a single hormone (insulin, glucagon, somatostatin, or pancreatic polypeptide). Spontaneous islet cell adenomas are relatively rare in rodents. Charles River Laboratories have shown from their historic databases (78–104 weeks of age) that in CD-1 (Crl:CD-1 (ICR)) mice, the incidence in the male is 0.14% and in the female is 0.25% (Giknis and Clifford 2005). They have also shown that in Wistar Han rats (104 weeks of age), the incidence in the male is 7.39% and in the female 1.77% (Giknis and Clifford 2003). In Sprague–Dawley (Crl:CD (SD)) rats, islet cell adenomas were present in males at an incidence of 6.91% and in females at 3.42% (Giknis and Clifford 2004). Based on these incidences, rats might be more prone to develop spontaneous islet cell adenomas. Islet cell adenomas are common in dogs and ferrets (Capen 2002). NHPs rarely develop islet cell adenomas (McClure and Chandler 1982; Beniashvili 1989; Capen 2002).

Islet cell carcinoma: An islet cell carcinoma is a malignant neoplasm of pancreatic islet cells with local invasion into the surrounding pancreatic exocrine tissue with potential vascular invasion (Figure 17.7d). The neoplasm is poorly demarcated, lacks a complete fibrous capsule, can have cellular atypia, and can metastasize to the liver and local draining lymph nodes (Capen 2002). Spontaneous islet cell carcinomas are extremely rare in rodents (Capen 2002). Charles River Laboratories (Giknis and Clifford 2005) historical databases showed (78–104 weeks of age) that in CD-1 (Crl:CD-1 (ICR)) mice, the incidence in males was 0.0% and in females is 0.03%. They also reported that in Wistar Han rats (104 weeks of age), the incidence in males is 0.36% and in females 0.18% (Giknis and Clifford 2003). In Sprague–Dawley (Crl:CD (SD)) rats, they were present in males at an incidence of 2.43% and in females at 0.04% (Giknis and Clifford 2004). Islet cell carcinomas are relatively rare in dogs, ferrets, and NHPs (McClure and Chandler 1982; Beniashvili 1989; Capen 2002).

17.7.5.1 Pancreatic Islet Cell Carcinogenesis

Pancreatic xenobiotic-induced carcinogenesis has been shown in rats with the following agents: diethylaminomethyl-4-hydroxyaminoquinoline-1-oxide, heliotrine, and azinophosmethyl. They primarily cause β-cell adenomas (Wilson and Longnecker 1999). Alloxan and STZ have also been shown to induce islet cell neoplasms in rats 7 months posttreatment. Nicotinamide, given with alloxan or STZ, can increase their incidence (Wilson and Longnecker 1999). Mice seem to be resistant to islet cell carcinogenesis (Wilson and Longnecker 1999).

17.7.6 ANIMAL MODELS OF DIABETES MELLITUS

Two commonly used rodent models of type 1 diabetes mellitus include the non-obese diabetic (NOD) mouse and the BB Wistar rat. Other less frequently used models include the Long Evans Tokushima Lean (LETL) rat and the derived KDP substrain and the LWE-iddm rat strain (Chatzigeorgiou et al. 2009). The NOD mouse strain was derived from selective breeding of JcI-ICR mice (Makino et al. 1980). Islet inflammation (insulitis) develops at 4–5 weeks of age and progresses with subsequent β-cell loss and decreases in serum insulin levels until the animals are clinically diabetic by 12–30 months of age. There is a bias for diabetes developing in females (90% incidence) more frequently than in males (60% incidence) (Atkinson and Leiter 1999). The BB Wistar rat is non-obese and derived from the Wistar strain. Severe lymphocytic insulitis develops in both sexes with onset at sexual maturity. The inflammation causes selective necrosis of β-cells and occurs within hours to days of onset, and within 7–21 days, islets lack β-cells, are generally sparse and small in size, and do not manifest inflammation (Marliss et al. 1982; Yale and Marliss 1984). Animals develop severe hyperglycemia, lack an insulin response to challenge, and can develop a neuropathy characterized by axonal atrophy. The pathogenesis is considered to be a cell-mediated autoimmune reaction against β-cells, though a humoral component is also probable (Yale and Marliss 1984). Chemically induced type 1 diabetes mellitus can be elicited in many animal model systems by treating with either streptozotocin (STZ) or alloxan. Both chemicals are either dosed intraperitoneally or intravenously. Clinical diabetes mellitus becomes evident when hyperglycemia occurs between 2 and 5 days after STZ or alloxan treatment (Deeds et al. 2011; Bugger and Abel 2009; Lenzen 2008; Kim and Steinberg 1984; Dunn et al. 1943). Based upon the mechanism of action of both of these chemicals, it is likely that this treatment regimen can be used to induce diabetes in any animal species following validation.

Commonly used rodent models of type 2 diabetes mellitus include the Zucker diabetic fatty (ZDF) rat, the Goto–Kakizaki (GK) rat, the *ob/ob* mouse, and the *db/db* mouse. An overview of less frequently utilized models is reported in Chatzigeorgiou et al. (2009). The ZDF rat is a commonly used model of type 2 diabetes mellitus. ZDF rats have a missense mutation in the leptin receptor gene (*Lepr* or *Fa*), which results in an inactive receptor and in hyperphagia leading to high circulating levels of triglycerides and obesity (Phillips et al. 1996). ZDF rats were derived by selective breeding of hyperglycemic ZF rats and have a second mutation in a β-cell–specific gene that results in hyperinsulinemia at 7–10 weeks of age in males. Females require a diabetogenic diet in order to become hyperglycemic. Male ZDF rats are obese, insulin resistant, hyperglycemic (starting at about 6 weeks of age), and hypertriglyceridemic and become hyperinsulinemic (peak insulin level at 7–10 weeks of age), after which the insulin levels decline markedly, correlating with the marked loss of β-cell mass (Nugent et al. 2008; Unger and Orci 2001; Unger 1997). Pancreatic islets become misshapen with loss of the islet cell patterns and the islet cell interactions that are seen in wild-type rodents (Figure 17.7e). Beta-cell vacuolation, degeneration, and apoptosis are prominent, with a temporal increase in the amount of islet fibrosis (Nugent et al. 2008; Unger and Orci 2001; Unger 1997). Alpha- and δ-cells remain at relatively stable numbers during diabetogenesis in this model. In obese ZDF rats, fat accumulates within islet cells leading to cellular overload and dysfunction/degeneration of β-cells (lipotoxicity), which is likely mediated by increased intracellular nitric oxide production (Unger 1997; Unger and Orci 2001). Blocking of triglyceride accumulation in β-cells also blocks the development of diabetes in this model (Unger 1997; Unger and Orci 2001).

The GK rat is a NOD rat strain that has primary β-cell defects and peripheral insulin resistance in both sexes (Portha 2005; Östenson 2001; Bisbis et al. 1993). The phenotype, spontaneous type 2 diabetes mellitus, is thought to be due to several mutations that are likely in genes that regulate fasting plasma glucose, fasting insulin levels, glucose tolerance, insulin secretion, and adiposity, including the Niddm1 locus on rat chromosome 1 (Galli et al. 1996; Gauguier et al. 1996). These mutations result in impaired insulin secretion from β-cells. Decreased β-cell neogenesis, which appears gestationally, is passed onto the offspring and results in acquired β-cell dysfunction with decreased β-cell differentiation due to chronic hyperglycemia (glucotoxicity). The phenotype of the GK rat is, therefore, dependent upon genetic as well as epigenetic factors (Portha 2005; Östenson 2001; Bisbis et al. 1993).

The *db/db* mouse is a model of obesity and type 2 diabetes mellitus. Obesity/diabetes in this model develops due to a lack of leptin (hypothalamic) action that is caused by a leptin receptor defect (Chen et al. 1996). A premature "stop" codon is inserted due to abnormal splicing of the leptin receptor transcript resulting in a short isoform of the receptor (*Ob-Ra*) (Lee et al. 1996). The strain develops obesity and severe diabetes mellitus by 8 weeks of age. The model also becomes hyperinsulinemic and hypertriglyceridemic (Buchanan et al. 2005; Chen et al. 1996; Lee et al. 1996).

The *ob/ob* mouse has recessive mutations in the leptin gene, which cause either a lack of mature leptin (*ob/ob²ᴶ* strain) or synthesis of a truncated leptin protein, which is degraded in the adipocyte (*ob/ob¹ᴶ* strain) (Zhang et al. 1994; Moon and Friedman 1997). Obesity and diabetes are caused by leptin deficiency, which results in long-term lack of hypothalamic appetite suppression, leading to hyperphagia. The mice are obese by 4 weeks of age, become hyperinsulinemic with impaired glucose tolerance, and develop type 2 diabetes mellitus by 15 weeks of age (Buchanan et al. 2005; Friedman and Halaas 1998; Moon and Friedman 1997).

Transgenic and knockout animals have been bred with some utility in the study of the pathogenesis of diabetes mellitus and as pharmacology models. These models include targeted disruption/deletion of genes such as insulin receptor substrate 1 (IRS1) (Tamemoto et al. 1994), insulin receptor substrate 2 (IRS2) (Withers et al. 1998), insulin receptor human transgene in muscle (Chang et al. 1994), and dominant-negative glucokinase (Grupe et al. 1995). These models have demonstrated postnatal survival, thus making them useful. Other genes such as glucokinase (Grupe et al. 1995) and insulin receptor (Joshi et al. 1996), when deleted, have resulted in perinatal death due to hyperglycemia and ketoacidosis. Genes (e.g., insulin receptor, PPARγ, GLUT4, and IGF1) have also been knocked out with tissue specificity (e.g., β-cells, muscle, liver, etc.), avoiding early death of the animals (Rees and Alcolado 2005).

REFERENCES

Adeghate E., Ponery A.S. (2002). Ghrelin stimulates insulin secretion from the pancreas of normal and diabetic rats. *J Neuroendocrinol* 14:555–60.

Aguzzi A., Wagner E.F., Williams R.L., Courtneidge S.A. (1990). Sympathetic hyperplasia and neuroblastomas in transgenic mice expressing polyoma middle T antigen. *New Biol* 2:533–43.

Akana S.F., Shinsako J., Dallman M.F. (1983). Drug-induced adrenal hypertrophy provides evidence for reset in the adrenocortical system. *Endocrinology* 113:2232–7.

Akanishi M., Sawamoto O., Kawashima M., Kuwamura M., Yamate J. (2004). Morphological changes in the parathyroid gland of rats with humoral hypercalcaemia of malignancy. *J Comp Pathol* 131:92–7.

Alison R.H., Capen C.C., Prentice D.E. (1994). Neoplastic lesions of questionable significance to humans. *Toxicol Pathol* 22:179–86.

Almeida H., Matos L., Ferreira J., Neves D. (2006). Age-related effects of dexamethasone administration in adrenal zona reticularis. *Ann N Y Acad Sci* 1067:354–60.

Anderson A.C. (1970). General pathology. In *The Beagle as an Experimental Dog* (A.C. Anderson and L.S. Good, eds.), pp. 520–46. Iowa State University Press, Ames.

Angelo G., Wood R.J., Mayer J. (2002). Novel intracellular proteins associated with cellular vitamin D action. *Nutr Rev* 60:209–11.

Asa S.L., Ezzat S. (1999). Molecular determinants of pituitary cytodifferentiation. *Pituitary* (3–4):159–68.

Atkinson M., Leiter E.H. (1999). The NOD mouse model of insulin dependent diabetes: as good as it gets? *Nat Med* 5:601–4.

Attia M.A. Cytological study on pituitary adenomas in senile untreated beagle bitches. Arch Toxicol 46(3–4):287–93

Axelrad A.A., Leblond C.P. (1955). Induction of thyroid tumors in rats by a low iodine diet. *Cancer* 8:339–67.

Baccarelli A., Pesatori A.C., Bertazzi P.A. (2000). Occupational and environmental agents as *endocrine disruptors: experimental and human evidence. J Endocrinol Invest* 23:771–81.

Bailey S.A., Zidell R.H., Perry R.W. (2004). Relationships between organ weight and body/brain weight in the rat: what is the best analytical endpoint? *Toxicol Pathol* 32:448–66.

Bani-Sacchi T., Bani D., Filipponi F., Michel A., Houssin D. (1990). Immunocytochemical and ultrastructural changes of islet cells in rats treated long-term with cyclosporine at immunotherapeutic doses. *Transplantation* 5:982–7.

Bedrak E., Chap Z., Brown R. (1983). Age-related changes in the hypothalamic-pituitary-testicular function of the rat. *Exp Gerontol* 18(2):95–104.

Beniashvili D.S. (1989). An overview of the world literature on spontaneous tumors in nonhuman primates. *J Med Primatol* 18:423–37.

Benitz K.F., Roberts G.K., Yusa A. (1967). Morphologic effects of minocycline in laboratory animals. *Toxicol Appl Pharmacol* 11:150–70.

Bielohuby M., Herbach N., Wanke R., Maser-Gluth C., Beuschlein F., Wolf E., Hoeflich A. (2007). Growth analysis of the mouse adrenal gland from weaning to adulthood: time- and gender-dependent alterations of cell size and number in the cortical compartment. *Am J Physiol Endocrinol Metab* 293(1): E139–46.

Bisbis S., Bailbe D., Tormo M.A., Picarel-Blanchot F., Derouet M., Simon J., Portha B. (1993). Insulin resistance in the GK rat: decreased receptor number but normal kinase activity in the liver. *Am J Physiol* 265:E807–13.

Bland M.L., Desclozeaux M., Ingraham H.A. (2003). Tissue growth and remodeling of the embryonic and adult adrenal gland. *Ann N Y Acad Sci* 995:59–72.

Blonz E.R., Stern J.S., Curry D.L. (1985). Dynamics of pancreatic insulin release in young Zucker rat: a heterozygote effect. *Am J Physiol* 248:E188–93.

Bonner-Weir S., O'Brien T.D. (2008). Perspectives in diabetes, islets in type 2 diabetes: in honor of Dr. Robert C. Turner. *Diabetes* 57:2899–904.

Borzelleca J.F., Capen C.C., Hallagan J.B. (1987). Lifetime toxicity/carcinogenicity study of FD & C Red No. 3 (erythrosine) in rats. *Food Chem Toxicol* 25:723–33.

Botts S., Jokinen M.P., Isaacs K.R., Meuten D.J., Tanaka N. (1991). Proliferative lesions of the thyroid and parathyroid glands. Guidelines for Toxicologic Pathology, 1–8.

Bourdeau A.M., Plachot J.J., Cournot-Witmer G., Pointillart A., Balsan S., Sachs C. (1987). Parathyroid response to aluminum in vitro: ultrastructural changes and PTH release. *Kidney Int* 31:15–24.

Brzoska M.M., Moniuszko-Jakoniuk J. (2005). Effect of low-level lifetime exposure to cadmium on calciotropic hormones in aged female rats. *Arch Toxicol* 79:636–46.

Buchanan J., Mazumder P.K., Hu P., Chakrabarti G., Roberts M.W., Yun U.J., Cookey R.C., Litwin S.E., Abel E.D. (2005). Reduced cardiac efficiency and altered substrate metabolism precedes the onset of hyperglycemia and contractile dysfunction in two mouse models of insulin resistance and obesity. *Endocrinology* 146:5341–9.

Bucher J.R., Huff J., Haseman J.K., Eustis S.L., Davis W.E., Jr., Meierhenry E.F. (1990). Toxicology and carcinogenicity studies of diuretics in F344 rats and B6C3F1 mice. 2. Furosemide. *J Appl Toxicol JAT* 10:369–78.

Buckingham J.C. (2008). The hypothalamo–pituitary–adrenocortical axis: endocrinology, pharmacology, pathophysiology and developmental effects. In *Adrenal Toxicology* (P.W. Harvey, D.J. Everett, C.J. Springall, eds.), pp. 77–107, Informa Healthcare, New York.

Bugger H., Abel E.D. (2009). Rodent models of diabetic cardiomyopathy. *Disease Models Mech* 2:454–66.

Burkhardt W.A., Guscetti F., Boretti F.S., Todesco A.I., Aldajarov N., Lutz T.A., Reusch C.E., Sieber-Ruckstuhl N.S. (2011). Adrenocorticotropic hormone, but not trilostane, causes severe adrenal hemorrhage, vacuolization, and apoptosis in rats. *Domest Anim Endocrinol* 40(3):155–64.

Butler P.C., Chou J., Carter W.B., Wang Y.N., Bu B.H., Chang D., Chang J.K., Rizza R.A. (1990). Effects of meal ingestion on plasma amylin concentration in NIDDM and nondiabetic humans. *Diabetes* 39:752–6.

Cabrera O., Berman D.M., Kenyon N.S., Ricordi C., Berggren P.-O., Caicedo A. (2006). The unique cytoarchitecture of human pancreatic islets has implications for islet cell function. *Proc Natl Acad Sci* 103(7):2334–9.

Capen C.C. (1983). Structural and biochemical aspects of parathyroid function in animals. In *Endocrine System* (T.C. Jones, U. Mohr, R.D. Hunt, eds.), pp. 217–47, Springer-Verlag, Berlin.

Capen C.C. (1994). Mechanisms of chemical injury of the thyroid gland. In *Receptor-Mediated Biological Processes: Implications for Evaluating Carcinogenesis*, pp. 173–91. Wiley-Liss, Inc. New York.

Capen C.C. (1997). Mechanistic data and risk assessment of selected toxic end points of the thyroid gland. *Toxicol Pathol* 25:39–48.

Capen C.C. (1998). Correlation of mechanistic data and histopathology in the evaluation of selected toxic endpoints of the endocrine system. *Toxicol Lett* 102–3, 405–9.

Capen C.C. (2001). Overview of structural and functional lesions in endocrine organs of animals. *Toxicol Pathol* 29:8–33.

Capen C.C. (2002). Tumors of the pancreatic islet cells. In *Tumors of Domestic Animals* (D.J. Meuten ed.), 4th edition, pp. 684–8, Iowa State Press, Ames, IA.

Capen C.C., Black H.E. (1974). Animal model of human disease. Medullary thyroid carcinoma, multiple endocrine neoplasia, Sipple's syndrome. Animal model: ultimobranchial thyroid neoplasm in the bull. *Am J Pathol* 74:377–80.

Capen C.C., Martin S.L. (1989a). The effects of xenobiotics on the structure and function of thyroid follicular and C-cells. *Toxicol Pathol* 17:266–93.

Capen C.C., Martin S.L. (1989b). Mechanisms that lead to disease of the endocrine system in animals. *Toxicol Pathol* 17:234–49.

Capen C.C., Rosol T.J. (1989). Recent advances in the structure and function of the parathyroid gland in animals and the effects of xenobiotics. *Toxicol Pathol* 17:333–45.

Capen C.C., DeLellis R.A., Yarrington J.T. (2002). Endocrine system. In *Handbook of Toxicologic Pathology* (W.M. Haschek, C. Rousseaux, M.A. Wallig, eds.), vol. 2, pp. 719–71, Academic Press, San Diego.

Carlson B.M. (1988). *The Digestive System in Patten's Foundations of Embryology*, 5th edition, pp. 518–20, McGraw Hill Publishing Company, New York.

Carlus M., Elies L., Fouque M.C., Maliver P., Schorsch F. (2011). Historical control data of neoplastic lesions in the Wistar Hannover Rat among eight 2-year carcinogenicity studies. *Exp Toxicol Pathol* 63:519–606.

Carney J.A. (1992). Adrenal gland. In *Histology for Pathologists* (S.S. Sternberg, ed.), Raven Press, New York.

Cejvan K., Coy D.H., Efendic S. (2003). Intra-islet somatostatin regulates glucagon release via type 2 somatostatin receptors in rats. *Diabetes* 52:1176–81.

Chamanza R., Marxfeld H.A., Blanco A.I., Naylor S.W., Bradley A.E. (2010). Incidences and range of spontaneous findings in control cynomolgus monkeys (*Macaca fascicularis*) used in toxicity studies. *Toxicol Pathol* 38:642–57.

Chang P.Y., Benecke H., Le Marchand-Brustel Y., Lawitts J., Moller D.E. (1994). Expression of a dominant-negative mutant human insulin receptor in the muscle of transgenic mice. *J Biol Chem* 269:16034–40.

Charollais A., Gjinovci A., Huarte J., Bauquis J., Nadal A., Martin F., Andreu A., Sanchez-Andres J.V., Calabrese A., Bosco D., Soria B., Wollheim C.B., Herrera P.L., Maeda P. (2000). Junctional communication of pancreatic beta cells contributes to the control of insulin secretion and glucose tolerance. *J Clin Invest* 106:235–43.

Chatzigeorgiou A., Halapas A., Kalafatakis K., Kamper E.F. (2009). The use of animal models in the study of diabetes mellitus. *In Vivo* 23(2):245–58.

Chen H., Charlat O., Tartaglia L.A., Woolf E.A., Weng X., Ellis S.J., Lakey N.D., Culpepper J., Moore K.J., Breitbart R.E., Duyk G.M., Tepper R.I., Morgenstern J.P. (1996). Evidence that the diabetes gene encodes the leptin receptor: identification of a mutation in the leptin receptor gene in db/db mice. *Cell* 84:491–5.

Chen H.J. (1984). Age and sex difference in serum and pituitary thyrotropin concentrations in the rat: influence by pituitary adenoma. *Exp Gerontol* 19(1):1–6.

Chen H., Hu B., Allegretto E.A., Adams J.S. (2000). The vitamin D response element-binding protein. A novel dominant-negative regulator of vitamin D-directed transactivation. *J Biol Chem* 275:35557–64.

Cheng L. (1980). Pheochromocytoma in rats: incidence, etiology, morphology and functional activity. *J Environ Pathol Toxicol* 4(5–6):219–28.

Chen-Pan C., Pan I.J., Yamamoto Y., Sakogawa T., Yamada J., Hayashi Y. (1999). Prompt recovery of damaged adrenal medullae induced by salinomycin. *Toxicol Pathol* 27:563–572.

Cheung C.C., Lustig R.H. (2007). Pituitary development and physiology. *Pituitary* 10(4):335–50.

Chevenne D., Trivin F., Porquet D. (1999). Insulin assays and reference values. *Diabet Metab (Paris)* 25:459–76.

Chronwall B.M., Millington W.R., Griffin W.S., Unnerstall J.R., O'Donohue T.L. (1987). Histological evaluation of the dopaminergic regulation of proopiomelanocortin gene expression in the intermediate lobe of the rat pituitary, involving in situ hybridization and [3H]thymidine uptake measurement. *Endocrinology* 120(3):1201–11.

Colby H.D., Longhurst P.A. (1992). Toxicology of the adrenal gland. In *Endocrine Toxicology* (C.K. Atterwill, J.D. Flack, eds.), pp. 243–281, Cambridge University Press, Cambridge.

Colagiovanni D.B., Drolet D.W., Dihel L., Meyer D.J., Hart K., Wolf J. (2006). Safety assessment of 4-thio-beta-d-arabinofuranosylcytosine in the beagle dog suggests a drug-induced centrally mediated effect on the hypothalamic–pituitary–adrenal axis. *Int J Toxicol* 25:119–26.

Colagiovanni D.B., Meyer D.J. (2008). Hypothalamic–pituitary–adrenal toxicity in dogs. In *Adrenal Toxicology* (P.W. Harvey, D.J. Everett, C.J. Springall, eds.), pp. 161–73, Informa Healthcare, New York.

Conaway D.H., Padgett G.A., Bunton T.E., Nachreiner R., Hauptman J. (1985). Clinical and histological features of primary progressive, familial thyroiditis in a colony of borzoi dogs. *Vet Pathol* 22:439–46.

Cónsole G.M., Jurado S.B., Rulli S.B., Calandra R.S., Gómez Dumm C.L. (2001). Ultrastructural and quantitative immunohistochemical changes induced by nonsteroid antiandrogens on pituitary gonadotroph population of prepubertal male rats. *Cells Tissues Organs* 169(1):64–72.

Cormack M.J. (1989). The endocrine system. In *Ham's Textbook of Histology*, 9th edition, pp. 611–5, Harper and Row, New York.

Craighead J.E., McLane M.F. (1968). Diabetes mellitus: induction in mice by encephalomyocarditis virus. *Science* 162:913–5.

Crofton K.M. (2008). Thyroid disrupting chemicals: mechanisms and mixtures. *Int J Androl* 31:209–23.

Curran P.G., DeGroot L.J. (1991). The effect of hepatic enzyme-inducing drugs on thyroid hormones and the thyroid gland. *Endocr Rev* 12:135–50.

De Koning E.J., Bodkin N.L., Hansen B.C., Clark A. (1993). Diabetes mellitus in *Macaca mulatta* monkeys is characterized by islet amyloidosis and reduction in beta cell population. *Diabetologia* 36:378–84.

Deeds M.C., Anderson J.M., Armstrong A.S., Gastineau D.A., Hiddinga H.J., Jahangir A., Eberhardt N.L., Kudva Y.C. (2011). Single dose streptozotocin-induced diabetes: considerations for study design in islet transplantation models. *Lab Anim* 45:131–40.

Deichmann W. B., Bernal E., Anderson W.A., Keplinger M., Landeen K., Macdonald W., McMahon R., Stebbins R. (1964). The chronic oral toxicity of oxytetracycline Hcl and tetracycline Hcl in the rat, dog and pig. *Ind Med Surg* 33:787–806.

DeLellis R.A., Wolfe H.J., Mohr U. (1987). Medullary thyroid carcinoma in the Syrian golden hamster: an immunohistochemical study. *Exp Pathol* 31:11–6.

DeLellis R.A., Nunnemacher G., Bitman W.R., Gagel R.F., Tashjian A.H., Jr., Blount M., Wolfe H.J. (1979). C-cell hyperplasia and medullary thyroid carcinoma in the rat. An immunohistochemical and ultrastructural analysis. *Lab Invest* 40:140–54.

Dempsey E.W. (1949). The chemical cytology of the thyroid gland. *Ann N Y Acad Sci* 50:336–57.

Dezaki K., Kakei M., Yada T. (2007). Ghrelin uses Galphai2 and activates voltage-dependent K+ channels to attenuate glucose-induced Ca2+ signaling and insulin release in islet beta cells: novel signal transduction of ghrelin. *Diabetes* 56:2319–27.

Diaz-Espiñeira M.M., Mol J.A., van den Ingh T.S., van der Vlugt-Meijer R.H., Rijnberk A., Kooistra H.S. (2008). Functional and morphological changes in the adenohypophysis of dogs with induced primary hypothyroidism: loss of TSH hypersecretion, hypersomatotropism, hypoprolactinemia, and pituitary enlargement with transdifferentiation. *Domest Anim Endocrinol* 35(1):98–111.

Dominick M.A., McGuire E.J., Reindel J.F., Bobrowski W.F., Bocan T.M., Gough A.W. (1993). Subacute toxicity of a novel inhibitor of acyl-CoA: cholesterol acyltransferase in beagle dogs. *Fundam Appl Toxicol* 20(2):217–24.

Donckier J.E., Michel L. (2010). Phaeochromocytoma: state-of-the-art. *Acta Chir Belg* 110(2):140–8.

Doppelt S.H., Neer R.M., Potts J.T., Jr. (1981). Human parathyroid hormone 1-34-mediated hypercalcemia in a rat model, and its inhibition by dichloromethane diphosphonate. *Calcif Tissue Int* 33:649–54.

Duffy P.H., Lewis S.M., Mayhugh M.A., Trotter R.W., Hass B.S., Latendresse J.R., Thorn B.T., Tobin G., Feuers R.J. (2008). Neoplastic pathology in male Sprague–Dawley rats fed AIN-93M diet ad libitum or at restricted intakes. *Nutr Res.* 28(1):36–42.

Dunn J.S., Sheenan H.L., McLetchie N.G.B. (1943). Necrosis of islets of Langerhans produced experimentally. *Lancet* 1:484–7.

El Etreby M.F., El Bab M.R. (1978a). Effect of 17 beta-estradiol on cells stained for FSH beta and/or LH beta in the dog pituitary gland. *Cell Tissue Res* 193(2):211–8.

El Etreby M.F., Fath El Bab M.R. (1978b). Effect of cyproterone acetate, d-norgestrel and progesterone on cells of the pars distalis of the adenohypophysis in the beagle bitch. *Cell Tissue Res* 191(2):205–18.

Elkahloun A.G., Powers J.F., Nyska A., Eisenhofer G., Tischler A.S. (2006). Gene expression profiling of rat pheochromocytoma. *Ann N Y Acad Sci* 1073:290–9.

Endo K., Katsumata K., Hirata M., Masaki T., Kubodera N., Nakamura T., Ikeda K., Ogata E. (2000). 1,25-Dihydroxyvitamin D3 as well as its analogue OCT lower blood calcium through inhibition of bone resorption in hypercalcemic rats with continuous parathyroid hormone-related peptide infusion. *J Bone Miner Res* 15:175–81.

Engeland W.C., Ennen W.B., Elayaperumal A., Durand D.A., Levay-Young B.K. (2005). Zone-specific cell proliferation during compensatory adrenal growth in rats. *Am J Physiol Endocrinol Metab* 288(2):E298–306.

Enochs W.S., Nilges M.J., Swartz H.M. (1993). The minocycline-induced thyroid pigment and several synthetic models: identification and characterization by electron paramagnetic resonance spectroscopy. *J Pharmacol Exp Ther* 266:1164–76.

Erdmann B., Denner K., Gerst H., Lenz D., Bernhardt R. (1995). Human adrenal CYP11B1: Localization by in situ-hybridization and functional expression in cell cultures. *Endocr Res* 21:425–35.

Esni F., Täljedal I., Perl A. et al. (1999). Neural cell adhesion molecule (NCAM) is required for cell type segregation and normal ultrastructure in pancreatic islets. *J Cell Biol* 144:325–37.

Fong A.C., Hardman J.M., Porta E.A. (1982). Immunocytochemical hormonal features of pituitary adenomas of aging Wistar male rats. *Mech Ageing Dev* 20(2):141–54.

Franklin I., Gromada J., Gjinovci A., Theander S., Wollheim C.B. (2005). Beta-cell secretory products activate alpha-cell ATP-dependent potassium channels to inhibit glucagon release. *Diabetes* 54:1808–15.

Friedman J.M., Halaas J.L. (1998). Leptin and the regulation of body weight in mammals. *Nature* 395:763–70.

Frith C.H., Chandra M. (1991). Incidence, distribution, and morphology of amyloidosis in Charles Rivers CD-1 mice. *Toxicol Pathol* 19:123–7.

Frith C.H., Botts S., Jokinen M.P., Eighmy J.J., Hailey J.R., Morgan S.J., Chandra M. (2000). Non-proliferative lesions of the endocrine system in rats. In: *Guides for Toxicologic Pathology*, pp 1–22, STP/ARP/AFIP, Washington, DC.

Fritz T.E., Zeman R.C., Zelle M.R. (1970). Pathology and familial incidence of thyroiditis in a closed beagle colony. *Exp Mol Pathol* 12:14–30.

Furth J., Ueda G., Clifton K.H. (1973). The pathophysiology of pituitaries and their tumors: methodological advances. In *Methods in Cancer Research* H. Busch, ed.), vol. 10, Academic Press, New York.

Galli J., Li L., Glaser A., Östenson C.G., Jiao H., Fakhrai-Rad H., Jacob H.J., Lander E.S., Luthman H. (1996). Genetic analysis of non-insulin dependent diabetes mellitus in the GK rat. *Nat Genet* 12:31–7.

Gauguier D., Froguel P., Parent V., Bernard C., Bihoreau M., Portha B., James M.R., Penicaud L., Lathrop M., Ktorza A. (1996). Chromosomal mapping of genetic loci associated with non-insulin dependent diabetes in the GK rat. *Nat Genet* 12:38–43.

Ghadially F.N. (1997). *Ultrastructural Pathology of the Cell and Matrix*, 4th edition, vol. 1, pp. 394–7, Butterworth-Heinemann Medical Publications, Boston, MA.

Giknis M.L.A., Clifford C.B. (2003). *Spontaneous Neoplasms and Survival in Wistar Han Rats: Compilation of Control Group Data*. Charles River Laboratories, Wilmington, MA.

Giknis M.L.A., Clifford C.B. (2004). *Compilation of Spontaneous Neoplastic Lesions and Survival in Crl:CD®(SD) Rats from Control Groups*. Charles River Laboratories, Wilmington, MA.

Giknis M.L.A., Clifford C.B. (2005). *Spontaneous Neoplastic Lesions in the Crl:CD-1 (ICR) Mouse in Control Groups from 18 Month to 2 Year Studies*. Charles River Laboratories, Wilmington, MA.

Giridharan N.V., Lakshmi C.N., Raghuramulu N. (1997). Identification of impaired-glucose-tolerant animals from a Wistar inbred rat colony. *Lab Anim Sci* 47:428–31.

Gittes R.F., Radde I.C. (1966). Experimental model for hyperparathyroidism: effect of excessive numbers of transplanted isologous parathyroid glands. *J Urol* 95:595–603.

Goedegebuure S.A., Hazewinkel H.A. (1986). Morphological findings in young dogs chronically fed a diet containing excess calcium. *Vet Pathol* 23:594–605.

Goelz M., Dixon D., Myers P., Clark J., Forsythe D. (1998). Ganglioneuroma in the adrenal gland of a rat. *Contemp Top Lab Anim Sci* 37(2):75–7.

Gomba S., Gautier A., Lemarchand-Beraud T., Gardiol D. (1976). Pigmentation and dysfunction of Gunn rat thyroid: correlation between morphological and biochemical data. *Virchows Arch B Cell Pathol* 20:41–54.

Gordon G., Sparano B.M., Kramer A.W., Kelly R.G., Iatropoulos M.J. (1984). Thyroid gland pigmentation and minocycline therapy. *Am J Pathol* 117:98–109.

Gosselin S.J., Capen C.C., Martin S.L. (1981). Histologic and ultrastructural evaluation of thyroid lesions associated with hypothyroidism in dogs. *Vet Pathol* 18:299–309.

Govendir M., Canfield P.J., Church D.B. (1999). Morphometric study of the β-cell volume of the canine pancreas with consideration of the axis of tissue transection. *Anat Histol Embryol* 28:351–4.

Greaves P. (2007). *Histopathology of Preclinical Toxicity Studies*. Academic Press, Amsterdam.

Greco D., Stabenfeldt G.H. (2007). Endocrine glands and their function. In *Textbook of Veterinary Physiology* (J.G. Cunningham, B.G. Klein, eds.), pp. 428–463. Elsevier, St. Louis.

Greim H., Hartwig A., Reuter U., Richter-Reichhelm H.B., Thielmann H.W. (2009). Chemically induced pheochromocytomas in rats: mechanisms and relevance for human risk assessment. *Crit Rev Toxicol* 39(8):695–718.

Grone A., Rosol T.J., Baumgartner W., Capen C.C. (1992). Effects of humoral hypercalcemia of malignancy on the parathyroid gland in nude mice. *Vet Pathol* 29:343–50.

Grupe A., Hltgren B., Ryan A., Ma Y.H., Bauer M., Stewart T.A. (1995). Transgenic knockouts reveal a critical requirement for pancreatic β cell glucokinase in maintaining glucose homeostasis. *Cell* 83:69–78.

Guberski D.L., Thomas V.A., Shek W.R. Like A.A., Handler E.S., Rossini A.A., Wallace J.E., Welsh R.M. (1991). Induction of type I diabetes by Kilham's rat virus in diabetes-resistant BB/Wor rats. *Science* 254: 1010–3.

Guzman R.E., Radi Z.A. (2007). Chronic lymphocytic thyroiditis in a cynomolgus macaque (*Macaca fascicularis*). *Toxicol Pathol* 35:296–9.

Haines D.C., Chattopadhyay S., Ward J.M. (2001). Pathology of aging B6;129 mice. *Toxicol Pathol* 29:653–61.

Hamlin M.H. 2nd, Banas D.A. (1990). *Pathology of the Fischer Rat, Reference and Atlas, Adrenal Gland* (G.A. Boorman, S.L. Eustis, M.R. Elwell, C.A. Montgomery Jr., W.F. MacKenzie, eds.), pp. 501–18. Academic Press, San Diego.

Hammer G.D., Parker K.L., Schimmer B.P. (2005). Minireview: transcriptional regulation of adrenocortical development. *Endocrinology* 146(3):1018–24.

Hannon J.P., Bossone C.A., Wade C.E. (1990). Normal physiological values for conscious pigs used in biomedical research. *Lab Anim Sci* 40:293–8.

Hardisty J.F., Boorman G. (1990). Thyroid gland. In *Pathology of the Fischer Rat: Reference and Atlas* (Boorman, G., Eustis, S.L., Elwell, M.R., Montgomery, C.A., and MacKenzie, W.F. eds.), pp. 519–34. Academic Press, San Diego.

Hardisty J.F., Boorman G. (1999). Thryoid and parathyroid. In *Pathology of the Mouse* (Maronpot, R., Boorman, G., and Gaul, B.W. eds.), pp. 537–52. Cache River Press, St. Louis.

Harvey P.W. (2005). Human relevance of rodent prolactin-induced non-genotoxic mammary carcinogenesis: prolactin involvement in human breast cancer and significance for toxicology risk assessments. *J Appl Toxicol* 25(3):179–83.

Harvey P.W. (2012). Hypothesis: prolactin is tumorigenic to human breast: dispelling the myth that prolactin-induced mammary tumors are rodent-specific. *J Appl Toxicol* Jan;32(1):1–9.

Harvey P.W., Everett D.J. (2003). The adrenal cortex and steroidogenesis as cellular and molecular targets for toxicity: critical omissions from regulatory endocrine disrupter screening strategies for human health? *J Appl Toxicol* 23(2):81–7. Review.

Harvey P.W., Sutcliffe C. (2010). Adrenocortical hypertrophy: establishing cause and toxicological significance. *J Appl Toxicol* 30(7):617–26.

Harvey P.W., Er J., Fernandes C., Rush K.C., Major I.R., Cockburn A. (1992). Corticosterone does not cause testicular toxicopathology in the rat: relevance to methylxanthines, ACTH and stress. *Hum Exp Toxicol* 11(6):505–9.

Harvey P.W., Everett D.J., Springall C.J. (2007). Adrenal toxicology: a strategy for assessment of functional toxicity to the adrenal cortex and steroidogenesis. *J Appl Toxicol* 27(2):103–15.

Heath J.E., Littlefield N.A. (1984). Morphological effects of subchronic oral sulfamethazine administration on Fischer 344 rats and B6C3F1 mice. *Toxicol Pathol* 12:3–9.

Hecker M., Newsted J.L., Murphy M.B., Higley E.B., Jones P.D., Wu R., Giesy J.P. (2006). Human adenocarcinoma (H295R) cells for rapid in vitro determination of effects on steroidogenesis: hormone production. *Toxicol Appl Pharmacol* 217(1):114–24.

Heider K. (1986). Spontaneous craniopharyngioma in a mouse. *Vet Pathol* 23(4):522–3.

Heimann P. (1966). Ultrastructure of human thyroid. A study of normal thyroid, untreated and treated diffuse toxic goiter. *Acta Endocrinol (Copenh)* 53(Suppl 110).

Helmchen U., Schmidt W.E., Siegel E.G., Creutzfeldt W. (1984). Morphological and functional changes of pancreatic B cells in cyclosporin A-treated rats. *Diabetologia* 27:416–8.

Helminski M., Solecki R., Petter H. (1989). Immunohistochemical studies on pituitary adenomas in Wistar rats. 1. Demonstration of ACTH, LH, neurophysin, oxytocin and vasopressin in the pituitary of Ico:WIST rats from chronic toxicity studies. *Arch Geschwulstforsch* 59(6):433–40.

Higley E.B., Newsted J.L., Zhang X., Giesy J.P., Hecker M. (2010). Assessment of chemical effects on aromatase activity using the H295R cell line. *Environ Sci Pollut Res Int* 17(5):1137–48.

Hill G.D., Pace V., Persohn E., Bresser C., Haseman J.K., Tischler A.S., Nyska A. (2003). A comparative immunohistochemical study of spontaneous and chemically induced pheochromocytomas in B6C3F1 mice. *Endocr Pathol* 14(1):81–91.

Hinson J.P., Raven P.W. (2006). Effects of endocrine-disrupting chemicals on adrenal function. *Best Pract Res Clin Endocrinol Metab* 20(1):111–20. Review.

Hodsman A.B., Bauer D.C., Dempster D.W., Dian L., Hanley D.A., Harris S.T., Kendler D.L., McClung M.R., Miller P.D., Olszynski W.P., Orwoll E., Yuen C.K. (2005). Parathyroid hormone and teriparatide for the treatment of osteoporosis: a review of the evidence and suggested guidelines for its use. *Endocr Rev* 26:688–703.

Hoffman B.B. (1987). Observations in New England Deaconess Hospital rats harboring pheochromocytoma. *Clin Invest Med* 10(6):555–60.

Hood A., Liu J., Klaassen C.D. (1999). Effects of phenobarbital, pregnenolone-16alpha-carbonitrile, and propylthiouracil on thyroid follicular cell proliferation. *Toxicol Sci Official J Soc Toxicol* 50:45–53.

Hood A., Allen M.L., Liu Y., Liu J., Klaassen C.D. (2003). Induction of T(4) UDP-GT activity, serum thyroid stimulating hormone, and thyroid follicular cell proliferation in mice treated with microsomal enzyme inducers. *Toxicol Appl Pharmacol* 188:6–13.

Hooth M.J., Herbert R.A., Haseman J.K., Orzech D.P., Johnson J.D., Bucher J.R. (2004). Toxicology and carcinogenesis studies of dipropylene glycol in rats and mice. *Toxicology* 204:123–40.

Hou J., Sheikh S., Martin D.L., Chatterjee N.K. (1993). Coxsackie virus B4 alters pancreatic glutamic decarboxylase expression in mice soon after infection. *J Autoimmun* 6:529–42.

Houston J.B., Humphrey M.J., Matthew D.E., Tarbit M.H. (1988). Comparison of two azole antifungal drugs, ketoconazole, and fluconazole, as modifiers of rat hepatic monooxygenase activity. *Biochem Pharmacol* 37(3):401–8.

Huff J., Cirvello J., Haseman J., Bucher J. (1991). Chemicals associated with site-specific neoplasia in 1394 long-term carcinogenesis experiments in laboratory rodents. *Environ Health Perspect* 93:247–70.

Ikezaki S., Takagi M., Tamura K. (2011). Natural occurrence of neoplastic lesions in young Sprague–Dawley rats. *J Toxicol Pathol* 24(1):37–40.

Imai T., Seo H., Murata Y., Ohno M., Satoh Y., Funahashi H., Takagi H., Matsui N. (1990). Alteration in the expression of genes for cholesterol side-chain cleavage enzyme and 21-hydroxylase by hypophysectomy and ACTH administration in the rat adrenal. *J Mol Endocrinol* 4(3):239–45.

Imaoka M., Satoh H., Furuhama K. (2007). Age- and sex-related differences in spontaneous hemorrhage and fibrosis of the pancreatic islets in Sprague–Dawley rats. *Toxicol Pathol* 35:388-94.

Imaoka M., Kato M., Tago S., Gotoh M., Satoh H., Manabe S. (2009). Effects of estradiol treatment and/or ovariectomy on spontaneous hemorrhagic lesions in the pancreatic islets of Sprague–Dawley rats. *Toxicol Pathol* 37:218–26.

Jaeger P., Jones W., Kashgarian M., Baron R., Clemens T.L., Segre G.V., Hayslett J.P. (1987). Animal model of primary hyperparathyroidism. *Am J Physiol* 252:E790–8.

Jain R., Lammert E. (2009). Cell–cell interactions in the endocrine pancreas. *Diabetes Obes Metab* 11(Suppl 4):159–67.

Jargin S.V. (2011). Validity of thyroid cancer incidence data following the Chernobyl accident. *Health Phys* 101:754–7.

Jeffery E.H., Abreo K., Burgess E., Cannata J., Greger J.L. (1996). Systemic aluminum toxicity: effects on bone, hematopoietic tissue, and kidney. *J Toxicol Environ Health* 48(6):649–65.

Johansson M.K., Sanderson J.T., Lund B.O. (2002) Effects of 3-MeSO2-DDE and some CYP inhibitors on glucocorticoid steroidogenesis in the H295R human adrenocortical carcinoma cell line. *Toxicol In Vitro* 16(2):113–21.

Jolette J., Wilker C.E., Smith S.Y., Doyle N., Hardisty J.F., Metcalfe A.J., Marriott T.B., Fox J., Wells D.S. (2006). Defining a noncarcinogenic dose of recombinant human parathyroid hormone 1-84 in a 2-year study in Fischer 344 rats. *Toxicol Pathol* 34(7):929–40.

Joshi R.L., Lamothe B., Cordonnier N., Mesbah K., Monthioux E., Jami J., Bucchini D. (1996). Targeted disruption of the insulin receptor gene in the mouse results in neonatal lethality. *EMBO J* 15:1542–7.

Jun H.-S., Yoon J.-W. (2003). A new look at viruses in type 1 diabetes. *Diabetes/Metab Res Rev* 19:8–31.

Kamel F., Kubajak C.L. (1987). Modulation of gonadotropin secretion by corticosterone: interaction with gonadal steroids and mechanism of action. *Endocrinology* Aug;121(2):561–8.

Kanno T., Gopel S., Roraman P. (2002). Cellular function in multicellular system for hormone-secretion: electrophysiological aspect of studies on a-, b-, and d-cells of the pancreatic islet. *Neurosci Res* 42:79–90.

Kanno J., Onodera H., Furuta K., Maekawa A., Kasuga T., Hayashi Y. (1992). Tumor-promoting effects of both iodine deficiency and iodine excess in the rat thyroid. *Toxicol Pathol* 20:226–35.

Kantham L., Quinn S.J., Egbuna O.I., Baxi K., Butters R., Pang J.L., Pollak M.R., Goltzman D., Brown E.M. (2009). The calcium-sensing receptor (CaSR) defends against hypercalcemia independently of its regulation of parathyroid hormone secretion. *Am J Physiol Endocrinol Metab* 297:E915–23.

Kasperlik-Załuska A.A., Zgliczyński W., Jeske W., Zdunowski P. (2005). ACTH responses to somatostatin, valproic acid and dexamethasone in Nelson's syndrome. *Neuro Endocrinol Lett* 26(6):709–12.

Kassim T.A., Clarke D.D., Mai V.Q., Clyde P.W., Mohamed Shakir K.M. (2008). Catecholamine-induced cardiomyopathy. *Endocr Pract* 14(9):1137–49.

Kast A., Peil H., Weisse I. (1994). Calcified foci at the junction between adrenal cortex and medulla of rhesus monkeys. *Lab Anim* 28(1):80–9.

Kater C.E., Biglieri E.G., Brust N., Chang B., Hirai J., Irony I. (1989). Stimulation and suppression of the mineralocorticoid hormones in normal subjects and adrenocortical disorders. *Endocr Rev* 10(2): 149–64.

Kato A., Suzuki M., Karasawa Y., Sugimoto T., Doi K. (2003). Histopathological study on the PTHrP-induced incisor lesions in rats. *Toxicol Pathol* 31:480–5.

Kato A., Suzuki M., Karasawa Y., Sugimoto T., Doi, K. (2005). Histopathological study of time course changes in PTHrP-induced incisor lesions of rats. *Toxicol Pathol* 33:230–8.

Kawamori D., Kurpad A.J., Hu J., Liew C.W., Shih J.L., Ford E.L., Herrera P.L., Polonsky K.S., McGuinness O.P., Kulkami R.N. (2009). Insulin signalling in alpha cells modulates glucagon secretion in vivo. *Cell Metab* 9:350–61.

Keenan K.P., Soper K.A., Smith P.F., Ballam G.C., Clark R.L. (1995a). Diet, overfeeding, and moderate dietary restriction in control Sprague–Dawley rats: I. Effects on spontaneous neoplasms. *Toxicol Pathol* 23(3):269–86.

Keenan K.P., Soper K.A., Hertzog P.R., Gumprecht L.A., Smith P.F., Mattson B.A., Ballam G.C., Clark R.L. (1995b) Diet, overfeeding, and moderate dietary restriction in control Sprague–Dawley rats: II. Effects on age-related proliferative and degenerative lesions. *Toxicol Pathol* 23(3):287–302.

Kim Y.T., Steinberg C. (1984). Immunologic studies on the induction of diabetes in experimental animals. Cellular basis for the induction of diabetes by streptozotocin. *Diabetes* 33:771–7.

Kitchen D.N., Todd G.C., Meyers D.B., Paget C. (1979). Rat lymphocytic thyroiditis associated with ingestion of an immunosuppressive compound. *Vet Pathol* 16:722–9.

Komatsu Y., Imai Y., Itoh F., Kojima M., Isaji M., Shibata N. (2005). Rat model of the hypercalcaemia induced by parathyroid hormone-related protein: characteristics of three bisphosphonates. *Eur J Pharmacol* 507:317–24.

Konstantinova I., Nikolova G., Ohara-Imaizumi M., Maeda P., Kucera T., Zarbalis K., Wurst W., Nagamatsu S., Lammert E. (2007). EphA-ephrin-A-mediated beta cell communication regulates insulin secretion from pancreatic islets. *Cell* 129:359–70.

Kumari M., Cover P.O., Poyse R.H., Buckingham J.C. (1997). Stimulation of the hypothalamo-pituitary–adrenal axis in the rat by three selective type-4 phosphodiesterase inhibitors: in vitro and in vivo studies. *Br J Pharmacol* 121:459–68.

La Perle K.M.D., Capen C.C. (2007). Endocrine system. In *Pathologic Basis of Veterinary Disease* (M.D. McGavin, J.F. Zachary, eds.), pp. 693–741. Elsevier, St. Louis.

Land C.E., Bouville A., Apostoaei I., Simon S. L. (2010). Projected lifetime cancer risks from exposure to regional radioactive fallout in the Marshall Islands. *Health Phys* 99:201–15.

Laroque P., Molon-Noblot S., Prahalada S., Stabinski L.G., Hoe C.M., Peter C.P., Duprat P., van Zwieten M.J. (1998). Morphological changes in the pituitary gland of dogs chronically exposed to exogenous growth hormone. *Toxicol Pathol* 26(2):201–6.

Latendresse J.R., Brooks C.L., Capen C.C.(1994). Pathologic effects of butylated triphenyl phosphate-based hydraulic fluid and tricresyl phosphate on the adrenal gland, ovary, and testis in the Fischer-344 rat. *Toxicol Pathol* 22(4):341–52.

Leav I., Schiller A.L., Rijnberk A., Legg M.A., der Kinderen P.J. (1976). Adenomas and carcinomas of the canine and feline thyroid. *Am J Pathol* 83:61–122.

Lee G.H., Proenca R., Montez J.M., Carroll K.M., Darvishzadeh J.G., Lee J.I., Friedman J.M. (1996). Abnormal splicing of the leptin receptor in diabetic mice. *Nature* 379:632–5.

Lenzen S. (2008). The mechanisms of alloxan- and streptozotocin-induced diabetes. *Diabetologia* 51:216–26.

Levine S., Saltzman A. (2004). Hydropic degeneration of the anterior pituitary gland (adenohypophysis) in uremic rats. *Toxicol Lett* 1;147(2):121–6.

Levine S., Saltzman A., Klein A.W. (2000). Proliferation of glial cells in vivo induced in the neural lobe of the rat pituitary by lithium. *Cell Prolif* 33(4):203–7.

Levine S., Saltzman A., Katof B., Meister A., Cooper T.B. (2002). Proliferation of glial cells induced by lithium in the neural lobe of the rat pituitary is enhanced by dehydration. *Cell Prolif* 35(3):167–72.

Levy B.M., Hampton S., Dreizen S., Hampton J.K., Jr. (1972). Thyroiditis in the marmoset (*Callithrix* spp. and *Saguinus* spp.). *J Comp Pathol* 82:99–103.

Liu S.K. (2002). Metabolic disease in animals. Semin *Musculoskelet Radiol* 6:341–6.

Lloyd R.V. (1983). Estrogen-induced hyperplasia and neoplasia in the rat anterior pituitary gland. An immuno-histochemical study. *Am J Pathol* 113(2):198–206.

Lloyd R.V., Mailloux J. (1987). Effects of diethylstilbestrol and propylthiouracil on the rat pituitary. An immunohistochemical and ultrastructural study. *J Natl Cancer Inst* 79(4):865–73.

Lloyd R.V., Jin L., Fields K., Kulig E. (1991). Effects of estrogens on pituitary cell and pituitary tumor growth. *Pathol Res Pract* 187(5):584–6.

Löhr M., Müller M.K., Goebell H., Klöppel. (1989). Prostaglandin analogue protects pancreatic B-cells against cyclosporin A toxicity. *Experientia* 45:351–4.

Lombardero M., Quintanar-Stephano A., Vidal S., Horvath E., Kovacs K., Lloyd R.V., Scheithauer B.W. (2009). Effect of estrogen on the blood supply of pituitary autografts in rats. *J Anat* 214(2):235–44.

Lorenzo A., Razzaboni B., Weir G.C., Yankner B.A. (1994). Pancreatic islet cell toxicity of amylin-associated with type-2 diabetes mellitus. *Nature* 368:756–60.

Lotinun S., Evans G.L., Bronk J.T., Bolander M.E., Wronski T.J., Ritman E.L., Turner R.T. (2004). Continuous parathyroid hormone induces cortical porosity in the rat: effects on bone turnover and mechanical properties. *J Bone Miner Res* 19:1165–71.

Lumbers E.R. (1999). Angiotensin and aldosterone. *Regul Pept* 80(3):91–100.

Lupulescu A., Potorac E., Pop A., Heitmanek C., Merculiev E., Chisiu N., Oprisan R., Neacsu C. (1968). Experimental investigations on immunology of the parathyroid gland. *Immunology* 14:475–82.

Lyle S.F., Wright K., Collins D.C. (1984). Comparative effects of tamoxifen and bromocriptine on prolactin and pituitary weight in estradiol-treated male rats. *Cancer* 1;53(7):1473–7.

Maita K., Hirano M., Harada T., Mitsumori K., Yoshida A., Takahashi K., Nakashima N., Kitazawa T., Enomoto A., Inui K., Shirasu Y. (1988) Mortality, major cause of moribundity, and spontaneous tumors in CD-1 mice. *Toxicol Pathol* 16:340–9.

Majeed S.K., Gopinath C. (1980). Calcification in the adrenals and ovaries of monkeys. *Lab Anim* 14(4):363–5.

Majeed S.K. (1993). Survey on spontaneous systemic amyloidosis in aging mice. *Arzneimittelforschung* 43:170–8.

Majka J.A., Solleveld H.A., Barthel C.H., Van Zwieten M.J. (1990). Proliferative lesions of the pituitary in rats. Guidelines for Toxicologic Pathology, STP/AFIP, Washington, DC, 1–8.

Makino S., Kunimoto K., Munaoko Y., Mizushima Y., Katagiri K., Tochino Y. (1980). Breeding of a non-obese diabetic strain of mice. *Exp Anim* 29:1–13.

Malendowicz L.K., Nussdorfer G.G. (1984). Sex differences in adrenocortical structure and function. XV. Cellular composition and quantitative ultrastructural study of adrenal cortex of adult male and female hamster. *J Submicrosc Cytol* 16(4):715–20.

Marliss E.B., Nakhooda A.F., Poussier P., Sima A.A.F. (1982). The diabetic syndrome of the "BB" Wistar rat: possible relevance to type 1 (insulin-dependent) diabetes in man. *Diabetologia* 22:225–32.

Marshall BioResources Reference Data Guide (2006). North Rose, NY, USA.

Mason J.I., Murry B.A., Olcott M., Sheets J.J. (1985). Imidazole antimycotics: inhibitors of steroid aromatase. *Biochem Pharmacol* 34(7):1087–92.

Matsushima S., Tsuchiya N., Fujisawa-Imura K., Hoshimoto M., Takasu N., Torii M., Ozaki K., Narana I., Kotani T. (2005). Ultrastructural and morphometrical evaluation of the parathyroid gland in iron-lactate-overloaded rats. *Toxicol Pathol* 33:533–9.

Mazzocchi G., Nussdorfer G.G. (1984). Long-term effects of captopril on the morphology of normal rat adrenal zona glomerulosa. A morphometric study. *Exp Clin Endocrinol* 84(2):148–52.

Mazzocchi G., Rebuffat P., Nussdorfer G.G. (1987). Atrial natriuretic factor (ANF) inhibits the growth and the secretory activity of rat adrenal zona glomerulosa in vivo. *J Steroid Biochem* 28(6):643–6.

McClain R.M. (1989). The significance of hepatic microsomal enzyme induction and altered thyroid function in rats: implications for thyroid gland neoplasia. *Toxicol Pathol* 17:294–306.

McClain R.M. (1992). Thyroid gland neoplasia: non-genotoxic mechanisms. *Toxicol Lett* 64–65(Spec No):397–408.

McClain R.M. (1995). Mechanistic considerations for the relevance of animal data on thyroid neoplasia to human risk assessment. *Mutat Res* 333:131–42.

McClure H.M., Chandler F.W. (1982). A survey of pancreatic lesions in nonhuman primates. *Vet Pathol* 19(Suppl 7):193–209.

McComb D.J., Kovacs K., Beri J., Zak F. (1984). Pituitary adenomas in old Sprague–Dawley rats: a histologic, ultrastructural, and immunocytochemical study. *J Natl Cancer Inst* 73(5):1143–66.

McComb D.J., Kovacs K., Beri J., Zak F., Milligan J.V., Shin S.H. (1985). Pituitary gonadotroph adenomas in old Sprague–Dawley rats. *J Submicrosc Cytol* 17(4):517–30.

McEwan P.E., Lindop G.B., Kenyon C.J. (1996). Control of cell proliferation in the rat adrenal gland in vivo by the renin-angiotensin system. *Am J Physiol* 271(1 Pt 1):E192–8.

Medeiros L.J., Federman M., Silverman M.L., Balogh K. (1984). Black thyroid associated with minocycline therapy. *Arch Pathol Lab Med* 108:268–9.

Mercado-Asis L.B., Yanovski J.A., Tracer H.L., Chik C.L., Cutler G.B. Jr. (1997). Acute effects of bromocriptine, cyproheptadine, and valproic acid on plasma adrenocorticotropin secretion in Nelson's syndrome. *J Clin Endocrinol Metab* 82(2):514–7.

Meuten D.J., Capen C.C., Thompson K.G., Segre G.V. (1984). Syncytial cells in canine parathyroid glands. *Vet Pathol* 21:463–8.

Miller M.D., Crofton K.M., Rice D.C., Zoeller R.T. (2009). Thyroid-disrupting chemicals: interpreting upstream biomarkers of adverse outcomes. *Environ Health Perspect* 117:1033–41.

Mirsky M.L., Sivaraman L., Houle C., Potter D.M., Chapin R.E., Cappon G.D. (2011). Histologic and cytologic detection of endocrine and reproductive tract effects of exemestane in female rats treated for up to twenty-eight days. *Toxicol Pathol* 39(4):589–605.

Mobine H.R., Baker A.B., Wang L., Wakimoto H., Jacobsen K.C., Seidman C.E., Seidman J.G., Edelman E.R. (2009). Pheochromocytoma-induced cardiomyopathy is modulated by the synergistic effects of cell-secreted factors. *Circ Heart Fail* 2(2):121–8.

Moller H., Rausing A. (1980). Methacycline hyperpigmentation: a five-year follow-up. *Acta Derm Venereol* 60:495–501.

Molon-Noblot S., Laroque P., Coleman J.B., Hoe C.M., Keenan K.P. (2003). The effects of ad libitum overfeeding and moderate and marked dietary restriction on age-related spontaneous pituitary gland pathology in Sprague–Dawley rats. *Toxicol Pathol* 31(3):310–20.

Moon B.C., Friedman J.M. (1997). The molecular basis of the obese mutation in ob2J mice. *Genomics* 42:152–6.

Morishita K., Okumura H., Ito N., Takahashi N. (2001). Primary culture system of adrenocortical cells from dogs to evaluate direct effects of chemicals on steroidogenesis. *Toxicology* 28;165(2–3):171–8.

Morohashi K., Honda S., Inomata Y, Handa O., Omura T. (1992). A common trans-acting factor, Ad4-binding protein, to the promoters of steroidogenic P-450s. *J Biol Chem* 267:17913-9.

Morohashi K.I., Omura T. (1996). Ad4BP/SF-1, a transcription factor essential for the transcription of steroidogenic cytochrome P450 genes and for the establishment of the reproductive function. *FASEB J* 10:1569–77.

Müller M.B., Preil J., Renner U., Zimmermann S., Kresse A.E., Stalla G.K., Keck M.E., Holsboer F., Wurst W. (2001). Expression of CRHR1 and CRHR2 in mouse pituitary and adrenal gland: implications for HPA system regulation. *Endocrinology* 142(9):4150–3.

Müller-Vieira U., Angotti M., Hartmann R.W. (2005). The adrenocortical tumor cell line NCI-H295R as an in vitro screening system for the evaluation of CYP11B2 (aldosterone synthase) and CYP11B1 (steroid-11beta-hydroxylase) inhibitors. *J Steroid Biochem Mol Biol* 96(3–4):259–70.

Mulrow P.J. (1998). Renin–angiotensin system in the adrenal. *Horm Metab Res* 30(6–7):346–9.

Mulrow P.J. (1999). Angiotensin II and aldosterone regulation. *Regul Pept* 80(1–2):27–32.

Mulrow P.J., Kusano E., Baba K., Shier D., Doi Y., Franco-Saenz R., Stoner G., Rapp J. (1988). Adrenal renin: a possible local hormonal regulator of aldosterone production. *Cardiovasc Drugs Ther* 2(4):463–71.

Musser E., Graham W. R. (1968). Familial occurrence of thyroiditis in purebred beagles. *Lab Anim Care* 18:58–68.

Naeser P. (1975). Structure of the adrenal glands in mice with the obese-hyperglycaemic syndrome (gene symbol ob). *Acta Pathol Microbiol Scand A* 83(1):120–6.

Nakachi K., Hayashi T., Hamatani K., Eguchi H., Kusunoki Y. (2008). Sixty years of follow-up of Hiroshima and Nagasaki survivors: current progress in molecular epidemiology studies. *Mutat Res* 659:109–17.

Neer R.M., Arnaud C.D., Zanchetta J.R., Prince R., Gaich G.A., Reginster J.Y., Hodsman A.B., Eriksen E.F., Ish-Shalom S., Genant H.K., Wang O., Mitlak B.H. (2001). Effect of parathyroid hormone (1-34) on fractures and bone mineral density in postmenopausal women with osteoporosis. *New Engl J Med* 344:1434–41.

Nickerson P.A. (1979). Adrenal cortex in retired breeder Mongolian gerbils (*Meriones unguiculatus*) and golden hamsters (*Mesocricetus auratus*). *Am J Pathol* 95(2):347–58.

Nikicicz H., Kasprzak A., Malendowicz L.K. (1984). Sex differences in adrenocortical structure and function. XIII. Stereologic studies on adrenal cortex of maturing male and female hamsters. *Cell Tissue Res* 235(2):459–62.

Nishizato Y., Imai S., Yabuki M., Kido H., Komuro S. (2010). Development of relevant assay system to identify steroidogenic enzyme inhibitors. *Toxicol In Vitro* 24(2):677–85.

Niwa J., Minase T., Hashi K., Mori M. (1987). Immunohistochemical, electron microscopic and morphometric studies of estrogen-induced rat prolactinomas after bromocriptine treatment. *Virchows Arch B Cell Pathol Incl Mol Pathol* 53(2):89–96.

Nolan L.A., Thomas C.K., Levy A. (2004). Permissive effects of thyroid hormones on rat anterior pituitary mitotic activity. *J Endocrinol* 180:35–43.

Nugent D.A., Smith D.M., Jones H.B. (2008). A review of islet of Langerhans degeneration in rodent models of type 2 diabetes. *Toxicol Pathol* 36:529–51.

Nussdorfer G.G., Mazzocchi G., Meneghelli V. (1988). Effect of atrial natriuretic factor (ANF) on the secretory activity of zona glomerulosa in sodium-restricted rats. *Endocr Res* 14(4):293–303.

Nussdorfer G.G. (1986). Cytophysiology of the adrenal cortex. *Int Rev Cytol* 98:1–405.

Nyska A., Maronpot R.R. (1999). Adrenal gland. In *Pathology of the Mouse* (Maronpot, R.R., Boorman, G.A., and Gaul, B.W. eds.), pp. 509–36, Cache River Press, Vienna, IL.

Ohshima M., Ward J.M. (1986). Dietary iodine deficiency as a tumor promoter and carcinogen in male F344/NCr rats. *Cancer Res* 46:877–83.

Okazaki K., Imazawa T., Nakamura H., Furukawa F., Nishikawa A., Hirose M. (2002). A repeated 28-day oral dose toxicity study of 17alpha-methyltestosterone in rats, based on the enhanced OECD Test Guideline 407′ for screening the endocrine-disrupting chemicals. *Arch Toxicol* 75(11–12):635–42.

Oksanen A. (1980). The ultrastructure of the multi-nucleated cells in canine parathyroid glands. *J Comp Pathol* 90:293–301.

Olsen J.H., Boice J.D. Jr., Jensen J.P., Fraumeni J.F. Jr. (1989). Cancer among epileptic patients exposed to anticonvulsant drugs. *J Natl Cancer Inst* 81:803–8.

Onodera T., Jenson A.B., Yoon J.W., Notkins A.L. (1978). Virus-induced diabetes mellitus: reovirus infection of pancreatic beta cells in mice. *Science* 301:529–31.

Östenson C.G. (2001). The Goto–Kakizaki rat. In *Animal Models of Diabetes, A Primer* (Sima, A.A.A.F., Shafrir, E. eds.), pp. 197–212. Harwood Academic Publishers, Newark, NJ.

Otis M., Campbell S., Payet M.D., Gallo-Payet N. (2005). Angiotensin II stimulates protein synthesis and inhibits proliferation in primary cultures of rat adrenal glomerulosa cells. *Endocrinology* 146(2):633–42.

Ozaki K., Haseman J.K., Hailey J.R., Maronpot R.R., Nyska A. (2002). Association of adrenal pheochromocytoma and lung phatology in inhalation studies with particulate compounds in the male F344 rat–the National Toxicology Program experience. *Toxicol Pathol* 30(2):263–70.

Ozawa H. (1991). Changing ultrastructure of thyrotrophs in the rat anterior pituitary after thyroidectomy as studied by immuno-electron microscopy and enzyme cytochemistry. *Cell Tissue Res* 263:405–12.

Pace V., Heider K., Persohn E., Schaetti P. (1997). Spontaneous malignant craniopharyngioma in an albino rat. *Vet Pathol* 34(2):146–9.

Pace V., Perentes E., Germann P.G. (2002). Pheochromocytomas and ganglioneuromas in the aging rats: morphological and immunohistochemical characterization. *Toxicol Pathol* 30(4):492–500.

Palotay J.L., Howard C.F.J. (1982). Insular amyloidosis in spontaneously diabetic non-human primates. *Vet Pathol* 19(Suppl. 7):181–92.

Pan F.C., Wright C. (2011). Pancreas organogenesis: from bud to plexus to gland. *Dev Dynam* 240:530–65.

Pascoe L., Jeunemaitre X., Lebrethon M.C., Curnow K.M., Gomez-Sanchez C.E., Gasc J.M., Saez J.M., Corvol P. (1995). Glucocorticoid-suppressible hyperaldosteronism and adrenal tumors occurring in a single French pedigree. *J Clin Invest* 96:2236–46.

Pasquale E.B. (2008). Eph-ephrin bidirectional signaling in physiology and disease. *Cell* 133:38–52.

Pataki A., Donatsch P., Hodel C., Rentsch G. (1975). Relevance of enzyme histochemistry of rat thyroid gland. *Acta Histochem Suppl* 14:159–65.

Patent G.J., Alfert M. (1967). Histological changes in the pancreatic islets of alloxan-treated mice, with comments on beta-cell regeneration. *Acta Anat* 66:504–19.

Patyna S., Arrigoni C., Terron A., Kim T.W., Heward J.K., Vonderfecht S.L., Denlinger R., Turnquist S.E., Evering W. (2008). Nonclinical safety evaluation of sunitinib: a potent inhibitor of VEGF, PDGF, KIT, FLT3, and RET receptors. *Toxicol Pathol* 36(7):905–16.

Paynter O.E., Burin G.J., Jaeger R.B., Gregorio C.A. (1988). Goitrogens and thyroid follicular cell neoplasia: evidence for a threshold process. *Regulat Toxicol Pharmacol RTP* 8:102–19.

Penhale W.J., Farmer A., McKenna R.P., Irvine W.J. (1973). Spontaneous thyroiditis in thymectomized and irradiated Wistar rats. *Clin Exp Immunol* 15:225–36.

Phillips M.S., Liu Q., Hammond H.A., Dugan V., Hey P.J., Caskey C.J., Hess J.F. (1996). Leptin receptor missense mutation in the fatty Zucker rat. *Nat Genet* 13:18–9.

Pont A., Williams P.L., Loose D.S., Feldman D., Reitz R.E., Bochra C., Stevens D.A. (1982). Ketoconazole blocks adrenal steroid synthesis. *Ann Intern Med* 97(3):370–2.

Portha B. (2005). Programmed disorders of β-cell development and function as one cause for type 2 diabetes? The GK rat paradigm. *Diabet/Metab Res Rev* 21:495–504.

Poteracki J., Walsh K.M. (1998). Spontaneous neoplasms in control Wistar rats: a comparison of reviews. *Toxicol Sci Official J Soc Toxicol* 45:1–8.

Pour P.M. (1983). Hyperplasia, parathyroid, hamster. In *Endocrine System* (Jones, T.C., Mohr, U., and Hunt, R.D. eds.), pp. 265–268. Springer-Verlag, Berlin.

Pour P.M., Wilson J.T., Salmasi S. (1983). Adenoma, carcinoma, parathyroid, rat. In *Endocrine System, Monographs on Pathology of Laboratory Animals* (Jones, T.C., Mohr, U., and Hunt, R.D. eds.), pp. 281–287. Springer-Verlag, Berlin.

Powers J.F., Picard K.L., Nyska A., Tischler A.S. (2008). Adrenergic differentiation and Ret expression in rat pheochromocytomas. *Endocr Pathol* Spring;19(1):9–16.

Pruett S., Lapointe J.M., Reagan W., Lawton M., Kawabata T.T. (2008). Urinary corticosterone as an indicator of stress-mediated immunological changes in rats. *J Immunotoxicol* 5(1):17–22.

Prysor-Jones R.A., Silverlight J.J., Jenkins J.S.. (1983). Hypothalamic dopamine and catechol oestrogens in rats with spontaneous pituitary tumours. *J Endocrinol* 96(2):347–52.

Rainey W.E. (1999) Adrenal zonation: clues from 11[beta]-hydroxylase and aldosterone synthase. *Mol Cell Endocrinol* 151:151.

Rainey W.E., Bird I.M., Mason J.I. (1994). The NCI-H295 cell line: a pluripotent model for human adrenocortical studies. *Mol Cell Endocrinol* 100(1–2):45–50. Review.

Ravier M., Güldenagel M., Charollais A., Gjinovci A., Caille D., Söhl G., Wollheim C.B., Willecke K., Henquin J.C., Maeda P. (2005). Loss of connexin36 channels alters beta-cell coupling, islet synchronization of glucose-induced Ca2+ and insulin oscillations, and basal insulin release. *Diabetes* 54:1798–807.

Rees D.A., Alcolado J.C. (2005). Animal models of diabetes mellitus. *Diabet Med* 22:359–70.

Reid J.D. (1983). The black thyroid associated with minocycline therapy. A local manifestation of a drug-induced lysosome/substrate disorder. *Am J Clin Pathol* 79:738–46.

Reimers T.J. (1998). Endocrine Reference Values for Normal Animals, unpublished data.

Reincke M., Beuschlein F., Menig G., Hofmockel G., Arlt W., Lehmann R., Karl M., Allolio B. (1998). Localization and expression of adrenocorticotropic hormone receptor mRNA in normal and neoplastic human adrenal cortex. *J Endocrinol* 156(3):415–23.

Reindel J.F., Dominick M.A., Bocan T.M., Gough A.W., McGuire E.J. (1994). Toxicologic effects of a novel acyl-CoA:cholesterol acyltransferase inhibitor in cynomolgus monkeys. *Toxicol Pathol* 22(5):510–8.

Remick A.K., Wood C.E., Cann J.A., Gee M.K., Feiste E.A., Kock N.D., Cline J.M. (2006). Histologic and immunohistochemical characterization of spontaneous pituitary adenomas in fourteen cynomolgus macaques (*Macaca fascicularis*). *Vet Pathol* 43(4):484–93.

Reznik G., Germann P.-G. (1996). Neuroblastoma, adrenal, rat. In *Monographs on Pathology of Laboratory Animals. Endocrine System* (Jones, T.C., Capen, C.C., and Mohr, U. eds.), 2nd edition, pp. 433–5. Springer, Berlin.

Reznik G., Ward J.M., Reznik-Schüller H. (1980). Ganglioneuromas in the adrenal medulla of F344 rats. *Vet Pathol* 17(5):614–21.

Ribelin W.E. (1984). The effects of drugs and chemicals upon the structure of the adrenal gland. *Fundam Appl Toxicol* 4(1):105–19.

Richardson T.A., Klaassen C.D. (2010a). Disruption of thyroid hormone homeostasis in Ugt1a-deficient Gunn rats by microsomal enzyme inducers is not due to enhanced thyroxine glucuronidation. *Toxicol Appl Pharmacol* 248:38–44.

Richardson T.A., Klaassen C.D. (2010b). Role of UDP-glucuronosyltransferase (UGT) 2B2 in metabolism of triiodothyronine: effect of microsomal enzyme inducers in Sprague–Dawley and UGT2B2-deficient Fischer 344 rats. *Toxicol Sci Official J Soc Toxicol* 116:413–21.

Rikihisa Y., Lin Y.C. (1989). Effect of gossypol on the thyroid in young rats. *J Comp Pathol* 100:411–7.

Rose N.R. (1985). The thyroid gland as source and target of autoimmunity. *Lab Invest* 52:117–9.

Rosen J.F., Chesney R.W., Hamstra A., DeLuca H.F., Mahaffey K.R. (1980). Reduction in 1,25-dihydroxyvitamin D in children with increased lead absorption. *N Engl J Med* 302(20):1128–31.

Rosenbaum J.S., Billingham M.E., Ginsburg R., Tsujimoto G., Lurie K.G., Hoffman B.B. (1988). Cardiomyopathy in a rat model of pheochromocytoma. Morphological and functional alterations. *Am J Cardiovasc Pathol* 1(3):389–99.

Rosol T.J., Yarrington J.T., Latendresse J., Capen C.C. (2001). Adrenal gland: structure, function, and mechanisms of toxicity. *Toxicol Pathol* 29(1):41–8. Review.

Rosol T.J., Capen C.C. (1989). Tumors of the parathyroid gland and circulating parathyroid hormone-related protein associated with persistent hypercalcemia. *Toxicol Pathol* 17:346–56.

Rosol T.J., Capen C.C., Weisbrode S.E., Horst R.L. (1986). Humoral hypercalcemia of malignancy in nude mouse model of a canine adenocarcinoma derived from apocrine glands of the anal sac. Biochemical, histomorphometric, and ultrastructural studies. *Lab Invest* 54:679–88.

Rudmann D.G., McNerney M.E., VanderEide S.L., Schemmer J.K., Eversole R.R., Vonderfecht S.L. (2004). Epididymal and systemic phospholipidosis in rats and dogs treated with the dopamine D3 selective antagonist PNU-177864. *Toxicol Pathol* 32(3):326–32.

Sam S., Frohman L.A. (2008). Normal physiology of hypothalamic pituitary regulation. *Endocrinol Metab Clin North Am* 37(1):1–22, vii. Review.

Sanchez A.R., Rogers R.S. 3rd, Sheridan P.J. (2004). Tetracycline and other tetracycline-derivative staining of the teeth and oral cavity. *Int J Dermatol* 43:709–15.

Sánchez-Criado J.E., de Las Mulas J.M., Bellido C., Navarro V.M., Aguilar R., Garrido-Gracia J.C., Malagón M.M., Tena-Sempere M., Blanco A. (2006). Gonadotropin-secreting cells in ovariectomized rats treated with different oestrogen receptor ligands: a modulatory role for ERbeta in the gonadotrope? *J Endocrinol* 188(2):167–77.

Sanderson J.T., Boerma J., Lansbergen G.W., van den Berg M. (2002). Induction and inhibition of aromatase (CYP19) activity by various classes of pesticides in H295R human adrenocortical carcinoma cells. *Toxicol Appl Pharmacol* 182(1):44–54.

Sandusky G.E., Van Pelt C.S., Todd G.C., Wightman K. (1988). An immunocytochemical study of pituitary adenomas and focal hyperplasia in old Sprague–Dawley and Fischer 344 rats. *Toxicol Pathol* 16(3):376–80.

Sankar B.R., Maran R.R., Sivakumar R., Govindarajulu P., Balasubramanian K. (2000). Chronic administration of corticosterone impairs LH signal transduction and steroidogenesis in rat Leydig cells. *J Steroid Biochem Mol Biol* 72(3–4):155–62.

Sasano H., White P.C., New M.I., Sasano N. (1988). Immunohistochemical localization of cytochrome P-450C21 in human adrenal cortex and its relation to endocrine function. *Hum Pathol* 19:181–5.

Sato M., Vahle J., Schmidt A., Westmore M., Smith S., Rowley E., Ma L.Y. (2002). Abnormal bone architecture and biomechanical properties with near-lifetime treatment of rats with PTH. *Endocrinology* 143:3230–42.

Satoh H., Kajimura T., Chen C.J., Yamada K., Furuhama K., Nomura M. (1997). Invasive pituitary tumors in female F344 rats induced by estradiol dipropionate. *Toxicol Pathol* 25(5):462–9.

Satoh H., Iwata H., Furuhama K., Enomoto M. (2000). Pituicytoma: primary astrocytic tumor of the pars nervosa in aging Fischer 344 rats. *Toxicol Pathol* 28(6):836–8.

Sawano F., Fujita H. (1981). Some findings on the cytochemistry of the thyroid follicle epithelial cell in rats and mice. *Arch Histol Jpn* 44:439–52.

Sayers A.C., Amsler H.A. (1977). Clozapine. In *Pharmacological and Biochemical Properties of Drug Substances* (Goldberg, M.E. ed.), vol. 1, pp. 1–31. American Pharmaceutical Association, Academy of Pharmaceutical Sciences, Washington, DC.

Schimmer B.P., Parke K.L. (1996). Adrenocorticotropic hormone; adrenocortical steroids and their synthetic analogs: inhibitors of the synthesis and actions of adrenocortical hormones. In *Goodman & Gilman's The Pharmacological Basis of Therapeutics* (Chapter 59) (Hardman, J.G., and Limbird, L.E. eds.), pp. 1459–85, McGraw-Hill, New York.

Schneider H.M., Storkel S., Will W. (1980). Das Amyloid der Langerhansschen Inseln und seine Beziehung zum Diabetes mellitus. *Dtsch med Wschr* 105:1143–7.

Sharawy M., Penney D.P., Dirksen T.R., Averill K. (1978). Changes in the adrenal cortex of the rat after chronic administration of the steroidogenic inhibitor U-8113. *Cell Tissue Res* 26;190(1):123–34.

Shirts S.B., Annegers J.F., Hauser W.A., Kurland L.T. (1986). Cancer incidence in a cohort of patients with seizure disorders. *J Natl Cancer Inst* 77:83–7.

Silverman D.A., Rose N.R. (1974). Neonatal thymectomy increases the incidence of spontaneous and methyl-cholanthrene-enhanced thyroiditis in rats. *Science* 184:162–3.

Silverman D., Rose N.R. (1975). Spontaneous and methylcholanthrene-enhanced thyroiditis in BUF rats. II. Induction of experimental autoimmune thyroiditis without completed Freund's adjuvant. *J Immunol* 114:148–50.

Sistare F.D., Morton D., Alden C., Christensen J., Keller D., DeJonghe S., Storer R.D., Reddy M.V., Kraynak A., Trela B., Bienvenue J.G., Bjurstrom S., Bosmans V., Brewster D., Colman K., Dominik M., Evans J., Hailey J.R., Kinter L., Liu M., Mahrt C., Marien D., Myer J., Perry R., Potenta D., Roth A., Sherratt P., Singer T., Slim R., Soper K., Fransson-Steen R., Stolz J., Turner O., Turnquist S., van Heerden M., Woicke J., DeGeorge J.J. (2011). An analysis of pharmaceutical experience with decades of rat carcinogenicity testing. Support for a proposal to modify current regulatory guidelines. *Toxicol Pathol* 39:716–44.

Son W.C., Bell D., Taylor I., Mowat V. (2010). Profile of early occurring spontaneous tumors in Han Wistar rats. *Toxicol Pathol* 38(2):292–6.

Sonino N., Boscaro M., Fallo F. (2005). Pharmacologic management of Cushing syndrome: new targets for therapy. *Treat Endocrinol* 4(2):87–94. Review.

Spady T.J., McComb R.D., Shull J.D. (1999). Estrogen action in the regulation of cell proliferation, cell survival, and tumorigenesis in the rat anterior pituitary gland. *Endocrine* 11(3):217–33.

Stefaneanu L., Kovacs K., Lloyd R.V., Scheithauer B.W., Young W.F. Jr, Sano T., Jin L. (1992). Pituitary lactotrophs and somatotrophs in pregnancy: a correlative in situ hybridization and immunocytochemical study. *Virchows Arch B Cell Pathol Incl Mol Pathol* 62(5):291–6.

Stocco D.M. (2001). StAR protein and the regulation of steroid hormone biosynthesis. *Annu Rev Physiol* 63:193–213.

Stokes W.S. (1986). Spontaneous diabetes mellitus in a baboon (*Papio cynocephalus* Anubis). *Lab Anim Sci* 36:529–33.

Strandberg J.D. (1996). Hyperplasia and pheochromocytoma, adrenal medulla, rat. In *ILSI Monograph on Pathology of Laboratory Animals, Endocrine System*, 2nd edition (Jones, T.C., Capen, C.C., and Mohr, U. eds.), pp. 411–21. Springer-Verlag, Berlin.

Szabo S., Lippe I.T. (1989). Adrenal gland: chemically induced structural and functional changes in the cortex. *Toxicol Pathol* 17(2):317–29.

Tajima K., Miyagawa J., Nakajima H., Shimizu M., Katayama S., Mashita K., Tarui S. (1985). Morphological and biochemical studies on minocycline-induced black thyroid in rats. *Toxicol Appl Pharmacol* 81:393–400.

Takagi A., Momma J., Aida Y., Takada K., Suzuki S., Naitoh K., Tobe M., Hasegawa R., Kurokawa Y. (1992). Toxicity studies of a synthetic antioxidant, 2,2'-methylenebis (4-ethyl-6-tert-butylphenol) in rats. 1. Acute and subchronic toxicity. *J Toxicol Sci* 17:135–53.

Takagi A., Takada K., Sai K., Momma J., Aida Y., Suzuki S., Naitoh K., Tobe M., Hasegawa R., Kurokawa Y. (1996). Chronic oral toxicity of a synthetic antioxidant, 2,2'-methylenebis(4-ethyl- 6-tert-butylphenol), in rats. *J Appl Toxicol JAT* 16:15–23.

Takayama S., Aihara K., Onodera T., Akimoto T. (1986). Antithyroid effects of propylthiouracil and sulfa-monomethoxine in rats and monkeys. *Toxicol Appl Pharmacol* 82:191–9.

Tamemoto H., Kadowaki T., Tobe K., Kagi T., Sakura H., Hayakawa T. Terauchi Y., Ueki K., Kaburagi Y., Satoh S., Sekihara H., Yoshioka S., Horikoshi H., Furuta Y., Ikawa Y., Kasuga M., Yazaki Y., Aizawa S. (1994). Insulin resistance and growth retardation in mice lacking insulin receptor substrate-1. *Nature* 372:182–6.

Taurog A., Dorris M.L., Doerge D.R. (1996). Minocycline and the thyroid: antithyroid effects of the drug, and the role of thyroid peroxidase in minocycline-induced black pigmentation of the gland. *Thyroid* 6:211–9.

Taylor C.G. (2005). Zinc, the pancreas, and diabetes: insights from rodent studies and future directions. *Biometals* 18:305–12.

Terao K., Ito E., Oarada M., Ishibashi Y., Legrand A.M., Yasumoto T. (1991). Light and electron microscopic studies of pathologic changes induced in mice by ciguatoxin poisoning. *Toxicon* 29(6):633–43.

Teshima T., Hara Y., Shigihara K., Takekoshi S., Nezu Y., Harada Y., Yogo T., Teramoto A., Osamura R.Y., Tagawa M. (2009). Coexistence of corticotroph adenoma and thyrotroph hyperplasia in a dog. *J Vet Med Sci* 71(1):93–8.

Thomas G.A., Williams E.D. (1994). Changes in structure and function of thyroid follicular cells. In *Pathobiology of the Aging Rat* (Mohr, U., Dungworth, D.L., and Capen, C.C. eds.), pp. 269–84. ILSI, Washington, DC.

Thomas G.A., Williams E.D. (1996). Changes in structure and function of thyroid follicular cells. In *Pathobiology of the Aging Mouse* (U. Mohr, D.L. Dungworth, C.C. Capen, J.P. Sundberg, J.M. Ward, eds.), pp. 87–102. ILSI, Washington, DC.

Thomas G.A., Williams E.D. (1999). Thyroid stimulating hormone (TSH)-associated follicular hypertrophy and hyperplasia as a mechanism of thyroid carcinogenesis in mice and rats. Species Differences in Thyroid, Kidney, and Urinary Bladder Carcinogenesis. *IARC Sci Publ* 147:45–59.

Thompson C.S. (2008). Animal models of diabetes mellitus: relevance to vascular complications. *Curr Pharm Design* 14:309–24.

Tischler A.S., DeLellis R.A., Perlman R.L., Allen J.M., Costopoulos D., Lee Y.C., Nunnemacher G., Wolfe H.J., Bloom S.R. (1985). Spontaneous proliferative lesions of the adrenal medulla in aging Long–Evans rats. Comparison to PC12 cells, small granule-containing cells, and human adrenal medullary hyperplasia. *Lab Invest* 53(4):486–98.

Tischler A.S. (1989). The rat adrenal medulla. *Toxicol Pathol* 17(2):330–2.

Tischler A.S., Sheldon W., Gray R. (1996). Immunohistochemical and morphological characterization of spontaneously occurring pheochromocytomas in the aging mouse. *Vet Pathol* 33(5):512–20.

Tischler A.S., Dichter M.D., Biales B. (1977). Neuroendocrine neoplasms and their cells of origin. *N Engl J Med* 296:919–25.

Tixier-Vidal A., Tougard C., Kerdelhue B., Jutisz M. (1975). Light and electron microscopic studies on immunocytochemical localization of gonadotropic hormones in the rat pituitary gland with antisera against ovine FSH, LH, LHalpha, and LHbeta. *Ann N Y Acad Sci* 254:433–61.

Todd G.C. (1986). Induction and reversibility of thyroid proliferative changes in rats given an antithyroid compound. *Vet Pathol* 23:110–7.

Tucker W.E., Jr. (1962). Thyroiditis in a group of laboratory dogs. A study of 167 beagles. *Am J Clin Pathol* 38:70–4.

Ullerås E., Ohlsson A., Oskarsson A. (2008). Secretion of cortisol and aldosterone as a vulnerable target for adrenal endocrine disruption—screening of 30 selected chemicals in the human H295R cell model. *J Appl Toxicol* 28(8):1045–53.

Ulrich-Lai Y.M., Figueiredo H.F., Ostrander M.M., Choi D.C., Engeland W.C., Herman J.P. (2006). Chronic stress induces adrenal hyperplasia and hypertrophy in a subregion-specific manner. *Am J Physiol Endocrinol Metab* 291(5):E965–73.

Unger R.H. (1997). How obesity causes diabetes in Zucker diabetic fatty rats. *Trends Endocrinol Metab* 8(7):276–82.

Unger R.H., Orci L. (2001). Diseases of liporegulation: new perspective on obesity and related disorders. *FASEB J* 15:312–21.

Vahle J.L., Sato M., Long G.G., Young J.K., Francis P.C., Engelhardt J.A., Westmore M.S., Linda Y., Nold J.B. (2002). Skeletal changes in rats given daily subcutaneous injections of recombinant human parathyroid hormone (1-34) for 2 years and relevance to human safety. *Toxicol Pathol* 30:312–21.

Vahle J.L., Long G.G., Sandusky G., Westmore M., Ma Y.L., Sato M. (2004). Bone neoplasms in F344 rats given teriparatide [rhPTH(1-34)] are dependent on duration of treatment and dose. *Toxicol Pathol* 32:426–38.

Vahle J.L., Sato M., Long G.G. (2007). Variations in animal populations over time and differences in diagnostic thresholds used can impact tumor incidence data. *Toxicol Pathol* 35:1045–6.

Vahle J.L., Zuehlke U., Schmidt A., Westmore M., Chen P., Sato M. (2008). Lack of bone neoplasms and persistence of bone efficacy in cynomolgus macaques after long-term treatment with teriparatide [rhPTH(1-34)]. *J Bone Miner Res* 23:2033–9.

van der Harst E., de Herder W.W., de Krijger R.R., Bruining H.A., Bonjer H.J., Lamberts S.W., van den Meiracker A.H., Stijnen T.H., Boomsma F. (2002). The value of plasma markers for the clinical behaviour of phaeochromocytomas. *Eur J Endocrinol* 147(1):85–94.

Van Zwieten M.J., Frith C.H., Nooteboom A.L., Wolfe H.J., Delellis R.A. (1983). Medullary thyroid carcinoma in female BALB/c mice. A report of 3 cases with ultrastructural, immunohistochemical, and transplantation data. *Am J Pathol* 110:219–29.

Vansell N.R., Muppidi J.R., Habeebu S.M., Klaassen C.D. (2004). Promotion of thyroid tumors in rats by pregnenolone-16alpha-carbonitrile (PCN) and polychlorinated biphenyl (PCB). *Toxicol Sci Official J Soc Toxicol* 81:50–9.

Vidal S., Horvath E., Kovacs K., Lloyd R.V., Smyth H.S. (2001). Reversible transdifferentiation: interconversion of somatotrophs and lactotrophs in pituitary hyperplasia. *Mod Pathol* 14(1):20–8.

Waechter F., Beilstein P., Burger A.G., O'Connell M., Fabreguettes C., Forster R., Weideli H. (1999). Subchronic toxicity study with ethylene-bis-(oxyethylene)-bis-(3-tert-butyl-4-hydroxy-5-methylhydrocinnamate) in the cynomolgus monkey: lack of stimulation of the pituitary–thyroid–liver axis. *Toxicol Sci* 51:36–43.

Wagner J.D., Carlson C.S., O'Brien T.D., Anthony M.S., Bullock B.C., Cefalu W.T. (1996). Diabetes mellitus and islet amyloidosis in cynomolgus monkeys. *Lab Anim Sci* 46:36–41.

Wagner J.D., Cline J.M., Shadoan M.K. et al. (2001). Naturally occurring and experimental diabetes in cynomolgus monkeys: a comparison of carbohydrate and lipid metabolism and islet pathology. *Toxicol Pathol* 29:142–8.

Wakefield L.M., Thordarson G., Nieto A.I., Shyamala G., Galvez J.J., Anver M.R., Cardiff R.D. (2003). Spontaneous pituitary abnormalities and mammary hyperplasia in FVB/NCr mice: implications for mouse modeling. *Comp Med* 53(4):424–32.

Westermark P., Wernstedt C., Heldin C.-H., Wilander E., Hayden D.W., O'Brien T.D., Johnson K.H. (1987). Amyloid fibrils in human insulinoma and islets of Langerhans of the diabetic cat are derived from a novel neuropeptide-like protein also present in normal islet cells. *Proc Natl Acad Sci USA* 84:3881–5.

Wieczorek G., Pospischil A., Perentes E. (1998). A comparative immunohistochemical study of pancreatic islets in laboratory animals rats, dogs, minipigs, nonhuman primates. *Exp Toxic Pathol* 50:151–72.

Wilhelm S., Prinz R.A. (2004). Editorial review of "Malignant progression from C-cell hyperplasia to medullary thyroid carcinoma in 167 RET germline mutations." *Surgery* 135:447–8.

Williams G. (1964). Amyloidosis in parabiotic mice. *J Pathol Bacteriol* 88:35–41.

Wilson G.L., Longnecker D.S. (1999). Pancreatic toxicology. In *Endocrine and Hormonal Toxicity* (P.W. Harvey, K.C. Rush, A. Cockburn, eds.), pp. 125–53. Wiley, London.

Withers D.J., Gutierrez J.S., Towery H., Burks D.J., Ren J.M., Previs S. Zhang Y., Bernal D., Pons S., Shulman G.I., Bonner-Weir S., White M.F. (1998). Disruption of IRS-2 causes type 2 diabetes in mice. *Nature* 391:900–4.

Wittkowski W. (1988). Tanycytes and pituicytes: morphological and functional aspects of neuroglial interaction. *Microsc Res Tech* 1;41(1):29–42.

Wolfgang G.H., Robertson D.G., Welty D.F., Metz A.L. (1995). Hepatic and adrenal toxicity of a novel lipid regulator in beagle dogs. *Fundam Appl Toxicol* 26(2):272–81.

Wynford-Thomas V., Wynford-Thomas D., Williams E.D. (1983). Experimental induction of parathyroid adenomas in the rat. *J Natl Cancer Inst* 70:127–34.

Xia Y., Wikberg J.E. (1996). Localization of ACTH receptor mRNA by in situ hybridization in mouse adrenal gland. *Cell Tissue Res* 286(1):63–8.

Yale J.F., Marliss E.B. (1984). Altered immunity and diabetes in the BB rat. *Clin Exp Immunol* 57(1):1–11.

Yanagisawa M., Hara Y., Satoh K., Tanikawa T., Sakatsume Y., Katayama S., Kawazu S., Ishii J., Komeda K. (1986). Spontaneous autoimmune thyroiditis in Bio Breeding/Worcester (BB/W) rat. *Endocrinol Jpn* 33:851–61.

Yarrington J.T., Huffman K.W., Gibson J.P. (1981). Adrenocortical degeneration in dogs, monkeys, and rats treated with alpha-(1,4-dioxido-3-methylquinoxalin-2-YL)-N-methylnitrone. *Toxicol Lett* 8(4–5):229–34.

Yarrington J.T., Loudy D.E., Sprinkle D.J., Gibson J.P., Wright C.L., Johnston J.O. (1985). Degeneration of the rat and canine adrenal cortex caused by alpha-(1,4-dioxido-3-methylquinoxalin-2-yl)-N-methylnitrone (DMNM). *Fundam Appl Toxicol* 5(2):370–81.

Yoon J.W., McClintock P.R., Onodera T., Notkins A.L. (1980). Virus-Induced diabetes mellitus. XVIII. Inhibition by a nondiabetogenic variant of encephalomyocarditis virus. *J Exp Med* 152:878–92.

Yoon J.W., Onodera T., Notkins A.L. (1978). Virus-induced diabetes mellitus. XV. Beta cell damage and insulin-dependent hyperglycemia in mice infected with coxsackie virus B4. *J Exp Med* 148:1068–80.

Yoshizawa K., Heatherly A., Malarkey D.E., Walker N.J., Nyska A. (2007). A critical comparison of murine pathology and epidemiological data of TCDD, PCB126, and PeCDF. *Toxicol Pathol* 35:865–79.

Yoshizawa K., Walker N.J., Nyska A., Kissling G.E., Jokinen M.P., Brix A.E., Sells D.M., Wyde M.E. (2010). Thyroid follicular lesions induced by oral treatment for 2 years with 2,3,7,8-tetrachlorodibenzo-p-dioxin and dioxin-like compounds in female Harlan Sprague–Dawley rats. *Toxicol Pathol* 38:1037–50.

Yu K.O., Narayanan L., Mattie D.R., Godfrey R.J., Todd P.N., Sterner T.R., Mahle D.A., Lumpkin M.H., Fisher J.W. (2002). The pharmacokinetics of perchlorate and its effect on the hypothalamus–pituitary–thyroid axis in the male rat. *Toxicol Appl Pharmacol* 182:148–59.

Zabka T.S., Fielden M.R., Garrido R., Tao J., Fretland A.J., Fretland J.L., Albassam M.A., Singer T., Kolaja K.L. (2011) Characterization of xenobiotic-induced hepatocellular enzyme induction in rats: anticipated thyroid effects and unique pituitary gland findings. *Toxicol Pathol* 39(4):664–77.

Zak M., Kovacs K., McComb D.J., Heitz P.U. (1985). Aminoglutethimide-stimulated corticotrophs. An immunocytologic, ultrastructural and immunoelectron microscopic study of the rat adenohypophysis. *Virchows Arch B Cell Pathol Incl Mol Pathol* 49(1):93–106.

Zayed I., van Esch E., McConnell R.F. (1998). Systemic and histopathologic changes in beagle dogs after chronic daily oral administration of synthetic (ethinyl estradiol) or natural (estradiol) estrogens, with special reference to the kidney and thyroid. *Toxicol Pathol* 26:730–41.

Zhang X., Yu R.M., Jones P.D., Lam G.K., Newsted J.L., Gracia T., Hecker M., Hilscherova K., Sanderson T., Wu R.S., Giesy J.P. (2005). Quantitative RT-PCR methods for evaluating toxicant-induced effects on steroidogenesis using the H295R cell line. *Environ Sci Technol* 15;39(8):2777–85.

Zhang Y., Proenca R., Maffei M., Barone M., Leoplold L, Friedman J.M. (1994). Positional cloning of the mouse obese gene and its human homologue. *Nature* 372:425–32.

18 Reproductive System and Mammary Gland

Justin D. Vidal, Michael L. Mirsky, Karyn Colman, Katharine M. Whitney, and Dianne M. Creasy

CONTENTS

18.1 INTRODUCTION

Compound-related effects on the reproductive system are often pivotal in pharmaceutical development. As with other organ systems, a pathologist's understanding of the physiology, background pathology, and species variations underlying the microscopic presentation of reproductive tissues can be critical to accurate risk assessment. However, the reproductive system has several unique features that require special attention, which includes dependence on hormones from the hypothalamus and pituitary, hormonal feedback, puberty, senescence, cyclicity in the female, stage-aware evaluation of spermatogenesis, and dramatic species differences. This requires the pathologist to be well versed in normal physiology and endocrinology, and in this chapter, we have included more information on normal anatomy, histology, physiology, and endocrinology than is typically provided in pathology textbooks. A firm grasp of the normal state will allow for better characterization of potential reproductive hazards and provide for the best possible risk assessment. In addition, we have considered the male and female reproductive systems together with the mammary gland as many basic concepts track across these organ systems. The reproductive organs cannot be effectively evaluated in isolation. For example, the testes, and spermatogenesis in particular, receive the most attention and are the most common target sites for male reproductive toxicants, but the epididymis and the hypothalamic–pituitary–gonadal (HPG) axis must also be considered. Sometimes they can be the primary site of toxicity, and changes in the testes occur as a secondary consequence. Similarly in the female, changes in the vaginal epithelium must be evaluated in conjunction with an understanding of the reproductive cycle, the HPG axis, and mammary gland. Background pathology and maturity status are confounding factors for identifying toxicity in all species, but especially in the male dog and female nonhuman primate (NHP; unless specified, NHP will refer to cynomologus macaque). Guidance is provided for recognizing and distinguishing these changes from drug-induced changes. Organ weights, sperm parameters, fertility, endocrine measurements, and reproductive cyclicity data are other important endpoints that can be used to evaluate reproductive toxicity and in some cases are more sensitive than histopathology for detecting toxicity. Although these parameters are not generally available to the pathologist from routine toxicity studies, it is important to understand their relevance and application for overall risk assessment.

18.2 MALE EMBRYOLOGY AND MATURATION

18.2.1 *In Utero* Development

The reproductive tract is derived from the mesonephros of the intermediate mesoderm. During embryogenesis (early in the second week of gestation for mouse), primordial germ cells (PGCs) (gonocytes) from the yolk sac wall near the developing allantois migrate through the dorsal hindgut mesentery to the mesonephros (Noden and De Lahunta 1985). The gonadal ridge forms as a ventromedial protrusion from the middle portion of the mesonephros and is populated by approximately 100 gonocytes. Epithelial cells, extending from the coelomic epithelium overlying the gonadal ridge

(Pelliniemi et al. 1993), cluster around the gonocytes, coalescing to form gonadal cords (primitive sex cords) extending from the coelomic epithelium to the mesonephric tubules. This array of gonadal cords comprises the indifferent gonad, destined by default to become an ovary unless the Sry (sex-related Y chromosomal) gene directs transcription of factors influencing male gonadogenesis. Under Sry-initiated guidance, gonadal cords are separated from the gonadal ridge coelomic epithelium by a mesenchymal sheet, the primordial tunica albuginea, the connective tissue structure that will serve as a scaffold for the future vascular supply to the testis. Gonadal cords become arranged as loops (approximately 20 to 30 in rat), with the ends of each cord connecting via the rete testis to the efferent ductules, both derived from mesonephric tubules. Gonocytes multiply during the second week of rodent gestation. The epithelial components (sustentacular cells, early Sertoli cells) of the gonadal cords multiply maximally during the second half of gestation in rodents, surrounding the centrally located gonocytes.

Leydig (interstitial) cells, the source of testosterone, reside in the intertubular interstitium and are derived from somatic progenitor cells of the gonadal ridge. Differentiation of fetal Leydig cells occurs after cord formation, starting from gestational day 15 in the rat with proliferation continuing to gestational day 19, followed by regression continuing to postnatal day (PND) 4 (Chen et al. 2010). High levels of testosterone produced by the fetal Leydig cells influence reproductive organogenesis late in gestation.

The mesonephric (Wolffian) ducts are aligned longitudinally within the intermediate mesoderm of the fetus, with mesonephric tubules extending medially. Under the influence of testosterone, mesonephric tubules fuse with gonadal cords to form the efferent ductules. The mesonephric duct forms the epididymis, vas deferens, and seminal vesicle. Anti-Müllerian hormone elaborated by Sertoli cells causes regression of the paramesonephric (Müllerian) ducts.

The prostate, coagulating and bulbourethral glands, and external genitalia are formed from the urogenital sinus, a midline invagination of mesenchymal and epithelial layers derived from mesoderm and endoderm, respectively. Rodent reproductive organogenesis commences approximately at gestational day 18 in response to androgens. Testosterone triggers expression of 5α-reductase to produce the more potent dihydrotestosterone (DHT) in target tissues. Isozymes of 5α-reductase are expressed in both epithelial and mesenchymal cells of the primordial glands (Berman et al. 1995). Prostate formation involves paired epithelial buds (future lobes) extending outward from the urethral portion of the urogenital sinus into the surrounding mesoderm, branching sequentially. Basal cells align along the basement membrane and columnar cells line the lumens. The surrounding mesenchyme forms smooth muscle and fibrous capsular components.

18.2.2 Postnatal Development

Postnatal testicular development varies among species, just as the timing of puberty varies. Among rodents (rats and mice having similar well-characterized timelines), there is a rapid succession of developmental steps commencing around PND 3 (Figure 18.1), when mitotic gonocytes migrate from the central position within gonadal cords toward the cord periphery (Clermont and Perey 1957; Nebel et al. 1961) and either degenerate or differentiate into type A spermatogonia by ~PND 9 in rat (Figure 18.2a). Sertoli cells continue to undergo mitosis until ~PND 15 to 18 in the rat (Orth 1982), by which time gonadal cords have become further populated by successive divisions of type A spermatogonia, generating intermediate and type B spermatogonia at the cord periphery, and preleptotene, leptotene, zygotene, and pachytene spermatocytes toward the cord center (Figure 18.2b). This beginning of the so-called first wave of spermatogenesis (Figure 18.1) represents an acceleration of the comparable progression from type A spermatogonium to pachytene spermatocyte that occurs in the adult over approximately 3 weeks (Russell 1992). After cessation of Sertoli cell mitotic divisions, initial formation of the Sertoli cell intercellular basolateral tight junctions that compose the blood–testis barrier (BTB) commences as a wave around PND 15 (Russell et al. 1989), occurring first in those cord segments containing pachytene spermatocytes. While the

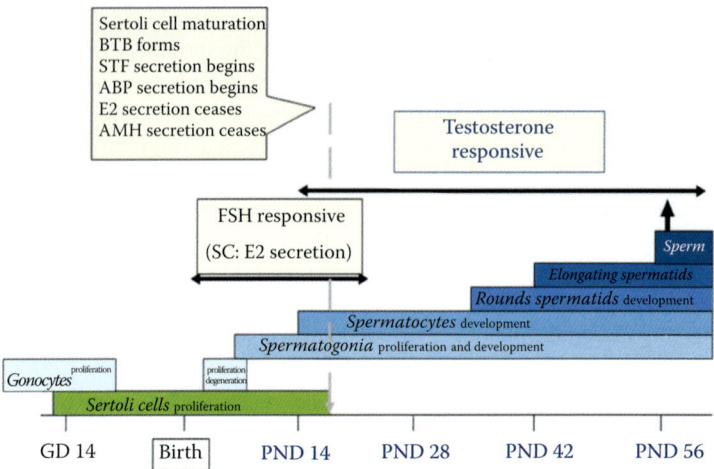

FIGURE 18.1   The major developmental events surrounding spermatogenesis are summarized in this figure. The timing of events relates to the rat. Sertoli cells undergo proliferation during gestation and up to PND 18 to establish the final Sertoli cell number. Sertoli cells are then unable to divide for the remainder of their life, even if damaged. Numerous maturation processes occur up to PND 18 including formation of the blood–testis barrier (BTB) and the beginning of seminiferous tubule fluid (STF) secretion. The follicle-stimulating hormone (FSH) is the major hormone regulating early spermatogenesis through stimulation of estradiol (E2) secretion by the Sertoli cell. Around PND 18, the luteinizing hormone (LH) begins to take over from FSH and stimulates Leydig cell production of testosterone, which then drives spermatogenesis and male sexual behavior. By PND 25, testosterone is the major hormone. Spermatogenesis starts under control of FSH and T but FSH decreases in importance and only acts to modulate/support spermatogenesis in the adult. Compounds that affect the developing testis often affect the adult testis in a totally different way because the regulatory processes are very different between the two.

BTB forms, many spermatocytes are subject to physiologic removal by apoptosis (Jahnukainen et al. 2004; Zheng et al. 2006), thereby balancing the ratio of germ cells to Sertoli cells. In general, the first representatives of a given germ cell type in the initial spermatogenic wave are subject to degeneration (Russell et al. 1987). The BTB is complete by ~PND 20, at which time Sertoli cells begin secretory function and the gonadal cord becomes a seminiferous tubule through formation of the central lumen (Morales et al. 2007) (Figure 18.2c). Round spermatids are first apparent by PND 26, followed by successive steps of elongating spermatids until mature step 19 spermatids are present at the seminiferous tubular lumen by PND 45, signifying (along with preputial separation at ~PND 43) rat puberty (Figure 18.2d).

After regression of the fetal population of Leydig cells, a new postnatal population derived from mesenchymal stem cells commences slow growth within the interstitium on ~PND 4. Committed progenitor Leydig cells are present by 2 weeks and immature Leydig cells capable of high level steroid metabolism start rapid growth in the fourth postnatal week (Chen et al. 2010). The immature Leydig cells undergo one or two mitotic divisions until PND 50 to 56, becoming fully differentiated into adult Leydig cells. Adult Leydig cells (~25 million per adult rat testis) are terminally differentiated, rarely dividing or dying, but replacements may be generated from an as yet undefined cell population such as undifferentiated mesenchymal progenitor cells, peritubular myoid cells, or vascular smooth muscle cells.

In juvenile studies with rats, it is important to be aware of the normal testicular morphology for each age, including (1) presence of gonocytes up to PND 9; (2) Sertoli cell mitoses up to PND 18; (3) accelerated first wave spermatogonial proliferation; (4) small numbers of Leydig cells early, followed by mitotic activity and increasing numbers; (5) increased spermatocytic apoptosis, especially

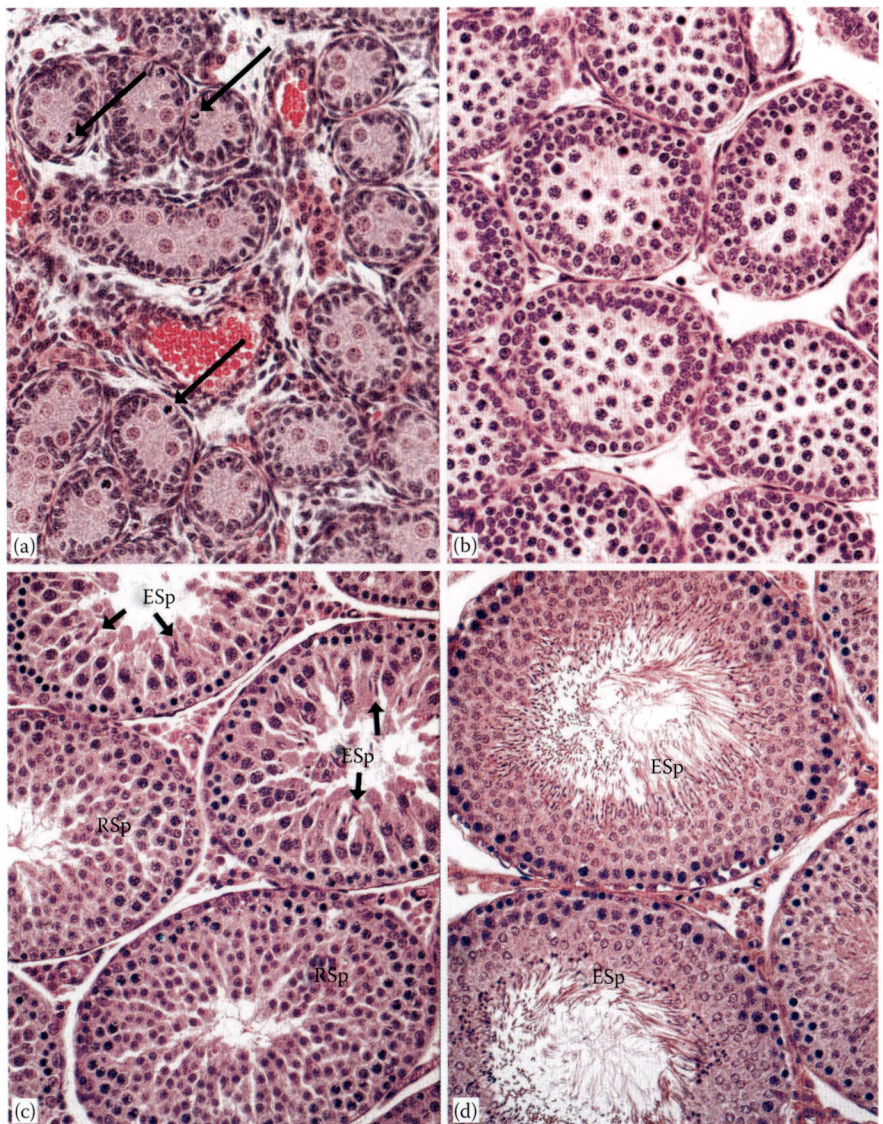

FIGURE 18.2 (a) PND 2 rat testis (top left) has large, pale, round gonocytes centrally located within the gonadal cords. Mitotic Sertoli cells are arrowed. (b) PND 22 rat testis (top right) has basal spermatogonia and early spermatocytes and central, more mature spermatocytes with an intervening palisade of Sertoli cell nuclei. There is a high attrition rate of germ cells during this first spermatogenic cycle. (c) PND 35 rat testis (lower left) has round spermatids (RSp) but no elongating spermatids in early stages and pachytene spermatocytes and a few early elongating spermatids (ESp) in late stages. (d) PND 70 rat testis (lower right) has mature seminiferous tubules with complete germ cell complements including mature elongating spermatids (ESp) in early-stage tubules that are approaching the point of spermiation.

PND 15 to 20; and (6) the specific sequential appearance of maturing germ cells. A familiarity with these age-related characteristics can help identify those changes related to test article administration.

Similar testicular developmental processes occur in other species with altered timing; events spanning days in rodents occupy weeks in dog and months to years in NHP and human, with substantial variability among individual animals (Table 18.1).

TABLE 18.1

Comparison of Pre- and Postnatal Testicular Development across Species

	Rat	Dog	Cynomolgus Monkey	Man
Primordial germ cell migration	GD 8–10			~6 weeks
Organogenesis	GD 6–17			3–7 weeks
Gonadogenesis	GD 12–15	GD 36		4–20 weeks
Fetal LCs evident	GD 16			8 weeks
Peak SC division	GD 19			
Development of genitalia				10–26 weeks
Peak T	GD 19			14–18 weeks
Peak LH	GD 21			12 weeks
Birth	GD 21	GD63	22 weeks	40 weeks
SC and gonocytes only	<PND 4	<16 weeks	<1 year	<2 months
LC nadir	PND 4			1.5 years
Increasing spermatogonia	PND 4–12	16 weeks		Birth to 10 years
Early spermatocytes	PND 9	20 weeks	36–48 months	
Adult LCs evident	PND 11	16 weeks		11 years
SC divisions stop	PND 15		~32 months	~15 years
BTB formation	PND 15–20	20 weeks	~34 months	Puberty
Testicular descent	PND 22	5–6 weeks	~36 months	Prenatal
Adult LC proliferation	PND 22			
Spermatids	PND 26	22 weeks	44–57 months	
Mature sperm	PND 45	~28 weeks	44–52 months	11–15 years

Sources: Clermont, Y. and Perey, B., *Am J Anat* 100:241–68, 1957; Cortes, D. et al., *Int J Androl* 10:589–96, 1987; Dang, D.C. and Meusy-Dessolle, N., *Arch Androl* 12(Suppl):43–51, 1984; Haruyama, E. et al., *A Toxicol Pathol* 40:935–42, 2012; Kawakami, E. et al., *J Vet Med Sci* 53:241–8, 1991; Marty, M.S. et al., *Birth Defects Res B Dev Reprod Toxicol* 68:125–36, 2003; Pryor, J.L. et al., *Environ Health Perspect* 108(Suppl 3):491–503, 2000.

18.3 TESTIS

18.3.1 FUNCTIONAL ANATOMY

The mature testis comprises compactly arrayed convoluted loops of seminiferous tubules separated by an interstitium containing Leydig cells, vasculature, macrophages, a protein- and testosterone-rich ultrafiltrate, and scant supporting stroma. In rodents, the seminiferous tubules are arranged circumferentially, whereas in dogs and primates, they are arranged in a lobular organization. The seminiferous epithelium is formed by basally located Sertoli cells supporting successive synchronized populations of maturing germ cells (spermatogonia, spermatocytes, round spermatids, and elongating spermatids). Seminiferous tubules are ensheathed by a basement membrane and an outer layer of contractile myoid cells and converge, through the tubuli recti at each end of the tubular loops, on the rete testis, which is continuous with the efferent ductules and epididymis. The mature testis resides in the extra-abdominal scrotal sac and is covered by the thick, fibrous tunica albuginea and the visceral vaginal tunic, continuous with the parietal peritoneum.

The testicular artery (branching from the aorta), which anastomoses with the artery of the ductus deferens (originating from the internal iliac artery), provides the vascular supply to the testis. The testicular vein forms an extensive (pampiniform) plexus around the artery within the spermatic cord, thereby creating a countercurrent heat exchange system to maintain the lower scrotal temperature. Vessels populate the tunica albuginea, traverse fibrous lamellae to the mediastinum in dog and NHP, and send branches (intertubular arterioles) to the interstitium, giving rise to intertubular and peritubular capillaries. In the rat, vessels radiate and arborize from the area of the rete testis on the caudodorsal aspect of the testis. A protein-rich filtrate escapes the interstitial capillaries (depending on the species) to lymphatic channels or the interstitium (Fawcett et al. 1973) to supply the seminiferous tubules. The transudate penetrates the myoid cell layer and seminiferous tubular basement membrane to reach the Sertoli cells and spermatogonia.

18.3.1.1 Germ Cells and Spermatogenesis

The germ cell types are distinctive in ploidy, morphology, and susceptibility to harmful influences, including certain pharmaceutical compounds. *Spermatogonia* are unique in being the sole proliferative cell population within the seminiferous epithelium and in residing outside of the protective BTB formed by tight junctions between Sertoli cells. Functionally, rodent spermatogonia are classified as stem cell, proliferative, or differentiating. Morphologically (based on increasing amounts of chromatin lining the nuclear envelope), they are described as type A, intermediate, and type B (Russell et al. 1990). The classifications and proliferative kinetics of spermatogonia vary among species (Clermont 1972). Spermatogonia are present in all tubular cross sections of a normal testis, although in variable numbers and sometimes inconspicuous in the course of the spermatogenic cycle.

Type B spermatogonia divide to generate preleptotene *spermatocytes*, which comprise the majority of cells in the prominent basal layer of stage VII rat tubules. Preleptotene spermatocytes move from the basalar compartment into the sequestered adluminal compartment by the shifting of Sertoli cell tight junctions; they also undergo DNA synthesis, becoming tetraploid, and initiate the meiotic process that proceeds over the next one and one-half spermatogenic cycles (approximately 20 days in rat) sequentially transforming into the various meiotic phases of primary spermatocytes. Like the other germ cell types, spermatocytes are susceptible to the variety of circumstances that may trigger apoptosis, including physiologic attrition as well as androgen deficiency and cytotoxic effects. Additionally, they can be targets of agents interfering with diakinesis. Primary spermatocytes ultimately divide twice (these two meiotic divisions occurring in rapid succession [rat stage XIV]) to form haploid round spermatids.

Spermatids, still linked by intercellular bridges established among their spermatogonial progenitors, undergo marked morphological transformation (spermiogenesis) from round to elongating forms, expanding and then condensing cytoplasm and shedding organelles, and depend on the Sertoli cell for successful terminal differentiation and release. The various morphological forms of spermatids are characterized as steps 1 through 19 in rat (steps 1 through 14 in the NHP and steps 1 through 12 in the dog) and are distinguished by the changing shape of the periodic acid–Schiff (PAS)-positive acrosome enclosing the haploid genetic cargo. Cohorts of round spermatids are present in each tubular cross section representing an early (pre-spermiation) stage. Mature (step 19 in rat) spermatids are released into the seminiferous tubular lumen (rat Stage VIII) in the Sertoli cell–coordinated process of spermiation. Residual bodies (condensed cytoplasmic remnants shed by spermatids during spermiation) are reabsorbed by Sertoli cells. Elongating spermatids are present in all tubular cross sections of a normal mature testis.

Spermatogenesis (Figure 18.3) is the process by which undifferentiated, stem cell spermatogonia become highly differentiated motile spermatozoa. This is accomplished by the spermatogonia undergoing a series of rapid mitotic divisions, which serves to massively increase their number. The final spermatogonial division produces the spermatocytes, which undergo meiosis, including DNA replication, chromosome pairing, chromosome condensation, and finally two rapid divisions, the first forming short-lived secondary spermatocytes and the second division forming the haploid round spermatid. The round spermatid then goes through a transformation, taking it from a

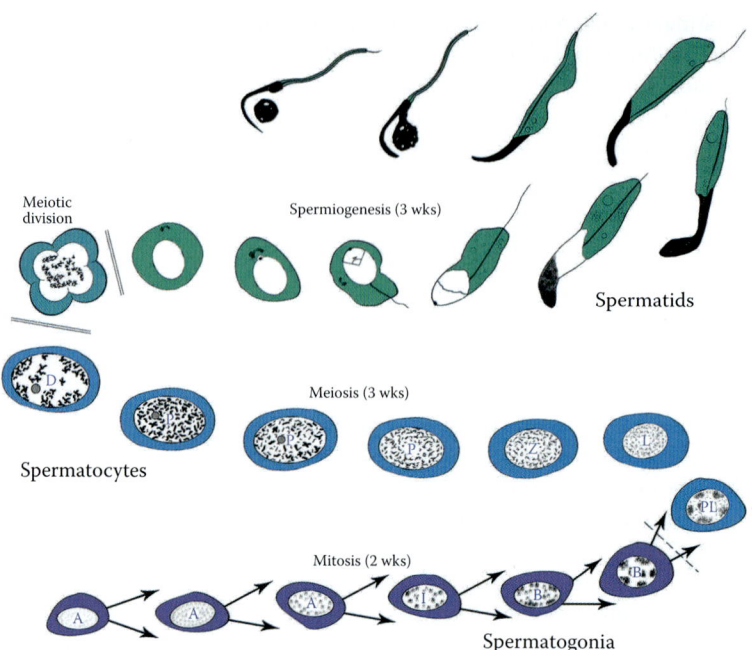

FIGURE 18.3 Spermatogenesis is the process whereby primitive stem cell spermatogonia develop into mature sperm. The process involves multiple mitotic divisions of the spermatogonia, which expands the progenitor cell population. Three types of spermatogonia can be morphologically distinguished: type A (A), intermediate (I), and type B (B). The final division produces the spermatocytes, which progress through meiotic prophase, comprising preleptotene (PL), leptotene (L), zygotene (Z), and pachytene (P), which can be split into early, mid, and late phases of development. After passing through diplotene and diakinesis (D), the tetraploid spermatocyte undergoes two rapid reduction divisions; the first produces diploid secondary spermatocytes and the second division produces the haploid round spermatid. The morphological transformation of the round spermatid into an elongated mature spermatid ready for release has been divided into 19 "steps of spermiogenesis" in the rat and the detailed characteristics of the developing spermatid are used to identify the 14 stages of spermatogenesis. The entire process takes 8 weeks in the rat with 2 weeks for spermatogonial divisions, 3 weeks for spermatocyte development, and 3 weeks for spermiogenesis.

regular-appearing round cell with round, centrally placed nucleus to an elliptical cell with a nucleus displaced to the cell periphery and finally ending up with a sickle-shaped, highly condensed nucleus that forms the head of the sperm attached to a whip-like tail comprising a mitochondrial lined flagellum surrounded by a thin coat of cytoplasm. This morphological transformation of the spermatid is termed "spermiogenesis" and it has been subdivided into a number of "steps of spermiogenesis" (19 in the rat, 16 in the mouse, 14 in the NHP, and 12 in the dog), which are used to identify the stages of the spermatogenic cycle (14 in the rat, 12 in the mouse, 12 in the NHP, and 8 in the dog) (Dreef et al. 2007; Russell et al. 1990).

As spermatogenesis proceeds, the successive developmental stages of germ cells move up through the seminiferous epithelium and each of the different cell types (spermatogonia, spermatocytes, and spermatids) form well-defined layers moving from base to lumen. The regularity of these layers and their precise cellular makeup is key to recognizing the "stages of the spermatogenic cycle" and also to identifying abnormalities in the spermatogenic process. Examination of any cross section of tubule will show four generations of cells developing at the same time and forming discrete layers. Each generation develops in total synchrony with the others, leading to defined cellular associations. For example, a section of tubule that contains mature elongating spermatids that are just on the point of release will always be accompanied by a round spermatid with an acrosome that covers half its nuclear membrane. Also present will be spermatocytes midway through pachytene development and preleptotene spermatocytes that have just formed from the final spermatogonial division. This specific cell association is one of the 14 cell associations that make up the stages of the spermatogenic cycle of the rat (Table 18.2). As each of the four generations of cells changes its morphology slightly, it enters the next stage in the cycle. The detailed morphological changes of the acrosome in the round spermatid as well as the changing shape of the elongating spermatid head (i.e., the steps of spermiogenesis) are used by the pathologist to define the precise stage of spermatogenesis for any given section of tubule.

In order to evaluate spermatogenesis in detail, the pathologist needs to have a very good knowledge of the spermatogenic cycle, its kinetics, and the morphological features of the different stages of the spermatogenic cycle. One also needs to understand species differences in the cycle. There are numerous comprehensive texts that provide excellent guidance on how to stage tubules (Clermont 1972; Creasy and Foster 2002; Dreef et al. 2007; Hess 1990; Leblond and Clermont 1952; Oakberg 1956; Russell et al. 1990) and the reader is encouraged to spend time studying the subject to obtain

TABLE 18.2

Rat Spermatogenesis

Stage	Basal Layer				Adluminal Layers		
	1			**2**	**3**		**4**
	Spermatogonia			**Spematocytes**	**Spermatids**		
IX		A_1 (mitosis)		L	P		Step 9
X		A_2		L	P		10
XI		A_2		L	P		11
XII		A_2 (mitosis)		L–Z	P		12
XIII		A_3		Z	D		13
XIV		A_3 (mitosis)		Z	Meiotic divisions		14
I	A	In		P		Step 1	15
II	A_1	In		P		2	16
III	A_1	In		P		3	17
IV	A_1	In (mitosis)		P		4	17
V	A_1	B		P		5	18
VI	A_1	B (mitosis)		P		6	19
VII	A_1		pL	P		7	19
VIII	A_1		pL	P		8	Spermiation

A, type A spermatogonium

In, intermediate spermatogonium

B, type B spermatogonium

pL, preleptotene spermatocyte

L, leptotene spermatocyte

Z, zygotene spermatocyte

P, pachytene spermatocyte

D, diplotene spermatocyte

Source: Leblond, C.P. and Clermont, Y., *Ann NY Acad Sci* 55:548–73, 1952.

Note: Germ cell development proceeds down the successive left to right columns, starting with type A spermatogonia and ending with release of step 19 spermatids at spermiation. Mitotic and meiotic divisions are indicated. Cell associations are indicated as rows corresponding to each stage. One complete column (one cycle), encompassing all stages, represents approximately 2 weeks. Adluminal layers are within the BTB formed by Sertoli cell tight junctions.

a clear understanding of the process. In reality, the majority of spermatogenic disturbances can be identified as long as the pathologist is familiar with approximately five or six different phases of germ cell development and with the appearance of tubules when they are at the beginning, in the middle, or at the end of the "spermatogenic cycle."

Morphologically, there are six easily distinguished phases of germ cell development: (1) early (type A and intermediate) spermatogonia, (2) late (type B) spermatogonia and early (preleptotene, leptotene, and zygotene) spermatocytes, (3) pachytene spermatocytes, (4) dividing spermatocytes, (5) round spermatids, and (6) elongating spermatids (Figures 18.4 and 18.5). Spermatogenesis is basically the same in all mammalian species, but there are detailed differences in the timing, regulation, staging classification, and morphological characteristics of the different cell types.

The timing of spermatogenesis is important to consider when evaluating the pattern of germ cell depletion and its recovery in toxicity studies of varying duration. Once committed to undergoing spermatogenesis, it takes approximately 8 weeks in the rat (timing is species specific) for spermatogonia to complete their development into spermatozoa that are ready to be released into the tubular lumen. This process involves an individual spermatogonium passing through four spermatogenic cycles (each cycle lasting approximately 2 weeks) as it develops into a mature spermatid. The practical implications of this process are important when evaluating spermatogenesis. If you were to follow the development of one spermatogonium, on day 1, it starts spermatogenesis as a type A spermatogonium, which is a pale staining, nondescript cell on the basal lamina. Two weeks later, it will become a preleptotene spermatocyte (prominent, darkly staining small spermatocyte, slightly off the basal lamina); another 2 weeks later, it will be a mid-pachytene spermatocyte (large spermatocyte with well-defined chromosomes, situated a third of the way up the epithelium). In another

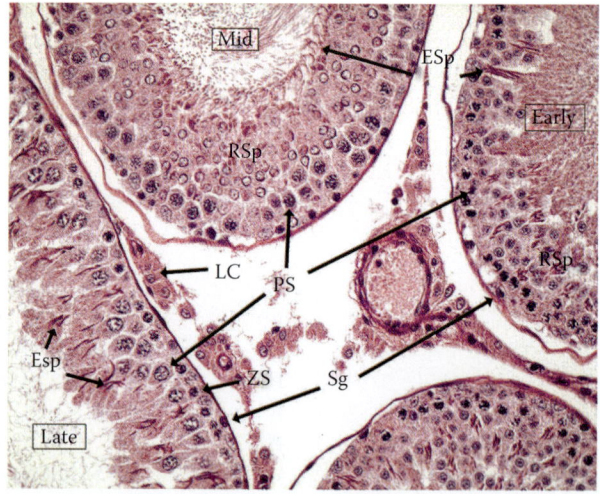

FIGURE 18.4 Normal cellular associations in early-, mid-, and late-stage tubules of rat testis. ESp, elongating spermatids; RSp, round spermatids; PS, pachytene spermatocytes; ZS, zygotene spermatocytes; Sg, spermatogonia; LC, Leydig cells. Early-stage tubules (stages I–VI) have elongating spermatids whose heads are embedded within the round spermatid population. The pachytene spermatocytes are early in their development and small in size. Mid-stage tubules (stages VII and VIII) have similar cell types to the early-stage tubules but the heads of the elongating spermatids form a luminal layer and are interspersed with residual bodies. The pachytene spermatocytes are midway through development and are larger. There is also an underlying layer of preleptotene spermatocytes. In the late-stage tubules (stages IX–XIV), there is only one generation of spermatids, which are elongating. The pachytene spermatocytes become larger as they approach meiotic division and the underlying prepachytene spermatocytes develop through leptotene and zygotene development. The interstitial space contains a blood vessel surrounded by Leydig cells.

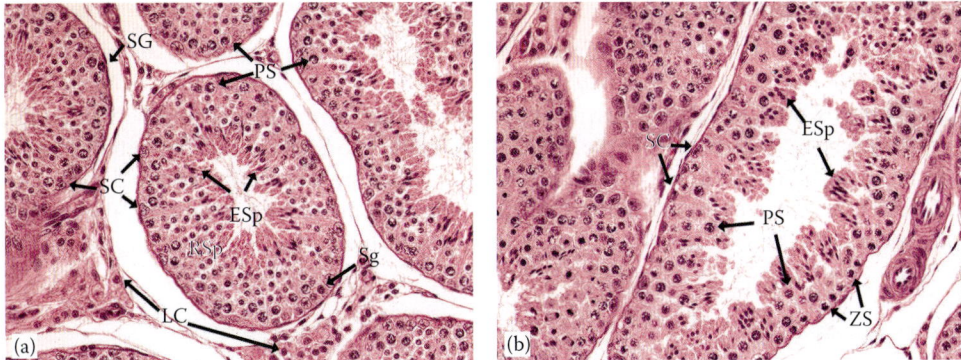

FIGURE 18.5 Normal cellular associations in early- and late-stage tubules in dog testes. (a) Early-stage tubules (stages I–V) contain a basal layer of Sertoli cell nuclei (SC) with large pale staining nuclei, interspersed with occasional intermediate spermatogonia (Sg), which are smaller and darker staining than Sertoli cell nuclei. The next layer of germ cells consists of pachytene spermatocytes (PS), which contain large nuclei with prominent chromosomal chromatin. The next germ cell layer comprises pale staining small round spermatids (RSp) lined by an adluminal layer of elongating spermatids (ESp). Note that the elongating spermatids have discrete short heads with relatively short "stumpy" tails that are partly embedded between the round spermatids. (b) Late-stage tubules (VI–VIII) contain two generations of spermatocytes, comprising a basal layer of small zygotene spermatocytes (ZS) and a more luminal layer of larger late pachytene spermatocytes (PS). There is only one layer of spermatids that are elongating (ESp).

2 weeks, it will be a round spermatid (pale staining, regular-appearing cell with an acrosomic cap, visible only by PAS, covering half the nucleus). At the end of another 2 weeks, the cell will have become a fully mature elongated spermatid (step 19) that is about to be released into the lumen. This timing is important when evaluating cell degeneration and depletion in studies of different durations.

18.3.1.2 Sertoli Cells

Sertoli cells are large, post-proliferative cells that make up approximately 10% of cells within the mature seminiferous epithelium and are essential to spermatogenesis. They are responsive to follicle-stimulating hormone (FSH) and serve multiple complex roles, including maintenance of the stem spermatogonial niche, simultaneous support of synchronous differentiation among four generations of germ cells, maintenance of the BTB, secretion of seminiferous fluid, production of secretory compounds (including anti-Müllerian hormone, androgen-binding protein, inhibin, growth factors, and endothelin), release of matured spermatids, and phagocytosis of residual bodies and apoptotic germ cell remnants (Gondos and Berndtson 1993). Maintenance of the BTB prevents penetration of toxicants and protects against immunologic exposure of antigens unique to adluminal germ cells. Sertoli cells subject to toxicant effects may manifest a variety of morphological changes, including effects on the germ cells they sustain. Mature Sertoli cells are less subject to apoptosis or necrosis in comparison to germ cells and are often the sole survivors within seminiferous epithelium in the face of a variety of injurious processes. Attached to the tubular basement membrane by hemidesmosomes, having abundant cytoplasm approximating a conical or pyramidal shape and having a large, basalar, folded nucleus with prominent nucleolus, the Sertoli cell has complex surface membrane formations, which are generally obscured by the germ cells it harbors. In the mouse, a single Sertoli cell can support approximately 50 germ cells (Radovsky et al. 1999), while in the NHP, the number is approximately half that of the mouse and varies widely among individual animals (Zhengwei et al. 1997) and daily sperm production in the respective species differs accordingly (Weinbauer and Nieschlag 1999).

18.3.1.3 Peritubular Cells

Peritubular myoid cells encircle the seminiferous tubules providing propulsive activity for move-ment of seminiferous fluid and spermatids. The spindloid myoid cells have thin, elongated nuclei, are closely apposed to the tubular basement membrane, and have gap junctions between adjacent cells making a small contribution to the BTB. Myoid cells, like Sertoli cells, have androgen recep-tors and respond to testosterone. Contractility is stimulated by endothelin, released cyclically by Sertoli cells (Tripiciano et al. 1996). Phosphodiesterase-5 produced by Leydig cells also stimulates myoid contractions. Myoid cells are susceptible to injury by histamine receptor antagonism (Franca et al. 2000).

18.3.1.4 Leydig Cells

Intratesticular androgen levels crucial to germ cell maintenance are sustained by Leydig cells, which reside in the intertubular interstitium. Leydig cells appear in clusters associated with the interstitial vasculature and have moderate amounts of eosinophilic, finely vacuolated cytoplasm, containing ample smooth endoplasmic reticulum consistent with their secretory activity and ovoid central nuclei. In response to luteinizing hormone (LH), Leydig cells synthesize testosterone and release it into the interstitial fluid for subsequent uptake by Sertoli cells and distribution into the systemic circulation via the spermatic vein. Relative numbers of Leydig cells and the degree of development of lymphatic vessels in the testicular interstitium vary among species (Fawcett et al. 1973).

18.3.1.5 Hormone Regulation

Overall control of male reproductive function occurs through endocrine regulation mediated through the HPG axis. Equally important, but less understood, is the regulation that occurs locally through paracrine and autocrine secretion of peptides and growth factors. The major androgenic steroid, testosterone, is synthesized primarily in the Leydig cells and has both intratesticular effects (on spermatogenesis) and peripheral effects (on accessory sex organs as well as nonreproductive organs such as muscle, skin, and bone to name but a few). The concentration of testosterone within the testis is much greater than that in the systemic circulation. For example, levels of the steroid in the testicular interstitial fluid can be up to 100-fold higher than that in the plasma and the con-centrations in the two compartments are not directly proportional to one another. Therefore, sam-pling plasma levels of testosterone does not provide a measure of intratesticular testosterone levels. Although these high intratesticular testosterone levels may be required to maintain quantitatively maximum spermatogenic potential, *qualitatively* normal spermatogenesis can be maintained with much lower intratesticular concentrations (Sharpe 1994).

The major stimulus for testosterone production comes from blood levels of LH from the pituitary. Feedback inhibition of LH and hypothalamic gonadotropin-releasing hormone (GnRH) is mediated through circulating levels of testosterone and its metabolites, DHT and estradiol. Aromatization of testosterone to estradiol takes place within the testis (indeed, estradiol is critically important for normal testis function) and also in many peripheral tissues such as adipose tissue and the cen-tral nervous system, whereas conversion to DHT through 5α-reductase activity occurs largely in androgen-dependent tissues such as the epididymis, prostate, and seminal vesicles, which utilize DHT rather than testosterone.

18.3.2 DISTINGUISHING DRUG-RELATED TOXICITY FROM BACKGROUND PATHOLOGY AND IMMATURITY

As with any other organ system, it is essential to have a good knowledge of the expected range of background pathology for the species being examined, so that drug-induced changes can be distin-guished from incidental findings. An additional factor that needs to be considered is the maturity status of the reproductive tissues. If a study is conducted where the animals are still immature at the end of dosing, then the study has not evaluated testicular toxicity and the possibility exists that the drug may be a testicular toxicant. If a study is conducted where the animals are peripubertal at the end of dosing, or there is a mixture of immature, peripubertal and mature animals, the study will be very difficult or impossible to interpret and runs the risk of indicating a false-positive or a false-negative result with regard to testicular toxicity.

Fortunately, there are relatively few background changes in the reproductive tract of young adult rodents, and with relatively large group sizes of 5–10 animals per group, confusion is not a common problem. Similarly, immaturity is rarely a confounding issue in rodent studies, since the animals mature early (8–10 weeks) and, on the basis of the standard starting age of rodents in toxicity studies (5–7 weeks of age), they will usually be adequately mature by the end of studies lasting 4 weeks or longer. However, problems can arise when this age of animal is used in studies lasting only 1–2 weeks.

A major problem exists when dealing with background pathology and immaturity in the beagle dog because there is a high incidence of degenerative lesions in the normal dog testis and it is common practice to use dogs that are only 5–6 months of age at study start, which results in dogs that are immature or peripubertal at the end of 4- or 13-week studies. Both issues (background pathology and immaturity) can seriously interfere with the ability of the pathologist to identify drug-induced toxicity.

18.3.2.1 Background Pathology in the Rat and Mouse

In studies of 6 months' duration or less, there are few background changes and very few age-related changes that will interfere with evaluation.

- Occasional atrophic tubules comprising one to a few (<5) affected tubular profiles per testis cross section, indicating a segmental germ cell depletion, is a common finding in rat testes. It is rarely seen as a drug-induced change, although the incidence of the finding can be increased as a developmental change in the F1 or F2 generation of animals that were exposed to a toxicant *in utero*. The finding is more common in mice and the affected tubules frequently show a patchy depletion.
- Multifocal or diffuse tubular degeneration/atrophy of varying severity is occasionally seen in the testes of normal rats and more commonly in the mouse. It may be unilateral or bilateral. Complete, unilateral atrophy is most likely secondary to efferent duct blockage (Figure 18.6b). It is unusual for more than one or two animals to show tubular degeneration/atrophy in an entire study, so if there is an apparent dose-related increased incidence, the finding should be considered potentially drug related. Similarly, an increased incidence of unilateral degeneration/atrophy may suggest a drug-related toxicity in the efferent ducts (discussed in more detail in Section 18.3.3.1.2.5).
- Diffuse tubular dilation of varying severity is occasionally seen as a unilateral or bilateral finding in testes of normal rats and mice (Figure 18.6a). It generally reflects partial obstruction of the efferent ducts and, if prolonged, or the blockage becomes worse, will progress to severe atrophy. It is rarely seen at incidences greater than one or two animals in a study. If the incidence is greater than this and particularly if there is an increased incidence of unilateral or bilateral severe tubular atrophy in some testes, drug-induced toxicity in the efferent ducts should be considered and studies should be undertaken to investigate this.
- Sperm granulomas in the epididymis are a relatively common finding in rats and mice and are due to extravasation of sperm from the duct into the surrounding interstitial tissue. They can occur anywhere in the epididymis but tend to be more frequent in the cauda. They can be induced by drugs and chemicals; hence, any dose-related increase in incidence should be noted.

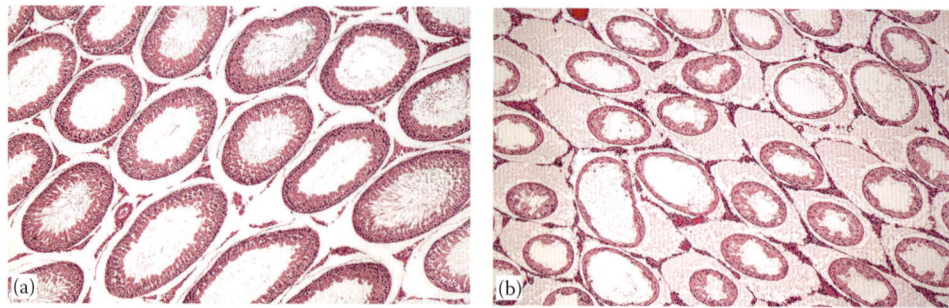

FIGURE 18.6   (a) Diffuse tubular dilation in the rat caused by granulomatous inflammation and obstruction of the efferent ducts. This can be unilateral or bilateral in distribution and can be a background finding or drug induced. Tubular dilation is caused by the backpressure of fluid in the tubular lumen and will generally progress to atrophy (b) where the atrophic tubules still have a dilated lumen but are lined only by Sertoli cells (owing to pressure atrophy). When efferent duct obstruction is drug induced, testes with tubular dilation and severe tubular atrophy are often seen at an increased incidence, often unilaterally.

- Epididymal sloughed (testicular) germ cells/luminal cell debris are present at a low level in mouse epididymides but are rare in rat epididymides, thereby providing a very sensitive indicator of spermatogenic disturbance. The head of the epididymis is often the most sensitive location to see sloughed cells. If they are consistently present and show a dose-related incidence and severity in the rat, they are almost certainly reflecting cell degeneration and loss from the testis, even though this may be difficult to see in the testis itself. The same is true in the mouse, except that there is a higher and more variable background level of sloughed cells in this species.
- Prostatic inflammatory cell infiltrate is commonly present in the rat and mouse. The severity is generally low. The infiltrate is generally interstitial and lymphocytic in the ventral prostate but intra-acinar/epithelial and neutrophilic in the dorsolateral prostate.

18.3.2.2   Background Pathology in the Dog

Compared with the rodent, spermatogenesis in the dog is relatively inefficient and less regular, with a high incidence of hypospermatogenesis (patchy depletion of germ cell layers reflecting reduced efficiency of spermatogenesis; Figure 18.7). In addition, some tubules are hypoplastic and contain no germ cells at all (tubular hypoplasia; Figure 18.7c). Both these lesions are commonly seen at a rate of 30% in normal beagle dogs 6 to 36 months old (Goedken et al. 2008; Rehm 2000). Degenerating (multinucleate or apoptotic) germ cells are present in almost all dog testes, albeit in low numbers. It is on this background of pathology with small group sizes of dogs that the pathologist must try to identify drug-induced changes. In the experience of these authors and Rehm (2000), these background changes are seen as frequently in dogs over 12 months of age as they are in dogs 10 months of age, but they are different from the changes associated with immaturity and peripuberty that are so often seen in dogs 7–10 months of age. It is important not to confuse hypospermatogenesis with immaturity because hypospermatogenesis can also be a drug-induced finding and needs to be consistently recorded in order to identify a treatment-related increase.

- Hypospermatogenesis: The characteristics of this change suggest that it is caused by an intermittent failure of spermatogonia to divide and produce progeny. It has all the characteristics of "maturation depletion." Typically in an affected tubule, one or more generations of germ cells (e.g., pachytene spermatocytes and round spermatids) will be almost completely missing but the luminal layer of elongating spermatids and the basal layer of

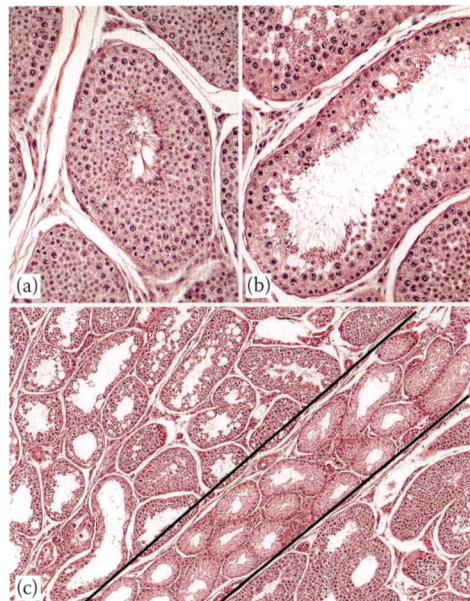

FIGURE 18.7 Background changes in dog testes. (a) Normal mid-stage (stage V) tubule at the point of spermiation with an adluminal layer of mature elongating spermatids, a layer of round spermatids, a layer of pachytene spermatocytes, and a basal layer of preleptotene spermatocytes. (b) The same stage tubule with partial depletion of the elongating spermatids, almost complete depletion of round spermatids, and partial depletion of pachytene spermatocytes but preleptotene spermatocytes are unaffected. Hypospermatogenesis in the dog testis is characterized by loss of one or more generations of germ cells, but with no significant increase in the numbers of degenerating (multinucleate) germ cells. (c) A central diagonal band of hypoplastic tubules separates normal tubules (lower right) from tubules with hypospermatogenesis (top left). The hypospermatogenesis is often accompanied by vacuolation as a background finding. The hypoplastic tubules are contracted, devoid of germ cells, and commonly located in a subcapsular, wedge-shaped area.

spermatogonia will be present (Figure 18.7b and c). Also, typically there is no increase in the numbers of degenerating germ cells, which supports the suggestion that this is caused by failure of spermatogonial division rather than active degeneration of cells. The intermittent nature of the spermatogonial failure results in different generations of germ cells being depleted in different tubules and since the change tends to be segmental, the hypospermatogenic tubules are scattered in a multifocal distribution. Almost all dog testes will have a few tubules that show this change but the severity can be quite marked in some dogs. In the experience of these authors, the change varies between different cohorts of dogs, is unrelated to age, and probably reflects a variable congenital inefficiency in spermatogenesis in this breed of dog. In more severely affected testes, the hypospermatogenesis may be accompanied by vacuolation and tubular atrophy.

It is important to record and grade this lesion consistently since it can also be induced or exacerbated by drugs that have an effect on spermatogonial proliferation. A dose-related increase in incidence or severity of hypospermatogenesis should be considered potentially drug induced.

Note that the term "hypospermatogenesis" has been applied to a similar change in rabbit testes (Morton et al. 1987) and has been used to describe rodent testes, apparently in reference to germ cell depletion or nonspecific degenerative changes; however, it is best reserved to indicate specifically the characteristic effect in dogs.

- Tubular hypoplasia is characterized by a group of tubules that are contracted with no or negligible lumen and have no germ cells in them (Figure 18.7c). The collection of tubules is typically wedge shaped with the base of the wedge in a subcapsular location, suggesting that the hypoplasia is affecting one or two tubules along their entire length. Most often, the area affected is small and single, frequently unilateral, but occasionally a large proportion of the testis can be affected.
- Multinucleate degenerating germ cells and occasionally apoptotic germ cells can be seen in most normal mature testes but they are generally infrequent. An increase in the numbers of such cells is often a very good indicator of toxicity because they represent an active degenerative process in the germ cells. A dose-related increase in the numbers of these degenerating cells should be considered likely to be drug related.
- Epididymal sloughed (testicular) germ cells/cell debris occur in most dogs and can be present in significant numbers, particularly in peripubertal dogs. Degenerative changes in the testis are usually accompanied by increased numbers of sloughed cells; thus, it is important to evaluate the background level in control animals and note when there is an increase.
- Decreased sperm content: Sperm content in the dog epididymis is quite variable, particularly in the cauda epididymis. Unlike the rat, sperm is not visible in the head or proximal corpus of the epididymis because it is too dilute. It only becomes visible part way down the corpus and gains significant density in the distal corpus (which is a good location to assess sperm content). Sperm in the cauda can be low or can sometimes fall out during processing. Care should be taken when assessing reductions in sperm.
- Sperm granuloma and sperm stasis: as with the rodent, sperm granulomas can be seen as a normal background finding. Sperm stasis, often associated with granulomatous inflammation, is also common in the efferent ducts, which in the dog are embedded in the initial segment of the epididymis. Sperm stasis at this site is due to a high incidence of blind-ending ductules in dogs (Foley et al. 1995; Hess 2002).
- Prostatic lymphohistiocytic inflammatory cell infiltrate and focal acinar atrophy as well as focal cystic acini are very common changes in the dog prostate (Dorso et al. 2008).

18.3.2.3 Background Pathology in the NHP

The majority of studies conducted in NHPs are in immature animals or a mixture of immature and mature animals. The problems associated with this variable maturity among NHPs are discussed in more detail below. Few background changes are seen in mature animals and spermatogenesis is more regular and easier to evaluate than in the dog. Occasional wedge-shaped groups of tubules (suggesting one or two affected tubules) may show dilation and patchy germ cell depletion and degeneration. This change often seems to occur in animals that have recently attained maturity. Focal or multifocal tubular vacuolation is also occasionally seen as a background finding. Sperm content in the epididymides of NHPs is more consistent than in dogs and there are relatively few sloughed germ cells in the lumen. Most current toxicity studies are conducted in the cynomolgus macaque, which is a nonseasonal breeding macaque, but it is important to recognize that the rhesus macaques are seasonal breeders, generally coming into seasonal activity around March. During the remainder of the year, the testes of rhesus macaques are likely to show varying degrees of regression (degeneration and atrophy), with oligo/aspermia in the epididymis; therefore, this macaque is not an appropriate model to use to evaluate male reproductive toxicity.

18.3.2.4 Immaturity in the Rat and Mouse

Rats mature at approximately 8–10 weeks of age but do not have a full complement of sperm in their cauda epididymis until at least 12 weeks of age. By 8 weeks of age, the testis generally has normal-appearing morphology, although there may be occasional tubules with reduced numbers of mature spermatids, a small amount of spermatid retention, and some degenerating elongating spermatids. The epididymis shows the most obvious changes at 8 weeks, having an increased number of sloughed degenerating germ cells (most noticeably in the cauda) and a relatively low content of sperm in the cauda epididymis. At 7 and 8 weeks of age, there may be variation in the caudal sperm content of individual rats; hence, it is important not to confuse this with drug-related changes; however, if there is an apparent dose relationship in the numbers of sloughed cells and reduced sperm in the epididymides of rats of this age, the change should be considered potentially drug related and the study should be repeated in older rats. A similar situation occurs in mice, but they mature earlier at around 6–8 weeks of age.

18.3.2.5 Immaturity in the Dog

Dogs present the biggest problem with respect to immaturity. Beagle dogs can mature anywhere between 7 and 12 months of age, although most are mature by 10 months of age (James and Heywood 1979; Kawakami et al. 1991). The age of maturation also varies depending on the supplier. Dorso et al. (2008) reported that 90% of dogs between 31 and 40 weeks of age supplied by Harlan France were sexually mature compared with only 10% of dogs of the same age that were supplied by Marshall Farms, USA. This difference was also reflected by a lower body weight of Marshall dogs compared with Harlan dogs of the same age. Testes will also show a massive weight range in a group of maturing dogs (e.g., 24–28 weeks of age), reflecting the varying status of spermatogenesis between individual animals.

The first cycle of spermatogenesis in the dog is relatively inefficient and not all tubules will mature at the same time. The result is that the peripubertal testis will have some tubules containing relatively few germ cells, others containing almost complete spermatogenesis, yet others with frequent degenerating cells, and there will be very few maturation-phase spermatids. The epididymis will have negligible or no sperm in the lumen but will likely contain significant numbers of sloughed testicular germ cells. This appearance is indistinguishable from testes undergoing germ cell loss and degeneration induced by a toxicant. The best way to avoid this uncertainty is to use dogs that are at least 10 months of age at necropsy. If younger dogs have been used and the pathologist is faced with the need to distinguish between immaturity and toxicant-induced changes, the best way is to examine the amount of sperm in the epididymis in conjunction with the relative diameter of the epididymal ducts. The distal corpus is often the most consistent region of the epididymis for evaluating sperm density and, along with the cauda, should be examined for the presence of sperm, for the presence of sloughed cell debris, and for expansion of the ducts. If sperm is present and the ducts appear expanded, then it should be assumed that the animal is mature and that any germ cell degeneration and depletion in the testis is either drug induced or due to background pathology. If the incidence or severity appears dose related, a drug-induced toxicity should be assumed. The secretory content of the prostate is not a reliable indicator of maturity since dogs with full testicular spermatogenesis and sperm in the epididymis can have immature-appearing prostates and vice versa.

18.3.2.6 Immaturity in the NHP

Most studies using NHPs are conducted using males that are totally immature or a mixture of immature, partially mature, and fully mature animals. Often, accurate birth dates are not available, resulting in variable maturation status in groups of animals purportedly of similar age. Male NHPs do not mature until they are at least 4.5 to 5 years of age and generally weigh >5 kg (Smedley et al. 2002). Although it is impractical to run all studies with mature animals, it should be an important consideration if testicular toxicity is suspected from other studies or if the class of drug has been associated with effects on spermatogenesis. During prepubertal development, it is quite common to see a small collection of tubules with advanced or even complete spermatogenesis while the remainder of tubules has not yet started spermatogenesis (Figure 18.8). This circumstance is normal in an immature NHP.

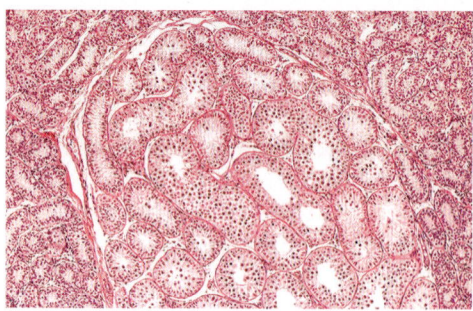

FIGURE 18.8 Prepubertal cynomolgus monkeys often show focal groups of tubules that have undergone maturation while the remaining tubules are totally immature.

18.3.3 TESTICULAR HISTOPATHOLOGY

18.3.3.1 Seminiferous Tubular Changes

18.3.3.1.1 Stage-Specific Changes

Often, early compound-related effects on the seminiferous epithelium can manifest as changes limited to a particular stage of the spermatogenic cycle. These changes frequently provide clues to the mechanism of action of the compound on the testis and are therefore important to recognize. Such stage-specific effects can be discerned in studies of 4 weeks' duration or less but will likely be obscured in studies of longer duration. In reporting such findings, it is important to note the stage(s) and germ cells affected.

18.3.3.1.1.1 Germ Cell Degeneration (Apoptosis)   Most germ cell death occurs through apoptosis, even though the morphological characteristics are not typical of apoptotic cells in general (Brinkworth et al. 1995; Lee et al. 1997). Germ cell degeneration is the term used to indicate morphological changes consistent with apoptosis in the absence of confirmatory special techniques (such as terminal deoxynucleotide dUTP nick end labeling or cleaved caspase-3 immunohistochemistry). Testicular germ cells are predisposed to programmed cell death as a result of a variety of influences (Blanco-Rodriguez and Martinez-Garcia 1998), including androgen deficiency (Troiano et al. 1994), growth factor inhibition (Brinkworth et al. 1995; Nurmio et al. 2007), antimitotic agents (Shinoda et al. 1999), cytotoxic agents, and proapoptotic mediators (Yan et al. 2000). The innate tendency for apoptotic demise of germ cells is a physiologic means of curtailing excessive progeny cell production and ensuring elimination of defective germ cells. Because of the nature of the apoptotic process (involving membrane-bound condensation of cytoplasmic and nuclear material and rapid resorption by Sertoli cells), the microscopically perceptible effects are subtle. When degenerating germ cells have a distribution pattern restricted to a particular stage and germ cell type, a test article effect is possible, and if substantiated, the mechanism of the injury can sometimes be inferred. A careful stage-aware examination of seminiferous tubules is therefore an important part of the toxicologic pathologist's assessment of testes from shorter-term studies (Creasy 1997). The germ cell type and the stage affected should be specified whenever relevant.

The morphological changes of cytoplasmic hypereosinophilia (Figure 18.9) and condensation, often conferring a homogeneous or hyalinized appearance to the affected individual cell, can be seen among spermatogonia, spermatocytes (Figure 18.10), and round spermatids undergoing degeneration; elongating spermatids may have misshapen nuclei (Figure 18.11). Cellular shrinkage results in a smooth, round profile often surrounded by a narrow clear space. The specific identity of a given degenerate germ cell may not be obvious owing to the rapid size decrease, loss of nuclear detail, and Sertoli cell phagocytosis resulting in a basalar shift in position within the seminiferous tubular

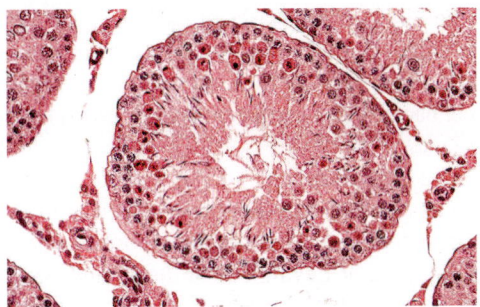

FIGURE 18.9 Numerous spermatocytes undergoing meiotic division in this stage XIV rat tubule have hypereosinophilic cytoplasm indicating degeneration. The underlying zygotene spermatocytes and overlying elongating spermatids are normal.

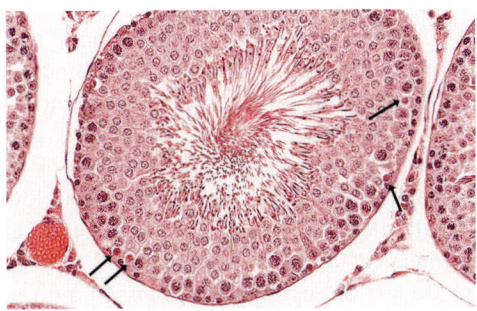

FIGURE 18.10 A rat stage VII tubule has degeneration of pachytene spermatocytes (arrows) attributable to decreased intratesticular testosterone levels. Note the atrophic Leydig cells with scant cytoplasm (compare with Figure 18.11).

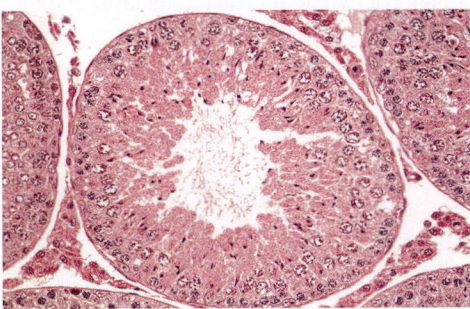

FIGURE 18.11 A late-stage (XIII) tubule in a rat testis has degeneration of elongating spermatids characterized by misshapen, fragmented, and condensed chromatin of spermatid heads.

strata. Care should be taken not to confuse residual bodies with degenerate germ cells; any germ cell degeneration diagnosed in rat stage IX or X should be judiciously considered.

Background attrition of germ cells is inconspicuous but common, particularly among peripubertal rodents and may be confused with compound-induced degeneration. Spermatogonia of rat stages XII to XIV are subject to removal by apoptosis as are spermatocytes undergoing meiotic division in rat stage XIV (Kerr 1992). Although similar, more pronounced stage- and cell-specific changes may be seen with test article administration, notably glycol ether administration affecting spermatocytes in diakinesis and in specific phases of pachytene development (Creasy et al. 1985), careful comparison against control testes is warranted to substantiate a compound-related effect. Normal adult NHPs reportedly have highly efficient conversion of early germ cells to spermatids (Zhengwei et al. 1997); hence, background germ cell degeneration is less likely to be a confounding factor in this species.

Perhaps the best example of germ cell degeneration is that occurring as a result of androgen deficiency. Degeneration of pachytene spermatocytes or round spermatids in rat stage VII/VIII tubules (Figure 18.10) is characteristic of decreased testosterone exposure, whether due to effects at the level of the hypothalamus, pituitary gland, or Leydig cell or due to androgen receptor blockade (Kerr et al. 1993; Russell et al. 1981; Sharpe 1994). Degeneration of occasional stage VII/VIII pachytene spermatocytes has also been noted among young, food-restricted rats as a result of low testosterone (Rehm et al. 2008).

Proliferating spermatogonia, as the only mitotically active class of germ cells and unprotected by the BTB, are particularly subject to apoptosis associated with administration of cytotoxic agents (Meistrich 1986).

18.3.3.1.1.2 Germ Cell Depletion   Substantial degeneration of a given germ cell type within a stage results in partial or complete loss of a cell layer. Sometimes, absent cells are made more obvious by a residual clear space indicating the Sertoli cell–lined niche previously occupied by the lost cell. Recognition of short-term germ cell depletion requires a familiarity of which cell layers should be present within a given tubular profile. Complete loss of the pachytene spermatocyte layer from a given stage can result in a tubular profile and an overall low magnification appearance that are not strikingly abnormal unless one has an awareness of the expected epithelial complement (Figure 18.12). With continued dosing, test article–related germ cell depletion becomes more obvious, as successive layers are lost through continued loss of a given germ cell type and failed development of the lost cells (maturation depletion). The term "maturation arrest" is misleading and not recommended to describe this loss of successive germ cell generations (Creasy and Foster 2002). Spermatogenesis is a sustained, continuous process; cells may die, but the process is not arrested unless stem cell spermatogonia are obliterated or Sertoli cell function is completely destroyed.

Whereas loss of the prominent pachytene spermatocyte layer and the adluminal spermatid layers can be fairly easily discerned, spermatogonial dropout can be more difficult to appreciate. The tubular stage immediately preceding spermiation (i.e., stage VII in rat) has a well-defined basal layer

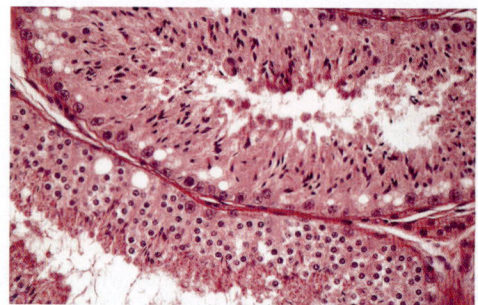

FIGURE 18.12   This is the appearance of dog testes after 4 weeks of dosing with a spermatogonial toxicant. The early-stage tubule (lower tubule) still has its round and elongating spermatids but is missing its pachytene and preleptotene spermatocytes. The late-stage tubule (upper tubule) contains elongating spermatids but is missing its zygotene and pachytene spermatocytes. This is termed "maturation depletion."

of germ cells comprising spermatogonia and preleptotene spermatocytes (Figures 18.4 and 18.11). Stage VII tubular profiles should be examined for completeness of the basal germ cell layer to exclude spermatogonial loss. Suspected depletion of a given germ cell type should prompt a search for evidence of precursor germ cell degeneration in preceding stages. Evidence of germ cell depletion accompanied by germ cell degeneration could best be described by the compound term germ cell degeneration/depletion. Four to six weeks of administration of a compound causing spermatogonial degeneration could result in tubules lined only by elongating spermatids and Sertoli cells. Chronic administration of agents affecting stem spermatogonia can result in Sertoli-only tubules (tubular atrophy).

Depending on the degree of involvement and chronicity, germ cell depletion may be associated with subtle to profound effects on testicular weights and sperm counts.

18.3.3.1.1.3   Spermatid Retention   Spermiation, the release of mature spermatids (rat: step 19; mouse: step 16; NHP: step 14; dog: step 12) into the tubular lumen, normally occurs at rat stage VIII. When mature spermatids remain attached at the tubular luminal surface (Figure 18.13) beyond stage IX, they are referred to as retained and represent failed spermiation. Such retained spermatids are subsequently phagocytosed by Sertoli cells and drawn toward the tubular basement membrane within the basal Sertoli cell cytoplasm, where the spermatid nuclei may appear with random orientation (Figure 18.13). Such irregularly arrayed basal spermatids are abnormal, regardless of stage and also considered retained. The rat stage IX–XI tubules are the rarest in histologic section, since they are of shortest duration, but it is important to identify and examine them for evidence of spermatid retention. Peripubertal animals may have sluggish spermiation (Lee et al. 1993) and occasional tubules in normal adult animals will have a few retained spermatids, so careful comparative examination of control animals is important to confirm a compound-related effect.

Retained spermatids may indicate Sertoli cell dysfunction or defective elongating spermatids. Spermatid retention is also a manifestation of androgen deficiency (Saito et al. 2000). Although the change is subtle, it is often associated with abnormal sperm parameters and decreased fertility. It is a change that is largely restricted to the rodent.

Among large animals (i.e., dog and NHP), the nuclear shape of more mature elongating spermatids is flattened (spatulate) compared to rodents' more needle-like configuration. Such spermatid nuclei in various planes relative to the section could mimic the appearance of more than one elongating spermatid population and thus spuriously resemble spermatid retention. In the dog, basal accumulations of phagocytized spermatids are frequently seen in tubules close to the centrally located rete as a background finding.

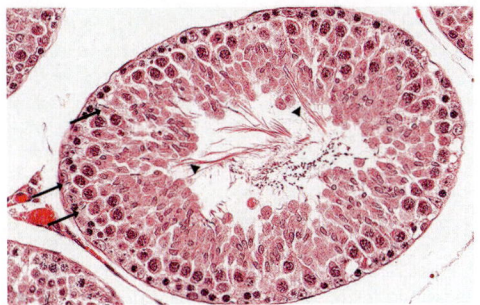

FIGURE 18.13   Retained spermatids are present basally (arrows) and attached to the luminal surface (arrowheads) of this stage X rat tubular cross section, caused by low testosterone levels (note Leydig cell atrophy).

18.3.3.1.2   Nonspecific Changes

Many factors can result in tubular changes that are not attributable to injury of a specific germ cell type and stage. Most causes of stage-specific effects can, with sufficient time, result in seminiferous tubules lacking clues to the initiating insult. Additionally, factors such as hypoxia, vascular injury, inflammation, and Sertoli cell toxicity may affect a broader spectrum of germ cells within multiple stages and manifest as a variety of morphological changes. Background pathology and changes after more than 4 weeks of treatment with a testicular toxicant frequently present as findings lacking stage specificity.

18.3.3.1.2.1   Tubular Degeneration/Atrophy   Germ cell degeneration, germ cell loss, and spermatid retention as well as vacuolation of Sertoli cell cytoplasm, formation of multinucleated germ cell syncytia, disorder within the germ cell layers, and exfoliation of germ cells into the tubular lumen can be seen individually or in any combination. Such variable patterns of change within one specimen can best be described generically as tubular degeneration (Figure 18.14). These changes are usually accompanied by the presence of cellular debris within the epididymal lumen and may be corroborated by decreased testis weights. When one morphological change predominates (generally in a shorter-term study), the corresponding more specific descriptive term could be used alone.

Degenerative tubular effects, with time, frequently result in tubules depleted of multiple germ cell types or lined only or predominantly by Sertoli cells, termed tubular atrophy (Figure 18.15a).

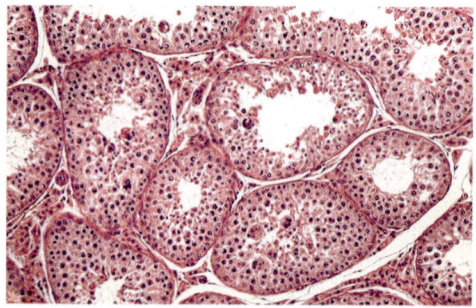

FIGURE 18.14   Although normal dog testes have occasional degenerating/multinucleate germ cells as a background finding, increased numbers of apoptotic and multinucleated degenerating germ cells are a good indication of a drug-induced degenerative change. If the numbers of degenerating cells are increased in a dose-related manner, the finding should be considered test article related.

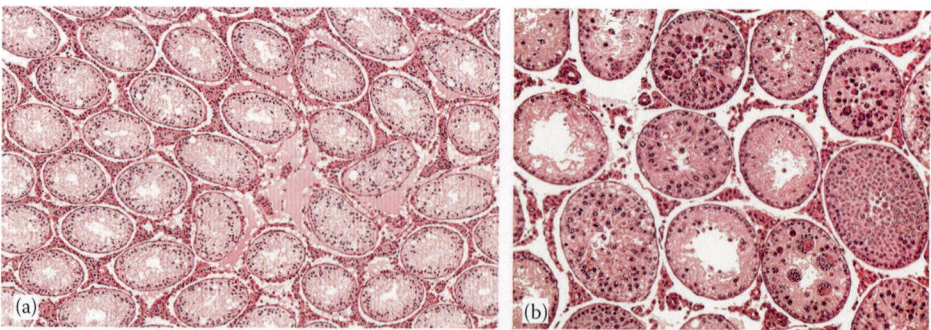

FIGURE 18.15   (a) Typical end-stage lesion caused by repeat dosing with a testicular toxicant in the rat. Tubules are contracted and lined by Sertoli cells with few remaining germ cells. Tubular atrophy is the recommended terminology. Note the relative increase in Leydig cells. (b) A mixture of tubules with germ cell degeneration, partial germ cell depletion, and total germ cell depletion are best described under the term "tubular degeneration/atrophy."

Isolated atrophic tubules are commonly encountered amid normal tubular profiles among control animals as well as animals administered test compound; to distinguish from more generalized compound-related effects, these spontaneous changes can be described as "focal" or "segmental" tubular atrophy. Atrophic tubules can also be found interspersed with tubules manifesting degenerative changes, demonstrating a continuum of effects, which can be described as "tubular degeneration/ atrophy" (Figure 18.15b).

Autolysis or artifacts of handling or poor fixation may be confused with tubular degeneration. Excessive pressure on unfixed tissue results in locally extensive cellular disorder and nuclear distortions without accompanying germ cell cytoplasmic tinctoral changes, multinucleated cells, or vacuolation; occasionally, artifactual telescoping of seminiferous epithelium within a tubule may be seen (Foley 2001). Poor fixation can cause subcapsular sloughing of germ cells into the tubular lumen, but other evidence of tubular degeneration would be absent. Autolysis manifests as loss of cellular and nuclear detail and individualization of Sertoli cells and germ cells with margination of nuclear chromatin (Bryant and Boekelheide 2007). In none of these confounding circumstances would germ cells be evident in the rete or epididymis.

18.3.3.1.2.2 Tubular Vacuolation   Compound-mediated effects on Sertoli cells can result in variably sized, small, clear cytoplasmic vacuoles, generally near the basement membrane (Figure 18.16). Larger clear spaces at variable levels within the seminiferous epithelium may occur owing to germ cell degenerative loss or failed adherence between germ cell and Sertoli cell. In small numbers, the latter form of vacuolation can be consistent with spontaneous physiologic germ cell attrition, justifying careful comparative review of the prevalence among control animals. Intracytoplasmic vacuoles may be due to impaired Sertoli cell fluid homeostasis or excessive lysosomal storage associated with phospholipidosis. Other common targets of phospholipidosis within the male reproductive system are testicular interstitial macrophages and epididymal epithelial cells. Vacuolation is frequently noted concurrently with other degenerative tubular changes, in which case tubular degeneration would be the preferred term.

18.3.3.1.2.3 Multinucleated Germ Cells   Through incomplete cytokinesis during mitosis, descendents of early spermatogonia form cohorts of synchronously developing germ cells joined by narrow cytoplasmic bridges, which are maintained by Sertoli cells. Injury to Sertoli cells can result in widening of the bridges and the formation of multinucleated giant cells (Figures 18.14 and 18.15b). Such syncytial cells or symplasts contain nuclei (up to 100 in rodents) of spermatocytes or round spermatids. The presence of large numbers of multinucleated germ cells in the absence of other degenerative changes is suggestive of primary Sertoli cell injury. More commonly, the syncytia are part of the tableau of changes associated with nonspecific tubular degeneration. Small numbers of giant cells

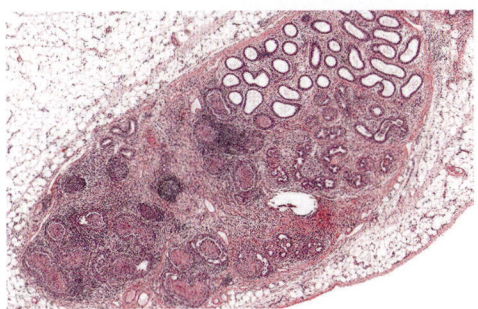

FIGURE 18.16   Granulomatous inflammation and obstruction of the efferent ducts causing obstruction to the outflow of fluid from the testis and resulting in tubular dilation or tubular atrophy in the connected testis. This can be a background or drug-induced finding.

can be present spontaneously, particularly among less mature animals. Multinucleated germ cells undergo degeneration and are phagocytosed by Sertoli cells or sloughed into the tubular lumen.

18.3.3.1.2.4 Necrosis Although apoptotic cell death is usual for germ cells, conditions (e.g., ischemia) resulting in decreased cellular energy can manifest morphologically as necrosis. The term "tubular necrosis" is applicable where there is extensive loss of cellular detail, encompassing all germ cell types and Sertoli cells, with maintenance of overall tubular architecture, consistent with coagulative necrosis. Vasoactive compounds such as serotonin or histamine can cause focal tubular necrosis (Creasy 2001). With loss of Sertoli cell integrity and consequent dissolution of the BTB, there is often accompanying inflammation as a result of exposed "immune-privileged" antigens. With profound ischemic effects (e.g., testicular torsion), interstitial elements including vasculature and Leydig cells are affected in addition to the tubules and the term testicular necrosis would apply.

18.3.3.1.2.5 Tubular Dilation Changes in tubular seminiferous fluid dynamics can result in increased luminal size or tubular dilation (Figure 18.6a). Decreased resorption of fluid or obstruction within the excurrent duct system (rete testis, efferent ductules, and epididymis) results in increased intratubular pressure, causing compression of the seminiferous epithelium. Despite the frequently narrowed tubular lining, all germ cell types are generally represented; however, severe instances of tubular dilation lead to germ cell loss and ultimately tubular atrophy (Figure 18.6b). The rete testis is often also distended, as can be the efferent ductules and epididymis, depending on the site of the underlying cause. Observation of rete testis dilation may be confounded by loss of seminiferous fluid with removal of the epididymis at necropsy (Foley 2001). Compounds decreasing the resorptive functions of the efferent ductules and epididymis can result in tubular dilation as can those decreasing peritubular myoid cell contractility (Yuan et al. 1994); however, dilation is frequently the spontaneous sequela of obstruction due to sperm stasis or sperm granuloma (La et al. 2011). Suprapharmacologic doses of a serotonin agonist to rats caused tubular dilation attributed to vasoconstriction within the mediastinum testis, resulting in decreased resorptive function in the rete and efferent ductules (Piner et al. 2002).

18.3.3.1.2.6 Sperm Stasis/Granuloma Impaired intratubular fluid secretion by Sertoli cells, excessive fluid uptake by efferent ductules, or decreased tubular motility owing to peritubular myoid cell dysfunction (Yuan et al. 1994) may predispose to impaction of mature spermatids. Sperm stasis frequently occurs within the seminiferous tubules near the rete testis, within the rete itself, or within the excurrent duct system. In rodents (notably mice), accumulations of sperm greater than two tubular diameters, termed spermatoceles, are not uncommon. Intratubular sperm aggregates result in atrophy of the seminiferous epithelium, occasionally breaching the basement membrane and inciting an inflammatory response to the exposed spermatids. Interstitial macrophages infiltrate and proliferate, resulting in a sperm granuloma. Mineralization and fibrosis are frequent sequelae.

An increased incidence of sperm stasis and granulomas among animals administered compound compared to control animals should prompt a review of the fluid dynamics within the testes and epididymides to corroborate or rule out a compound-related effect.

18.3.3.1.2.7 Germ Cell Exfoliation Individualized, nondegenerate germ cells may appear in the seminiferous tubular lumen, rete testis, and epididymis as a result of loss of adherence between germ cells and their supporting Sertoli cells. This finding has been associated with a toxic effect on Sertoli cells, for example, colchicines, vinblastine, or carbendazim, causing microtubule disruption (Creasy and Foster 2002).

18.3.3.2 Leydig Cell Changes
18.3.3.2.1 Atrophy
Decreased size of Leydig cells occurs with decreased LH stimulation (Keeney et al. 1988). Affected Leydig cells have lesser amounts of smooth endoplasmic reticulum and impaired steroidogenesis;

however, numbers of Leydig cells are not depleted. Decreased gonadotropin release can result from GnRH antagonists, as well as from androgen, estrogen, and progesterone receptor agonists (O'Connor et al. 2002). Rats administered an aromatase inhibitor (formestane) sustained Leydig cell atrophy, which is the opposite of what occurred in dogs, which show Leydig cell hypertrophy/hyperplasia owing to the important role of estrogen in gonadotropin control (Juniewicz et al. 1988; Junker-Walker and Nogues 1994). Antagonism of Leydig cell LH receptors could also plausibly result in Leydig cell atrophy.

The alkylating agent ethane dimethyl sulfonate causes necrosis and loss of adult Leydig cells after a single administration in rats (Bartlett et al. 1986; Molenaar et al. 1986), with subsequent increases in LH and FSH and regeneration of Leydig cells from mesenchymal precursor cells. Administration of corticosterone to rats causes apoptosis of Leydig cells (Gao et al. 2002).

Leydig cell atrophy manifests as small cells associated with interstitial vasculature and having decreased cytoplasm and increased space between individual cells (Figures 18.10 and 18.13). Because of decreased androgen levels associated with Leydig cell atrophy, decreased sizes and weights of androgen-dependent tissues (excurrent ducts and accessory sex glands) are common concomitant observations, as are the seminiferous tubular changes (stage VII/VIII spermatocyte/round spermatid degeneration, spermatid retention) seen with testosterone deficiency.

18.3.3.2.2 Hypertrophy
Adult Leydig cells rarely divide but can be renewed from mesenchymal precursor cells. In initial response to LH, adult Leydig cells hypertrophy with increased smooth endoplasmic reticulum and enhanced steroidogenic capability. Diffuse hypertrophy of Leydig cells due to gonadotropic stimulation can resemble an increase in numbers of Leydig cells and is frequently diagnosed as hyperplasia or hypertrophy/hyperplasia. Actual Leydig cell hyperplasia can only be confirmed using unbiased quantitative analysis, requiring prospective tissue sampling. Men with seminiferous tubular atrophy associated with nonobstructive azoospermia have been shown to have Leydig cell hypertrophy but not hyperplasia (Tash et al. 2002). Tubular atrophy within the testis results in an increased proportion of Leydig cells within testicular tissue, with interstitial aggregates bridging circumferentially around tubular profiles (Figure 18.15a) rather than restricted to smaller triangular areas among adjacent tubules (Figure 18.4). In the absence of confirmatory quantitative analyses (requiring stereologic methods), such histologic presentations are most accurately referred to as hypertrophy rather than hyperplasia (Mendis-Handagama 1992). Focal Leydig cell hypertrophy can accompany focal tubular atrophy; a paracrine influence on Leydig cell sensitivity to LH has been proposed as a mechanism for this effect (Aoki and Fawcett 1978). Hypertrophied nonhyperplastic Leydig cells can occur in young animals and have increased eosinophilic cytoplasm but, in rats, lack lipid droplets associated with hyperplastic cells.

18.3.3.3 Vascular Changes
18.3.3.3.1 Polyarteritis and "Beagle Pain" Syndrome
The testis and epididymis are sites of predilection for the spontaneous inflammatory vasculitides of rat and dog, polyarteritis nodosa and juvenile polyarteritis syndrome (Snyder et al. 1995; Son 2004), respectively. Polyarteritis (periarteritis) nodosa affects aging rats, involving the pancreatic, spermatic, and mesenteric arteries most commonly with inflammation and degeneration of media and adventitia, fibrinoid necrosis of the media and intima, and disruption of the elastic lamina and possible thrombosis of small- to medium-sized arteries (Berg 1967).

Cadmium causes endothelial necrosis within the testis and epididymis (Gunn et al. 1963); however, the changes associated with the resulting testicular necrosis overshadow the vascular changes.

18.3.3.4 Proliferative Changes
18.3.3.4.1 Leydig Cell Hyperplasia and Adenoma
Proliferative changes of Leydig cells are common among older rats, in contrast to mice and men. Leydig cell tumors occur with near 100% incidence among aging F344 rats and 1% to 5% incidence

among Sprague–Dawley rats. Among men, testicular tumors are uncommon and Leydig cell tumors are extremely rare with an estimated incidence of less than 3 per million. Rats can have increased incidence of Leydig cell tumors with chronic exposures to compounds causing inhibition of testosterone synthesis (e.g., vinclozolin), inhibition of conversion of testosterone to DHT (e.g., finasteride), androgen receptor antagonism (e.g., flutamide), or dopaminergic agonism (e.g., mesulergine) (Clegg et al. 1997). Certain biological distinctions of rats contribute to the increased incidence of Leydig cell proliferation including the absence of sex hormone–binding globulin in circulation to modulate free testosterone levels and increased sensitivity of Leydig cells to hormonal stimulation due to increased numbers of LH receptors and the presence of luteinizing hormone releasing hormone (LHRH) receptors (Cook et al. 1999). Because of these characteristics unique to rats, increased incidences of Leydig cell tumors in rats chronically exposed to nongenotoxic compounds are generally not considered relevant to man (Alison et al. 1994).

Leydig cell hyperplasia is an increase in numbers of Leydig cells in one or more foci or (less commonly) throughout the entire testis and is distinguished from Leydig cell adenoma by standardized but arbitrary size criteria. Hyperplastic Leydig cells are usually also hypertrophied compared to normal Leydig cells, having larger nuclei and expanded cytoplasm containing lipid droplets (Ettlin et al. 1992). Vacuolated hyperplastic Leydig cells should be distinguished from vacuolated interstitial macrophages, which may be a manifestation of phospholipidosis and can be present among younger animals. The accumulations of hyperplastic Leydig cells do not compress adjacent tubules and occupy an area less than three tubular cross sections, according to the Society of Toxicologic Pathologists (STP) criteria for distinction from Leydig cell adenomas. The apparent size of the examined cellular proliferation necessarily depends on the plane of section in each case, potentially further blurring the distinction between hyperplasia and adenoma.

Leydig cell adenomas range from small nodular foci to large masses replacing the gonad. The cells are generally monomorphic, having abundant eosinophilic vacuolated cytoplasm, a central round (in contrast to more ovoid in normal and hyperplastic Leydig cells) nucleus with a single nucleolus. Cells are polygonal or occasionally spindloid in shape forming nests or cords aligned on vasculature, which may form distended blood-filled spaces. Adenomas may contain collagenous stroma and may have areas of hemorrhage, necrosis, or mineralization. Leydig cell tumors containing glandular or tubular structures have been reported in rats (Kanno et al. 1987; Qureshi et al. 1991). Compression of adjacent tissue can cause seminiferous tubular atrophy.

Compared to rats, mice normally have larger and more numerous Leydig cells. What is frequently termed diffuse Leydig cell hyperplasia in mice may more accurately be described as Leydig cell hypertrophy. Leydig cell tumors in mice are uncommon but occur particularly in association with increased estrogen levels (Huseby 1980). Transgenic mice expressing excess aromatase have circulating estrogen levels twice that of wild type mice and frequently develop Leydig cell tumors (Fowler et al. 2000). A spontaneous Leydig cell tumor in a mouse occurred in association with a Sertoli cell tumor presumed to express estrogen (Franks 1968). Whereas the compounds known to induce Leydig cell tumors in rats do not have the same effect in mice, estrogen agonists (e.g., diethylstilbestrol, estradiol, ethinylestradiol) do cause an increased incidence of murine Leydig cell tumors (Cook et al. 1999). Leydig cell tumors also have been reported to occur spontaneously in epididymides from aged mice in the absence of analogous testicular tumors (Mitsumori et al. 1989); however, differentiation of Leydig cell tumors from tumors of adrenal rests can be problematic (Mostofi and Bresler 1976). Malignant Leydig cell tumors are rare in rodents and have features of anaplasia and abnormal mitotic figures in addition to evidence of invasion or metastasis. Malignant Leydig cell tumors are described for mice exposed prenatally to diethylstilbestrol (Newbold et al. 1987) but may also occur spontaneously (Ohnuma et al. 2010).

Leydig cell tumors are not uncommon among older dogs; they are, however, rare in the context of chronic studies using purpose-bred beagles. Aromatase inhibitors administered to dogs have resulted in Leydig cell hypertrophy and hyperplasia (Junker-Walker and Nogues 1994).

18.3.3.4.2   Rete Testis Hyperplasia, Adenoma, and Carcinoma

Proliferative changes of the rete testis are generally spontaneous and occur more commonly among mice than rats. Exposure to diethylstilbestrol *in utero* has been shown to produce neoplastic lesions of the murine rete testis (Newbold et al. 1985) and cadmium chloride has been associated with rete adenocarcinoma in rats (Rehm and Waalkes 1988). Spontaneous tumors in mice are also described (Yoshitomi and Morii 1984). Hyperplasia of the rete testis manifests as focal or multifocal increased epithelial cellularity with papillary intraluminal projections supported by scant stroma. Adenomas are distinguished by the compression of adjacent tissue and more extensive stroma. Carcinomas display cellular pleomorphism, more numerous mitotic figures and hemorrhage, necrosis, and dense collagenous stroma, and invasion may be evident.

18.3.3.4.3   Mesothelioma

The testicular tunica vaginalis, the mesothelial covering of the tunica albuginea, is a common site for mesothelioma to occur and may be a primary site of tumor development in rats but not in mice. Fibrous and epithelial cellular components are represented in the tumor architecture, forming solid sheets, tubuloalveolar structures, or papillary processes (Tanigawa et al. 1987). Papillary structures arising from the tunica vaginalis propria of the testis, epididymides, and spermatic cord with or without involvement of the peritoneal cavity were reported in one cohort of F344 rats (Gould 1977).

18.3.3.4.4   Other Testicular Tumors

Other proliferative changes of the testis, unrelated to compound administration, occur with a rarity precluding extensive discussion in this setting (Maekawa and Hayashi 1992). Seminomas (Kerlin et al. 1998; Kim et al. 1985; Nyska et al. 1993), Sertoli cell tumors (Boorman et al. 1987; Rehm and Waalkes 1988; Wakui et al. 2008), and teratomas (Jamadagni et al. 2011; Sawaki et al. 2000; Tani et al. 1997) have been described.

18.3.4   Nonmorphological Endpoints for Assessing Toxicity

18.3.4.1   Organ Weights

Organ weights are an important adjunct to morphology for assessing drug-related toxicity. In particular, the weights of the accessory sex organs (prostate and seminal vesicles) are a very important indicator of overall androgen status and are a more sensitive indicator than histopathologic evaluation in rodents (Creasy 2008a). When weighing the prostate and seminal vesicles, it is important to include all the secretions since these comprise much of the weight and are a measure of the functional activity of the gland. In the case of the testes, it is important to use absolute weight or weight relative to brain weight and not use body weight relative values, because like the brain, testis growth and size are maintained despite body weight loss. In most cases of body weight loss, testis weight (relative to body weight) will increase compared with controls. If there is a significant decrease in absolute testis weight, the most likely microscopic correlate will be decreased numbers of germ cells and contraction (due to reduced seminiferous tubule fluid) of the seminiferous tubules. In most cases, histomorphologic examination will be more sensitive than organ weight loss, but fluid content (seminiferous tubule fluid or interstitial fluid) can decrease with little morphological evidence. In general, the pattern of organ weight change seen in the epididymis will reflect that in the testis, since up to 50% of the epididymal weight is made up of sperm and fluid.

Testicular weight can also increase as a drug-related response and is invariably caused by an increase in fluid content, generally due to increased seminiferous tubule fluid and accompanied by tubular dilation. Increased weight of the accessory sex organs can occur in response to administration of exogenous androgens or can be seen with hyperprolactinemia. Expulsion of secretion can also be inhibited by α adrenergic receptor antagonists and result in increased weight and acinar/vesicle dilation owing to secretory accumulation. Changes in testis weight and prostate weight are less sensitive in dogs and NHPs owing to interanimal variation. In particular, prostate weight can vary quite markedly between individual dogs of similar age (Dorso et al. 2008). For additional discussion of the importance of accessory sex organ weights, see Section 18.5.2.1.

18.3.4.2 Sperm Parameters

Sperm parameters are generally not measured in routine safety evaluation studies on drugs. Instead, they are generally conducted in fertility studies where histopathology is usually not performed. Adding sperm measurements to a study designed to investigate reproductive toxicity can be very useful and provide unique information, not available from histopathology alone. Measuring caudal sperm count provides an integrated measure of testicular sperm output and transit time through the epididymis. A more direct measure of sperm output from the testis can be achieved by measuring testicular spermatid head count (homogenization resistant spermatid count). This measures a specific subpopulation of the mature elongating spermatids (steps 16–19) in the testis, which can be expressed as a function of the time taken for their development (daily sperm production). The value will go down when spermatogenesis is decreased but can go up in situations of spermatid retention. Testicular spermatid head count is an easily performed quantitative measurement of testicular spermatogenesis and is greatly preferred over manual counting of cells by the pathologist via the microscope. Its biggest disadvantage is that it requires one testis for the assay, which is then unavailable for histopathologic evaluation. Sperm motility and sperm morphology are the other two main parameters measured. Sperm motility is a measure of function while morphology is a measure of sperm quality. Sperm motility can be altered by direct toxicity to the epididymis, resulting in disturbed maturation of the sperm, but can also be caused by disturbances in testicular spermatogenesis. Sperm morphology is a sensitive endpoint in rodents because of the normally very low incidence of abnormal sperm (generally <2%–3%). Increases in abnormal sperm generally reflect disturbances in testicular spermatogenesis. Depending on the nature of the toxicity, sperm measurements can often provide a more sensitive and quantitative endpoint for establishing a NOEL (no-observed-effect level) for a drug-induced change. For example, if the main change caused by a drug was degeneration or malformation of elongating spermatids, recognized by misshapen condensed spermatid heads in the testis, it is likely that the change would be much easier to detect and quantify using sperm motility and morphology, rather than trying to evaluate these cells in a testicular section.

Sperm collection is a terminal procedure in rodents owing to the production of the copulatory plug, which prevents collection of usable, ejaculated sperm. In dogs and NHPs, sperm can be collected and monitored before, during, and at the end of dosing as well as during a recovery period. This availability can be very useful for monitoring functional effects of toxicity and rate of recovery. It can also be useful for confirming sexual maturity in dogs and NHPs. Collection of good samples can be a challenge in large animals, and variability between animals and between different ejaculates from the same animal can also cause problems for evaluation.

18.3.4.3 Clinical Pathology: Hormone Measurements and Biomarkers

Although measuring hormone levels appears an easy and attractive option for investigating possible endocrine-mediated mechanisms of toxicity or demonstrating hormone changes as a potential biomarker of toxicity for the clinic, the procedure requires careful study design. The main hormones of interest (FSH, LH, and testosterone) are pulsatile in their secretion. In rodents, the pulsatility is very irregular, demonstrated by the fact that a testosterone pulse only occurs after a series of closely spaced pulses of LH, which occur irregularly (Ellis and Desjardins 1982). There is large variability in the hormone profile of one rat on different occasions and between individual rats on the same occasion. On the basis of the coefficients of variation in the various hormones in rats, it is calculated that group sizes of 20–30 rats are necessary to provide a reasonable chance (80% chance of seeing a 25% change) in testosterone, whereas FSH and LH are somewhat less variable and a similar power can be gained from using group sizes of 10–20, and for prolactin, 15–20 rats per group (Chapin et al. 2011). If smaller group sizes of 5–10 rats per group are used, the results can provide very misleading conclusions.

In dogs, the hormones are still pulsatile but the pulses are more regular, with LH pulsing once every 1–1.5 h and testosterone pulsing approximately 50 min afterward. On the basis of the coefficients of variation of the various hormones in dogs, similar numbers would be needed (20 per group) to stand any chance of detecting changes using a single sample time point. This group size is obviously impractical; a much more sensible way of approaching the problem is to pool multiple samples over a 2 h period (Chapin et al. 2011).

In the case of NHPs, their LH and testosterone secretion patterns are similar to dogs but they have a marked circadian rhythm where the highest hormone levels are at night and this needs to be taken into consideration. The problem of hierarchy and dominance also needs to be considered because the dominant male will suppress testosterone levels and spermatogenesis in the lower-ranking males. This can be dramatic and result in marked decreases in testosterone levels and decreases in testicular volume of up to 45% in subordinate males when NHPs are group housed (Czoty et al. 2009; Niehoff et al. 2010).

Inhibin B has received much attention as a possible biomarker for spermatogenic damage and Sertoli cell function [reviewed by Buzzard et al. (2004), Chapin et al. (2011), and Meachem et al. (2001)]. Until recently, there was no method of easily measuring Inhibin B in the serum of rats since the only commercially available enzyme-linked immunosorbent assay did not cross-react with rat or dog hormone. A new Beckman Coulter assay for Inhibin B has recently been released and appears to be able to detect Inhibin B in rat serum but does not work in dogs (Chapin et al. 2011). In humans, Inhibin B has proved most useful for placing individuals into treatment categories for therapeutic purposes but has shown limited ability to predict fecundity or as a useful indicator of spermatogenic health (Chapin et al. 2011; Mabeck et al. 2005; Meachem et al. 2001).

Hormone changes can be due to direct, drug-induced effects on the endocrine system, but they can also be secondary responses to drug-induced disturbances in spermatogenesis. Distinguishing between the two responses is important with regard to understanding the significance of any hormone perturbations.

Apart from hormones and sperm parameters, currently there are very few other useful biomarkers of damage, either in nonclinical or in clinical studies (Chapin 2011).

18.3.4.4 Toxicogenomics

There have been relatively few reports on the successful use of "-omics" for investigation of mechanisms of testicular toxicity. It is possible to develop a "signature gene" response of a compound or a class of compounds, but currently there is little evidence on how that relates to the morphological features or the functional consequences of a drug-induced lesion. The alterations in testicular gene expression have been documented for four well-characterized testicular toxicants (cyclophosphamide, 2,5-hexanedione, ethylene glycol monomethyl ether [EGME], and sulfasalazine), 6 h after dosing, which was mostly prior to the development of morphological changes. There was differential gene expression for the four toxicants that could be related to the known morphological characteristics of the lesions, and three spermatogenesis-related genes (heat shock protein 70-2, insulin growth factor binding protein 3, and glutathione *S*-transferase pi) were affected by all the compounds and proposed as potential biomarkers of testicular toxicity (Fukushima et al. 2005; Rouquie et al. 2009). Using the well-characterized anti-androgen flutamide, Rouquie et al. (2009) evaluated the changes in the expression of selected genes (those known to be functionally associated with the testicular lesion) and showed that the no-observed-adverse-effect level (NOAEL) based on transcript changes was the same as the NOAEL based on morphological and hormone changes in a standard 28-day toxicity study design.

18.3.5 Expected Effects of Testicular Toxicity in Other Organs

Most disturbances in testicular spermatogenesis will result in changes in sperm parameters and frequently in the appearance of sloughed germ cells in the epididymis. Decreased sperm output may or may not be detectable by qualitative evaluation. If testosterone production by the Leydig cells is affected, then changes (organ weight decrease or atrophic changes) will generally be seen in the accessory sex organs. Primary or secondary endocrine disturbances will result in increased or decreased secretion of gonadotropins from the pars distalis of the pituitary. When the hormone perturbation is marked or prolonged, this may involve morphologically detectable hypertrophy of gonadotrophs in the pituitary and possible weight change, but in general, these changes are difficult to see without using quantitative immunohistochemistry. The male mammary gland in the rat is a surprisingly sensitive indicator of endocrine disturbance and can be used as an additional endpoint to confirm suspected anti-androgenic activity or hyperprolactinemia (Creasy 2008b, see also this chapter).

18.4 EPIDIDYMIS AND EFFERENT DUCTS

18.4.1 FUNCTIONAL ANATOMY

18.4.1.1 Efferent Ducts

The efferent ducts connect the rete testis with the epididymis for transport of spermatozoa. They comprise multiple (approximately 6 in rat and 14 in dog) coiled, small-caliber tubules lined by low, ciliated epithelium (Ilio and Hess 1994). In the rat, these multiple ducts take a long tortuous course through the epididymal fat pad before merging into a single common duct that enters the initial segment of the epididymis. In the dog, the ducts remain separate and are much shorter in length and partly embedded within the connective tissue of the initial segment. Each ductule makes an independent junction with the epididymal duct or forms a blind-ended structure that may predispose to sperm accumulations and granulomas (Foley et al. 1995). Consistent with their mesonephric tubular origin, the efferent ducts have absorptive capabilities analogous to renal tubules, reabsorbing 90% of the seminiferous tubule fluid. Resorption of fluid involves active transport mediated through a sodium chloride ion-exchange mechanism and removal of fluid by an adequate blood supply. Estrogen is an important regulator of fluid resorption and endothelin is also thought to be involved in the process (Harneit 1997; Hess 2002).

18.4.1.2 Epididymides and Vas Deferens

Each epididymis comprises a single, coiled duct (three meters long in rat) lined by pseudostratified epithelium with occasional ciliated cells. Three major regions of the epididymis (caput [head], corpus [body], and cauda [tail]) are morphologically evident and may be further subdivided on the basis of functional activity. The transition from efferent ductule to epididymal caput is abrupt with an increase in both lumen diameter and epithelial height. Continuing distally, the epithelial height decreases and luminal diameter increases. The cell types (principal, basal, narrow, clear, and halo) making up the epididymal epithelium also change along the course of sperm transport. The epididymal epithelium is variably secretory or absorptive along its course, maintaining an environment for sperm maturation. Junctions between adjacent epithelial cells maintain a hematologic barrier similar to, but less stringent than, that of the Sertoli cells. The epididymal barrier function allows for adjustment of luminal fluid components appropriate for maturational phase of the transported sperm as well as maintaining their immunologic sequestration. The expanded lumen of the cauda facilitates storage of mature sperm, 1 to 2 weeks after leaving the testis; caudal smooth muscle layers, continuing and increasing in thickness in the vas deferens, enable sperm propulsion. The vas deferens conducts the sperm to the urethra, joining the secretions from other accessory sex glands at the ampulla.

18.4.2 EFFERENT DUCT AND EPIDIDYMAL HISTOPATHOLOGY

18.4.2.1 Efferent Duct Changes

The efferent ducts are not routinely examined in toxicity studies but they can be a target for toxicity and, if affected, will often result in secondary lesions in the testis, which need to be recognized. The major function of the efferent ducts is the resorption of seminiferous tubule fluid. Drugs can interfere with this process, either causing excessive resorption, which leads to sperm stasis, or inhibiting resorption, which results in dilation of the ducts. In either case, the lesions can progress to the breakdown of the tight junctions between the epithelial cells and loss of the blood–epithelial barrier that separates the antigenically foreign sperm from the inflammatory cells of the host. The result is a progressive granulomatous inflammation, which will obstruct the ductules (Figure 18.17). If sufficient ductules are blocked, or the distal common duct becomes blocked, pressure builds up in the testis and the seminiferous tubular lumens become dilated. This pressure can rapidly lead to atrophy of the tubular epithelium, leaving a testis that contains totally atrophic tubules, which generally have dilated lumens. Unless the efferent ducts are sampled, the cause of the testicular atrophy is not evident, but a characteristic of this mechanism of toxicity is that the tubular dilation or the tubular atrophy is frequently unilateral. This frequent unilateral involvement is due to the fact that dilation or atrophy only occurs once sufficient ductules have become blocked or if the final common duct is affected, and this frequently only occurs in one testis.

There are a number of mechanisms through which efferent duct blockage can occur. A 5-hydroxy-tryptamine agonist has been shown to cause vasoconstriction of the blood vessels overlying the rete testis and efferent ducts, resulting in inhibition of fluid resorption and dilation of the seminiferous tubules, rete testis, and efferent ducts (Piner et al. 2002). La et al. (2011) have demonstrated a very close correlation between efferent duct inflammation and testicular dilation and atrophy (which was largely unilateral) with a leukotriene A4 hydrolase inhibitor. Similarly, Tani et al. (2005) described predominantly unilateral testicular atrophy associated with sperm granulomas in the efferent ducts and initial segment of the epididymis in mice in a 2-year bioassay with 2-methylimidazole. One of the best characterized examples of efferent duct toxicants with testicular atrophy secondary to impaired fluid reabsorption is the fungicide benomyl and its metabolite, carbendazim (Gotoh et al. 1999; Hess and Nakai 2000; Nakai et al. 1992). Efferent duct dilation and seminiferous tubule dilation occurred in mice administered an estrogen antagonist, and a similar effect is seen in the estrogen receptor knockout mouse (Hess et al. 2002).

This profile of changes has only been described in rodents, and it is likely that the anatomical layout of the efferent ducts (which are long and tortuous and merge into a single common duct) make rodents much more susceptible to complete obstruction and backpressure of fluid into the testis than most other mammals. In contrast, the efferent ducts of larger mammals, including dogs, NHPs, and humans, are either very short or embedded within the initial segment of the epididymis and have multiple entry points into the initial segment of the epididymis (La et al. 2011).

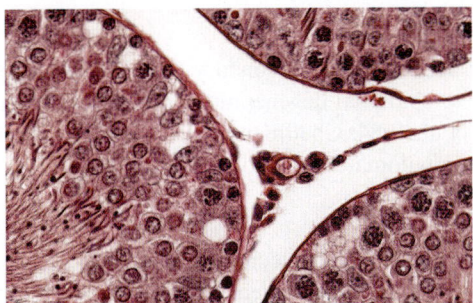

FIGURE 18.17   Tubular vacuolation can take many forms. In most cases, it represents vacuoles within or between Sertoli cells. It is generally an early indication of Sertoli cell damage but can sometimes represent the space left by an apoptotic germ cell, as in this rat testis.

18.4.2.2 Epididymis Changes

18.4.2.2.1 Epithelial Apoptosis

Epithelial apoptosis occurs in response to decreased testosterone levels. After testosterone reduction, the apoptosis moves in a wave down the epididymis, starting in the initial segment, and then moves to the head, corpus, and finally the cauda (Ezer and Robaire 2002; Robaire and Fan 1998). Epithelial apoptosis is an early change to low testosterone; epididymal atrophy is the end-stage lesion.

18.4.2.2.2 Epithelial Vacuolation

Epithelial vacuolation can be seen in response to a number of different mechanisms of toxicity. It generally occurs in specific segments of the epididymis, probably reflecting disturbances in the cell physiology of functionally specific regions of the epididymis. In most cases, the content of the vacuoles is undetermined and such changes are generally readily reversible. Drugs that cause phospholipidosis in other tissues may sometimes produce a foamy vacuolation in the epididymal epithelium. Intracellular vacuoles are frequently seen in the rat and dog epididymis at the junction between the corpus and cauda, and sometimes these may form a cribriform appearance. They are commonly seen in controls and generally are not drug related, although they may become more pronounced if sperm content decreases. Cribriform change in the caput epididymis in conjunction with aspermia is frequently associated with obstruction of the efferent ducts.

18.4.2.2.3 Epithelial Degeneration

Epithelial degeneration is uncommon as a drug-induced change. It has been described after dosing with methyl chloride (Chapin et al. 1984) where it was followed by an inflammatory response and the formation of sperm granulomas.

18.4.2.2.4 Sperm Granulomas

Sperm granulomas can occur as a background incidental lesion but can also be drug or chemically induced. Ligation or obstruction of the vas deferens will result in almost 100% incidence of sperm granulomas in the epididymis (Flickinger and Howard 2002). In most cases, induced sperm granulomas appear to be region specific. 2-Methyl imidazole–induced sperm granulomas occurred in the proximal caput and efferent ducts (Tani et al. 2005), while methyl chloride produced them in the cauda (Chapin et al. 1984). With guanethidine, they occur at the cauda–vas junction and are thought to be due to inhibition of adrenergic receptors in the smooth muscle of the vas (Evans et al. 1977). High doses of L-cysteine produced them mostly in the corpus and cauda (Sawamoto et al. 2003). In most cases, the mechanism is unknown, but in a number of cases, the sperm granuloma appears to be caused by initial damage to the epididymal epithelium resulting in rupture of the ductal lining and leakage of sperm into the interstitium.

18.4.2.2.5 Inflammation and Edema

Inflammation and edema may be primary or secondary to epithelial degeneration. Inflammation has been described secondary to epithelial degeneration with methyl chloride and prior to sperm granuloma formation (Chapin et al. 1984; Chellman et al. 1986). L-Cysteine also produces edema prior to development of sperm granulomas (Sawamoto et al. 2003).

18.4.2.2.6 Atrophy

Atrophy is a common secondary response to decreased spermatogenesis and seminiferous fluid production from the testis. It will also result from decreased testosterone levels since the epididymis is an androgen-dependent tissue. It is characterized by contraction of the ductal lumens and attenuation of the epithelial lining. In the case of decreased testosterone, atrophy will typically be preceded by epithelial apoptosis and accompanied by decreased weight of the accessory sex organs.

18.4.2.2.7 Luminal Cell Debris/Sloughed Testicular Germ Cells

Luminal germ cell debris/sloughed testicular germ cells in the rat are a very sensitive indicator of spermatogenic disturbance in the testis. In the normal adult rat, there are very few sloughed cells intermixed with the sperm and so any increase generally reflects loss of cells from the testis. This debris can sometimes be a more sensitive endpoint than actual histomorphologic changes in spermatogenesis (also see Section 18.3.2.1). The numbers of sloughed cells in the epididymis generally will be significantly increased in normal peripubertal animals.

18.4.2.2.8 Proliferative Changes

There are very few proliferative changes seen in the epididymis, and none have been described as drug induced. Hyperplasia has not been described as a lesion. Leydig cell adenomas have been described as a rare tumor in the B6C3F1 mouse, but their derivation of this is obscure since Leydig cells are not normally found in the epididymis. Histiocytic sarcoma has also been described as a primary tumor in the epididymis of the mouse (Baldrick and Reeve 2007; Yano et al. 2008).

18.5 ACCESSORY SEX GLANDS

18.5.1 FUNCTIONAL ANATOMY

18.5.1.1 Prostate Gland and Coagulating Glands

The prostate gland is an accessory sex gland present in all species routinely used in toxicologic studies. The compound tubuloalveolar gland, derived from buds off the pelvic urethra, is lined by columnar epithelium and surrounds the urethra at the neck of the urinary bladder, releasing serous fluid containing proteolytic enzymes into the urethra through multiple ducts. Among rodents, there are multiple lobes (paired ventral, dorsal, and lateral) as well as paired coagulating glands (anterior lobes) adjacent to the seminal vesicles. The epithelium lining the acini (or alveoli) comprises numerous columnar secretory cells and small numbers of nonsecretory basal cells, lymphocytes, and macrophages. In the dog, the prostate gland has two closely apposed lobes divided into lobules by trabeculae extending from the capsule. Smooth muscle fibers are present within the capsule. Development and maintenance of the prostate gland (as well as the epididymis and seminal vesicles) are dependent on androgen stimulation. In the adult, DHT, formed from testosterone by 5α-reductase activity within epithelial cells of the target tissue, is the effector androgen.

18.5.1.2 Seminal Vesicles

The seminal vesicles form as outpouchings from the mesonephric duct distal to the vas deferens. In the species having them (e.g., rat, mouse, rabbit, and NHP), the seminal vesicular secretions make up the largest portion of the ejaculate. The paired, curved, saccular structures have a pseudostratified columnar or columnar epithelial lining with infoldings forming a honeycombed mucosa and produce a viscous, alkaline secretory product discharged into the urethra through the ejaculatory duct.

18.5.2 SEMINAL VESICLE AND PROSTATE HISTOPATHOLOGY

18.5.2.1 Atrophy and Decreased Secretory Product

Atrophy and decreased secretory product are the main changes likely to be seen as a drug-induced effect. This change can be a primary effect owing to decreased androgen stimulation or may be secondary owing to a drug-induced deterioration in the animal's clinical condition leading to decreased testosterone levels. In most cases, organ weight will be more sensitive than histopathology for detecting decreased functional activity (Creasy 2008a). Although atrophy is mediated in part by epithelial apoptosis, this is not an obvious feature of the atrophic process in rodents. It is more obvious in dogs, at least in the early stages of prostatic atrophy. In rodents, the prostatic acini are filled with secretion and the epithelial cells are tall and columnar with a small pale apical secretory droplet. Significant decreases in organ weight are mostly due to decreased amounts of stored secretion within the prostatic acini or vesicular sacs of the seminal vesicles, but because of the size variation between acini and the variable sectioning of the seminal vesicles, this change may not be readily apparent by morphological assessment. In the case of the dog, there is no stored secretory product and the apical secretory droplets are much more prominent and intensely staining. Any decrease in intracellular secretory content is more readily apparent and generally accompanied by an increased rate of apoptosis. However, the amount of secretory granules and background apoptosis in the dog prostatic epithelium shows regional variation, which can confuse evaluation. Organ weight changes are not a sensitive indicator of functional status in the dog and NHP owing to interanimal variation and small group sizes. Atrophy in the NHP prostate is also difficult to evaluate since there is only a small amount of stored secretion and the height of the secretory epithelium of the prostate and seminal vesicles is relatively low compared with dogs and rodents.

18.5.2.2 Inflammation

Although it is common to see interstitial and acinar mononuclear inflammatory cell infiltrate in the prostate of rodents, especially as an aging change, inflammation of the prostate can be drug induced by estrogenic compounds. The dorsolateral prostate is particularly prone to this response.

18.5.2.3 Proliferative Changes

The most common proliferative change seen in the prostate and seminal vesicles is a reactive hyperplasia of the acinar or vesicular epithelium in response to inflammation, often secondary to urogenital infections. Preneoplastic hyperplasia and tumors of the prostate are uncommon as background lesions in rodents but have been described in association with administration of exogenous DHT and some carcinogens. Prostatic hyperplasia in the dog has been used as an experimental model for studying benign prostatic hyperplasia in humans by administering mixtures of androgens and estrogens (Mahapokai et al. 2000). An unusual "mesenchymal proliferative response" has been described in the seminal vesicles of mice. It comprises focal aggregates of atypical and sometimes highly pleomorphic epithelioid cells in the submucosa of the gland. It is more commonly seen in the urinary bladder of mice and is also discussed in Chapter 12. Although its origins are unknown, it bears many similarities to the decidual response sometimes seen in the uterus; currently, it is not considered a neoplastic response.

18.6 RELEVANCE OF MALE REPRODUCTIVE SYSTEM CHANGES TO HUMANS

Because of the lack of any reliable biomarkers of testicular toxicity in humans, there are very few known testicular toxicants in animals that have been confirmed in man. In the few cases where sufficient epidemiological evidence has been assimilated (e.g., glycol ethers, lead, 1,2-dibropmochloropropane), there is good concordance between the animal models and man. Most toxicity studies are conducted in rat and, to a lesser extent, in dog and even fewer in NHP. The efficiency of spermatogenesis and the overall fecundity of these species is much greater than that of humans; this is particularly so for the rat. In general, the regulatory viewpoint is that any detectable, drug-induced change in spermatogenesis or sperm parameters is considered adverse, regardless of whether the change affects fertility in the test species. This perspective is based on the fact that, taken as a species, humans are considered borderline for fertility and a small functional deficit can push a proportion of exposed individuals from being barely fertile to infertility. It will also generally be assumed that any change in the test species will occur in humans at a similar exposure level, unless good evidence can be provided to prove otherwise. Because of the difficulties in demonstrating mechanisms of toxicity in the testis, it is generally unlikely that such evidence will be forthcoming. Very often, testicular toxicants will demonstrate species differences between rat and dog, with one being sensitive and the other showing no effect. Since spermatogenesis and its regulation are basically similar between mammalian species, neither species is considered more or less relevant to man than the other. In this respect, the NHP is not considered any more relevant to man than rat or dog and regardless of how many species are resistant versus sensitive, risk assessment will generally be based on the most sensitive species.

18.7 FEMALE EMBRYOLOGY AND FUNCTIONAL ANATOMY

18.7.1 EMBRYOLOGY

The development of the female reproductive tract begins with formation of the PGCs in the yolk sac. The PGCs subsequently migrate to and colonize the genital ridge where they stimulate the splanchnic mesoderm of the genital ridge to develop into the gonad. In females, failure of PGCs to colonize the genital ridge results in a small ovary containing only stromal elements in the adult (McLaren 1991). In the developing ovary, the PGCs continue to proliferate, develop into oogonia, and enter into meiosis I, arresting in the dictyate stage before birth. In the absence of Sry expression (which activates the male differentiation pathway), the secondary sex cords develop in the developing gonad, giving rise to pre-granulosa cells that associate with the oocytes to form primordial follicles (McLaren 1991; Pepling 2006). A review of ovarian development and differentiation, with an emphasis on current knowledge of the molecular mechanisms associated with these processes, has recently been published (Edson et al. 2009). In the absence of androgenic stimulation, the mesonephric (Wolffian) duct degenerates and the upper portion of the female reproductive tract (uterine tubes, uterus, cervix, and anterior vagina) develops from the paramesonephric (Müllerian) duct. The lower portion of the tract, including the posterior vagina, vulva, and clitoris, are derived from the urogenital sinus.

18.7.2 OVARY

In the rodent and the dog, the broad ligament (or mesovarium) attaches the ovary to the dorsal body wall near the kidneys and the infundibulum of the uterine tube and the mesovarium form a bursa that encloses and isolates the ovary from the abdominal cavity (Walker and Homberger 1997; Wimsatt and Waldo 1945). In contrast, the ovary of the human and NHP is located within the pelvis and lacks an ovarian bursa (Beck 1972; Buse et al. 2008; Yuan and Foley 2002). In the mature, normally cycling rodent and dog, the ovary has an irregular shape caused by the protrusion of multiple follicles or corpora lutea from its surface, while in the NHP, the ovary has a more regular appearance with a single dominant structure (follicle or corpus luteum). Histologically, the ovary is covered by a single layer of peritoneal mesothelium, also referred to as the ovarian surface epithelium. In general, this mesothelial layer is flattened to cuboidal, though its appearance may change over the course of the cycle in response to systemic hormones or locally produced ovarian factors (Gaytán et al. 2005). In dogs, this epithelium also gives rise to the subsurface epithelial structures (SESs) within the cortex of the ovary by infolding or invagination (O'Shea 1966). The outer portion of the ovary, the cortex, contains the ovarian follicles and corpora lutea, while the inner or central portion, the medulla, contains interstitial glands and larger-caliber blood vessels and nerve fibers that enter at the hilus. The margins of the cortex and medulla in the normally cycling rodent are often indistinct but are readily observed in the dog and the NHP; however, the dominant cycling structure(s) (follicle or corpus luteum) may occupy a significant portion of the ovary with extension into the medulla. The ovarian stroma consists of ovoid or spindle-shaped mesenchymal cells, collagen fibers, and ground substance that form a highly mutable matrix able to accommodate repeated cycles of follicular and luteal growth and regression, which are detailed below. The rete ovarii are remnants of embryonic mesonephric tubules and appear as tubular structures lined by cuboidal to columnar epithelium within the ovarian medulla or hilus, with variable extension into the surrounding tissues (Wenzel and Odend'hal 1985). Other mesonephric remnants may also persist in the mesovarium and mesosalpinx.

The smallest follicles, the primordial follicles, are generally located in the outer portion of the cortex and consist of a small oocyte, arrested at the dictyate stage of meiosis I, encircled by a single layer of flattened, pre-granulosa cells and an outer basal lamina. The factors maintaining the primordial follicles in their arrested state of development are not well understood. During each estrous cycle, a small cohort of primordial follicles is "activated" and begins to enlarge as primary follicles; growth of the oocytes is initiated and the pre-granulosa cells become cuboidal, begin to display receptors for FSH, and start to proliferate. With continued growth, the secondary follicle develops as two or more layers of granulosa cells that now encircle the enlarging oocyte and a thick coat of glycoproteins (the zona pellucida) is secreted between the oocyte and adjacent granulosa cells (Wassarman et al. 1999). In response to factors released by the growing follicle, elongated cells recruited from the surrounding stroma form a sheath, the theca, outside of the follicular basement membrane (Magoffin 2005). Those cells nearest the follicular basement membrane, the theca interna, exhibit ultrastructural features of steroid-secreting cells consistent with their role in androgen production. The outermost thecal cells (the theca externa) are a loosely organized band of non-steroidogenic cells with ultrastructural features of fibroblasts and smooth muscle cells (Magoffin 2005; O'Shea 1981; Young and McNeilly 2010). At the end of this stage, the follicle becomes increasingly dependent on gonadotropins (and particularly FSH) for continued growth. In the absence of sufficient stimulation, granulosa cells begin to degenerate and the follicle undergoes atresia (Kumar et al. 1997; Markström et al. 2002; Messinis et al. 2010; Osmun 1985). As the atretic follicles regress, residual cells of the theca interna form the interstitial glands and these may contain remnants of the zona pellucida. Interstitial glands of the mouse are generally more prominent than those of the rat. Cells of the interstitial glands retain their steroidogenic function and serve as a source of androgens and other growth factors under the regulation of LH, prolactin, and catecholamines (Peluso 1992). In those follicles that continue to grow, granulosa cell proliferation continues and clefts begin to form in the zona granulosa; these spaces eventually coalesce, producing a single, fluid-filled antrum and the tertiary follicle is formed. The oocyte has now reached its maximum size and remains encircled by granulosa cells (the cumulus oophorus) that form a stalk extending into the antral cavity. The layer of cumulus cells immediately adjacent to the zona pellucida, the corona radiata, will remain with the oocyte after ovulation. The theca interna cells of the tertiary follicle may be enlarged, ovoid to polygonal in shape and more prominent with vacuolated cytoplasm. Only a single (in the NHP) or small number of follicles (in rodent and dog) are at the appropriate developmental stage to respond to rapidly rising levels of FSH and it is these follicles that are recruited to continue to develop into preovulatory (Graafian) follicle(s) (Fortune 1994). As the preovulatory follicle grows and the antral space continues to enlarge, the cumulus oophorus breaks down and the oocyte and attached corona radiata are released from their mural attachment. Under the influence of FSH, the mural granulosa cells produce increasing levels of estrogen and display receptors for LH, which further drives granulosa cell proliferation and estrogen production (Edson et al. 2009). On the day of proestrus, increasing levels of estrogen feed back to the hypothalamus and trigger the LH surge, which initiates the final phase of follicular preparation for ovulation. Release of the oocyte early on the morning of estrus is followed by collapse of the follicle wall, breakdown of the basement membrane with intermingling of the granulosa and thecal cells, and rapid ingrowth of the thecal microvasculature (Stouffer 2006). Subsequent enlargement of the corpus luteum occurs mainly through differentiation and hypertrophy of the luteinized cells, with only a minor contribution through cell proliferation (Stouffer 2006).

In NHP, a single corpus luteum is present on one of the two ovaries, but in rodents and dogs, multiple corpora lutea are present on each ovary. In dogs and NHPs, luteal regression occurs prior to the start of the next cycle; however, in rodents, follicles and corpora lutea from different cycles are present simultaneously, creating a complicated histologic picture. A number of publications are available detailing follicular and luteal development, physiology, morphology, and classification in the rodent (Boling 1942; Hirshfield and Midgley 1978; Hirshfield and Schmidt 1987; Kagabu and Umezu 2004; Niswender et al. 2000; Oakberg 1979; Pedersen and Peters 1968; Rajkovic et al. 2006; Stouffer 2006). In rodents, each generation of corpora lutea persists in the ovary for three to four estrous cycles and these may be distinguished by size, appearance, and histochemical characteristics (Boling 1942; Guraya 1975; Westwood 2008). The maximum size of the most recent corpus luteum is attained by diestrus and maintained through the next metestrus. In the rodent, the corpus luteum of the most recent ovulation undergoes predictable changes in appearance that reflect the day of the estrous cycle. At the next ovulation, a new generation of corpora lutea forms and the preceding cohort regresses through apoptotic depletion (Matsuyama et al. 1996). As complete luteal regression requires repeated exposures to prolactin (Bowen and Keyes 2000), three to four generations of corpora lutea are evident in the ovaries of mature, regularly cycling rodents. The regressing corpora lutea gradually decrease in size and contain lightly eosinophilic luteal cells, macrophages, increased collagen, and varying quantities of yellow-brown pigment. Eventually, regression results in the disappearance of the corpus luteum, leaving no remnant in the ovary.

18.7.3 Uterine Tube

The uterine tube (or oviduct) is subdivided into three major segments: the infundibulum (adjacent to the ovary and including the fimbriae), the ampulla, and the isthmus (which joins the uterine horn), on the basis of regional differences in structure (Lee et al. 1976). All segments of the uterine tube are composed of a mucosa, lamina propria, and tunica muscularis and covered by serosa. After ovulation, the fimbriae and infundibulum collect the oocyte and convey it to the ampulla where fertilization typically occurs in the mated animal.

18.7.4 Uterus

The rodent uterus is duplex, consisting of two discrete horns that fuse along the midline as they approach the cervix, but each retaining its own cervical opening into the vagina, giving the cervix the appearance of a single cervix grossly with two cervical canals microscopically. The canine uterus is bicornuate with two horns uniting caudally into a single, short body before the cervix. The NHP uterus is simplex and is anatomically similar to the human uterus. The uterine wall is composed of three layers: the endometrium, the myometrium, and the serosa. The endometrium consists of a single layer of simple cuboidal to columnar epithelium resting on a bed of well-vascularized endometrial stroma. Varying numbers of endometrial glands, continuous with the luminal epithelium and lined by cuboidal epithelium, penetrate the stroma. The myometrium consists of two layers of smooth muscle: the inner circular layer and the outer longitudinal layer. The size, weight, and microscopic appearance of the uterus change considerably over the course of the reproductive cycle, reflecting its response to changes in the levels of circulating ovarian hormones. Both epithelial and stromal cells express hormone receptors and, in general, epithelial proliferation is regulated by stromal receptors, while functional differentiation is mediated through epithelial receptors (Cunha et al. 2004).

18.7.5 Cervix

In the rodent, the mucosal lining of the cervix at the uterine junction is tall cuboidal to columnar and blends with the endometrium. Posteriorly, the mucosa becomes stratified squamous epithelium. The stroma throughout the cervix contains a mixture of dense collagen and smooth muscle fibers, and a thick septum of smooth muscle extending from the myometrium separates the two cervical canals. During the estrous cycle, changes in the cervix are most obvious in the squamous epithelium and are generally similar to those occurring in the vagina, though less pronounced.

In the dog, the uterine body communicates caudally with the cervix, which is approximately 1.5 to 2 cm long and is thickened and firm, relative to the uterus and vagina. The cervical canal is open during proestrus and estrus, during parturition, and in the immediate postpartum period. At all other times, it is usually closed. Histologically, the cervix consists of a superficial epithelium, occasionally with ciliated cells, overlying a lamina propria containing cervical (mucous) glands and blood vessels and surrounded by prominent smooth muscle tissue. Increases in the thickness of the epithelium, together with hypertrophy of the muscularis, are seen during estrus, while increases in the size and number of glands, as well as venous blood vessels, occur during diestrus (Goericke-Pesch et al. 2010).

In the cynomolgus macaque, the uterine cervix has a single, tortuous, endocervical canal with numerous glandular colliculi and a prominent exocervix that protrudes into the vagina. The endocervical canal and glandular colliculi are lined by mucus-secreting columnar epithelial cells, while the exocervix is lined by stratified squamous epithelial cells. A distinct squamocolumnar junction (SCJ) separates the two epithelial types and the location of the SCJ varies with age and endocrine status (Wood 2008).

18.7.6 VAGINA

The vaginal mucosa consists of a stratified squamous epithelium resting on a thin collagenous lamina propria. The remainder of the wall consists of a poorly defined muscularis of smooth muscle fibers and an outer adventitia attached dorsally to the rectum and ventrally to the urethra. At the cranial aspect of the rodent vagina, the two separate cervical ostia open into the common vaginal canal. The cervical ostia extend a short distance into the vaginal canal, resulting in short, peripheral recesses or fornices that may be mistaken for the cervical canals if sectioning at the junction of these two organs is suboptimal. The vagina of the dog is a muscular tube with longitudinal folds, averaging 10 to 14 cm in length in an 11.4 kg dog, which runs from the vestibule to the cervix, where it narrows because of a dorsal median fold of mucosa. The vaginal wall undergoes significant alterations in appearance during estrus, becoming swollen and turgid under the influence of estrogens and may be mistaken for an abnormal gross finding. The microscopic appearance of the vagina changes dramatically across the estrous cycle in the rodent and the dog and is a useful, reliable histologic indicator of the stage of the estrous cycle (Rehm et al. 2007b; Westwood 2008). This is in contrast to the NHP, where cyclic changes in the vagina are more difficult to appreciate.

18.8 GENERAL PHYSIOLOGY AND MATURATION

18.8.1 RODENTS

Laboratory rats and mice are continuously polyestrous mammals and ovulate every 4–5 days throughout the year. The age at which female rodents attain sexual maturity is heavily influenced by strain, but in general, mice are sexually mature at 5–7 weeks and rats are sexually mature at 5–8 weeks of age. The estrous cycle of the laboratory rodent has been divided into four stages of unequal duration, on the basis of hormonally induced changes in the reproductive tract. These stages have been described *in vivo* using vaginal cytology and *ex vivo* using histologic examination of the reproductive tract (Allen 1922; Goldman et al. 2007; Long and Evans 1922; Westwood 2008). The cycle begins with proestrus (follicular phase), followed by estrus (ovulation), metestrus, and diestrus (luteal phase). In general, diestrus is the phase with the most variable duration and, therefore, the greatest impact on the length of the normal estrous cycle (Allen 1922; Mandl 1951).

As rodents age, estrous cycles begin to become irregular and increase in length. The specific causes for this lengthening are unclear but appear to be related to changes in the hypothalamus that govern responses to estrogen and the release of GnRH (Downs and Wise 2009). The resulting hormonal perturbations may differ somewhat by species (Downs and Wise 2009; Maffucci and Gore 2006; Nelson et al. 1981). In the mouse, increasing cycle length is generally associated with prolongation of diestrus (Nelson et al. 1981). In the rat, increased cycle length often involves prolongation of proestrus, though increased duration of diestrus may be observed (LeFevre and McClintock 1988; Nass et al. 1984; Peluso and Gordon 1992). In both rats and mice, increasing cycle length progresses to the development of estrous cycle irregularities including persistent estrus, repeated pseudopregnancy, and, eventually, persistent anestrus late in life (Felicio et al. 1984; Peluso and Gordon 1992; vom Saal et al. 1994). The age at which these senescent changes begin and the sequence in which they occur vary and are influenced by species, strain, and husbandry (Felicio 1984; LeFevre and McClintock 1991; vom Saal et al. 1994). Persistent estrus refers to a state, which may last for months, in which the vaginal epithelium remains cornified in association with low circulating progesterone, tonic secretion of estradiol, and an absence of LH surges. These endocrine findings reflect the presence of numerous follicular cysts in the ovary, ongoing follicular development, and an absence of corpora lutea (vom Saal et al. 1994). Repeated pseudopregnancy refers to repeated periods of vaginal diestrus, often lasting approximately 14 days, which may be separated by brief intervals of estrus or proestrus. This condition occurs when corpora lutea persist in the ovaries of the non-gravid animal and is associated with high levels of circulating progesterone with normal diestrus levels of estrogen and slightly increased prolactin. Persistent corpora lutea in animals exhibiting repeated pseudopregnancy typically lack the basophilia seen during the normal estrous cycle and may contain areas that are hypocellular or acellular (Peluso and Gordon 1992). Persistent anestrus is the final stage of ovarian decline in which cyclical activity is absent, circulating levels of estrogen and progesterone are low, and vaginal cytology is dominated by leukocytes. Histologic findings in the reproductive tract at this stage include an absence of corpora lutea with limited or no follicular development and small uteri with atrophic glands (Peluso and Gordon 1992; vom Saal et al. 1994).

18.8.2 Dogs

The reproductive biology of canids, including the domestic dog, is highly unusual for mammals in several ways. Beagle dogs housed indoors under carefully controlled lighting and temperature conditions such as are seen in the laboratory environment are nonseasonal (i.e., they can have ovulatory cycles at any time of year) with a prolonged period of inactivity or anestrus (ranging from 3 to 12 months) between successive ovulatory cycles. At ovulation, the primary oocytes are not ready for fertilization and must undergo maturation within the oviduct for a period up to 72 h (Reynaud et al. 2005). Lastly, the duration of diestrus (progesterone influence) is prolonged in the nonpregnant dog, lasting at least as long as in the pregnant state. Heape (1900) referred to the dog as having four stages within the estrous cycle (proestrus, estrus, metestrus, and anestrus), and this terminology has been used and widely accepted over the years. The metestrus stage is, however, more accurately termed diestrus owing to the active hormonal milieu at this time (Johnston et al. 2001) and is referred to as such in this chapter. The identification of the phases of the estrous cycle has traditionally been related to behavioral or clinical observations rather than to hormonal or cytological characteristics, and for the purposes of this chapter, the stages will be matched with endocrinologic and morphological characteristics in line with the principal endpoints of toxicologic studies. The hormonal changes occurring through the estrous cycle from prepuberty or anestrus through proestrus, estrus, and diestrus have been reported for the dog in detail (Concannon 2011; Concannon et al. 1989; Gräf 1978; Johnston et al. 2001).

Puberty in beagle dogs generally begins around 6 months of age with the first "cycle" (i.e., commencement of first proestral phase) observed between 8 and 14 months of age (Wildt et al. 1981). Therefore, in standard toxicology studies in dogs, the females are frequently peripubertal at study start and even at the time of necropsy in short-term studies (≤6 months' duration). This is an important consideration in the interpretation of possible effects observed after treatment with xenobiotics as spurious imbalances in cyclic activity may be seen simply related to the age of the dogs utilized. In pubertal bitches, the duration and character of the proestrus–estrus phases may be less predictable than that in mature dogs (>18 months of age), with shorter duration or decreased or variable patterns of serum estradiol, LH, and progesterone levels, resulting in such behavior patterns as "split heats," "false heats," or "silent heats" (Johnston et al. 2001). A split or false heat occurs when the bitch shows clinical characteristics of proestrus with serosanguinous discharge, swelling, and even attraction to males but then does not transition to a true estrus period with ovulation. The clinical signs subside with, in the case of a split heat, a return to estrus behavior and ovulation several days or weeks later. In a false heat or the first phase of a split heat, ovulation does not occur and the follicles do not become luteinized. This is thought to result from increasing estradiol levels due to follicular development at puberty, which may be responsible for the clinical signs, though the exact cause is still not known. In a "silent heat," the bitch manifests no clinical signs, including vulvar swelling, in relation to ongoing follicular development, luteinization, and hormonal changes, but ovulation does occur and the internal reproductive organs show classic morphology related to the true phase of the cycle. Hence, in pubertal bitches used in toxicology studies, *in vivo* clinical observations may not be reliable indicators of the hormonal status or cyclic activity of the dog.

The female dog is, for the most part, a very poor model for the effects of xenobiotics on the human reproductive tract, particularly when it comes to hormonal effects on the cycle and organs. In addition, the duration of the estrus cycle with a prolonged anestrus period and the age of dogs used in standard toxicology studies, combined with a low number of dogs assigned to groups, make interpretation and risk assessment of possible changes problematic. In short-term studies, the dogs may not be mature enough to have begun estrus activity or have sufficient time to complete a single estrus cycle, and because of the variability between dogs in the age of puberty and duration of the various stages, an imbalance in the stages observed may be seen as part of normal biological variation.

18.8.3 Nonhuman Primates

The cynomolgus macaque has a menstrual cycle and endocrine profile that is generally similar to that of the human female. The cynomolgus macaque reaches sexual maturity at 2.5–4 years with menopause at 20–25 years. The menstrual cycle has an average length of 30 days and can be subdivided into follicular, periovulatory, luteal, and menstrual phases. The cynomolgus macaque demonstrates cyclicity year-round, while the rhesus macaque displays a strong seasonality, which may complicate interpretation of potential reproductive findings. Both rhesus and cynomolgus macaques display evidence of sex skin swelling and erythema around the time of ovulation; however, this finding varies with season in rhesus and is inconsistent, is variable, and may be absent in some cynomolgus macaques (Engelhardt et al. 2005; Ghosh and Sengupta 1992). The length of acclimation and social interactions in group housing can have dramatic effects on the menstrual cycle of macaques. Newly group-housed cynomolgus macaques demonstrate an increase in cycle length in the 6 months after the housing change (Weinbauer et al. 2008) and subordinate animals in established groups have fewer ovulatory cycles and more luteal phase defects when compared to dominant animals (Adams et al. 1985).

18.9 HORMONAL BASIS OF THE OVARIAN CYCLE

18.9.1 Rodents

The neuroendocrine regulation of the estrous cycle in the female laboratory rodent, with emphasis on the rat, has been described in detail (Freeman 2006). In the female rodent, the hypothalamus integrates numerous physiological signals with environmental cues to regulate the production and release of GnRH (also referred to as LHRH). On proestrus, rising levels of estrogen, in combination with permissive neural stimulation related to photoperiod, facilitate the release of a surge of GnRH. The GnRH surge, in turn, stimulates the anterior pituitary to release high levels of LH and FSH that drive follicular growth and steroidogenesis in the ovary. A number of factors other than ovarian steroids and photoperiod also influence gonadotropin secretion including pheromones (Dudley et al. 1996; Kelliher and Wersinger 2009), energy balance (Martin et al. 2008; McShane and Wise 1996; Nakanishi et al. 1976), stress (Brann and Mahesh 1991; Rivier and Rivest 1991; Tilbrook et al. 2002), immunologic/inflammatory responses (Kalra et al. 1998; Karsch et al. 2002), and xenobiotics (Mattison 1993). The proestrus surge of LH sets in motion the machinery that prepares the follicle for ovulation and stimulates cells of the theca interna to increase androgen production (particularly androstenedione) that serves as substrate for the production of estradiol. A concurrent surge in FSH stimulates the growth and proliferation of granulosa cells in growing follicles and, in antral follicles, stimulates increased production of estrogens and inhibin and upregulates expression of LH receptors by granulosa cells. A second peak of FSH secretion early on the morning of estrus is thought to promote the selection of pre-antral follicles that will develop for the next ovulation (Hoak and Schwartz 1980). This second FSH peak may be a consequence of follicular rupture and a rapid decline in serum inhibin levels (Rivier et al. 1990). After ovulation and through early diestrus, ovarian estrogen and inhibin feed back to the hypothalamus and pituitary gland to further inhibit LH and FSH release. In late diestrus and early proestrus, estrogen levels once again begin a rapid rise that sets the stage in the hypothalamus for the next cycle. Estrogen and progesterone produced in the ovary are responsible for the physiological and morphological changes that take place in the tubular organs of the tract.

During the rodent estrous cycle, progesterone is produced by both the ovarian follicle and the corpus luteum. After the LH surge in proestrus, granulosa cells of the follicle produce an initial peak of progesterone that prepares the follicle for ovulation and contributes to the suppression of gonadotropin release by the pituitary gland (Freeman 2006). Inhibition of either progesterone production or signaling through the progesterone receptor at this stage will impair ovulation (Robker et al. 2009). A second peak in circulating progesterone occurs in late metestrus/early diestrus owing to secretion by the newly formed corpus luteum (Smith et al. 1975). In the gravid female, progesterone prepares the endometrium for implantation of the embryo, inhibits myometrial contractility, and inhibits the maternal immune response to fetal antigens throughout pregnancy (McCracken et al. 1999).

In the absence of cervical stimulation, the newly formed corpus luteum of the rodent has been described as being "nonfunctional" as it is limited in its capacity to produce progesterone and is incapable of supporting uterine decidualization (Freeman 2006). The corpus luteum of the non-mated rodent produces progesterone for 1–2 days after ovulation, but levels fall thereafter and the predominant progestin released is 20α-hydroxyprogesterone (20α-OHP), which will not support uterine decidualization or inhibit gonadotropin release (Ichikawa et al. 1974; Smith et al. 1975). The early decline in progesterone production serves as the basis for the short estrous cycle in the rodent. In contrast, in rodents in which the cervix is stimulated artificially or by mating, the corpus luteum is "rescued" by a neuroendocrine reflex that initiates diurnal release of prolactin from the pituitary gland for the next 10–11 days (Smith and Neill 1976). This prolactin stimulates the development and hypertrophy of the luteal cells, upregulates expression of LH-R required for continued progesterone production, and suppresses expression of 20α-hydroxysteroid dehydrogenase, the enzyme that mediates the conversion of progesterone to 20α-OHP (Risk and Gibori 2001). In the sterile-mated or artificially stimulated rodent, this temporary development of the corpus luteum (pseudopregnancy) (Figure 18.18a) ends with the discontinuation of prolactin support from the pituitary gland. After a fertile mating, placental lactogen produced by the conceptus replaces prolactin in the second half of gestation to maintain the function of the corpus luteum.

While prolactin plays a critical role in support of the rodent corpus luteum, it also plays a key role in its demise. During proestrus, rising levels of estrogen induce pituitary lactotrophs to release increased levels of prolactin, which contributes to luteal regression. Inhibition of this prolactin surge on proestrus will impair regression of the corpora lutea, resulting in their accumulation in the ovary (Rehm et al. 2007c; Smith et al. 1975). It has been suggested that luteal regression induced by prolactin is due to T-lymphocyte-mediated apoptosis of luteal cells through a Fas/FasL-mediated

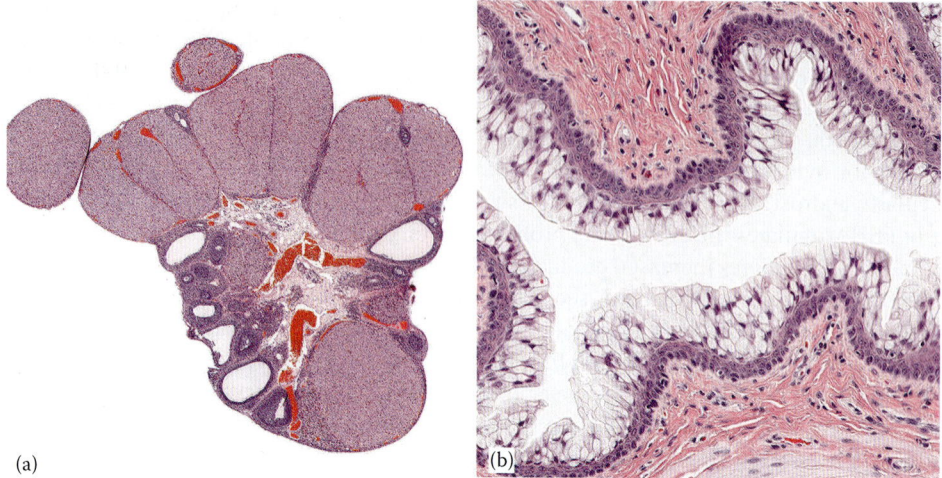

(a)

(b)

FIGURE 18.18 Tissues from a pseudopregnant rat. (a) Multiple large corpora lutea are present. (b) Vaginal mucification. Note the lack of a stratum corneum, which would be present during normal proestrus.

pathway, accompanied by the local expression of chemotactic factors and an influx of macrophages into the corpus luteum (Bowen et al. 1996; Risk and Gibori 2001).

18.9.2 Dogs

Clinically, proestrus is defined as the stage where observations of the dog's behavior or external genitalia signify that estrus is about to occur. Signs include a serosanguinous vaginal discharge and progressive swelling of the vulva. The duration of this phase is variable, ranging from 0 to 27 days, with an average of around 9 days. During this time, FSH levels fall as estrogen levels rise to a peak in line with follicular development in the ovary. Toward the end of proestrus, the estrogen levels decrease and progesterone levels start to rise, related to the luteinization (preovulatory) of the follicles and replacement of granulosa cells by luteal cells (Concannon et al. 1977). During late proestrus, serum testosterone levels are also elevated, peaking at the time of the LH surge, with levels observed that are similar to those in intact male dogs (Concannon and Castracane 1985; Olson et al. 1984). Approximately 2–3 days before ovulation, there is an LH surge that can last from 24 to 96 h (Phemister et al. 1973). A temporary increase in FSH is also seen around the time of the LH peak (Olson et al. 1982; Reimers et al. 1978) and increased androstenedione (a steroid precursor to estradiol or testosterone and produced by theca cells) also increases during proestrus, peaking around the time of the LH peak and then decreasing through estrus (Concannon and Castracane 1985).

In the dog, estrus is generally considered to begin when the female will first allow the male to mate and end when she will no longer allow coitus to occur. It can last from 4 to 24 days, with an average of around 9 days. This phase usually coincides with ovulation, which can occur over a period of 72 h, but can be quite variable beginning some days before or some days after the LH peak. Behavior during estrus is, however, strongly associated with decreasing estrogen levels combined with rapidly increasing progesterone levels. Testosterone levels decrease to basal levels after the LH peak and LH levels are lower than at any other time in the estrus cycle, owing to a depletion of pituitary LH (Fernandes et al. 1987). A variable serosanguinous or straw-colored vaginal discharge and vulval swelling are present during estrus.

Clinically, diestrus begins when the female no longer accepts the male; however, some authors prefer to define it through vaginal cytology (Holst and Phemister 1974) and, for the purposes of staging the ovarian cycle in toxicology studies, it would seem prudent to use vaginal and ovarian morphology as the defining factors. At this time, the vulva decreases in size and the vaginal discharge dries up. As the luteal phase takes over with the development of the corpora lutea, progesterone levels rise until around 2 to 4 weeks after the LH surge and then gradually decline over a period of 5 to 6 weeks with a similar profile observed for androstenedione. In dogs, during the luteal phase, progesterone and androstenedione levels are similar regardless of the pregnancy status of the animal (Concannon et al. 1989). Prolactin levels gradually rise during the luteal phase and mammary gland development is frequently seen clinically toward the end of diestrus. Lactation may be observed in nonpregnant animals and correlates with the decreased progesterone and increased prolactin. LH levels increase somewhat in both pregnant and nonpregnant dogs in late diestrus. Clinically, in nonpregnant bitches, the end of diestrus is not apparent as the bitch moves silently into a period of anestrus.

During anestrus, the external genitalia are small with no discharge observed and females are not attractive to males at this time. The duration of this phase can vary from 1 month to 2 years (Allen 1992) but is usually around 4 to 6 months (Bouchard et al. 1994; Sokolowski 1977). Although this is considered to be a quiet or inactive phase of the cycle, hormonally this is not the case. Levels of FSH increase during anestrus, and in late anestrus, they are as high as that seen in the preovulatory surge in estrus (Olson et al. 1982). LH levels increase in a pulsatile manner in late anestrus and may be responsible for initiating the next proestrus phase (Concannon et al. 1986; Olson et al. 1982; Shille et al. 1987). Estrogen concentrations fluctuate during anestrus and are reported to rise, at least in some dogs, approximately 7 weeks before the onset of proestrus (Jeffcoate 1992; Mellin et al. 1976; Olson et al. 1982). These changes in estradiol levels could be related to follicular development and may also be responsible for so-called split or false heats.

18.9.3 Nonhuman Primates

The menstrual cycle of the NHP is similar to the human menstrual cycle and typically lasts between 28 and 32 days with ovulation occurring at the midway point around day 14. The first half of the cycle is termed the follicular phase, and during this period, there are low levels of gonadotropins and rising levels of estradiol stemming from the developing dominant follicle (Weinbauer et al. 2008; Zeleznik and Pohl 2006). Inhibin B levels are highest during the early follicular phase and decrease as ovulation approaches (Fraser et al. 1999; Shimizu et al. 2002). Estradiol levels continue to rise until around day 12, which is followed by a sharp increase in the levels of FSH and LH leading to ovulation of the Graafian follicle (Weinbauer et al. 2008; Zeleznik and Pohl 2006). During this periovulatory period, progesterone levels begin to rise and may play a role in oocyte maturation, ovulation, and luteinization (Borman et al. 2004; Chaffin and Stouffer 2002). After ovulation, the luteal phase begins, estradiol and gonadotropin levels decrease rapidly, and progesterone and inhibin A levels continue to rise as the corpus luteum develops (Suresh and Medhamurthy 2009). During the luteal phase, gonadotropin levels remain low, and unlike the human, the NHP does not have elevated luteal phase estradiol levels (Shimizu 2008). Circulating progesterone reaches a maximum level around day 22, and in the absence of maternal recognition of pregnancy, corpus luteum function declines and the menstrual phase begins (Weinbauer et al. 2008). During the menstrual phase, progesterone and inhibin A levels decrease and there is a brief increase in FSH levels to support follicular recruitment for the next cycle (Gougeon 1996; Jabbour et al. 2006; Weinbauer et al. 2008; Zeleznik and Pohl 2006).

18.10 HISTOLOGY OF THE FEMALE REPRODUCTIVE SYSTEM

18.10.1 Rodents

The histology of the reproductive tract during the estrous cycle is similar in normally cycling rats and mice and has been previously described in detail (Greaves 2007; Li and Davis 2007; Westwood

TABLE 18.3

Key Histologic Features of Female Reproductive Organs at Various Stages of the Estrous Cycle in the Rodent

	Immature–Juvenile	Proestrus	Estrus	Metestrus	Diestrus
Ovary					
Follicles	Primordial, primary, secondary, and tertiary (antral) follicles. Antral follicles increase with approach of puberty. Atretic follicles present.	Primordial, primary, secondary, plus early and late (tertiary) antral follicles. Atretic follicles present.	Primordial, primary, secondary, and early antral follicles. Few large antral follicles often atretic.	Primordial, primary, and growing secondary follicles. Few growing antral follicles. Atretic follicles present.	Primordial, primary, secondary, and growing tertiary follicles. Atretic follicles present.
Corpora lutea	Absent	3–4 generations. Largest (most recent) slightly eosinophilic; may exhibit vacuolar degeneration or apoptotic cells. Early generations are smaller, eosinophilic, and generally lack apoptosis.	3–4 generations. Most recent small, with densely basophilic spindle-shaped cells, mitotic figures, sometimes central cavity. Earlier generations eosinophilic with apoptotic cells	3–4 generations. Most recent are basophilic, usually solid though some contain central cavity. A few mitotic figures are present. Older generations eosinophilic.	3–4 generations. Most recent have attained maximum size. Cells are lightly basophilic with foamy cytoplasm. No apoptotic cells present. Older generations eosinophilic.
Uterine Tube			Cumulus-oocyte complex and mucinous material may be present.	Cumulus-oocyte complex and mucinous material may be present.	
Uterus					
Endometrium	Lumen narrow. Little endometrial area; glands present. Epithelium cuboidal without mitotic figures. Stroma compact. Myometrium thin.	Lumen dilated, lined by hypertrophied cuboidal or columnar epithelium with mitotic figures common. Stromal edema may be prominent (especially in mouse). Neutrophils may be variable.	Lumen collapsed, lined by tall columnar epithelium, glandular epithelium cuboidal. Prominent epithelial degeneration and apoptosis. Few mitotic figures. Numerous stromal granulocytes may be present in glands. In mice, stromal edema may be present.	Lumen narrow, lined by low columnar epithelium with a few mitotic figures and scattered apoptotic debris. Glandular epithelium large cuboidal with numerous mitoses. Many stromal granulocytes; may be present in glands.	Lumen narrow, lined by low columnar cells; mitoses increase from early to late. Glands lined by cuboidal epithelium. Stroma relatively dense, usually with decreased numbers of granulocytes.
Vagina					
Epithelium	Low, simple, or stratified cuboidal epithelium, 2–3 layers thick.	Stratified squamous with stratum granulosum and stratum mucification early; stratum corneum late. Basal mitotic figures common.	Early: Stratum mucification separates from surface; often absent. Stratum corneum prominent. Late: Stratum corneum separates from surface. Generally few mitotic figures.	Stratum corneum absent. Progressive loss of stratum granulosum and superficial stratum germinativum, with variable infiltrates of neutrophils and lymphocytes. In mice, leukocytic infiltrates may be florid.	Early: Epithelium is thinnest in appearance; becomes progressively thicker. Late: superficial, lightly basophilic polygonal cells with early mucification but no stratum granulosum. Granulocytes decrease from early to late.

Note: All features of a specific stage may not be present owing to variability in the stage of cycle or the plane of histologic section.

2008; Yoshida et al. 2009; Yuan and Carlson 1985; Yuan and Foley 2002). Therefore, the major changes at each stage of the cycle are only briefly summarized. The key to determining the stage of the cycle using histology is appreciating the predictable and synchronous changes occurring in each of the organs that reflect the hormonal milieu when the samples were obtained (Table 18.3). It should be kept in mind that all features of a specific stage may not be present because of variability in the stage of cycle and the plane of histologic section. Because the rodent estrous cycle is entrained to photoperiod, it is also important to recognize that the time of day at which samples are obtained can significantly influence the histologic appearance of the tissues of the reproductive tract (Yuan and Carlson 1985).

18.10.1.1 Proestrus

In the ovary, preovulatory follicles are present as are the large corpora lutea of the most recent cycle, which contain sporadic apoptotic cells and, occasionally, larger areas of vacuolar degeneration (Figure 18.19a). The uterine lumen is variably, but often obviously, dilated. The uterine luminal

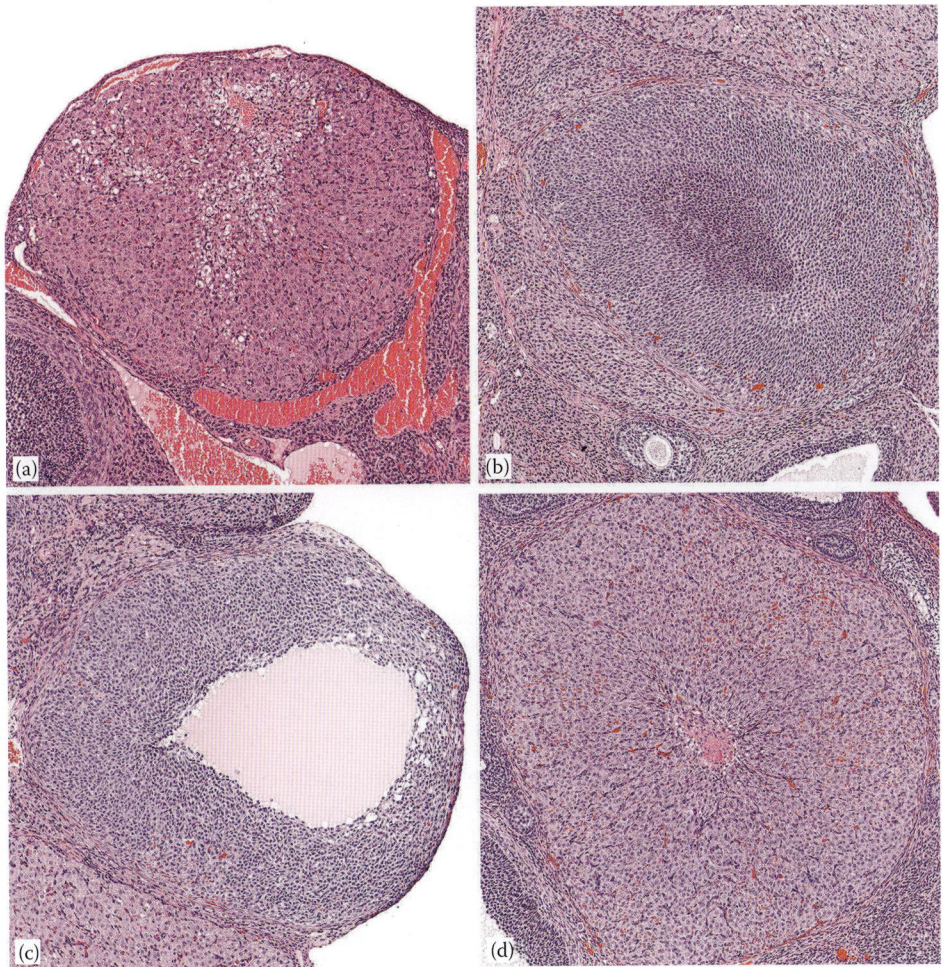

FIGURE 18.19 The morphological features of the rat corpus luteum throughout the estrus cycle. (a) Proestrus. Large corpus luteum from the prior cycle with apoptosis and vacuolar degeneration. (b) Estrus. Newly formed basophilic corpus luteum. (c) Metestrus. Developing and enlarging basophilic corpus luteum with a central cavity. (d) Diestrus. Large, slightly basophilic corpus luteum with small amounts of central fibrous connective tissue.

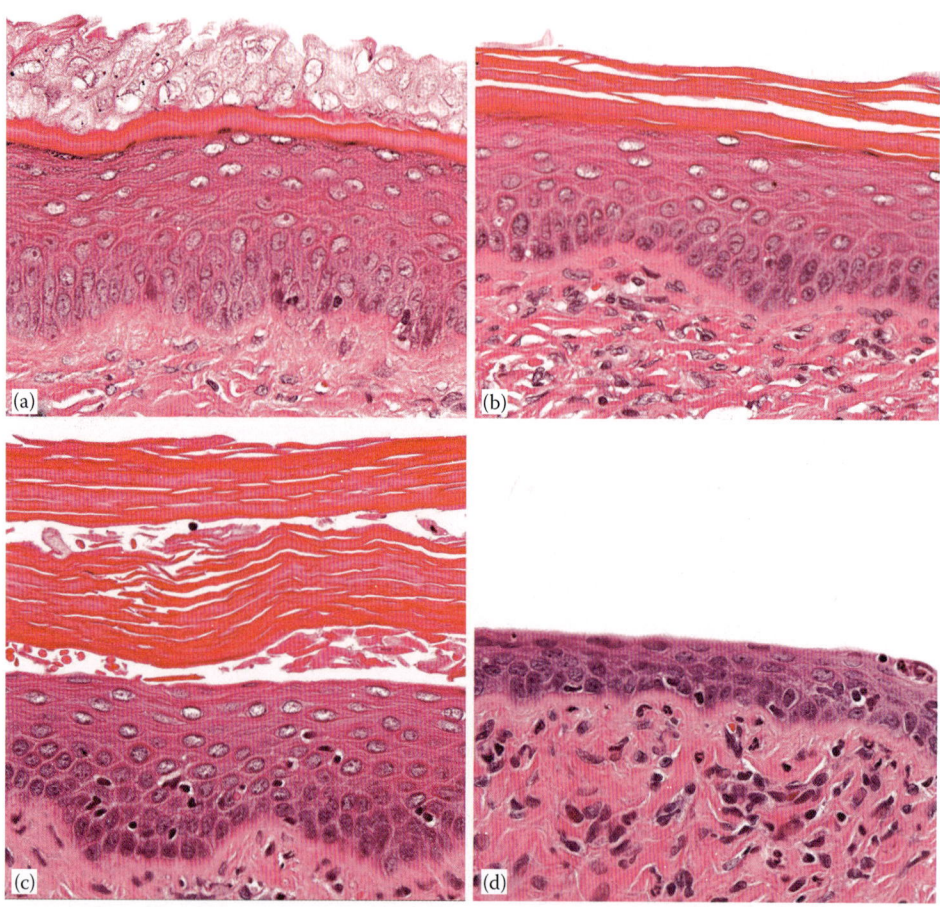

FIGURE 18.20 The morphological features of the rat vagina throughout the estrus cycle. (a) Proestrus (late). Tall stratified squamous epithelium with a stratum corneum and superficial mucification. (b) Estrus. Stratified squamous epithelium with prominent stratum corneum and complete loss of superficial mucification. (c) Metestrus. There is loss of the stratum corneum and stratum granulosum with prominent intraluminal sloughed debris and some influx of intraepithelial neutrophils and lymphocytes. (d) Diestrus. The vaginal epithelium reaches its thinnest point with some intraepithelial neutrophils and lymphocytes.

epithelium is columnar (though it may be compressed) and usually contains a few mitotic figures without evidence of apoptosis; endometrial glands may be distorted or dilated and are lined by cuboidal epithelium. In the mouse, endometrial stromal edema is often pronounced, while this is usually less apparent in the rat. The vaginal epithelium is stratified squamous with cornified (stratum corneum) and mucified (stratum mucification) layers of cells present on the surface (Figure 18.20a). A useful marker for the onset of proestrus is formation of the stratum granulosum (Westwood 2008).

18.10.1.2 Estrus

The ovary contains characteristic early basophilic corpora lutea (Figure 18.19b), occasionally with a central cavity and a few atretic antral follicles. Corpora lutea of earlier generations contain numerous degenerated/apoptotic cells. The uterine tube may contain one or more cumulus–oocyte complexes and mucinous material from the recent ovulation. The uterine lumen is collapsed, luminal epithelium is typically tall columnar, the glandular epithelium is cuboidal, and both show prominent evidence of degeneration and apoptosis. Granulocytes are often numerous in the stroma and may be present in the glands; in the mouse, slight stromal edema may persist. The vaginal stratum mucification has been sloughed from the epithelium, but the stratum corneum is present (Figure 18.20b) and begins to slough at the end of this phase.

18.10.1.3 Metestrus

In the ovary, basophilic corpora lutea have enlarged and most are solid, though central cavities may still be observed (Figure 18.19c). Cumulus–oocyte complexes may still be observed in the uterine tubes. The uterine lumen is now narrow and lined by columnar epithelium containing a few mitotic figures and scattered foci of vacuolar degeneration or apoptotic remnants; endometrial glandular epithelium is often large cuboidal, with numerous mitotic figures. Granulocytes are often numerous within the endometrial stroma and may be observed in the endometrial glands. The vaginal epithelium has lost the stratum corneum and stratum granulosum (Figure 18.20c) and there is often mild to moderate infiltration of the epithelium by neutrophils and lymphocytes.

18.10.1.4 Diestrus

The most recent basophilic corpora lutea in the ovary have attained their greatest diameter (Figure 18.19d). Apoptotic cells are not present in the corpora lutea and this may help distinguish diestrus from proestrus. The uterine lumen is narrow and lined by low columnar epithelial cells and mitotic figures are common; granulocytes tend to be less prominent in the endometrial stroma. At the end of metestrus and beginning of diestrus, the vaginal epithelium has reached its thinnest appearance and consists of 3–6 layers of the stratum germinativum (Figure 18.20d). As diestrus progresses, the epithelium increases in thickness to 8–10 layers and the superficial layers of cells start to become polygonal and slightly basophilic as early mucification occurs.

18.10.2 Dogs

The histology of the reproductive tract during the estrous cycle of the dog has been recently reviewed (Barrau et al. 1975; Chandra and Adler 2008; Fowler et al. 1971; Rehm et al. 2007b; Steinhauer et al. 2004) and basic changes are described below and in Table 18.4 (see also Figures 18.21 through 18.26).

18.10.2.1 Proestrus

During proestrus, numerous antral follicles begin to form within the cortex (Figure 18.23a and b). If the dog has cycled previously, atretic corpora lutea may be present. During proestrus and into estrus, the uterine vessels become progressively more prominent and the walls of the uterus become noticeably thicker as the lumen begins to form an "X-like" shape when viewed in cross section. Extravasation of red blood cells (RBCs) occurs into the uterine lumen (Figure 18.23e) and free RBCs can also be seen in the superficial endometrium, thought to emanate from the venule rather than superficial capillaries (Walter et al. 2011). The surface and endometrial glandular cells proliferate, resulting in more tortuous glands and the cells have a homogeneous, eosinophilic cytoplasm. Under estrogenic stimulation, the vaginal epithelium becomes progressively thicker and more stratified squamous, with hypertrophy and mitoses observable in the basal layers. At the beginning of proestrus, the vaginal mucosa is non-keratinized (Figure 18.23f), but by the end of proestrus, the epithelium is keratinized with prominent stratum granulosum and stratum corneum up to 20 or 30 cells thick.

18.10.2.2 Estrus

The antral follicles increase in size with the appearance of distinct folds in the granulosa layer prior to ovulation; the canine granulosa cells start to become luteinized and begin to produce progesterone (Figure 18.24a). Ovulation occurs from the luteinized follicles over a period of 72 h and the ova are

TABLE 18.4

Histologic Features of Female Reproductive Organs at Various Stages of the Estrus Cycle in the Dog

	Immature	Proestrus	Estrus	Diestrus	Anestrus
Ovary					
Follicles	Primordial, primary, and secondary (early antral) Polyovular follicles frequent Atretic follicles	Primordial, primary plus early and late (tertiary) antral follicles	Primordial, primary plus preovulatory luteinized follicles Vascularized theca	Primordial and primary	Primordial, primary, and secondary (late anestrus)
Corpora lutea (cortical)	Absent	Absent	Present (late estrus): cavitated May have central fluid and RBCs	Prominent (cavitated in early diestrus). Late (day 20+): Regression with vacuolation and apoptosis	Present: highly vacuolated with macrophages and lipofuscin
Corpora albicans (adjacent to medulla)	Absent	Present, if already cycled	Present, if already cycled	Present, if already cycled	Present, if already cycled
Uterine Tubes					
Mucosa (infundibulum/cranial)	Cuboidal epithelium. Undeveloped lamina propria/stroma	Columnar epithelium Increasing submucosal edema Increasingly complex epithelial folds	Tall, columnar epithelium with prominent ciliated and secretory differentiation Submucosal edema (early) Prominent epithelial folds/glands	Combination of differentiated and undifferentiated epithelial cells Reducing epithelial folds/glands	Low cuboidal epithelium Compact, cell-rich stroma Simple epithelial infoldings
Mucosa (caudal isthmus)	Cuboidal epithelium	Cuboidal epithelium	Columnar epithelium Occasional ciliated cells	Cuboidal epithelium Rare ciliated cells	Cuboidal epithelium

Uterus					
Endometrium	Few glands Little stroma	Proliferation of superficial and, later, basal glands Increasing stromal edema Extravasation of RBCs into lumen and subepithelial hemorrhage	Proliferation and maturation of superficial and basal glands Glandular secretion Decreasing stromal edema Decreasing hemorrhage/ extravasation with pigmented macrophages	Prominent glandular endometrium with two zones: 1. Basal coiled glands 2. Luminal crypts Late (after day 21): Decreasing stromal collagen; endometrial apoptosis	Quiescent glandular tissue
Myometrium	Undeveloped	Hypertrophy Edema	Proliferation and hypertrophy	Hypertrophied	Quiescent
Cervix					
Epithelium—cranial	Cuboidal—1 layer	Cuboidal—1–2 layers	Cuboidal—2–3 layers	Cuboidal—2–3 layers (early)	Cuboidal—1–2 layers
caudal	Cuboidal—1–2 layers	Cuboidal—multilayered	Stratified—multilayered	Cuboidal—multilayered	Cuboidal—multilayered
Stroma	Undeveloped, few glands	Dense, cellular. Few glands	Edematous. Increasing glandular development	Increased glands. Increased vascularity	Dense, cellular. Few glands
Vagina					
Epithelium	Stratified, non-keratinized, squamous Approximately 2–3 layers	Stratified, non-keratinized, squamous Approximately 5–7 layers and increasing	Early: Stratified, squamous with thick keratin layer Late: Desquamation of keratin layer	Cuboidal to columnar, pseudostratified Approximately 3–5 layers. Mucus cells may be present (early to mid) Neutrophilic infiltration	Cuboidal to squamous Approximately 1–2 layers
Stroma	Loose connective tissue	Increasing edema. Increased collagen	Thickened with dense collagen	Neutrophilic infiltration Progressive regression	Reduced
Muscularis	Thin	Increasing hypertrophy	Hypertrophy	Progressive reduction	Thin

Note: All features of a specific stage may not be present owing to variability in the stage of cycle or the plane of histologic section.

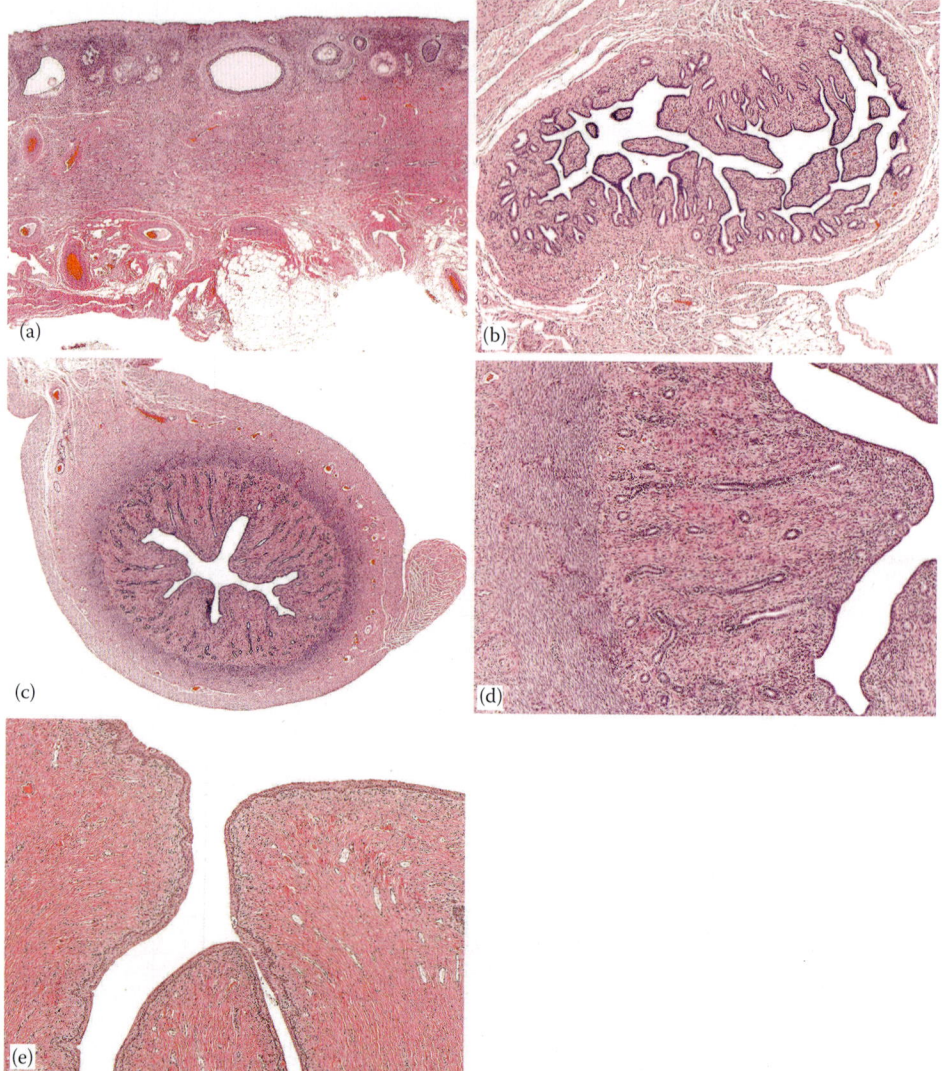

FIGURE 18.21   (a) Immature ovary with secondary and early tertiary follicles, and prominent follicular atresia (dog). Note the absence of corpora albicans. (b) Immature uterine tube (dog). (c) Immature uterus (dog, low power). (d) Immature uterus (dog, higher power). Note the absence of glandular development. (e) Immature vagina (dog). Note the thin, stratified squamous epithelium.

extruded via the surface of the ovary into the bursa, where they remain for a few hours before moving into the ovarian tubes (Concannon 2011).

In the uterus during estrus, as the estrogen levels fall and progesterone rises, the edema is reduced and glands become even more numerous and complex (Figure 18.24d and e). Some extravasation of RBCs can still be seen but become progressively fewer and less obvious while pigment-laden macrophages are frequently seen in their place. The keratinized vaginal epithelium reaches maximal thickness, the submucosa becomes progressively more thickened and expanded by edema, and the muscularis is hypertrophic (Figure 18.24f). Toward the end of estrus, the keratinized epithelium starts to slough into the lumen and the mucosa starts to shrink as fluid leaves the stroma.

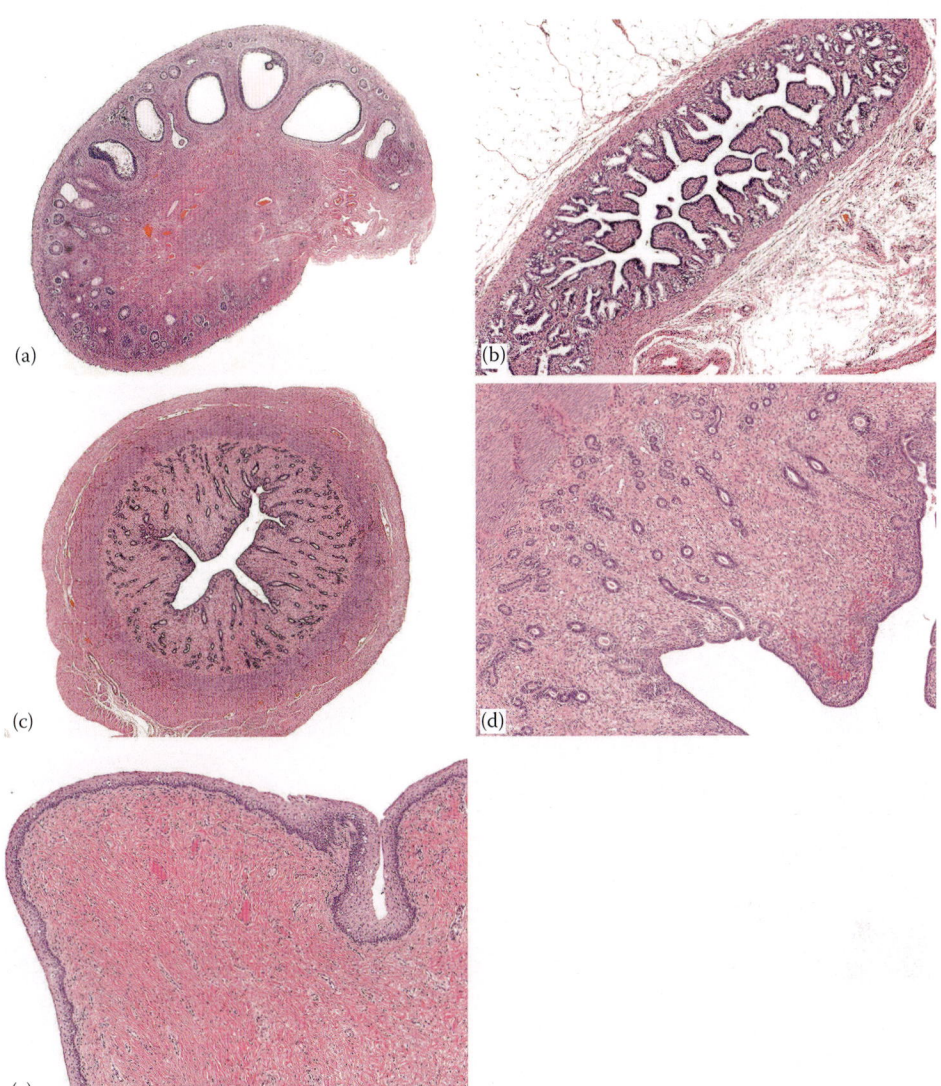

FIGURE 18.22 (a) Peripubertal ovary with prominent tertiary follicles and some follicular atresia (dog). Note the absence of corpora lutea and late/large tertiary follicles. (b) Peripubertal uterine tube with early ciliated and secretory cell development, similar to early proestrus (dog). (c) Peripubertal uterus (dog, low power). Note the increased thickness of endometrium and the more prominent myometrium, similar to early proestrus. (d) Peripubertal uterus (dog, higher power). Note the presence of red cell extravasation/hemorrhage within the superficial endometrium, similar to proestrus (not always present). (e) Peripubertal vagina, similar to early proestrus (dog).

18.10.2.3 Diestrus

After ovulation, the follicles do not collapse, but rather start to fill from the outside in, with a proliferation of luteal tissue forming corpora lutea (Figure 18.25a and b) (England and Allen 1989). The cavity of the corpus luteum is generally filled in by approximately 20 days after ovulation; thus, in early diestrus, normal corpora lutea will have a central cavity while true luteal cysts are rare in beagle dogs (Andersen and Simpson 1973). The maximal size and weight of the uterus is seen in diestrus, approximately 7 to 9 weeks after the onset of estrus. The uterus assumes a characteristic

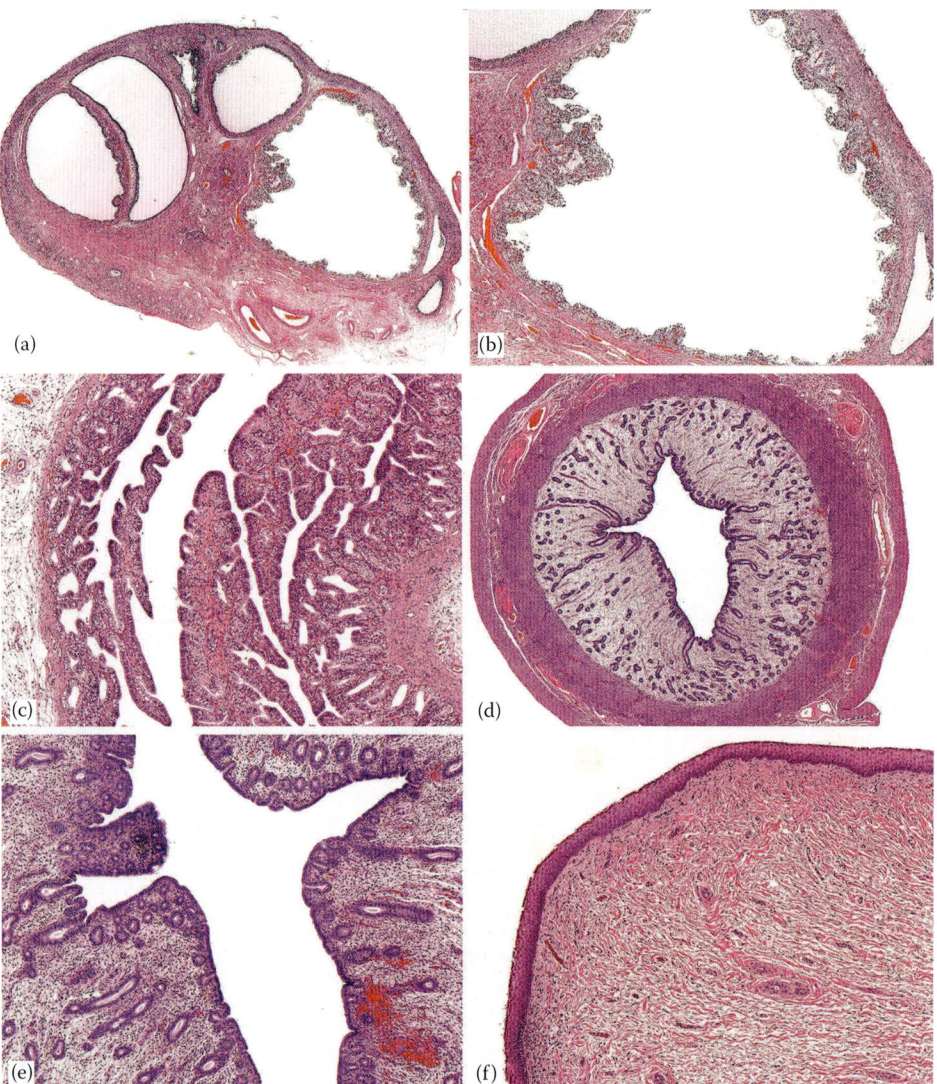

FIGURE 18.23 (a) Late proestrus ovary with large (late) tertiary follicles showing preovulatory luteinization (dog). (b) Preovulatory, luteinized follicle in the proestrus ovary (dog). (c) Proestrus uterine tube (dog). Note the presence of secretory cells and increased infolding/complexity. (d) Proestrus uterus (dog, low power). Note the endometrial edema, proliferation of superficial glands, and increased prominence of myometrium. (e) Proestrus uterus with glandular proliferation, edema, and superficial red cell extravasation/hemorrhage (dog, higher power). (f) Proestrus vagina with subepithelial edema and thickened, squamous epithelium.

twisted ("corkscrew") appearance during diestrus (Figure 18.25c), related to the maximal influence of progesterone and glandular proliferation. Under the increasing influence of progesterone from the corpora lutea, the glands continue to proliferate and two layers of the endometrium become apparent (Figure 18.25d). An inner zone is seen with many superficial crypts and elongated villous projections extending into the uterine lumen covered by a vacuolated epithelium, while the outer zone contains many secretory and somewhat dilated glands within a loose stroma. As the progesterone levels decrease in late diestrus, regression of the endometrium occurs through progressive apoptosis of glandular tissue (Chu et al. 2006, 2002; Van Cruchten et al. 2003) with degeneration and

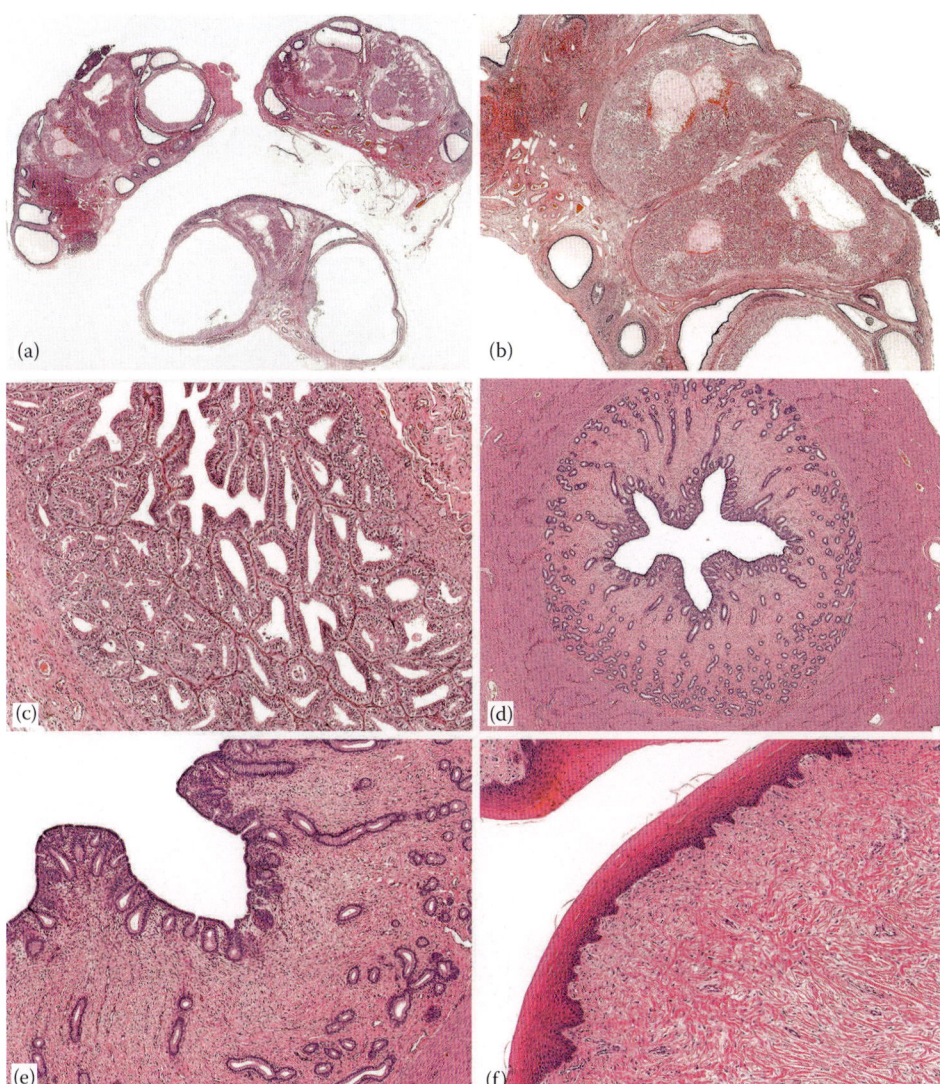

FIGURE 18.24   (a) Estrus ovary with large tertiary follicles showing preovulatory luteinization, and ovulated follicles showing varying degrees of luteinization (dog). (b) Ovulated, progressively luteinizing follicles/cavitated corpora lutea with central fluid and RBCs in the estrus ovary (dog). (c) Estrus uterine tube (dog). Note the presence of secretory and ciliated cells with prominent infolding/complexity. (d) Estrus uterus (dog, low power). Note the reduced endometrial edema, proliferation of superficial and deep endometrial glands, and myometrial proliferation/hypertrophy. (e) Estrus uterus (dog, higher power). (f) Estrus vagina with desquamation of keratinized squamous epithelium.

desquamation of the superficial layer, and by the end of diestrus, the uterus is small and inactive. By the onset of diestrus, the vaginal epithelium is reduced to around three to six cells thick (Figure 18.25f) and is columnar in appearance, with prominent infiltration of granulocytes both within the epithelium and lamina propria. By mid-diestrus, the vagina resembles that of anestrus.

18.10.2.4   Anestrus

Luteolysis occurs slowly in the female dog, with clear signs of degeneration occurring only after approximately 60 days (Hoffmann et al. 2004). The precise mechanism through which regression

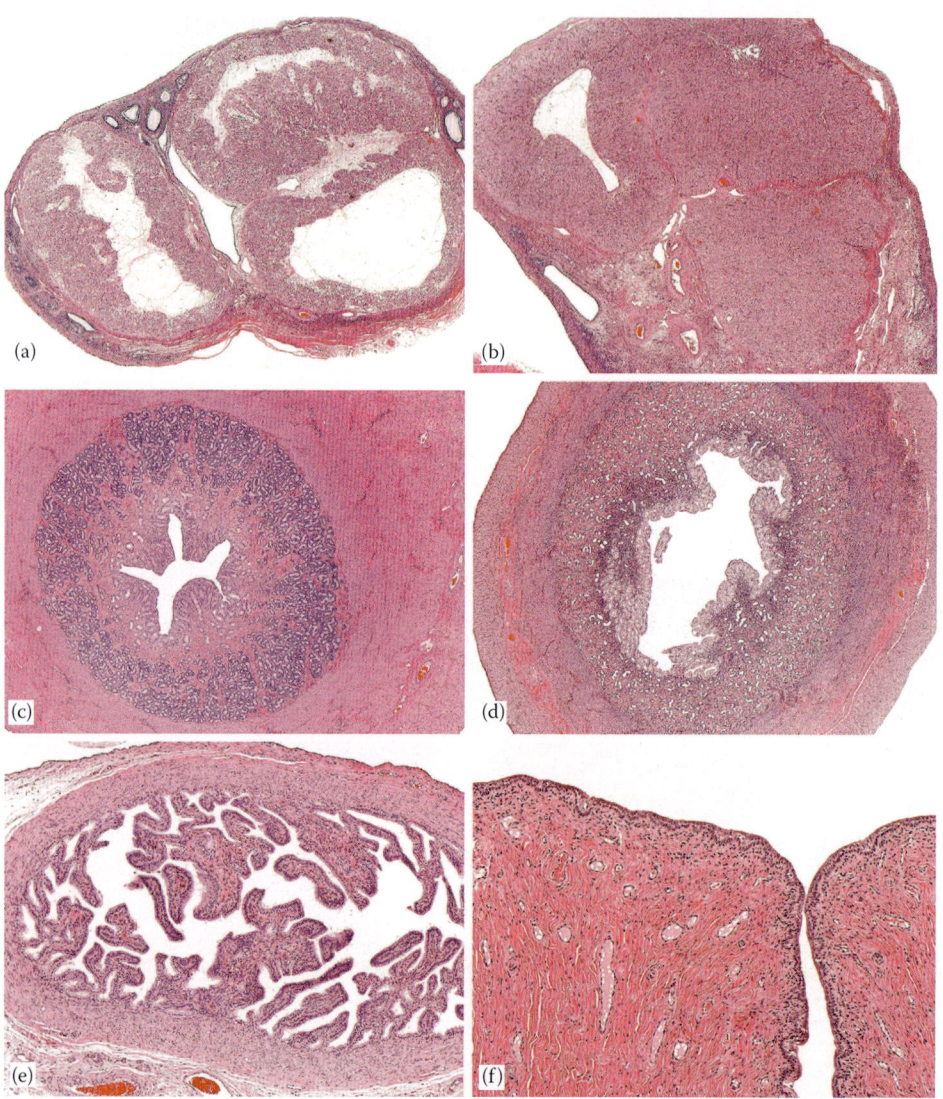

FIGURE 18.25 (a) Early diestrus ovary with early, cavitated corpora lutea (dog). (b) Mid diestrus with mature corpora lutea (dog). Note that one is still cavitated even at this stage. (c) Early diestrus uterus with superficial and deep glandular proliferation and hypertrophied myometrium (dog). (d) Mid diestrus uterus (dog). Note the reduced myometrial hypertrophy and two distinct endometrial zones. (e) Diestrus uterine tube (dog). Note the decreased folding and combination of differentiated/undifferentiated epithelial cells. (f) Diestrus vagina with pseudostratified epithelium (with mucus cells) and inflammatory cell infiltration.

occurs is still not known (Concannon 2011; Hoffmann et al. 2004; Kowalewski et al. 2006; Luz et al. 2006). Full regression of the subsequent inactive corpora albicans occurs slowly and remnants can be seen throughout the anestrus period (Figure 18.26a) and may remain through up to two further estrus cycles (Dore 1989). During anestrus, small primary follicles are present as a narrow band in the peripheral cortex (Figure 18.26a) overlying the deeper, regressing corpora albicans. Throughout anestrus, the uterus is small and inactive with sparse glandular tissue and a cuboidal to low columnar surface epithelium, similar to that seen in prepubertal female dogs, but not quite as undeveloped (Figure 18.26c and d). The vaginal epithelium has a quiescent appearance with two to three layers

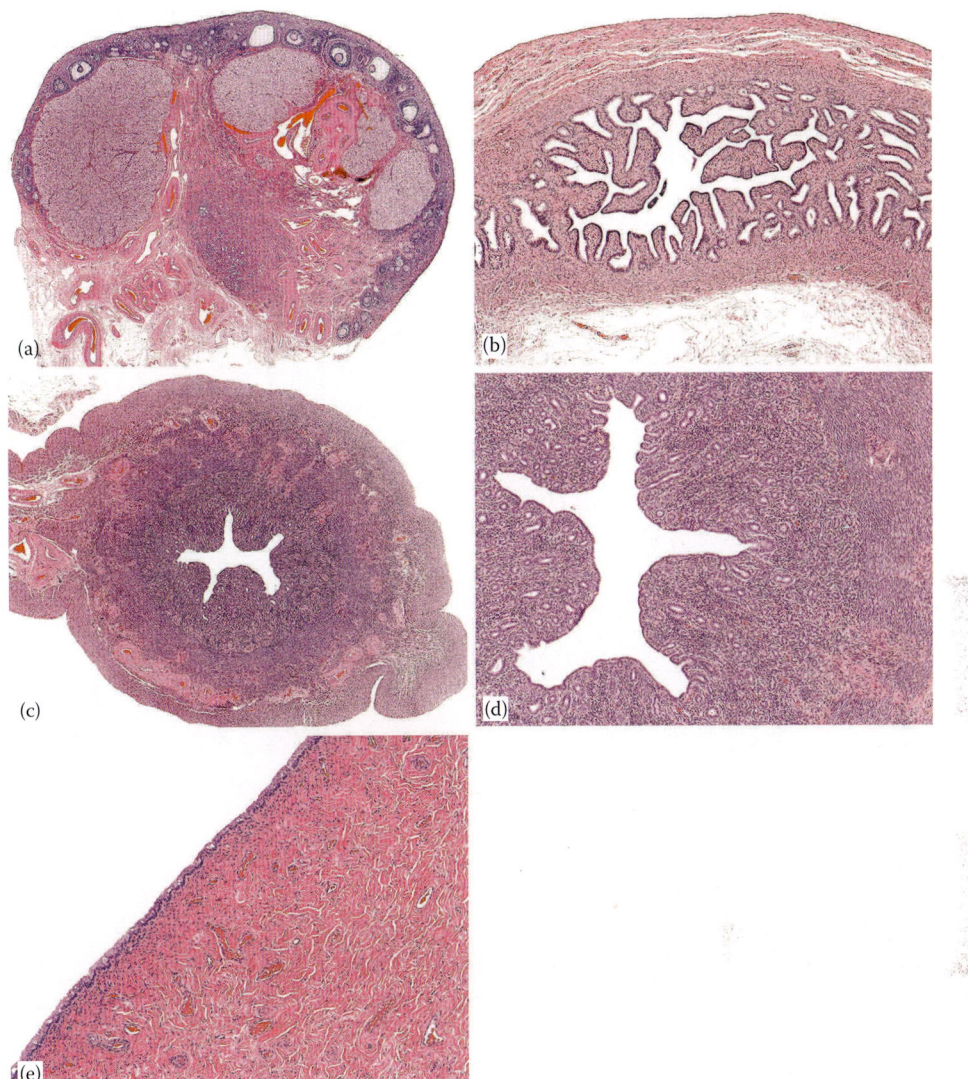

FIGURE 18.26 (a) Anestrus ovary with early antral follicles, and corpora lutea/albicans (dog). (b) Anestrus uterine tube (dog). (c) Anestrus uterus (dog, low power). (d) Anestrus uterus (dog, higher power). Note the presence of quiescent glandular tissue and compact myometrium. (e) Anestrus vagina (dog). Note the thin epithelium with subepithelial mononuclear cell infiltration.

of cuboidal cells (Figure 18.26e), the outer layer appearing pseudostratified in some cases, with a dense, thin subepithelial stroma and a well-defined smooth muscle wall (muscularis).

18.10.3 Nonhuman Primates

The histology of the reproductive tract during the menstrual cycle is, in general, similar in both NHP and women and has been previously reviewed (Bartelmez 1951; Brenner and Slayden 1994; Buse et al. 2008; Koering 1969; Poonia et al. 2006; Watanabe et al. 2006; van Esch et al. 2008). The major histologic changes during the menstrual cycle of a normally cycling NHP are described below and in Table 18.5, but since many animals in a nonclinical toxicology setting are prepubertal or

TABLE 18.5

Key Histologic Features of Female Reproductive Organs at Various Stages of the Menstrual Cycle in the NHP

	Prepubertal/Immature	Follicular Phase	Periovulatory Phase	Luteal Phase	Menstrual Phase	Repair Phase/Early Follicular Phase
Ovary	Multiple small- to medium-sized variably atretic antral follicles. Primordial and primary follicles are numerous and often form a distinctive band within the cortex. No evidence of a corpus luteum.	A single large dominant follicle becomes evident within one of the ovaries and the remaining smaller follicles display varying amounts of atresia. There may be evidence of a large regressing corpus luteum from the prior cycle and smaller remnants of corpora lutea from past cycles.	A single large dominant follicle that can occupy a large portion of one ovary or a newly forming corpus luteum often with a central cavity and hemorrhage.	Large active corpus luteum will be present on one of the two ovaries. During the early luteal phase, there may be a small central cavity with or without hemorrhage, and as the luteal phase progresses, the central cavity can contain fibrous connective tissue.	Large corpus luteum present on one of the ovaries but showing signs of regression.	Regressing corpus luteum.
Uterus						
Endometrium	Compact with dense stroma and few small straight glands.	Endometrial height increases dramatically; stromal edema is often prominent; glands are straight with numerous mitotic figures and pseudostratification.	Variable and features of both follicular and luteal phase may be present. Basal glands become more tortuous and sacculated; subnuclear vacuoles may be present.	Glands begin to become more tortuous and sacculated and this change progresses though the luteal phase to include both basal and superficial glands; subnuclear vacuoles may be present within the glands; glands often contain secretory material; numerous spiral arteries present.	Distinct sacculated glands; superficial stroma will begin to separate and small pools of blood form and large areas of the superficial endometrium begin to slough and multiple large foci of hemorrhage are present; large numbers of inflammatory cells present.	Endometrium will be small and compact with straight glands
Vagina						
Epithelium	Generally thin, but as puberty approaches, it may be thick and keratinized with rete pegs.	Thick stratified squamous with a prominent keratin layer.	Thick stratified squamous with a prominent keratin layer.	Thick stratified squamous epithelium, but the keratin layer may be absent or less obvious.	Thick stratified squamous epithelium, but the keratin layer may be absent or less obvious; variable amounts of hemorrhage and debris can be observed.	Thick stratified squamous but the keratin layer may be absent or less obvious.

Note: All features of a specific stage may not be present owing to variability in the stage of cycle or the plane of histologic section.

just reached menarche (see Section 18.14), the histologic appearance may not be as described for a cycling animal. In the NHP, the ovaries and endometrium are the most useful organs for evaluating the cycling status as histologic changes are pronounced and easily recognized at low magnification. The cyclic changes in the vagina and cervix are less obvious with routine histology.

18.10.3.1 Prepubertal/Immature

The ovaries typically contain multiple, small- to medium-sized variably atretic antral follicles without evidence of corpora lutea, suggesting that ovulation has not occurred to date (Figure 18.27b). Primordial and primary follicles are numerous and often form a distinctive band within the cortex. The uterus is small and the endometrium is compact with dense stroma and few small straight glands (Figure 18.28a). The vagina is typically thin and the cervix is inactive in immature NHP when compared to a cycling animal; however, as puberty approaches, waves of estradiol from developing

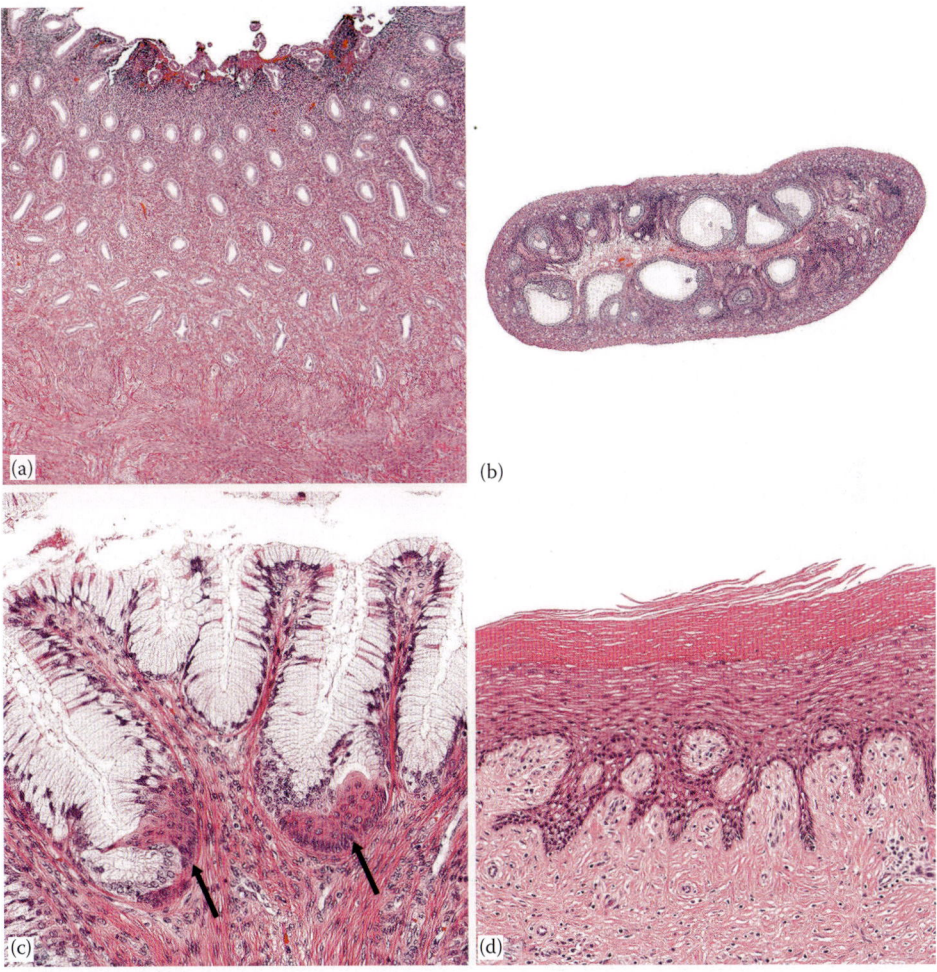

FIGURE 18.27 Typical appearance and spontaneous changes present in the female reproductive tract of young NHPs. (a) Small amounts of hemorrhage and glandular/stromal breakdown within the superficial endometrium with a weakly proliferative phase appearance to the endometrium without the secretory phase pattern and endometrial shedding characteristic of normal menses. (b) Ovary with multiple small- to medium-sized variably atretic tertiary follicles and no evidence of an active or regressing corpus luteum. (c) Squamous metaplasia of the endocervical glands (arrows). (d) Vagina with prominent keratin layer and rete pegs.

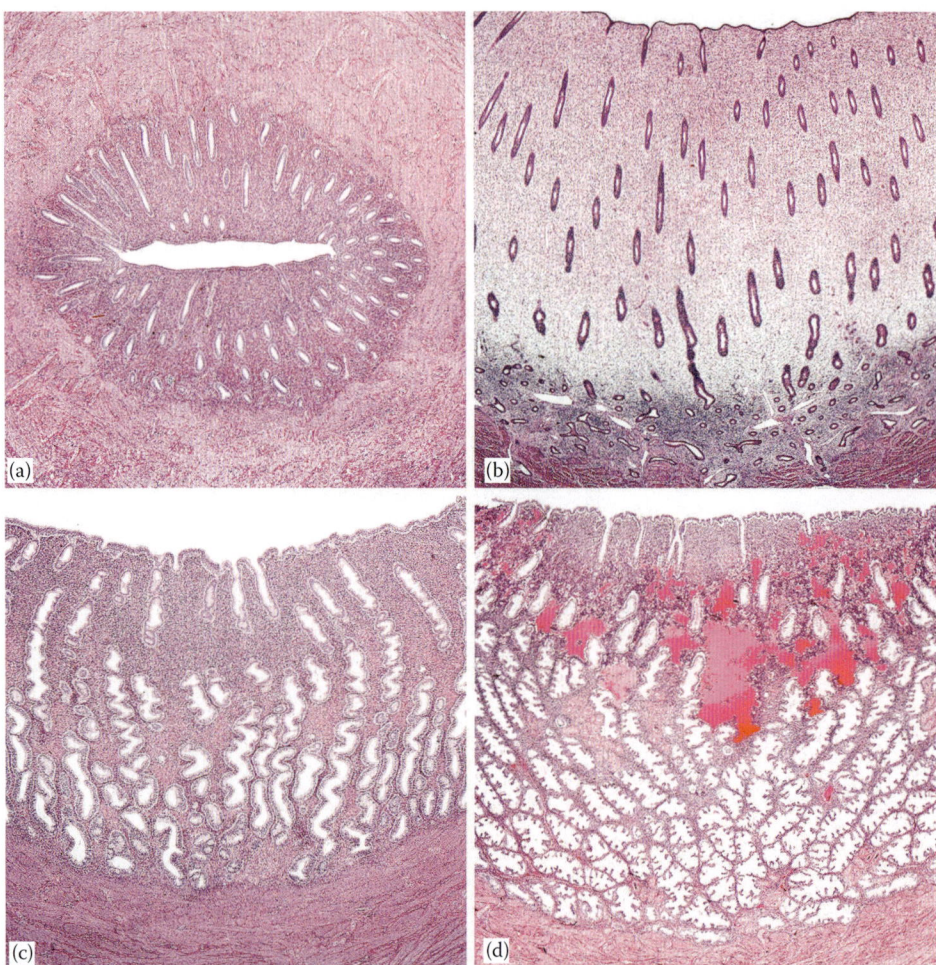

FIGURE 18.28 The morphological features of the NHP endometrium during the menstrual cycle. (a) Prepubertal. Short, compact endometrium with dense stroma and few small straight glands. (b) Follicular phase. Markedly expanded endometrium when compared to the prepubertal state (same magnification) with straight glands and stromal edema. (c) Luteal phase. The endometrial glands become progressively more tortuous and sacculated. (d) Menstrual phase. The endometrial glands are extensively sacculated and the superficial endometrium begins to slough with multiple foci of hemorrhage.

follicles may induce a hyperplasia with rete peg formation and a keratin layer in the vagina (Figure 18.27d) and foci of squamous metaplasia within the cervix (Figure 18.27c).

18.10.3.2 Follicular Phase

The ovaries typically contain multiple, small- to medium-sized antral follicles, and as the follicular phase progresses, a single, large, dominant follicle becomes evident within one of the ovaries and the remaining smaller follicles display varying amounts of atresia. There may be evidence of a regressing corpus luteum from the prior cycle. The endometrium expands dramatically and stromal edema is often prominent (Figure 18.28b). The glands are straight with numerous mitotic figures and display pseudostratification. Because of the large number of mitotic figures, the follicular phase endometrium is often referred to as the proliferative phase. The vagina is thick stratified squamous with a prominent keratin layer.

18.10.3.3 Periovulatory Phase

The changes during the periovulatory period in the NHP are more variable than those described in the human. In the human endometrium, glandular sacculation and subnuclear vacuoles are considered hallmarks of recent ovulation; however, in the NHP, these changes can be evident prior to ovulation. As a result of this variability, the late follicular phase and early luteal phase can be combined into a single periovulatory phase for ease of evaluation.

18.10.3.4 Luteal Phase

A large active corpus luteum will be present on one of the two ovaries. During the early luteal phase, there may be a small central cavity, with or without hemorrhage (corpus hemorrhagicum). As the luteal phase progresses, the central cavity can contain fibrous connective tissue. The endometrial glands display distinct progressive changes throughout the luteal phase. The basal glands begin to become tortuous and sacculated during the periovulatory period (Figure 18.28c), and this change progresses though the luteal phase to include both basal and superficial glands. During the early to mid-luteal phase, subnuclear vacuoles may be present within the glands, and although this is a characteristic change described in the human literature, it is variable in NHP. Throughout the luteal phase, the glands often contain secretory material, and as a result, the luteal phase endometrium is often referred to as the secretory phase. Numerous spiral arteries are developing during this time. The vagina is still a thick stratified squamous epithelium, but the keratin layer may be absent or less obvious.

18.10.3.5 Menstrual Phase

A large corpus luteum will still be present on one of the ovaries but will begin showing signs of regression. The endometrium has distinct sacculated glands, and the superficial stroma will begin to separate, forming small pools of blood (Figure 18.28d). As the menstrual phase progresses, large areas of the superficial endometrium begin to slough and multiple large foci of hemorrhage are present. There are often large numbers of inflammatory cells present. Within the lumen of the cervix and vagina, variable amounts of hemorrhage and debris are observed.

18.10.3.6 Repair Phase/Early Follicular Phase

After menstruation, the endometrium will undergo repair as the next cycle begins. The endometrium will be small and compact with straight glands. While the endometrium is not always distinct from a prepubertal animal or anovulatory cycle, the presence of a recently regressing corpus luteum distinguishes this normal phase of the cycle.

18.10.4 SAMPLING OF THE REPRODUCTIVE TRACT FOR EXAMINATION

Ideally, representative sections of all the major organs (ovaries, uterine tubes, uterus, cervix, and vagina) should be included in a histologic evaluation of the female reproductive tract. At a minimum, ovaries, uterus, and vagina should be examined to evaluate the status of the cycle and synchrony of the tissues. Examination of the mammary gland and anterior pituitary gland may provide additional useful information for interpreting treatment-related findings in the female reproductive tract. Recommended methods for selection and trimming of tissue sections for evaluation of the rodent and NHP reproductive tracts have been published (Kittel et al. 2004; van Esch et al. 2008). For all tissues, consistency in sample selection and sectioning is important to facilitate interpretation. When evaluating the tubular organs of the tract, all layers including mucosa, muscularis, and serosa/adventitia should be present. In the rodent, examination of the anterior portion of the vagina [segments 4 and 5 per Berger et al. (2005)] is recommended as cyclical changes may be inconsistent along the anteroposterior axis of the mucosa and the posterior vaginal epithelium is covered continuously by cornified epithelium (Yuan and Foley 2002). This can be accomplished with a consistently oriented transverse section as described above or a horizontally oriented longitudinal section extending from the uterine body through the cervix to the posterior vagina. Because of the inherent variability in normal ovarian morphology related to follicular and luteal dynamics, sections of the ovary for routine histologic examination should target the greatest cross-sectional area. This practice will help avoid tangential sections that may not fully represent the population of ovarian structures present and is most likely to include portions of the medulla for examination.

18.11   NONMORPHOLOGICAL ENDPOINTS FOR ASSESSING TOXICITY

18.11.1   Organ Weights

Evaluation of ovarian weights can provide useful additional information when evaluating the female reproductive system in repeat-dose toxicity studies (Ohtake et al. 2009; Rehm et al. 2007c; Tsujioka et al. 2009). In all species, age and stage of the cycle can have a marked impact on the weight of the ovaries and ovarian weights are best evaluated in conjunction with the histopathology data. In rodents and dogs, care must be taken to remove the bursa and uterine tubes as these structures can contribute significantly to the overall weight. Uterine weights are not a typical endpoint on most repeat-dose toxicity studies but can be useful when evaluating compounds expected to have a direct effect on the tubular tract (Tsujioka et al. 2009). Like ovarian weights, uterine weights are subject to large changes throughout the cycle. In rodents, fluid within the lumen is an important part of the estrogen-driven weight increase and is easily lost without careful dissection. Because of large variability during the cycle, uterine weights can be used most effectively in an investigative setting using immature or ovariectomized animals.

18.11.2   Vaginal Cytology/Vaginal Swabs

Evaluation of daily vaginal cytology samples in rodents is a simple and effective way to monitor the hypothalamo–hypophyseal–ovarian axis (Goldman et al. 2007), but because of the need for mature animals prior to study start for baseline data collection and the need for extra animals to replace those with abnormal cycles, vaginal cytology is not often used or recommended in standard repeat-dose toxicity studies. Vaginal cytology is a critical and sensitive endpoint when characterizing findings observed in the female reproductive system and can be used as needed for compounds with known class effects. The strength of vaginal cytology lies in the longitudinal assessment of the estrus cycle and to ensure that animals used on a study are cycling normally at the onset of dose administration. Care must be taken to ensure that the procedure does not cause cervical stimulation and result in pseudopregnancy.

In dogs, vaginal cytology can be used to track the estrous cycle, but the long length and variability of the canine cycle make this impractical in most nonclinical toxicology settings.

In NHPs, daily vaginal swabs can be a useful method to ensure the use of mature females and to track the length and frequency of the menstrual cycle (Weinbauer et al. 2008). Multiple cycles of baseline data are required prior to test article administration to ensure that mature, normally cycling animals are used. Despite the relative ease of the procedure, detection of test article–related effects and interpretation of the data may be difficult in standard repeat-dose toxicity studies owing to the small sample size and high incidence of irregular cycles in NHPs.

18.11.3   Follicle Counts

Quantitative assessment of primordial and primary follicles can be performed manually with hematoxylin and eosin or immunohistochemistry or by the use of a semiautomated approach using immunohistochemistry (Picut et al. 2008; Regan et al. 2005). Follicle counting has been recommended as a method to detect changes to follicular reserves, but there is considerable variability in this technique, it is very labor intensive, and most cases of early follicular degeneration/depletion will manifest with repeated dosing and can be detected histologically using qualitative endpoints. As a result, follicular counting is recommended to be used as a second-tier methodology to provide further characterization of findings if necessary (Regan et al. 2005).

18.11.4 Hormone Measurements

Another approach to evaluating effects on the hypothalamo–hypophyseal–ovarian axis is to measure various hormones throughout the reproductive cycle. This approach is more labor intensive than the other described techniques and is not recommended as an add-on in standard repeat-dose toxicology studies. Because of the cyclic nature and rapid changes over short periods, measuring hormones during the female reproductive cycle needs to be timed carefully and anchored with daily vaginal cytology or vaginal swabs to ensure that samples are collected in a controlled fashion. In rodents, estradiol, progesterone, LH, FSH, and prolactin are most typically used and can be measured in proestrus, estrus, and diestrus, but this requires a large number of animals. When multiple samples cannot be collected or handling stress is anticipated to induce acute endocrine changes, collection of trunk blood after decapitation at specific cycle stages may be helpful.

In NHPs, estradiol, progesterone, LH, and FSH measurements are of greatest value and a typical profile would include several samples spaced 2–3 days apart during the follicular and luteal phases with daily samples between days 10 and 16 to evaluate periovulatory surges in gonadotropins.

18.12 OVARIAN HISTOPATHOLOGY

18.12.1 Nonproliferative Changes

18.12.1.1 Hypoplasia

A failure of the PGCs to migrate to the genital ridge *in utero* results in a small ovary with stromal elements only. Without primordial follicles, there is no development of cycling structures (follicles or corpora lutea), systemic levels of estradiol and progesterone are low, and the uterus and vagina resemble a prepubertal state. Elevations in gonadotropins secondary to decreased negative feedback may stimulate the ovarian stroma. Ovarian hypoplasia has been observed on occasion (Vidal, personal observation) in nonclinical toxicology studies in both dogs and NHPs.

18.12.1.2 Atrophy

Ovarian atrophy is most easily recognized when it has reached an advanced stage and includes a number of features including small size, prominent stroma and interstitial glands, and an absence of antral follicles or corpora lutea. Small follicles may also be decreased or absent in senescence or menopause, but as long as there is a follicular reserve, growing pre-antral follicles may be evident as their development may occur independently of gonadotropin stimulation (McGee and Hsueh 2000).

Atrophy is the final stage observed in reproductive senescence or menopause but may also occur as a result of xenobiotic treatment that impairs or inhibits the normal production of gonadotropins and ovarian steroids. Atrophy may also result from direct damage to oocytes and granulosa cells, particularly in the small follicles, although less common in pharmaceutical development. This process has been well described as a consequence of exposure to both direct- and indirect-acting toxicants (Davis and Heindel 1998; Mattison 1993). Because the oocytes enclosed in the primordial follicles formed at birth are a nonrenewable population, agents that damage primordial follicles diminish the reproductive life span of the animal (Hirshfield 1997). Furthermore, the degree of damage to this population determines the rapidity with which follicular depletion and ovarian failure occur (Lohff et al. 2006). In short-term toxicity studies in rodents, early stages of xenobiotic-induced atrophy such as reduced follicular or luteal number or size may not be readily recognized in standard sections of the ovary (Yuan and Foley 2002). However, atrophy of the interstitial cells may be a useful indicator for hormonal dysregulation (Mirsky et al. 2011; Yuan and Foley 2002). In the dog, ovarian atrophy can be observed as an induced change after suppression of the estrus cycle by xenobiotics inhibiting FSH/LH secretion or activity such as by administration of progestogens (Murakoshi et al. 2000; Sahara et al. 1994), cell proliferation (important for follicular and luteal development), and estrogen modulators such as selective estrogen receptor modulators (SERMs) like tamoxifen or idoxifene (Brown et al. 1999a; Rehm et al. 2007a); however, clearly distinguishing between normal anestrus and xenobiotic-induced ovarian atrophy in the dog may be difficult or impossible in a standard nonclinical toxicology study. In the NHP, ovarian atrophy typically consists of a lack of dominant cycling structure (tertiary follicle or corpora luteum) with multiple variably atretic small follicles and as a result may look similar to non-ovulatory cycles.

Xenobiotic administration resulting in ovarian atrophy accompanied by uterine and vaginal atrophy suggests that there is inhibition of the production or actions of either gonadotrophs or ovarian steroids, or accelerated loss of oocytes and follicles. In contrast, the administration of exogenous hormones or their analogs may induce ovarian atrophy owing to feedback inhibition of gonadotroph secretion, while proliferative or hypertrophic responses are seen in the uterus or vagina in association with hormone receptor activation (Cartwright and Moreland 2008; Yuan and Foley 2002).

18.12.1.3   Follicular Atresia

As discussed earlier, follicles that fail to progress to ovulation undergo atresia and, indeed, this is the fate of the majority of developing ovarian follicles. A number of authors have discussed the morphology, classification, and progression of follicular atresia in the rodent (Braw and Tsafriri 1980; Byskov 1974; Hirshfield 1988; Osmun 1985). In the normal rodent ovary, follicular atresia occurs most commonly at the early antral stage (approximately 200–400 µm diameter in the rat) (Hirshfield and Midgley 1978) and the earliest light microscopic evidence of follicular atresia is the presence of individual apoptotic cells or pyknotic nuclei among the mural granulosa cells or within the antral space. Progression of atresia in granulosa cells is associated with an increase in apoptotic DNA fragmentation as well as a decrease in proliferative capacity as measured by bromodeoxyuridine incorporation (Durlinger et al. 2000). In NHPs, follicular atresia most often involves tertiary follicles and, to a lesser extent, secondary follicles (Buse et al. 2008), and as a result, follicular atresia is readily observed in the NHP and can be easily mistaken for a test article–related finding.

While follicular atresia is a normal part of ovarian physiology, it may also be seen as a result of xenobiotic treatment through a variety of mechanisms. Atresia of small (primordial or primary) follicles is not commonly observed in adult rodents (Fenwick and Hurst 2002) and is rarely encountered in pharmaceutical development. However, small ovarian follicles have been shown to be susceptible to damage by a number of cytotoxic and mutagenic agents used as chemotherapeutics, heavy metals, industrial chemicals, and irradiation (Generoso et al. 1971; Hooser et al. 1994; Hoyer 2004; Junaid et al. 1997; Nozaki et al. 2009; Plowchalk and Mattison 1992; Sakurada et al. 2009).

In contrast, atresia of larger growing follicles as a consequence of xenobiotic treatment is a relatively common event. Treatment-related atresia of medium or large antral follicles was recently reported in rats as a consequence of 2 or 4 weeks of treatment with a variety of ovarian toxicants exerting effects directly on follicular elements (e.g., cisplatin and cyclophosphamide) or indirectly as a result of metabolic or hormonal follicular dysregulation (e.g., indomethacin, EGME, tamoxifen, and mifepristone) (Sanbuissho et al. 2009).

18.12.1.4   Mineralization

In NHPs, focal or multifocal mineralization of primary follicles can often be seen as an incidental finding within the ovarian cortex and has no known functional significance (Cline et al. 2008; Majeed and Gopinath 1980).

18.12.1.5   Cysts

Cysts in and around the ovary are common background findings that have been well described in a variety of species (Cline et al. 2008; Cooper and Gabrielson 2007; Davis et al. 1999; Maekawa et al.

1996; Marr-Belvin et al. 2010; Montgomery and Alison 1987; Peluso and Gordon 1992). The incidence of ovarian cysts in rodents is strain dependent and increases with age. Cysts can arise from cycling ovarian structures (follicles or corpora lutea), rete ovarii, surface epithelium, SESs, ovarian bursa, or embryonic remnants.

The dominant features of follicular cysts include an enlarged antrum with an attenuated lining of one to several layers of flattened to cuboidal granulosa cells with varying degrees of degeneration. The antrum may appear to be empty or contain homogeneous, pale, acidophilic residue or blood; scattered cell debris; a degenerate oocyte; or vacuolated or pigment-laden macrophages. The theca is often recognizable in smaller cysts but, with enlargement, the theca becomes obscure and the cyst is encircled by a thin fibrous coat. In large follicular cysts, the antrum may be lined by a single layer of flattened cells lacking any features indicative of a follicular origin.

The majority of cysts observed in cycling female rodents are derived from ovarian follicles that fail to ovulate and transitional stages have been described (Brawer et al. 1989). While non-ovulatory follicular cysts are sporadically seen in young females, they become more common in middle age as hormonal dysregulation leads to lengthening of the estrous cycle and the onset of periods of persistent estrus. These follicular cysts form against a background of altered responsiveness of GnRH regulatory pathways to ovarian steroids and delay or attenuation of the LH surge (Gore et al. 2000; Lederman et al. 2010; Neal-Perry and Santoro 2006; Peluso et al. 1979; Temel et al. 2002). A low level of ongoing cell proliferation in combination with decreased expression of apoptotic factors may contribute to the persistence of follicular cysts once formed (Salvetti et al. 2009). In aged (≥18 months) female rodents, cysts derived from other structures become more common as the growth and development of the remaining follicles wane in the final stages of reproductive senescence. When cysts are observed in the ovary, their origin (the structure from which they developed) should be determined, if possible, as this may aid in identifying the mechanism underlying their development. In some cases, particularly in aged rodents, the origin of the cyst may not be obvious and it may be termed a "Cyst, NOS" or "cyst, not otherwise specified."

When the majority of cells lining the lumen of a follicular cyst are luteinized, the cyst may be referred to as a luteinized follicular cyst or luteinized unruptured follicle. These luteinized non-ovulatory follicular structures appear to be steroidogenically active in rodents as in other species (Plas-Roser 1984; Westfahl 1993).

True corpus luteum cysts (also referred to as luteal cysts or cystic corpora lutea) that arise after ovulation and that are also steroidogenically active are rarely observed as spontaneous findings in rodents (Montgomery and Alison 1987); however, normally developing corpora lutea of metestrus often display a central cavity (Westwood 2008), and in rare cases, these central cavities may persist into diestrus in control rats (Yoshida et al. 2009). In addition, luteolysis during a normal proestrus may give the appearance of a central cavity and mimic a cystic change. In some cases, these changes may be difficult to distinguish from luteinized follicles and true cystic corpora lutea. When an oocyte is evident within the lumen of the luteinized structure, recognizing its origin as a non-ovulatory or anovulatory follicle is straightforward. McEntee (1990b) used the presence of a zone of fibrous tissue between the luteal cells and cyst lumen to classify cystic luteinized structures as corpus luteum cysts; however, non-ovulatory luteinized follicular cysts and incomplete corpora lutea in rodents may exhibit a similar appearance (Walker et al. 1988; Yuan and Foley 2002). When it is not possible to clearly distinguish corpus luteum cysts and luteinized follicular (non-ovulatory) cysts in routine histologic sections, use of the term "luteinized cyst" may be more appropriate.

Follicular cysts have been reported after treatment with a number of xenobiotics having distinct actions (Figure 18.29). While most of these xenobiotics alter the normal estrous cycle, there is no single factor that has been consistently reported to underlie cyst development, but dysregulation of circulating gonadotropin levels (particularly LH), an increased estrogen/progesterone ratio,

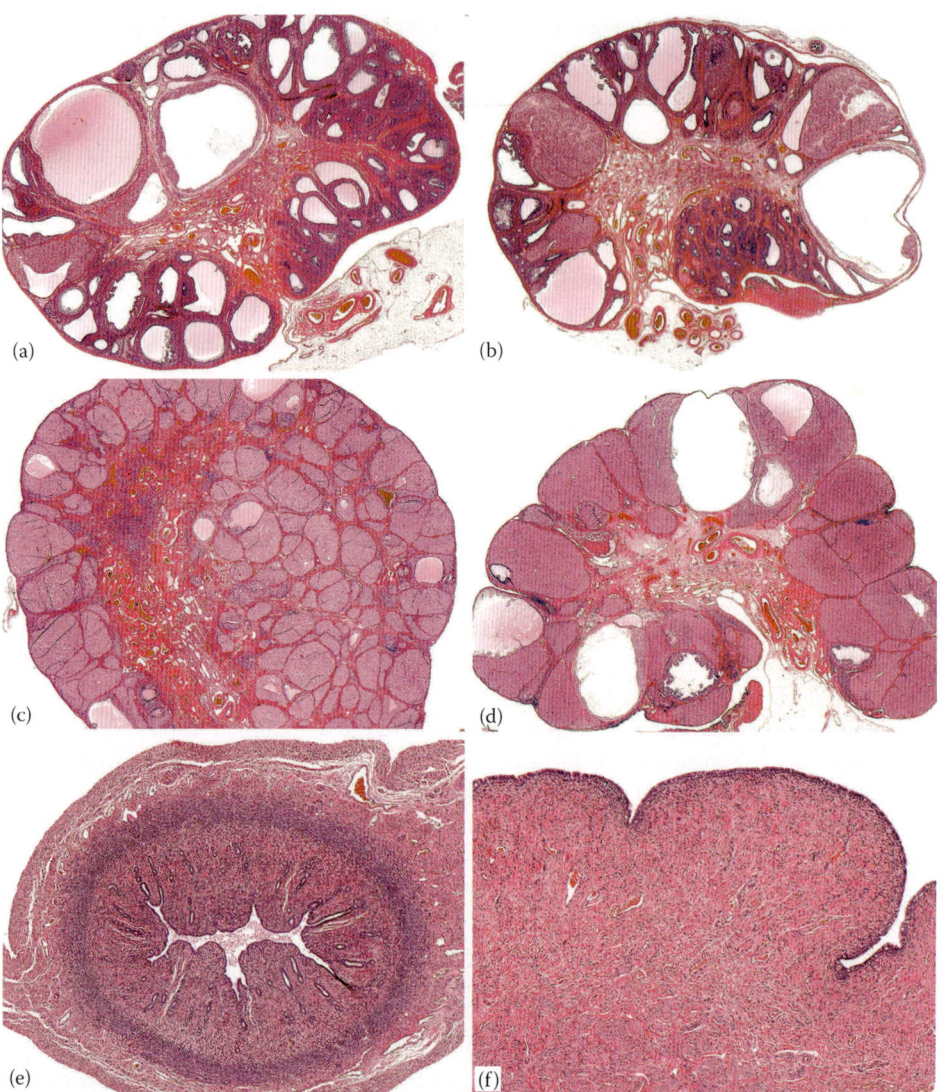

FIGURE 18.29 (a–d) Canine ovaries after various doses of an aromatase inhibitor for 6 months, with varying degrees of abnormal follicular development, cystic follicles, luteal cysts, and abnormal corpora lutea. (e) Canine uterus after 6 months' administration of an aromatase inhibitor showing lack of endometrial glands, myometrial atrophy, and a small amount of proteinaceous luminal content. (f) Canine vagina after 6 months' administration of an aromatase inhibitor—anestrus appearance.

and increased levels of circulating androgens commonly occur in association with cyst formation. Aromatase inhibitors that prevent the conversion of androgens to estrogens consistently induce the development of follicular cysts in rodents and dogs and are generally associated with increased circulating LH, FSH, and androgens and decreased estradiol and progesterone (Arthur et al. 1989; Kafali et al. 2004; Matsuda et al. 1997; Shirai et al. 2009). In contrast, cysts induced by the estrogen analog, estradiol valerate, were associated with low LH in association with high levels of FSH similar to those expected at proestrus (Grosser et al. 1987). Other classes of xenobiotics that induce ovarian cysts include dopamine antagonists (Ishii et al. 2009; Ota et al. 1986), dopamine agonists (Greaves 2007), nonsteroidal anti-inflammatory drugs (NSAIDs) (Gaytán et al. 2003; Tsubota et al.

2009; Walker et al. 1988), SERMs (Cohen et al. 2000; Tsujioka et al. 2009), progesterone receptor antagonists (van der Schoot et al. 1987), and platinum-based chemotherapeutics (Borovskaya et al. 2004; Yeh et al. 2009). Most of these types of compounds clearly have the capacity to alter follicular development through disruption of hormonal regulation or the metabolic responses thereto. When prominent luteinization of non-ovulatory follicular cysts is observed, this may indicate effects on pathways regulating ovulation, as noted with progesterone receptor antagonists, NSAIDs, and peroxisome proliferator-activated receptor agonists (Gaytán et al. 2003; Kim et al. 2008; Sánchez-Criado et al. 1993; Sato et al. 2009; Tsubota et al. 2009).

Cysts derived from embryonic remnants of the mesonephric tubules (rete ovarii) or mesonephric ducts are commonly observed in many species (Cline et al. 2008; Long 2002; McEntee 1990b; Marr-Belvin et al. 2010; Wenzel and Odend'hal 1985). Cysts arising from the rete ovarii are lined by cuboidal to columnar and sometimes ciliated epithelium surrounded by fine fibrous connective tissue and are often observed within the medulla/hilus but may extend into the adjacent mesovarium and fat. Cysts arising from the mesonephric ducts are similar in appearance but confined to the mesovarium and surrounded by a thin layer of smooth muscle fibers and are often referred to as parovarian or paraovarian cysts. Cysts may vary in size from microscopic dilation with little functional consequence to large macroscopically evident structures that distort or even obliterate normal ovarian architecture. Cysts arising from embryonic remnants are especially common in NHPs and aging mice (Cline et al. 2008; Long 2002). Cysts arising from vestiges of the paramesonephric duct system may also be observed in the mesosalpinx and broad ligament of the uterus.

Epithelial inclusion cysts, lined by a single layer of cuboidal or flattened epithelium, may be located in the center of the ovary or in the cortex and like other cysts are more frequently observed in older rodents. Some of these cysts may be derived from invaginations of the ovarian surface epithelium, but more recent observations suggest that the majority are continuous with the rete duct system (Burdette et al. 2007; Davis et al. 1999; Fleming et al. 2007; Long 2002; Peluso and Gordon 1992).

In dogs, cysts arising from the surface epithelium and SESs are observed in the outer cortex, are usually rather small (approximately 5 mm), and are lined by a thin, single-layered cuboidal epithelium. SES cysts are sensitive to hormonal influences and, therefore, may potentially be seen as an induced change.

Cysts may arise from the ovarian bursa in rodents and dogs and are more common in aged animals. These can most easily be observed macroscopically as tissue handling and processing may cause collapse of the bursal cyst.

Epidermoid cysts have been infrequently reported in rodents, though Maekawa et al. (1996) considered these to be common in mice. Epidermoid cysts are lined by stratified squamous epithelium and are usually filled with keratin. An association with teratomas has been reported by some authors (Davis et al. 1999; Greaves 2007). In humans, these cysts have been considered to be of heterogeneous origin, possibly arising as highly differentiated or poorly sampled teratomas, metaplastic foci originating from ovarian surface epithelium, or areas of metaplasia in foci of endometriosis (Khedmati et al. 2009; Nogales and Silverberg 1976).

18.12.1.6 Polyovular Follicles

Ovarian follicles containing more than one oocyte are occasionally observed in a wide range of mammalian species (Mossman and Duke 1973). The mechanism underlying the formation of these polyovular (or multi-oocyte) follicles is not clear, but they are occasionally observed in some strains of mice, young dogs, and rhesus macaques. In the rodent, follicles are formed in the perinatal period as germ cell nests break down and individual oocytes associate with somatic pre-granulosa cells. It has been suggested that follicles containing more than one oocyte arise through incomplete separation of germ cell nests or because of developmental differences in oocytes and somatic cells at the time of segregation (Bristol-Gould and Woodruff 2006). Polyovular follicles have been reported in transgenic mice overexpressing the inhibin α subunit (McMullen et al. 2001) as well as disruption of Dmrt4, a zinc finger-like DNA binding motif (Balciuniene et al. 2006). Increased polyovular

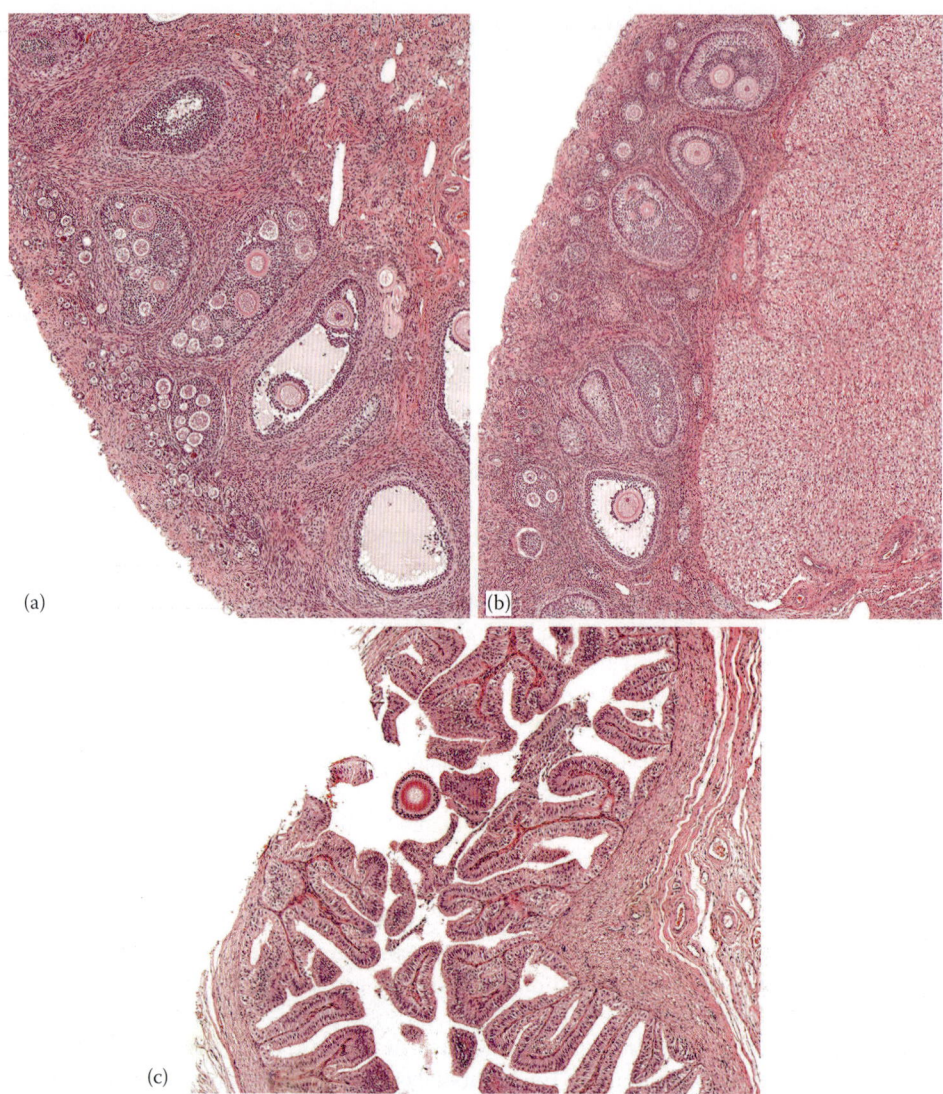

(a)

(b)

(c)

FIGURE 18.30 (a) Polyovular follicles—immature ovary (dog). (b) Polyovular follicles—anestrus (dog). Note the presence of corpus luteum/albicans. (c) Mature ovum within uterine tube during late estrus/early diestrus (dog).

follicles have been reported after xenobiotic exposure that induces hormonal dysregulation during the fetal or perinatal period and, in particular, disruption of estrogen signaling pathways (Iguchi et al. 1986, 1988; Jefferson et al. 2007; Kirigaya et al. 2009; Rodriguez et al. 2010). In dogs, developing follicles may contain more than one oocyte, particularly in the early stages of follicular development (Figure 18.30a and b). In younger animals, the incidence of growing follicles containing two or more oocytes ranges between 14% and 40%, in bitches of 1 to 2 years of age (McDougall et al. 1997; Payan-Carreira and Pires 2008; Telfer and Gosden 1987). In rhesus macaques, the number of polyovular follicles increases after exposure to exogenous FSH (van Wagenen and Simpson 1973).

18.12.1.7   Absence of Recent (Basophilic) Corpora Lutea

Differences in the appearance of the most recent cohort of corpora lutea and those of earlier cohorts in the rodent have been discussed above. In the evaluation of short-term nonclinical studies, the absence of recent corpora lutea can be an early feature of hormonal dysregulation. Reliable detection of this finding usually requires that treatment be sustained for at least 5 days to ensure that all animals have gone through an entire estrous cycle. In routine sections, basophilic corpora lutea may not be observed in individual animals owing to variability in sampling and slide preparation. However, an absence of basophilic corpora lutea in most or all animals of a treated cohort is suggestive of anovulation as an effect of treatment and frequently occurs in association with noncyclical changes in the vaginal epithelium.

18.12.1.8 Changes in Size/Number of Corpora Lutea

Increased size/numbers of corpora lutea may be indicative of altered regulation of prolactin secretion. As discussed earlier, the surge of prolactin during proestrus induces regression of previous generations of corpora lutea (Rehm et al. 2007c; Wuttke and Meites 1971). Inhibition of the proestrus prolactin surge using bromocriptine or other dopamine agonists will result in the accumulation of increased numbers of corpora lutea without an increase in luteal size (Kumazawa et al. 2009; Rehm et al. 2007c; Wuttke and Meites 1971). As prolactin is also luteotrophic, xenobiotics that induce sustained increases in prolactin levels, such as dopamine antagonists, will also increase the numbers of corpora lutea in the ovary. As these corpora lutea are actively producing progesterone, they often attain a size greater than the corpora lutea of the regularly cycling female rodent (Ishii et al. 2009; Rehm et al. 2007c; Taketa et al. 2011). The presence of increased and enlarged functional corpora lutea has also been observed in rodents after treatment with chemicals such as EGME or atrazine (Davis et al. 1997; Taketa et al. 2011). Recent evidence suggests that EGME promotes luteal survival and progesterone production indirectly through upregulation of prolactin secretion while the effects of atrazine appear to be independent of prolactin (Taketa et al. 2011).

18.12.1.9 Degeneration and Hemorrhage within Corpora Lutea

Normal morphological development and endocrine function of the corpus luteum are dependent on the rapid ingrowth of thecal blood vessels that occurs after ovulation (Ferrara et al. 1998). Inhibition of angiogenesis has been shown to lead to both morphological and functional alterations in the corpus luteum with secondary effects in the uterus and vagina (Ferrara et al. 1998; Patyna et al. 2008; Ryan et al. 1999). In the rat, this has resulted in lower ovarian weight and decreased numbers of corpora lutea, often with central degeneration/necrosis in the most recent cohort of corpora lutea (Figure 18.31a) (Ferrara et al. 1998; Patyna et al. 2008). In the rat, care should be taken to distinguish central degeneration/necrosis from newly formed corpora lutea during estrus/metestrus, luteinized follicular cysts, luteal cysts, and luteolysis during normal proestrus (Figures 18.19 and 18.31). In the NHP, absence of active corpora lutea, decreased numbers of developing follicles, and increased numbers of atretic follicles in the ovaries were observed with associated uterine atrophy (Patyna et al. 2008; Ryan et al. 1999). Pharmacologic inhibition of angiogenesis, as well as other oncology targets, often involves inhibition of a spectrum of receptor tyrosine kinases with differing effects on corpus luteum function and development (Yaghmaei et al. 2009). In these cases, the corpora lutea can be enlarged with an increase in ovarian weight, may be fewer in number, and often contain varying amounts of central hemorrhage (Figure 18.31c), with or without interstitial or bursal hemorrhage (Sleer and Taylor 2007; Yaghmaei et al. 2009).

18.12.1.10 Interstitial Glands

The interstitial glands (or secondary interstitial cells) formed from the theca-interstitial cells that persist after follicular atresia remain responsive to LH stimulation and continue to produce androstenedione (Erickson et al. 1985). In normally cycling rodents, the interstitial glands are composed of small polygonal cells with eosinophilic lightly granular cytoplasm that are arranged in solid nests or cords. After xenobiotic-induced hormone disruption, these cells may rapidly atrophy, becoming small with elongated condensed nuclei and scant cytoplasm (Mirsky et al. 2011; Yuan and Foley 2002). Hypertrophy and hyperplasia of interstitial cells are common findings in the ovaries of aging rodents (Alison et al. 1990; Davis et al. 1999). Interstitial cell hypertrophy and hyperplasia may occur after the administration of anti-estrogens owing to increased levels of gonadotropins and

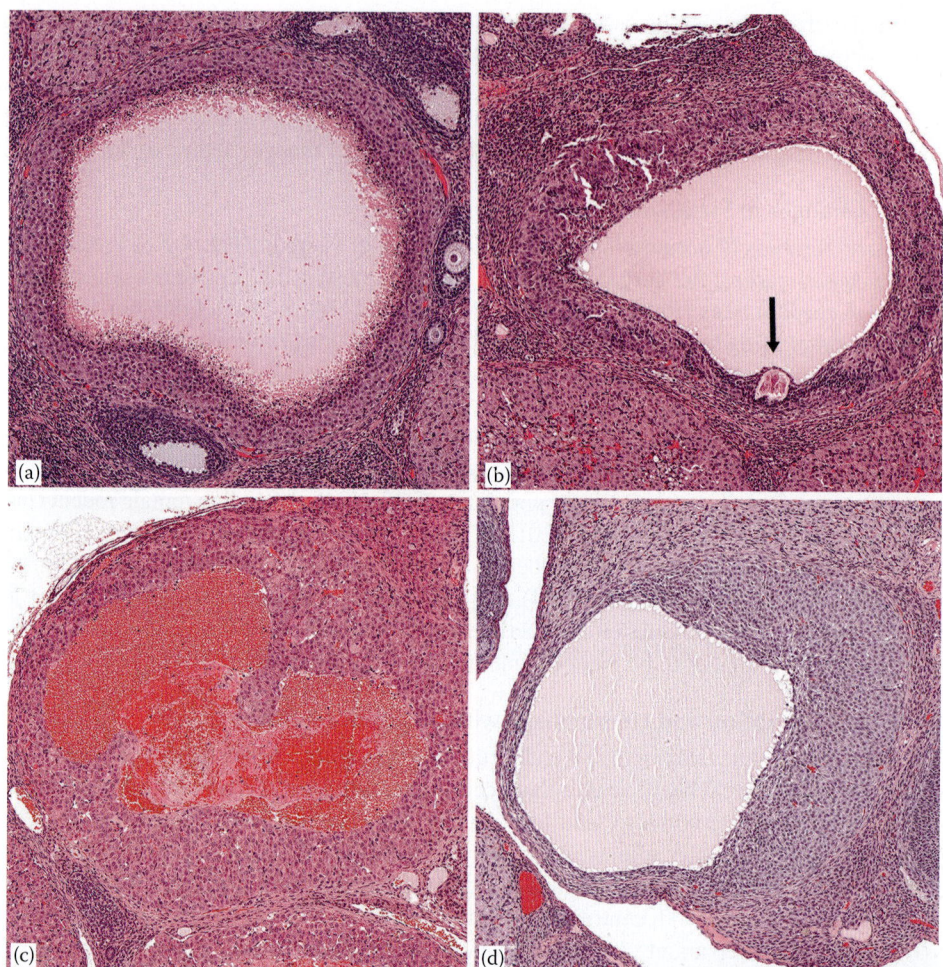

FIGURE 18.31 (a) Corpus luteum with prominent central degeneration from a rat given a vascular endothelial growth factor inhibitor. (b) Luteinized follicular cyst. Note the variable luteinization of the granulosa cells and the presence of an oocyte (arrow). (c) Corpus luteum with prominent central hemorrhage from a rat given a receptor tyrosine kinase inhibitor. (d) Luteal cyst.

other alterations of the hypothalamic–pituitary–ovarian axis (Peluso and Gordon 1992; Sourla et al. 1997). Vinclozolin (a pesticide with anti-androgenic properties) has also been reported to cause ovarian interstitial cell hyperplasia in the absence of detectable effects on gonadotropins or ovarian steroids, but in association with decreased thyroid hormones (Matsuura et al. 2005).

18.12.2 PROLIFERATIVE CHANGES

Hyperplastic and neoplastic changes in the ovary are generally classified according to the cell of origin and include those arising from the epithelium, sex cord stroma, or germ cells.

18.12.2.1 Epithelial Proliferative Changes

Hyperplastic and neoplastic lesions of epithelial origin can arise from the surface epithelium and often form multiple papillary fronds and cystic structures. These changes can range from focal papillary hyperplasia to cystadenomas and cystadenocarcinomas. Cystadenomas/adenocarcinomas are frequently observed in mice but are uncommon in rats (Alison et al. 1987; Lewis 1987).

Hyperplasia of the surface epithelium with or without papillary infoldings has been reported fairly consistently in dogs given estrogenic compounds and is often associated with ovarian atrophy (Brown et al. 1999a; Rehm et al. 2007a). This change may also be seen in the uterus of dogs with effects observed in the ovaries.

In mice, an epithelial proliferative lesion may be observed with an admixed population of stromal elements and is termed tubulostromal hyperplasia/adenoma/adenocarcinoma (Alison et al. 1987). This change consists of downgrowths of surface epithelium with interspersed aggregates of variably luteinized stromal cells. Tubulostromal adenomas/adenocarcinomas are commonly reported as both a spontaneous and xenobiotic-induced finding in mice and may be related to elevations in gonadotropins as germ cell–deficient mice develop tubulostromal adenomas at a younger age than controls (Alison et al. 1987; Dixon et al. 1999; Duncan and Chada 1993).

18.12.2.2 Sex Cord-Stromal Proliferative Changes

Proliferative changes arising from sex cord-stromal elements are one of the most common types observed in nonclinical species (Alison et al. 1987; Dixon et al. 1999; Lewis 1987). Stromal hyperplasia, with varying degrees of luteinization, is a commonly observed age-related change and can be seen secondary to elevations in gonadotropins during anestrus or menopause. Tumors arising from sex cord stroma often have distinct features and may be classified on the basis of cell of origin and include granulosa cell tumors, thecal cell tumors, and Sertoli cell tumors. Granulosa cell tumors are the most commonly observed primary ovarian tumor in rodents and have also been observed in dogs and NHPs (Alison et al. 1987; Cline et al. 2008; Dixon et al. 1999; Kennedy et al. 1994; Lewis 1987). Granulosa cell tumors can rarely be seen in bitches as young as 14 months and are observed on occasion as spontaneous ovarian tumors in toxicology studies (Figure 18.32) (McEntee 1990a).

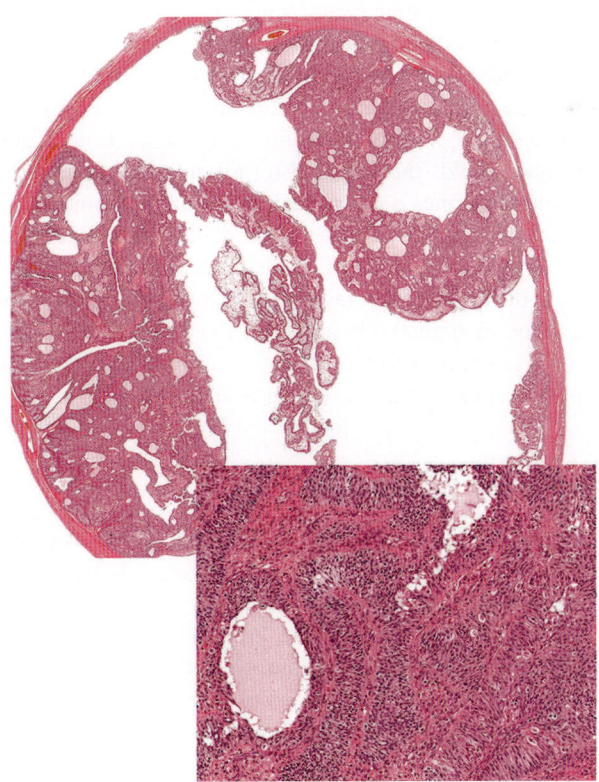

FIGURE 18.32 Ovary—benign granulosa cell tumor (Sertoli cell type) in a young beagle dog.

The majority (approximately 80%) are benign (Dow 1960; Norris et al. 1970) and unilateral. In practice, it may be difficult to distinguish these different subclassifications and a diagnosis of mixed sex cord-stromal tumor can be used.

18.12.2.3 Germ Cell Tumors

Tumors arising from germ cells include teratomas, dysgerminomas, and yolk sac carcinomas. Most germ cell tumors are only sporadically observed, but teratomas have occasionally been reported in most species (Alison et al. 1987; Cline et al. 2008; Dixon et al. 1999; Kennedy et al. 1994; Lewis 1987).

18.12.2.4 Other Proliferative Changes

A variety of other proliferative changes can be identified in the ovary including rete hyperplasia/adenoma, hemangioma, fibroma, and mesothelioma. Fibromas, an unusual tumor type in the canine ovary, have been seen with an increased incidence in old dogs given mibolerone (a non-progestational androgenic steroid) for over 9 years at efficacious doses, though not at suprapharmacologic doses (Seaman 1985). The tumors were observed as single or multiple firm, rounded or sometimes bilateral nodular masses in the medulla or hilar region of the ovary. In addition, proliferative changes have been identified in the smooth muscle extending from the hilus of the ovary into the mesovarium, and rats treated with various β-receptor agonists have developed mesovarial leiomyomas (Gopinath and Gibson 1987; Jack et al. 1983).

18.13 HISTOPATHOLOGY OF THE UTERINE TUBE

The anatomy of the uterine tube poses some problems for routine examination in nonclinical toxicity studies. Because of its coiled structure and segmental variability, even slight differences in tissue trimming and preparation make consistent examination of the uterine tube difficult. This inconsistency decreases the likelihood that subtle treatment-related changes will be recognized and, indeed, morphological effects of xenobiotic treatment in the rodent uterine tube have been infrequently reported. However, the uterine tube expresses receptors for ovarian steroids and prolactin and receptor expression changes with development and functional state (Okada et al. 2003; Shao et al. 2008). Therefore, hormone disruption holds the potential for altering the appearance of the uterine tube. The administration of chlorcyclizine, a compound with antihistamine and hypocholesterolemic properties, induced atrophy of the uterine tube in association with other changes consistent with hormonal dysregulation (Hruban et al. 1972). Estrogen receptor modulators have also been shown to cause various changes in the uterine tube; tamoxifen induced epithelial vacuolation, while clomiphene administration resulted in epithelial hyperplasia and apoptosis (Brown et al. 1999b; Shao et al. 2009). Methotrexate can cause inflammation of the uterine tube in association with changes in estrogen and progesterone receptor expression (Yang et al. 2009).

18.14 HISTOPATHOLOGY OF THE UTERUS

The physiology and function of the uterus and vagina are largely driven by ovarian steroids. Receptors for estrogen, progesterone, and androgens have been identified in the epithelium, stroma, and smooth muscle of the rodent uterus and vagina, and their expression across the estrous cycle has been detailed (Ohta et al. 1993; Pelletier et al. 2000; Pessina et al. 2006; Tibbetts et al. 1998; Wang et al. 2000). Furthermore, mice with defined mutations in the genes for these hormone receptors have been developed to better understand both the actions mediated by the various steroid hormones and their analogs as well as the role that the various receptor isoforms play in the reproductive tract (Hewitt and Korach 2003; Mulac-Jericevic and Conneely 2004; Walters et al. 2010). As a result of this hormonal dependence, most of the changes typically observed in these organs as a result of aging or toxicity are secondary to hormonal dysregulation.

18.14.1   Nonproliferative Changes

18.14.1.1   Uterine Atrophy

Atrophy of the uterus is a common finding in association with reproductive senescence and ovarian failure, resulting in the loss of ovarian steroids; ovariectomy will induce a similar change. The uterus is decreased in size and weight and the endometrium and myometrium are attenuated; the luminal epithelium is low columnar, endometrial glands are decreased in number or absent, smooth muscle cells of the myometrium are decreased in size, and, over time, there is progressive replacement of the endometrial stroma by collagen (Alison et al. 1990; Davis et al. 1999). Atrophy of the uterus may also occur as a result of xenobiotic damage. Agents that damage follicles directly, such as cyclophosphamide, may induce uterine atrophy secondary to ovarian failure (Plowchalk and Mattison 1992). Other compounds may prevent the production of ovarian steroids or inhibit their receptor binding. Aromatase inhibitors prevent the conversion of androgens to estrogens and induce uterine atrophy when administered to rodents (Steele et al. 1987; Yano et al. 1996). SERMs may also induce uterine atrophy in mice and rats, though there are differences in the affected uterine compartments on the basis of species, dose, and duration of administration (Carthew et al. 1996; Greaves et al. 1993; Nephew et al. 2000). Long-term administration of progestational compounds has also been shown to induce uterine atrophy (Bhowmik and Mukherjea 1988).

18.14.1.2   Uterine Luminal Dilation

The uterine lumen in rodents is normally dilated on the day of proestrus as a result of fluid accumulation. Fluid accumulation occurs in response to increasing levels of estrogen beginning in late diestrus while increasing progesterone on proestrus promotes fluid resorption, and these effects are mediated through steroid-driven changes in ion transport (Armstrong 1968; Salleh et al. 2005). Pathological luminal dilation (hydrometra) is a fairly common finding in aged rodents in association with altered hormonal regulation of the reproductive tract (Brown and Leininger 1992; Maekawa and Maita 1996). On occasion, treatment with xenobiotics may induce uterine luminal dilation as a result of systemic hormonal dysregulation, progesterone receptor antagonism, and direct modulation of the ion transporter mechanisms (Gopinath 1992; Mirsky et al. 2011; van der Schoot et al. 1987; Walker et al. 1988). In young adult rodents (<6 months of age) in particular, effects of treatment must be distinguished from normal cyclical changes in the uterus.

18.14.1.3   Endometrial Glandular Dilation

Focal dilation of uterine glands is occasionally observed as a spontaneous finding in rodents. Typically, only a small number of glands are affected, but this change may be extensive in association with dilation of the uterine lumen during proestrus. Affected glands are lined by attenuated or flattened epithelium because of luminal distension by serous or proteinaceous residue. Differentiation from cystic glandular hyperplasia is based on the absence of glandular epithelial proliferation.

18.14.1.4   Inflammation

The endometrium normally contains neutrophils, lymphocytes, and macrophages within the stroma. In rodents, the numbers of these inflammatory cells vary with the stage of the estrous cycle, and studies in ovariectomized rodents have shown that they increase in response to estrogen and decrease in response to progesterone (Tibbets et al. 1998). The influx of inflammatory cells, particularly neutrophils, in response to estrogen during estrus and metestrus may be rather florid and should not be misinterpreted as endometritis (Cartwright and Moreland 2008; Yuan and Carlson 1985). In NHPs and humans, unique granular lymphocytes termed endometrial lymphocytes or endometrial granulocytes increase in numbers during the luteal phase (King et al. 1996; van Esch et al. 2008). In addition, varying amounts of inflammation normally occur within the endometrium during menses. Inflammation of the uterus is an unusual finding in nonparous laboratory animals in nonclinical toxicology studies, though it has been reported in association with endometrial hyperplasia or persistent vaginal septum (Brown and Leininger 1992; De Schaepdrijver et al. 1995; Lezmi et al. 2010). Administration of compounds with hormonal activity, particularly estrogens, may induce endometritis and pyometra (Cline et al. 2004; Gopinath 1992; Greenman and Fullerton 1986; Ramos et al. 2005).

18.14.1.5 Anovulatory and Irregular Cycles in NHPs

The cycles after menarche are often long and irregular, and in rhesus macaques, only 15% are reported to have ovulated in the first five cycles after menarche (Resko et al. 1982). These anovulatory cycles may be associated with uterine bleeding, which, while not often clinically apparent, may be observed using vaginal swabs, during histologic evaluation of the uterus, or as contamination of a urine sample, and mistaken for menses. Histologically, there are often small amounts of hemorrhage in the endometrium or uterine lumen with a weakly proliferative phase appearance to the endometrium without the secretory phase pattern and endometrial shedding characteristic of normal menses (Figure 18.27a). This is similar to the glandular and stromal breakdown with hemorrhage that is commonly observed during anovulatory cycles around menarche in humans (Strickland and Wall 2003). In addition, there is a lack of a regressing corpus luteum suggesting anovulation and often the ovary will display multiple small- to medium-sized variably atretic tertiary follicles (Figure 18.27b). This appearance of the ovaries and endometrium is especially common in NHPs used in a nonclinical toxicology setting as many are young and have only recently reached menarche.

Anovulatory cycles and cycle irregularity also occur in mature cycling female NHPs and are often related to social interactions. Subordinate animals have a higher incidence of anovulatory cycles and luteal phase defects, and randomization prior to study start will disrupt established hierarchy. In one study, changes from single to group housing increased cycle length from 31 to 46 days for a period of 6 months (Weinbauer et al. 2008). Histologically, this can be observed as animals lacking a clear menstrual phase, endometria with a weak secretory phase pattern, or as described above for anovulatory cycles.

18.14.1.6 Squamous Metaplasia of the Endometrium

Squamous metaplasia occurs as a spontaneous finding in aging rats and mice and is often observed in association with endometrial hyperplasia or uterine inflammation (Baldrick and Reeve 2007; Brix et al. 2005; Gopinath 1992; Maekawa and Maita 1996). Glandular epithelium is more commonly affected, though luminal epithelium may also be involved, particularly in association with suppurative endometritis. In young rats, squamous metaplasia has been reported in the glandular or luminal epithelium in the transition zone of the endocervix (Cartwright and Moreland 2008); however, this may represent normal variation in the anatomy of this zone during the estrous cycle. Squamous metaplasia of the endometrium has also been recognized in rodents as a result of vitamin A deficiency, or in response to treatment with estrogens, the anti-estrogen tamoxifen, or oral contraceptive drugs (Greaves 2007; Karlsson et al. 1998; Mäntylä et al. 1996). Recent work in transgenic mice suggests that estrogen-mediated metaplasia of the uterine epithelium is related to altered expression and regulation of transcription factor p63 and beta-catenin (Kurita 2011).

In dogs, squamous metaplasia of the surface or glandular epithelium, inflammation, edema, increased endometrial collagen, luminal dilation, glandular atrophy, and cystic glands have all been reported in varying combinations with xenobiotics having estrogenic activity on the canine uterus (Brown et al. 1999a; Jabara 1962; Rehm et al. 2007a).

18.14.1.7 Uterine Adenomyosis

Adenomyosis is the presence of otherwise normal-appearing clusters of endometrial glands deep within the myometrium. The glands do not extend beyond the uterine serosa, differentiating this condition from endometriosis in primates. Adenomyosis is infrequent in rats but may be seen with some frequency in certain strains of mice (Maekawa and Maita 1996). For instance, CD-1 mice are reported to have a high incidence of uterine adenomyosis after 6 months of age (Greaves and White 2006). The development of adenomyosis in adult rodents has been attributed, at least in part, to disruption of the hormonal regulation of the uterus, but the pathogenesis of the condition is not well understood (Greaves and White 2006). Adenomyosis has often been reported in rodents after the exposure of neonates to estrogens, anti-estrogens, or other endocrine-disrupting compounds. Adult rodents appear to be more resistant to developing adenomyosis in response to xenobiotics, though it has been induced after prolonged exposure to exogenous estrogen or high levels of progestins or prolactin (Greaves and White 2006; Lipschutz et al. 1967; Mori et al. 1991). In NHPs, small foci of adenomyosis may occur as an isolated spontaneous finding or may be present in conjunction with endometriosis. Adenomyosis may also occur secondary to chronic administration of hormonally active xenobiotics including estrogens and the androgenic anabolic steroid nandrolone decanoate (Baskin et al. 2002; Obasanjo et al. 1998). In dogs, adenomyosis has been reported as an infrequent spontaneous finding in the beagle (Kim et al. 2010); it has also been reported accompanying cystic endometrial hyperplasia induced by chronic progestin administration (Johnson 1989).

18.14.1.8 Endometriosis

Endometriosis is a common disorder in rhesus and cynomolgus macaques and is defined as the presence of endometrial glands and stroma exterior to the uterus. Hysterectomy and chronic treatment with estrogens have been demonstrated to increase the incidence of endometriosis in rhesus macaques (Hadfield et al. 1997). Although endometriosis has been reported in some colonies with an incidence as high as 30% (Ami et al. 1993; Zondervan et al. 2004), it is rarely observed in young cynomolgus macaques that are used in nonclinical toxicology testing.

18.14.2 PROLIFERATIVE CHANGES

18.14.2.1 Decidual Reaction of the Uterus (Deciduoma)

Decidual reactions (deciduomas) are non-neoplastic growths occurring in the uterus of the nonpregnant rodent (Brown and Leininger 1992; Elcock et al. 1987; Gopinath 1992; Maekawa and Maita 1996; Ohta 1987). Decidual reactions are dependent on a progesterone-dominant hormonal milieu and usually occur in response to mechanical irritation of the endometrium (which may include palpation). Most decidual reactions occur during early pseudopregnancy when the endometrium is primed for stromal differentiation and epithelial proliferation. However, a low incidence of decidual reactions has been reported to occur spontaneously. In the rodent, decidual reactions are nodular, polypoid, or diffuse growths with a highly organized structure similar to the metrial gland of pregnancy that may extend into the myometrium (Elcock et al. 1987; Picut et al. 2009; Velardo et al. 1953). Though rare in nonclinical safety studies, decidual reactions have sporadically occurred in young rats in studies of up to 6 months' duration, as well as in aged mice. Once formed, decidual reactions in the rat typically persist for 8–14 days, after which they regress.

18.14.2.2 Endometrial Hyperplasia

Cystic endometrial hyperplasia is a fairly common spontaneous finding in older rats and mice. The incidence of this finding is related to strain in both species, increases with age, and, in mice, may approach 100% by early middle age in genetically predisposed animals (Brix et al. 2005; Brown and Leininger 1992; Davis et al. 1999). In rats, cystic endometrial hyperplasia is usually diffuse and the development of this lesion has been described by Leininger and Jokinen (1990). Early changes include an increase in the size and number of glands lined by crowded epithelium with many mitoses. With progression, the glands become tortuous and dilated, the stroma becomes increasingly collagenous, and, finally, the epithelium becomes somewhat attenuated and less crowded, though the glandular cysts remain. In mice, similar changes occur though mitotic activity is variable and stratification of the glandular epithelium has also been described (Davis et al. 1999; Maekawa and

Maita 1996). Adenomyosis may occur in association with cystic endometrial hyperplasia, particularly in mice. In aging rats, development of spontaneous cystic endometrial hyperplasia appears to be related to prolonged hormonal stimulation and is frequently observed in association with ovarian cysts; in aging mice, a relationship to prolonged estrogen stimulation is less clear (Davis et al. 1999; Greaves and Faccini 1984). The development of xenobiotic-induced cystic endometrial hyperplasia in rodents has largely been recognized and studied in animals exposed *in utero*, prepubertally, or after ovariectomy (Kumasaka et al. 1994; Tang et al. 1984; Wordinger and Morrill 1985). In adult mice, cystic endometrial hyperplasia was reported after chronic treatment with diethylstilbestrol or 17β-estradiol (Greenman and Fullerton 1986; Greenman et al. 1983; Highman et al. 1978). In short-term studies of 1–3 months in adult rats, compounds with estrogenic activity typically induce hypertrophy of the luminal or glandular epithelium (mainly increased epithelial height) in association with myometrial hypertrophy, increased uterine weight, decreased ovarian weight, and increased vaginal epithelial thickness (Andrews et al. 2002; Attia and Zayed 1989; Biegel et al. 1998; Okazaki et al. 2001; Yamasaki et al. 2002). In rhesus and cynomolgus macaques, endometrial hyperplasia has been reported as a common finding secondary to administration of various estrogenic xenobiotics (Baskin et al. 2002; Cline et al. 2008).

Endometrial stromal hyperplasia is a common spontaneous finding in aged mice and has also been reported in F344 rats (Leininger and Jokinen 1990; Reuber et al. 1981). Histologically, the endometrium is hypercellular because of an increase in spindle- or stellate-shaped stromal cells; mitotic figures may be prominent. Typically, the endometrial architecture is otherwise normal, though endometrial glands may be widely separated and stromal collagen may be increased.

18.14.2.3 Cystic Endometrial Hyperplasia/Pyometra in Dogs

18.14.2.3.1 Diffuse Endometrial Hyperplasia

Diffuse cystic endometrial hyperplasia, with or without mucometra, is a common observation in dogs related to repeated progestogenic stimulation that can be exacerbated by a previous estrogenic influence. Administration of combined (estrogenic + progestogenic) or progestogenic contraceptives, progestin estrus inhibitors (e.g., medroxyprogesterone acetate, megestrol acetate, or chlormadinone acetate), or other agents resulting in prolonged increases in serum progesterone invariably induces cystic endometrial hyperplasia (El Etreby 1979; Johnson 1989; Murakoshi et al. 2000; Sahara et al. 1994; Sokolowski and Zimbelman 1973; Von Berky and Townsend 1993).

18.14.2.3.2 Segmental Endometrial Hyperplasia

In dogs, an unusual spontaneous lesion that is frequently confused with pregnancy or pseudopregnancy has been described. It can occur in young dogs and is seen from time to time in toxicology studies. Grossly, it appears as a focal swelling of the uterus ranging from approximately 1 cm up to around 4 cm in diameter. The term "deciduoma" has been used in some references, but a more accurate term is a segmental or focal cystic endometrial hyperplasia. Histologic characteristics are similar to a site of placentation but without the conceptus or any fetal placental tissue (Koguchi et al. 1995; Schlafer and Gifford 2008) and is not, therefore, an indication of a pregnancy or a site of placentation, but rather a form of localized or segmental cystic endometrial hyperplasia.

18.14.2.3.3 Pyometra

Pyometra is a well-documented condition seen in aging dogs during diestrus as a sequel to persistent cystic endometrial hyperplasia that has not often been reported as a spontaneous change in young dogs such as those used in toxicology studies. In one survey, the earliest age of onset in untreated beagle dogs in a breeding colony was 4 years (Fukuda 2001). Dogs treated with estrogenic or progestogenic compounds that stimulate the endometrium and cause cystic endometrial hyperplasia can also produce classic pyometra, particularly after chronic administration (Goyings et al. 1977; Nelson and Kelly 1976; Noakes et al. 2001; Withers and Whitney 1967).

18.14.2.4 Endometrial Polyp

Endometrial polyps are a common, benign, age-related, spontaneous finding in rats and mice and can also be observed in rhesus and cynomolgus macaques (Chandra and Frith 1992; Cline et al. 2008; Dixon et al. 1999; Goodman and Hildebrandt 1987b; Kaspareit et al. 2007; Poteracki and Walsh 1998). Endometrial polyps are either sessile or pedunculated mass lesions that contain varying amounts of glands or stroma. In rhesus and cynomolgus macaques, the incidence of polyps increases with exposure to endogenous or exogenous estrogens (Baskin et al. 2002; Cline et al. 2008).

18.14.2.5 Endometrial Adenoma/Adenocarcinoma

Endometrial adenomas or adenocarcinomas are, in general, an uncommon tumor in most common strains and species used in nonclinical toxicology testing with the exception of the Han-Wistar rat and the rabbit, which have high incidences of endometrial carcinomas (Deerberg et al. 1981; Elsinghorst et al. 1984). Endometrial adenomas have been induced in mice by a number of xenobiotics including estrogens, bromoethane, chloroethane, and ethylene oxide, administered either chronically or during critical windows of development (Highman et al. 1978; Newbold et al. 1990; Picut et al. 2003).

18.14.2.6 Leiomyoma

Leiomyomas are common, benign, age-related spontaneous expansile masses arising within the smooth muscle of the uterus. These tumors have been widely reported in aging rodents, dogs, NHPs, and women (Chandra and Frith 1992; Cline et al. 2008; Dixon et al. 1999; Kennedy et al. 1994). In humans, uterine leiomyomas are often referred to as fibroids. Long-term administration of estrogenic compounds (7+ years) has been reported to induce smooth muscle tumors (leiomyoma and leiomyosarcoma) in the uterus and vagina of dogs (Johnson 1989).

18.14.2.7 Stromal Sarcoma

Stromal sarcomas have been reported in mice and rats but are rarely reported in other nonclinical species (Goodman and Hildebrandt 1987c; Reuber et al. 1981).

18.15 CHANGES IN THE CERVIX AND VAGINA

In rats and mice, the appearance of the vaginal epithelium changes remarkably during each phase of the estrous cycle, while changes in the cervical epithelium are less remarkable. Epithelial proliferation and cornification during the estrous cycle occur under the influence of estrogen, and this responsiveness is an extremely sensitive indicator of compounds with estrogenic activity (Reel et al. 1996). Development of the mucified layer of cells normally observed in proestrus requires the influence of progesterone in combination with estrogen (Barker and Walker 1966). These mucified cells are typically cuboidal to cylindrical and clear to basophilic, with cytoplasmic vacuoles containing sialomucins (Warren and Spicer 1961).

18.15.1 NONPROLIFERATIVE CHANGES

18.15.1.1 Atrophy

In the absence of estrogenic stimulation, as seen after ovariectomy or during the late stage of reproductive senescence (anestrus), the vaginal and cervical epithelium atrophy and become thin, with only two to three layers of cuboidal cells present, usually without evidence of mucification. Atrophy may also occur as a consequence of debilitation, presumably due to decreased gonadotropin secretion (Maekawa and Maita 1996; Yuan and Foley 2002). Atrophy of the vaginal or cervical epithelium may be observed owing to any xenobiotic-induced endocrine disruption affecting the production or actions of estrogen (Luo et al. 1998; Matsuda et al. 1997; Yuan and Foley 2002).

18.15.1.2   Mucification

Vaginal and cervical epithelial cells formed under the influence of progesterone hypertrophy and produce clear to basophilic mucinous material contained within cytoplasmic vacuoles (Barker and Walker 1966). When the formation of these mucin-filled cells is excessive or inappropriate without a relationship to the estrous cycle, it is referred to as mucification (Figure 18.18b). Mucification normally occurs under the influence of progesterone and is observed spontaneously during pregnancy, pseudopregnancy, and as a manifestation of reproductive senescence in association with persistent diestrus and a decreased estrogen:progesterone ratio. Typically, the stratum basale consists of one to two layers of cells with two to four superficial layers of hypertrophied, cuboidal, or cylindrical cells containing clear to basophilic mucinous material that stains histochemically with PAS or alcian blue stains. Epithelial mucification of the vagina and, to a lesser extent, the cervix is a common feature of endocrine disruption in the intact rodent and has been reported after treatment with exogenous progestins, gonadotropins, androgens (including non-aromatizable androgens), anti-estrogens, aromatase inhibitors, and compounds that increase prolactin levels (Brown et al. 1999b; Daly and Kramer 1998; Lotz and Krause 1978; Mirsky et al. 2011; Rehm et al. 2007c; Sourla et al. 1998b). It is important that mucification due to endocrine disruption be distinguished from the normal cyclical appearance of the vaginal epithelium at proestrus. Noncyclical mucification may accompany atrophy or hyperplasia of the vaginal epithelium and usually occurs in the absence of an underlying stratum granulosum or stratum corneum.

18.15.1.3   Inflammation

It is not unusual to see scattered infiltrates of varying types of inflammatory cells within the wall or lumen of the cervix and vagina. In rodents, an increase in neutrophils is commonly seen during estrus into early diestrus and should not be mistaken for inflammation. This increase in neutrophils is largely driven by estrogens and decreases in estrogen can cause a decrease in neutrophil influx. In NHPs, it is normal to see lymphoid aggregates and lymphoid follicles within the vagina (Cline et al. 2008).

18.15.1.4   Endocervical Squamous Metaplasia

Varying degrees of squamous metaplasia of the endocervical glands is often observed in young NHPs (Cline et al. 2008). Squamous metaplasia tends to occur within the basal compartment of the cervical mucus glands secondary to waves of estradiol from developing follicles in peripubertal animals, and some degree of cervical squamous metaplasia is considered to be normal in 2- to 4-year-old NHPs (Figure 18.27c) (Cline et al. 2008; Graham 1970; Wood 2008). Despite the common occurrence of cervical squamous metaplasia in young NHPs, the cervix can be a site of test article–related changes and cervical squamous metaplasia has been reported with estrogenic compounds and dioxin (Graham 1970; Scott et al. 2001).

18.15.1.5   Cysts

Cysts in the wall of the cervix or vagina are infrequently seen in rodents. Squamous epithelial cysts are occasionally seen in rodents of all ages (Leininger and Jokinen 1990; Yuan and Lund 1991). These cysts are typically located beneath the mucosal epithelium, lined by squamous epithelium, and often filled with keratin. Additionally, the appearance of the epithelium may vary with the stage of the estrous cycle. Cystic dilation of the vaginal fornix with luminal accumulation of inspissated material has rarely been reported in aged rats, presumably as a strain-specific finding (Yoshitomi 1990).

18.15.2   Proliferative Changes

18.15.2.1   Hyperplasia/Hyperkeratinization

Elevations of endogenous estrogens (persistent estrus during reproductive senescence) or administration of exogenous estrogens may induce hyperplasia and hyperkeratosis of the cervical and vaginal epithelium in rodents (Cartwright and Moreland 2008; Greenman and Fullerton 1986). In mice, adenosis, a proliferative downgrowth of the cervical and vaginal epithelium, has been described as a consequence of estrogenic stimulation in mice (Greaves 2007; Highman et al. 1978). Treatment with mifepristone (RU486), a progesterone receptor antagonist, induces vaginal epithelial hyperplasia and hyperkeratosis because of the unopposed activity of estrogen in the vagina despite increased levels of circulating progesterone (van der Schoot et al. 1987). Hyperplasia of the cervical and vaginal epithelium has also been reported in rats after treatment with a nucleoside analog for treatment of retroviral infections (Woicke et al. 2007). In dogs, any agent that has estrogenic activity will produce cervical and vaginal epithelial and stromal changes consistent with those seen in estrus (Heywood and Wadsworth 1981). This includes a thickened, multilayered, squamous epithelium with keratinization (Rehm et al. 2007b). Since there is a close link in the activity of estrogen receptors in the stromal and epithelial cells, stromal changes such as edema and hypertrophy of the muscularis are also observed (Vermeirsch et al. 2002).

18.15.2.2 Squamous Papilloma/Carcinoma

Squamous papillomas and carcinomas can arise within the vagina or cervix and have similar features to those arising from skin (Dixon et al. 1999; Goodman and Hildebrandt 1987a).

18.15.2.3 Vaginal Polyp

Vaginal polyps are pedunculated lesions that project into the vaginal lumen. There is typically a squamous epithelium overlying a fibrous or fibromuscular central core (Dixon et al. 1999).

18.15.2.4 Granular Cell Tumor

Granular cell tumors can range from small aggregates of granular cells to well-demarcated expansile masses and are typically found within the cervical or vaginal wall of rats (Dixon et al. 1999; Markovits and Sahota 2000a). Granular cells are of unknown histogenesis but typically have pale abundant eosinophilic cytoplasm and are PAS positive (diastase resistant) and S100 positive (Markovits and Sahota 2000a). Granular cell tumors can occur at a relatively high frequency in rats and the incidence has been shown to decrease with administration of aromatase inhibitors, suggesting a role of endogenous estrogens (Markovits and Sahota 2000b).

18.16 RELEVANCE OF FEMALE REPRODUCTIVE SYSTEM CHANGES TO HUMANS

When evaluating the potential effects of a test article on the female reproductive system in a nonclinical general toxicology study, extrapolation to humans can be a challenge owing to the differences in anatomy, physiology, and reproductive strategies across species. Despite the dramatic species differences described throughout this chapter, when test article–related changes are identified in the female reproductive tract in nonclinical general toxicity studies, they are often relevant to women, as many of the basic mechanisms (GnRH-induced release of gonadotropins, LH-induced ovulation, steroid hormone feedback mechanisms, etc.) are conserved across species. However, the anatomic and physiologic differences between species may mean that the given change observed in animals may not be the actual hazard for women, but rather serve as an indication of the underlying mechanism. For example, the spectrum of pseudopregnancy-like changes (hypertrophy of corpora lutea, vaginal mucification, and mammary hyperplasia) seen in rats given dopamine receptor antagonists are not relevant to humans with a menstrual cycle, but the underlying dopaminergic control of prolactin production is conserved across species and is relevant to humans who may present with galactorrhea or amenorrhea secondary to hyperprolactinemia. Therefore, identification of end-organ toxicity in the female reproductive system must be evaluated with the endocrine axis and associated organs in order to truly characterize the hazard and understand the potential risk to women.

A greater challenge is present when test article–related changes are not identified in a general toxicology setting. Does the absence of findings in animals translate to women? Recent work has suggested that 2- or 4-week general toxicology studies can detect most reproductive toxicants (Sanbuissho et al. 2009); however, these studies employed a number of endpoints (estrous cyclicity, additional sections of ovary, immunohistochemistry) not typically used in most general toxicity studies. These endpoints are labor intensive and may complicate other aspects of the study and are not typically recommended or used in routine studies. Standard general toxicology studies are very useful for identifying end-organ toxicity, but organ weight and pathology evaluation take place at a single time point in animals that are not synchronized, and without baseline and longitudinal cycle evaluation, detection of cycle irregularities (which is a very sensitive endpoint for endocrine disruption) is difficult. In addition, unlike female fertility studies, general toxicology studies do not allow for evaluation of corpus luteum function as the corpora lutea of cycling rats are essentially nonfunctional without cervical stimulation, and fertility studies are the only method to detect effects on gamete transport, fertilization, implantation, and early embryonic development. As a result, data from general toxicity studies are best used along with available target biology information and data from genetic and reproductive toxicology studies to develop a weight of evidence for the potential risk to women of childbearing potential and not used as a stand-alone data set.

18.17 MAMMARY GLAND EMBRYOLOGY AND FUNCTIONAL ANATOMY

The mammary gland has evolved as a modification of an apocrine gland to supply nourishment to offspring (Lefèvre et al. 2010). In the last 50 years, much interest has been focused on the mammary gland in an effort to try to better understand the origin, biology, and pathophysiology of human breast cancer. However, morphological assessment of the mammary gland also plays an important part in the safety evaluation of new drugs and chemicals. Because the function of the mammary gland is regulated by the same hormones important for reproduction function, it can serve as a sensitive indicator of hormonal disruption that may have relevance for human risk assessment.

Much of what we know about the mammary gland has been learned from its study in rodents. There are, however, differences among species in terms of the development, histology, and hormonal regulation of the mammary gland. For species-specific information on the histology of the mammary gland during growth and lactation, a number of useful references are available for the mouse (Daniel and Silberstein 1987; Richert et al. 2000), rat (Masso-Welch et al. 2000; Russo et al. 1989), dog (Chandra et al. 2010; Nelson and Kelly 1974; Rehm et al. 2007b; Turner and Gomez 1934), and macaque (Cline 2007).

The mammary glands are paired structures located to either side of the midline and the number of glands present varies with the species. Normally, there are six pairs of glands in the rat (two thoracic, two abdominal, and one inguinal), five pairs in the mouse (three cervicothoracic, one abdominal, and one inguinal), five pairs in the dog (two thoracic, two abdominal, and one inguinal), and one pair of pectoral glands in the NHP. The embryonic and fetal development of the mammary gland has been most extensively studied in the rodent and serves as a useful model for other species (Hovey et al. 1999; Sakakura 1987; Topper and Freeman 1980). Briefly, primitive mammary ectoderm migrates in the embryo to form the milk lines extending bilaterally from the cervical to the inguinal region. Focal condensations of this ectoderm form milk buds that associate with the epidermal nipple anlage. Proliferation and cavitation of each milk bud form a rudimentary duct system extending into the underlying mesenchyme (the future mammary fat pad) prior to birth. After birth, there is little growth of the juvenile mammary gland in mice, dogs, or macaques while some limited ductal growth does occur in rats (Cline 2007; Imagawa et al. 1990; Turner and Gomez 1934). At puberty, with the onset of ovarian function, the mammary duct system undergoes allometric growth and elongation to fill the mammary fat pad. After puberty, further development of the mammary gland in the virgin female is relatively limited, with some limited additional branching and formation of terminal ductules and some alveoli occurring under the influence of the hormonal fluctuations of the ovarian cycle.

18.18   STRUCTURE OF THE MAMMARY GLAND

From the nipple, the lactiferous ducts open into large main or primary ducts that branch into smaller secondary and tertiary ducts eventually giving rise to terminal ductules and the secretory alveoli. With the exception of the lactiferous duct in the nipple, which is partially lined by stratified squamous epithelium, ducts of all sizes and alveoli are typically lined by two layers of simple epithelium. Cells lining the lumen vary from cuboidal to columnar in ducts to cuboidal in alveoli; attenuation may occur with secretion. The layer of cells beneath the luminal layer and adjacent to the basement membrane consists of flattened, stellate, myoepithelial cells that produce the basement membrane around the ducts and alveoli and are responsible for contraction of alveoli and ducts during milk ejection (Masso-Welch et al. 2000; Richert et al. 2000). In general, mammary epithelial cells express cytokeratin intermediate filaments, particularly 8, 18, and 19, while myoepithelial cells express keratin 14, as well as vimentin and smooth muscle actin (Masso-Welch et al. 2000; Sorenmo et al. 2010; Tsubura et al. 1991; Wood et al. 2007). The epithelial basement membrane is continuous and contains laminin and collagen type IV, and the identification of these proteins may be useful in characterizing invasive carcinomas (Masso-Welch et al. 2000). During growth of the mammary gland, the terminal end buds (TEBs) are responsible for duct elongation, branching, and production of the alveolar buds (Hovey et al. 2002). TEBs, composed of immature basophilic epithelial cells, have a solid or cavitary club-shaped appearance and are most numerous at puberty, declining in number thereafter (Russo and Russo 1994; Sorenmo et al. 2010; Wood et al. 2007). TEBs should not be confused histologically with foci of ductular or alveolar hyperplasia (Lucas et al. 2007). At the distal extent of the duct system in the rodent, the terminal ductules and their associated alveolar buds comprise the lobuloalveolar unit (LAU) and form the secretory lobule during lactation (Cardiff and Wellings 1999). The analogous structure in the primate is called the terminal ductal lobular unit (TDLU) and both the LAU and TDLU are the major sites responsive to hormonal stimulation (Cardiff and Wellings 1999). The epithelium of the mammary gland is supported by a connective tissue stroma consisting of varying proportions of adipose tissue and collagen, blood vessels, nerve fibers, and cells of the immune system. In the rodent, the stroma consists mainly of adipose tissue with relatively scant collagen generally forming a thin layer investing ducts and alveoli. In comparison, collagen forms a much greater proportion of the mammary gland in dogs and NHPs. In addition to its supportive role, the stroma is now recognized as being integral to normal mammary development, growth, and function through numerous paracrine interactions with the epithelium (Hovey and Aimo 2010; Hovey et al. 1999; Imagawa et al. 2002; Parmar and Cunha 2004).

In the male, development of the mammary gland remains relatively rudimentary in comparison with the female. In rodents, testosterone from the developing testis induces mesenchymal cells expressing the androgen receptor to destroy the growing mammary stalk (Dürnberger and Krotochwil 1980). As a consequence, many strains of male mice lack nipples and the duct system largely deteriorates, while in rats, the mammary duct system remains intact but lacks communication with the exterior (Sakakura 1987). In the male rat, dog, and NHP, growth of the mammary duct system during the juvenile period is limited as in females. In the NHP, transient gynecomastia has been reported in young peripubertal males, but it is unclear if this is similar to that reported in young boys (Cline 2008). In the rat, there are significant androgen-driven changes at puberty, while in the dog and NHP, there is relatively little growth after puberty (Ahrén and Etienne 1957; Cline and Wood 2008; Turner and Gomez 1934). Despite its lack of development in the male dog and NHP, the mammary gland remains responsive to exogenous hormones (Biegel et al. 1998; Daane and Lyons 1954) and can be a useful marker of estrogenic endocrine disruption (Latendresse et al. 2009). In the rat, the mammary gland exhibits a unique dimorphism (Figure 18.33). This unique sex-dependent morphology of the mammary gland in the rat has led to the glandular structure in the female being referred to as "tubuloalveolar" as it consists of scattered branched tubular ducts and fewer alveoli and that of the male being referred to as "lobuloalveolar" as it consists of large contiguous lobules of alveoli with fewer ducts (Lucas et al. 2007). After puberty, the epithelium of

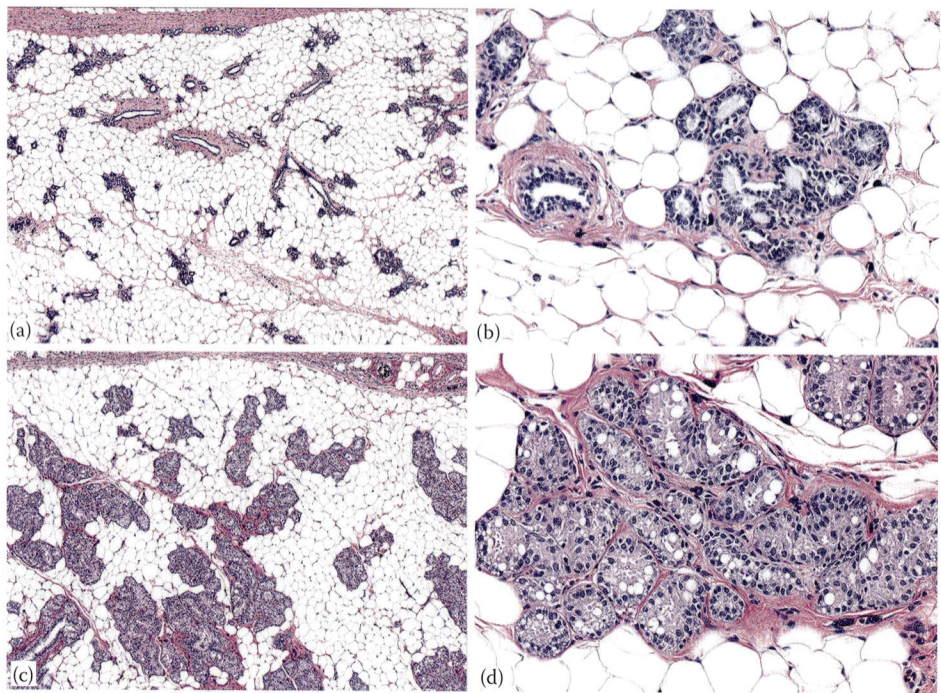

FIGURE 18.33 Dimorphic morphology of the rat mammary gland. The mammary gland of the adult female rat (a and b) has a tubuloalveolar appearance with numerous ducts and a few lobules, lined by cuboidal epithelial cells, scattered within the fat pad. In the adult male rat (c and d), the mammary gland has a lobuloalveolar architecture with large, contiguous lobules of alveoli and fewer ducts lined by hypertrophied, cuboidal to columnar, sometimes vacuolated epithelial cells.

the male rat mammary gland hypertrophies under the influence of androgens and becomes vacuolated, often obscuring the lumen in ducts and alveoli (Ahrén and Etienne 1957; Cardy 1991; Lucas et al. 2007). Generally, this "male" morphology predominates, though it is not unusual to find areas in which ducts with the tubuloalveolar appearance of the prepubertal male or virgin female are present, particularly at terminal branches or periphery of the gland (Creasy 2008b). In young peripubertal rats, reports by Ahrén and Etienne (1957) and Latendresse et al. (2009) have indicated that some male rats will exhibit a mainly tubuloalveolar morphology and suggested that the predominant growth pattern observed may be related to the age of the animal at the time of sampling.

18.19 REGULATION OF MAMMARY GLAND GROWTH AND FUNCTION

The development and structure of the mammary gland are intimately tied to and highly dependent on the interactions of a number of steroid and protein hormones and growth factors. Much of our knowledge of the endocrine regulation of mammary gland development has been derived from rodent models in which hormones were administered alone or in combination to animals from which various endocrine organs have been removed. More recently, the use of mouse models in which hormone or hormone receptor genes are disrupted has contributed greatly to refining our understanding of the molecular basis of mammary growth.

During puberty, the ovarian follicles begin to produce estrogen that stimulates the TEBs to advance into the mammary fat pad resulting in elongation of the duct system. The activities of estrogen on the mammary epithelium are mediated by signaling through ERα expressed on the epithelium (Mallepell et al. 2006). While ERβ is also expressed in the mammary gland, it is not required for duct growth (Förster et al. 2002). Optimal growth and branching of the ducts under the influence of estrogen also require growth hormone (GH), which exerts its effects by inducing stromal production of insulin-like growth factor-1 (IGF-1) (Kleinberg 1998; Sternlicht 2006). Glucocorticoids appear to play a role in duct growth by facilitating epithelial cell proliferation, but their precise role has yet to be determined (Brisken and Rajaram 2006; Nandi 1958). Progesterone and prolactin are also important, particularly for lactational development of the normal mammary gland, but they play a relatively limited role in mammary development in the virgin female. Progesterone, acting mainly through PRβ expressed on duct epithelium, is required for formation of side branches and alveologenesis (Brisken and O'Malley 2010). Both estrogen and progesterone appear to act through paracrine mechanisms in stimulating duct growth and morphogenesis (Brisken et al. 1998; Mallepell et al. 2006). Prolactin is not directly required for the growth or branching of mammary ducts, though it plays an indirect role in branching by promoting progesterone synthesis (Ben-Jonathan et al. 2008). However, prolactin is essential for lobuloalveolar differentiation and lactation (Ben-Jonathan et al. 2008). Prolactin receptors are expressed in both the mammary epithelium and stroma, and increased receptor expression is seen in the epithelium during pregnancy and lactation (Camarillo et al. 2001). Androgen receptors are expressed by the mammary gland, play a role in mammary biology, and are implicated in toxicological effects of treatment with xenobiotics (Lucas et al. 2007; Pelletier 2000; Yeh et al. 2003). The importance of epithelial–stromal interactions in the development and function of the mammary gland has been recognized for some time (Daniel and Silberstein 1987; Sakakura 1987). Recent work has started to identify some of the mediators of these interactions including growth factors, cytokines, and paracrine hormones, as well as the signaling pathways regulating their functions (Hynes and Watson 2010; Imagawa et al. 2002; Kariagina et al. 2010; Kleinberg et al. 2009; Watson and Khaled 2008). A review of the hormonal regulation of lactation is beyond the scope of this chapter and the interested reader is referred to several useful discussions of this topic (Anderson et al. 2007; Neville 2006; Neville et al. 2002).

18.20 CONSIDERATIONS IN THE EXAMINATION OF THE MAMMARY GLAND

Examination of the mammary gland should be undertaken with knowledge of its normal structure, an appreciation of the expected glandular volume and distribution, and a degree of tolerance for its normal variability. Samples of mammary gland should be obtained from the same location to ensure consistency in glandular architecture and density within and across studies and an adequate quantity of mammary tissue should be available for examination. Inclusion of an anatomical marker in the section, such as the inguinal lymph node, helps ensure consistency in both location and interpretation (Lucas et al. 2007). Some variability in mammary structure may be encountered in the rat and the dog depending upon the gland obtained for examination and the manner in which it is sectioned (Chandra et al. 2010; Hvid et al. 2010; Russo et al. 1989). A standardized recommendation for trimming of the mammary gland for histologic examination has been published by the Registry of Industrial Toxicology Animal-data (Ruehl-Fehlert et al. 2003). Within a species, the degree of glandular development and hormone responsiveness among individual animals and strains may vary considerably (Harvell et al. 2000; Imagawa et al. 1990; Naylor and Ormandy 2002; Topper and Freeman 1980). Furthermore, differences in the histology of the gland have been associated with the various stages of the ovarian cycle (Chandra et al. 2010; Cline 2007; Nelson and Kelly 1974; Rehm et al. 2007b; Schedin et al. 2000; Strange et al. 2007). In the virgin rodent and NHP, these features are relatively subtle, but in the bitch, they are more obvious as ovulation is normally followed by a prolonged luteal phase with secretion of progesterone and development of mammary tissue in preparation for lactation. Age will also affect the appearance of the gland and, while the mammary gland of young mature intact virgin female rodents is similar to that of aged animals, branching, alveolar buds, and size of lobules tend to increase with age (Russo et al. 1989).

18.21   HISTOPATHOLOGY OF THE MAMMARY GLAND

18.21.1   Non-Neoplastic Changes

18.21.1.1   Atrophy

Loss of estrogen (or antagonism of the estrogen receptor) may lead to atrophy of the mammary gland, resulting in a decrease of glandular tissue and a reduction in the size of the epithelium lining these structures (Figure 18.34). Mammary gland atrophy has been reported in intact male and female rodents treated with potent anti-estrogens such as fulvestrant (ICI 182,780), EM-800, and tamoxifen (Chan et al. 2001; Kennel et al. 2003; Luo et al. 1998). The androgen receptor antagonist flutamide has been shown to induce atrophy of the mammary gland in male rats (Toyoda et al. 2000). Furthermore, it has been suggested that any compound decreasing circulating testosterone might induce atrophy of the mammary gland in the male, though this has not been demonstrated experimentally (Creasy 2008b; Lucas et al. 2007; Rudmann et al. 2005). Atrophy of the mammary gland in intact female dogs or NHPs as a result of xenobiotic treatment is not common.

18.21.1.2   Sex-Dependent Alterations in the Mammary Gland of the Rat

Under conditions of inappropriate hormonal stimulation, the characteristic appearance of the mammary epithelium in the rat may be altered to resemble that of the opposite sex. In the male rat, compounds with estrogenic activity or those that increase prolactin levels (such as dopamine antagonists) cause loss of the normal lobuloalveolar architecture resulting in the acquisition of a more female-like tubuloalveolar structure (Andrews et al. 2002; Biegel et al. 1998; Cardy 1991; Wang et

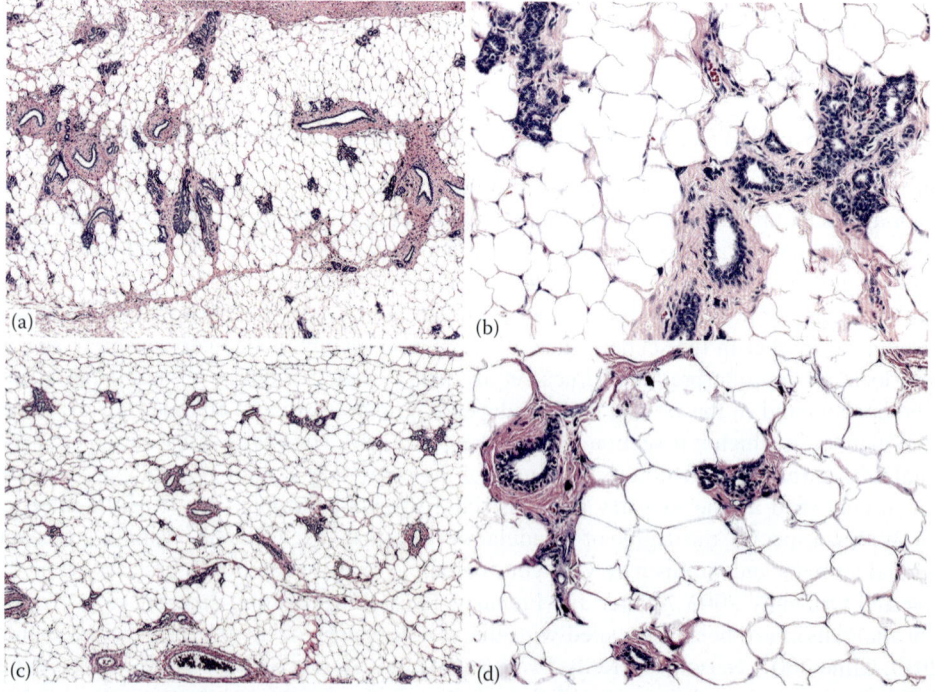

FIGURE 18.34   In comparison with mammary tissue from a control female at diestrus (a and b), atrophy of the mammary gland in a female rat treated for 4 weeks with a GnRH antagonist (c and d) is characterized by reduced numbers and size of ducts and alveoli, epithelial attenuation, and a corresponding increase in the relative amount of space occupied by the fat pad.

al. 2006). Because the morphology of the male mammary gland prior to androgen stimulation at puberty is similar to that of the female, loss of androgen stimulation also results in a morphology that is again similar to the female. As a result, this is often referred to as "feminization," but this rat-specific phenomenon should not be confused with gynecomastia and should be carefully conveyed to clinicians and regulators. This "feminization" of the male gland may be more correctly described as atrophy because of the dramatic decrease in the volume of lobuloalveolar tissue and conversion to the female acinar pattern (Creasy 2008b). Weak hormonal modulators or low doses of strong hormonal modulators can produce a mixture of male and female differentiation, but the altered structures should be spread throughout the gland (Creasy 2008b; Latendresse 2009).

In the female rat, acquisition of lobuloalveolar morphology (male phenotype) occurs after the administration of androgens (e.g., DHT, dehydroepiandrosterone, testosterone, 17α methyl testosterone) and some SERMs such as LY2066948, which not only are potent estrogen receptor antagonists but also cause hyperandrogenemia (Creasy 2008b; Rudmann et al. 2005). The acquisition of the male phenotype has been shown to be due to direct androgenic action on the mammary gland since it can be blocked using the androgen receptor blocker flutamide (Rudmann et al. 2005; Sourla et al. 1998a). The lobuloalveolar hyperplasia seen in females in response to exogenous androgen administration may be difficult to distinguish from that induced by estrogenic compounds or aromatase inhibitors secondary to endogenous elevations in androgens (Creasy 2008b; Mirsky et al. 2011).

18.21.1.3 Inflammation

Inflammation of the mammary gland (or mastitis) is a rare finding in nonclinical safety studies but may be encountered in breeding animals as a consequence of bacterial infections during or after lactation. Inflammation has been reported as a consequence of release of secretory material from the duct system into the mammary stroma (Boorman et al. 1990). In older female beagle dogs, lymphocytic inflammation may be observed in the mammary stroma as a spontaneous finding (Cameron and Faulkin 1971). It should be noted that in normally cycling female dogs, the histology of the mammary gland during the first estrus/metestrus may mimic an inflammatory reaction as the gland is enlarged with stromal proliferation characterized by a loose, swirling pattern of fibroblasts against an edematous or myxomatous background accompanied by foci of extravasated erythrocytes and scattered lymphocytes (Chandra et al. 2010; Rehm et al. 2007b).

18.21.1.4 Dilation of Ducts and Acini

A number of terms including cyst, dilation, ectasia, and galactocele have been used to describe dilation of the secretory system within the mammary gland. Dilated ducts are typically lined by flattened to cuboidal epithelium with a thin connective tissue wall and the lumen contains proteinaceous residue, cell debris, and sometimes inflammatory cells. Marked dilation of ducts or alveoli may be visible grossly as white secretion-filled cysts termed galactoceles (van Zwieten et al. 1994). In rodents, duct dilation is a fairly common finding, particularly in older females, but has been described in up to 5% of males in 2-year bioassays using Sprague–Dawley rats (van Zwieten et al. 1994). In macaques, cystic changes in lobular or ductal elements of the mammary gland are a common incidental finding usually observed in parous females (Cline 2007). While dilation of the mammary duct system has been reported in the general canine population (Hampe and Misdorp 1974; Miller et al. 2001), this finding is not a commonly observed spontaneous finding in nonclinical studies, possibly because of the relatively young age of the animals. Dilation of mammary ducts has occasionally been reported as an effect of treatment in nonclinical safety studies, as with the administration of thalidomide to dogs (Teo et al. 2001) or mice treated with keratinocyte growth factor (Yi et al. 1994). Cystic dilation of ducts or alveoli with secretion may be a general indicator of a disturbance of the HPG axis as it has been observed after the administration of estrogenic or progestogenic components of combination steroid contraceptives and in response to hyperprolactinemia (Creasy 2008b).

18.21.1.5 Fibrosis

Fibrosis, as a pathologic change in the mammary gland, is likely more easily observed in mice and rats than in large animals in nonclinical toxicology studies because of the relatively greater proportion of adipose tissue present relative to collagenous connective tissue. Spontaneous fibrosis is often observed in older rats, mainly around large ducts, though it may also occur in intralobular or interlobular areas (Boorman et al. 1990). In mice, fibrosis at the expense of adipose tissue is reported in older animals in association with decreased size of the mammary gland (Kenney et al. 1996). Fibrosis of the mammary gland may be induced experimentally and has been reported in association with iodine deficiency (Eskin et al. 1995) or prenatal exposure to organochlorines (Foster et al. 2004) in rats and accompanying duct proliferation in mice treated with epidermal growth factor (Molinolo et al. 1998). Fibrosis and inflammation may also be seen in association with the testing of implants of foreign materials (Greaves 2007).

18.21.2 Proliferative Changes

18.21.2.1 Hyperplasia

The term "hyperplasia" has been applied to a variety of changes in the mammary gland. In part, this stems from the need to find an objective term to convey a physiological response (e.g., lobuloalveolar hyperplasia caused by hormonal treatment), while in others, it has been used to indicate the presence of an abnormal proliferative lesion within the tissue. The lack of clarity around the term in veterinary pathology has arisen for a variety of reasons, including real differences in morphology owing to species and strain, the use of inconsistent or imprecise terminology often borrowed from human medicine, and a lack of descriptive clarity in the literature (Cline 2007; Greaves 2007). Much of the work done to understand the nature of mammary hyperplasia has been done in rodents and humans. Many, if not all, hyperplasias and mammary tumors are thought to arise in the proliferative compartments of the gland, including the TEB or terminal ducts in rodents and TDLU of humans (Allred et al. 2001; Cardiff 1998; Russo and Russo 1996). Additionally, there is considerable evidence that hyperplasia is often part of a continuum leading up to the development of cancers (Allred et al. 2001; Bombonati and Sgroi 2011). Therefore, recognition and appropriate characterization of mammary gland hyperplasia in nonclinical safety studies can have considerable importance for human risk assessment. In laboratory animals, mammary hyperplasias are generally divided into lobular and ductal forms. Lobular hyperplasias are focal or multifocal and characterized by enlargement of the lobular unit (relative to surrounding tissue) with maintenance of the normal relationships between cell types and structures, an absence of or minimal atypia, and the presence of a scant fibrous stroma separating acini. Ductal hyperplasias (DHs) arise in the epithelium of inter- or intralobular ducts and are characterized by three or more layers of epithelium (including myoepithelium), which may form solid or papillary structures lying above the basement membrane. When features such as anisocytosis, anisokaryosis, piling or crowding of epithelium, or loss of cellular polarity are present, the hyperplasia may be classified as atypical.

18.21.2.1.1 Rat

Hyperplasia of the mammary gland in the male and female rat has been reported after the administration of a diverse set of agents including progesterone, estrogens and estrogen agonists, androgens and androgen agonists, and compounds that increase serum levels of prolactin (Biegel et al. 1998; Chambô-Filho et al. 2005; Laqueur and Fluhmann 1942; Okazaki et al. 2001; Rehm et al. 2007c; Selye 1940). This xenobiotic-induced hyperplasia is usually multifocal or diffuse and tends to resemble mammary gland development during pregnancy or lactation (Figure 18.35). Typically, there is an increase in the number of ducts and alveoli per unit area, occasionally associated with duct dilation, with or without secretory material in ducts and alveoli (Creasy 2008b). In aging rats, focal lobular hyperplasia is characterized as an increase in lobular size with relatively normal-appearing

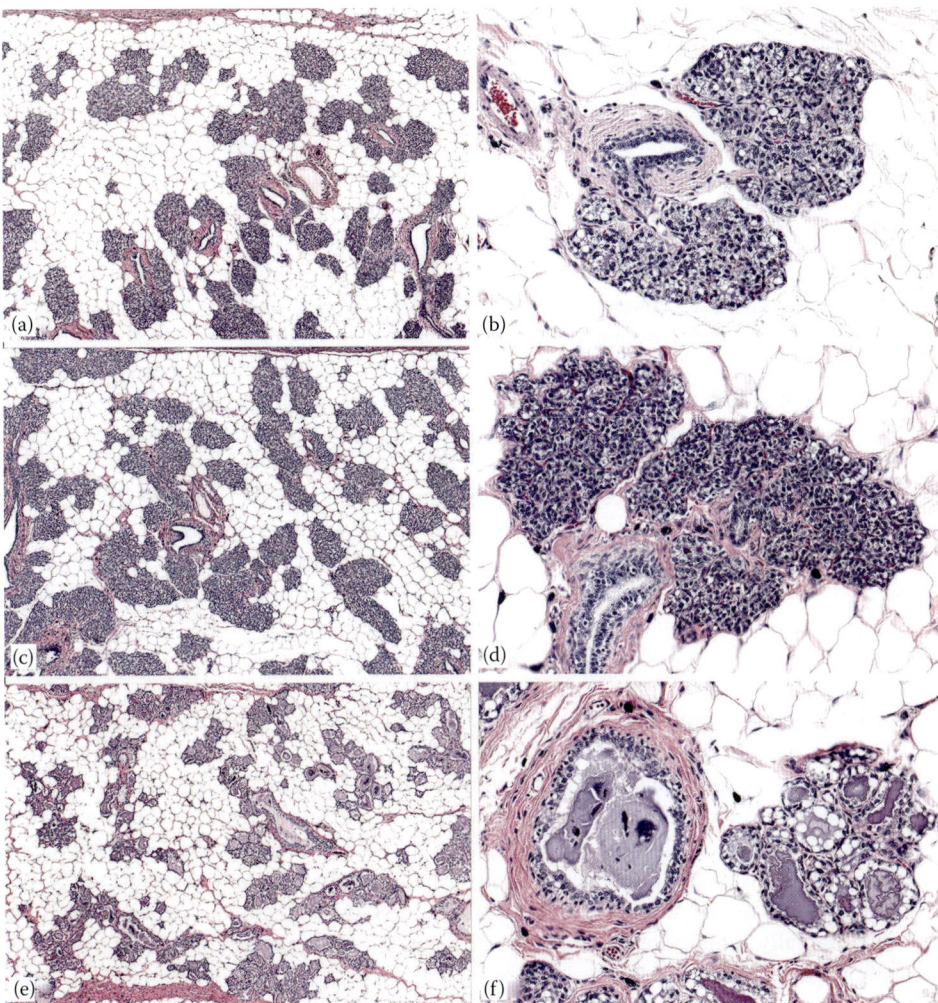

FIGURE 18.35 Lobular hyperplasia in the mammary gland in female rats treated for 4 weeks with a dopamine antagonist (a and b), progesterone (c and d), or a progesterone receptor antagonist (e and f).

alveoli lined by a single layer of well-differentiated epithelium, while atypical hyperplasia involves focal irregular proliferation of the epithelium within ducts or alveoli (Mann et al. 1996; van Zwieten et al. 1994). In these atypical foci, the epithelial cells are usually enlarged with hyperchromatic nuclei and basophilic cytoplasm and the proliferating cells may assume a variety of arrangements extending into the lumen. Although hyperplasia of the ductal epithelium is a common response to hormonal disturbance in man and NHP, it is not a common change in rats except after chronic exposure to xenobiotics or as an age-related change (Creasy 2008b).

18.21.2.1.2 Mouse

Several forms of mammary gland hyperplasias have been described in the mouse including keratinized nodules, hyperplastic alveolar nodules (HANs), plaques, and DHs. With the exception of keratinized nodules, murine mammary hyperplasias are generally considered to be precursors of mammary carcinomas (Medina 2002). The keratinized nodule is a nonpalpable lesion that appears grossly as gray-white keratin-filled foci and histologically consists of a few alveoli completely filled with desquamated cells and keratinized material accompanied by stromal mononuclear cell infiltration and fibrosis (Tsubura et al. 2007). HANs as described by Tsubura et al. (2007) are focal alveolar hyperplasias that may be recognized in the nonpregnant mammary gland as milky-white 1- to 2-mm nodules with histology closely resembling that of the pregnant mammary gland. Luminal epithelial cells of the HAN contain prominent lipid granules and may express mouse mammary tumor virus (MMTV) antigen (depending on the strain of mouse), while associated myoepithelial cells express α-smooth muscle actin, are distributed around the luminal cells, and rest upon a basement membrane expressing type IV collagen. HAN may be induced by mammary tumor viruses, chemical carcinogens, irradiation, or prolonged hormone stimulation (Medina 2008). The mechanism underlying the development of the HAN depends on its inciting cause. MMTV-associated HANs frequently exhibit insertional mutagenesis with activation of *wnt, fgf,* or *notch* genes; chemically induced HANs are often associated with *ras* activation; and spontaneous HANs usually exhibit alterations in the regulation of the cell cycle (Medina 2008). Plaques are flat, palpable disc-shaped lesions composed of radiating ducts in a delicate connective tissue stroma that are filled with proliferating cells containing fewer lipid granules and less MMTV expression than HANs. Myoepithelial cells expressing keratin 14 are usually absent from these foci. A unique characteristic of the plaque is its appearance and regression in response to hormonal stimulation (Tsubura et al. 2007). The third type of hyperplasia, DH, is characterized by an increase in small tertiary ducts and proliferation of intraluminal ductal epithelium and has been induced by chemical carcinogens, irradiation, and progestins *in vivo* (Medina 2002). DH is unassociated with MMTV infection and has morphological features similar to carcinoma *in situ* in humans (Medina 2002).

18.21.2.1.3   Dog

Canine mammary hyperplasias are either lobular or ductal, on the basis of the criteria discussed earlier (Cameron and Faulkin 1971; Misdorp et al. 1999). Recently, efforts have been made to apply classification schemes from human breast pathology (on the basis of histology and immunohistochemistry) to canine lesions for comparative analysis and clinical prognosis (Ferreira et al. 2010, 2011; Mouser et al. 2010). The utility of using such an approach in nonclinical safety testing is unknown at the present time. Spontaneous hyperplasias are infrequently observed in dogs in nonclinical safety studies as the animals in these studies are usually less than 4 years of age (Warner 1976). Experimentally, female dogs administered exogenous estrogens exhibit duct proliferation and ectasia without increased alveolar development, while exposure to progestins induces mammary lobuloalveolar growth and neoplasia (Bhatti et al. 2007; Concannon et al. 1981; El Etreby and Gräf 1979). Progestins stimulate GH production in the canine mammary gland as well as increased circulating GH and IGF-1, and it has been suggested that paracrine effects of GH (and local GH-induced IGF-1) may lead to mammary epithelial proliferation (Selman et al. 1994).

18.21.2.1.4   Nonhuman Primate

Spontaneous hyperplasias have been sporadically reported in macaques, and comprehensive reviews discussing their epidemiology and features have been recently published (Cline 2007; Wood et al. 2006). Focal or multifocal lobular hyperplasia, similar to that in dogs and rats, occurs fairly commonly in older macaques with enlargement of one or more lobules with relatively normal lobular architecture and cellular arrangement against a background of atrophic lobules (Cline 2007). Borrowing criteria from human breast pathology, atypical lobular hyperplasia has also been described, in which <50% of acini in the affected lobule are distended and distorted by atypical epithelial cells (O'Malley 2010; Wood et al. 2007). DH has been reported in intact or hormone-treated, ovariectomized, middle-aged or older macaques and subdivided as "conventional" (implying an absence of atypia) or "atypical" (Wood et al. 2006). The frequency of intraductal hyperplasia varies in macaques depending on the age and sectioning pattern but has been reported in up to 42% of control animals in chronic studies (Cline 2007; Tavassoli et al. 1988; Valerio 1989). The systemic administration of hormonal agents or growth factors may induce relatively widespread changes in the mammary gland of the NHP. In intact female rhesus macaques chronically administered high doses of estrogen, diffuse hyperplasia of the mammary gland with multilayered ductal epithelium was evident after 2–4 weeks, full lobular development with ducts lined by one to two layers of epithelium was evident by 10 weeks, and morphology similar to pseudopregnancy with large lobules containing secretory alveoli was evident after 5 months of treatment (Geschickter and Hartman 1959). An intact male treated in this same study responded similarly to the females though the response was somewhat delayed (Geschickter and Hartman 1959). While it has not been demonstrated that progestins alone induce changes in mammary gland morphology in NHPs, combining progestins with estrogen does result in increased lobular and ductular proliferation (Cline 2007). GH or IGF-1 alone or in combination induced proliferation of mammary lobules in aged female rhesus macaques, while epidermal growth factor induced mild ductal and acinar proliferation in female and male cynomolgus macaques (Ng et al. 1997; Reindel et al. 2001).

18.21.2.2 Neoplastic Lesions

In nonclinical toxicology, mammary tumors are usually encountered in the setting of chronic toxicity or carcinogenicity testing of rodents, and much of our data come from these assays.

In all species, a number of factors may play a role in susceptibility to treatment-related development of mammary tumors. For instance, in mice, the incidence of mammary tumors is heavily influenced by the presence or absence of MMTV. In general, strains positive for MMTV have high lifetime incidences of mammary tumors. In strains negative for MMTV, the incidence of mammary tumors is variable, ranging from 0% to approximately 50% in control females in carcinogenicity studies (Rehm and Liebelt 1996). In rodents in particular, other factors such as age at the time of exposure, sex, hormone status, and nutrition have been shown to influence whether or not exposure to a xenobiotic or physical agent such as radiation induces the development of mammary tumors. The impacts of these factors in the development of mammary tumors in various species of laboratory animals have been recently reviewed (Cline 2007; Greaves 2007).

Several decades of chemical and pharmaceutical safety testing, clinical assessment of spontaneous tumors in veterinary species, and experimental work on the biology of breast cancer have led to the publication of a number of detailed reviews of the classification, histological features, and biological characteristics of mammary tumors in the rat (Boorman et al. 1990; Mann et al. 1996; Mohr 1993; Russo et al. 1989; van Zwieten et al. 1994), mouse (Bruner et al. 2001; Cardiff and Wellings 1999; Medina 1982; Rehm and Liebelt 1996), dog (Benjamin 2001; Goldschmidt et al. 2011; Misdorp 2002; Misdorp et al. 1999), and macaque (Cooper and Gabrielson 2007; Tarara 2007; Wood et al. 2006). Additional online resources for mammary tumors of the rodent include the Registry of Industrial Toxicology Animal-data database and a document on diagnostic terminology being developed by the International Harmonization of Nomenclature and Diagnostic Criteria for Lesions in Rats and Mice (INHAND) initiative. Additionally, a number of genetically modified mouse strains have been developed for the study of mammary biology and neoplasia and many of these have recently been reviewed (Cardiff et al. 2007).

As would be expected, there is variability among laboratory animal species with respect to the types, morphology, and biological behavior of mammary tumors. Despite this heterogeneity, mammary tumors in all species are generally amenable to classification using a relatively simple system, based first on whether they are of epithelial or stromal (mesenchymal) origin and, second, on whether they exhibit benign or malignant features. In the dog in particular, epithelial mammary tumors are further subclassified as "simple," if the proliferative component is limited to tubular or alveolar structures, or "complex," if there is proliferation of both glandular structures and myoepithelial elements in a myxoid stroma.

18.21.2.2.1 Adenoma

Adenomas are described in all species as expansile, well-demarcated masses, consisting mainly of epithelial structures supported by scant connective tissue stroma. The neoplastic epithelial cells are relatively well differentiated and arranged in one or two layers lining tubules or acinar-like structures and sometimes containing secretory material. "Basaloid" adenomas, composed of neoplastic cells resembling basal cells, were described in dogs as a result of treatment with contraceptive steroids; this morphology has been recently clarified (Goldschmidt et al. 2011; Kwapien et al. 1977). In some adenomas, the neoplastic cells may be arranged in papillary fronds on delicate cores of collagen extending into the lumen of multilocular or cystic structures separated by collagen trabeculae (papillary adenoma, papillary cystadenoma). Benign papillary tumors are reported to occur more commonly in rodents.

18.21.2.2.2   Fibroadenoma

Fibroadenomas have been reported in rodents, dogs, and macaque, and a similar finding termed "fibroadenomatous change" is also described in macaques (Wood et al. 2006). In fibroadenomas, the neoplastic cells are well differentiated and typically arranged in tubular or alveolar structures separated by abundant collagen containing well-differentiated fibrocytes. In larger tumors, the fibrous component may predominate, making differentiation from fibroma problematic. Some authors have taken the position that fibroadenomas are fibromas arising within the mammary gland that displace and eventually destroy resident glandular tissue (Greaves 2007).

18.21.2.2.3   Carcinoma

In all species, malignant epithelial tumors or adenocarcinomas may exhibit a number of different morphologies even within the same tumor. The most commonly recognized of these subtypes include tubular (mostly tubular or alveolar), papillary (predominance of papillary structures, lined by or filled with neoplastic cells), cribriform (sieve-like pattern with spaces separating the tumor cells), and solid (dense cords or sheets of tumor cells with scant stroma) carcinomas. Some carcinomas may contain areas of squamous differentiation and, if extensive, may be termed an adenosquamous carcinoma. Carcinomas may also be subdivided on the basis of intralobular versus intraductal development and then subdivided as noninvasive (lacking penetration of the basement membrane; carcinoma *in situ*) or invasive (demonstrable penetration of the basement membrane). In general though, classifying mammary adenocarcinomas by subtypes in routine rodent carcinogenicity studies has not been demonstrated to be biologically meaningful (Greaves 2007; van Zwieten 1994). In the case of well-differentiated tumors, mammary carcinomas may be difficult to distinguish from adenomas, which contain limited areas of cellular atypia. As in other tissues, histologic criteria of malignancy include loss of cellular polarity, piling of epithelium within lumina, cellular and nuclear pleomorphism, nuclear hyperchromasia, increased mitotic figures, and evidence of local tissue or vascular invasion or distant metastasis. In the rat, carcinomas tend to be expansile and locally invasive, but metastasis is relatively uncommon. Spontaneous mammary carcinomas typically occur in older rats but have been sporadically reported in control females as young as 10 weeks (Oishi et al. 1995). In strains of mice commonly used in toxicology studies, carcinomas are relatively uncommon (Greaves 2007). In contrast to rats, mammary carcinomas in mice metastasize with some frequency, usually via the blood, to the lung (Medina 2008). In purpose-bred beagle dogs, Benjamin (2001) observed that spontaneous mammary carcinomas usually occur in females older than 5 years, with the peak incidence at 8–10 years. Additionally, data from this cohort indicated that metastasis is fairly common in female beagle dogs with mammary carcinoma and that histologic type is related to metastasis with ductal carcinomas demonstrating more aggressive behavior than other tumors (Benjamin 2001). In macaques, ductal carcinomas have been most frequently reported (Wood et al. 2006). The relatively monomorphic appearance of ductal carcinoma *in situ* may aid in distinguishing this tumor. Invasive ductal carcinomas may be associated with scirrhous reaction, local invasion, and distant metastasis. Lobular carcinomas *in situ* may appear very similar to atypical lobular hyperplasias but are distinguished by a greater proportion of acini (>50%) containing atypical cells (Wood et al. 2006). In comparison with other laboratory animal species, the lifetime incidence of mammary tumors in female macaques appears to be low (<10%) (Wood et al. 2006).

18.21.2.2.4   Fibroma/Fibrosarcoma

Both fibromas and fibrosarcomas have been reported in the mammary gland and are similar in appearance to their counterparts observed in other tissues and particularly the skin.

18.21.2.2.5   Benign/Malignant Mixed Mammary Tumors

Mixed mammary tumors are fairly common in the female dog and infrequently observed in other species. Histologically, these tumors consist of at least one epithelial and one mesenchymal component in addition to collagen (e.g., cartilage or bone). In the rat, the adenolipoma, a tumor consisting of glandular and mature-appearing adipose tissue, would fall into this category. In the benign mixed category, both components of the tumor lack features of malignancy, while in the malignant mixed category, at least one of the components exhibits features of malignancy. In the event that both components display a sufficient degree of atypia or evidence of invasive behavior, the tumor may be classified as a carcinosarcoma.

18.22   RELEVANCE OF MAMMARY GLAND CHANGES TO HUMANS

When evaluating the potential effects of a test article on the mammary gland in a nonclinical general toxicology study, extrapolation to humans can be a challenge owing to the differences in anatomy, physiology, and reproductive biology across species. As was discussed in the female reproductive system, a number of the common changes identified in the mammary gland may be relevant to humans, not because of the nature of the nonclinical finding but rather because of the underlying mechanism. For example, identification of atrophy in the male rat mammary gland could be easily dismissed as being nonrelevant, as atrophy is not a risk to men who do not normally undergo mammary gland development. However, the morphological finding in the male rat mammary gland may be indicative of an underlying decrease in androgen production/action resulting in glandular atrophy, which is relevant across species. Therefore, identification of end-organ toxicity in the mammary gland must be evaluated together with changes involving the endocrine axis and entire reproductive tract in order to truly characterize the hazard and understand the potential risk to humans. In some cases, clear identification of an underlying mechanism may not be possible. This can be especially true of proliferative lesions identified in chronic studies. In these cases, a clear understanding of the animal model is critical before beginning to develop a weight of evidence for the potential risk to humans. For example, the strain of rat or mouse, the timing of reproductive senescence in rats, the underlying role of local GH production in dogs, and the age of NHP all can have a significant impact on how one interprets potential test article–related findings in the mammary gland. In addition, available target biology information and data from genetic and reproductive toxicology studies are critical to develop a weight of evidence for the potential risk to humans.

REFERENCES

Adams, M.R., J.R. Kaplan, and D.R. Koritnik. 1985. Psychosocial influences on ovarian endocrine and ovulatory function in *Macaca fascicularis*. *Physiol Behav* 35:935–40.

Ahrén, K., and M. Etienne. 1957. The development of the mammary gland in normal and castrated male rats after the age of 21 days. *Acta Physiol Scand* 41:283–300.

Alison, R.H., C.C. Capen, and D.E. Prentice. 1994. Neoplastic lesions of questionable significance to humans. *Toxicol Pathol* 22:179–86.

Alison, R.H., K.T. Morgan, J.K. Haseman, and G.A. Boorman. 1987. Morphology and classification of ovarian neoplasms in F344 rats and (C57BL/6 X C3H)F1 mice. *J Natl Cancer Inst* 78(6):1229–43.

Alison, R.H., K.T. Morgan, and C.A. Montgomery. 1990. Ovary. In *Pathology of the Fischer Rat*, ed. G.A. Boorman, S.L. Eustis, M.R. Elwell, C.A. Montgomery, and W.F. MacKenzie, 429–42. San Diego: Academic Press.

Allen, E. 1922. The oestrus cycle in the mouse. *Am J Anat* 30:297–371.

Allen, W.E. 1992. Physiology of the reproductive cycle: 2.6 Anestrus. In *Fertility and Obstetrics in the Dog*, 10–11. Oxford: Blackwell Scientific Publications.

Allred, D.C., S.K. Mohsin, and S.A.W. Fuqua. 2001. Histological and biological evolution of human premalignant breast disease. *Endocr Relat Cancer* 8:47–61.

Ami, Y., Y. Suzaki, and N. Goto. 1993. Endometriosis in cynomolgus monkeys retired from breeding. *J Vet Med Sci* 55:7–11.

Andersen, A.C., and M.E. Simpson. 1973. *The Ovary and Reproductive Cycle of the Dog (Beagle)*. Los Altos, CA: Geron-X, Inc.

Anderson, S.M., M.C. Rudolph, J.L. McManaman, and M.C. Neville. 2007. Secretory activation in the mammary gland: it's not just about milk protein synthesis! *Breast Cancer Res* 9:204–17.

Andrews, P., A. Freyberger, E. Hartmann et al. 2002. Sensitive detection of the endocrine effects of the estrogen analogue ethinylestradiol using a modified enhanced subacute rat study protocol (OECD Test Guideline no. 407). *Arch Toxicol* 76:194–202.

Aoki, A., and D.W. Fawcett. 1978. Is there a local feedback from the seminiferous tubules affecting activity of the Leydig cells? *Biol Reprod* 19:144–58.

Armstrong, D.T. 1968. Hormonal control of uterine lumen fluid retention in the rat. *Am J Physiol* 214:764–71.

Arthur, A.T., G.G. McCormick, J.W. Rickig et al. 1989. Toxicology evaluation of an aromatase inhibitor CGS 18320B in dogs. *Toxicologist* 9:253.

Attia, M.A., and I. Zayed. 1989. Thirteen-weeks subcutaneous treatment with high dose of natural sex hormones in rats with special reference to their effect on the pituitary–gonadal axis. I. Oestradiol. *Dtsch Tierarztl Wschr* 96:438–45.

Balciuniene, J., V.J. Bardwell, and D. Zarkower. 2006. Mice mutant in the DM domain gene Dmrt4 are viable and fertile but have polyovular follicles. *Mol Cell Biol* 26:8984–91.

Baldrick, P., and L. Reeve. 2007. Carcinogenicity evaluation: comparison of tumor data from dual control groups in the CD-1 mouse. *Toxicol Pathol* 35:562–9.

Barker, T.E., and B.E. Walker. 1966. Initiation of irreversible differentiation in vaginal epithelium. *Anat Rec* 154:149–60.

Barrau, M.D., J.H. Abel, H.G. Verhage, and W.J. Tietz. 1975. Development of the endometrium during the estrus cycle in the bitch. *Am J Anat* 142:47–65.

Bartelmez, G.W. 1951. Cyclic changes in the endometrium of the rhesus monkey (*Macaca mulatta*). *Contrib Embryol Carnegie Institut* 34:99–146.

Bartlett, J.M.S., J.B. Kerr, and R.M. Sharpe. 1986. The effect of selective destruction and regeneration of rat Leydig cells on the intratesticular distribution of testosterone and morphology of the seminiferous epithelium. *J Androl* 7:240–53.

Baskin, G.B., S.M. Smith, and P.A. Marx. 2002. Endometrial hyperplasia, polyps, and adenomyosis associated with unopposed estrogen in rhesus monkeys (*Macaca mulatta*). *Vet Pathol* 39:572–5.

Beck, L.R. 1972. Comparative observation on the morphology of the mammalian periovarial sac. *J. Morphol* 136:247–54.

Benjamin, S.A. 2001. Epithelial mammary gland neoplasia in beagles: lifetime morbidity and mortality. In *Pathobiology of the Aging Dog*, ed. U. Mohr, W.W. Carlton, D.L. Dungworth, S.A. Benjamin, C.C. Capen, and F.F. Hahn, 179–87. Ames: Iowa State University Press.

Ben-Jonathan, N., C.R. LaPensee, and E.W. LaPensee. 2008. What can we learn from rodents about prolactin in humans? *Endocr Rev* 29:1–41.

Berg, B.N. 1967. Longevity studies in rats. II. Pathology of ageing rats. In *Pathology of Laboratory Rats and Mice*, ed. E. Cotchin and F.J.C. Roe, 749–86. Oxford: Blackwell Scientific Publications.

Berger, L., M. El-Alfy, C. Martel, and F. Labrie. 2005. Effects of dehydroepiandrosterone, premarin, and acolbifene on histomorphology and sex steroid receptors in the rat vagina. *J Steroid Biochem Mol Biol* 96:201–15.

Berman, D.M., H. Tian, and D.W. Russell. 1995. Expression and regulation of steroid 5 alpha-reductase in the urogenital tract of the fetal rat. *Mol Endocrinol* 9:1561–70.

Bhatti, S.F.M., N.A.S. Rao, A.C. Okkens et al. 2007. Role of progestin-induced mammary-derived growth hormone in the pathogenesis of cystic endometrial hyperplasia in the bitch. *Dom Anim Endocrinol* 33:294–312.

Bhowmik, T., and M. Mukherjea. 1988. Changes in the ovary and uterus of rat after injectable contraceptive therapy. *Contraception* 37:529–38.

Biegel, L.B., J.A. Flaws, A.N. Hirshfield et al. 1998. 90-day feeding and one-generation reproduction study in Crl:CD BR rats with 17 beta-estradiol. *Toxicol Sci* 44:116–42.

Blanco-Rodriguez, J., and C. Martinez-Garcia. 1998. Apoptosis pattern elicited by several apoptogenic agents on the seminiferous epithelium of the adult rat testis. *J Androl* 19:487–97.

Boling, J.L. 1942. Growth and regression of corpora lutea during the normal estrous cycle of the rat. *Anat Rec* 82:131–45.

Bombonati, A., and D.C. Sgroi. 2011. The molecular pathology of breast cancer progression. *J Pathol* 223: 307–17.

Boorman, G.A., D.P. Abbott, M.R. Elwell, and S.L. Eustis. 1987. Sertoli's cell tumor, testis, rat. In *Monographs on Pathology of Laboratory Animals, Genital System*, ed. T.C. Jones, U. Mohr, and R.D. Hunt, 212–17. New York: Springer.

Boorman, G.A., J.T. Wilson, M.J. van Zwieten, and S.L. Eustis. 1990. Mammary gland. In *Pathology of the Fischer rat*, ed. G.A. Boorman, S.L. Eustis, M.R. Elwell, C.A. Montgomery, Jr., and W.F. MacKenzie, 295–313. San Diego: Academic Press.

Borman, S.M., C.L. Chaffin, K.M. Schwinof, R.L. Stouffer, and M.B. Zelinski-Wooten. 2004. Progesterone promotes oocyte maturation, but not ovulation, in nonhuman primate follicles without a gonadotropin surge. *Biol Reprod* 71:366–73.

Borovskaya, T.G., V.E. Goldberg, T.I. Fomina et al. 2004. Morphological and functional state of rat ovaries in early and late periods after administration of platinum cytostatics. *Bull Exp Biol Med* 137:331–5.

Bouchard, G., R.S. Youngquist, and C.S. Reddy. 1994. Estrus induction in the bitch using DES. In *Proceedings of the Annual Meeting of the Society for Theriogenology, Kansas City, MO, August 25–27*, 176–184. Nashville: Society for Theriogenology.

Bowen, J.M, and P.L. Keyes. 2000. Repeated exposure to prolactin is required to induce luteal regression in the hypophysectomized rat. *Biol Reprod* 63:1179–84.

Bowen, J.M., P.L. Keyes, J.S. Warren, and D.H. Townson. 1996. Prolactin-induced regression of the rat corpus luteum: expression of monocytes chemoattractant protein-1 and invasion of macrophages. *Biol Reprod* 54:1120–7.

Brann, D.W., and V.B. Mahesh. 1991. Role of corticosteroids in female reproduction. *FASEB J* 5:2691–8.

Braw, R.H., and A. Tsafriri. 1980. Effect of PMSG on follicular atresia in the immature rat ovary. *J Reprod Fertil* 59:267–72.

Brawer, J., M. Richard, and R. Farookhi. 1989. Pattern of human chorionic gonadotropin binding in the polycystic ovary. *Am J Obstet Gynecol* 161:474–80.

Brenner, R.M., and O.D. Slayden. 1994. Cyclic changes in the primate oviduct and endometrium. In *The Physiology of Reproduction*, 2nd edition, ed. E. Knobil and J.D. Neill, 1213–314. New York: Raven Press.

Brinkworth, M.H., G.F. Weinbauer, S. Schlatt, and E. Nieschlag. 1995. Identification of male germ cells undergoing apoptosis in male rats. *J Reprod Fertil* 105:25–33.

Brisken, C., and B. O'Malley. 2010. Hormone action in the mammary gland. *Cold Spring Harbor Perspect Biol* 2:a003178.

Brisken, C., S. Park, T. Vass, J.P. Lydon, B.W. O'Malley, and R.A. Weinberg. 1998. A paracrine role for the epithelial progesterone receptor in mammary gland development. *Proc Natl Acad Sci USA* 95:5076–81.

Brisken, C., and R.D. Rajaram. 2006. Alveolar and lactogenic differentiation. *J Mammary Gland Biol Neoplasia* 11:239–48.

Bristol-Gould, S., and T.K. Woodruff. 2006. Folliculogenesis in the domestic cat (*Felis catus*). *Theriogenology* 66:5–13.

Brix, A., A. Nyska, J.K. Haseman, D.M. Sells, M.P. Jokinen, and N.J. Walker. 2005. Incidences of selected lesions in control female Harlan Sprague–Dawley rats from two-year studies performed by the National Toxicology Program. *Toxicol Pathol* 33:477–83.

Brown, A.P., R.L. Morrissey, J.A. Crowell, and B.S. Levine. 1999a. Thirteen-week oral toxicity study of difluoromethylornithine in combination with tamoxifen citrate in female dogs. *Cancer Chemother Pharmacol* 43:479–88.

Brown, A.P., R.L. Morrissey, J.A. Crowell, and B.S. Levine. 1999b. Difluoromethylornithine in combination with tamoxifen in female rats: 13-week oral toxicity study. *Cancer Chemother Pharmacol* 44:475–83.

Brown, H.R., and J.R. Leininger. 1992. Alterations of the uterus. In *Pathobiology of the Aging Rat*, ed. U. Mohr, D.L. Dungworth, and C.C. Capen, Vol. 1, 377–88. Washington, DC: ILSI Press.

Bruner, R., K. Küttler, R. Bader et al. 2001. Integumentary system. In *International Classification of Rodent Tumors: The Mouse*, ed. U. Mohr, 1–22. Berlin: Springer-Verlag.

Bryant, B.H., and K. Boekelheide. 2007. Time-dependent changes in post-mortem testis histopathology in the rat. *Toxicol Pathol* 35:665–71.

Burdette, J.E., R.M. Oliver, V. Ulyanov et al. 2007. Ovarian epithelial inclusion cysts in chronically superovulated CD1 and Smad2 dominant-negative mice. *Endocrinol* 148:3595–604.

Buse, E., M. Zöller, and E. van Esch. 2008. The macaque ovary, with special reference to the cynomolgus macaque (*Macaca fascicularis*). *Toxicol Pathol* 36:24S–66S.

Buzzard, J.J., K.L. Loveland, M.K. O'Bryan et al. 2004. Changes in circulating and testicular levels of inhibin A and B and activin A during postnatal development in the rat. *Endocrinology* 145:3532–41.

Byskov, A.G. 1974. Cell kinetic studies of follicular atresia in the mouse ovary. *J Reprod Fertil* 37:277–85.

Camarillo, I.G., G. Thordarson, J.G. Moffat et al. 2001. Prolactin receptor expression in the epithelia and stroma of the rat mammary gland. *J Endocrinol* 171:85–95.

Cameron, A.M., and L.J. Faulkin. 1971. Hyperplastic and inflammatory nodules in the canine mammary gland. *J Nat Cancer Inst* 47:1277–87.

Cardiff, R.D. 1998. Are the TDLU of the human the same as the LA of mice? *J Mammary Gland Biol Neopl* 3:3–5.

Cardiff, R.D., R.J. Munn, and J.J. Galvez. 2007. The tumor pathology of genetically engineered mice: a new approach to molecular pathology. In *The Mouse in Biomedical Research, Volume II, Diseases*, 2nd edition, ed. J.G. Fox, S.W. Barthold, M.T. Davisson, C.E. Newcomer, F.W. Quimby, and A.L. Smith, 581–622. San Diego: Academic Press.

Cardiff, R.D., and S.R. Wellings. 1999. The comparative pathology of human and mouse mammary glands. *J Mammary Gland Biol Neoplasia* 4:105–22.

Cardy, R.H. 1991. Sexual dimorphism of the normal rat mammary gland. *Vet Pathol* 28:139–45.

Carthew, P., R.E. Edwards, B.M. Nolan, E.A. Martin, and L.L. Smith. 1996. Tamoxifen associated uterine pathology in rodents: relevance to women. *Carcinogenesis* 17:1577–82.

Cartwright, J., and S. Moreland. 2008. Endocrine disruption: a guidance document for histologic evaluation of endocrine and reproductive tests. Part 3e: female reproductive system. Morphological patterns of endocrine disruption. Organization of Economic Cooperation and Development. http://www.oecd.org/dataoecd/30/19/43754876.pdf.

Chaffin, C.L., and R.L. Stouffer. 2002. Local role of progesterone in the ovary during the periovulatory interval. *Rev Endocr Metab Disord* 3:6–72.

Chambô-Filho, A., A.F. Camargos, and F.E.L. Pereira. 2005. Morphological changes induced by testosterone in the mammary glands of female Wistar rats. *Braz J Med Biol Res* 38:553–8.

Chan, T.W., M. Pollack, and H. Huynh. 2001. Inhibtion of insulin-like growth factor signaling pathways in mammary gland by pure antiestrogen ICI 182,780. *Clin Cancer Res* 7:2545–54.

Chandra, M., and C.H. Frith. 1992. Spontaneous neoplasms in aged CD-1 mice. *Toxicol Lett* 61:67–74.

Chandra, S.A., and R.A. Adler. 2008. Frequency of different estrus stages in purpose-bred beagles: a retrospective study. *Toxicol Pathol* 36:944–9.

Chandra, S.A., J.M. Cline, and R.R. Adler. 2010. Cyclic morphological changes in the beagle mammary gland. *Toxicol Pathol* 38:969–83.

Chapin, R.E. 2011. Whither the resolution of testicular toxicity. *Birth Defects Res (Part B)*. 92:504–7.

Chapin, R.E., D.M. Creasy, and J.C. O'Conner. 2011. The measurement of male reproductive hormones in laboratory animals. *Toxicol Pathol* (in press).

Chapin, R.E., R.D. White, K.T. Morgan, and J.S. Bus. 1984. Studies of lesions induced in the testis and epididymis of F-344 rats by inhaled methyl chloride. *Toxicol Appl Pharmacol* 76:328–43.

Chellman, G.J., K.T. Morgan, J.S. Bus, and P.K. Working. 1986. Inhibition of methyl chloride toxicity in male F-344 rats by the anti-inflammatory agent BW-755C. *Toxicol Appl Pharmacol* 85:365–79.

Chen, H., E. Stanley, S. Jin, and B. Zirkin. 2010. Stem Leydig cells: from fetal to aged animals. *Birth Defects Res (Part C)* 90:272–83.

Chu, Po-yin, C.S. Lee, and P.J. Wright. 2006. Degeneration and apoptosis of endometrial cells in the bitch. *Theriogenology* 66:1545–9.

Chu, Po-yin, P.J. Wright, and C.S. Lee. 2002. Apoptosis of endometrial cells in the bitch. *Reprod Fertil Dev* 14:297–305.

Clegg, E.D., J.C. Cook, R.E. Chapin, P.M.D. Foster, and G.P. Daston. 1997. Leydig cell hyperplasia and adenoma formation: mechanisms and relevance to humans. *Reprod Toxicol* 11:107–21.

Clermont, Y. 1972. Kinetics of spermatogenesis in mammals: seminiferous epithelium cycle and spermatogonial renewal. *Physiol Rev* 52:198–236.

Clermont, Y., and B. Perey. 1957. Quantitative study of the cell population of the seminiferous tubules in immature rats. *Am J Anat* 100:241–68.

Cline, J.M. 2007. Assessing the mammary gland of nonhuman primates: effects of endogenous hormones and exogenous hormonal agents and growth factors. *Birth Defects Res (Part B)* 80:126–46.

Cline, J.M., A.A. Franke, T.C. Register, D.L. Golden, and M.R. Adams. 2004. Effects of dietary isoflavone aglycones on the reproductive tract of male and female mice. *Toxicol Pathol* 32:91–9.

Cline, J.M., and C.E. Wood. 2008. The mammary glands of macaques. *Toxicol Pathol* 36:130S–41S.

Cline, J.M., C.E. Wood, J.D. Vidal, R.P. Tarara, E. Buse, G.F. Weinbauer, E.P.C.T. de Rijk, and E. van Esch. 2008. Selected background findings and interpretation of common lesions in the female reproductive system in macaques. *Toxicol Pathol* 36:142S–163S.

Cohen, I., M.L. Sims, M.R. Robbins, M.C. Lakshmanan, P.C. Francis, and G.G. Long. 2000. The reversible effects of raloxifene on luteinizing hormone levels and ovarian morphology in mice. *Reprod Toxicol* 14:37–44.

Concannon, P.W. 2011. Reproductive cycles of the bitch. *Anim Reprod Sci* 124:200–10.

Concannon, P.W., and V.D. Castracane. 1985. Serum androstenedione and testosterone concentrations during pregnancy and nonpregnant cycle in dogs. *Biol Reprod* 33:1078–83.

Concannon, P.W., W. Hansel, and K. McEntee. 1977. Changes in LH, progesterone and sexual behavior associated with preovulatory luteinization in the bitch. *Biol Reprod* 17:604–13.

Concannon, P.W., J.P. McCann, and M. Temple. 1989. Biology and endocrinology of ovulation, pregnancy and parturition in the dog. *J Reprod Fert Suppl* 39:3–25.

Concannon, P.W., T.R. Spraker, H.W. Casey, and W. Hansel. 1981. Gross and histopathologic effects of medroxyprogesterone acetate and progesterone on the mammary glands of adult beagle bitches. *Fertil Steril* 36:373–87.

Concannon, P.W., S. Whaley, and S.P. Anderson. 1986. Increased LH pulse frequency associated with termination of anestrus during the ovarian cycle of the dog [Abstract]. *Biol Reprod Suppl* 34:119.

Cook, J.C., G.R. Klinefelter, J.F. Hardisty, R.M. Sharpe, and P.M.D. Foster. 1999. Rodent Leydig cell tumorigenesis: a review of the physiology, pathology, mechanisms, and relevance to humans. *Crit Rev Toxicol* 29:169–261.

Cooper, T.K., and K.L. Gabrielson. 2007. Spontaneous lesions in the reproductive tract and mammary gland of female non-human primates. *Birth Defects Res B Dev Reprod Toxicol* 80:149–70.

Cortes, D., J. Müller, and N.E. Skakkebæk. 1987. Proliferation of Sertoli cells during development of the human testis assessed by stereological methods. *Int J Androl* 10:589–96.

Creasy, D. 2008a. Endocrine disruption: a guidance document for histologic evaluation of endocrine and reproductive tests. Part 2: male reproductive system. Organization of Economic Cooperation and Development. http://www.oecd.org/dataoecd/29/35/43754701.pdf.

Creasy, D. 2008b. Endocrine disruption: a guidance document for histologic evaluation of endocrine and reproductive tests. Part 4: mammary gland. Organization of Economic Cooperation and Development. http://www.oecd.org/dataoecd/30/20/43754898.pdf.

Creasy, D.M. 1997. Evaluation of testicular toxicity in safety evaluation studies: the appropriate use of spermatogenic staging. *Toxicol Pathol* 25:119–31.

Creasy, D.M. 2001. Pathogenesis of male reproductive toxicity. *Toxicol Pathol* 29:64–76.

Creasy, D.M., J.C. Flynn, T.J.B. Gray, and W.H. Butler. 1985. A quantitative study of stage-specific spermatocyte damage following administration of ethylene glycol monomethyl ether in the rat. *Exp Mol Pathol* 43:321–36.

Creasy, D.M., and P.M.D. Foster. 2002. Male reproductive system. In *Handbook of Toxicologic Pathology*, ed. W.M. Haschek, C.G. Rousseaux, and M.A. Wallig, 785–846. San Diego: Academic Press.

Cunha, G.R., P.S. Cooke, and T. Kurita. 2004. Role of stromal–epithelial interactions in hormonal responses. *Arch Histol Cytol* 57:41–34.

Czoty, P.W., R.W. Gould, and M.A. Nader. 2009. Relationship between social rank and cortisol and testosterone concentration in male cynomolgus monkeys (*Macaca fascicularis*). *J Neuroendocrinol* 21:68–76.

Daane, T.A., and W.R. Lyons. 1954. Effect of estrone, progesterone and pituitary mammotropin on the mammary glands of castrated C3H male mice. *Endocrinology* 55:191–9.

Daly, T.J., and B. Kramer. 1998. Alterations in rat vaginal histology by exogenous gonadotrophins. *J Anat* 193:469–72.

Dang, D.C., and N. Meusy-Dessolle. 1984. Quantitavtive study of testis histology and plasma androgens at onset of spermatogenesis in the prepubertal laboratory-born macaque (*Macaca fascicularis*). *Arch Androl* 12(Suppl):43–51.

Daniel, C.W., and G.B. Silberstein. 1987. Postnatal development of the rodent mammary gland. In *The Mammary Gland*, ed. M.C. Neville and C.W. Daniel, 3–36. New York: Plenum Press.

Davis, B., J. Almekinder, N. Flagler, G. Travlos, R. Wilson, and R.R. Maronpot. 1997. Ovarian luteal cell toxicity of ethylene glycol monomethyl ether and methoxy acetic acid in vivo and in vitro. *Toxicol Appl Pharmacol* 142:328–37.

Davis, B.J., D. Dixon, and R.A. Herbert. 1999. Ovary, oviduct, uterus, cervix, and vagina. In *Pathology of the Mouse*, ed. R.R. Maronpot, 409–43. Vienna, IL: Cache River Press.

Davis, B.J., and J.J. Heindel. 1998. Ovarian toxicants: multiple mechanisms of action. In *Reproductive and Developmental Toxicology*, ed. K.S. Korach, 373–95. New York: Marcel Dekker.

Deerberg, F., S. Rehm, and W. Pittermann. 1981. Uncommon frequency of adenocarcinomas of the uterus in virgin Han:Wistar rats. *Vet Pathol* 18:707–13.

De Schaepdrijver, L.M., J.L. Fransen, E.S. Van der Eycken, and W.C. Coussement. 1995. Transverse vaginal septum in the specific-pathogen-free Wistar rat. *Lab Anim Sci* 45:181–3.

Dixon, D., J.R. Leininger, M.G. Valerio, A.N. Johnson, L.G. Stabinski, and C.H. Frith. 1999. Proliferative lesions of the ovary, uterus, vagina, cervix and oviduct in rats. URG-5. In *Guides for Toxicologic Pathology*. Washington, DC: STP/ARP/AFIP.

Dore, M.A. 1989. Structural aspects of luteal function and regression in the ovary of the domestic dog. *J Reprod Fertil Suppl* 39:41–53.

Dorso, L., F. Chanut, P. Howroyd, and R. Burnett. 2008. Variability in weight and histologic appearance of the prostate of beagle dogs used in toxicology studies. *Toxicol Pathol* 36:917–25.

Dow, C. 1960. Ovarian abnormalities in the bitch. *J Comp Pathol* 70:59–69.

Downs, J.L., and P.M. Wise. 2009. The role of the brain in female reproductive aging. *Mol Cell Endocrinol* 299:32–8.

Dreef, H.C., E. van Esch, and E.P.C.T. de Rijk. 2007. Spermatogenesis in the cynomolgus monkey (*Macaca fascicularis*): a practical guide for routine morphological staging. *Toxicol Pathol* 35:395–404.

Dudley, C.A., G. Rajendren, and R.L. Moss. 1996. Signal processing in the vomeronasal system: modulation of sexual behavior in the female rat. *Crit Rev Neurobiol* 10:265–90.

Duncan, M.K. and K.K. Chada. 1993. Incidence of tubulostromal adenoma of the ovary in aged germ cell-deficient mice. *J Comp Pathol* 109(1):13–9.

Durlinger, A.L., P. Kramer, B. Karels et al. 1999. Control of primordial follicle recruitment by anti-Mullerian hormone in the mouse ovary. *Endocrinology* 140:5789–96.

Durlinger, A.L., P. Kramer, B. Karels, J.A. Grootegoed, J.T. Uilenbroek, and A.P. Themmen. 2000. Apoptotic and proliferative changes during induced atresia of pre-ovulatory follicles in the rat. *Hum Reprod* 15:2504–11.

Dürnberger, H., and K. Kratochwil. 1980. Specificity of tissue interaction and origin of mesenchymal cells in the androgen response of the embryonic mammary gland. *Cell* 19:465–71.

Edson, M.A., A.K. Nagaraja, and M.M. Matzuk. 2009. The mammalian ovary from genesis to revelation. *Endo Rev* 30:624–712.

El Etreby, M.F. 1979. Effect of cyproteroneacetate, levorgenestrol and progesterone on adrenal glands and reproductive organs in the beagle bitch. *Cell Tissue Res* 200:229–43.

El Etreby, M.F., and K.-J. Gräf. 1979. Effect of contraceptive steroids on mammary gland of beagle dog and its relevance to human carcinogenicity. *Pharmacol Ther* 5:369–402.

Elcock, L.H., B.P. Stuart, R.E. Mueller, and H.E. Hoss. 1987. Deciduoma, uterus, rat. In *Genital System*, ed. T.C. Jones, U. Mohr, and R.D. Hunt, 140–6. Berlin: Springer.

Ellis, G.B. and C. Desjardins. 1982. Male rats secrete luteinizing hormone and testosterone episodically. *Endocrinology* 110:1618–27.

Elsinghorst, T.A., H.J. Timmermans, and H.G. Hendriks. 1984. Comparative pathology of endometrial carcinoma. *Vet Q* 6:200–8.

Engelhardt, A., J.K. Hodges, C. Niemitz, and M. Heistermann. 2005. Female sexual behavior, but not sex skin swelling, reliably indicates the timing of the fertile phase in wild long-tailed macaques (*Macaca fascicularis*). *Horm Behav* 47:195–204.

England, G.C., and W.E. Allen. 1989. Ultrasonographic and histological appearance of the canine ovary. *Vet Rec* 125:555–6.

Erickson, G.F., D.A. Magoffin, C.A. Dyer, and C. Hofeditz. 1985. The ovarian androgen producing cells: a review of structure/function relationships. *Endocr Rev* 5:371–99.

Eskin, B.A., C.E. Grotkowski, C.P. Connolly, and W.R. Ghent. 1995. Different tissue responses for iodine and iodide in rat thyroid and mammary glands. *Biol Trace Elem Res* 49:9–19.

Ettlin, R.A., S.R. Qureshi, E. Perentes et al. 1992. Morphological, immunohistochemical, stereological and nuclear shape characteristics of proliferative Leydig cell alterations in rats. *Pathol Res Pract* 188:643–8.

Evans, B., B.J. Gannon, J.W. Heath, and G. Burnstock. 1977. Long lasting damage to the internal male genital organs and their adrenergic innervations in rats following chronic treatment with the antihypertensive drug guanethidine. *Fertil Steril* 23:657–67.

Ezer, N., and B. Robaire. B. 2002. Androgenic regulation of the structure and function of the epididymis. In *The Epididymis: from Molecules to Clinical Practice*, ed. B. Robaire and B.T. Hinton, 297–316. New York: Kluwer Academic/Plenum Publishers.

Fawcett, D.W., W.B. Neaves, and M.N. Flores. 1973. Comparative observations on intertubular lymphatics and the organization of the interstitial tissue of the mammalian testis. *Biol Reprod* 9:500–32.

Felicio, L.S., J.F. Nelson, and C.E. Finch. 1984. Longitudinal studies of estrous cyclicity in aging C57BL/6J mice: II. Cessation of cyclicity and the duration of persistent vaginal cornification. *Biol Reprod* 31:446–53.

Fenwick, M.A., and P.R. Hurst. 2002. Immunohistochemical localization of active caspase-3 in the mouse ovary: growth and atresia of small follicles. *Reproduction* 124:659–65.

Fernandes, P.A., R.A. Brown, A.C. Kostas, H.R. Sawyer, T.M. Nett, and P.N. Olson. 1987. Luteal function in the bitch: changes during diestrus in pituitary concentration of and the number of luteal receptors for luteinizing hormone and prolactin. *Biol Reprod* 37:804–11.

Ferrara, N., H. Chen, T. Davis-Smyth, H.P Gerber, T.N. Nguyen, D. Peers, V. Chisholm, K.J. Hillan, and R.H. Schwall. 1998. Vascular endothelial growth factor is essential for corpus luteum angiogenesis. *Nat Med* 4:336–40.

Ferreira, E., H. Gobbi, B.S. Saraiva, and G.D. Cassali. 2010. Columnar cell lesions of the canine mammary gland: pathological features and immunophenotypic analysis. *BMC Cancer* 10:61–7.

Ferreira, E., H. Gobbi, B.S. Saraiva, and G.D. Cassali. 2011. Histological and immunohistochemical identifiecation of atypical ductal mammary hyperplasia as a preneoplastic marker in dogs. *Vet Pathol* DOI:10.1177/0300985810396105.

Fleming, J.S., H.J. McQuillan, M.J. Millier, C.R. Beaugié, and V. Livingstone. 2007. E-cadherin expression and bromodeoxyuridine incorporation during development of ovarian inclusion cysts in age-matched breeder and incessantly ovulated CD-I mice. *Reprod Biol Endocrinol* 5:14.

Flickinger, C.J., and S.S. Howard. 2002. Consequences of obstruction on the epididymis. In *The Epididymis: from Molecules to Clinical Practice*, ed. B. Robaire and B.T. Hinton, 503–22. New York: Kluwer Academic/Plenum Publishers.

Foley, G.L. 2001. Overview of male reproductive pathology. *Toxicol Pathol* 29:49–63.

Foley, G.L., N. Bassily, and R.A. Hess. 1995. Intratubular spermatic granulomas of the canine efferent ductules. *Toxicol Pathol* 23:731–5.

Förster, C., S. Mäkela, A. Wärri et al. 2002. Involvement of estrogen receptor beta in terminal differentiation of mammary gland epithelium. *Proc Natl Acad Sci USA* 99:15578–83.

Fortune, J.E. 1994. Ovarian follicular growth and development in mammals. *Biol Reprod* 50:225–32.

Foster, W.G., E.V. Younglai, O. Boutross-Tadross, C.L. Hughes, and M.G. Wade. 2004. Mammary gland morphology in Sprague–Dawley rats following treatment with an organochlorine mixture in utero and neonatal genistein. *Toxicol Sci* 77:91–100.

Fowler, E.H., M.K. Feldman, and W.F. Loeb. 1971. Comparison of histologic features of ovarian and uterine tissues with vaginal smears of the bitch. *Am J Vet Res* 32:327–34.

Fowler, K.A., K. Gill, N. Kirma, D.L. Dillehay, and R.R. Tekmal. 2000. Overexpression of aromatase leads to development of testicular Leydig cell tumors. *Am J Pathol* 156:347–53.

Franca, L.R., M.C. Leal, E. Sasso-Cerri, A. Vasconcelos, L. Debeljuk, and L.D. Russell. 2000. Cimetidine (Tagamet) is a reproductive toxicant in male rats affecting peritubular cells. *Biol Reprod* 63:1403–12.

Franks, L.M. 1968. Spontaneous interstitial and Sertoli cell tumors of a testis in a C3H mouse. *Cancer Res* 28:125–7.

Fraser, H.M., N.P. Groome, and A.S. McNeilly. 1999. Follicle-stimulating hormone-inhibin B interactions during the follicular phase of the primate menstrual cycle revealed by gonadotropin-releasing hormone antagonist and antiestrogen treatment. *J Clin Endocrinol Metab* 84:1365–9.

Freeman, M.E. 2006. Neuroendocrine control of the ovarian cycle in the rat. In *Knobil and Neill's Physiology of Reproduction*, 3rd edition, ed. J.D. Neill, 2327–88. San Diego: Elsevier.

Fukuda, S. 2001. Incidence of pyometra in colony-raised beagle dogs. *Exp Anim* 50:325–9.

Fukushima, T., T. Yamamoto, R. Kikkawa et al. 2005. Effects of male reproductive toxicants on gene expression in rat testes. *J Toxicol Sci* 30:195–206.

Gao, H.-B., M.-H. Tong, Y.-Q. Hu, Q.-S. Guo, R. Ge, and M.P. Hardy. 2002. Glucocorticoid induces apoptosis in rat Leydig cells. *Endocrinology* 143:130–8.

Gaytán F., C. Bellido, M. Gaytán, C. Morales, and J.E. Sánchez-Criado. 2003. Differential effects of RU486 and indomethacin on follicle rupture during the ovulatory process in the rat. *Biol Reprod* 69(1):99–105.

Gaytán, M., M.A. Sánchez, C. Morales et al. 2005. Cyclic changes of the ovarian surface epithelium in the rat. *Reproduction* 129:311–21.

Generoso, W.M., S.K. Stout, and S.W. Huff. 1971. Effects of alkylating chemicals on reproductive capacity of adult female mice. *Mutat Res* 13:171–84.

Geschickter, C.F., and C.G. Hartman. 1959. Mammary response to prolonged estrogenic stimulation in the monkey. *Cancer* 12:767–81.

Ghosh, D., and J. Sengupta. 1992. Patterns of ovulation, conception and preimplantation embryo development during the breeding season in rhesus monkeys kept under semi-natural conditions. *Acta Endocrinol (Copenh)* 127:168–73.

Goedken, M.J., R.L. Kerlin, and D. Morton. 2008. Spontaneous and age-related testicular findings in beagle dogs. *Toxicol Pathol* 36:465–71.

Goericke-Pesch, S., B. Schmidt, K. Failing, and A. Wehrend. 2010. Changes in the histomorphology of the canine cervix through the oestrus cycle. *Theriogenology* 74:1075–81.

Goldman, J. M., A.S. Murr, and R.L. Cooper. 2007. The rodent estrous cycle: characterization of vaginal cytology and its utility in toxicological studies. *Birth Defects Res B* 80:84–97.

Goldschmidt, M., L. Peña, R. Rasotto, and V. Zappulli. 2011. Classification and grading of canine mammary tumors. *Vet Pathol* 48:117–31.

Gondos, B., and W.E. Berndtson. 1993. Postnatal and pubertal development. In *The Sertoli Cell*, ed. L.D. Russell and M.D. Griswold, 115–54. Clearwater: Cache River Press.

Goodman, D.G., and P.K. Hildebrandt. 1987a. Squamous cell carcinoma, endometrium/cervix, rat. In *Monographs on Pathology of Laboratory Animals. Genital System*, eds. T.C. Jones, U. Mohr, and R.D. Hunt, 82–83. Berlin, Heidelberg, New York, Tokyo: Springer.

Goodman, D.G., and P.K. Hildebrandt. 1987b. Stromal polyp, endometrium, rat. In *Monographs on Pathology of Laboratory Animals. Genital System*, eds. T.C. Jones, U. Mohr, and R.D. Hunt, 146–148. Berlin, Heidelberg, New York, Tokyo: Springer.

Goodman, D.G., and P.K. Hildebrandt. 1987c. Stromal sarcoma, endometrium, rat. In *Monographs on Pathology of Laboratory Animals. Genital System*, eds. T.C. Jones, U. Mohr, and R.D. Hunt, 70–72. Berlin, Heidelberg, New York, Tokyo: Springer.

Gopinath, C. 1992. Susceptibility of the uterus to toxic substances. In *Pathobiology of the Aging Rat*, ed. U. Mohr, D.L. Dungworth, and C.C. Capen, Vol. 1, 389–94. Washington, DC: ILSI Press.

Gopinath, C., and W.A. Gibson. 1987. Mesovarian leiomyomas in the rat. *Environ Health Perspect* 73:107–13.

Gore, A.C., T. Oung, S. Yung, R.A. Flagg, and M.J. Woller. 2000. Neuroendocrine mechanisms for reproductive senescence in the female rat. *Endocrine* 13:315–23.

Gotoh, Y., J. Netsu, M. Nakai, and T. Nasu. 1999. Testicular damage after exposure to carbendazim depends on the number of patent efferent ductules. *J Vet Med Sci* 61:755–60.

Gougeon, A. 1996. Regulation of ovarian follicular development in primates: facts and hypotheses. *Endocr Rev* 17:121–55.

Gould, D.H. 1977. Mesotheliomas of the tunica vaginalis propria and peritoneum in Fischer rats. *Vet Pathol* 14:372–9.

Goyings, L.S., J.H. Sokolowski, R.G. Zimbelman, and S. Geng. 1977. Clinical, morphologic, and clinicopathologic findings in beagles treated for two years with melengestrol acetate. *Am J Vet Res* 38:1923–31.

Gräf, K.J. 1978. Serum oestrogen, progesterone and prolactin concentrations in cyclic, pregnant and lactating beagle dogs. *J Reprod Fertil* 52:9–14.

Graham, C.E. 1970. Response of the rhesus monkey uterine cervix to chronic estrogenic stimulation. *Am J Obstet Gynecol* 108:1192–96.

Greaves, P. 2007. *Histopathology of Preclinical Toxicity Studies*, 3rd edition. New York: Academic Press.

Greaves, P., and J.M. Faccini. 1984. *Rat Histopathology. A Glossary for Use in Toxicity and Carcinogenicity Studies*, 171–86. Amsterdam: Elsevier.

Greaves, P., R. Goonetilleke, G. Nunn, J. Topham, and T. Orton. 1993. Two-year carcinogenicity study of tamoxifen in Alderley Park Wistar-derived rats. *Cancer Res* 53:3919–24.

Greaves, P., and I.N.H. White. 2006. Experimental adenomyosis. *Best Pract Res Clin Obst Gynaecol* 20:503–10.

Greenman, D.L., and F.R. Fullerton. 1986. Comparison of histological responses of BALB/c and B6C3F1 female mice to estradiol when fed purified or natural-ingredient diets. *J Toxicol Environ Health* 19:531–40.

Greenman, D.L., D. Gaylor, B. Highman, J. Farmer, M.J. Norvell, and G. Gass. 1983. Nonneoplastic changes induced in female C3H mice by chronic exposure to diethylstilbestrol or 17 beta-estradiol. *J Toxicol Environ Health* 11:843–56.

Grosser, P.M., G.F. McCarthy, B. Robaire, R. Farookhi, and J.R. Brawer. 1987. Plasma patterns of LH, FSH and prolactin in rats with a polycystic ovarian condition induced by oestradiol valerate. *J Endocr* 114:33–9.

Gunn, S.A., T.C. Gould, and W.A.D. Anderson. 1963. The selective injurious response of testicular and epididymal blood vessels to cadmium and its prevention by zinc. *Am J Pathol* 42:685–702.

Guraya, S.S. 1975. Histochemical observations on the lipid changes in the rat corpus luteum during various reproductive states. *J Reprod Fertil* 42:59–65.

Hadfield, R.M., P.L. Yudkin, C.L. Coe, J. Scheffler, H. Uno, D.H. Barlow, J.W. Kemnitz, and S.H. Kennedy. 1997. Risk factors for endometriosis in the rhesus monkey (*Macaca mulatta*): a case–control study. *Hum Reprod Update* 3:109–15.

Hampe, J.F., and W. Misdorp. 1974. IX. Tumors and dysplasias of the mammary gland. *Bull WHO* 50:111–33.

Harneit, S., H.J. Paust, A.K. Mukhopadhyay, and S. Ergun. 1997. Localization of endothelin 1 and endothelin receptors A and B in human epididymis. *Mol Hum Reprod* 3:579–84.

Harvell, D.M.E., T.E. Strecker, M. Tochacek et al. 2000. Rat strain-specific actions of 17β-estradiol in the mammary gland: correlation between estrogen-induced lobuloalveolar hyperplasia and susceptibility to estrogen-induced mammary cancers. *Proc Natl Acad Sci USA* 97:2779–84.

Heape, W. 1900. The sexual season of mammals and the relationship of "pro-estrus" to menstruation. Part I. *Q J Microbiol Sci* 44:1–70.

Hess, R.A. 1990. Quantitative and qualitative characteristics of the stages and transitions in the cycle of the rat seminiferous epithelium: light microscopic observation of perfusion-fixed and plastic embedded testes. *Biol Reprod* 43:525–42.

Hess, R.A. 2002. The efferent ductules: structure and function. In *The Epididymis: From Molecules to Clinical Practice*, ed. B. Robaire and B.T. Hinton, 49–80. New York: Kluwer Academic/Plenum Publishers.

Hess, R.A., and M. Nakai. 2000. Histopathology of the male reproductive system induced by the fungicide benomyl. *Histol Histopathol* 15:207–24.

Hess, R.A., Q. Zhou, and R. Nie. 2002. The role of estrogens in the endocrine and paracrine regulation of the efferent ductules, epididymis and vas deferens. In *The Epididymis: from Molecules to Clinical Practice*, ed. B. Robaire and B.T. Hinton, 317–38. New York: Kluwer Academic/Plenum Publishers.

Hewitt, S.C., and K.S. Korach. 2003. Oestrogen receptor knockout mice: roles for oestrogen receptors α and β in reproductive tissues. *Reproduction* 125:143–9.

Heywood, R., and P.F. Wadsworth. 1981. The experimental toxicology of estrogens. In *Pharmacology of Estrogens. International Encyclopedia of Pharmacology and Therapeutics, Section 106*, ed. R.R. Chaudhury, 63–80. New York: Pergamon Press.

Highman, B., M.J. Norvell, and T.E. Shellenberger. 1978. Pathological changes in female C3H mice continuously fed diets containing diethylstilbestrol or 17beta-estradiol. *J Environ Pathol Toxicol* 1:1–30.

Hirshfield, A.N. 1988. Size-frequency analysis of atresia in cycling rats. *Biol Reprod* 38:1181–8.

Hirshfield, A.N. 1997. Overview of ovarian follicular development: considerations for the toxicologist. *Environ Mol Mutagen* 29:10–5.

Hirshfield, A.N., and A.R. Midgley, Jr. 1978. Morphometric analysis of follicular development in the rat. *Biol Reprod* 19:597–605.

Hirshfield, A.N., and W.A. Schmidt. 1987. Kinetic aspects of follicular development in the rat. *Adv Exp Med Biol* 219:211–36.

Hoak, D.C., and N.A.B. Schwartz. 1980. Blockade of recruitment of ovarian follicles by suppression of the secondary surge of follicle-stimulating hormone with porcine follicular fluid. *Proc Natl Acad Sci USA* 77:4953–6.

Hoffmann, B., F. Büsges, E. Engel, M.P. Kowalewski, and P. Papa. 2004. Regulation of corpus luteum-function in the bitch. *Reprod Dom Anim* 39:232–40.

Holst, P.A., and R.D. Phemister. 1974. Onset of diestrus in the beagle bitch: definition and significance. *Am J Vet Res* 35:401–6.

Hooser, S.B., D.P. Douds, D.G. DeMerell, P.B. Hoyer, and I.G. Sipes. 1994. Long-term ovarian and gonadotropin changes in mice exposed to 4-vinylcyclohexene. *Reprod Toxicol* 8:315–23.

Hovey, R.C., and L. Aimo. 2010. Diverse and active roles for adipocytes during mammary gland growth and function. *J Mammary Gland Biol Neoplasia* 15:279–90.

Hovey, R.C., T.B. McFadden, and R.M. Akers. 1999. Regulation of mammary gland growth and morphogenesis by the mammary fat pad: a species comparison. *J Mammary Gland Biol Neoplasia* 4:53–68.

Hovey, R.C., J.F. Trott, and B.K. Vonderhaar. 2002. Establishing a framework for the functional mammary gland: from endocrinology to morphology. *J Mammary Gland Biol Neoplasia* 7:17–38.

Hoyer, P.B. 2004. Ovarian toxicity in small pre-antral follicles. In *Ovarian Toxicology*, ed. P.B. Hoyer, 17–40. Boca Raton: CRC Press.

Hruban, Z., T.-W. Wong, and E. Hopkins. 1972. Chlorcyclizine-induced changes in the ovaries and the uterus of rats. *J Reprod Fert* 31:463–7.

Huseby, R.A. 1980. Demonstration of a direct carcinogenic effect of estradiol on Leydig cells of the mouse. *Cancer Res* 40:1006–13.

Hvid, H., I. Thorup, M.B. Oleksiewicz, I. Sjögren, and H.E. Jensen. 2010. An alternative method for preparation of tissue sections from the rat mammary gland. *Exp Toxicol Pathol* DOI:10.1016/j.etp.2010.02.005.

Hynes, N.E., and C.J. Watson. 2010. Mammary gland growth factors: roles in normal development and cancer. *Cold Spring Harbor Perspect Biol* 2:a003186.

Ichikawa, S., T. Sawada, Y. Nakamura, and H. Morioka. 1974. Ovarian secretion of pregnane compounds during the estrous cycle and pregnancy in rats. *Endocrinology* 94:1615–20.

Iguchi, T., N. Takasugi, H.A. Bern, and K.T. Mills. 1986. Frequent occurrence of polyovular follicles in ovaries of mice exposed neonatally to diethylstilbestrol. *Teratology* 34:29–35.

Iguchi, T., R. Todoroki, N. Takasugi, and Y. Petrow. 1988. The effects of an aromatase inhibitor and a 5 alpha-reductase inhibitor upon the occurrence of polyovular follicles, persistent anovulation, and permanent vaginal stratification in mice treated neonatally with testosterone. *Biol Reprod* 39:689–97.

Ilio, K.Y. and R.A. Hess. 1994. Structure and function of the ductuli efferentes: a review. *Microsc Res Technol* 29:432–67.

Imagawa, W., G.K. Bandyopadhyay, and S. Nandi. 1990. Regulation of mammary epithelial cell growth in mice and rats. *Endocr Rev* 11:494–523.

Imagawa, W., V.K. Pedchenko, J. Helber, and H. Zhang. 2002. Hormone/growth factor interactions mediating epithelial/stromal communication in mammary gland development and carcinogenesis. *J Steroid Biochem Mol Biol* 80:213–30.

Inoue, S., H. Watanabe, H. Saito, M. Hiroi, and A. Tonosaki. 2000. Elimination of atretic follicles from the mouse ovary: a TEM and immunohistochemical study in mice. *J Anat* 196:103–10.

Ishii, S., M. Ube, M. Okada et al. 2009. Collaborative work on evaluation of ovarian toxicity. 17. Two- or four-week repeated-dose studies and fertility study of sulpiride in female rats. *J Toxicol Sci* 34:SP175–88.

Jabara, A.G. 1962. Some tissue changes in the dog following stilboestrol administration. *Austral J Exp Biol* 40:293–308.

Jabbour, H.N., R.W. Kelly, H.M. Fraser, and H.O. Critchley. 2006. Endocrine regulation of menstruation. *Endocr Rev* 27:17–46.

Jack, D., D. Poynter, and N.W. Spurling. 1983. Beta-adrenoceptor stimulants and mesovarian leiomyomas in the rat. *Toxicology.* 27:315–20.

Jahnukainen, K., D. Chrysis, M. Hou, M. Parvinen, S. Eksborg, and O. Söder. 2004. Increased apoptosis occurring during the first wave of spermatogenesis is stage-specific and primarily affects midpachytene spermatocytes in the rat testis. *Biol Reprod* 70:290–6.

Jamadagni, S.B., P.S. Jamadagni, S.N. Upadhyay, S.N. Gaidhani, and J. Hazra. 2011. A spontaneous teratocarcinoma in the testis of a Swiss albino mouse. *Toxicol Pathol* 39:414–7.

James, R.W., and R. Heywood. 1979. Age-related variations in the testes and prostate of beagle dogs. *Toxicology* 12:273–9.

Jeffcoate, I.A. 1992. Concentrations of luteinizing hormone and oestradiol in plasma and response to injection of gonadotrophin-releasing hormone analogue at selected stages of anoestrus in domestic bitches. *J Reprod Fertil* 94:423–9.

Jefferson, W.N., E. Padilla-Banks, and R.R. Newbold. 2007. Disruption of the developing female reproductive system by phytoestrogens: genistein as an example. *Mol Nutr Food Res* 51:832–44.

Jöchle, W., and A.C. Andersen. 1977. The estrus cycle in the dog: a review. *Theriogenology* 7:113–40.

Johnson, A.N. 1989. Comparative aspects of contraceptive steroids—effects observed in beagle dogs. *Toxicol Pathol* 17:389–95.

Johnston, S.D., M.V. Root Kustritz, and P.N. Olson. 2001. The canine estrus cycle. In *Canine and Feline Theriogenology*, 16–31. Philadelphia: Saunders.

Junaid, M., D.K. Chowdhuri, R. Narayan, R. Shanker, and D.K. Saxena. 1997. Lead-induced changes in ovarian follicular development and maturation in mice. *J Toxicol Environ Health* 50:31–40.

Juniewicz, P.E., J.E. Oesterling, J.R. Walters, R.E. Steele, G.D. Niswender, D.S. Coffee, and L.L. Ewing. 1988. Aromatase inhibition in the dog. I. Effect on serum LH, serum testosterone concentrations, testicular secretions and spermatogenesis. *J Urology* 139:827–31.

Junker-Walker, U., and V. Nogues. 1994. Changes induced by treatment with aromatase inhibitors in testicular Leydig cells of rats and dogs. *Exp Toxicol Pathol* 46:211–3.

Kafali, H., M. Iriadam, I. Ozardah, and N. Demir. 2004. Letrozole-induced polycystic ovaries in the rat: a new model for cystic ovarian disease. *Arch Med Res* 35:103–8.

Kagabu, S., and M. Umezu. 2004. Histological analysis of the 'critical point' in follicular development in mice. *Reprod Medical Biol* 3:141–5.

Kalra, P.S., T.G. Edwards, B. Xu, M. Jain, and S.P. Kalra. 1998. The anti-gonadotropic effects of cytokines: the role of neuropeptides. *Dom Anim Endocrinol* 15:321–32.

Kanno, J., C. Matsuoka, K. Furuta, H. Onodera, A. Maekawa, and Y. Hayashi. 1987. Glandular changes associated with the spontaneous interstitial cell tumor of the rat testis. *Toxicol Pathol* 15:439–43.

Kariagina, A., J. Xie, J.R. Leipprandt, and S.Z. Haslam. 2010. Amphiregulin mediates estrogen, progesterone, and EGFR signaling in the normal rat mammary gland in hormone-dependent rat mammary cancers. *Horm Cancer* 1:229–44.

Karlsson, S., M.J. Iatropoulos, G.M. Williams, L. Kangas, and L. Nieminen. 1998. The proliferation in uterine compartments of intact rats of two different strains exposed to high doses of tamoxifen or toremifene. *Toxicol Pathol* 26:759–68.

Karsch, F.J., D.F. Battaglia, K.M. Breen, N. Debus, and T.G. Harris. 2002. Mechanisms for ovarian cycle disruption by immune/inflammatory stress. *Stress* 5:101–12.

Kaspareit, J., S. Friderichs-Gromoll, E. Buse, and G. Habermann. 2007. Spontaneous neoplasms observed in cynomolgus monkeys (*Macaca fascicularis*) during a 15-year period. *Exp Toxicol Pathol* 59:163–9.

Kawakami, E., T. Tsutsui, and A. Ogasa. 1991. Histoloogical observations of the reproductive organs of the male dog from birth to sexual maturity. *J Vet Med Sci* 53:241–8.

Keeney, D.S., S.M. Mendis-Handagama, B.R. Zirkin, and L.L. Ewing. 1988. Effect of long term deprivation of luteinizing hormone on Leydig cell volume, Leydig cell number, and steroidogenic capacity of the rat testis. *Endocrinology* 12:2906–15.

Kelliher, K.R., and S.R. Wersinger. 2009. Olfactory regulation of the sexual behavior and reproductive physiology of the laboratory mouse: effects and neural mechanisms. *ILAR J* 50:28–42.

Kennedy, P.C., J.M. Cullen, J.F. Edwards et al. 1994. *Histological Classification of Tumors of the Genital System of Domestic Animals*. Washington, DC: Armed Forces Institute of Pathology.

Kennel, P., C. Pallen, E. Barale-Thomas, G. Espuña, and R. Bars. 2003. Tamoxifen: 28-day oral toxicity study in the rat based on the Enhanced OECD Test Guideline 407 to detect endocrine effects. *Arch Toxicol* 77:487–99.

Kenney, N.J., H. Hosick, E. Herrington, and G.H. Smith. 1996. The aged mammary gland. In *Pathobiology of the Aging Mouse*, Vol. 2, ed. U. Mohr, D.L. Dungworth, C.C. Capen, W.W. Carlton, J.P. Sundberg, and J.M. Ward, 369–79. Washington, DC: ILSI Press.

Kerlin, R.L., A.R. Roesler, A.B. Jakowski, G.G. Boucher, D.L. Krull, and W.H. Appel. 1998. A poorly differentiated germ cell tumor (seminoma) in a Long Evans rat. *Toxicol Pathol* 26:691–4.

Kerr, J.B. 1992. Spontaneous degeneration of germ cells in normal rat testis: assessment of cell types and frequency during the spermatogenetic cycle. *J Reprod Fertil* 95:825–30.

Kerr, J.B., M. Millar, S. Maddocks, and R.M. Sharpe. 1993. Stage-dependent changes in spermatogenesis and Sertoli cells in relation to onset of spermatogenic failure following withdrawal of testosterone. *Anat Rec* 235:547–59.

Khedmati, F., C. Chirolas, and J.D. Seidman. 2009. Ovarian and paraovarian squamous-lined cysts (epidermoid cysts): a clinicopathologic study of 18 cases with comparison to mature cystic teratomas. *Int J Gynecol Pathol* 28:193–6.

Kim, H.S., S.C. Kang, H.S. Zhang, J.S. Kang, J.H. Kim, K.H. Kim, B.H. Kang, and B.I. Yoon. 2010. Uterine adenomyosis in beagle dogs. *Lab Anim Res* 26:211–3.

Kim, J., M. Sato, Q. Li et al. 2008. Peroxisome proliferator-activated receptor gamma is a target of progesterone regulation in the preovulatory follicles and controls ovulation in mice. *Mol Cell Biol* 28:1770–82.

Kim, S.-N., J.E. Fitzgerald, and F.A. de la Iglesia. 1985. Spermatocytic seminoma in the rat. *Toxicol Pathol* 13:215–21.

King, A., T. Burrows, and Y.W. Loke. 1996. Human uterine natural killer cells. *Nat Immunol* 15:41–52.

Kirigaya, A., H. Kim, S. Hayashi, P. Chambon, H. Watanabe, T. Iguchi, and T. Sato. 2009. Involvement of estrogen receptor beta in the induction of polyovular follicles in mouse ovaries exposed neonatally to diethylsilbestrol. *Zoolog Sci* 26:704–12.

Kittel, B., C. Ruehl-Fehlert, G. Morawietz et al. 2004. Revised guides for organ sampling and trimming in rats and mice—Part 2: a joint publication of the RITA and NACAD groups. *Exp Toxicol Pathol* 55:413–31.

Kleinberg, D.L. 1998. Role of IGF-I in normal mammary development. *Breast Cancer Res* 47:201–8.

Kleinberg, D.L., T.L. Wood, P.A. Furth, and A.V. Lee. 2009. Growth hormone and insulin-like growth factor-I in the transition from normal mammary development to preneoplastic mammary lesions. *Endocr Rev* 30:51–74.

Koering, M.J. 1969. Cyclic changes in ovarian morphology during the menstrual cycle in *Macaca mulatta*. *Am J Anat* 126(1):73–101.

Koguchi A., K. Nomura, T. Zujiwara, Y. Kawai, and A. Okaniwa. 1995. Maternal placenta-like endometrial hyperplasia in a beagle dog (canine deciduoma). *Exp Anim* 44:251–3.

Kowalewski, M.P., G. Schuler, A. Taubert, E. Engel, and B. Hoffmann. 2006. Expression of cyclooxygenase 1 and 2 in the canine corpus luteum during diestrus. *Theriogenology* 66:1423–30.

Kumar, T.R., Y. Wang, N. Lu, and M.M. Matzuk. 1997. Follicle stimulating hormone is required for ovarian follicle maturation but not male fertility. *Nat Genet* 15:201–4.

Kumasaka, T., E. Itoh, H. Watanabe et al. 1994. Effects of various forms of progestin on the endometrium of the estrogen-primed, ovariectomized rat. *Endocr J* 41:161–9.

Kumazawa, T., A. Nakajima, T. Ishiguro et al. 2009. Collaborative work on evaluation of ovarian toxicity. 15. Two- or four-week repeated-dose studies and fertility study of bromocriptine in female rats. *J Toxicol Sci* 34:SP157–65.

Kurita, T. 2011. Normal and abnormal epithelial differentiation in the female reproductive tract. *Differentiation* doi:10.1016/j.diff.2011.04.008.

Kwapien, R.P., R.C. Giles, R.G. Geil, and H.W. Casey. 1977. Basaloid adenomas of the mammary gland in beagle dogs administered investigational contraceptive steroids. *J Natl Cancer Inst* 59:933–9.

La, D.K., C.A. Johnson, D.M. Creasy, R.A. Hess, E. Baxter, M. Pereira, and S.S. Snook. 2011. Efferent duct toxicity with secondary testicular changes in rats following administration of a novel leukotriene A4 hydrolase inhibitor. *Toxicol Pathol* 40:705–14.

Laqueur, G.L., and C.F. Fluhmann. 1942. Effects of testosterone propionate in immature and adult female rats. *Endocrinology* 30:93–101.

Latendresse, J.R., T.J. Bucci, G. Olson et al. 2009. Genistein and ethinyl estradiol dietary exposure in multigenerational and chronic studies induce similar proliferative lesions in mammary gland of male Sprague–Dawley rats. *Reprod Toxicol* 28:342–53.

Leblond, C.P., and Y. Clermont. 1952. Definition of the stages of the cycle of the seminiferous epithelium in the rat. *Ann NY Acad Sci* 55:548–73.

Lederman, M.A., D. Lebesgue, V.V. Gonzalez et al. 2010. Age-related LH surge dysfunction correlates with reduced responsiveness of hypothalamic anteroventral periventricular nucleus kisspeptin neurons to estradiol positive feedback in middle-aged rats. *Neuropharmacology* 58:314–20.

Lee, J.-H., M. Sugimura, and N. Kudo. 1976. Segmentation of the rat oviduct. *Jpn J Vet Res* 24:77–86.

Lee, J., J.H. Richburg, S.C. Younkin, and K. Boekelheide. 1997. The Fas system is a key regulator of germ cell apoptosis in the testis. *Endocrinology* 138:2081–88.

Lee, K.-P., S.R. Frame, G.P. Sykes, and R. Valentine. 1993. Testicular degeneration and spermatid retention in young male rats. *Toxicol Pathol* 21:292–302.

Lefèvre, C.M., J.A. Sharp, and K.R. Nicholas. 2010. Evolution of lactation: ancient origin and extreme adaptation of the lactation system. *Ann Rev Genomics Hum Genet* 11:219–38.

LeFevre, J., and M.K. McClintock. 1988. Reproductive senescence in female rats: a longitudinal study of individual differences in estrous cycles and behavior. *Biol Reprod* 38:780–9.

LeFevre, J., and M.K. McClintock. 1991. Isolation accelerates reproductive senescence and alters its predictors in female rats. *Horm Behav*. 25:258–72.

Leininger, J.R., and M.P. Jokinen. 1990. Oviduct, uterus, and vagina. In *Pathology of the Fischer Rat*, ed. G.A. Boorman, S.L. Eustis, M.R. Elwell, C.A. Montgomery, and W.F. MacKenzie, 443–59. San Diego: Academic Press.

Lewis, D.J. 1987. Ovarian neoplasia in the Sprague–Dawley rat. *Environ Health Perspect* 73:77–90.

Lezmi, S., K. Thibault-Duprey, A. Bidaut et al. 2010. Spontaneous metritis related to the presence of vaginal septum in pregnant Sprague Dawley Crl:CD(SD) rats: impact on reproductive toxicity studies. *Vet Pathol* DOI: 10.1177/0300985810391113.

Li, S., and B. Davis. 2007. Evaluating rodent vaginal and uterine histology in toxicity studies. *Birth Defects Res (Part B)* 80:246–52.

Lipschutz, A., R. Iglesias, V.I. Panasevich, and S. Salinas. 1967. Pathological changes induced in the uterus of mice with the prolonged administration of progesterone and 19-nor-contraceptives. *Br J Cancer* 21:160–5.

Lohff, J.C., P.J. Christian, S.L. Marion, and P.B. Hoyer. 2006. Effect of duration of dosing on onset of ovarian failure in a chemical-induced mouse model of perimenopause. *Menopause* 13:482–8.

Long, G.G. 2002. Apparent mesonephric duct (rete anlage) origin for cysts and proliferative epithelial lesions in the mouse ovary. *Toxicol Pathol* 30:592–8.

Long, J.A., and H.M. Evans. 1922. The oestrous cycle in the rat and its associated phenomena. *Memoirs Univ Calif* 6:1–148.

Lotz, W., and R. Krause. 1978. Correlation between the effects of neuroleptics on prolactin release, mammary stimulation and the vaginal cycle in rats. *J Endocrinol* 76:507–15.

Lucas, J.N., D.G. Rudmann, K.M. Credille, A.R. Irizarry, A. Peter, and P.W. Snyder. 2007. The rat mammary gland: morphologic changes as an indicator of systemic hormonal perturbations induced by xenobiotics. *Toxicol Pathol* 35:199–207.

Luo, S., A. Sourla, C. Labrie et al. 1998. Effect of twenty-four-week treatment with the antiestrogen EM-800 on estrogen-sensitive parameters in intact and ovariectomized mice. *Endocrinology* 139:2645–56.

Luz, M.R., M.D. Cesário, M. Binelli, and M.D. Lopes. 2006. Canine corpus luteum regression: apoptosis and caspase-3 activity. *Theriogenology* 66:1448–53.

Mabeck, L.M., M.S. Jensen, G. Toft, M. Thulstrup, M. Andersson, T.K. Jensen, A. Giwercman, J. Olsen, J.P. Bonde, and the Danish First Pregnancy Planners Study Team. 2005. Fecundability according to male serum inhibin B—a prospective study among first pregnancy planners. *Hum Reprod* 20(10):2909–15.

Maekawa, A., and Y. Hayashi. 1992. Neoplastic lesions of the testis. In *Pathobiology of the Aging Rat*, ed. U. Mohr, D.L. Dungworth, and C.C. Capen, 413–8. Washington DC: ILSI Press.

Maekawa, A., and K. Maita. 1996. Changes in the uterus and vagina. In *Pathobiology of the Aging Mouse*, ed. U. Mohr, D.L. Dungworth, C.C. Capen, W.W. Carlton, J.P. Sundberg, and J.M. Ward, Vol. 1, 469–80. Washington, DC: ILSI Press.

Maekawa, A., K. Maita, and J.H. Harleman. 1996. Changes in the ovary. In *Pathobiology of the Aging Mouse*, ed. U. Mohr, D.L. Dungworth, C.C. Capen, W.W. Carlton, J.P. Sundberg, and J.M. Ward, Vol. 1, 451–67. Washington, DC: ILSI Press.

Maffucci, J.A., and A.C. Gore. 2006. Age-related changes in hormones and their receptors in animal models of female reproductive senescence. In *Handbook of Models for Human Aging*, ed. P.M. Conn, 533–52. San Diego: Elsevier.

Magoffin, D.A. 2005. Ovarian theca cell. *Int J Biochem Cell Biol* 37:1344–9.

Mahapokai, W., F.J. Van Sluijs, and J.A. Schalken. 2000. Models for studying benign prostatic hyperplasia. *Prostate Cancer Prostatic Dis* 3:28–33.

Majeed, S.K., and C. Gopinath. 1980. Calcification in the adrenals and ovaries of monkeys. *Lab Anim* 14:363–5.

Mallepell, S., A. Krust, P. Chambon, and C. Brisken. 2006. Paracrine signaling through the epithelial estrogen receptor alpha is required for proliferation and morphogenesis in the mammary gland. *Proc Natl Acad Sci USA* 103:2196–201.

Mandl, A.M. 1951. The phases of the oestrous cycle in the adult white rat. *J Exp Biol* 28:576–84.

Mann, P.C., G.A. Boorman, L.O. Lollini, D.N. McMartin, and D.G. Goodman. 1996. Proliferative lesions of the mammary gland in rats, IS-2. In *Guides for Toxicologic Pathology*. Washington, DC: STP/ARP/AFIP.

Mäntylä, E.T.E., S.H. Karlsson, and L.S. Nieminen. 1996. Induction of endometrial cancer by tamoxifen in the rat. In *Hormonal Carcinogenesis II. Proceedings of the Second International Symposium*, ed. J.J. Li, S.A. Li, J.A. Gustafsson, S. Nandi, and L.I. Sekely, 442–5. New York: Springer Verlag.

Markovits, J.E., and P.S. Sahota. 2000a. Granular cell lesions in the distal female reproductive tract of aged Sprague–Dawley rats. *Vet Pathol* 37:439–48.

Markovits, J.E., and P.S. Sahota. 2000b. Aromatase inhibitors prevent spontaneous granular cell tumors in the distal female reproductive tract of Sprague–Dawley rats. *Toxicol Pathol* 28:799–801.

Markström, E., E.C. Svensson, R. Shao, B. Svangerg, and H. Billig. 2002. Survival factors regulating ovarian apoptosis—dependence on follicle differentiation. *Reproduction* 123:23–30.

Marr-Belvin, A.K., C.C. Bailey, H.L. Knight, S.A. Klumpp, S.V. Westmoreland, and A.D. Miller. 2010. Ovarian pathology in rhesus macaques: a 12-year retrospective. *J Med Primatol* 39:170–6.

Martin, B., E. Golden, O.D. Carlson, J.M. Egan, M.P. Mattson, and S. Maudsley. 2008. Caloric restriction: impact upon pituitary function and reproduction. *Ageing Res Rev* 7:209–24.

Marty, M.S., R.E. Chapin, L.G. Parks, and B.A. Thorsrud. 2003. Development and maturation of the male reproductive system. *Birth Defects Res B Dev Reprod Toxicol* 68:125–36.

Masso-Welch, P.A., K.M. Darcy, N.C. Stangle-Castor, and M.M. Ip. 2000. A developmental atlas of rat mammary gland histology. *J Mammary Gland Biol Neoplasia* 5:165–85.

Matsuda, A., K. Higuchi, M. Karasawa, S. Yoneyama, J. Deguchi, and M. Miyamoto. 1997. Fourteen-day oral combination dose toxicity study of CGS 16949 A (aromatase inhibitor) with 5-fluorouracil or tamoxifen in rats. *J Toxicol Sci* 22:1–24.

Matsuura, I., T. Saitoh, M. Ashina et al. 2005. Evaluation of a two-generation reproduction toxicity study adding endpoints to detect endocrine disrupting activity using vinclozolin. *J Toxicol Sci* 30(Special Issue):163–88.

Matsuyama, S., K.T. Chang, H. Kanuka et al. 1996. Occurrence of deoxyribonucleic acid fragmentation during prolactin-induced structural luteolysis in cycling rats. *Biol Reprod* 54:1245–51.

Mattison, D.R. 1993. Sites of female reproductive vulnerability: implications for testing and risk assessment. *Reprod Toxicol* 7(Suppl 1):53–62.

McCracken, J.A., E.E. Custer, and J.C. Lamsa. 1999. Luteolysis: a neuroendocrine-mediated event. *Physiol Rev* 79:263–323.

McDougall, K., M.A. Hay, K.L. Goodrowe, C.J. Gartley, and W.A. King. 1997. Changes in the number of follicles and of oocytes in ovaries of prepubertal, peripubertal and mature bitches. *J Reprod Fertil Suppl* 51:25–31.

McEntee, K. 1990a. Ovarian neoplasms. In *Reproductive Pathology of Domestic Mammals*, 69–93. San Diego: Academic Press.

McEntee, K. 1990b. Cysts in and around the ovary. *Reproductive Pathology of Domestic Mammals*, 52–68. San Diego: Academic Press.

McGee, E.A., and A.J.W. Hsueh. 2000. Initial and cyclic recruitment of ovarian follicles. *Endocr Rev* 21:200–14.

McLaren, A. 1991. Development of the mammalian gonad: the fate of the supporting cell lineage. *Bioessays* 13:151–6.

McMullen, M.L., B.N. Cho, C.J. Yates, and K.E. Mayo. 2001. Gonadal pathologies in transgenic mice expressing the rat inhibin alpha-subunit. *Endocrinology* 142:5005–14.

McShane, T.M., and P.M. Wise. 1996. Life-long moderate caloric restriction prolongs reproductive life span in rats without interrupting estrous cyclicity: effects on the gonadotropin-releasing hormone/luteinizing hormone axis. *Biol Reprod* 54:70–5.

Meachem, S.J., E. Nieschlag, and M. Simoni. 2001. Inhibin B in male reproduction: pathophysiology and clinical relevance. *Eur J Endocrinol* 145:561–71.

Medina, D. 1982. Mammary tumors. In *The Mouse in Biomedical Research. Volume IV. Experimental Biology and Oncology*, ed. H.L. Foster, J.D. Small, and J.G. Fox, 373–96. New York: Academic Press.

Medina, D. 2002. Biological and molecular characteristics of the premalignant mouse mammary gland. *Biochim Biophys Acta* 1603:1–9.

Medina, D. 2008. Premalignant and malignant mammary lesions induced by MMTV and chemical carcinogens. *J Mammary Gland Biol Neoplasia* 13:271–7.

Meistrich, M.L. 1986. Components of testicular function and sensitivity to disruption. *Biol Reprod* 34:17–28.

Mellin, T.N., G.P. Orczyk, M. Hichens, and H.R. Behrman. 1976. Serum profiles of luteinizing hormone, progesterone and total estrogens during the canine estrus cycle. *Theriogenology* 5:175–87.

Mendis-Handagama, S.M. 1992. Estimation error of Leydig cell numbers in atrophied testes due to the assumption of spherical nuclei. *J Microsc* 168:25–32.

Messinis, I.E., C.I. Messini, and K. Dafopoulos. 2010. The role of gonadotropins in the follicular phase. *Ann NY Acad Sci* 1205:5–11.

Miller, M.A., S.J. Kottler, L.A. Cohn et al. 2001. Mammary duct ectasia in dogs: 51 cases (1992–1999). *J Am Vet Med Assoc* 218:1303–7.

Mirsky, M.L., L. Sivaraman, C. Houle, D.M. Potter, R.E. Chapin, and G.D. Cappon. 2011. Histologic and cytologic detection of endocrine and reproductive tract effects of exemestane in female rats treated for up to twenty-eight days. *Toxicol Pathol* 39:589–605.

Misdorp, W. 2002. Tumors of the mammary gland. In *Tumors in Domestic Animals*, 4th edition, ed. D.J. Meuten, 575–606. Ames: Iowa State Press.

Misdorp, W., R.W. Else, E. Hellmén, and T.P. Lipscomb. 1999. *Histological Classification of Mammary Tumors of the Dog and the Cat*, 2nd series, Vol VII, 1–59. Washington, DC: AFIP.

Mitsumori, K., F.A. Talley, and M.R. Elwell. 1989. Epididymal interstitial (Leydig) cell tumors in B6C3F1 mice. *Vet Pathol* 26:65–9.

Mohr, U. 1993. Integumentary system. In *International Classification of Rodent Tumors: Part I. The Rat*, ed. U. Mohr. Lyons: International Agency for Research on Cancer.

Molenaar, R., D.G. de Rooij, F.F. Rommerts, and H.J. van der Molen. 1986. Repopulation of Leydig cells in mature rats after selective destruction of the existent Leydig cells with ethylene dimethane sulfonate is dependent on luteinizing hormone and not follicle-stimulating hormone. *Endocrinology* 118:2546–54.

Molinolo, A., M. Simian, S. Vanzulli et al. 1998. Involvement of EGF in medroxyprogesterone acetate (MPA)-induced mammary gland hyperplasia and its role in MPA-induced mammary tumors in BALB/c mice. *Cancer Lett* 126:49–57.

Montgomery, C.A., and R.H. Alison. 1987. Non-neoplastic lesions of the ovary in Fischer 344 rats and B6C3F1 mice. *Environ Health Perspect* 73:53–75.

Morales, A., F. Mohamed, and J.C. Cavicchia. 2007. Apoptosis and blood–testis barrier during the first spermatogenic wave in the pubertal rat. *Anat Rec* 290:206–14.

Mori, T., T. Singtripop, and S. Kawashima. 1991. Animal model of uterine adenomyosis: is prolactin a potent inducer of adenomyosis in mice? *Am J Obstet Gynecol* 165:232–4.

Morton, D.G., S.E. Weisebrode, W.E. Wyder, J.K. Maurer, and C.C. Capen. 1987. Spermatid giant cells, tubular hypospermatogenesis, spermatogonial swelling, and cytoplasmic vacuoles in testes of laboratory rabbits. In *Monographs on Pathology of Laboratory Animals, Genital System*, ed. T.C. Jones, U. Mohr, and R.D. Hunt, 212–7. New York: Springer.

Mossman, H.W., and K.L. Duke. 1973. *Comparative Morphology of the Mammalian Ovary*. Madison, WI: University of Wisconsin Press.

Mostofi, F.K., and V.M. Bresler. 1976. Tumours of the testis. In *Pathology of Tumours in Laboratory Animals, Vol. 1. Tumours of the Rat*, ed. V.S. Turusov, 135–50. Lyon: International Agency for Research on Cancer.

Mouser, P., M.A. Miller, E. Antuofermo, S.S. Badve, and S.I. Mohammed. 2010. Prevalence and classification of spontaneous mammary intraepithelial lesons in dogs without clinical mammary disease. *Vet Pathol* 47:275–84.

Mulac-Jericevic, B., and O.M. Conneely. 2004. Reproductive tissue selective actions of progesterone receptors. *Reprod* 128:139–46.

Murakoshi, M., R. Ikeda, M. Tagawa, T. Iwasaka, and T. Nakayama. 2000. Histopathalogical study of female beagle dogs for four year treatment with subcutaneous implantation of chlormadinone actetate (CMA). *J Exp Clin Med* 25:87–91.

Nakai, M., R.A. Hess, B.J. Moore, R.F. Guttroff, L.F. Strader, and R.E. Linder. 1992. Acute and long-term effects of a single dose of the fungicide carbendazim (methyl 2-benzimidazole carbamate) on the male reproductive system in the rat. *J Androl* 13:507–18.

Nakanishi, Y., J. Mori, and H. Nagasawa. 1976. Recovery of pituitary secretion of gonadotrophins and prolactin during re-feeding after chronic restricted feeding in female rats. *J Endocrinol* 69:329–39.

Nandi, S. 1958. Endocrine control of mammary-gland development and function in the C3H/He Crgl mouse. *J Natl Cancer Inst* 21:1039–63.

Nass, T.E., P.S. LaPolt, H.L. Judd, and J.K.H. Lu. 1984. Alterations in ovarian steroid and gonadotrophin secretion preceding the cessation of regular oestrous cycles in ageing female rats. *J Endocrinol* 100:43–50.

Naylor, M.J., and C.J. Ormandy. 2002. Mouse strain-sepecific patterns of mammary epithelial ductal side branching are elicited by stromal factors. *Dev Dyn* 225:100–5.

Neal-Perry, G., and N.F. Santoro. 2006. Aging in the hypothalamic–pituitary–ovarian axis. In *Knobil and Neill's Physiology of Reproduction*, 3rd edition, ed. J.D. Neill, 2729–55. San Diego: Elsevier.

Nebel, B.R., A.P. Amarose, and E.M. Hackett. 1961. Calendar of gametogenic development in the prepuberal male mouse. *Science* 134:832–3.

Nelson, J.F., L.S. Felicio, H.H. Osterburg, and C.E. Finch. 1981. Altered profiles of estradiol and progesterone associated with prolonged estrous cycles and persistent vaginal cornification in aging C578L/6J mice. *Biol Reprod* 24:784–94.

Nelson, L.W., and W.A. Kelly. 1974. Changes in canine mammary gland histology during the estrous cycle. *Toxicol Appl Pharmacol* 27:113–22.

Nelson, L.W., and W.A. Kelly. 1976. Progestogen-related gross and microscopic changes in female beagles. *Vet Pathol* 13:143–56.

Nephew, K.P., E. Osborne, R.A. Lubet, C.J. Grubbs, and S.A. Khan. 2000. Effects of oral administration of tamoxifen, toremifene, dehydroepiandrosterone, and vorozole on uterine histomorphology in the rat. *Proc Soc Exp Biol Med* 223:288–94.

Neville, M.C. 2006. Lactation and its hormonal control. In *Knobil and Neill's Physiology of Reproduction*, Vol. 2, 3rd edition, ed. J.D. Neill, 2993–3054. St. Louis: Elsevier.

Neville, M.C., T.B. McFadden, and I. Forsyth. 2002. Hormonal regulation of mammary differentiation and milk secretion. *J Mammary Gland Biol Neoplasia* 7:49–66.

Newbold, R.R., B.C. Bullock, and J.A. McLachlan. 1985. Lesions of the rete testis in mice exposed prenatally to diethylstilbestrol. *Cancer Res* 45:5145–50.

Newbold, R.R., B.C. Bullock, and J.A. McLachlan. 1987. Testicular tumors in mice exposed in utero to diethylstilbestrol. *J Urol* 138:1446–50.

Newbold, R.R., B.C. Bullock, and J.A. McLachlan. 1990. Uterine adenocarcinoma in mice following developmental treatment with estrogens: a model for hormonal carcinogenesis. *Cancer Res* 50:7677–81.

Ng, S.T, J. Zhou, O.O. Adesanya, J. Wang, D. LeRoith, and C.A. Bondy. 1997. Growth hormone treatment induces mammary gland hyperplasia in aging primates. *Nat Med* 3:1141–4.

Niehoff, M.O., M. Bergmann, and G.F. Weinbauer. 2010. Effects of social housing of sexually mature male cynomolgus monkeys during general and reproductive toxicity evaluation. *Reprod Toxicol* 29:57–67.

Niswender, G.D., J.L. Juengel, P.J. Silva, M.K. Rollyson, and E.W. McIntush. 2000. Mechanisms controlling the function and life span of the corpus luteum. *Physiol Rev* 80:2–29.

Noakes, D.E., G.K. Dhaliwal, and G.C.W. England. 2001. Cystic endometrial hyperplasia/pyometra in dogs: a review of the causes and pathogenesis. *J Reprod Fert Suppl* 57:395–406.

Noden, D.M. and A. De Lahunta. 1985. *Embryology of Domestic Animals*. Baltimore: Williams and Wilkins.

Nogales, F.F., Jr., and S.G. Silverberg. 1976. Epidermoid cysts of the ovary: a report of five cases with histogenetic considerations and ultrastructural findings. *Am J Obstet Gynecol* 124:523–8.

Norris, H.J., F.M. Garner, and H.B. Taylor. 1970. Comparative pathology of ovarian neoplasms. IV. Gonadal stromal tumours of canine species. *J Comp Pathol* 80:399–405.

Nozaki, Y., E. Furubo, T. Matsuno et al. 2009. Collaborative work on evaluation of ovarian toxicity. 6. Two- or four-week repeated-dose studies and fertility study of cisplatin in female rats. *J Toxicol Sci* 34:73–81.

Nurmio, M., J. Toppari, F. Zaman et al. 2007. Inhibition of tyrosine kinases PDGFR and c-kit by imatinib mesylate interferes with postnatal testicular development in the rat. *Int J Androl* 30:366–76.

Nyska, A., A. Harmelin, J. Sandbank, M. Scolnik, and T. Waner. 1993. Intratubular spermatic seminoma in a Fischer-344 rat. *Toxicol Pathol* 21:397–401.

O'Connor, J.C., J.C. Cook, M.S. Marty, L.G. Davis, A.M. Kaplan, and E.W. Carney. 2002. Evaluation of Tier 1 screening approaches for detecting endocrine-active compounds (EACs). *Crit Rev Toxicol* 32:521–49.

O'Malley, F.P. 2010. Lobular neoplasia: morphology, biological potential and management in core biopsies. *Mod Pathol* 23:S14–S25.

O'Shea, J.D. 1966. Histochemical observations on mucin secretion by subsurface epithelial structures in the canine ovary. *J Morphol* 120:347–58.

O'Shea, J.D. 1981. Structure–function relationships in the wall of the ovarian follicle. *Aust J Biol Sci* 34:379–94.

Oakberg, E. 1956. A description of spermiogenesis in the mouse, and its use in the analysis of the cycle of the seminiferous epithelium and germ cell renewal. *Am J Anat* 99:391–413.

Oakberg, E.F. 1979. Follicular growth and atresia in the mouse. *In Vitro* 15:41–9.

Obasanjo, I.O., J.M. Cline, S. Schmotzer, and D.S. Weaver. 1998. Nandrolone decanoate causes pathologic changes in the uterus of surgically postmenopausal female cynomolgus macaques. *Menopause* 5:163–8.

Ohnuma, A., T. Yoshida, N. Takahashi et al. 2010. Malignant Leydig cell tumor with spindle-shaped cells in a male CD-1 mouse. *J Vet Med Sci* 72:661–4.

Ohta, Y. Age-related decline in deciduogenic ability of the rat uterus. 1987. *Biol Reprod* 37:779–85.

Ohta, Y., T. Sato, and T. Iguchi. 1993. Immunocytochemical localization of progesterone receptor in the reproductive tract of adult female rats. *Biol Reprod* 48:205–13.

Ohtake, S., M. Fukui, and S. Hisada. 2009. Collaborative work on evaluation of ovarian toxicity. 1. Effects of 2- or 4-week repeated-dose administration and fertility studies with medroxyprogesterone acetate in female rats. *J Toxicol Sci* 34(Suppl 1):SP23–9.

Oishi, Y., K. Yoshizawa, J. Suzuki et al. 1995. Spontaneously occurring mammary adenocarcinoma in a 10-wk-old female rat. *Toxicol Pathol* 23:696–700.

Okada, A., Y. Ohta, S. Inoue, H. Hiroi, M. Muramatsu, and T. Iguchi. 2003. Expression of estrogen, progesterone and androgen receptors in the oviduct of developing, cycling and pre-implantation rats. *J Mol Endocrinol* 30:301–15.

Okazaki, K., S. Okazaki, S. Nishimura, H. Nakamura, and Y. Kitamura. 2001. A repeated 28-day oral dose toxicity study of methoxychlor in rats, based on the 'Enhanced OECD Test Guideline 407' for screening endocrine-disrupting chemicals. *Arch Toxicol* 75:513–21.

Olson, P.N., R.A. Bowen, M.D. Behrendt, J.D. Olson, and T.M. Nett. 1982. Concentrations of reproductive hormones in canine serum throughout late anestrus, proestrus and estrus. *Biol Reprod* 27:1196–1206.

Olson, P.N., R.A. Bowen, M.D. Behrendt, and T.M. Nett. 1984. Concentrations of testosterone in canine serum throughout late anestrus, proestrus, estrus and early diestrus. *Am J Vet Res* 45:145–8.

Orth, J.M. 1982. Proliferation of Sertoli cells in fetal and postnatal rats: a quantitative autoradiographic study. *Anat Rec* 203:485–92.

Osmun, P. 1985. Rate and course of atresia during follicular development in the adult cyclic rat. *J Reprod Fertil* 73:261–70.

Ota, H., A. Wakizaka, and M. Fukushima. 1986. Modulation of ovarian LH receptor and serum hormone levels in rats with hyperprolactinemia induced by administration of ovine prolactin or sulpiride. *Tohoku J Exp Med* 148:213–27.

Parmar, H., and G.R. Cunha. 2004. Epithelial–stromal interactions in the mouse and human mammary gland *in vivo*. *Endocr Rel Cancer* 11:437–58.

Patyna, S., C. Arrigoni, A. Terron, T.W. Kim, J.K. Heward, S.L. Vonderfecht, R. Denlinger, S.E. Turnquist, and W. Evering. 2008. Nonclinical safety evaluation of sunitinib: a potent inhibitor of VEGF, PDGF, KIT, FLT3, and RET receptors. *Toxicol Pathol* 36:905–16.

Payan-Carreira, R., and M.A. Pires. 2008. Multioocyte follicles in domestic dogs: a survey of frequency of occurrence. *Theriogenology* 69:977–82.

Pedersen, T., and H. Peters. 1968. Proposal for a classification of oocytes and follicles in the mouse ovary. *J Reprod Fertil* 17:555–7.

Pelletier, G. Localization of androgen and estrogen receptors in rat and primate tissues. 2000. *Histol Histopathol* 15:1261–70.

Pelletier, G., C. Labrie, and F. Labrie. 2000. Localization of oestrogen receptor alpha, oestrogen receptor beta and androgen receptors in the rat reproductive organs. *J Endocrinol* 165:359–70.

Pelliniemi, L.J., K. Fröjdman, and J. Parank. 1993. Embryological and prenatal development and function of Sertoli cells. In *The Sertoli Cell*, ed. L.D. Russell and M.D. Griswold, 87–114. Clearwater: Cache River Press.

Peluso, J.J. 1992. Morphologic and physiologic features of the ovary. In *Pathobiology of the Aging Rat*, ed. U. Mohr, D.L. Dungworth, and C.C. Capen, Vol. 1, 337–49. Washington, DC: ILSI Press.

Peluso, J.J., and L.R. Gordon. 1992. Nonneoplastic and neoplastic changes in the ovary. In *Pathobiology of the Aging Rat*, ed. U. Mohr, D.L. Dungworth, and C.C. Capen, Vol. 1, 351–64. Washington, DC: ILSI Press.

Peluso, J.J., R.W. Steger, H. Huang, and J. Meites. 1979. Pattern of follicular growth and steroidogenesis in the ovary of aging cycling rats. *Exp Aging Res* 5:319–33.

Pepling, M.E. 2006. From primordial germ cell to primordial follicle: mammalian female germ cell development. *Genesis* 44:622–32.

Pessina, M.A., R.F. Hoyt, I. Goldstein, and A.M. Traish. 2006. Differential regulation of the expression of estrogen, progesterone, and androgen receptors by sex steroid hormones in the vagina: immunohistochemical studies. *J Sex Med* 3:804–14.

Phemister, R.D., P.A. Holst, J.S. Spano, and M.L. Hopwood. 1973. Time of ovulation in the beagle bitch. *Biol Reprod* 8:74–82.

Picut, C.A., H. Aoyama, J.W. Holder, L.S. Gold, R.R. Maronpot, and D. Dixon. 2003. Bromoethane, chloroethane and ethylene oxide induced uterine neoplasms in B6C3F1 mice from 2-year NTP inhalation bioassays: pathology and incidence data revisited. *Exp Toxicol Pathol* 55:1–9.

Picut, C.A., C.L. Swanson, K.L. Scully, V.C. Roseman, R.F. Parker, and A.K. Remick. 2008. Ovarian follicle counts using proliferating cell nuclear antigen (PCNA) and semi-automated image analysis in rats. *Toxicol Pathol* 36:674–9.

Picut, C.A., C.L. Swanson, R.F. Parker, K.L. Scully, and G.A. Parker. 2009. The Metrial gland in the rat and its similarities to granular cell tumors. *Toxicol Pathol* 37:474–80.

Piner, J., M. Sutherland, M. Millar, K. Turner, D. Newall, and R.M. Sharpe. 2002. Changes in vascular dynamics of the adult rat testis leading to transient accumulation of seminiferous tubule fluid after administration of a novel 5-hydroxytryptamine (5HT) agonist. *Reprod Toxicol* 16:141–50.

Plas-Roser, S., M.T. Kauffmann, and C. Aron. 1984. Progesterone secretion by luteinized unruptured follicles in mature female rats. *J Steroid Biochem* 20:441–4.

Plowchalk, D.R., and D.R. Mattison. 1992. Reproductive toxicity of cyclophosphamide in the C57BL/6N mouse: 1. Effects on ovarian structure and function. *Reprod Toxicol* 6:411–21.

Poonia, B., L. Walter, J. Dufour, R. Harrison, P.A. Marx, and R.S. Veazey. 2006. Cyclic changes in the vaginal epithelium of normal rhesus macaques. *J Endocrinol* 190:829–35.

Poteracki, J., and K.M. Walsh. 1998. Spontaneous neoplasms in control Wistar rats: a comparison of reviews. *Toxicol Sci* 45:1–8.

Pryor, J.L., C. Hughes, W. Foster, B.F. Hales, and B. Robaire. 2000. Critical windows of exposure for children's health: the reproductive system in animals and humans. *Environ Health Perspect* 108(Suppl 3):491–503.

Qureshi, S.R., E. Perente, R.A. Ettlin, M. Kolopp, D.E. Prentice, and A. Frankfurter. 1991. Morphologic and immunohistochemical characterization of Leydig cell tumor variants in Wistar rats. *Toxicol Pathol* 19:280–6.

Radovsky, A., K. Mitsumori, and R.E. Chapin. 1999. Male reproductive tract. In *Pathology of the Mouse, Reference and Atlas*, ed. R.R. Maronpot, G.A. Boorman, and B.W. Gaul, 381–407. Vienna, IL: Cache River Press.

Rajkovic, A., S.A. Pangas, and M.M. Matzuk. 2006. Follicular development: mouse, sheep, and human models. In *Knobil and Neill's Physiology of Reproduction*, ed. Neill, J.D., 3rd edition, 383–423. San Diego: Elsevier.

Ramos, A.M.G., S. Perazzio, A.F. de Camargos, and F.E.L. Pereira. 2005. Spontaneous inflammatory pelvic disease in adult non-castrated female rats treated with estrogen. *Braz J Inf Dis* 9:6–8.

Reel, J.R., J.C. Lamb, IV, and B.H. Neal. 1996. Survey and assessment of mammalian estrogen biological assays for hazard characterization. *Fund Appl Toxicol* 34:288–305.

Regan, K.S., J.M. Cline, C. Creasy et al. 2005. STP position paper: ovarian follicular counting in the assessment of rodent reproductive toxicity. *Toxicol Pathol* 33:409–12.

Rehm, S. 2000. Spontaneous testicular lesions in purpose-bred beagle dogs. *Toxicol Pathol* 28:782–7.

Rehm, S., and A.G. Liebelt. 1996. Nonneoplastic and neoplastic lesions of the mammary gland. In *Pathobiology of the Aging Mouse*, Vol. 2, ed. U. Mohr, D.L. Dungworth, C.C. Capen, W.W. Carlton, J.P. Sundberg, and J. M. Ward, 381–98. Washington, DC: ILSI Press.

Rehm, S., H.A. Solleveld, S.T. Portelli, and P.J. Wier. 2007a. Histologic changes in ovary, uterus, vagina, and mammary gland of mature beagle dogs treated with the SERM idoxifene. *Birth Defects Res B Dev Reprod Toxicol* 80:225–32.

Rehm, S., D.J. Stanislaus, and A.M. Williams. 2007b. Estrous cycle-dependent histology and review of sex steroid receptor expression in dog reproductive tissues and mammary gland and associated hormone levels. *Birth Defects Res B Dev Reprod Toxicol* 80:233–45.

Rehm, S., D.J. Stanislaus, and P.J. Wier. 2007c. Identification of drug-induced hyper- or hypoprolactinemia in the female rat based on general and reproductive toxicity study parameters. *Birth Defects Res B Dev Reprod Toxicol* 80:253–7.

Rehm, S., and M.P. Waalkes. 1988. Mixed Sertoli–Leydig cell tumor and rete testis adenocarcinoma in rats treated with CdCl2. *Vet Pathol* 25:163–6.

Rehm, S., T.E. White, E.A. Zahalka, D.J. Stanislaus, R.W. Boyce, and P.J. Weir. 2008. Effects of food restriction on testis and accessory glands in maturing rats. *Toxicol Pathol* 36:687–94.

Reimers, T.J., R.D. Phemister, and G.D. Niswender. 1978. Radioimunological measurement of follicle stimulating hormone and prolactin in the dog. *Biol Reprod* 19:673–9.

Reindel, J.F., A.W. Gough, G.D. Pilcher, W.F. Bobrowski, G.P. Sobocinski, and F.A. de la Iglesia. 2001. Systemic proliferative changes and clinical signs in cynomolgus monkeys administered a recombinant derivative of human epidermal growth factor. *Toxicol Pathol* 29:159–73.

Resko, J.A., R.W. Goy, J.A. Robinson, and R.L. Norman. 1982. The pubescent rhesus monkey: some characteristics of the menstrual cycle. *Biol Reprod* 27:354–61.

Reuber, M.D., G. Vlahakis, and W.E. Heston. 1981. Spontaneous hyperplastic and neoplastic lesions of the uterus in mice. *J Gerontol* 36:663–73.

Reynaud, K., A. Fontbonne, N. Marseloo, S. Thournire, M. Chebrout, C.V. de Lesegno, and S. Chastant-Maillard. 2005. In vivo meiotic resumption, fertilization and early embryonic development in the bitch. *Reproduction* 130:193–201.

Richert, M.M., K.L. Schwertfeger, J.W. Ryder, and S.M. Anderson. 2000. An atlas of mouse mammary gland development. *J Mammary Gland Biol Neoplasia* 5:227–41.

Risk, M., and G. Gibori. 2001. Mechanisms of luteal cell regulation by prolactin. In *Prolactin*, ed. N.D. Horseman, 265–95. Boston: Kluwer Academic Publishers.

Rivier, C., H. Meunier, V. Roberts, and W. Vale. 1990. Inhibin: role and secretion in the rat. *Rec Prog Hormone Res* 46:231–59.

Rivier, C., and S. Rivest. 1991. Effect of stress on the activity of the hypothalamic–pituitary–gonadal axis: peripheral and central mechanisms. *Biol Reprod* 45:523–32.

Robaire, B., and X. Fan. 1998. Regulation of apoptotic cell death in the rat epididymis. *J Reprod Fertil Supp* 153:211–4.

Robker, R.L., L.K. Akison, and D.L. Russell. 2009. Control of oocyte release by progesterone receptor-regulated gene expression. *Nuclear Receptor Signaling* 7:e012. DOI:10.1621/nrs.07012.

Rodriguez, H.A., N. Santambrosio, C.G. Santamaria, M. Muñoz-de-Toro, and E.H. Lugue. 2010. Neonatal exposure to bisphenol A reduces the pool of primordial follicles in the rat ovary. *Reprod Toxicol* 30:550–7.

Rouquie, D., C. Friry-Santini, F. Schorsch, H. Tinwell, and R. Bars. 2009. Standard and molecular NOAELs for rat testicular toxicity induced by flutamide. *Toxicol Sci* 109:59–65.

Rudmann, D.G., I.R. Cohen, M.R. Robbins, D.E. Coutant, and J.W. Henck. 2005. Androgen dependent mammary gland virilism in rats given the selective estrogen receptor modulator LY2066948 hydrochloride. *Toxicol Pathol* 33:711–9.

Ruehl-Fehlert, C., B. Kittel, G. Morawietz et al. 2003. Revised guides for organ sampling and trimming in rats and mice—Part 1: a joint publication of the RITA and NACAD groups. *Exp Toxicol Pathol* 55:91–106.

Russell, L.D. 1992. Normal development of the testis. In *Pathobiology of the Aging Rat*, ed. U. Mohr, D.L. Dungworth, and C.C. Capen, 395–405. Washington, DC: ILSI Press.

Russell, L.D., L.E. Alger, and L.G. Nequin. 1987. Hormonal control of pubertal spermatogenesis. *Endocrinology* 120:1615–32.

Russell, L.D., A. Bartke, and J.C. Goh. 1989. Postnatal development of the Sertoli cell barrier, tubular lumen, and cytoskeleton of Sertoli and myoid cells in the rat, and their relationship to tubular fluid secretion and flow. *Am J Anat* 184:179–89.

Russell, L.D., R.A. Ettlin, A.P. SinhaHikim, and E.D. Clegg. 1990. *Histological and Histopathological Evaluation of the Testis*. Clearwater: Cache River Press.

Russell, L.D., J.P. Malone, and S.L. Karpas. 1981. Morphologic pattern elicited by agents affecting spermatogenesis by disruption of its hormonal stimulation. *Tissue Cell* 13:369–80.

Russo, I.H., and J. Russo. 1994. Aging of the mammary gland. In *Pathobiology of the Aging Rat*. Vol. 2, ed. U. Mohr, D.L. Dungworth, and C.C. Capen, 447–58. Washington, DC, ILSI Press.

Russo, I.H., and J. Russo. 1996. Mammary gland neoplasia in long-term rodent studies. *Env Health Perpect* 104:938–67.

Russo, I.H., M. Tewari, and J. Russo. 1989. Morphology and development of the rat mammary gland. In: *Monographs on Pathology of Laboratory Animals. Integument and Mammary Glands*, ed. T.C. Jones, U. Mohr, and R.D. Hunt, 233–52. Berlin: Springer-Verlag.

Russo, J., I.H. Russo, M.J. van Zwieten, A.E. Rogers, and B.A. Gusterson. 1989. Classification of neoplastic and nonneoplastic lesions of the rat mammary gland. In *Monographs on Pathology of Laboratory Animals. Integument and Mammary Glands*, ed. T.C. Jones, U. Mohr, and R.D. Hunt, 275–304. Berlin: Springer-Verlag.

Ryan, A.M., D.B. Eppler, K.E. Hagler, R.H. Bruner, P.J. Thomford, R.L. Hall, G.M. Shopp, and C.A. O'Neill. 1999. Preclinical safety evaluation of rhuMAbVEGF, an antiangiogenic humanized monoclonal antibody. *Toxicol Pathol* 27:78–86.

Sahara, K., M. Murakoshi, T. Nishina, H. Kino, and T. Tsutsui. 1994. Pathologic changes related to subcutaneous implantation of chlormadinone acetate for preventing estrus in bitches. *J Vet Med Sci* 52:425–7.

Saito, K., L. O'Donnell, I. McLachlan, and D.M. Robertson. 2000. Spermiation failure is a major contributor to early spermatogenic suppression caused by hormone withdrawal in adult rats. *Endocrinology* 141:2779–85.

Sakakura, T. 1987. Mammary embryogenesis. In *The Mammary Gland*, ed. M.C. Neville and C.W. Daniel, 37–66. New York: Plenum Press.

Sakurada, Y., S. Kudo, S. Iwasaki, Y. Miyata, M. Nishi, and Y. Masumoto. 2009. Collaborative work on evaluation of ovarian toxicity. 5. Two- or four-week repeated-dose studies and fertility study of busulfan in female rats. *J Toxicol Sci* 34:65–72.

Salleh, N., D.L. Baines, R.J. Naftalin, and S.R. Milligan. 2005. The hormonal control of uterine luminal fluid secretion. *J Membrane Biol* 206:17–28.

Salvetti, N.R., C.G. Panzani, E.J. Gimeno, L.G. Neme, N.S. Alfaro, and H.H. Ortega. 2009. An imbalance between apoptosis and proliferation contributes to follicular persistence in polycystic ovaries in rats. *Reprod Biol Endocrinol* 7:68.

Sanbuissho, A., M. Yoshida, S. Hisada et al. 2009. Collaborative work on evaluation of ovarian toxicity by repeated-dose and fertility studies in female rats. *J Toxicol Sci* 34:SP1–22.

Sánchez-Criado, J., A. Sánchez, A. Ruiz, and F. Gaytán. 1993. Endocrine and morphological features of cystic ovarian condition in antiprogesterone RU486-treated rats. *Acta Endocrinol* 129:237–45.

Sato, N., K. Uchida, M. Nakajima, A. Watanabe, and T. Kohira. 2009. Collaborative work on evaluation of ovarian toxicity. 13. Two- or four-week repeated dose studies and fertility study of PPAR alpha/gamma dual agonist in female rats. *J Toxicol Sci* 34:SP137–46.

Sawaki, M., K. Shinoda, S. Hoshuyama, F. Kato, and K. Yamasaki. 2000. Combination of a teratoma and embryonal carcinoma of the testis in SD IGS rats: a report of two cases. *Toxicol Pathol* 28:832–5.

Sawamoto, O., J. Yamate, M. Kuwamura, T. Kotani, and Z. Kurisu. 2003. Development of sperm granulomas in the epididymides of L-cysteine-treated rats. *Toxicol Pathol* 31:281–9.

Schedin, P., T. Mitrenga, and M. Kaeck. 2000. Estrous cycle regulation of mammary epithelial cell proliferation, differentiation, and death in the Sprague–Dawley rat: a model for investigating the role of estrous cycling in mammary carcinogenesis. *J Mammary Gland Biol Neoplasia* 5:211–25.

Schlafer, D.H., and A.T. Gifford. 2008. Cystic endometrial hyperplasia, pseudoplacentational endometrial hyperplasia, and other cystic conditions of the canine and feline uterus. *Theriogenology* 70:349–358.

Scott, M.A., R.P. Tarara, A.G. Hendrickx, K. Benirschke, J.W. Overstreet, and B.L. Lasley. 2001. Exposure to the dioxin 2,3,7,8-tetrachlorodibenzo-*p*-dioxin (TCDD) induces squamous metaplasia in the endocervix of cynomolgus macaques. *J Med Primatol* 30:156–60.

Seaman, W.J. 1985. Canine ovarian fibroma associated with prolonged exposure to mibolerone. *Toxicol Pathol* 13:177–80.

Selman, P.J., J.A. Mol, G.R. Rutteman, and E. van Garderen. 1994. Progestin-induced growth hormone excess in the dog originates in the mammary gland. *Endocrinology* 134:287–92.

Selye, H. 1940. Effect of chronic progesterone over-dosage on the female accessory sex organs of normal, ovariectomized and hypophysectomized rats. *Anat Rec* 78:253–71.

Shao, R., M. Nutu, B. Weijdegård et al. 2008. Differences in prolactin receptor (PRLR) in mouse and human fallopian tubes: evidence for multiple regulatory mechanisms controlling PRLR isoform expression in mice. *Biol Reprod* 79:748–57.

Shao, R., M. Nutu, B. Weijdegård et al. 2009. Clomiphene citrate causes aberrant tubal apoptosis and estrogen receptor activation in rat fallopian tube: implications for tubal ectopic pregnancy. *Biol Reprod* 80:1262–71.

Sharpe, R.M. 1994. Regulation of spermatogenesis. In *The Physiology of Reproduction*. 2nd edition, eds. E. Knobil and J.D. Neil, 1363–434. New York: Raven Press.

Shille, V.M., M.J. Thatcher, and M.L. Lloyd. 1987. Concentrations of LH and FSH during selected periods of anestrus in the bitch. *Biol Reprod Suppl* 36:184.

Shimizu, K. 2008. Reproductive hormones and the ovarian cycle in macaques. *J Mammal Ova Res* 25:122–6.

Shimizu, K., C. Kojima, M. Kondo, W.Z. Jin, M. Ito, G. Watanabe, N.P. Groome, and K. Taya. 2002. Circulating inhibin A and inhibin B in normal menstrual cycle during breeding seasons of Japanese monkeys. *J Reprod Dev* 48:335–61.

Shinoda, K., K. Mitsumori, K. Yasuhara et al. 1999. Doxorubicin induces male germ cell apoptosis in rats. *Arch Toxicol* 73:274–81.

Shirai, M., K. Sakurai, W. Saitoh et al. 2009. Collaborative work on evaluation of ovarian toxicity. 8. Two- or four-week repeated-dose studies and fertility study of Anastrozole in female rats. *J Toxicol Sci* 34:SP91–9.

Sleer, L.S., and C.C. Taylor. 2007. Platelet-derived growth factors and receptors in the rat corpus luteum: localization and identification of an effect on luteogenesis. *Biol Reprod* 76:391–400.

Smedley, J.V., S.A. Bailey, R.W. Perry, and C.M. O'Rourke. 2002. Methods for predicting sexual maturity in male cynomolgus macaques on the basis of age, body weight, and histologic evaluation of the testes. *Contemp Top Lab Anim Sci* 41:18–20.

Smith, M.S., M.E. Freeman, and J.D. Neill. 1975. The control of progesterone secretion during the estrous cycle and early pseudopregnancy in the rat: prolactin, gonadotropin and steroid levels associated with rescue of the corpus luteum of pseudopregnancy. *Endocrinology* 96:219–26.

Smith, M.S., and Neill, J.D. 1976. Termination at midpregnancy of the two daily surges of plasma prolactin initiated by mating in the rat. *Endocrinology* 98:696–701.

Snyder, P.W., E.A. Kazacos, J.C. Scott-Moncrieff et al. 1995. Pathologic features of naturally occurring juvenile polyarteritis in beagle dogs. *Vet Pathol* 32:337–45.

Sokolowski, J.H. 1977. Reproductive patterns in the bitch. *Vet Clin North Am* 7:653–66.

Sokolowski, J.H., and R.G. Zimbelman. 1973. Canine reproduction: effects of a single injection of medroxy-progesterone acetate on the reproductive organs of the bitch. *Am J Vet Res* 34:1493–9.

Son, W.-C. 2004. Idiopathic canine polyarteritis in control beagle dogs from toxicity studies. *J Vet Sci* 5:147–50.

Sorenmo, K.U., R. Rasotto, V. Zappulli, and M.H. Goldschmidt. 2010. Development, anatomy, histology, lymphatic drainage, clinical features, and cell differentiation markers of canine mammary neoplasms. *Vet Pathol* 48:85–97.

Sourla, A., M. Flamand, A. Bélanger, and F. Labrie. 1998b. Effect of dehydroepiandrosterone on vaginal and uterine histomorphology in the rat. *J Steroid Biochem Mol Biol* 66:137–49.

Sourla, A., S. Luo, C. Labrie, A. Bélanger, and F. Labrie. 1997. Morphological changes induced by 6-month treatment of intact and ovariectomized mice with tamoxifen and the pure antiestrogen EM-800. *Endocrinology* 138:5605–17.

Sourla, A., C. Martel, C. Labrie, and F. Labrie. 1998a. Almost exclusive androgenic action of dehydroepi-androsterone in the rat mammary gland. *Endocrinology* 139:753–64.

Steele, R.E., L.B. Mellor, W.K. Sawyer, J.M. Wasvary, and L.J. Browne. 1987. In vitro and in vivo studies demonstrating potent and selective estrogen inhibition with the nonsteroidal aromatase inhibitor CGS 16949A. *Steroids* 50:147–61.

Steinhauer, N., A. Boos, and A.R. Günzel-Apel. 2004. Morphological changes and proliferative activity in the oviductal epithelium during hormonally defined stages of the oestrus cycle in the bitch. *Reprod Dom Anim* 39:110–9.

Sternlicht, M.D. 2006. The cues that regulate ductal branching morphogenesis. *Breast Cancer Res* 8:201–11.

Stott, G.G. 1974. Granulosa cell islands in the canine ovary: histogenesis, histomorphologic features and fate. *Am J Vet Res* 35:1351–5.

Stouffer, R.L. 2006. Structure, function, and regulation of the corpus luteum. In *Knobil and Neill's Physiology of Reproduction*, 3rd edition, ed. J.D. Neill, 475–526. San Diego: Elsevier.

Strange, R., K.C. Westerlind, A. Ziemiecki, and A.-C. Andres. 2007. Proliferation and apoptosis in mammary epithelium during the rat estrous cycle. *Acta Physiol* 190:137–49.

Strickland, J.L., and J.W. Wall. 2003. Abnormal uterine bleeding in adolescents. *Obstet Gynecol Clin North Am* 30:321–35.

Suresh, P.S. and R. Medhamurthy. 2009. Dynamics of circulating concentrations of gonadotropins and ovarian hormones throughout the menstrual cycle in the bonnet monkey: role of inhibin A in the regulation of follicle-stimulating hormone secretion. *Am J Primatol* 10:817–24.

Taketa, Y., A. Inomata, S. Hosokawa et al. 2011. Histopathological characteristics of luteal hypertrophy induced by ethylene glycol monomethyl ether with a comparison to normal luteal morphology in rats. *Toxicol Pathol* 39:372–80.

Tang, F.Y., T.A. Bonfiglio, and L.K. Tang. 1984. Effect of estrogen and progesterone on the development of endometrial hyperplasia in the Fischer rat. *Biol Reprod* 31:399–413.

Tani, Y., P.M. Foster, R.C. Sills, P.C. Chan, S.D. Peddada, and A. Nyska. 2005. Epididymal sperm granuloma induced by chronic administration of 2-methyoimidazole in B6C3F1 mice. *Toxicol Pathol* 33:313–9.

Tani, Y., S. Murat, N. Maeda, J. Fukushige, and T. Hosokawa. 1997. A spontaneous testicular teratoma in an ICR mouse. *Toxicol Pathol* 25:317–20.

Tanigawa, H., H. Onodera, and A. Maekawa. 1987. Spontaneous mesotheliomas in Fischer rats—a histological and electron microscopic study. *Toxicol Pathol* 15:157–63.

Tarara, R.P. 2007. Review of mammary gland neoplasia in nonhuman primates. *Breast Dis* 28:23–7.

Tash, J.A., S. McCallum, M.P. Hardy, B. Knudsen, and P.N. Schlegel. 2002. Men with non-obstructive azoospermia have Leydig cell hypertrophy but not hyperplasia. *J Urol* 168:1068–70.

Tavassoli, F.A., H.W. Casey, and N.J. Norris. 1988. The morphologic effects of synthetic reproductive steroids on the mammary gland of rhesus monkeys. Mestranol, ethynerone, mestranol-ethynerone, chloroethynyl norgestrel-mestranol, and anagestone acetate-mestranol combinations. *Am J Pathol* 131:213–34.

Telfer, E., and R.G. Gosden. 1987. A quantitative cytological study of polyovular follicles in mammalian ovaries with particular reference to the domestic bitch (*Canis familiaris*). *J Reprod Fert* 81:137–47.

Temel, S., W. Lin, S. Lakhlani, and L. Jennes. 2002. Expression of estrogen receptor-alpha and cFos in norepinephrine and epinephrine neurons of young and middle-aged rats during the steroid-induced luteinizing hormone surge. *Endocrinology* 143:3974–83.

Teo, S.K., M.G. Evans, M.J. Brockman et al. 2001. Safety profile of thalidomide after 53 weeks of oral administration in beagle dogs. *Toxicol Sci* 59:160–8.

Tibbetts, T.A., M. Mendoza-Meneses, B.W. O'Malley, and O.M. Conneely. 1998. Mutual and intercompartmental regulation of estrogen receptor and progesterone receptor expression in the mouse uterus. *Biol Reprod* 59:1143–52.

Tilbrook, A.J., A.I. Turner, and I.J. Clarke. 2002. Stress and reproduction: central mechanisms and sex differences in non-rodent species. *Stress* 5:83–100.

Topper, Y.J., and C.S. Freeman. 1980. Multiple hormone interactions in the developmental biology of the mammary gland. *Physiol Rev* 60:1049–106.

Toyoda, K., M. Shibutani, T. Tamura, T. Koujitani, C. Uneyama, and M. Hirose. 2000. Repeated dose (28 days) oral toxicity study of flutamide in rats, based on the draft protocol for the 'Enhanced OECD Test Guideline 407' for screening for endocrine-disrupting chemicals. *Arch Toxicol* 74:127–32.

Tripiciano, A., A. Filippini, Q. Giustiniani, and F. Palombi. 1996. Direct visualization of rat peritubular myoid cell contraction in response to endothelin. *Biol Reprod* 55:25–31.

Troiano, L., M.F. Fustini, E. Lovato et al. 1994. Apoptosis and spermatogenesis: evidence from an in vivo model of testosterone withdrawal in the adult rat. *Biochem Biophys Res Comm* 202:1315–21.

Tsubota, K., K. Kushima, K. Yamauchi et al. 2009. Collaborative work on evaluation of ovarian toxicity. 12. Effects of 2- or 4-week repeated dose studies and fertility study of indomethacin in female rats. *J Toxicol Sci* 34:SP129–36.

Tsubura, A, T. Hatano, S. Hayama, and S. Morii. 1991. Immunophenotypic difference of keratin expression in normal mammary glandular cells from five different species. *Acta Anat* 140:287–93.

Tsubura, A., K. Yoshizawa, N. Uehara, T. Yuri, and Y. Matsuoka. 2007. Multistep mouse mammary tumorigenesis through preneoplasia to neoplasia and acquisition of metastatic potential. *Med Mol Morphol* 40:9–17.

Tsujioka, S., Y. Ban, L.D. Wise et al. 2009. Collaborative work on evaluation of ovarian toxicity. 3. Effects of 2- or 4-week repeated dose toxicity and fertility studies with tamoxifen in female rats. *J Toxicol Sci* 34:SP43–51.

Turner, C., and E. Gomez. 1934. The normal development of the mammary gland of the male and female albino mouse. *Mo Agr Exp Stn Res Bull* 182:3–20.

Valerio, M.G. 1989. Comparative aspects of contraceptive steroids: effects observed in the monkey. *Toxicol Pathol* 17:401–10.

Van Cruchten S., W. Van den Broeck, L. Duchateau, and P. Simoens. 2003. Apoptosis in the canine endometrium during the estrous cycle. *Theriogenology* 60:1595–608.

van der Schoot, P., G.H. Bakker, and J.G.M. Klijn. 1987. Effects of the progesterone antagonist RU486 on ovarian activity in the rat. *Endocrinology* 121:1375–82.

van Esch, E., J.M. Cline, E. Buse, and G.F. Weinbauer. 2008. The macaque endometrium, with special reference to the cynomolgus monkey (*Macaca fascicularis*). *Toxicol Pathol* 36:67S–100S.

van Wagenen, G., and M.E. Simpson. 1973. Postnatal development of the ovary in *Homo sapiens* and *Macaca mulatta* and induction of ovulation in the macaque. New Haven, CT: Yale University Press.

van Zwieten, M.J., H. HogenEsch, J.A. Majka, and G.A. Boorman. 1994. Nonneoplastic and neoplastic lesions of the mammary gland. In *Pathobiology of the Aging Rat*, Vol. 2., ed. U. Mohr, D.L. Dungworth, and C.C. Capen, 459–76. Washington, DC: ILSI Press.

Velardo, J.T., A.B. Dawson, A.G. Olsen, and F.L. Hisaw. 1953. Sequence of histological changes in the uterus and vagina of the rat during prolongation of pseudopregnancy associated with the presence of deciduomata. *Am J Anat* 93:273–305.

Vermeirsch, H., W. Van Den Broeck, and P. Simeons. 2002. Immunolocalization of sex steroid hormone receptors in canine vaginal and vulvar tissue and their relation to sex steroid hormone concentrations. *Reprod Fertil Dev* 14:251–8.

vom Saal, F.S., C.E. Finch, and J.F. Nelson. 1994. Natural history and mechanisms of reproductive aging in humans, laboratory rodents, and other selected vertebrates. In *The Physiology of Reproduction*, 2nd edition, ed. E. Knobil and J.D. Neill, 1213–314. New York: Raven Press.

Von Berky, A.G., and W.L.Townsend. 1993. The relationship between the prevalence of uterine lesions and the use of medroxyprogesterone acetate for canine population control. *Aust Vet J* 70:249–50.

Wakui, S., T. Muto, Y. Kobayashi et al. 2008. Sertoli–Leydig cell tumor of the testis in a Sprague–Dawley rat. *J Am Assoc Lab Anim Sci* 47:67–70.

Walker, R.F., L.W. Schwartz, and J.M. Manson. 1988. Ovarian effects of an anti-inflammatory–immunomodulatory drug in the rat. *Toxicol Appl Pharmacol* 94:266–75.

Walker, W.F. Jr., and D.G. Homberger. 1997. *Anatomy & Dissection of the Rat*, 3rd edition, 65–78. New York: W.H. Freeman and Co.

Walter, I., G. Galabova, D. Dimov, and M. Helmreich. 2011. The morphological basis of proestrus endometrial bleeding in canines. *Theriogenology* 75:411–20.

Walters, K.A., U. Simanainen, and D.J. Handelsman. 2010. Molecular insights into androgen actions in male and female reproductive function from androgen receptor knockout models. *Hum Reprod Update* 16:543–58.

Wang, H., H. Eriksson, and L. Sahlin. 2000. Estrogen receptors alpha and beta in the female reproductive tract of the rat during the estrous cycle. *Biol Reprod* 63:1331–40.

Wang, X.J., E. Bartolucci-Page, S.E. Fenton, and L. You. 2006. Altered mammary gland development in male rats exposed to genistein and methoxychlor. *Toxicol Sci* 91:93–103.

Warner, M.R. 1976. Age incidence and site distribution of mammary dysplasia in young beagle bitches. *J Natl Cancer Inst* 57:57–61.

Warren, L., and S.S. Spicer. 1961. Biochemical and histochemical identification of sialic acid containing mucins of rodent vagina and salivary glands. *J Histochem Cytochem* 9:400–8.

Wassarman, P., J. Chen, N. Cohen et al. 1999. Structure and function of the mammalian egg zona pellucida. *J Exp Zool* 285:251–8.

Watanabe, D., T. Hoshiya, J. Sato, Y. Yamaguchi, K. Horiguchi, Y. Nagashima, A. Okaniwa, and H. Yoshikawa. 2006. Changes in the reproductive organs depending on phases of reproductive cycle and aging in female cynomolgus monkeys. *J Toxicol Pathol* 19:169–77.

Watson, C.J., and W.T. Khaled. 2008. Mammary development in the embryo and adult: a journey of morphogenesis and commitment. *Development* 135:995–1003.

Weinbauer, G.F., M. Niehoff, M. Niehaus, S. Srivastav, A. Fuchs, E. Van Esch, and J.M. Cline. 2008. Physiology and endocrinology of the ovarian cycle in macaques. *Toxicol Pathol* 36:7S–23S.

Weinbauer, G.F., and E. Nieschlag. 1999. Testicular physiology of primates. In *Reproduction in Nonhuman Primates*, ed. G.F. Weinbauer and R. Korte, 13–26. Münster: Wasmann Verlag.

Wenzel, J.G., and S. Odend'hal. 1985. The mammalian rete ovarii: a literature review. *Cornell Vet* 75:411–25.

Westfahl, P.K. 1993. Comparison of luteinized unruptured follicles and corpora lutea: steroid hormone production and response to luteolytic and luteotropic agents. *Biol Reprod* 48:807–14.

Westwood, F.R. 2008. The female rat reproductive cycle: a practical histological guide to staging. *Toxicol Pathol* 36:375–84.

Wildt, D.E., S.W.J. Seager, and P.K. Chakraborty. 1981. Behavioral, ovarian and endocrine relationships in the pubertal bitch. *J Anim Sci* 53:182–91.

Wimsatt, W.A., and C.M. Waldo. 1945. The normal occurrence of a peritoneal opening in the bursa ovarii of the mouse. *Anat Rec* 93:47–57.

Withers, A.R., and J.C. Whitney. 1967. The response of the bitch to treatment with medroxyprogesterone acetate. *J Small Anim Pract* 8:265–71.

Woicke, J., S.K. Durham, and M.G. Mense. 2007. Lobucavir-induced proliferative changes in mice. *Exp Toxicol Pathol* 59:197–204.

Wood, C.E. 2008. Morphologic and immunohistochemical features of the cynomolgus macaque cervix. *Toxicol Pathol* 36:119S–29S.

Wood, C.E., J.M. Hester, and J.M. Cline. 2007. Mammary gland development in early pubertal female macaques. *Toxicol Pathol* 35:793–803.

Wood, C.E., A.L. Usborne, M.F. Starost et al. 2006. Hyperplastic and neoplastic lesions of the mammary gland in macaques. *Vet Pathol* 43:471–83.

Wordinger, R.J., and A. Morrill. 1985. Histology of the adult mouse oviduct and endometrium following a single prenatal exposure to diethylstilbestrol. *Virchows Arch B Cell Pathol Incl Mol Pathol* 50:71–9.

Wuttke, W., and J. Meites. 1971. Luteolytic role of prolactin during the estrous cycle of the rat. *Proc Soc Exp Biol Med* 137:988–91.

Yaghmaei, P., K. Parivar, and F. Jalalvand. 2009. Effect of Imatinib on the oogenesis and pituitary–ovary hormonal axis in female Wistar rat. *Int J Fertil Steril* 3:11–6.

Yamasaki, K., M. Sawaki, S. Noda, N. Imatanaka, and M. Takatsuki. 2002. Subacute oral toxicity study of ethynylestradiol and bisphenol A, based on the draft protocol for the 'Enhanced OECD Test Guideline no. 407.' *Arch Toxicol* 76:65–74.

Yan, W., M. Samson, B. Jegou, and J. Toppari. 2000. Bcl-w forms complexes with Bax and Bak, and elevated ratios of Bax/Bcl-w and Bak/Bcl-w correspond to spermatogonial and spermatocyte apoptosis in the testis. *Mol Endocrinol* 14:682–99.

Yang, X.-J., H.-C.Wang, Y.-P. Chen, J. Zhao, and F.-Y. Zheng. 2009. Examination of the effects of methotrexate on histological and steroid receptor changes in the endosalpinx of the rat. *Eur J Obstet Gynecol Reprod Biol* 146:193–9.

Yano, B.L., J.F. Hardisty, J.C. Seely, B.E. Butterworth, E.E. McConnell, J.A. Swenberg, G.A. Williams, K.E. Stebbins, B.B. Gollapudi, and D.L. Eisenbrandt. 2008. Nitrapyrin: a scientific advisory group review of the mode of action of carcinogenicity in B6C3F1 mice. *Regul Toxicol Pharmacol* 51:53–65.

Yano, S., Y. Ikegami, and K. Nakao. 1996. Studies on the effect of the new non-steroidal aromatase inhibitor fadrozole hydrochloride in an endometriosis model in rats. *Arzneim Forsch* 46:192–5.

Yeh, J., B.S. Kim, Y.J. Liang, and J. Peresie. 2009. Gonadotropin stimulation as a challenge to calibrate cisplatin induced ovarian damage in the female rat. *Reprod Toxicol* 28:556–62.

Yeh, S., Y.C. Hu, P.H. Wang et al. 2003. Abnormal mammary gland development and growth retardation in female mice and MCF7 breast cancer cells lacking androgen receptor. *J Exp Med* 198:1899–908.

Yi, E.S., A.A. Bedoya, H. Lee et al. 1994. Keratinocyte growth factor causes cystic dilation of the mammary glands of mice. *Am J Pathol* 145:1015–22.

Yoshida, M., A. Sanbuissho, S. Hisada, M. Takahashi, Y. Ohno, and A. Nishikawa. 2009. Morphological characterization of the ovary under normal cycling in rats and its viewpoints of ovarian toxicity detection. *J Toxicol Sci* 34:SP189–97.

Yoshitomi, K. 1990. Cystic dilatation of the vaginal fornix in aged female Crj:F344/Du rats. *Vet Pathol* 27:282–4.

Yoshitomi, K., and S. Morii. 1984. Benign and malignant epithelial tumors of the rete testis in mice. *Vet Pathol* 21:300–3.

Young, J.M., and A.S. McNeilly. 2010. Theca: the forgotten cell of the ovarian follicle. *Reproduction* 140:489–504.

Yuan, Y.-D., and R.G. Carlson. 1985. Structure, cyclic change, and function vagina and vulva, rat. In *Genital System*, ed. T.C. Jones, U. Mohr, and R.D. Hunt, 161–8. Berlin: Springer-Verlag.

Yuan, Y.-D., and G.L. Foley. 2002. Female reproductive system. In *Handbook of Toxicologic Pathology*, 2nd edition, ed. W.M. Haschek, C.G. Rousseaux, and M.A. Wallig, Vol. 2, 847–94. San Diego: Academic Press.

Yuan, Y.-D., and J.E. Lund. 1991. Vaginal epithelial inclusion cyst in a rat. *Lab Anim Sci* 41:175–7.

Yuan, Y.D., A.H. Kennedy, and R. Ochoa. 1994. Testicular toxicity of theophylline in rats. *Toxicol Pathol* 22:655 (abstract).

Zeleznik, A.J. and C.R. Pohl. 2006. Control of follicular development, corpus luteum function, the maternal recognition of pregnancy, and the neuroendocrine regulation of the menstrual cycle in higher primates. In *Knobil and Neill's Physiology of Reproduction*, ed. J.D. Neill, 2449–510. St. Louis, MO: Elsevier.

Zheng, S., T.T. Turner, and J.L. Lysiak. 2006. Caspase 2 activity contributes to the initial wave of germ cell apoptosis during the first round of spermatogenesis. *Biol Reprod* 74:1026–33.

Zhengwei, Y., R.I. McLachlan, W.J. Bremner, and N.G. Wreford. 1997. Quantitative (stereological) study in the adult monkey (*Macaca fascicularis*). *J Androl* 18:681–7.

Zondervan, K.T., D.E. Weeks, R. Colman, L.R. Cardon, R. Hadfield, J. Schleffler, A.G. Trainor, C.L. Coe, J.W. Kemnitz, and S.H. Kennedy. 2004. Familial aggregation of endometriosis in a large pedigree of rhesus macaques. *Hum Reprod* 19:448–55.

19 Skin

Zbigniew W. Wojcinski, Lydia Andrews-Jones,
Daher Ibrahim Aibo, and Robert Dunstan

CONTENTS

19.1 INTRODUCTION, EMBRYOLOGY, AND ANATOMY OF SKIN

19.1.1 INTRODUCTION

In drug development, cutaneous toxicity may be the result of direct or indirect causes and may occur after topical application or systemic administration. Mechanisms of cutaneous toxicity may involve chemical toxicity, immune-mediated causes, or photosensitization. The chemical structure (e.g., ultraviolet [UV] absorption) and characteristics (e.g., lipophilicity and antigenicity) of a compound, bioavailability (including metabolism and distribution to skin), skin location, and species can influence the potential for dermatotoxicity and pattern of associated histopathologic changes observed.

Since skin characteristics vary between species (and strain within a species), selection of the appropriate animal model can significantly influence the predictivity of preclinical testing of new chemical entities when assessing their potential for safety in humans. Cutaneous responses may also be affected by age, gender, nutritional or hormonal status, disease state, and genetic background (Feingold and Elias 1988; Greaves 2000).

Permeation of the intact skin usually occurs through three main routes: the majority of compounds permeate via intercellular lipid domains; the others enter via skin appendages or the keratin bundles in the stratum corneum (Godin and Touitou 2007). Although well recognized as a protective barrier to the external environment, the skin is also a dynamic organ capable of biotransformation. This is of particular concern for certain chemicals or drugs that may elicit toxicity through the production of reactive metabolites resulting from bioactivation. A comparative review of metabolizing enzymes in the human, rat, and pig skin has been reviewed by Oesch et al. (2007). Some drug-metabolizing enzymes were specific to the skin, and most were located within the epidermis, most commonly in the differentiated layers. Drug-induced dermal toxicity must also be differentiated from infectious disease, spontaneous inflammatory conditions, vascular thrombotic disease, or iatrogenic causes (e.g., injury from excessive blood sampling) (Greaves 2000).

Cutaneous responses to injury can vary depending on the nature of the initial insult and may range from a mild acute inflammatory response to chronic inflammation and induration. Inflammatory and immune responses can alter the permeability characteristics of the skin, and chronic cutaneous irritation can also lead to proliferation of various cell types. Skin is capable of repair and regeneration, but an uncontrolled response can lead to scarring, production of excessive proliferative tissue, or cutaneous neoplasia. Since both local and systemic disease conditions may be reflected in skin, histopathologic evaluation of skin constitutes an integral component of any diagnostic evaluation.

The predictivity of animal models for dermatotoxicity has been the subject of much debate owing to the differences in skin characteristics between species. Animal models have included mice, rats, rabbits, guinea pigs, swine (pigs), and monkeys. Of all these species, swine skin is most structurally comparable to human skin (see below and Section 19.2.1.2). Swine and humans have comparable stratum corneum, epidermal thickness, and hair follicle density and have similar chemical composition of the stratum corneum (Godin and Touitou 2007; Swindle et al. 2012). Rodents have much thinner skin (especially epidermis) with greater permeation compared to humans (Bartek et al. 1972; Wester et al. 1989).

The responses of skin to chemical insult can be derived from a basic understanding of its embryology and functional anatomy.

19.1.2 EMBRYOLOGY

The epidermis, hair follicles, sweat and sebaceous glands, and nervous tissue are derived from the ectoderm, whereas the dermis and vasculature originate from the mesoderm. Melanocytes are derived from embryonic neural crest cells.

19.1.3 FUNCTIONAL ANATOMY

The skin is composed of epidermis, underlying dermis, subcutis, and appendages, including hair follicles, sebaceous glands, sweat glands, and nails (Figure 19.1). Skin characteristics vary across species in epidermal pattern, type and distribution of hair follicles, sweat glands and sebaceous glands, and presence or absence of a superficial vascular plexus (Table 19.1).

Skin constitutes the largest organ of the body (15%–20% of total mass), providing a protective covering for underlying soft tissues against mechanical injury, irradiation from sunlight, and noxious agents. Skin thickness varies with species (Figure 19.2a–f) and in different locations on the body and is regulated by epidermal mitotic activity (Bullough 1972). In general, skin is thicker over dorsal and lateral surfaces and thinnest on ventral and medial surfaces. Areas of skin that contact the ground (e.g., footpads and heels) have the thickest epidermis. In addition to its protective barrier function, skin has several additional functions including thermoregulation, sensation (e.g., touch,

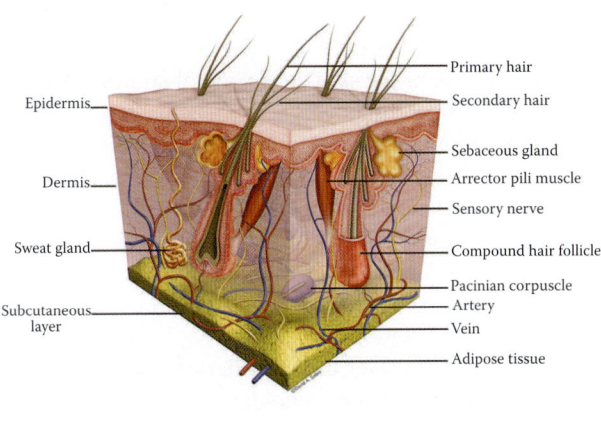

Skin

FIGURE 19.1 Drawing of the structure of mammalian skin providing an overview of the major anatomic structures.

TABLE 19.1

Comparison of Skin Components across Species

	Human/ Nonhuman Primate	Pig	Dog	Rat	Mouse
Epidermal pattern	Epidermal	Epidermal	Largely infundibular[a]	Largely infundibular[a]	Largely infundibular[a]
Compound hair follicles	No	No	Yes (except for vibrissae)	No[b]	No[b]
Sweat glands	Eccrine glands over entire body; apocrine in genitals, underarms	Eccrine glands in carpal glands; apocrine glands associated with all follicles	Eccrine glands in footpad, nose; apocrine glands associated with all follicles, and in the perianal region where they drain into the anal sac	Eccrine glands in footpads; no apocrine glands	Eccrine glands in footpads; no apocrine glands
Sebaceous glands	Associated with all follicles	Associated with all follicles	Associated with all follicles	Associated with all follicles	Associated with all follicles
Superficial vascular plexus	Yes	Yes	Yes	Yes	No

[a] Because of the density of follicles, most of the epidermis in these species is largely composed of infundibular epithelium.

[b] In rodents, there is retention of old telogen hairs from a single follicle, often giving the appearance of a compound hair. This is, however, different from the compound hair seen in dogs where the hair shafts are formed by multiple follicles that enter into a common infundibulum.

temperature, and pain.), excretion (e.g., sweat), synthesis of vitamin D (via absorption of UV radiation), and phosphorus and calcium metabolism. The protective function of skin is provided by a relatively impermeable layer of keratin, as well as the inflammatory and immune responses of its cellular constituents.

19.1.3.1 Epidermis

The epidermis is the outermost layer of the skin consisting of stratified squamous keratinizing epithelium (i.e., keratinocytes) and non-keratinocytes (i.e., melanocytes, Langerhans cells, and Merkel cells). The thickness of the epidermis varies with species and anatomic location; it is thinner in haired areas where hair serves as the major structural protective barrier and thicker in non-hairy areas, such as footpads and mucocutaneous junctions (Table 19.2).

The keratinized epithelium is arranged in four principal layers or strata supported by an epidermal cell cytoskeleton, although clear differentiation of these layers may not be present in hairy mammals, especially rodents where the normal epidermis may be two to three nucleated cell layers thick.

The basal cell layer is the innermost layer of the epidermis resting on the basal lamina or basement membrane. It consists of a single layer of cuboidal cells containing a large nucleus and basophilic cytoplasm. Basal cells are mitotically active stem cells and replenish the overlying epithelial cells that are continually sloughed from the surface; this replacement cycle is approximately 27 days for healthy, middle-aged humans. Basal cells contain numerous desmosomes that connect adjacent basal cells to the overlying cells of the spinous cell layer. The basal cells are anchored to the

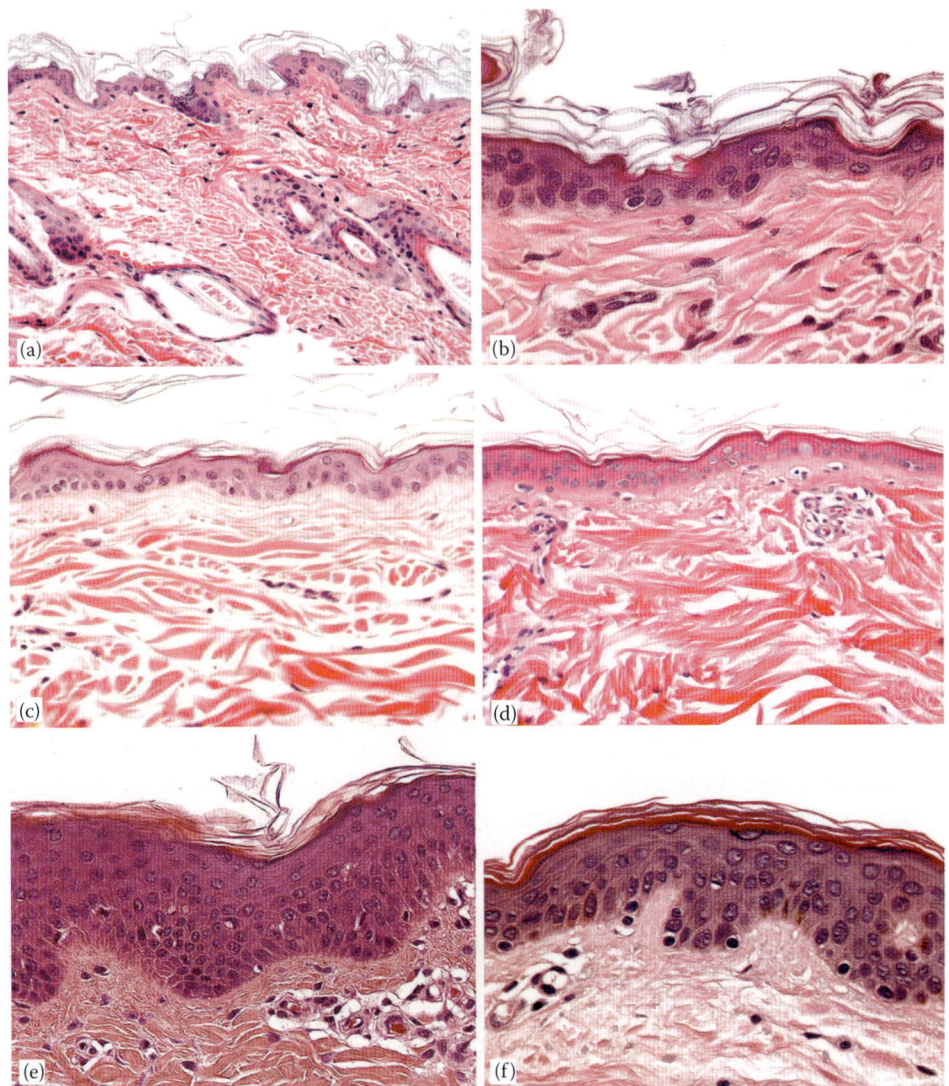

FIGURE 19.2 Comparative histology of normal skin: (a) mouse; (b) rat; (c) dog; (d) monkey; (e) pig; and (f) human.

basal lamina by hemidesmosomes. Ultrastructurally, basal cells contain numerous free ribosomes, a small amount of rough endoplasmic reticulum (RER), and a small Golgi complex. The lateral desmosomes and basal hemidesmosomes contain numerous single and bundles of intermediate filaments called tonofilaments. Cells of this layer synthesize three types of keratin (keratins 5, 14, and 15) that can be used to differentiate epidermal layers from each other (Moll et al. 2008; Porter 2006).

The spinous cell layer overlies the basal cell layer and is the thickest layer of the epidermis. It is composed of polyhedral to flattened cells containing large numbers of desmosomes that interdigitate with each other via intercellular bridges, giving this layer a "prickle cell" or "spinous" appearance. Similar to basal cells, cells of the spinous cell layer contain free ribosomes, RER, and a Golgi apparatus, but in contrast to basal cells, they contain more tonofilaments (i.e., cytokeratin) that radiate outward from the perinuclear area to the interdigitated cellular processes that bridge

TABLE 19.2

Comparative Thickness of the Stratum Corneum and Epidermis and Number of Cell Layers from the Back (Thoracolumbar Area) of Nine Species

Species	Stratum Corneum (μm) Mean ± SE	Epidermis (μm) Mean ± SE	Number of Cell Layers Mean ± SE
Cat	5.84 ± 1.02	12.97 ± 0.93	1.28 ± 0.13
Cow	8.65 ± 1.17	36.76 ± 2.95	2.22 ± 0.11
Dog	5.56 ± 0.85	21.16 ± 2.55	1.89 ± 0.16
Horse	7.26 ± 1.04	33.59 ± 2.16	2.50 ± 0.25
Monkey	12.05 ± 2.30	26.87 ± 3.14	2.67 ± 0.24
Mouse	2.90 ± 0.12	13.32 ± 1.19	1.75 ± 0.08
Pig	12.28 ± 0.72	51.89 ± 1.49	3.94 ± 0.13
Rabbit	6.56 ± 0.37	10.85 ± 1.00	1.22 ± 0.11
Rat	5.00 ± 0.85	21.66 ± 2.23	1.83 ± 0.17
Human[a]	15.11 ± 1.543[b]	86.18 ± 6.832[b]	4–5

Source: Modified from Monteiro-Riviere, N.A. et al., *Journal of Investigative Dermatology*, 95(5):582–6, 1990.

Note: Animal studies, n = 6; human study, n = 20; SE, standard error.

[a] Source: Liu, Y. et al., *Comparative Medicine*, 60(2):142–8, 2010.

[b] Mean ± standard deviation.

the intercellular spaces. As keratinocytes of the spinous cell layer move outward, they continue to produce tonofilaments that collect together to form tonofibrils contributing to the eosinophilic appearance of these cells. These keratinocytes also contain cytoplasmic membrane-coated granules (also known as lamellar granules), which are flattened vesicles containing complex lipids, proteases, and lipases (the latter of which are involved in desquamation) and are typically arranged in a lamellar pattern (Fartasch 2004). In general, keratinocytes in the basal levels of the spinous cell layer are mitotically active only when the skin is responding to injury; thus, suprabasilar mitoses are indicative of ongoing epidermal proliferation and are characteristic of certain chronic skin conditions.

Above the spinous cell layer resides the granular cell layer, which is the outermost layer of the epidermis still containing nuclei. Cells of the granular cell layer contain keratohyalin granules, which are large, irregular, and coarse but are not membrane bound. The keratohyalin granules give these cells a more basophilic appearance. These cells contain membrane-coated granules, also called lamellar bodies that release lipid-rich substances or proteases by exocytosis, and contribute to the waterproof barrier of the skin and antimicrobial defenses (Fartasch 2004; Madison 2003). Spinous cells also contain the protein filaggrin, which contributes to the assembly of keratin filaments into coarse bundles. These cells are also permeable to calcium ions and involved in the cross-linking of involucrum and other proteins, which serve to form a thick, tough layer under the plasmalemma known as the cornified envelope.

The most superficial layer of the epidermis is the stratum corneum, which is also referred to as the "horny layer" owing to its morphological characteristics. The stratum corneum is the major skin barrier to water loss and penetration of substances that come into contact with the skin, including topically applied pharmaceuticals (Bouwstra et al. 2003; Freinkel and Woodley 2001). This layer is composed of numerous layers of flattened dead cells ("squames") that are keratinized and do not contain nuclei or organelles, within a continuous extracellular lipid matrix, a so-called brick-and-mortar arrangement (Freinkel and Woodley 2001). Cells deeper in this layer contain desmosomes that are progressively lost as the cells move to the surface and are sloughed (desquamated). Internally, these cells contain numerous 10 nm keratin filaments in an amorphous matrix (Fuchs 1995).

The growth and development of epidermal cells, termed keratinocytes, are under the influence of epidermal growth factor (EGF) and interleukin (IL)-1α, whereas transforming growth factor (TGF)-β suppresses proliferation and differentiation. Cyclic adenosine monophosphate, protein kinase C, inositol phosphate, lymphokines, and p63 gene expression also contribute to epidermal homeostasis. Apoptosis is influenced by UV radiation. Keratinocytes characteristically elaborate cytokines, chemotactic polypeptides, and adhesion molecules (Bos and Kapsenberg 1993). In addition to keratinocytes, several types of cells with antigen-presenting capabilities are also present in the epidermis including melanocytes, Langerhans cells, and Merkel cells.

19.1.3.1.1 Melanocytes

Melanocytes are present in the skin of pigmented animals and contain melanin granules that are responsible for the color of skin and hair. Melanin can nonspecifically bind some xenobiotics (Ono et al. 2003); hence, pigment can become a consideration in the development or toxicity of some pharmaceuticals. The influence of drugs on skin pigmentation is described in subsequent sections.

Melanocytes are located in the basal cell layer and lower layers of the spinous cell layer, as well as in the superficial dermis. Melanocytes are stellate or elongated in shape with long, undulating processes that extend through the intercellular spaces of the spinous cell layer. Melanocytes contain RER, which produces tyrosinase that is packaged by the Golgi apparatus into round or oval granules (melanosomes). Ultrastructurally, melanocytes are identified by the presence of melanosomes, which can be abnormal in some pathologies (Cheville 1994). In the melanosomes, tyrosinase (which is activated by UV light) converts the amino acid tyrosine into melanin by the reactions of 3,4-dihydroxyphenylalanine (DOPA, methyl DOPA) and dopaquinone (Hirobe 2011). Melanosomes move to the tips of the long processes and are transferred to the cytoplasm of keratinocytes of the spinous cell layer through a process of cytocrine secretion. Melanosomes are then transported to the supranuclear area to form a protective cap above the nucleus, thereby providing protection from UV radiation penetrating the skin surface. Over a period of several days, melanin pigment is degraded by lysosomes in these cells and the number of melanin granules decreases as cells move toward the surface of the epidermis. The size of melanosomes and the amount of tyrosinase activity, rather than the number of melanocytes, determines the degree of pigmentation. Continued exposure to UV radiation will eventually result in an increase in the number and size of melanosomes. The distribution of melanosomes within the cell will also influence the degree of pigmentation. Variation in skin pigmentation may be influenced by the amount and composition (i.e., color) of melanin in the epidermis, as well as melanosome size (Alaluf et al. 2002a).

Melanosomes may be identified by characteristic immunostaining for tyrosinase activity or transmission electron microscopy (TEM). Hypopigmentation may be due to either an absence of melanocytes or an inability of melanocytes to produce melanin. Certain compounds that are chemically related to tyrosine and DOPA (i.e., precursors of melanin), such as p-tertiary butylcatechol, p-tertiary butyphenol, and hydroquinone, may cause hypopigmentation, while other chemicals may induce hyperpigmentation. 4-S-Cysteaminylphenol (4-S-CAP) exhibits selective cytotoxicity on follicular melanocytes in the black mouse, causing swelling and lysis of melanocytes, leading to the depigmentation of black hair follicles. Similar changes are not observed in albino mice, indicating that active melanin and tyrosinase synthesis are key to melanocytotoxicity of 4-S-CAP (Ito and Jimbow 1987).

The principal function of melanocytes and melanin production is to protect cutaneous structures from harmful UV radiation from sunlight, and they are particularly efficient in blocking the most damaging shorter wavelength ranges (Rees 2003). Other less critical functions in animals include camouflage or, conversely, the drawing of attention from congeners (Rees 2003). The greater the amount of melanin in skin, the greater the protective potential against the aging and carcinogenic effects of UV radiation (Miyamura et al. 2007). Melanin scatters incident UV radiation and serves as a filter that reduces the penetration of UV through the epidermis layers (Kadekaro et al. 2003). In addition, melanin scavenges radical oxygen species produced by UV exposure that are responsible for DNA damage in epidermal cells (Kadekaro et al. 2003). Keratinocyte-derived factors such as α-melanocyte-stimulating hormone (α-MSH) and adrenocorticotropic hormone (ACTH) are important in the regulation of skin pigmentation (Yamaguchi and Hearing 2009). Both α-MSH and ACTH interact with melanocortin 1 receptor (MC1R) on melanocytes (Yamaguchi and Hearing 2009). MC1R is responsible for the level and type of melanin produced in the human as well as in the mouse (Rees 2004). Eumelanin is the most common type in dark-skinned humans, while pheomelanin is more common in light-skinned humans of Celtic or northern European descent (Freinkel and Woodley 2001). Interestingly, an association between MC1R protein sequence changes and various skin cancers (including squamous cell carcinoma [SCC] and melanoma) has been observed and several authors have ascribed this association to the loss of the UV radiation–shielding role of eumelanin subsequent to MC1R sequence change, though other theories have also been advanced (Rees 2003). The most critical transcription factor in the regulation of melanocyte differentiation and melanogenesis (and in that respect downstream target of MC1R) is the microphthalmia transcription factor (Lin and Fisher 2007).

Other factors involved in skin pigmentation homeostasis include those derived from dermal fibroblasts and act as inhibitors (Dickkopf1 or DKK1 and TGF-β1) or activators (basic fibroblast growth factor or bFGF, stem cell factor or SCF, or hepatocyte growth factor or HGF) (Yamaguchi and Hearing 2009). Estrogen increase usually drives an increase in skin pigmentation while androgen increase has the opposite effect (Tadokoro et al. 2003). Pigmentation increase or decrease is a condition that sometimes follows skin inflammation and is characterized microscopically by an increase or decrease in the number of melanocytes as well as melanin production (Costin and Hearing 2007; Ruiz-Maldonado and Orozco-Covarrubias 1997). Arachidonate derivatives (prostaglandins E2 and F2α, leukotrienes C4 and D4, and thromboxane B2) seem to be involved in the inflammation-associated pigmentation as these substances activate melanocytes (Costin and Hearing 2007). The influence of drugs on skin pigmentation is described in subsequent sections.

19.1.3.1.2 Langerhans Cells

Since Langerhans cells are a key component of the immune function of skin, they are discussed in detail in the skin immunology section (Section 19.1.3.7).

19.1.3.1.3 Merkel Cells

Merkel cells are scattered among the keratinocytes of the basal cell layer and function as mechanoreceptors. They are attached by desmosomes to keratinocytes and have processes that interdigitate with proximal keratinocytes. Merkel cells have nuclei that are deeply indented with dense cytoplasm containing intermediate cytokeratin filaments. A characteristic feature of Merkel cells is the presence of dense-core vesicles located in the perinuclear zone and cytoplasmic processes near nerve fibers. Unmyelinated sensory nerve fibers penetrate the basal lamina to lie adjacent to Merkel cells forming Merkel cell–neuron complexes that serve as mechanoreceptors. Merkel cells may also release neurocrine-like substances (e.g., serotonin and substance P). Positive immunoreactivity for cytokeratin 20 is highly specific for Merkel cells in skin (Halata et al. 2003).

19.1.3.2 Dermis

The epidermis is separated from the dermis by a basement membrane consisting of type IV collagen, laminin, entactin, fibrillin, and perlecan. The junction between the epidermis and dermis is typically smooth in areas protected by a dense hair coat; however, in areas where the skin is subjected to mechanical stress (e.g., footpads, lips), interdigitation of epidermal projections with dermal papillae and ridges is very prominent. These interdigitations form rete pegs in larger mammalian species. The epidermis is bound to the dermis by anchoring fibers composed of type IV collagen.

The dermis is composed of two layers: a superficial papillary layer and a deeper reticular layer. It varies in thickness depending on its anatomical location (i.e., thin in the eyelids, thicker in footpads). Adnexa, nerves, blood vessels (superficial, middle, and deep vascular plexi), and lymphatic vessels are present in the dermis.

The superficial papillary layer of the dermis is composed of a loose network of connective tissue consisting largely of type II collagen fibers (reticular fibers) and elastic fibers in a matrix of glycosaminoglycan. The papillary layer also contains a variety of cell types including fibroblasts, macrophages, mast cells, dermal dendritic cells, plasma cells, and lymphocytes, and occasionally, chromatophores and fat cells. Fibroblasts produce collagen and cytokines. Numerous capillary loops (superficial vascular plexi), which serve to nourish the avascular epidermis and play a role in thermoregulation, are present in the papillary dermis. Meissner's corpuscles, which function as mechanoreceptors, are located in the dermal papillae, in areas of the skin sensitive to tactile stimulation.

The superficial papillary layer is contiguous with the deeper reticular layer with no well-defined interface. The reticular layer is composed of dense irregular connective tissue consisting of type I collagen fibers, packed in large bundles and oriented parallel to the surface of the skin. Thick elastic fibers and fine reticulum are intermingled with the collagen bundles. The interstices of the reticular layer contain proteoglycans (i.e., dermatan sulfate) that hold water, adding moisture to the dermis. There are fewer cells in the reticular layer than in the papillary layer of the dermis, and it may include fibroblasts, macrophages, mast cells, lymphocytes, and occasionally fat cells (in the deeper layers). In addition to their role as a source of dermal collagen, fibroblasts serve as resident sentinel cells capable of producing inflammatory chemokines in response to tissue injury or in response to infection or other environmental factors (Smith et al. 1997). Smooth muscle cells arranged in groups are present in the deeper reticular layer and function to wrinkle the skin in areas where they are present. Skeletal muscle fibers in the skin (panniculus carnosus) penetrate the dermis and allow for voluntary movement (Rose et al. 1977). Skeletal muscle fibers may also be associated with large facial sinus hairs. The reticular layer also contains hair follicles, sweat glands, and sebaceous glands. Arrector pili muscles are attached to hair follicles and, when stimulated by cold, contract, causing piloerection. Pacinian corpuscles and Ruffini corpuscles, which respond to tensile forces, are also located in the deeper reticular layer of the dermis. The reticular dermis also contains middle and deep vascular plexi.

19.1.3.3   Subcutis

The subcutis (hypodermis) contains abundant fat and loose connective tissue (collagen and elastic fibers) that connect the dermis to the underlying fascia, skeletal muscle, or bone. Fat cells may be arranged in small clusters or large masses (i.e., panniculus adiposus). The prominence of the subcutis varies by anatomic location and nutritional status. Adipose tissue is especially prominent in the footpads where it functions as a "shock absorber" and as an insulating layer (Lafontan 2012). The role of adipocytes in the subcutis has been expanding during the last decade and now includes regulation of metabolism and energy homeostasis, as well as roles in angiogenesis and immune function (Lafontan 2012; Miner 2004). These cells secrete lipoprotein lipase that hydrolyzes triglycerides into very low-density lipoproteins and chylomicrons, or complement-related proteins including adipsin (or complement factor D). Adipocyte-derived hormones can have pro-inflammatory (IL-6, tumor necrosis factor alpha [TNF-α], plasminogen activator inhibitor-1, angiotensinogen, resistin, C-reactive protein) or anti-inflammatory (adiponectin and nitric oxide) activities (Lau et al. 2005; Miner 2004).

The leptin hormone is probably the most widely investigated adipocyte-derived molecule (Mantzoros et al. 2011). This hormone maintains appetite and food intake and a fall in leptin levels results in increased appetite and decreased energy expenditure, decreased thyroid hormone production (which slows metabolic rates), decreased reproductive hormones (energy saving), decreased insulin growth factor 1 (which reduces growth rate), and increased growth hormone (which mobilizes energy), as well as in increased cortisol levels in humans (Dardeno et al. 2010).

19.1.3.4   Hair Follicle

The hair follicle is composed of the hair shaft, hair bulb, dermal papilla, matrix cells, and outer root sheath (Paus and Cotsarelis 1999). Hairs originate from invaginations of the epidermis into the dermis and hypodermis (subcutis) forming hair follicles. Hair follicles have a thickened basement membrane ("glassy membrane") that separates the dermis from the epithelium of the hair follicle and are surrounded by dense bands of dermal connective tissue composed of collagen and elastic fibers. The base of the hair follicle is enlarged to form an indented hair root that contains the dermal papilla, sometimes also called the follicular papilla to distinguish it from the dermal papilla beneath the epidermis. Together, the hair root and dermal papilla form the hair bulb. The dermal papilla is highly innervated and vascularized and controls the physiological functions of the hair follicle (Cotsarelis 1997). The hair root is composed of proliferating hair matrix cells organized in an external root sheath (subtending the basement membrane) and an internal root sheath. Although hair matrix cells show some similarity to regular epidermal germinative cells in their capacity to proliferate, they do however differ in that they produce hard keratin (as opposed to the soft keratin of skin epidermis) and exhibit intermittent mitotic activity and keratinization in contrast to the continuous mitotic activity and keratinization of regular epidermal cells. Hair growth occurs in three phases: anagen (growth phase), catagen (involution period), and telogen (resting phase during which hair shedding occurs). The rate of hair growth and duration of the growth cycle vary in different areas of the body and are influenced by sex hormones and growth factors. Hair growth may also be influenced by nutritional status or certain drugs, and alteration of the hair cycle can be a therapeutic target, such as in treatments for male pattern baldness.

The external root sheath consists of a single layer at the level of the hair bulb and several layers of cells similar to the spinous cell layer nearer to the skin surface. The internal root sheath extends only as far as the opening of the sebaceous gland and consists of an outer single layer of cuboidal cells (Henle's layer), one to three layers of flattened epithelial cells (Huxley's layer) containing trichohyalin granules, and the cuticle layer (the innermost layer of the internal root sheath). The internal root sheath of larger follicles is corrugated and forms several follicular folds at the level of the sebaceous gland opening but then becomes thinner with cells fusing to become part of the sebum.

The hair shaft consists of an inner medulla of loose cuboidal or flattened cells, a cortex of densely packed keratinized cells, and an outer cuticle layer. The cuticle is composed of a single layer of overlapping, flat keratinized cells, resembling roof shingles. The medulla is solid in the root but has air vacuoles in between the cells in the shaft. The surface pattern of cuticular cells and the arrangement of cells in the medulla are species specific and allow for species identification. The distinctive layers of the hair shaft arise from different layers of the hair root matrix. The central most matrix cells form the medulla, whereas matrix cells peripheral to these progressively give rise to the cortex, cuticle, and internal root sheath. Cells of the cortex are connected by desmosomes and produce keratin filaments and trichohyalin granules that coalesce to form an amorphous matrix. Melanocytes are present in the matrix and transfer melanosomes to cortical cells via long dendritic processes. Hair color is determined by the amount of melanin present in the cortical cells. With age, melanocytes lose the ability to produce tyrosinase and melanin, resulting in loss (graying) of hair color. Arrector pili muscles (smooth muscle) are anchored to the papillary layer of the dermis by elastic fibers and attach at an oblique angle to the connective tissue sheath surrounding the hair follicles. These muscles are innervated by autonomic nerve fibers and, upon contraction, cause the hair to "bristle." The small air spaces that form when these muscles contract are thought to contribute to the insulating capacity of the hair coat.

Hair follicles in animals are classified on the basis of morphological appearance and organization in the skin. Primary hair follicles are characterized by a large diameter, deeply rooted in the dermis, and usually have sebaceous and sweat glands and arrector pili muscles. Secondary follicles have a smaller diameter, rooted more superficially in the dermis, and may have associated sebaceous glands but not sweat glands or arrector pili muscles. Single or simple follicles have only one emergent hair, whereas compound follicles have several hairs emerging from one opening at the skin surface. Each hair of a compound follicle arises from its own papilla but then fuse at the level of the opening of the sebaceous gland to form a single orifice with multiple hair shafts. The types of hair follicles differ with animal species. For example, in dogs, compound follicles are composed of a single large primary follicle surrounded by numerous smaller secondary follicles with as many as 15 hairs emerging from a single opening. A knock-out mouse model lacking TGF-α has been developed as an animal model of abnormal hair development ("waved hair" phenotype) (Cotsarelis 1997).

19.1.3.5   Sweat Glands

Sweat glands are classified into two types on the basis of morphological appearance and functional characteristics: apocrine and eccrine (merocrine).

Apocrine glands are simple sac-like or tubular glands with a coiled secretory component connected to a straight duct that opens to the hair follicle just below the opening at the skin surface. The secretory component has a large lumen lined by flattened cuboidal to low columnar epithelial cells containing lipid, glycogen, or pigment granules. In general, secretory activity is manifested by cytoplasmic profusions (secretory blebs) at the apical surface of these cells. Myoepithelial cells surround the secretory portion of the gland, which is innervated by postganglionic fibers of the sympathetic nervous system. The ductal segment has a narrow lumen lined by two layers of flattened cells. Apocrine glands are distributed throughout the skin of most mammals in contrast to humans where they are principally found in the axillary, pubic, and perianal areas (thought to represent vestigial scent glands) or in rodents where they are only present in the plantar areas. In animals, apocrine glands may become specialized, such as the anal sac glands of dogs and cats, the ceruminous glands of the external ear canal, and the glands of Moll in the eyelids.

The eccrine (merocrine) glands are also simple, coiled, tubular glands with a straight duct connecting directly to the surface of the epidermis rather than to a hair follicle. In humans, eccrine sweat glands are found throughout the body, but in animals, these glands are limited to the footpads of carnivores and rodents, the nasolabial area in pigs and ruminants, and the carpal region in pigs. Two distinct cuboidal cell types are present in the secretory epithelium: dark (mucoid) cells in the shape of an inverted cone containing numerous glycoprotein droplets in the apical portion of the cell, and clear cells that do not contain secretory granules but do contain abundant glycogen and are involved in fluid transport. The secretion of the dark cells is mucoid whereas the clear cells produce a watery secretion. Intercellular canaliculi coursing from the base of the epithelium to the lumen are present between adjacent clear cells. The entire secretory unit is surrounded by myoepithelial cells containing myosin filaments and actin filaments and is innervated by postganglionic sympathetic fibers. The straight duct is composed of two layers of cuboidal cells overlying a basement membrane and opens directly to the surface of the skin.

19.1.3.6   Sebaceous Glands

Sebaceous glands produce sebum by holocrine secretion and may be simple, branched, or compound alveolar glands. They are derived from the external root sheath of the hair follicle and penetrate the dermis. Sebaceous glands are most often associated with hair follicles but may also be found at mucocutaneous junctions. The secretory unit of the sebaceous glands is composed of a solid mass of epithelial cells, surrounded by a connective tissue sheath. A single layer of low cuboidal cells lines the basal lamina at the periphery of the secretory unit and constitutes the germinative layer. As cells proliferate, they move inward and enlarge, taking on a polyhedral shape and accumulating lipid droplets. The composition of sebum is very species specific, consisting of an oily mixture of different cholesterol esters, triglycerides, wax esters, and cellular debris. It is extruded through short ducts lined by stratified squamous epithelium, either into the lumen of the hair follicle or directly onto the skin surface at the mucocutaneous junctions. In certain species, sebaceous glands may be arranged in clusters or may be associated with modified sweat glands, such as in the anal sacs of cats.

Similar to epidermal keratinocytes, sebocytes of murine and human skin are involved in inflammatory and immune responses through the elaboration of cytokines and expression of receptors including TNF-α, vascular intestinal peptide, and proopiomelanocortin (POMC) (Bohm and Luger 1998). Zymbal's gland is a specialized sebaceous gland of rodents located at the base (anteroventral aspect) of the external ear canal (Haines and Eustis 1990). Cells of this gland contain cytochrome P450 isoenzymes and peroxidases and are capable of chemical metabolism.

19.1.3.7 Skin Immunology

Immune defense mechanisms of the skin can be subdivided into physical barrier and innate and adaptive immunity. Barrier mechanisms include epidermal relative resistance to injury and UV radiation, water impermeability of the stratum corneum, and the presence of antioxidant as well as antimicrobial molecules. The innate and adaptive immunologic functions of skin are served by Langerhans cells, keratinocytes, mast cells, dermal dendritic cells, and various blood-derived cells such as T cells and macrophages (Clark 2010; DiMeglio et al. 2011; Ilkovitch 2011). This section will focus on reviewing well-established knowledge about key effector cells in skin as an immune organ, known differences between human and animal models, and known areas where skin immunology can affect development or the toxicity of xenobiotics.

Skin immune function varies on the basis of the distribution, regional density, and age effects. These cells may participate in various skin defense reactions including hypersensitivity reactions and graft rejection and in the pathogenesis of disease such as psoriasis. Scientists seeking to modulate skin immune function through therapeutic intervention need to be aware of species-specific differences in skin immunologic function between humans and animal models such as mice (DeMeglio et al. 2011).

Mast cells are skin-resident perivascular dermal cells with important roles in skin inflammation and immune modulation. Beta-tryptase in the cytoplasmic granules of mast cells has pro- or anti-inflammatory properties (Harvima and Nilsson 2011). Beta-tryptase promotes angiogenesis and pro-inflammatory cytokines production and leads to autoactivation of mast cells. Mast cells can produce pro-inflammatory cytokines such as TNF-α, interferon-γ, and IL-6. Beta-tryptase and chymase can cleave chemokines and neuropeptides leading to the inhibition of their activity and termination of the inflammatory process. Mast cells can also produce anti-inflammatory cytokines such as IL-10. In mice, mast cells are classified according to their location into mucosal mast cell or connective tissue mast cell, both types of cell located in the skin (Heib et al. 2008), while in humans, mast cells are segregated on the basis of their chemical content as tryptase-containing cells, usually found in the intestinal and nasal mucosa and alveolar wall, and tryptase- and chymase-containing cells, located in the skin (and intestinal submucosa). Spontaneous accumulations of mast cells have been reported in the subcutaneous tissues of various mouse strains including C3H, Balb/c, and CFW/L1 (Moskalewski et al. 1988).

Langerhans cells are the key players in skin immune function. Langerhans cells (dendritic cells) are bone marrow derived and found primarily in the spinous cell layer as well as in the dermis. They constitute 2%–4% of the epidermal non-keratinocyte populations. These cells are recognized by their dense nucleus, pale cytoplasm, and long slender processes that radiate from the cell body into the intercellular spaces between keratinocytes, giving these cells their characteristic dendritic appearance. Ultrastructurally, Langerhans cells have a polymorphous nucleus; the cytoplasm is electron lucent, containing few mitochondria, RER, and no intermediate filaments, but numerous lysosomes, multivesicular bodies, and small vesicles. A characteristic feature of Langerhans cells is the presence of membrane-bound Birbeck granules formed from clathrin-associated endocytosis, but of undetermined function (Itagaki et al. 1995; Romani et al. 2003). Langerhans cells are negative to immunoreactive lysozyme, in contrast to tissue macrophages that stain intensely for lysozyme (Moore 1986). Human Langerhans cells are identified using the CD1, major histocompatibility complex (MHC) II, and CD207 (or langerin) molecules (Ricklin et al. 2010). In the canine and porcine skin, Langerhans cells also exhibit a similar profile with expression of CD1 and MHC II molecules. Langerin (CD207), a more recently discovered lectin, is becoming the standard in identification of these cells by immunohistochemistry and has been detected in the Langerhans cells of mice, pigs, and humans (Valladeau et al. 2002) (Figure 19.3a). Although capable of mitosis, Langerhans cells originate and are continually replenished from bone marrow, migrating from the bloodstream into the epidermis where they differentiate from precursor cells. Langerhans cells contain antibody (Fc) and complement (C3) cell-surface receptors and are capable of phagocytizing and processing foreign antigens (Berman et al. 1983). They function as antigen-presenting cells in the epidermis, migrating to local lymph nodes where epitopes of processed foreign antigen are presented to T lymphocytes to initiate the immune response (Toews et al. 1980). Langerhans cells are very potent stimulators of CD4+ and CD8+ responses by T cells and play an important role not only in immunosurveillance against viruses and neoplastic cells but also in skin allograft reactions; they also induce contact hypersensitivity reaction after exposure to epicutaneous antigens (Stoitzner 2010; Zanni et al. 1998). Langerhans cells also have a role in immune tolerance to self-antigens (Steinman et al. 2003) and downregulation of immune mechanisms through activation of regulatory T cells (Romani et al. 2012). Experiments in mice have revealed that Langerhans cells were dispensable and could be efficiently replaced by lymph node–derived dermal dendritic cells for antigen processing and presentation (Bosnjak et al. 2005).

Normal human skin harbors ~20 billion T cells (~1 million/cm²), which is twice the number present in the circulation. The vast majority of these skin-resident T cells were found to be T helper (Th)1 effector memory cells with smaller contingents of Th2 cells, central memory cells, and FOXP3-positive T regulatory cells (Clark 2010). In mice, some intraepidermal resident $\gamma\delta$ T cells specialize

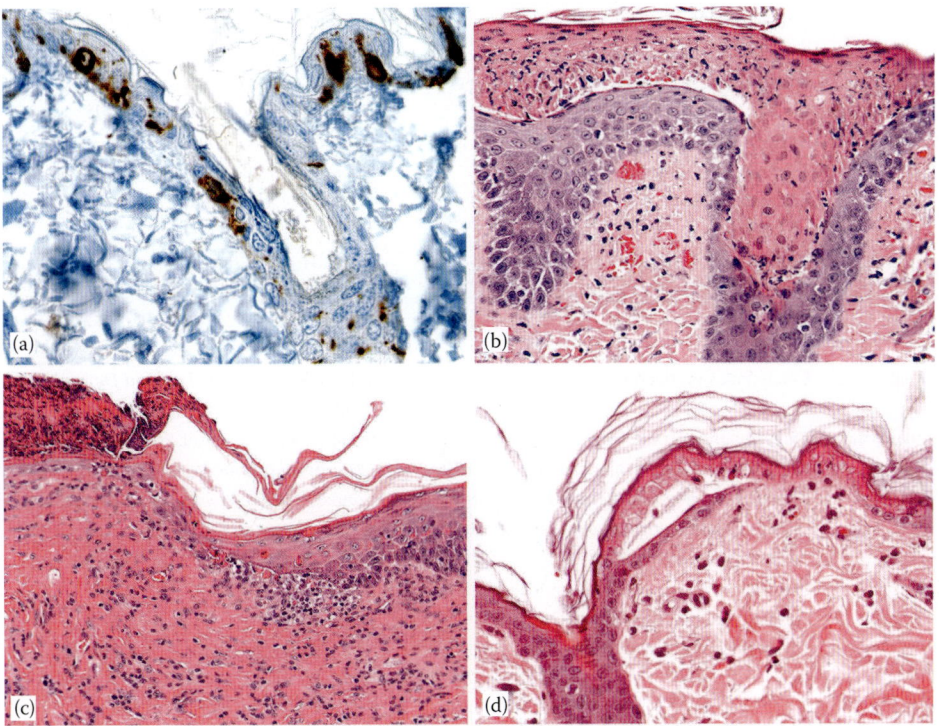

FIGURE 19.3   (a) Murine skin stained immunohistochemically with Langerin (CD207) for identification of Langerhans cells. (b) Epidermal necrosis in a case of non-immunologic cytotoxicity in a mouse. Eosinophilic coagulation necrosis is subtended by a viable regenerated epidermis. These lesions are most often associated with an "outside–in" injury such as a chemical burn. (c) Immunologic dermatotoxicity in graft-versus-host disease. Note the individual necrosis of keratinocytes in the epidermis and subtle clefting at the dermal-epidermal junction. (d) Intraepidermal vesiculation in the skin of a rat characterized by a well-delineated cleft between layers of the epidermis.

in the processing of antigens from skin-resident bacteria or dysregulated local self-antigens (Strid et al. 2009). Memory (Th1 polarized) effector skin-resident cells can proliferate locally and can carry effector functions, including induction of epidermal proliferation in models of psoriasis (Nestle et al. 2005). Regulatory T cells are responsible for tolerance to the local skin flora and are involved in the control of inflammatory processes. Mice deficient in the transcription factor FOXP3 can, for instance, develop autoimmune-like disease while the reintroduction of wild-type T regulatory cells prevents overt activation of the immune system in these animals (Khattri et al. 2003). In addition, these cells are involved in tolerance to tumor cells, and half the T cells present in some skin SCCs in humans were found to be T regulatory cells. The latter cells are under active scrutiny for their

TABLE 19.3

Selected Skin-Resident or Induced Immune Cell Functions

Cells	Immune Functions	References
Keratinocyte, follicular epithelial cells	Barrier function: proteases and protease inhibitors	See references in text
	Antimicrobial peptide secretion; cytokine/chemokines secretion	See references in text and Frohm, M. et al., *Journal of Biological Chemistry* (1997); Marchini et al., *British Journal of Dermatology* (2002); Takahashi, M. et al., *Experimental Dermatology* (2004)
	Activation of Langerhans cell	See references in text and Wood, G.S. et al., *Journal of Investigative Dermatology* (1986)
	Chemokines for T cells, eosinophils, monocytes	See references in text and Tokura, Y. et al., *Experimental Dermatology* (2008)
Langerhans cells	Antigen processing and presentation	See references in text
	Tolerance to self-antigens and immune dampening through induction of regulatory T cells	See reference in text and Romani, N. et al., *Journal of Investigative Dermatology* (2012)
	Activation of Th17 cells, induction of IL-22 producing CD4 T cells	Fujita, H. et al., *Proceedings of the National Academy of Sciences of the United States of America* (2009); Igyarto, B.Z. et al., *Immunity* (2011)
	Chemokines production	Tokura, Y. et al., *Experimental Dermatology* (2008)
Dermal dendritic cells	Three subgroups of dermal dendritic cells, antigen presentation, and priming of T cells	Schakel, K. and Hansel, A., *Current Opinion in Allergy and Clinical Immunology* (2011)
	Plasmacytoid dendritic cells express Toll-like receptors that recognize nucleic acids and secrete type I interferons	Conrad, C. et al., *Seminars in Immunology* (2009)
T cells	In mice, intraepidermal $\gamma\delta$ T cells respond to a limited number of pathogen motifs or dysregulated self-antigens	See references in text
	T effector memory cells in the dermis	See references in text
	T regulatory cells in the dermis, immune tolerance, control of local inflammation, escape mechanisms for cancer cells	See references in text
	Th17 cells in the dermis produce Th17 cytokines dependent on IL-23 stimulation: control of infections, roles in autoimmunity	See references in text

pro-tumorigenic role (Clark 2010). Finally, a small contingent of Th17 cells is located in the skin and has been involved in skin infection control and autoimmunity. The proliferation and survival of these cells depend on the local production of IL-23, and they secrete IL-17A, IL-17F, TNF-α, or IL-22 (van der Fits et al. 2009). In mice, the skin application of imiquimod, a toll-like receptor 7/8 ligand, causes a psoriasis-like syndrome (van der Fits 2009). These investigators showed that the imiquimod-induced syndrome was dependent on IL-23 stimulation of Th17 cells and subsequent IL-22 production by these cells.

Keratinocytes possess immunologic capabilities through their protein secretion capacities and interaction with T cells as antigen irrelevant signal transducers, antigen/superantigen-specific accessory and presenting cells, and as antigen-specific target cells (Nickoloff 2006; Nickoloff and Turka 1993; Strid et al. 2009). Upon stimulation, keratinocytes upregulate synthesis and secretion of antimicrobial and signaling peptides including cathelicidins, defensins, and S100 proteins or proteases and protease inhibitors such as LEKT1 involved in skin impermeabilization (Schauber and Gallo 2008; Strid et al. 2009). Keratinocytes also secrete cytokines and chemokines such as CCL17, CCL20, CCL27, or IL-15 that are involved in the homing of T cells and neutrophils to the skin or serve as keratinocyte autocrine factors and T cell and monocyte differentiation factors (Strid et al. 2009). Finally, keratinocytes express MHC I and could be induced to express MHC II, although the subsequent induction of immune-competent cells through this expression is still being debated (Salmon et al. 1994). Activated keratinocytes upregulate the expression of adhesion molecules, such as intercellular adhesion molecule 1, which interacts with integrins on the surface of T lymphocytes. Such activation has been demonstrated in various diseases, including psoriasis and hypersensitivity (Salmon et al. 1994). Major skin immune cells and their most prominent functions are listed in Table 19.3.

Skin also contains a complex neuromediator network that plays a significant role in the regulation of inflammatory and immune responses in the skin as well as in the maintenance of tissue integrity (Luger 2002). Cutaneous neuromediators include acetylcholine, catecholamines, and neuropeptides such as substance P, calcitonin gene-related peptide, vasointestinal peptide, and POMC-derived peptides (e.g., α-MSH [Luger 2002]). Loss of cutaneous innervation is a class effect of some drugs or chemicals (so-called stocking-and-glove injury; peripheral neuropathy).

19.2 DERMATOLOGIC DRUG DEVELOPMENT

19.2.1 Special Considerations in Dermatologic Drug Development

The skin is the first line of defense against most external insults and is quite efficient at preventing entry into the body. The complexity of this barrier function, and its many components, must be taken into account for any compound (including cosmetics) intended to be applied topically, and the formulation of that compound, depending upon the desired absorption rate and characteristics. The skin is a physiologically active and dynamic organ involved in the regulation of hormonal, thermal, and immune function, with an ability to metabolize compounds (Phase I and II). Therefore, the defensive and metabolizing properties of the skin must also be taken into account in the design of studies to test the safety of pharmaceutical agents and cosmetics. Although dermal irritation is a key consideration with any topically applied substance, potential systemic toxicity after cutaneous administration is also an important consideration in drug development. Skin lesions can also reflect serious systemic disease conditions such as disseminated intravascular coagulation, vasculitis, and septicemia associated with life-threatening bacterial infections (Kingston and Mackey 1986; Louden et al. 2006).

Since skin has a large surface area exposed to the external environment, it is of particular concern as a target for exogenous noxious substances and chemicals from the environment and can become an entry point for systemic toxicity. If the physical barrier function of the skin (i.e., the stratum corneum) becomes compromised through abrasion or disease, or if the biological functions of the skin are overwhelmed, the chance of systemic toxicity resulting from cutaneous absorption may be increased. The skin can also be a target organ of systemic toxicity or immune reaction, especially if compounds are metabolized within the skin. The expression and inducibility of cytochrome P450 isozymes have been shown in human organotypic skin models (Neis et al. 2010).

The stratum corneum is the primary barrier to percutaneous absorption of many topically applied compounds. The thickness of the stratum corneum varies widely in different areas of the body (e.g., the face versus the footpads) and between species. This variation in thickness must be taken into account when designing studies and especially when interpreting and attempting to put into context the absorption data from animal models.

The stratum corneum is composed of protein-rich, lipid-depleted, cornified keratinocytes embedded in a largely hydrophobic lipid, extracellular matrix (ECM) in a so-called brick-and-mortar arrangement (Freinkel and Woodley 2001). The stratum corneum is also hydrated (i.e., 20% water residing in corneocyte proteins), and the water content may increase after prolonged immersion in water or occlusion, which may affect its permeability. Thus, the entire composition of the topical formulation, including permeability enhancers, surfactants, and excipients in addition to lipophilicity, ionization state, and molecular size of the drug substance, must all be taken into consideration in dermatotoxicity testing. A change in formulation of a topically applied compound can have profound effects on the rate, depth, or extent of absorption, and thus alter the pharmacokinetics of the compound, both locally and systemically.

Dermatokinetic modeling can be used to estimate topical substance uptake in the skin. The rate and extent of uptake will depend on the formulation (i.e., conventional vehicles versus microemulsions), solute concentration, solubility, duration of exposure, application surface area, and site of application on the body (Kreilgaard et al. 2000). Solvent extraction of selective skin lipids has been shown to increase transepidermal water loss, providing an alternative to repeated tape stripping of skin in pigs (a method to reduce the thickness of the stratum corneum) and suggesting an alternate strategy for improving absorption of topically administered substances (Monteiro-Riviere et al. 2001). Additional factors affecting percutaneous absorption include hydrophobicity (i.e., the ability to partition into epidermal lipid as measured by the octanol/water partitioning ratio, K_{ow}), the rate of diffusion through the epidermis, and molecular size or molecular volume. Low-molecular-weight hydrophobic compounds permeate skin better than hydrophilic or high-molecular-weight compounds.

Although adnexal structures in the skin (e.g., pilosebaceous units and sweat/sebaceous glands) constitute only a fraction of the surface area, they represent another portal of entry of chemicals into the body and can be a therapeutic target as in the treatment of acne. Hair follicle density and glandular anatomy can, therefore, have a profound effect on the predictability of some animal models for some compounds. Swine have a more similar density of hair follicles to humans than common laboratory animals, and thus would be a more appropriate model for compounds where this is a concern. Different strains of minipig have different follicular density (see Section 19.2.1.2), which may be a factor in strain selection. There are hairless rodent and guinea pig models, but the reason for the hairless condition must be taken into account when designing studies or interpreting results from these models. For example, hr/hr mice are immunologically competent, but their hairlessness is caused by entrapment of the growing hairs within the subcutis. This results in the formation of follicular cysts and a granulomatous foreign body response to the entrapped hair (Jackson Labs information sheet, and personal observations of one of the authors). Clearance of drug substances from the skin is influenced by the extent of vascularity, rate of blood flow, and metabolism within the skin. Saturation of the stratum corneum can occur as a result of the slow rate of transfer of hydrophobic agents into the aqueous phase of the deeper layers of the epidermis, resulting in depot formation and prolonged exposure to a chemical substance long after application. Certain chemicals may bind to collagen in the underlying dermis or melanocytes.

Skin-related toxicity from chemical application must be differentiated from spontaneous or husbandry-related skin lesions, which may be attributed to environmental conditions or husbandry practices (International Harmonization of Nomenclature and Diagnostic Criteria for Lesions in Rats and Mice [INHAND] 2012). The latter include bite wounds, self-mutilations, ringtail (associated with low humidity and high temperature), infectious etiologies (e.g., dermatomycoses and mites), pressure sores, and ulcerative pododermatitis (associated with cage wire flooring) (INHAND 2012). Adequate controls may be necessary to differentiate a test article–related versus an environment-related lesion, especially under conditions that are unique to the study under question.

Owing to the importance of histopathologic diagnoses as an indicator of toxicity, and in order to allow comparative assessments, standardization of the nomenclature used in histopathologic terminology is under development with global expert input (Nishikawa et al. 2010). A pathology thesaurus intended for global use is in preparation by the INHAND and the Global Editorial and Steering Committee.

19.2.1.1 Species Selection

Selection of the appropriate animal model can be influenced by the size of the animal, skin thickness, hair density, and pigmentation status. Details on the effects of pigmentation were previously described under melanocytes in the anatomy section. For clinical entities that bind to melanin, comparison of metabolic and kinetics may require assessment in albino and pigmented strains.

19.2.1.1.1 Animal Models

The primary goal of nonclinical safety testing is to determine a safe starting dose for initiation of clinical trials and identify potential adverse effects to monitor. For many years, animal models have been shown to be reasonably effective predictors of human safety in the course of drug development but do not always predict toxicities (Greaves et al. 2004; Olson et al. 2000). Unfortunately, of all tissues, in both of two recent reviews, skin has the lowest rate of concordance between human and animal toxicities seen, with skin hypersensitivity reactions being the most common nonpredicted human toxicity (Greaves et al. 2004; Olson et al. 2000). Greaves et al. (2004) showed that dogs and monkeys had a concordance rate of ~10%–15% for true positives, but 50%–60% for false negatives (pigs were not reviewed). This illustrates the importance of selection of the most appropriate animal model for nonclinical safety studies to support clinical trials especially for compounds intended for topical application. As in other areas of drug development, cutaneous toxicity may be attributed to intrinsic (direct) toxic effects or to an exaggerated pharmacodynamic effect. Vehicle (either systemic or topically applied) reactions must also be considered, such as hypersensitivity reactions to the surfactant cremophor EL (Dorr 1994; Lorenz et al. 1982).

Many factors have been evaluated in determining the most appropriate animal models for assessment of dermal tolerance, including body size, handling, ethical use of animals, skin morphology, and permeability characteristics. In terms of cutaneous permeability from greatest to least permeable, the order established is rabbit > rat > pig > human. Although the rodent is still used for dermal toxicity testing, the minipig is now considered the animal model of choice for assessing dermal toxicity on the basis of the anatomical and physiological similarities between pig and human skin. The guinea pig is also considered an acceptable animal model for assessing cutaneous effects comparable to the rabbit, but its use is most often limited to evaluation of sensitization (Nixon et al. 1975). A good understanding of comparative anatomy and species- or strain-specific differences or variations is crucial to selecting an appropriate species, strain, and animal model for the concept under study.

19.2.1.1.2 Hairlessness

Particular consideration should be given to hairless animal models. These models are attractive because of their ease of use, especially the ability to observe skin changes more easily, and are extensively used in dermatologic research. However, hairlessness is an abnormality of the skin of these species, and therefore, the reason for the hairless condition must be taken into account when designing studies or interpreting results from these models. For example, hr/hr mice are immunologically competent, but their hairlessness is caused by entrapment of the growing hairs within the subcutis. These results in the formation of follicular cysts and a granulomatous foreign body response to the entrapped hair (Jackson Labs information sheet: http://jaxmice.jax.org/strain/000673.html, and personal observations of one of the authors).

Hairless guinea pigs (Crl: IAF(HA)BR, a mutant from the Hartley strain) have skin morphology similar to humans in terms of skin thickness, distinct strata, serrated/non-serrated basal keratinocytes, shallow dermal papillae, and few vellus hair follicles, thus providing an animal model that may be better than haired guinea pigs or other rodent models for investigating cutaneous toxicity and experimental pathology (Sueki et al. 2000).

Another hairless mouse (Skh:Hairless-1) has been developed as a model for assessing the chronic toxicity of topically applied drugs and cosmetics, as well as for investigating photodamage after UV irradiation (Kligman and Kligman 1998; Wilson and Agin 1982).

Mexican hairless dogs provide a suitable model for investigating dermatotoxic effects of topically applied agricultural chemicals, treatment of comedones, pigmentation, and alopecia, and for evaluating skin reactions to UV irradiation (Kimura 1996; Kimura et al. 1998).

A hairless rat model derived from Wistar rats, whose dermal histology is well characterized, has been developed (Itagaki et al. 1995). The Charles River (CR) hairless rat possesses a phenotype that is distinct from the hairless mouse allele hr/hr (Panteleyev and Christiano 2001). Skin from the CR hairless rat is characterized by abnormal keratinization of the hair shaft; formation of a thick, dense layer of keratinocytes in the stratum corneum; hair follicle degeneration; and atrophic hair follicles.

19.2.1.2   Comparative Anatomy (Human, Monkey, Pig, Dog, Rabbit, Rat, and Mouse)

19.2.1.2.1   Rodent

Regulatory agencies request that preclinical safety assessments for topical drug candidates be conducted in two species (one rodent and one nonrodent), and both topical and systemic effects must be assessed. Rats are commonly selected as the rodent species for repeated-dose studies. If the minipig is selected for evaluation of dermal tolerance, the rat is only required for evaluation of systemic toxicity, which may be by either cutaneous or oral route of administration. The oral route of administration is often selected for the rat, contingent on bioavailability. Rodents are also the species of choice for evaluation of potential carcinogenicity and photo-cocarcinogenicity. Other nonrodent species, such as dogs or nonhuman primates, are rarely used unless required to address differences in drug metabolism (McAnulty et al. 2011; Swindle et al. 2012).

19.2.1.2.2   Minipigs

On the basis of their sensitivity to a wide variety of drugs and chemicals, and their anatomic, metabolic, and physiologic similarities to humans, minipigs are generally preferred over dogs or nonhuman primates for safety assessment of topically applied compounds (McAnulty et al. 2011; Simon and Maibach 2000; Swindle et al. 2012; van der Laan et al. 2010). Since pigs are larger, more test compound may be needed than for the dog or monkey. The development of minipigs has produced an animal model of more manageable size (McAnulty et al. 2011; Svendsen 2006), although full-sized domestic pigs are still used for some applications.

Of all the commonly used laboratory species, minipigs have skin that is most comparable to humans. Similar to humans, minipig skin is covered by only sparse hair. The skin surface is textured with fine intersecting lines and has variable thickness over different parts of the body. Most significantly, the thickness of the epidermis ranges from 70 to 140 µm in minipigs, which is more comparable to the thickness of human epidermis (50–120 µm) than the 10–20 µm in rats (McAnulty et al. 2011). The need for an animal model such as the minipig with comparable anatomy is due to the fact that skin thickness and follicular density can greatly affect the rate of percutaneous absorption of topically applied compounds and thus influence topical bioavailability. For example, there is approximately 100% percutaneous absorption of haloprogin in rats and rabbits, but only 10%–20% in humans and pigs (Bartek et al. 1972; McAnulty et al. 2011). Other similarities between human and minipig skin include the presence of large amounts of elastic tissue in the dermis and Langerhans cells in the epidermis (McAnulty et al. 2011) and skin that is tightly adhered to underlying tissues as opposed to the loose skin of laboratory rodents or dogs.

Of the commercially available minipig strains, the Gottingen is used most often in drug development, followed by the Yucatan, Sinclair, and Hanford strains (Table 19.4). Strain considerations include skin color, hair growth pattern, and growth rates. Gottingen minipigs have the slowest growth rate and pale pink skin. Yucatan minipigs have little or no hair but are darkly pigmented and larger. A micro-Yucatan strain that is only slightly larger than the Gottingen has been developed. Sinclair minipigs have variable hair and color (McAnulty et al. 2011). The Hanford strain is also pale pink in color and has a hair follicle density similar to humans. Strain comparisons and origins are extensively reviewed in McAnulty et al. (2011). Micropigs (cross mixture of four breeds of pigs: Tamworth, Potbellied, Gloucester Old Spot, and Kune Kune) are now also commercially available and are an attractive alternative on the basis of their smaller body size (adult micropigs weigh approximately 18 to 40 kg [Internet search]).

As with any toxicology, familiarity with background histopathologic changes is an important consideration in determining potential drug-induced versus spontaneous lesions. For example, a generalized condition of spontaneous cutaneous purpura has been reported in Gottingen minipigs (Maratea et al. 2006). Vascular lesions associated with thrombocytopenic purpura syndrome (i.e., platelet counts < 20,000/µL) were observed in Gottingen minipigs ranging in age from 7 weeks to 1 year and are of unknown etiopathogenesis. Histopathologically, degenerative vascular lesions with morphological features of arteriosclerosis were described in small- to medium-sized muscular arteries and arterioles in the skin and various parenchymatous organs. Perivascular hemorrhages and associated accumulations of small aggregates of extracellular and intrahistiocytic hemosiderin pigment were present. Lesions in the small- to medium-sized arteries noted histopathologically were luminal stenosis, circumferential neointimal proliferation, medial thickening, thrombosis, necrosis of the tunica media, deposits of alcian blue–positive myxoid material in the media, and disruption/fragmentation of the internal elastic lamina. Histopathologic findings in the arterioles

TABLE 19.4
Minipig Strain Comparisons

Strain	Gottingen	Yucatan	Micro-Yucatan	Hanford	Sinclair (Minn Min)	Micropig (Teacup Pig)
Size, birth (kg)	0.45	0.50–0.90	0.60–0.70	0.73	0.59	0.50
Size, adult (kg)	45	70–83	55–70	80–95	55–70	18–40
Color	White	Black, gray (minimal hair)	Black, gray, some white (minimal hair)	White (follicle density closest to human)	Black, red, white, roan	White, spotted, black, brown
Origin	59% Vietnam PB, 33% Sinclair, 8% German Landrace	Mexico and Central America	From Yucatan, selective breeding	Palouse, Pitman–Moore, feral LA swamp hog, Yucatan	49% Piney woods, 22% Ras-n-lansa, 16% Catalina island feral hog, 13% guinea hog	Tamworth, PB, Gloucester Old Spot, Kune Kune
Foundation	1961	1960	1985	1958	1949	1996
Available from	Marshall Bioresources	Sinclair, Cerdo Micro	Sinclair Bioresources	Sinclair Bioresources	Sinclair Bioresources	Pet Trade

Source: McAnulty, P.A. et al. (eds.), *The Minipig in Biomedical Research*, CRC Press, Boca Raton, FL, 2011.

consisted of concentric laminar ("onion-skin" pattern) thickening of vessel walls, accumulation of amphophilic matrix between layers of hyperplastic and vacuolated smooth muscle cells, endothelial cell hypertrophy, necrosis of the tunica media, luminal stenosis, and thrombosis. Perivascular mild to moderate lymphocytic and histiocytic infiltrates with fewer neutrophils and eosinophils were present around the affected blood vessels (Maratea et al. 2006).

19.2.1.2.3 Macaques

Topical application of test compounds to macaques often requires special handling, including jacketing to prevent the animals from interfering with the application site. Macaque skin is not as good a model for human skin, especially the pharmacokinetic aspects, as is pig skin. Therefore, unless there is a unique characteristic of the test compound that requires its testing in this species, macaques are not commonly used for topical studies. As with any species, the skin can be a target of a systemically administered compound, and they can have reactions at injection sites. Laboratory-housed macaques can also have cutaneous manifestations of several diseases unique to these species, some of which are of concern for human health. These include herpes B virus (www.cdc.gov/herpesbvirus/index.html), leprosy, and measles. Any researcher working with these animals needs to be familiar with these and other diseases with zoonotic potential.

A unique feature of the skin of macaques is the presence of sex skin and estrus-related swelling that is present around the base of the tail and perineum in females and extending to the backs of the thighs and dorsal and ventral midline to the level of the forelimbs in both sexes (Lowenstine 2003). Histologically, the sex skin in these areas is edematous and highly vascularized, which may appear similar to hemangioma. Administration of hormone-modulating compounds to macaques may cause florid hyperplasia (Lowenstine 2003). Age spots (1–3 mm pink to red) and benign angiomas have been observed in older macaques (Lowenstine 2003).

19.2.1.2.4 Rabbit

Traditionally, the albino rabbit has been the animal model for assessment of local irritation and for the evaluation of systemic toxicity. However, on the basis of the higher sensitivity to cutaneous irritants and the greater permeability of rabbit skin relative to human skin, the relevance of this animal model for the evaluation of topical agents has led to consideration of other animal models. Testing of irritancy potential in rabbit skin has shown a good correlation with effects in humans for severe irritants and nonirritants but failed to predict mild or moderate skin irritants (Phillips et al. 1972).

19.2.1.2.5 Guinea Pig

The hairless guinea pig was discussed earlier in Section 19.2.1.1.1.

19.2.1.2.6 Dogs

Beagle dogs are often used as the nonrodent species for toxicity studies in drug development. Drug-induced cutaneous toxicity must be differentiated from nonspecific histopathologic findings in endocrine skin disorders of dogs, which may manifest as epidermal hyperkeratosis, follicular keratosis, follicular dilation or atrophy, empty hair follicles, predominantly telogen hair follicles, sebaceous gland atrophy, or epidermal melanosis (Scott 1982).

19.2.1.3 Specific Conditions

19.2.1.3.1 Androgenic Alopecia (Male Pattern Baldness)

Several animal models have been developed to study androgenic alopecia, including the stumptailed macaque (*Macaca arctoides*), testosterone-induced alopecia in B6C3F1AF1 mice, human-to-mouse xenografts in nude *Hfh11^{nu}/Hfh11^{nu}* mice and SCID *prkdc^{scid}/prkdc^{scid}* mice, and testosterone-primed nude mouse xenografts (Sundberg et al. 1999). Skin grafts of alopecic skin to

C3H/HeJ provide a model of alopecia areata involving immune system activation before the onset of overt hair loss (McElwee et al. 2003b).

19.2.1.3.2   Radiation Exposure

Repeated β-irradiation in mice produced 100% skin tumors histologically classified as SCCs, basal cell carcinomas, fibrosarcomas, and osteosarcomas (Ootsuyama and Tanooka 1988). Depending on the mode of application, ionizing radiation may act as an initiator and promoter of carcinogenesis. In this animal model, mouse skin more closely resembles human skin in its response to radiation than rat skin. Nude $Ng^{-/-}$ mice exposed to long-term UV irradiation have been used as a model of human actinic elastosis, a condition associated with chronic sunlight exposure (Berger et al. 1980).

19.2.1.4   Methods in Dermatotoxicity Testing

19.2.1.4.1   In Vitro

Alternatives to the use of animals for cutaneous toxicity testing have been under investigation for many years in line with efforts to replace, reduce, and refine animal usage ("3 Rs"). *In vitro* alternatives included cell, tissue, and organ cultures (Carere et al. 2002; Helman et al. 1986; Nemecek and Dayan 1999; Rogers and McDougal 2002; Semlin et al. 2011). Cell culture assays have been used to evaluate release of cytokines and other mediators in assessing irritation, corrosivity, and contact sensitization potential of chemical substances (Liebsch and Spielmann 2002; Ryan et al. 2001; Spielmann and Liebsch 2001). Rodent skin organ cultures have demonstrated a good correlation with *in vivo* lesions on the basis of similarity of the histopathologic and biochemical (e.g., leakage of intracellular enzymes) changes observed (Kao et al. 1983). Skin organ cultures, including reconstituted human skin (e.g., Epiderm™ 606), have also been used for evaluation of irritancy potential, cutaneous absorption, and metabolism of drugs (Jacobs et al. 2002; Kao et al. 1985; Monti et al. 2008) and are commercially available. On the basis of organ culture studies comparing mouse, rat, rabbit, guinea pig, marmoset, and human, it was determined that diffusional and metabolic (i.e., cutaneous first pass metabolism) properties must be taken into consideration for topically-applied compounds (Kao et al. 1985). Exposure of human skin organ cell cultures to various known contact irritants (all-*trans* retinoic acid, sodium lauryl sulfate [SLS], and benzalkonium chloride) resulted in histologic changes characterized by epidermal hyperplasia, incomplete keratinization, loss of granular cell layer, necrosis, and acantholysis (Varani et al. 2007). Reconstructed human epidermis models (e.g., EpiDerm and EpiSkin) have been developed to assess irritancy potential *in vitro* and have demonstrated concordance with *in vivo* irritancy in humans (Jirova et al. 2010). A genetically modified human skin equivalent has been developed that incorporates a therapeutic gene linked to a multidrug-resistant gene in keratinocytes via a bicistronic retroviral vector providing a long-term *in vitro* model for investigating gene therapy (Therrien et al. 2008). A combination of analysis of IL-1α and IL-8 expression and release, together with the *in vitro* MTT cytotoxicity assay in reconstructed human epidermis, has been shown to provide discrimination and classification of potential *in vivo* irritant and sensitizing agents in a single *in vitro* assay (Coquette et al. 2003).

Hair follicles have been shown to be long-term reservoirs for topically applied substances and a target for drug delivery. Pig ear skin has proved to be superior to human skin for evaluating *in vitro* follicular penetration of topically applied substances since, unlike human skin, it does not contract after excision (Lademann et al. 2010).

In vitro tests have also been applied for assessment of phototoxicity and immunotoxicity. The 3T3 NRU assay is used to determine the phototoxic potential of compounds that absorb radiation in the UVA and visible light range. An *in vitro* test has been developed to assess delayed hypersensitivity that involves binding of the test compound to Langerhans cells, activation of Langerhans cells, and subsequent lymphocyte blastogenesis.

Although numerous attempts have been made, there is no single *in vitro* test that can replace *in vivo* dermatotoxicity testing on the basis of the complexity of response in the whole animal that cannot be fully replicated *in vitro*. However, skin organ cell cultures together with skin cell monolayer cultures can be utilized as an initial method of screening compounds for potential irritancy and corrosivity (Varani et al. 2007), as well as percutaneous absorption characteristics.

19.2.1.4.2   In Vivo

For *in vivo* dermatotoxicity testing, consideration must be given to selection of the appropriate animal model (species and strain) and the objective of the test (Auletta 2004). Dermatotoxicity testing endpoints most often include acute irritation/dermal tolerance, chronic toxicity, carcinogenicity, immunotoxicity, and photosafety. Several guidance (see CDER, ICH, and EMA websites) documents are available. Consideration must be given to dose (often expressed as concentration, milligram per milliliter, or milligram per square centimeter), dose volume, area of application, type of vehicle (formulation), duration of application and occlusion/semi-occlusion, and prevention of oral ingestion via grooming behavior of the test animal. Assessment of systemic exposure and toxicity are a function of skin permeability, which may influence selection of intact or abraded skin in the test system. For practical reasons, the site of application is limited to 10% body surface area.

Skin irritation tests are designed to assess the degree of adverse cutaneous effects of compounds and differentiate among minor irritants that may produce mild and reversible inflammation, major irritants that cause severe inflammation, and corrosive agents that cause massive destruction or necrosis of the skin (Fielder et al. 1987). The assessment of the degree of cutaneous irritation most commonly used in animal testing and accepted by regulatory agencies (i.e., Code of Federal Regulations 1980) is the Draize technique (Zbinden 1987). Other techniques include the mouse ear model, including evaluation of acute response parameters such as ear thickness, vascular permeability, changes in blood flow, and cellular infiltration (Patrick et al. 1985). Clinical irritancy can be assessed by the human skin patch test.

Traditionally, skin sensitization assays have utilized three guinea pig tests, including the guinea pig maximization test, the occluded patch test, and the open epicutaneous test (Kimber et al. 2001). More recently, the local lymph node assay (LLNA) has provided a more sensitive method for providing quantitative estimation of skin-sensitizing potency for risk assessment (Kimber et al. 2001).

In recent years, it has become apparent that changes in the total number of cells within a histologic section may be a critical endpoint in the toxicopathologic evaluation of drugs or environmental toxins (Collan 1998). To this end, stereologic methods have been refined to discern subtle changes in cell numbers within a designated volume of tissue. The thickness of sections may be estimated by confocal microscopy or by the method of Gschwendtner et al. (1994). An estimate of total cell numbers may then be determined using the formula of Ebbeson and Trang (1965). Stereology can be used, in association with biochemical methods, to determine correlations between reactive cells and elaboration of a certain active peptide in comparison to unreactive cells as has been applied to studies of oncogene amplification (Collan 1998).

Quantitative analysis of skin reflectance or lightness (using a gray scale of 0 [black] to 100 [white]), red to green color saturation (+60 to −60), and yellow to blue color saturation (+60 to −60) provide an objective measure of melanin in the epidermis (Alaluf et al. 2002b).

19.2.1.5   Criteria for Grading Skin Lesions

The Draize test principally utilizes rabbits and guinea pigs and consists of application of the test substance to the test site(s) on the dorsum (shaved) of the test species. Solutions are applied directly to the test site whereas solids are dissolved in an appropriate solvent prior to administration. In certain circumstances, the skin may be abraded prior to application of the test substance. Test sites are evaluated grossly at 4, 24, and 72 h and graded on the degree of erythema, eschar, and edema formation (Table 19.5). Although not often conducted for screening of cosmetics or household substances, such as soaps, histopathologic evaluation of test sites can provide additional information on the nature of the grossly observed changes.

TABLE 19.5

Grading Values for Skin Reactions after Topical Application of Potential Primary Irritants (Draize Scale)

Skin Reaction	Grade
Erythema and Eschar Formation	
No erythema	0
Very slight erythema	1
Well-defined erythema	2
Moderate to severe erythema	3
Severe erythema to slight eschar formation	4
Edema Formation	
No edema	0
Very slight edema (barely perceptible)	1
Slight edema (raised edges of area well defined)	2
Moderate edema (raised approximately 1 mm)	3
Severe edema (raised more than 1 mm and extending beyond the area of exposure)	4

Source: Modified from the National Academy of Sciences Committee for the Revision of NAS Publication 1138, *Principles and Procedures for Evaluating the Toxicity of Household Substances*, National Academy of Science, Washington, DC, pp. 23–59, 1977.

High-resolution laser Doppler perfusion imaging is an effective new method for characterizing and grading skin irritation (i.e., inflammatory response) after single exposure to a chemical irritant (Fullerton et al. 2002).

19.2.1.6 Photosafety

19.2.1.6.1 Basic Principles in Assessing Photosafety

Photoirritation (phototoxicity) is a light-induced, non-immunologic response to a photoreactive chemical resembling primary skin irritation. A single application of the test compound in the presence of light may be sufficient to elicit a reaction (Maurer 1987). Examples of photosensitizing drugs include fluoroquinolones, tetracycline, amiodarone, naproxen, psoralens, and retinoids (Ferguson 2002). Mechanisms are reviewed in Section 19.3.6. Regulatory agencies have issued guidance documents (CDER/ICH) for photosafety testing to avoid such untoward effects clinically (Jacobs et al. 2004). Chemicals may absorb light variably in the UV spectrum: UVB, 290–320 nm; UVA, 320–400 nm; visible wavelength, >400 nm. An *in vitro* assay, the 3T3 NRU assay, has been developed to assess potential phototoxicity for compounds that absorb in the UVA and visible light range. Unfortunately, this assay will not support UVB-absorbing compounds owing to the cytotoxic nature of UVB irradiation on cell cultures. In the 3T3 NRU assay, Balb/c 3T3 cells are incubated with different concentrations of test substance and either exposed to solar simulated light or maintained in the dark. Cell viability is assessed after 24 h by the vital dye neutral red, measuring optical density (Charles River Laboratories [CRL] 2009). The phototoxic potential of the test substance is determined by comparison of the IC_{50} (i.e., the concentration of test substance that reduces cell viability by 50%), with and without solar simulated light exposure, and is expressed as the photoirritancy factor (PIF) as follows:

$$PIF = \frac{IC_{50}(-UVA)}{IC_{50}(+UVA)}.$$

The mean photo effect (MPE), defined as the weighted average across a representative set of photo effect values, can be calculated from comparison of the concentration–response curves. The

MPE can provide a measure of the phototoxic potential in cases where two equally effective (IC_{50}) concentrations in dark (−UVA) and light (+UVA) cannot be determined.

On the basis of the ICH guidance, the phototoxicity potential of the test substance is interpreted from the following table:

PIF	MPE	Phototoxic Potential
<2	<0.1	Non-phototoxic
>2 and <5	>0.1 and <0.15	Probably phototoxic
>5	>0.15	Phototoxic

In vivo, several animal models for phototoxicity testing have been developed including guinea pig (Lovell and Sanders 1992) and hairless mouse or rat models, Balb/Crj (Balb/c) mouse auricular skin model, and the hairless pigmented dog model (all described further in Section 19.2.1.1). The test compound is applied to a designated area on the back of the test species and the application site is exposed to UV irradiation from a solar simulator. The response is graded for irritation potential using a Draize scale. In a review of concordance of toxicity of pharmaceuticals in humans and animals, phototoxicity response in guinea pigs correlated well with that in humans (Olson et al. 2000).

19.2.1.7 Wound Healing

Wound healing is a complex process that requires the coordination of many physiologic processes turning on and off in a coordinated fashion for an optimal result. It is also the only physiologic process other than reproduction that requires neovascularization in a healthy adult. Normal wound healing involves four overlapping physiologic stages: hemostasis, inflammation, proliferation, and remodeling. Abnormal wound healing can be the result of excessive healing as in keloids, or hypertrophic scars, or the result of insufficient healing as in chronic ulcers (Grey et al. 2006; Shih et al. 2010). Improving the outcome of wound healing is a focus of many therapeutic strategies (Gibran et al. 2007). Adverse effects on the ability of a wound to heal are a potential concern for many therapeutics or toxicants, especially anything that affects the processes of inflammation, neovascularization, or remodeling of connective tissue.

Many factors, both local and systemic, have been implicated in impeding wound healing, so these must also be considered (Braiman-Wiksman et al. 2007). Local factors include size and depth of the wound, location, inadequate blood supply, excess mobility, wound dehiscence, foreign body reaction, and persistent infection. Systemic factors include age, malnutrition, vitamin deficiency, malignancy, chemotherapy or immunosuppressant drugs, impaired macrophage activity, and inherited neutrophil disorders. Bacterial infection of a wound leading to an inflammatory response can inhibit wound healing (Corsetti et al. 2010). Wound healing is a complex process involving several phases including (1) hemostasis, (2) inflammation, (3) proliferation, and (4) remodeling. The phase of hemostasis involves platelet aggregation and fibrin clot formation at the site of injury to control bleeding. This is followed by the inflammatory phase in which cell debris and bacteria are removed by phagocytosis and numerous cytokines including TGFs, fibroblast-derived growth factor, platelet-derived growth factor, IL-1, TNF-α, colony-stimulating factor 1, and vascular endothelial factor, all released to affect cell division and migration (Singer and Clark 1999). In the proliferative phase, angiogenesis, granulation tissue formation, collagen deposition, epithelialization, and wound contraction occur. Fibroblasts provide collagen and fibronectin to form a provisional ECM over which epithelial cells proliferate. Myofibroblasts provide the mechanism for wound contraction and ultimately undergo apoptosis when their role is complete. In the remodeling phase, collagen is realigned along the lines of tension.

Skin wound models fall into broad categories, partial- and full-thickness excisional wounds, incisional wounds, and burn wounds. There are many *in vitro* models available, from which valuable information can be obtained, but they cannot mimic the entirety of the physiologic processes necessary for wound healing, or the effects of systemic factors on the ability of an organism

In intact skin, nanoparticles less than 1 μm can penetrate the epidermis, particularly in areas of flexed skin in motion, but rarely reach the dermis. Systemic exposure to nanoparticles may be increased by dermabrasion, damaged skin, or skin wounds.

Systemic exposure to nanoparticles applied topically can be affected by many factors, including skin thickness, which may affect the choice of test species. Studies in minipigs of sunscreen containing TiO_2 nanoparticles applied to intact skin demonstrated no systemic exposure on the basis of the lack of evidence for increased levels of TiO_2 concentrations in liver or lymph nodes. Polyethylene glycol–coated cadmium selenide quantum dot nanoparticles were shown to reach liver levels of 2% of the cadmium applied to dermally abraded skin. Hairless mice did have systemic exposure after topical application of TiO_2 nanoparticles, indicating that species-specific systemic exposure may be related to skin thickness. Additionally, other constituents of topical formulations may influence skin penetration of nanoparticles. Aqueous formulations tend to reduce penetration of TiO_2 nanoparticles, whereas oily formulations may enhance penetration.

In addition to concerns over systemic exposure, nanoparticles may potentially interact with antigen-presenting cells in the skin. Regulatory guidances for the evaluation of nanoparticle immunotoxicity are still being developed (Dobrovolskaia et al. 2009).

19.2.3.1.1 Detection of Nanoparticles in Skin Sections

The use of conventional stains and light microscopy methods may be inadequate for visualization of nanoparticles in skin sections. Nanoparticles do not react with conventional histologic stains, high-power magnification is required, the nanoparticles may be highly dispersed within the tissues, and the depth of field on conventional light microscopes is limiting (e.g., 0.2 μm depth of field at 100× numerical aperture magnification captures only 1/25 of the thickness of a 5 μm section at any one time) (Hubbs et al. 2011). Special labeling techniques have been developed to enhance detection of nanoparticles by microscopy including colloidal gold labeling, silver enhancement of gold labeling, and use of fluorescent indicators.

Tissue reactions may help guide detection but can be extremely subtle if the particle is designed to be inert. Histopathologic studies of the toxic effects of nanoparticles have largely focused on the lungs after inhalation, where the principal changes observed were granulomatous inflammation and fibrosis, with pleural thickening and dilation of lymphatics. Reactions seen in the skin of minipigs after particle-mediated delivery of a DNA vaccine were mild local skin irritation, low-grade perivascular mononuclear cell infiltrates in the superficial dermis, and a few phagocytosed gold particles (Pilling et al. 2002).

While conventional scanning electron microscopy has been shown to be a useful means for demonstrating micrometer-sized particles, it has proved less than optimal for nanoparticles. Field emission scanning electron microscopy has significantly improved resolution for detecting nanoparticles owing to its unique "cold" cathode design, which produces low-voltage images with negligible electrical charging to produce high-quality images.

19.2.3.2 Implanted Biomaterials

Implanted biomaterials are typically inert, solid materials such as plastics, polymeric materials, metals, and alloys, often employed as medical devices (Darby 1987). With emergent technologies, biomaterials now include biopolymers, self-assembled systems, nanoparticles, carbon nanotubes, and quantum dots (Williams 2009). Medical devices constitute a diverse range of products with similarly divergent uses. These biomaterials typically do not elicit a pharmacologic response (unless in combination with a drug), and reactions are time dependent rather than dose dependent. Potential safety risks associated with implanted biomaterials may be associated with the type of material used, leachables from the implant, and local or systemic response (Jacobs and Urban 1996). As such, local tissue responses (e.g., irritation, sensitization) are considered key parameters in the safety evaluation of biomaterial implants.

Similar to pharmaceuticals, medical devices are also subject to classification and regulatory approval prior to use in humans (Anderson and Langone 1999). The principal guidance used in biocompatibility testing is provided by the Biological Evaluation of Medical Devices Technical Committee of the ISO, which is accepted by most industrialized countries. The ISO 10993 standards document (2007) contains 20 sections pertinent to the safety evaluation of medical devices. These documents define the testing requirements based on the intended use of the product. On the basis of these documents, the Food and Drug Administration's Center for Devices and Radiologic Health (FDA CDRH 2007) has adopted a flow diagram for testing procedures.

Preclinical testing is intended to assess potential safety risks from contact and interaction of the device, or components of the device, with tissues. *In vitro* procedures may be used as screening tools, but *in vivo* studies are needed for full testing. Preclinical evaluation may include testing for cytotoxicity; sensitization; irritation (or intracutaneous reactivity); acute, subchronic, or chronic systemic toxicity; genotoxicity; implantation; hemocompatibility; carcinogenicity; reproductive/developmental toxicity; pyrogenicity; and biodegradation. In *in vivo* testing, intramuscular implantation is most frequently used, and animal models include rabbits, rats, and mice. The site of implantation is evaluated clinically, grossly at necropsy, and microscopically.

Reaction to implanted biomaterials is time dependent rather than dose dependent as is more typically seen with pharmaceuticals. The tissue response to implanted biomaterials is most often inflammatory and reparative in nature; however, on occasion, an immunologic reaction may be triggered by the device. Histopathologic assessment may include a morphological evaluation of the reaction as well as use of scoring protocols to assess the degree of change (e.g., necrosis, inflammatory cell infiltrates that include polymorphonuclear neutrophils, lymphocytes, plasma cells, macrophages, giant cells, fibroblasts, vascularity, and fibrosis) in comparison to controls. The principal response to implanted materials is a foreign body inflammatory reaction, which may range from acute to chronic, depending on the nature of the implanted material and the duration of implantation at the time of sampling. Degeneration, necrosis, and edema of the surrounding tissues may be followed by reparative processes, including granulomatous inflammation, multinucleated giant cells, and fibrosis. Both the immune and vascular systems are involved with infiltration of cells and release of secretory factors, including cytokines, chemokines, complement, and tissue and vascular growth factors. For some biomaterials (e.g., latex), an immune response consistent with a delayed-type hypersensitivity reaction may be elicited. Chronic immune dysfunction may be observed with certain medical devices such as silicone breast implants, with potentially severe systemic manifestations (Hajdu et al. 2011; Shoenfeld and Agmon-Levin 2011). Carbon-overlayed Millipore filters, implanted subcutaneously in dogs for 28 days for administration of a specific thromboxane receptor antagonist (ICI 185,282), developed foreign body granulomas associated with enlarged epithelioid macrophages and altered fibroplasia and monocyte infiltrates at the site of implantation (Westwood et al. 1995). It was postulated that the granulomatous response was due to a drug-induced disturbance of the macrophage response to the subclinical inflammation or an atypical response to the stimuli of macrophage activity (Westwood et al. 1995).

Cytochemical methods (e.g., lysozomal activity) may be used to further characterize local responses. Evaluation of hematologic and clinical biochemistry parameters may assist in determination of systemic effects.

A skin irritation test may be used for devices that interact with the skin whereby the test article (or an extract) is applied directly to the skin (intact or abraded) of the animal model (e.g., rabbit). At 72 h after application, the skin is scored for erythema and edema.

Biomaterials can be carcinogenic. Malignant tumors, including fibrosarcomas and sarcomas, have been described in rat and guinea pig carcinogenicity studies after exposure to metal alloys used in prostheses (Sunderman 1989). In transgenic p53+/− mice, implanted transponders were associated with capsule membrane endothelialization, inflammation, mesenchymal basophilia, dysplasia, and sarcoma (Blanchard et al. 1999). Subcutaneous inflammatory, fibrotic, or neoplastic (mostly sarcomas) lesions have been associated with implanted identification microchips in chronic bioassays in mice and rats (Elcock et al. 2001; Le Calvez et al. 2006; Tillmann et al. 1997).

19.2.3.3 Carcinogenicity

Chronic administration of any drug by either parenteral or topical administration has the potential to induce a carcinogenic response. Therefore, the evaluation of carcinogenic potential must be included in the safety evaluation of drugs intended for chronic use. Carcinogenicity testing is typically conducted by topical administration of the test article (e.g., mouse skin painting tests) to rodents for assessment of both topical and systemic effects (Bibby 1981). Mice and rats are the conventional animal models typically used in carcinogenicity bioassays, although other species, such as hairless mice and rats, hamsters, or transgenic mice, may be used. Conventional mouse strains that are used in carcinogenicity studies include B6C3F1, BALB/c, CD-1, and C3H, whereas transgenic mice have included p53+/−,Tg.AC, and RasH2, and XPA$^{-/-}$ mice. Lynch et al. (2007) specifically reviewed three mouse strains used for dermal carcinogenic hazard identification: SENCAR (SENsitivity to CARcinogenicity), Tg.AC, and RasH2 mice (Tennant et al. 1998). These models make good short-term screening tools for carcinogenicity, but results must be interpreted in light of what is known about the compound and the model, especially where the compound is irritating to the skin. The utility and predictability of these various models for replacement of 2-year carcinogenicity bioassays are still being evaluated. Ideally, they must show positivity for carcinogens, and negativity for noncarcinogens, ideally with no false negatives (Cohen 2001; Jacobson-Kram et al. 2004; Pritchard et al. 2003; Sistare et al. 2002; Storer et al. 2010).

The SENCAR mouse is an outbred strain (not genetically engineered) that was selected specifically for increased skin tumor multiplicity and decreased tumor latency in response to known dermal carcinogens, which has a low incidence of spontaneous cutaneous tumors (Aldaz et al. 1987).

The Tg.AC mouse is "genetically initiated" via a v-Ha-ras coding sequence that is linked to a globulin promoter and a simian virus 40polyA signal sequence; the ras transgene is expressed in induced papillomas, but not in normal skin. Mutation and activation of the ras^{Ha} gene is an early event in keratinocyte transformation leading to development of a benign tumor (Yuspa 1998). Subsequent upregulation of *fos* gene and AP-1 transcriptional activity is associated with malignant conversion of benign tumors (Yuspa 1998). The utility of this model for carcinogenicity testing has been subject to multiple reviews (Cohen 2001; Jacobson-Kram et al. 2004; Pritchard et al. 2003; Sistare et al. 2002). The Tg.AC transgenic mouse model is no longer recommended for carcinogenicity testing of topical agents owing to a high level of false positives associated with cutaneous irritation of test articles. Pigmented rodent strains (e.g., C57BL/6 mice) and metallotheionein-I(MT)/ret transgenic mice may be used for evaluation of melanocytic tumors (Kato et al. 1998).

Methodology used in cutaneous carcinogenicity testing includes application of the test article daily to the shaved area on the back of the animal model for 104 weeks. Multiple dose levels are investigated with the highest dose used being the maximum tolerated dose, a dose that does not produce severe or irreversible lesions (e.g., necrosis) as determined from dose-range finding studies.

Mouse skin has been used extensively in the investigation of multistage carcinogenesis (Argyris 1982; Hecker 1987; Yuspa 1998). In the two-stage model of chemical carcinogenesis, initiation and promotion can be assessed in mouse and rat models (Schweizer et al. 1982). In the promotion assay, initiating agents such as 7,12-dimethylbenz[a]anthracene (DMBA), urethane, benzo(a)pyrene, or UV light are applied to skin. Initiating agents cause DNA damage to keratinocytes, which appear visibly normal but retain the capacity to proliferate unlike terminally differentiated skin cells. The chemical under investigation is then applied repeatedly for several weeks to the initiated skin to assess promotion. Phorbol esters (e.g., 12-O-tetradecanoyl 13-acetate) are commonly used as a positive promoter control. A positive response in this assay is the development of skin papillomas, which may progress to carcinomas. To detect the initiating potential of chemicals, the test article is applied to skin prior to the application of a promoting agent such as phorbol ester. Administration of DMBA and phorbol 12-myristate 13-acetate to SENCAR mice in a multistage model of carcinogenesis produces skin papillomas (Aldaz et al. 1987). Histopathologic and cytogenetic analyses determined a positive correlation between the degree of aneuploidy and the aggressiveness and atypia of the papillomas.

PUVA (psoralen + UVA) therapy is a combination of treatment with 8-methoxypsoralen (8-MOP) and UVA (320–400 nm) radiation intended to treat chronic skin diseases such as psoriasis and vitiligo through a photosensitizing mechanism but has been associated with an increased risk of skin cancer. Gavage administration of 8-MOP followed by UVA irradiation for up to 8 months to C3H/HeN-hr hairless mice caused an erythematous phototoxic reaction and scarring but did not result in tumors (Langner et al. 1977). However, PUVA treatment of HRA/Skh mice resulted in a significant increase in hyperplastic skin lesions and cutaneous SCC (Lambertini et al. 2005). Analysis of skin changes in these mice demonstrated increased protein expression of p53 and PCNA (proliferating cell nuclear antigen) in hyperplastic lesions and SCC and an increased mutation frequency of p53 suppressor gene (but not H-ras gene) in SCC. It is proposed that p53 mutation leads to inactivation of p53 protein and subsequent tumor development (Lambertini et al. 2005).

19.3 MECHANISMS OF DERMATOTOXICITY

19.3.1 TOPICAL DERMATOTOXICITY

Topical application of certain chemicals can damage the surface of the skin and manifests as irritant dermatitis. The degree or severity of cutaneous irritation is influenced by many factors including the type, amount, and strength of the noxious agent, the duration of exposure, and skin susceptibility. Several different mechanisms may be involved in skin damage including direct toxicity (e.g., chemical burns from strong acids or alkalis), immune-mediated reactions (i.e., allergic reactions), phototoxic or photoallergic reactions, and genotoxicity. Direct toxicity that is associated with reversible injury is termed "irritation" while irreversible skin injury (i.e., full-thickness necrosis of the epidermis) is referred to as "corrosion" (INHAND 2012).

19.3.2 SYSTEMIC DERMATOTOXICITY

Systemic dermatotoxicity may be the result of percutaneous absorption of chemicals or their metabolites causing systemic side effects, or primary systemic toxicity can manifest as cutaneous lesions (Merk 2009). Certain compounds may be absorbed to a greater degree through the skin than through the gastrointestinal tract. The degree of lipophilicity and hydrophilicity of a compound will influence its penetration through the stratum corneum and passage through the viable epidermis and dermis, respectively. Hexachlorophene, used to treat staphylococcal infections topically, has been shown to be neurotoxic in animal experiments and, depending on the age of exposure, to be a developmental neurotoxicant. Topical application of corticosteroids to rats causes body weight gain suppression, increases in total cholesterol and triglycerides, atopic lymphatic tissue, and adrenal and renal lesions. While some topically applied chemicals may cause a localized hypersensitivity (e.g., urticaria), other chemicals may cause a more severe anaphylactic type of reaction.

Cutaneous lesions as a manifestation of primary systemic toxicity may be the result of non-immunologic or immunologic reactions, which may manifest as cutaneous responses (Alanko and Hannuksela 1998; Wintroub and Stern 1985).

Non-immunologic causes may include anticancer agents, corticosteroids, drugs that may induce vasoconstriction of the dermal vasculature, photosensitizing drugs, or endocrine disruptors. The responses seen with anticancer drugs include inflammation, ulceration, and, in some cases, epithelial proliferation, the result of toxic effects on epidermal cells or secondary to cytokine release. Prolonged use of corticosteroids is manifested by atrophic effects on the skin and adnexal structures, whereas vasoconstrictive agents may cause overt necrosis as a result of ischemia. Distribution of drugs or metabolites to the skin that are photoreactive may result in a photosensitizing reaction when the affected skin is exposed to sunlight or UV radiation. Certain endocrine disruptors may cause pigmentary changes in the skin by affecting melanogenesis or mineralization as a consequence of an imbalance of calcium homeostasis.

Immunologic reactions in the skin may be secondary to a generalized systemic response (i.e., anaphylactic reaction) or to a reaction with hapten–carrier complexes in the skin, or the result of an idiosyncratic reaction. There are numerous examples of adverse skin reactions to drugs adminis-tered systemically, including penicillin and trimethoprim-sulfamethoxazole.

Idiosyncratic drug reactions (IDRs) are a major concern with the safety of pharmaceuticals that can manifest as severe cutaneous reactions. These are discussed in more detail in Section 19.3.5.

19.3.3 Non-Immunologic Dermatotoxicity

Non-immunologic cutaneous lesions are attributed to direct damage as a result of trauma (e.g., abrasion), chemical burns (e.g., strong acids and alkalis, oxidizing agents) (Figure 19.3b), or exacer-bation of preexisting dermatologic disease (Wintroub and Stern 1985). Skin irritation is more com-mon than chemical burns, and rashes are the most common adverse reactions to drugs (Bigby et al. 1986). Chemicals such as croton oil, SLS, and benzalkonium chloride are known to be skin irritants. The degree of skin irritation is influenced by the type of chemical, rate of penetration and time course of inflammatory response, and nature of the inflammatory process (cellular and vascular reactions). However, the chemical structure may not necessarily correlate with the degree of irrita-tion observed. The pathophysiology of skin irritation is not well understood, and many chemicals may share common effector pathways. Non-immunologic activation of the effector pathway (e.g., interaction with mast cells, activation of complement, alteration of arachidonic metabolism) has been proposed as one possible mechanism (Haschek et al. 2010). In some cases, skin irritation may occur without morphological manifestations. For example, genotoxic agents via DNA alkylation may cause mutations in the proliferative cell population of the epidermis.

19.3.4 Immunologic Dermatotoxicity

Immunologic mechanisms constitute an important and common pathway in cutaneous diseases and for cutaneous reaction to foreign agents (Breathnach and Katz 1986). Immune responses in the skin are associated with a network of signaling pathways of skin-associated lymphoid tissues (SALTs) (Streilein 1989). SALT consists of interactions of Langerhans cells, keratinocytes, skin-seeking T cells, and mast cells (Streilein 1989).

Immunologic reactions may involve humoral or cellular components. Humoral reactions include skin anaphylaxis (type I hypersensitivity reaction mediated via IgE) and immunocomplex reac-tions (type III hypersensitivity reaction mediated via IgG, IgM, complement; Arthus reaction). Cell-mediated immunotoxicity is a delayed-type response (type IV hypersensitivity reactions) often observed 24–96 h after application of the test article or as occurs in graft-versus-host reac-tion (Figure 19.3c). Contact allergic reactions are delayed-type hypersensitivity reactions and involve the capture and metabolism of antigens by keratinocytes and Langerhans cells and the formation of the hapten–protein complexes (Khan et al. 2006). At the same time, keratinocytes or Langerhans cells secrete cytokines (IL-1β, TNFα, IL-18, etc.) important for the migration of Langerhans cells to the local lymph nodes. These Langerhans cells upregulate receptors (CCR7, etc.) important for interaction with these cytokines and their homing to the lymph nodes. In the lymph nodes, Langerhans cells present the antigen to the resident T cells resulting in their activa-tion and proliferation and migration to the skin. Upon re-exposure of the antigen, dermal dendritic cells or keratinocytes present the antigen to the T memory cells in the skin, which then release cytokines (IFN-γ, IL-17, etc.) and recruit macrophages that produce more cytokines and elicit an inflammatory reaction. With lipid-soluble antigens that can cross the cell membrane, intracellular processing and modification lead to their presentation linked to MHC I and elicitation of cyto-toxic T cells and the killing of the eliciting cell. Chemicals such as 2,4-dinitrofluorobenzene and picryl chloride are associated with allergic contact dermatitis. Clinical manifestations of delayed hypersensitivity include exanthemas, erythema multiforme, and Stevens-Johnson syndrome (SJS) or toxic epidermal necrolysis (TEN). Erythema multiforme and TEN represent severe, often life-threatening forms of immune-mediated diseases. Inappropriate activation of cytotoxic CD8+ T cells has been implicated as a cause of these diseases (Haschek et al. 2010). A broad spectrum of drugs has been associated with development of erythema multiforme and TEN, including sulfon-amides, penicillins, cephalosporins, ivermectin, aurothioglucose, griseofulvin, propylthiouracil, D-limonene, anticonvulsant drugs, minoxidil, and nonsteroidal anti-inflammatory drugs (NSAIDs) (Haschek et al. 2010; Karaoui and Chahine-Chakhtoura 2009; Paul et al. 1998).

Sensitization is assessed *in vivo* utilizing guinea pigs and involves both induction and challenge phases (Andersen 1987). Several factors may influence contact sensitization including the antigenic potency of the chemical, vehicle, total dose, surface concentration, size of the skin area of applica-tion, anatomical characteristics of site of application, skin disease (trauma), degree of percutane-ous penetration, draining lymph nodes in the area, number of exposures, and effects of occlusion (Boukhman and Maibach 2001). Delayed hypersensitivity reactions are determined by the second application of test substance to previously sensitized skin. The initial sensitizing application is by either topical or intradermal administration for a period of 3 weeks. The second application (chal-lenge) occurs after a 2-week rest period and the response is evaluated 24–48 h after the second application. A positive response is determined if the irritation after the second application is more severe than the initial application.

Allergic cutaneous drug reactions can be seen in human patients after nontopical (systemic) delivery of a compound, especially antibiotics, blood products, and inhaled mucolytics; the anti-biotics amoxicillin, trimethoprim–sulfamethoxazole, and ampicillin have some of the highest reaction rates (Khan et al. 2006). Drugs that cause cutaneous drug reactions may be low-molecular-weight molecules, but they are believed to undergo bioactivation to reactive metabolites that bind covalently to cellular macromolecules, thus generating haptenated proteins that initiate an immune response. For the cutaneous reaction to occur, the sensitizing molecule must transit to the skin. Bioactivation can occur in the liver, or in the systemic circulation with subsequent delivery to the skin, or bioactivation may occur in the skin itself (Khan et al. 2006). Although these drugs have the potential for these reactions, the vast majority of patients receiving the drugs do not develop cutaneous drug reactions (< 1%, and 1:100,000–1:1,000,000 for severe reactions). Therefore, other factors are also involved such as genetic predisposition and environmental factors, particularly viral infections (Khan et al. 2006). Clinical presentations of other forms of hypersensitivity include type I reactions with presentations ranging from urticaria, angioedema, to anaphylactic shock. Immune complex reactions or type III hypersensitivity are usually seen in the skin as vasculitis and purpura.

Drug-induced cutaneous immune reactions must be differentiated from autoimmune skin dis-eases such as pemphigus vulgaris, pemphigus foliaceous, pemphigus vegetans, bullous pemphigoid, pemphigoid erythematosus, systemic lupus erythematosus, and discoid lupus erythematosus (all of which have been reported to occur in dogs) (Parker 1981). For instance, pemphigus-like reactions have been associated with sulfhydryl groups containing drugs, with captopril or D-penicillamine, while lupus erythematosus–like syndrome was observed in patients treated with isoniazid, hydrala-zine, or procaine, with a role for autoantibodies against histones demonstrated in several cases (Merk et al. 2001).

19.3.5 IDIOSYNCRATIC DRUG REACTIONS

IDRs are considered type B adverse drug reactions in that they are unpredictable and are not related to the known pharmacologic properties of the drug. Clinically, IDRs are relatively uncom-mon (6%–10% of all adverse drug reactions) but are of considerable concern because of their unpredictability and the serious nature of the adverse reaction, which can result in death. IDRs may manifest in systemic disease (e.g., hepatotoxicity, hemolytic anemia, agranulocytosis) and sometimes in severe cutaneous manifestations (e.g., erythema multiforme, TEN, or SJS). IDRs share many clinical and pathological attributes with other diseases, which may preclude diagnosis on the findings alone. Most IDR-induced skin rashes cannot be readily differentiated from other skin disorders unless they present specific diagnostic features pathognomonic for IDRs, as described for fixed drug reactions and TEN.

The mechanisms involved in IDRs are uncertain but have been generally classified as either non-immune or immune mediated. Several mechanistic hypotheses have been proposed for the development of IDRs. In the hapten hypothesis, the drug and its reactive metabolite are not immunogenic themselves but may become immunogenic when covalently bound to endogenous protein. The reactive metabolite hypothesis proposes that reactive metabolites may act as haptens when detoxification systems (e.g., glutathione) are overwhelmed or depleted. The characteristic delay in onset of adverse reactions after initiation of drug administration and the reduced delay after rechallenge favor an immune-mediated mechanism for most IDRs. There is circumstantial evidence that metabolites play a key role in both non-immune and immune-mediated IDRs. Since most drugs do not bind covalently to proteins, metabolism of a drug is considered critical to hapten formation. There is a strong correlation between the formation of certain types of reactive metabolites and the risk of developing an idiosyncratic reaction with several examples including sulfonamides, isoniazid, and halothane. Drugs that possess sulfhydryl, arylamine, or other readily oxidizable moieties are especially susceptible to forming reactive metabolites after oxidation of the parent molecule.

IDRs have been reported in animals (e.g., sulfonamide toxicity in dogs); however, similar to humans, the unpredictable nature of IDRs has hampered the development of animal models. Nevertheless, animal models still are considered the best approach for understanding the mechanisms involved in IDRs. Two animal models under investigation, sulfonamide-induced hypersensitivity in dogs and nevirapine-induced skin rash in rats, are of particular interest with respect to drug-induced skin IDRs (Funk-Keenan et al. 2012; Lavergne et al. 2006; Ng et al. 2012; Uetrecht 2006).

19.3.5.1 Sulfonamide

In humans, sulfonamide hypersensitivity is a well-recognized phenomenon characterized by fever, dermatopathy (i.e., rash), lymphadenopathy, and, occasionally, eosinophilia, agranulocytosis, thrombocytopenia, or aplastic anemia (Cribb et al. 1996). Sulfonamide hypersensitivity has also been reported in various dog breeds, manifested by cutaneous drug eruptions, as well as hepatotoxicity, polyarthritis, fever, and blood dyscrasias. In dogs, the onset of clinical signs may range from 5 to 36 days after initiation of treatment and has a more rapid onset upon rechallenge, consistent with an immune-mediated mechanism (Cribb 1989; Trepanier et al. 2003). The occurrence of antidrug, anti-myeloperoxidase, and anti-cathepsin G antibodies in sulfonamide-induced hypersensitivity in dogs lends further support to an immune-mediated reaction (Lavergne et al. 2006). It is believed that the immune response is initiated by the metabolism of sulfonamide to hydroxylamines, which, upon further oxidation to nitroso derivatives, may form protein adducts that trigger an antibody or cell-mediated immune response (Lavergne et al. 2008).

19.3.5.2 Nevirapine

Nevirapine is a non-nucleoside reverse transcriptase inhibitor that has been used for the treatment of human immunodeficiency virus 1 infections (Popovic et al. 2010). Its use clinically has been associated with a high incidence of skin rash and hepatotoxicity. Clinically, the incidence of skin rash has been reported to range from 17% to 48% depending on the dosing regimen, and up to 0.3% of rashes have been considered severe (i.e., SJS, SJS/TEN transition syndrome, and a syndrome of drug reaction with eosinophilia and systemic symptoms). Skin rash has been reported to occur in patients within 6 weeks of initiation of nevirapine administration (Pollard et al. 1998). In rats, the incidence and severity of nevirapine-induced skin rash is strain and gender related (Uetrecht 2006). Skin rash has been observed in Brown Norway rats and Sprague–Dawley rats given nevirapine, but Lewis rats appear to be resistant. This finding not only supports the idiosyncratic nature of the skin reaction in rats but also suggests that genetic factors are involved. Nevirapine-induced skin rash occurs with a higher incidence in female Brown Norway rats than in males at the same dose, which is considered to be related to the more rapid metabolism of nevirapine in male rats compared to female rats. The onset of skin lesions is observed 2–3 weeks after initiation of treatment, with reappearance of skin rash earlier and more severe after rechallenge (Popovic et al. 2006). The skin lesions in rats are characterized histopathologically by an inflammatory infiltrate of predominantly CD4+ and CD8+ T lymphocytes and macrophages (Shenton et al. 2003). Mechanistic investigations have demonstrated that depletion of CD4+ T cells, but not CD8+ T cells, was partially protective (Shenton et al. 2005). Furthermore, it was shown that sensitivity could be transferred from sensitized rats to naïve rats via CD4+ T cells but not CD8+ T cells.

Additionally, tolerance could be induced in Brown Norway rats if low doses of nevirapine were given to rats prior to higher doses known to induce rash. It has been determined that the development of skin rash is related to the 12-hydroxylation of nevirapine, rather than the parent drug (Popovic et al. 2010). It has been postulated that the 12-hydroxy metabolite is converted to a reactive quinone methide metabolite by sulfation, and since sulfotransferases are present in the skin, this provides a plausible explanation for the development of nevirapine-induced skin rashes. Initiation of the immune response may be triggered by these metabolites and it is thought that a similar mechanism occurs in humans that develop nevirapine-induced skin rash.

19.3.6 Phototoxicity

Numerous topically and systemically administered drugs of many different classes, including NSAIDs, antimicrobials, anticonvulsants, antihypertensive agents, and diuretics, have been associated with photosensitization in humans and animals. Some examples of photosensitizing drugs are phenothiazine, tetracyclines, sulfonamides, chlorpromazine, nalidixic acid, and fluorocoumarins (psoralens). Some compounds have been developed specifically for their photosensitizing properties for use in photodynamic therapy. For example, methyl aminolevulinate hydrochloride is cytotoxic to precancerous and cancer cells upon activation by appropriate wavelength light (Health Canada 2009).

Photosensitization may involve either non-immune (i.e., photoirritation) or immune-mediated (i.e., photoallergy) mechanisms. Photoallergic reactions have been associated with administration of sulfonamides, phenothiazides, coumarin derivatives, and glyceryl *p*-aminobenzoic acid.

The targets for the photochemical reaction are the chromophores in the drug product or the DNA of skin cells. The cutaneous response observed, which is triggered by photoactivation of the parent drug or metabolite upon exposure to sunlight or UV irradiation, has a histopathologic response similar to that seen with other skin toxicities. Cutaneous photoirritation reactions are similar in character to primary irritation reactions. Photoirritation reactions may occur after a single exposure whereas photoallergic reactions require a period of induction for a reaction to occur. Acute photoirritation may manifest as mild erythema (resembling sunburn) or, in more severe cases, as blistered skin with skin sloughing. Phototoxic lesions were induced in albino Balb/c mice by oral administration of quinolone antibacterial agents followed by UVA irradiation (Shimoda et al. 1993). Auricular lesions in mice were characterized by degeneration of epidermal cells, dermal edema, neutrophilic infiltration, and degenerated fibroblasts that became progressively more severe with time. Photoallergic reactions are immune mediated and most often idiosyncratic. It should be noted that compounds causing photoirritancy may also be associated with photoallergenic reactions. Examples include benzocaine, *p*-aminobenzoic acid, and promethazine (Johnson and Grimwood 1994).

Some photoirritants have been associated with UV-induced skin carcinogenesis (e.g., 8-MOP). Treatment of psoriasis by photochemotherapy (PUVA) with oral methoxsalen, a psoralen, in conjunction with UVA radiation, is associated with an increased risk of irregular pigmented skin lesions, SCC, and malignant melanoma (Stern et al. 1997). Other compounds may enhance UV-associated carcinogenesis by indirect mechanisms by decreasing the protective properties of the skin through alteration of the optical or structural features or biological functions of the skin.

19.3.6.1 Fluoroquinolones

Toxicity of the quinolone class of antibacterial agents manifested as adverse effects on the central nervous system, peripheral nervous system, and cardiovascular, gastrointestinal, and musculoskeletal systems, and phototoxicity in particular is well established in humans and animals. Fluoroquinolones are potent photosensitizing agents attributed to halogenation at the C8 position on the molecule. In addition to causing initial phototoxicity reactions, fluoroquinolones may also sensitize an individual to subsequent photoallergic reactions. Severe skin rashes with fluoroquinolones are also attributed to hypersensitivity reactions. While most quinolone-associated phototoxic reactions are mild and self-limiting, serious life-threatening photosensitizing reactions, including SJS, TEN, and Sweet's syndrome, have been reported with fluoroquinolones. Fluoroquinolone phototoxicity is characterized by cutaneous erythema (similar to sunburn), edema, painful blistering, and sloughing of skin. Phototoxic and photoallergic reactions of quinolones have been investigated in guinea pigs and mice. The morphological changes observed in the auricular skin of Balb/c mice administered quinolones orally, followed by UVA irradiation, included degeneration of basal cells in the epidermis, dermal edema, degeneration of dermal fibroblasts (with dense, irregularly shaped nuclei and eosinophilic granules), and neutrophilic infiltration in the dermis (Shimoda et al. 1993).

Chronically administered photosensitizing quinolones have been associated with an increased risk of development of skin tumors (Stern 1998). Prolonged oral administration of fluoroquinolones in combination with UVA irradiation to Skh hairless mice caused an increased incidence of benign skin tumors compared to mice exposed to UVA irradiation alone (Makinen et al. 1997). Neoplastic progression from solar keratosis (characterized by cellular atypia, nuclear enlargement, and hyperchromasia), keratoacanthoma, and benign papillomas to SCCs was observed.

19.4 BIOMARKERS OF DERMATOTOXICITY

A biomarker is a measurable characteristic that is an indicator of normal biologic processes, pathogenic processes, or biological responses to a xenobiotic. Biomarkers can include structural features (molecular to gross), biochemical measurements, or organ system functional tests (Draft Guidance for Industry; Use of Histology in Biomarker Qualification Studies Dec. 2011; www.fda.gov/Drugs/GuidanceComplianceRegulatoryInformation/Guidances). Ideally, biomarkers will be highly sensitive (no false negatives) and specific (no false positives) to the process or tissue being studied, will have measurable changes that are proportional to the extent of injury and coincide with onset or progression of the process, and will translate across multiple species; any sampling will be minimally invasive, and the sampling procedure will be rapid, simple, and inexpensive. Realistically, at this time, many biomarkers are neither sensitive nor specific, but this is a rapidly expanding field with ongoing discovery and characterization of novel biomarkers. Any biomarker data must be interpreted in context with the entirety of the data available.

Since the skin is readily available for sampling or examination, it can serve as a portal to test for internal disease or local cutaneous disease, and some new techniques such as micropatch microneedle devices (information on Internet) are being developed to sample the skin for biomarkers or for drug delivery. Biomarkers of specific skin diseases, as with other organ diseases, are also being developed, which can be detected in systemic samples such as blood or urine (Paczesny et al. 2010). Structural biomarkers in skin that indicate various disease processes can be detected.

Cytochemical techniques have been used for determining enzyme activity in inflammatory lesions in skin. Increased lysosomal enzyme activity has been demonstrated in association with macrophages and giant cells, whereas succinic and lactate dehydrogenase enzyme activities may be inhibited by more toxic chemicals (Greaves 2000). A variety of antibodies have been developed to aid in the characterization of intermediate filaments, including vimentin, desmin, glial fibrillary acidic protein, neurofilament polypeptide, and human keratin polypeptides (Virtanen et al. 1981). Although there are currently no qualified biomarkers of endothelial cell activation, von Willebrand factor propeptide, E-selectin, asymmetric dimethyl arginine, and circulating endothelial cells are considered specific for activated endothelial cells in assessments of drug-induced vascular injury (Zhang et al. 2010). Lectins may also serve as markers for endothelial cells and monkeys have the greatest histochemical similarity with humans, followed by pig and cattle, then cats, dogs, and sheep (Roussel and Dalion 1988). The DOPA reaction may be reduced in the affected areas with chemicals that cause hypopigmentation (Greaves 2000). Analysis of skin residues can serve as a biomarker for exposure to insecticides (e.g., Aldicarb) (Anwar 1997).

In vitro techniques have been developed as an alternative to whole animal experimentation for assessing potential irritancy of chemicals, as described previously, and can be used to generate biomarker data.

More recently, transcriptomics and proteomics have been used to assess mRNA and protein expression of human keratinocytes exposed to chemicals (Rogers et al. 2009). When exposed to SLS, human keratinocytes showed altered expression of 20 proteins, including downregulation of small heat shock protein 27 (HSP27) and superoxide dismutase (Cu–Zn), and upregulation of cofilin-1. The most significant alteration in both protein and mRNA levels was noted for HSP27 and was accompanied by nuclear translocation. Similar results were obtained after exposure of keratinocyte to other acidic and basic chemicals. IL-1 production was also increased in keratinocytes by irritation. Thus, these proteins may be useful biomarkers for skin hazard assessment and may lead to a better understanding of mechanistic pathways in skin irritation.

Plucked human hair follicles have been used as surrogates for tumor tissue to which immuno-histochemical biomarkers, including Ki67, EGFR, phosphor-p27, phosphor-histone H3, phosphor-MAPK, and phosphor-Rb, have been used to assess the pharmacodynamic effects of drugs (Randall and Foster 2007).

19.5   NON-NEOPLASTIC SKIN CHANGES

19.5.1   Pathologic Findings in Dermatotoxicity

19.5.1.1   Epidermis

19.5.1.1.1   Clinical Manifestations

The external position of skin on the body lends itself to clinical evaluation more readily than internal organs. Changes from the normal appearance of skin can be easily visualized and morphologically described. Although the etiopathogenesis of skin lesions may be difficult to establish from clinical observation, the character, severity, and extent may serve to determine a differential diagnosis and possibly be of prognostic value. An initial adverse effect in the skin may be a color change manifested as pallor, blanching, erythema (redness), hypopigmentation, or hyperpigmentation. Effects on adnexal structures may be present as hypertrichosis, hypotrichosis, alopecia, oily skin, or dry skin. More severe skin lesions may present as macules, papules, plaques, nodules, wheals (urticaria), vesicles, bullae, erosions, ulcers, pustules, cysts, atrophy, scars, sclerosis, scaling, crusts, fissures, or gangrene.

19.5.1.1.2   Clinical Pathology

Changes in clinical pathology parameters associated with skin lesions may be reflected in alterations in hematology parameters, such as increased white blood cell counts and neutrophilia in an acute (non-immunologic) inflammatory response. Immunologic skin reactions are often accompanied by changes in lymphocyte subsets and immunoglobulin levels, depending on the type of immune reaction. In atopic dermatitis (type I hypersensitivity reaction), the anaphylactic response is mediated by increased IgE levels, which instigate degranulation of mast cells and basophils with subsequent release of histamine, serotonin, and other mediators of acute inflammation. The Arthus reaction in skin (type III hypersensitivity reaction) is also an antibody-mediated response involving complement-fixing IgG and IgM. In this reaction, antigen and antibody form complexes that precipitate in the bloodstream and become lodged in the microvasculature where they trigger complement activation and consequent release of cytokines, chemokines, and vasoactive factors. In delayed-type reactions (type IV hypersensitivity reaction), small-molecule antigens bound to carrier proteins interact with antigen-presenting cells (e.g., Langerhans cells), which present the modified antigen to T lymphocytes. This reaction is manifested by increased lymphocyte counts. Erythema multiforme and TEN are associated with increased levels of cytotoxic (CD8+) T cells against keratinocytes. The severe cutaneous lesions of TEN are also associated with increased levels of TNF and IL-6.

19.5.1.1.3 Gross Pathology

Gross pathologic findings in most cases are similar to clinical observations. Color changes in the skin may be the result of effects on cutaneous vasculature such as erythema in acute irritation or after inflammatory episodes, may be due to pigmentary changes from local effects on melanin, or may be secondary to systemic effects as may occur with jaundice. The basic skin lesions include macules, papules, plaques, nodules, wheals, vesicles, bullae, erosions, ulcers, pustules, cysts, atrophy, excoriations, fissures, scars, sclerosis, scaling, crusts, or gangrene (Table 19.6).

TABLE 19.6
Basic Macroscopic Skin Lesions

Gross Change	Definition
Macule	Flat, well-delineated hypo- or hyperpigmented lesion. Change in color owing to vascular disturbance, capillary dilation, or infarction
Papule	Small solid skin elevation < 1 cm
Plaque	Elevated lesion often formed by the confluence of papules
Nodule	Raised, solid lesion that is characterized by its palpability and depth of skin involvement (i.e., epidermal, epidermal–dermal, dermal, dermal–subdermal, and subcutaneous)
Wheal	Flattened papule or plaque of variable size (3–4 mm to 10–12 cm) that has sharp borders
Vesicle	Elevated, well-delineated lesion of <0.5 cm diameter with a thin, often translucent wall that contains fluid (e.g., serum, lymph, blood, or extracellular fluid)
Bulla	Morphologically similar to a vesicle but is >0.5 cm
Erosion	Circumscribed, moist lesion that is usually depressed from the surface of the skin owing to the loss of a portion of the epidermis
Ulceration	Deep destruction of the epidermis and penetration into the papillary dermis
Pustule	Well-delineated lesion that contains a purulent exudate composed of leukocytes, cellular debris, and the presence or absence (sterile) of bacteria
Cyst	Sac-like oval or spherical nodule or papule that contains fluid or cellular material
Atrophy	Thinning of the skin affecting both the epidermis and dermis
Excoriation	Superficial loss of epidermis that may be linear or punctuate in appearance, typically the result of an abrasion
Fissure	Linear crack in the skin, often located on the hands or feet as a result of excessive drying
Scar	Result of healing of a wound or ulcer. May be hypertrophic, atrophic, or sclerotic (sclerosis)
Crust	Composed of dried blood, serum, or purulent exudates. Variable thickness and color
Gangrene	Well-demarcated, blue–black discoloration of the skin, often the result of bacterial infection with vascular occlusion and subsequent necrosis and sloughing

19.5.1.1.4   Histopathology

For current specific descriptions of histopathologic terms in rodents, the reader is referred to the ongoing effort of the INHAND working group (INHAND 2012). Histopathologic changes in the epidermis are often a reflection of disturbances of cell kinetics, cell differentiation, or cell coherence. In normal skin, there is a homeostatic balance between proliferation, differentiation, and desquamation. Conditions that alter the balance in favor of proliferation lead to a thickening of the epidermis (i.e., acanthosis), while a decrease in proliferation rate (e.g., due to corticosteroids) results in a thinning of the epidermis (i.e., atrophy). In atrophy, the thickness of all non-keratinized layers is reduced and there are fewer nucleated epidermal cells accompanied by a loss of distinction of the nucleated strata (INHAND 2012). With acanthosis, there are multiple architectural changes in the epidermis including hyperkeratosis or orthohyperkeratosis of the stratum corneum, increased numbers of mitotic figures in the germinative layer, and elongation of the rete ridges with a consequent increase in the surface area of the epidermal–dermal interface. Incomplete differentiation and maturation of epidermal cells may lead to parakeratosis characterized by retention of pyknotic nuclei in multiple, loose layers of the stratum corneum and a thinning of the granular cell layer. Premature cornification of individual cells results in dyskeratosis, which is often associated with acantholysis and is indicative of irreversible epidermal injury. Since keratinocytes follow an organized process of programmed cell death in keratinization, differentiation from apoptosis can be difficult, and the term dyskeratosis is used to describe apoptotic keratinocytes (INHAND 2012). Dyskeratotic cells are characterized by large, round cells containing abundant eosinophilic cytoplasm (packed with keratin filaments) and pyknotic nuclei. Single-cell necrosis is described in spontaneous conditions such as erythema multiforme (INHAND 2012).

Loss of epidermal coherence from dissociation of desmosomes (acantholysis) and loss of intercellular substance can lead to fluid accumulation in the epidermis. Fluid may be derived from the dermis (i.e., serous exudate) or the result of leukocyte infiltration of the epidermis. The simplest form of intercellular fluid accumulation is termed spongiosis in which epidermal cells still remain in contact with each other but the epidermis takes on a sponge-like appearance. With progressive fluid accumulation, cell contact is broken, individual cells lyse, and fluid collects in a cavity or vesicle (Figure 19.3d). Enlargement of the vesicle or confluence of several vesicles can result in a blister or bulla formation. Epicutaneous administration of hexane, toluene, carbon tetrachloride, and 2-chloroethanol can cause nuclear pyknosis, spongiosis (toluene and carbon tetrachloride), and separation of the junction between the basal cells and the basement membrane (Kronevi et al. 1979).

Loss of the superficial epidermal cell layers from trauma or abrasion is termed erosion. Extension of epidermal loss involving the entire thickness of the epidermis as well as the superficial dermis is termed ulceration (Figure 19.4a). Chemical substances that are irritating or corrosive (e.g., strong acids or alkalis) can cause degeneration and necrosis leading to erosion or ulceration, depending on the severity of the insult to the skin. Repair of erosions occurs by proliferation of epidermal cells from the edges of the lesion and extension (i.e., "creeping") over the affected area. Ulcers initially heal by formation of granulation tissue, which precedes epidermal proliferation to cover the wound. Acute inflammation of the epidermis may be a secondary outcome of trauma, infection, direct cytotoxicity, or an immune reaction. Histopathologically, acute inflammation is characterized by infiltration of neutrophils that may be diffuse or that accumulate in pockets forming microabscesses or pustules. Pustules containing rounded, nucleated keratinocytes, such as observed in pemphigus-type diseases, are termed "acantholytic pustules" (INHAND 2012). Chronic inflammation may be the result of non-immunologic or immunologic mechanisms and is characterized by a predominance of lymphocytic and histiocytic cell types.

Hyperplastic changes of the epidermis may be due to numerous causes, including response to chronic irritation or stimulation from growth factors (e.g., EGF, somatotropin) (Figure 19.4b and c). Administration of urinary human EGF to cynomolgus monkeys for 4 weeks resulted in cutaneous desquamation and epidermal hyperplasia (Maraschin et al. 1995). Topical application of

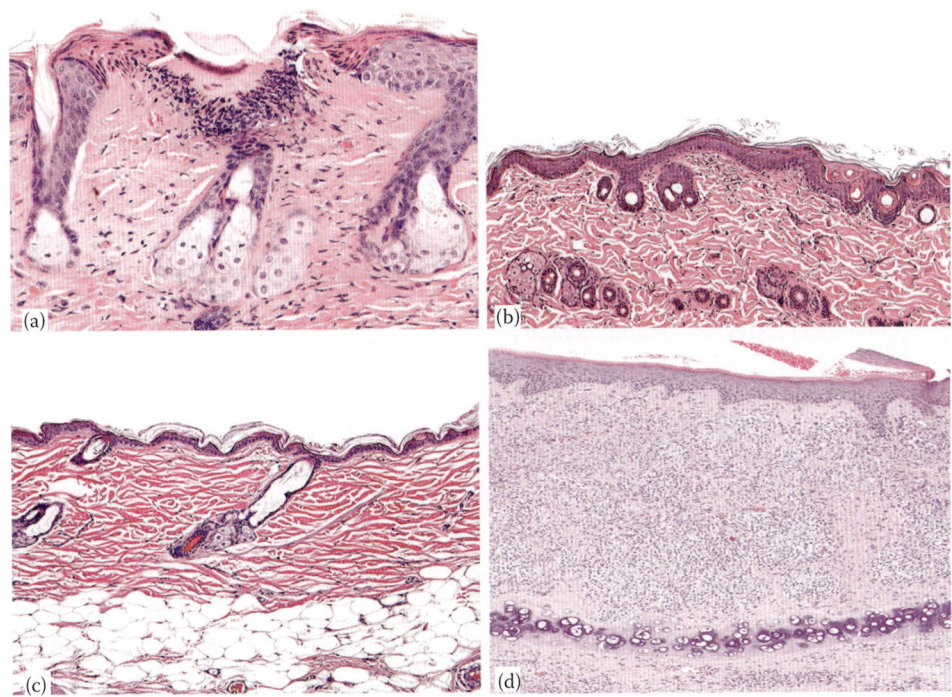

FIGURE 19.4   (a) Focal ulceration in the skin of a mouse with transmural epidermal necrosis and superficial dermal involvement. (b and c) Epidermal hyperplasia (b) characterized by moderate thickening of the epidermis and hyperkeratosis compared to normal mouse skin (c). (d) Granulomatous inflammation in the ear of a nonhuman primate. A dense, mixed mononuclear cell infiltrate consisting largely of macrophages with associated fibrosis present between the overlying epidermis and the deeper auricular cartilage.

hydrocarbon constituents of JP-8 jet fuel to pig skin caused erythema and an increase in epidermal thickness and the number of cell layers (Muhammad et al. 2005).

Epidermal inclusion cysts are a common, spontaneous, nonneoplastic lesion reported in aged F344 rats and Osborne–Mendel rats (Goodman et al. 1979, 1980). Squamous cysts occur in the upper dermis, characterized by a wall consisting of stratified keratinizing epithelium and a cavity filled with concentrically arranged lamellar keratin (INHAND 2012).

19.5.1.2 Dermis

19.5.1.2.1   Histopathology

The dermis forms the supporting structure of the epidermis and consists of a network of collagen and elastic fibers integrated into an ECM, resident histiocytes, and supported by a vasculature that projects upward to the superficial dermis. The vascular network of the skin is a key component of dermal lesions, providing a conduit for inflammatory cells to the area, but also serving as a target tissue. Acute inflammation of the dermis is characterized by an inflammatory infiltrate consisting of polymorphonuclear leukocytes, lymphocytes, fibroblasts, and histiocytes; vascular dilation; accumulation of red blood cells in capillaries; and edema. Depending on the severity, these changes correlate to clinical manifestations of erythema, urticaria, wheals, and papules. In type I hypersensitivity reactions after release of cellular mediators from the IgE-activated mast cells, vasodilation and edema are the prominent features with fewer leukocytes and histiocytes being involved.

Cutaneous necrotizing vasculitis may affect blood vessels of all sizes and occur in all areas of the dermis. It is characterized by a neutrophilic infiltrate and deposition of fibrillar and amorphous material in the wall of affected blood vessels. As necrosis of the vessel wall and leukocytolysis progress, cellular and nuclear debris are observed in the vessel wall and red blood cells may be found in the perivascular tissue (i.e., perivascular hemorrhage). The later appearance of lymphocytes and histiocytic cells is indicative of a repair process.

Lymphocytic infiltrates are a component of most inflammatory conditions in the skin but, in some instances, may be the predominant cell type. Perivascular infiltrates in the superficial dermis may extend to involve the overlying epidermis. Lymphoid cuffing of venules in the dermis may occur in drug eruptions and is associated with dermal edema, but with minimal involvement of the epidermal–dermal interface. Accumulation of atypical lymphocytes in the dermis is indicative of a neoplastic process.

The predominant cell type in granulomatous inflammation is the histiocyte (Figure 19.4d). A granuloma is an aggregation of histiocytic cells and may include multinucleated giant cells. Granulomas can be very destructive lesions leading to atrophy, fibrosis, and scarring. Granulomatous inflammation can result from systemic administration such as with the thromboxane receptor antagonist ICI 185,282 in dogs or intradermal administration of Hylan, a modified hyaluronan, in guinea pigs (Sasaki et al. 2003; Westwood et al. 1995).

Lesions in the dermis may also affect the reticular fibers and ECM. Dense packing and homogenization of collagen bundles, with concomitant loss of elastic fibers, are key features of scleroderma. Subcutaneous administration of porcine growth hormone to beagle dogs caused a dose-related increased thickness of dermal collagen manifested as large skin folds on the forehead and face and was considered a pharmacologic effect (Prahalada et al. 1998). Solar elastosis is the result of sun damage to skin (Knowles and Hargis 1986) or may be induced in rats by chronic exposure to UV irradiation (Berger et al. 1980; Fisher et al. 2002; Nakamura and Johnson 1968; Tsukahara et al. 2012). It is characterized by aggregates of thick, basophilic elastic fibers in the superficial dermis. Elastosis may also be chemically induced by penicillamine (used to treat Wilson's disease) characterized by increased amounts of soluble collagen, alterations of elastic fibers, and protrusions that establish themselves perpendicular to the long axis of elastic fibers (Smith 1994). Amyloid deposits, characterized by pale eosinophilic material that has apple-green dichroism when stained with Congo red and viewed under polarizing light, may be found anywhere in the dermis and are often associated with systemic amyloidosis (Faccini et al. 1990).

19.5.1.3 Subcutis

19.5.1.3.1 Histopathology

Inflammatory changes may also be observed in the subcutis and typically involve fat cells or the vasculature. Subcutaneous injection of saline into the dorsal skin of Sprague–Dawley rats did not significantly affect histomorphology at the injection site (Wells et al. 2010). Although spontaneous acellular intimal thickening was observed in untreated males and females, an increased incidence of intimal hyperplasia was observed in males only, suggesting an increased sensitivity of male rats to saline injection or physical trauma at the injection site. Degeneration and fat necrosis from various causes (e.g., trauma, injection, perivascular inflammation) lead to the liberation of fatty acids, which are strong stimuli for attracting inflammatory cells such as neutrophils and macrophages, resulting in steatitis. Sequential infections with unrelated viruses (lymphocytic choriomeningitis virus and vaccinia virus) have been associated with extensive necrosis of pelvic, mesenteric, and perirenal fat in C3H/St male mice (Yang et al. 1985). The delayed-type hypersensitivity reaction observed supports the use of this animal model for Weber–Christian disease in which inflammatory nodules are observed in the subcutaneous fat. Phagocytosis of degenerate fat can lead to formation of lipogranulomas. Subcutaneous injection of olive oil, a solubilizing agent for lipophilic compounds, in Sprague–Dawley rats resulted in lipogranuloma formation at the injection site (Ramot et al. 2009).

Mineralization may occur secondary to inflammation in the subcutis or may be associated with high dietary levels of calcium. Dihydrotachysterol causes mineralization of subcutaneous tissues by a mechanism involving mobilization of calcium stores.

Certain chemicals can have a direct effect on subcutaneous fat. Recombinant human leptin produces atrophy of both white and brown fat in C57BL/6 mice (Sarmiento et al. 1997), whereas troglitazone increases brown fat but decreases white fat in mice (Breider et al. 1999). Cynomolgus monkeys administered recombinant human IL-3 develop extramedullary hematopoeisis at the injection site in the subcutis (Khan et al. 1996).

19.5.1.4 Adnexa

19.5.1.4.1 Histopathology

Hair, scales, feathers, nails, claws, and horns are all derived from skin and thus have a similar response to toxic agents as epidermis. Hair follicles may respond to a toxicant with loss (hypotrichosis, alopecia), proliferation (hypertrichosis), or a color change. Depilatory agents, such as eflornithine HCl (Vaniqa™), have been developed as treatments for excessive hair (Hickman et al. 2001). In toxic alopecia, the effect on the hair follicle will depend on the stage of hair growth (i.e., anagen, telogen, or catagen). At the anagen stage, chemical toxicity is the result of inhibition of mitotic activity of proliferating cells in the hair bulb. The effect on hair with this type of toxicity is manifested within days or weeks and may occur with colchicine (antigout agent) or chemotherapeutic agents (e.g., doxorubicin) (Figure 19.5a). The telogen phase toxicity occurs by different mechanisms and may appear over a period of several months. For example, chronic exposure to the heavy metal thallium (previously used in rodenticides) causes alopecia, ulceration, and hyperkeratosis and parakeratosis of skin and hair epithelia through a mechanism of inhibition of cysteine incorporation into keratin and interference with energy production in hair bulb cells, resulting in premature telogen and consequent hair shedding (Cavanagh and Gregson 1978). Other toxicants that cause alopecia from chronic exposure by a similar mechanism include copper, mercury, cadmium, and arsenic (Haschek et al. 2010; Pierard 1979). The list of toxic chemicals that may cause alopecia is quite extensive, including retinoids, interferons, lithium, heparin, coumarins, β-adrenergic blockers, androgens, progesterone–estrogen combination, cytotoxic drugs (e.g., acyclovir), bromocriptine, selenium, mimosine, iodine, propanolol, triparanol, phenylglycidyl ether, and dixyrazine (Haschek et al. 2010; Moore et al. 1983). Administration of a progesterone–estrogen combination (i.e., quingestanol acetate and quinesterol) to female Wistar rats caused hair loss, which did not recover during the 30-week observation period after cessation of treatment (Lumb et al. 1985). A suppurative to pyogranulomatous infundibular folliculitis has been described in rats after oral administration of canertinib, an irreversible inhibitor of the EGF receptor (Brown et al. 2008). Methoxychlor and its metabolites (mono-OH methoxychlor and bis-OH methoxychlor) inhibit growth and induce atresia of antral follicles in rodents and baboons (Gupta et al. 2007).

In determining the relationship of alopecia to drug exposure, other causes of hair loss such as infectious disease, excessive grooming, systemic disease, or hormonal imbalance as occurs in hyperadrenocorticism (Cushing's disease) (Figure 19.5b) must be ruled out (Militzer and Wecker 1986). The cause of alopecia areata has not been fully elucidated but is believed to involve a disturbance of the immune system (i.e., autoimmunity), genetic factors (i.e., HLA class II), and, possibly, psychogenic (i.e., stress) and environmental factors (McDonagh and Messenger 1994, 1996). The C3H/HeJ strain of mice is a spontaneous model of human alopecia areata and develops circumscribed hair loss associated with nonscarring inflammation of dystrophic anagen hair follicles (Carroll et al. 2002; McDonagh and Messenger 1994; McElwee et al. 2003a). In this mouse model, gene array profiling and immunomodulation studies confirmed the role of CD4+- and CD8+-expressing cells in the cell-mediated immune response involved in the pathogenesis of alopecia areata. Up to 70% of Dundee Experimental Bald Rats (DEBR) develop a nonscarring, inflammatory hair loss similar to human alopecia, which is believed to have an autoimmune pathogenesis (McElwee et al. 2003a).

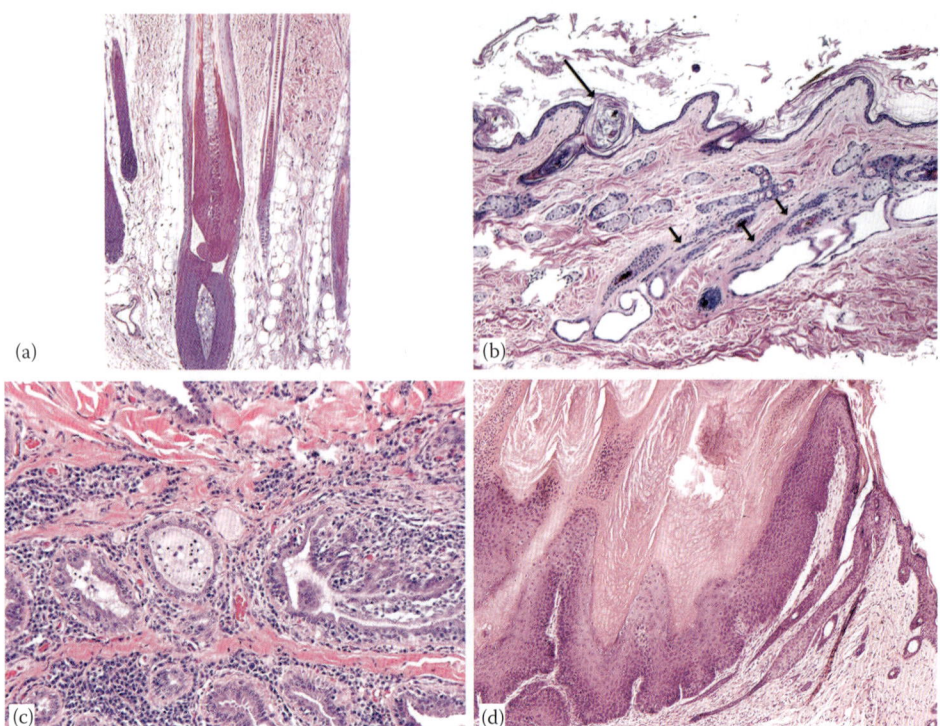

FIGURE 19.5   (a) An example of anagen defluxion in the skin of a rat after doxorubicin administration. The follicle is in anagen (the active growth phase of the hair cycle), but there is a "pinching" of the follicle just above the bulb owing to a transient decrease in mitotic activity that affected the formation of the hair shaft while the follicle remained in anagen. (b) Alopecia associated with hyperadrenocorticism in a dog. There is profound follicular atrophy in which infundibula are largely devoid of hair shafts (long arrow) and hair follicles are no more than cords of epithelial cells (short arrows). (c) Hidradenitis in a dog. Note the dilation of apocrine glands, some of which contain abundant luminal secretion intermixed with inflammatory cells. There is also periglandular inflammation composed primarily of plasma cells. (d) Keratoacanthoma, a benign tumor of follicular epithelium that is well delineated, with a "cup-shaped" cavity containing abundant compact keratin (B6C3F1 mouse).

Administration of the nucleoside analog BW 134U to beagle dogs resulted in loss of nails and footpad erosions associated with radiomimetic defects in the stratum germinativum (Szczech and Tucker 1985). Similarly, chronic oral administration of the nucleoside analog acyclovir to Beagle dogs for 1 year caused erosion of the footpads, cracking, splitting, and loosening of nails, although healing of the footpads and nail regeneration occurred during the course of the study and all footpads and nails were normal at study termination (Tucker at al. 1983).

Several chemicals may cause increased hair growth. Excessive hair growth in areas other than those governed by androgens is termed hypertrichosis, whereas excessive growth of coarse hair in females is called hirsutism. Cyclosporin A, which causes hypertrichosis of the face and back of human transplant patients, produces a similar effect in nude mice by a postulated mechanism of induction of abnormal keratinization of hair follicles (Greaves 2000). Hirsutism has been associated with increased prolactin levels.

Chloracne is a severe form of acne in humans caused by exposure to halogenated aromatic hydrocarbons such as polychlorinated biphenyls, tetrachlorodibenzo-*p*-dioxin, and naphthalenes (Tindall 1985). Clinically, chloracne is manifested by comedones and cysts around the eyes, ears, back, and genitalia; hyperpigmentation; conjunctivitis; and ocular discharge. There is distension and dilation of the follicular infundibulum, progressive degeneration of sebaceous glands, keratinization of sebaceous gland cells, hyperkeratosis of the follicular canal, and comedo and pustule formation. Skin effects vary across species; a review of animal models was included in Panteleyev and Bickers (2006). Similar histopathologic findings have been observed in Skh:HR-1 and HRS/J mouse strains, with the exception of hyperkeratinization of the sebaceous glands, which is considered pathognomonic for human chloracne and was not consistently observed with the chloracnegens tested (Puhvel et al. 1982).

Sweat gland toxicity may be caused by numerous compounds including cytostatic agents (e.g., cytarabine, bleomycin), formaldehyde, arsenic, lead, fluorine, and thallium. Neutrophilic eccrine hidradenitis is a selective toxicity of eccrine sweat glands caused by cytotoxic agents used in cancer chemotherapy such as cytarabine and bleomycin and is characterized by acute periductal neutrophilic inflammation and necrosis and squamous metaplasia of the eccrine duct cells (Haschek et al. 2010; Scallan et al. 1988) (Figure 19.5c).

The hamster flank organ has been used for studying the modulating effects of drugs and hormones on sebaceous glands (Gomez 1975; Greaves 2000; Plewig and Luderschmidt 1977). Antiandrogenic agents cause atrophy of the hamster flank organ similar to the effect observed after castration. The initial change is degeneration of sebaceous cells sparing cells at the edge of the gland with progression of atrophy to where the flank organ has the appearance of small sebaceous glands of normal hamster skin. Spironolactone and retinoids produce similar effects on this organ, whereas testosterone administration to intact male or immature castrated female hamsters has the opposite effect with an increase in size and pigmentation of the flank organ (Gomez 1975; Greaves 2000; Luderschmidt et al. 1982). The guinea pig flank model has been used to evaluate cutaneous irritation and vascular responses to pyrethroids (McKillop et al. 1987).

19.5.1.5 Pigmentation

19.5.1.5.1 Histopathology

Mechanisms of skin hyperpigmentation include increased melanocyte numbers and increased synthesis of melanin through modulation of enzyme activity or the activation/inhibition of regulation mechanisms (e.g., loss of the inhibitory feedback mechanisms and increased production of POMC-derived hormones such as MSH, ACTH, or β-lipotropin), as well as dominant mutations of the MC1R gene (Fistarol and Itin 2010). Hyperpigmentation can also occur when there is interference or blockade of melanin removal mechanisms in macrophages by the deposition of non-melanin pigment (drug or metabolites, endogenous pigments such as lipofuscin, or the products of drug/metabolite interaction with endogenous molecules) in the skin structures.

Hyperpigmentation of skin has been associated with a variety of both topically and systemically administered drugs. Drugs such as oral contraceptive drugs, cancer chemotherapeutics (e.g., bleomycin), cytotoxic drugs (e.g., Busulfan), and antimalarial agents may increase melanin production either by a direct effect on melanocytes or indirectly by modulation of the pituitary (Greaves 2000; Hendrix and Greer 1992). NSAIDs (e.g., acetaminophen, salicylates, or oxicam derivatives) and other drugs (e.g., barbiturates, tetracycline) can cause a syndrome called fixed drug eruption that includes hyperpigmentation (Dereure 2001). It is believed that these drugs haptenize melanocyte protein, resulting in specific immune reactions against the hapten–protein complex and increased pigmentation. In carcinogenicity studies in Long–Evans rats, medroxalol hydrochloride, a β1/β2 adrenergic antihypertensive agent, caused graying of pigmented hair attributed to melanin binding of the drug (Sells and Gibson 1987).

Numerous mechanisms have been postulated for decreased pigmentation, including a reduction in number of melanocytes per unit area, inhibition of melanin synthesis, abnormal melanization, failure of melanin transfer to keratinocytes, or interaction with melanin synthetic pathway enzymes (Bolognia and Pawelek 1988; Walsh and Gough 1989). For example, 4-*n*-butylresorcinol (Rucinol) is a potent inhibitor of tyrosinase and TRP-1, effectively inhibits melanin production in B16 melanoma cells without causing cytotoxicity, and has been shown in the clinic to reduce the hyperpigmentation of cutaneous liver spots (Katagiri et al. 2001). The antithyroid agent methimazole causes depigmentation of the ears of brown guinea pigs when applied topically, which is attributed to its inhibitory effect on peroxidase activity and plays a critical role in melanogenesis (Kasraee 2002). The platelet aggregation inhibitor PD-89454 caused loss of pigmentation of perioral pigmented skin in Long–Evans rats and skin of the nose, perioral and periocular skin, and oral mucous membranes of Beagle dogs after 4 weeks of treatment (Walsh and Gough 1989). Microscopically, melanin was decreased or absent in melanocytes and keratinocytes in the hair follicles of the affected areas of skin of rats or the skin of dogs as demonstrated by Fontana–Masson stain. Ultrastructurally, melanocytes in affected areas appeared globoid with small dendritic processes and reduced numbers of melanosomes that were smaller and incompletely pigmented. The postulated mechanism is uncertain but, on the basis of the ultrastructural findings, is suggestive of interference with either formation of melanosomes or melanization of melanosomes. Modulation of the molecular pathways involved in melanin synthesis by various drugs or chemicals has also been reported. Agents that specifically target melanocytes include vaccines developed by targeting melanoma-associated antigens, which result in anti-melanocyte immune reactions (a similar mechanism has also been reported for some chemicals, including 4-tertiary butyl phenol and triglycidyl-*p*-aminophenol) or imiquinod (Solano et al. 2006).

Depigmenting agents, such as hydroquinone, retinoic acid, tretinoin, kojic acid, phenols/catechols, and linoleic acid have been developed to specifically treat acquired hyperpigmentary disorders (e.g., melasma, solar lentigo) (Briganti et al. 2003).

Melanocytotoxic agents such as cysteaminylphenol and cysteinylphenol, intended for the treatment of melanoma, caused depigmentation of black hair follicles or skin when administered subcutaneously to C57BL/6J mice or topically to black guinea pigs (Ito et al. 1987). Microscopically, swelling, lysis, and necrosis of melanocytes were evident in pigmented hair follicles of C57BL/6J mice and decreased melanin pigment in various layers of epidermis of black guinea pigs. In contrast, no degenerative changes were observed in albino A/J mice. The mechanism of depigmentation involved destruction of the membranous organelles in melanocytes, decreased synthesis of melanosomes, and a reduction in the number of functional melanocytes (Ito et al. 1987).

19.6 HYPERPLASTIC, PRENEOPLASTIC, AND NEOPLASTIC SKIN CHANGES

19.6.1 Skin

The incidence and type of spontaneous tumors in rodents are typically low but increase with age, and will vary with species and strain. In B6C3F1 and CD-1 mice, the most common spontaneous skin tumors include fibroma, fibrosarcoma, fibrous histiocytoma, hemangiosarcoma, histiocytic sarcoma, and undifferentiated sarcomas. In Fisher 344/N, Wistar, Han Wistar, Osborne–Mendel, Long–Evans, and Sprague–Dawley rats, fibroma, fibrosarcoma, keratoacanthoma, squamous cell papilloma, SCC, and lipoma are most often observed (Baldrick 2005; Baldrick and Reeve 2007; Brix et al. 2005; Dinse et al. 2010; Goodman et al. 1979; Haseman et al. 1998; Maekawa et al. 1983; Sommer 1997; Son et al. 2010; Son and Gopinath 2004). Preneoplastic intraepithelial lesions include solar/actinic keratosis. Pseudocarcinomatous hyperplasia of the prepuce and penile mucosa has been observed as a spontaneous lesion in cynomolgus monkeys (Chamanza et al. 2010). It is characterized by marked epidermal hyperplasia with prominent rete pegs, hyperpigmentation, and severe inflammation (lymphoplasmacytic cells and eosinophils) of the epidermis with extension into the underlying tissues. Continuous prolonged exposure to sunlight is considered the most important etiologic factor in the development of skin tumors in domestic animals (Madewell 1981).

Chemically induced skin tumors have been associated with numerous topically applied and systemically administered compounds. Peroxisome proliferator-activated receptor agonists have been associated with the development of hemangiosarcomas in mice and hamsters and liposarcomas and fibrosarcomas in rats (Hardisty et al. 2007). Although uncommon in dogs, solar elastosis has been reported to be associated with cutaneous SCC and hemangioma (Knowles and Hargis 1986).

The histomorphological appearance of selected skin tumors and their differential diagnosis is presented in the following sections.

19.6.1.1 Epidermis

19.6.1.1.1 Squamous Cell Hyperplasia

Squamous cell hyperplasia is often found associated with chronic inflammatory conditions involving the epidermis. The lesion is characterized by a highly variable growth pattern that may exhibit regular, irregular, or papillary features, with hyperkeratosis and prominent rete ridge formation. The non-keratinized layers are increased and there are increased numbers of cells in the spinous cell layer. Differential diagnoses include basal cell hyperplasia, squamous cell papilloma, and SCC (Bruner et al. 2001; goRENI 2012; INHAND 2012).

19.6.1.1.2 Squamous Cell Papilloma

Squamous cell papillomas are benign neoplastic changes of the epidermis (Aldaz et al. 1987). They may be flat (endophytic) or pedunculated (exophytic) with a distinct border of basal cells. The growth pattern of squamous cell papillomas is endophytic, exophytic, or papillary, with variable hyperkeratosis, some parakeratosis, and, occasionally, dyskeratosis (i.e., premature keratinization of individual cells). The stroma is highly vascularized and lined by acanthotic epithelium with small foci of keratinization. Cells may be fusiform or columnar and stain darkly. Mitotic figures are rarely observed. The pedunculated form has a characteristic narrow stalk, whereas the flat form is more expansive and forms a poorly demarcated, continuous transition with adjacent hyperplastic epithelium. Hyperplastic sebaceous glands may occasionally be present. Differential diagnoses include squamous cell hyperplasia, keratoacanthoma, SCC, and fibroma/fibropapilloma (Bruner et al. 2001; goRENI 2012; INHAND 2012).

19.6.1.1.3 Keratoacanthoma

Keratoacanthoma is a benign tumor believed to arise from the epithelium of hair follicles (Ramselaar et al. 1980). They are typically well demarcated, but not encapsulated, with single or multiple "cup-shaped" cavities filled with lamellated, concentrically arranged whorls ("lamellated horn pearls") or homogeneous keratin (Figure 19.5d). Cavities are lined by several layers of well-differentiated or acanthotic squamous epithelial cells exhibiting features of abortive hair follicle formation. Characteristically, the granular cell layer is absent. The nuclear-to-cytoplasmic ratio is low and mitotic figures may be observed (Bruner et al. 2001; goRENI 2012; INHAND 2012). Whorls of keratin may fuse to form larger masses. In skin grafting studies in immunoincompetent nude (nu/nu) mice, the rapid growth and regression of keratoacanthomas appear to follow the hair growth cycle, with growth during the anagen phase and regression during the telogen phase, rather than immune mediated (Ramselaar et al. 1980). Differential diagnoses include cysts, benign hair follicle tumors (e.g., trichofolliculoma), squamous cell papilloma, and SCC. Induced keratoacanthomas may regress in mice but not in rats (Bruner et al. 2001).

19.6.1.1.4 Squamous Cell Carcinoma

SCC is a malignant tumor of the epidermis characterized by variable squamous differentiation, nuclear atypia, loss of intercellular bridges, penetration of the basal lamina, and invasion of the dermis or underlying striated muscles by cords or nests of neoplastic cells. Keratinizing forms of SCCs have cells arranged in cords or whorls with central keratinization, often referred to as "lamellated horn pearls" (Figure 19.6a). There is dyskeratosis and hyperkeratosis with variable degrees of keratinization. Occasionally, nests of cells may be present without keratinization. In the pseudoglandular form of SCC, a tubular or alveolar pseudoglandular pattern may be evident as a result of acantholysis, with the lumen occupied by desquamated acantholytic cells and debris. The lumen may be lined by one or several layers of epithelial cells with varying degrees of keratinization. In the non-keratinizing form of SCC, there is little evidence of keratinization. Cells appear atypical, polygonal, or spindle shaped with eosinophilic cytoplasm. There are numerous mitotic figures that may appear atypical or bizarre. Nuclear atypia is evident and the nuclei may be giant, fragmented,

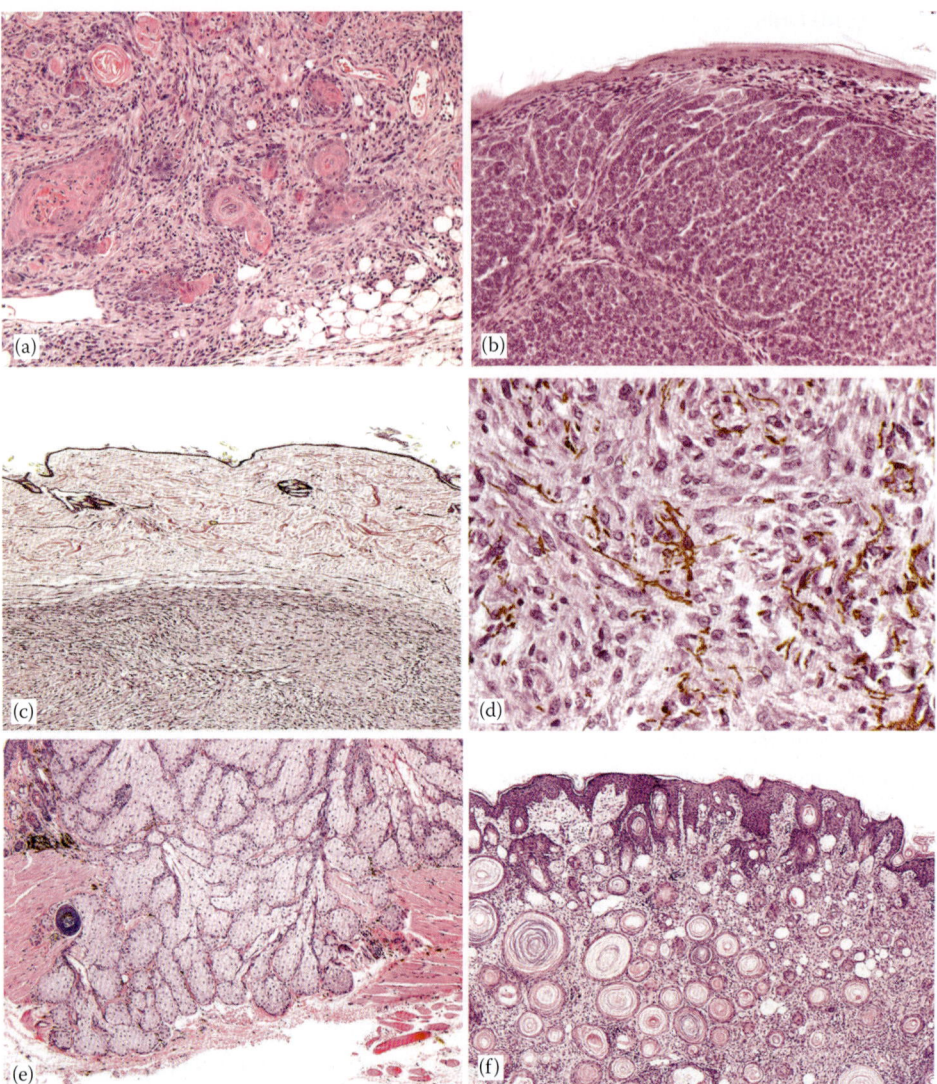

FIGURE 19.6   (a) SCC, invasive, with variable squamous differentiation, nuclear atypia, and characteristic whorls of keratin ("lamellated horny pearls") (Tg:AC hemizygous mouse [FBV/N]). (b) Basal cell tumor (trichoblastoma), a benign tumor arising from the matrix cells of the hair follicle. This example is composed of ribbons and trabeculae of small keratinocytes (F344/N rat). (c) Fibroma, a well-demarcated nodule of fusiform cells and interwoven bands of mature collagen (B6C3F1 mouse). (d) Malignant melanoma is characterized by anaplastic, spindle, polygonal, epithelioid, and pigmented dendritic cells (B6C3F1 mouse). (e) Sebaceous gland adenoma consisting of multiple coalescing lobules of sebocytes that demonstrate otherwise normal holocrine differentiation with drainage into associated ducts (B6C3F1 mouse). (f) Trichoepithelioma, a benign hair follicle tumor demonstrating largely differentiation reminiscent of the infundibular and isthmic region of the hair follicle. The tumor is characterized by multiple cysts containing keratin in patterns that range from basketweave to laminated to compact (B6C3F1 mouse).

or multiple. Inflammation and ulceration may be evident. Differential diagnoses include squamous cell papilloma, keratoacanthoma, basal cell carcinoma, and malignant mammary adenoacanthoma (adenosquamous carcinoma) (Bruner et al. 2001; goRENI 2012; INHAND 2012). SCC has been associated with chronic dermatosis in beagle dogs (Hargis et al. 1977). SCC of the lip has been described in cynomolgus monkeys (Chamanza et al. 2010).

19.6.1.1.5   Basal Cell Tumor (Benign)

Benign basal cell tumors arise from the epidermis or epidermal appendages. They are well demarcated, often multilobulated, and composed of uniform sheets or strands of closely packed cells (Figure 19.6b). Basal cell tumors do not penetrate the basement membrane. Cells resemble typical basal cells of the epidermis with scant cytoplasm. Nuclei are round to oval and the cytoplasm is scant and stains intensely basophilic. Mitotic figures are rarely observed. Keratinization, sebaceous cells, or hair follicle formation may be evident. Basal cell tumors may be classified as basosquamous (i.e., foci of keratinization present), trichoblastoma (i.e., foci of sebaceous cells/trichogenesis present), or granular (i.e., contain PAS-positive granules) types. Differential diagnosis includes basal cell carcinoma (Bruner et al. 2001; goRENI 2012; INHAND 2012).

19.6.1.1.6   Basal Cell Carcinoma

Basal cell carcinomas are malignant tumors arising from the epidermis or epidermal appendages. They consist of heterogeneous sheets or strands of closely packed cells that may exhibit palisading at the periphery. The extent of demarcation is quite variable, and there may be extensive local invasion but rarely metastasis. Neoplastic cells resemble basal cells of the epidermis or appendages in that they are small, with scant slightly basophilic cytoplasm and dark blue nuclei. Mitotic figures may be numerous. Basal cell carcinomas may present in a solid form with necrotic areas in the center ("pseudocyts") or as a basosquamous form incorporating squamous cells. Desmoplasia may be evident in the surrounding mesenchymal tissue. Differential diagnoses include benign basal cell tumor, benign hair follicle tumor, and sebaceous cell carcinoma (Bruner et al. 2001; goRENI 2012; INHAND 2012). The Sonic Hedgehog signaling pathway has been implicated in the development of human basal cell carcinomas through activation of the Patched gene by mutations in Smoothened, which acts as a proto-oncogene (Xie et al. 1998). Basal cell carcinomas occur in transgenic mice overexpressing mutated smoothened transmembrane protein (Xie et al. 1998).

19.6.1.2   Dermis/Subcutis (Mesenchymal)

19.6.1.2.1   Fibroma

Fibromas are subcutaneous, moderately well-defined solid nodules or masses of dense interwoven bands of mature collagen, occasionally containing foci of myxomatous degeneration (Ernst et al. 2001; Greaves 2000; Zackheim 1973) (Figure 19.6c). Cells are typically fusiform containing elongated hyperchromatic or vesicular nuclei with one or more prominent nucleoli (Ernst et al. 2001). A few small fibroblast-like or stellate cells may be interspersed throughout the tumor, but these neoplasms are typically uniform in appearance, lacking pleomorphism or mitotic figures (Ernst et al. 2001; Greaves 2000). Differential diagnoses include reactive fibrosis or scars, benign fibrous histiocytoma, leiomyoma, benign Schwannoma, and fibrosarcoma (Ernst et al. 2001; Zackheim 1973).

19.6.1.2.2   Fibrosarcoma

Fibrosarcomas are malignant tumors composed of pleomorphic spindle-shaped cells, often arranged in a characteristic "herring-bone" pattern, with variable amounts of collagen interspersed between bands of cells (Ernst et al. 2001; Zackheim 1973). Numerous mitotic figures may be evident, as well as areas of hemorrhage and necrosis. Tumors may be locally aggressive, but metastases rarely occur. Differential diagnoses include fibroma, hemangiosarcoma, malignant fibrous histiocytoma (MFH), leiomyosarcoma, and malignant Schwannoma. Transplantable mouse fibrosarcomas that have histologic (i.e., well differentiated with storiform pattern) and ultrastructural features resembling human MFH have been developed; these may serve as control tumors in chemical carcinogenicity investigations (Becker et al. 1982; Brooks 1986).

19.6.1.2.3   Benign Fibrous Histiocytoma

Fibrous histiocytoma is a benign tumor of pluripotential mesenchymal stem cells characterized by fibroblast-like cells, admixed with histiocytic cells (Ernst et al. 2001). Cells are arranged in characteristic storiform or cartwheel patterns interspersed with thin bundles of collagen. Neoplastic cells are well differentiated, exhibiting little pleomorphism or mitoses. Tumors may contain scattered inflammatory cells. Differential diagnoses include fibroma, benign Schwannoma, and MFH (Ernst et al. 2001).

Canine cutaneous histiocytoma (CCH) is a benign tumor of the skin in young dogs characterized by pleomorphic monocyte–macrophage cell types (Cockerell and Slauson 1979; Kelly 1970; Taylor et al. 1969). These tumors are often solitary, do not metastasize, and often regress spontaneously. Infiltrating lymphocytes are considered a characteristic feature of CCH. Tumor cells are characterized by the presence of irregular nuclei, lysosomal granules, and perinuclear filaments and are α-naphthyl acetate esterase positive, consistent with a mononuclear–phagocyte system origin (Glick et al. 1976).

19.6.1.2.4   MFH/Histiocytic Sarcoma

MFH, also referred to as undifferentiated pleomorphic sarcoma, are tumors composed of cells with features resembling histiocytes and fibroblasts. MFHs have been reported in dogs, cats, and rats and occur in the subcutis on the head, trunk, or limbs (Choi et al. 2011; Gleiser et al. 1979; Goodman et al. 1980; Renlund and Pritzker 1984). Four subtypes of MFH have been described on the basis of histopathologic appearance, including storiform-pleomorphic, myxoid, giant cell, and inflammatory (Choi et al. 2011). The subtype of MFH may affect prognosis. In dogs, the giant cell variant of MFH is associated with a higher rate of local recurrence and metastasis to subcutaneous tissues, lymph nodes, lung, and liver (Choi et al. 2011). In rats, spontaneous fibrous histiocytic tumors are highly malignant and metastasize (Greaves and Faccini 1981). A study in Sprague–Dawley rats on the development of MFH at the site of implanted Millipore filters suggests that these tumors arise from pluripotential mesenchymal stem cells rather than from mononuclear/phagocytic cells. It is postulated that MFH in this animal model is due to chronic inflammation and scarring, which are both predisposing factors for tumor development (Greaves et al. 1985). Although the immunohistochemistry of MFH is not well characterized in animals, MFH cells are often vimentin positive and CD-18 negative (Choi et al. 2011; Helm et al. 1993). MEP-1 is a monoclonal antibody specific against fibroblast-like MFH cells. In a study of DMBA-induced MFH in rats using immunohistochemical quantitative staining, it was shown that the majority of positive cells were fibroblast-like cells and that the histiocyte-like cells were most likely infiltrating macrophages (Tsuchiya et al. 1993). Spontaneous histiocytic tumors in rats were variably positive immunohistochemically for α1-antitrypsin, α1-chymotrypsin, muramidase, desmin, neuron-specific enolase, S100, glial fibrillary acid protein, and vimentin (Wright et al. 1991).

19.6.1.2.5   Sarcoma

Sarcoma is a malignant tumor of pluripotential mesenchymal stem cells consisting of sheets of undifferentiated spindle-shaped cells whose microscopic morphological characteristics preclude definitive categorization (Ernst et al. 2001). Differential diagnoses include pleomorphic liposarcoma, fibrosarcoma, leiomyosarcoma, malignant Schwannoma, and rhabdomyosarcoma (Ernst et al. 2001). Single subcutaneous injection of DMBA to neonatal rats induced sarcoma (Taguchi et al. 2006).

19.6.1.2.6   Mast Cell Tumor/Mastocytoma

Mastocytomas are benign or malignant tumors of mast cells often forming nodules in the subcutis (Frith et al. 2001). Mastocytomas are composed of well-differentiated mast cells containing characteristic metachromatic granules (i.e., toluidine blue or Giemsa stained). Tumors may contain varying amounts of collagen and are characteristically infiltrated by eosinophils. The principal differential diagnosis is histiocytic sarcoma (Frith et al. 2001). Canine mastocytomas often occur in the dermis and exhibit collagen necrosis (Hottendorf and Nielsen 1966). Two distinct histologic subtypes have been identified in cats: one consisting of solitary, discrete tumors in the dermis consisting of slightly atypical mast cells, and the other characterized by multiple, discrete subcutaneous nodules of histiocytic-like cells with few toluidine blue cytoplasmic granules (Wilcock et al. 1986). Spontaneous regression was observed in some cats within a 2-year period.

19.6.1.3 Melanocytic

19.6.1.3.1 Nevi

Numerous variants of melanocytic dysplasia have been reported in humans, occasionally referred to as dysplastic nevi (Cook and Robertson 1985). They may be solitary or multiple and form a variety of patterns, including lentiginous, predominantly spindle cell, or non-lentiginous. Melanocytic dysplasia most often develops into benign intradermal melanonevi but occasionally may progress to malignant melanomas.

19.6.1.3.2 Benign Melanoma

Benign melanomas are nodular masses of pigmented cells present in the dermis and may be associated with the overlying epidermis. Tumor cells vary in shape (e.g., polygonal, epithelioid, or spindle shaped) and degree of pigmentation (i.e., intracytoplasmic dark brown pigment granules). The principal differential diagnosis is malignant melanoma (INHAND 2012). Benign melanoma has been reported in a variety of domestic and laboratory animals, including dogs, cats, and pigs, but is exceedingly rare in mice and rats (Garma-Avina et al. 1981; INHAND 2012).

19.6.1.3.3 Malignant Melanoma

Malignant melanoma is characterized by dense clusters of dermal melanocytes containing variable amounts of intracytoplasmic, dark brown pigment granules. Cells may be spindle shaped, polygonal, epithelioid, or anaplastic and are typically pleomorphic (Figure 19.6d). Spindle cell variants are most commonly observed in mice. These tumors are locally invasive. Differential diagnosis includes basal cell carcinoma (Bruner et al. 2001; goRENI 2012; INHAND 2012). Numerous classification systems have been proposed for malignant melanoma (McGovern et al. 1986). The nucleic acid index (i.e., calculated by measuring the fluorescence intensities of acridine orange in nuclei relative to the surrounding cytoplasm that reflects the concentration of DNA to RNA) has been used as a method for analyzing nucleic acid derangements in histological sections, thereby providing a quantitative measure for grading malignancy (i.e., melanocytic dysplasia) of melanomas (Berman et al. 2005). Malignant melanomas are also classified according to size and vertical and horizontal growth phases, with elevation above the skin considered an indicator of invasive potential with probability of metastases (Drepper et al. 1980; Elder et al. 1980). Malignant melanomas have been induced in C57BL/6 mice after treatment with DMBA and croton oil (Berkelhammer and Oxenhandler 1987). An animal model of malignant skin melanoma has been developed in transgenic mice via the Tyr-SV40E transgene, which targets expression of simian virus 40 oncogene sequences in transgenic mice (Mintz et al. 1993). Spontaneous amelanotic melanomas have been reported in male and female F344/N rats involving the ears, eyelids, scrotum, and perianal regions with metastases to the lungs and mandibular lymph nodes (Yoshitomi et al. 1995). These tumors originate from the dermis and are characterized by predominantly spindle-shaped cells (rarely epithelioid cells), arranged in an interlacing fascicular pattern with a perivascular orientation. Ultrastructurally, cells contain numerous intracytoplasmic premelanosomes that are devoid of melanin (Yoshimoto et al. 1995). A spontaneous occurrence of amelanotic melanoma (epithelioid cell type) has been described in F344 rat (Nakashima et al. 1996). Spontaneous cutaneous melanomas in Sinclair miniature swine are considered to be similar to human melanomas in histopathologic appearance and patterns of metastases and regression (Oxenhandler et al. 1982).

19.6.2 Adnexa

19.6.2.1 Sebaceous Cell Hyperplasia

Sebaceous cell hyperplasia has been reported more commonly in rats than in mice. This lesion is characterized by an abundance of sebaceous cells that still retain the normal glandular architecture. Differential diagnosis is the sebaceous cell adenoma (Bruner et al. 2001; goRENI 2012; INHAND 2012).

19.6.2.2 Sebaceous Cell Adenoma

Sebaceous cell adenoma is characterized by a loss of regular sebaceous gland architecture while maintaining a clear, glandular, acino-lobular pattern (Figure 19.6e). The tumor may manifest an endophytic (i.e., small, flat, subepidermal nodules) or exophytic (i.e., protruding papillomatous nodules) growth pattern. Acinar cells exhibit variable degrees of maturation and are typically small with abundant, foamy, and clear cytoplasm and pyknotic nuclei. Large numbers of immature germinative, basiloid cells may be present at the periphery or predominate in some acini or lobules. Mitotic figures vary in number. Differential diagnoses include sebaceous cell hyperplasia, sebaceous cell carcinoma, and benign basal cell tumor (Bruner et al. 2001; goRENI 2012; INHAND 2012).

19.6.2.3 Sebaceous Cell Carcinoma

In sebaceous cell carcinoma, there is a significant distortion of the sebaceous gland architecture, but with retention of a glandular, acino-lobular pattern. Neoplastic cells are poorly differentiated, with irregular size and shape and significant nuclear atypia. Occasionally, cells may be well-differentiated focally, and there may be squamous cell differentiation and single-cell necrosis. The size of the intra-cytoplasmic lipid vacuoles is highly variable. The tumor is highly invasive locally and metastasis may occur. Differential diagnoses include sebaceous cell adenoma and basal cell carcinoma (Bruner et al. 2001; goRENI 2012; INHAND 2012). In humans, SCCs show a distinct pattern and extent of chromosome loss compared to basal cell carcinoma (Quinn et al. 1994).

19.6.2.4 Benign Hair Follicle Tumor (Trichofolliculoma, Pilomatricoma, Trichoepithelioma, Tricholemmoma)

Benign hair follicle tumors arise from the pilosebaceous unit. They are well demarcated and may exhibit different stages of hair formation or contain single or multiple cysts. Benign hair follicle tumors are typically noninvasive and nonencapsulated. Trichofolliculomas contain anagen hair follicles as well as single or multiple cysts or well-differentiated hair shafts. Pilomatricomas also contain all components of anagen hair follicles and cysts and are differentiated by the presence of large numbers of "ghost cells" and multinucleated cells. Trichoepitheliomas demonstrate abrupt keratinization but do not contain an infundibulum, mature hair shafts, or ghost cells (Figure 19.6f). In tricholemmomas, only basal cells, hair matrix cells, and cells of the outer sheath are present. Outer sheath cells are vacuolated and contain glycogen. Differential diagnoses include cysts, benign basal cell tumors, keratoacanthoma, and basal cell carcinoma (Bruner et al. 2001; goRENI 2012; INHAND 2012). Epitheliomas, described as "wart-like" lesions around the eyes, mouth, and perianal regions, have been reported in LVG hamsters associated with infection by an unclassified hamster papovavirus (Coggin et al. 1985).

REFERENCES

Alaluf, S., Atkins, D., Barrett, K. et al. 2002a. Ethnic variation in melanin content and composition in photo-exposed and photoprotected human skin. *Pigment Cell Research*. 15(2):112–8.

Alaluf, S., Atkins, D., Barrett, K. et al. 2002b. The impact of epidermal melanin on objective measurements of human skin colour. *Pigment Cell Research*. 15(2):119–26.

Alanko, K., and M. Hannuksela. 1998. Mechanisms of drug reactions. In: Kauppinen, K., Alanko, K., Hannuksela, M., and Maibach, H.I. (eds.). *Skin Reactions to Drugs*. CRC Press, Boca Raton, FL.

Aldaz, C.M., Conti, C.J., Klein-Szanto, A.J. et al. 1987. Progressive dysplasia and aneuploidy are hallmarks of mouse skin papillomas: relevance to malignancy. *Proceedings of the National Academy of Sciences of the United States of America*. 84(7):2029–32.

Andersen, K.E. 1987. Testing for contact allergy in experimental animals. *Pharmacology and Toxicology*. 61(1):1–8.

Anderson, J.M. and J.J. Langone. 1999. Issues and perspectives on the biocompatibility and immunotoxicity evaluation of implanted controlled release systems. *Journal of Controlled Release*. 57:107–13.

Anwar, W.A. 1997. Biomarkers of human exposure to pesticides. *Environmental Health Perspectives*. 105 Suppl 4:801–6.

Argyris, T.S. 1982. Tumor promotion by regenerative epidermal hyperplasia in mouse skin. *Journal of Cutaneous Pathology*. 9(1):1–18.

Auletta, C.S. 2004. Current in vivo assays for cutaneous toxicity: local and systemic toxicity testing. *Basic and Clinical Pharmacology and Toxicology*. 95(5):201–8.

Baldrick, P. 2005. Carcinogenicity evaluation: comparison of tumor data from dual control groups in the Sprague–Dawley rat. *Toxicologic Pathology*. 33(2):283–91.

Baldrick, P., and L. Reeve. 2007. Carcinogenicity evaluation: comparison of tumor data from dual control groups in the CD-1 mouse. *Toxicologic Pathology*. 35(4):562–9.

Bartek, M.J., LaBudde J.A., and H.I. Maibach. 1972. Skin permeability *in vivo*: comparison in rat, rabbit, pig and man. *Journal of Investigative Dermatology*. 58(3):114–23.

Becker, F.F., Nevares, D., and B. Mackay. 1982. Transplantable lines of spontaneous mouse fibrosarcomas. *Veterinary Pathology*. 19(2):206–9.

Berger, H., Tsambaos, D., and G. Mahrle. 1980. Experimental elastosis induced by chronic ultraviolet exposure. Light- and electron-microscopic study. *Archives of Dermatological Research*. 269(1):39–49.

Berkelhammer, J., and R.W. Oxenhandler. 1987. Evaluation of premalignant and malignant lesions during the induction of mouse melanomas. *Cancer Research*. 47(5):1251–4.

Berman, B., France, D.S., Martinelli., G.P. et al. 1983. Modulation of expression of epidermal Langerhans cell properties following in situ exposure to glucocorticosteroids. *Journal of Investigative Dermatology*. 80(3):168–71.

Berman, D.M., Wincovitch, S.S. Garfield, S.S. et al. 2005. Grading melanocytic dysplasia in paraffin wax embedded tissue by the nucleic acid index. *Journal of Clinical Pathology*. 58(11):1206–10.

Bibby, M.C. 1981. The specificity of early changes in the skin during carcinogenesis. *British Journal of Dermatology*. 104(4):485–8.

Bigby, M., Jick, S., Jick, H., and K. Arndt. 1986. Drug-induced cutaneous reactions. A report from the Boston Collaborative Drug Surveillance Program on 15,438 consecutive inpatients, 1975 to 1982. *JAMA*. 256(24):3358–63.

Blanchard, K.T., Barthel, C., French, J.E. et al. 1999. Transponder-induced sarcoma in the heterozygous p53+/− mouse. *Toxicologic Pathology*. 27(5):519–27.

Bohm, M., and T.A. Luger. 1998. The pilosebaceous unit is part of the skin immune system. *Dermatology*. 196(1):75–9.

Bolognia, J.L., and J.M. Pawelek. 1988. Biology of hypopigmentation. *Journal of the American Academy of Dermatology*. 19(2 Pt 1):217–55.

Bos, J.D., and M.L. Kapsenberg. 1993. The skin immune system: progress in cutaneous biology. *Immunology Today*. 14(2):75–8.

Bosnjak, I.L., Miranda-Saksena, M., Koelle, D.M. et al. 2005. Herpes simplex virusinfection of human dendritic cells induces apoptosis and allows crosspresentation via uninfected dendritic cells. *Journal of Immunology*. 174:2220–7.

Boukhman, M.P., and H.I. Maibach. 2011. Thresholds in contact sensitization: immunologic mechanisms and experimental evidence in humans—an overview. *Food and Chemical Toxicology*. 39(12):1125–34.

Bouwstra, J.A., Honeywell-Nguyen P.L., Gooris, G.S. et al. 2003: Review: structure of the skin barrier and its modulation by vesicular formulations. *Progress in Lipid Research*. 42:1–36.

Braiman-Wiksman, L., Solomonik, I., Spira, R. et al. 2007. Novel insights into wound healing sequence of events. *Toxicologic Pathology*. 35(6):767–79.

Breathnach, S.M., and S.I. Katz. 1986. Cell-mediated immunity in cutaneous disease. *Human Pathology*. 17(2):161–7.

Breider, M.A., Gough, A.W., Haskins, J.R. et al. 1999. Troglitazone-induced heart and adipose tissue cell proliferation in mice. *Toxicologic Pathology*. 27(5):545–52.

Briganti, S., Camera, E., and M. Picardo. 2003. Chemical and instrumental approaches to treat hyperpigmentation. *Pigment Cell Research*. 16(2):101–10.

Brix, A.E., Nyska, A., Haseman, J.K. et al. 2005. Incidences of selected lesions in control female Harlan Sprague–Dawley rats from two-year studies performed by the National Toxicology Program. *Toxicologic Pathology*. 33(4):477–83.

Brooks, J.J. 1986. The significance of double phenotypic patterns and markers in human sarcomas. A new model of mesenchymal differentiation. *American Journal of Pathology*. 125(1):113–23.

Brown, A.P., Dunstan, R.W., Courtney, C.L. et al. 2008. Cutaneous lesions in the rat following administration of an irreversible inhibitor of erbB receptors, including the epidermal growth factor receptor. *Toxicologic Pathology*. 36(3):410–9.

Bruner, R., Kuttler, K., Bader, R. et al. 2001. Integumentary system. In: Mohr, U. (ed.). *International Classification of Rodent Tumors. The Mouse*. Springer-Verlag, Heidelberg, pp. 1–22.

Bullough, W.S. 1972. The control of epidermal thickness. 2. *British Journal of Dermatology*. 87(4):347–54.

Campbell, R.L., and R.D. Bruce. 1981. Comparative dermatotoxicology. I. Direct comparison and human primary skin irritation responses to isopropylmyristate. *Toxicology and Applied Pharmacology*. 59:555–63.

Carere, A., Stammati, A., and F. Zucco. 2002. In vitro toxicology methods: impact on regulation from technical and scientific advancements. *Toxicology Letters*. 127(1–3):153–60.

Carroll, J.M., McElwee, K.J.E., King, L. et al. 2002. Gene array profiling and immunomodulation studies define a cell-mediated immune response underlying the pathogenesis of alopecia areata in a mouse model and humans. *Journal of Investigative Dermatology*. 119(2):392–402.

Cavanagh, J.B., and M. Gregson. 1978. Some effects of a thallium salt on the proliferation of hair follicle cells. *Journal of Pathology*. 125(4):179–91.

CDER (Center for Drug Evaluation and Research): http://www.fda.gov/Drugs/GuidanceComplianceRegulatory Information/Guidances/ucm065014.htm, date of publication.

Chamanza, R., Marxfeld, H.A., Blanco, A.I. et al. 2010. Incidences and range of spontaneous findings in control cynomolgus monkeys (*Macaca fascicularis*) used in toxicity studies. *Toxicologic Pathology*. 38(4):642–57.

Cheville, N. 1994. *Ultrastructural Pathology. An Introduction to Interpretation*. Iowa State University Press, Ames, IA.

Choi, H., Kwon, Y., Chang, J. et al. 2011. Undifferentiated pleomorphic sarcoma (malignant fibrous histiocytoma) of the head in a dog. *Journal of Veterinary Medical Science*. 73(2):235–9.

Clark, R.A. 2010. Skin-resident T cells: the ups and downs of on site immunity. *Journal of Investigative Dermatology*. 130(2):362–70.

Cockerell, G.L., and D.O. Slauson. 1979. Patterns of lymphoid infiltrate in the canine cutaneous histiocytoma. *Journal of Comparative Pathology*. 89(2):193–203.

Coggin, J.H. Jr., Hyde, B.M., Heath, L.S. et al. 1985. Papovavirus in epitheliomas appearing on lymphoma-bearing hamsters: lack of association with horizontally transmitted lymphomas of Syrian hamsters. *Journal of the National Cancer Institute*. 75(1):91–7.

Cohen, S.M. 2001. Alternative models for carcinogenicity testing: weight of evidence evaluations across models. *Toxicologic Pathology* 29(Suppl.):183–190.

Collan, Y. 1998. Alternatives for morphometric and stereologic analysis in toxicopathology. *Toxicology Letters*. 102–3:393–7.

Conrad, C., Meller, S., and M. Gilliet. 2009. Plasmacytoid dendritic cells in the skin: to sense or not to sense nucleic acids. *Seminars in Immunology*. 21(3):101–9.

Cook, M.G., and I. Robertson. 1985. Melanocytic dysplasia and melanoma. *Histopathology*. 9(6):647–58.

Coquette, A., Berna, N., Vandenbosch, A. et al. 2003. Analysis of interleukin-1alpha (IL-1alpha) and interleukin-8 (IL-8) expression and release in in vitro reconstructed human epidermis for the prediction of in vivo skin irritation and/or sensitization. *Toxicology In Vitro*. 17(3):311–21.

Corsetti, G., D'Antona, G., Dioguardi, F.S., and R. Rezzani. 2010. Topical application of dressing with amino acids improves cutaneous wound healing in aged rats. *Acta Histochemica*. 112(5):497–507.

Costin, G.E., and V.J. Hearing. 2007. Human skin pigmentation: melanocytes modulate skin color in response to stress. *FASEB Journal*. 21(4):976–94.

Cotsarelis, G. 1997. The hair follicle: dying for attention. *American Journal of Pathology*. 151(6):1505–9.

Cribb, A.E. 1989. Idiosyncratic reactions to sulfonamides in dogs. *Journal of the American Veterinary Medical Association*. 195(11):1612–4.

Cribb, A.E., Lee, B.L., Trepanier, L.A. et al. 1996. Adverse reactions to sulphonamide and sulphonamide-trimethoprim antimicrobials: clinical syndromes and pathogenesis. *Adverse Drug Reactions and Toxicology Reviews*. 15:9–50.

CRL (Charles River Laboratories) Technical Sheet. 2009. The 3T3 Neutral Red Uptake in vitro Photoirritation Test. http://www.criver.com/SiteCollectionDocuments/pc_dis_3T3_NRU_Test.pdf.

Darby, T.D. 1987. Safety evaluation of polymer materials. *Annual Review of Pharmacology and Toxicology*. 27:157–67.

Dardeno, T.A., Chou, S.H., Moon, H.S. et al. 2010. Leptin in human physiology and therapeutics. *Frontiers in Neuroendocrinology*. 31(3):377–93.

Davidson, J.M. 1998. Animal models for wound repair. *Archives of Dermatological Research*. 290(Suppl.):S1–11.

Dereure, O. 2001. Drug-induced skin pigmentation. *American Journal of Clinical Dermatology*. 2(4):253–62.

DiMeglio, P., Perer, G.K., and F.O. Nestle. 2011. Review: the multitasking organ: recent insights into skin immune function. *Immunity*. 35(6):857–69.

Dinse, G.E., Peddada, S.D., Harriset S.F. et al. 2010. Comparison of NTP historical control tumor incidence rates in female Harlan Sprague Dawley and Fischer 344/N rats. *Toxicologic Pathology*. 38(5):765–75.

Dobrovolskaia, M.A., Germolec, D.R., and J.L. Weaver. 2009. Evaluation of nanoparticle immunotoxicity. *Nature Nanotechnology*. 4(7):411–4.

Dorr, R.T. 1994. Pharmacology and toxicology of Cremophor EL diluent. *The Annals of Pharmacotherapy*. 28(5 Suppl):S11–4.

Drepper, H., Lindemann, M., and D. Obst. 1980. A new classification of malignant melanoma proposed according to the TNM-system. *Journal of Cancer Research and Clinical Oncology*. 96(3):223–9.

Ebbeson, S.O.E. and D. Tang. 1965. A method for estimating the number of cells in histological sections. *Journal of Microscopy*. 84:449.

Elcock, L.E., Stuart B.P., Wahle, B.S. et al. 2001. Tumors in long-term rat studies associated with microchip animal identification devices. *Experimental and Toxicologic Pathology*. 52(6):483–91.

Elder, D.E., Jucovy, P.M., Tuthillet, R.J. et al. 1980. The classification of malignant melanoma. *American Journal of Dermatopathology*. 2(4):315–20.

EMA (European Medicines Agency): http://www.ema.europa.eu/ema/index.jsp?curl=pages/regulation/general/general_content_000397.jsp&mid=WC0b01ac058002956f.

Ernst, H., Carlton, W.W., Courntey, C. et al. 2001. Soft tissue and skeletal muscle. In: Mohr, U. (ed.). *International Classification of Rodent Tumors. The Mouse*. Springer-Verlag, Heidelberg, pp. 361–88.

Faccini, J.M., Abbott, D.P., and G.J.J. Paulus. 1990. *Mouse Histopathology. A Glossary for Use in Toxicity and Carcinogenicity Studies*. Elsevier, Amsterdam.

Fang, R.C., and T.A. Mustoe. 2008. Animal models of wound healing: utility in transgenic mice. *Journal of Biomaterials Science, Polymer Edition*. 19(8):989–1005.

Fartasch, M. 2004. The epidermal lamellar body: a fascinating secretory organelle. *Journal of Investigative Dermatology*. 122(5):XI–XII.

FDA CDRH (Center for Devices and Radiologic Health). 2007. Blue Book Memorandum #695-1. http://www.fda.gov/MedicalDevices/DeviceRegulationandGuidance/GuidanceDocuments/ucm080742.htm.

Feingold, K.R., and P.M. Elias. 1988. Endocrine–skin interactions. Cutaneous manifestations of adrenal disease, pheochromocytomas, carcinoid syndrome, sex hormone excess and deficiency, polyglandular autoimmune syndromes, multiple endocrine neoplasia syndromes, and other miscellaneous disorders. *Journal of the American Academy of Dermatology*. 19(1 Pt 1):1–20.

Ferguson, J. 2002. Photosensitivity due to drugs. *Photodermatology, Photoimmunology and Photomedicine*. 18(5):262–9.

Fielder, R.J., Gaunt, I.F., Rhodes, C. et al. 1987. A hierarchical approach to the assessment of dermal and ocular irritancy: a report by the British Toxicology Society Working Party on Irritancy. *Human Toxicology*. 6(4):269–78.

Fisher GJ, Kang S, Varani J, Bata-Csorgo Z, Wan Y, Datta S, Voorhees JJ 2002. Mechanisms of photoaging and chronological skin aging. *Archives of Dermatology*. 138:1462–70.

Fistarol, S.K., and P.H. Itin. 2010. Disorders of pigmentation. *Journal der Deutschen Dermatologischen Gesellschaft*. Mar;8(3):187–201.

Freinkel, R.K., and D.T. Woodley, eds. 2001. *The Biology of the Skin*. Parthenon Publishing Pearl River, New York.

Frith, C.H., Ward, J.M., Harleman, J.H. et al. 2001. Hematopoietic system. In: Mohr, U. (ed.). *International Classification of Rodent Tumors. The Mouse*. Springer-Verlag, Heidelberg, pp. 417–51.

Frohm, M., Agerberth, B., Ahangari, G. et al. 1997. The expression of the gene coding for the antibacterial peptide LL-37 is induced in human keratinocytes during inflammatory disorders. *Journal of Biological Chemistry*. 272(24):15258–63.

Fuchs, E. 1995. Keratins and the skin. *Annual Review of Cell and Developmental Biology*. 11:123–53.

Fujita, H., Nograles, K.E., Kikuchi, T. et al. 2009. Human Langerhans cells induce distinct IL-22-producing CD4+ T cells lacking IL-17 production. *Proceedings of the National Academy of Sciences USA*. 106(51):21795–800.

Fullerton, A., Rode, B., and J. Serup. 2002. Skin irritation typing and grading based on laser Doppler perfusion imaging. *Skin Research and Technology*. 8(1):23–31.

Funk-Keenan, J., Sacco, J., Amos Wong, Y.Y., Rasmussen, S., Mosting-Reif A., and L.A. Trepanier. 2012. Evaluation of Polymorphisms in the sulfonamide detoxification genes CYB5A and CYB5R3 in dogs with sulfopnamide hypersensitivity. *J Veterinary Internal Medicine* 26:1126–33.

Garma-Avina, A., Valli, V.E., and J.H. Lumsden. 1981. Cutaneous melanomas in domestic animals. *Journal of Cutaneous Pathology*. 8:3–24.

Gibran, N.S., Boyce, S., and D.G. Greenhalgh. 2007. Cutaneous wound healing. *Journal of Burn Care and Research*. 28(4):577–9.

Gleiser, C.A., Raulston, G.L., Jardine, J.H. et al. 1979. Malignant fibrous histiocytoma in dogs and cats. *Veterinary Pathology*. 16(2):199–208.

Glick, A.D., Holscher, M., and G.R. Campbell. 1976. Canine cutaneous histiocytoma: ultrastructural and cyto-chemical observations. *Veterinary Pathology.* 13(5):374–80.

Godin, B., and E. Touitou. 2007. Transdermal skin delivery: predictions for humans from *in vivo*, ex vivo and animal models. *Advanced Drug Delivery Reviews.* 59:1152–61.

Gomez, E.C. 1975. Hamster flank organ: relevance of studies with topically applied antiandrogens. In: Maibach, H.I. (ed.). *Animal Models in Dermatology.* Churchill Livingstone, New York.

Goodman, D.G., Ward, J.M., Squire, R.A. et al. 1979. Neoplastic and nonneoplastic lesions in aging F344 rats. *Toxicology and Applied Pharmacology.* 48(2):237–48.

Goodman, D.G., Ward, J.M., Squire, R.A. et al. 1980. Neoplastic and nonneoplastic lesions in aging Osborne–Mendel rats. *Toxicology and Applied Pharmacology.* 55(3):433–47.

goRENI (global open RENI—the standard reference for nomenclature and diagnostic criteria in toxicologic pathology) website: http://www.goreni.org/. 2012.

Greaves, P. 2000. *Histopathology of Preclinical Toxicity Studies. Interpretation and Relevance in Drug Safety Evaluation.* 2nd ed. Elsevier, New York.

Greaves, P., and J.M. Faccini. 1981. Spontaneous fibrous histiocytic neoplasms in rats. *British Journal of Cancer.* 43(3):402–11.

Greaves, P., Martin, J.M., and Y. Rabemampianina. 1985. Malignant fibrous histiocytoma in rats at sites of implanted millipore filters. *American Journal of Pathology.* 120(2):207–14.

Greaves, P., Williams, A., and M. Eve. 2004. First dose of potential new medicines to humans: how animals help. *Nature Reviews, Drug Discovery.* 3:226–36.

Grey, J.E., Enoch, S., and K.G. Harding. 2006. ABC of wound healing. Wound assessment. *British Medical Journal.* 332:285–8.

Gschwendtner, A., Lorenz, A., and T. Mairinger. 1994. How thick is your section?—A simple method to evaluate the thickness of paraffin sections. *Analytical Cellular Pathology.* 6:201.

Gupta, R.K., Aberdeen, G., Babus, J.K. et al. 2007. Methoxychlor and its metabolites inhibit growth and induce atresia of baboon antral follicles. *Toxicologic Pathology.* 35(5):649–56.

Haines, D.C., and S.L. Eustis. 1990. Specialized sebaceous glands. In: Boorman, G.A. et al. (eds.). *Pathology of the Fischer Rat Reference and Altas. Vol. II.* Academic Press, San Diego, pp. 279–93.

Hajdu, S.D., Agmon-Levin, N., and Y. Shoenfel. 2011. Silicone and autoimmunity. *European Journal of Clinical Investigation.* 41(2):201–11.

Halata, Z., Grim, M., and K.I. Bauman. 2003. Friedrich Sigmund Merkel and his "Merkel cell" morphology, development, and physiology: review and new results. *Anatomical Record. Part A, Discoveries in Molecular, Cellular, and Evolutionary Biology.* 271(1):225–39.

Hardisty, J.F., Elwell, M.R., Ernst, H. et al. 2007. Histopathology of hemangiosarcomas in mice and hamsters and liposarcomas/fibrosarcomas in rats associated with PPAR agonists. *Toxicologic Pathology.* 35(7):928–41.

Hargis, A.M., Thomassen, R.W., and R.D. Phemister. 1977. Chronic dermatosis and cutaneous squamous cell carcinoma in the beagle dog. *Veterinary Pathology.* 14(3):218–28.

Harvima, I.T. and G. Nilsson. 2011. Mast cells as regulators of skin inflammation and immunity. *Acta Dermato-Venereologica.* 91(6):644–50.

Haschek, W.M., Rousseaux, C.G., and M.A. Wallig. 2010. Skin and oral mucosa. In: Haschek, W.M., Rousseaux, C.G., and M.A. Wallig (eds.). *Fundamentals of Toxicologic Pathology.* 2nd ed. Academic Press, New York, pp. 135–61.

Haseman, J.K., Hailey, J.R., and R.W. Morris. 1998. Spontaneous neoplasm incidences in Fischer 344 rats and B6C3F1 mice in two-year carcinogenicity studies: a National Toxicology Program update. *Toxicologic Pathology.* 26(3):428–41.

Health Canada. Health Products and Food Branch. 2009. Summary Basis of Decision (SBD) PrMetvix™. Submission Control Number: 110853.

Hecker, E. 1987. Three stage carcinogenesis in mouse skin—recent results and present status of an advanced model system of chemical carcinogenesis. *Toxicologic Pathology.* 15(2):245–58.

Heib, V., Becker, M., Taube, C. et al. 2008. Advances in the understanding of mast cell function. *British Journal of Haematology.* 142(5):683–94.

Helm, K.F., Helm, T., and F. Helm. 1993. Palisading cutaneous fibrous histiocytoma. An immunohistochemical study demonstrating differentiation from dermal dendrocytes. *American Journal of Dermatopathology.* 15(6):559–61.

Helman, R.G., Hall, J.W., and J.Y. Kao. 1986. Acute dermal toxicity: in vivo and in vitro comparisons in mice. *Fundamental and Applied Toxicology.* 7(1):94–100.

Hendrix, J.D., Jr., and K.E. Greer. 1992. Cutaneous hyperpigmentation caused by systemic drugs. *International Journal of Dermatology.* 31(7):458–66.

Hickman, J.G., Huber, F., and M. Palmisano. 2001. Human dermal safety studies with eflornithine HCl 13.9% cream (Vaniqa), a novel treatment for excessive facial hair. *Current Medical Research and Opinion.* 16(4):235–44.

Hirobe, T. 2011. How are proliferation and differentiation of melanocytes regulated? *Pigment Cell and Melanoma Research.* 24(3):462–78.

Hottendorf, G.H. and S.W. Nielsen. 1966. Collagen necrosis in canine mastocytomas. *American Journal of Pathology.* 49(3):501–13.

Hubbs, A.F., Mercer, R.R., Benkovic, S.A. et al. 2011. Nanotoxicology—a pathologist's perspective. *Toxicologic Pathology.* 39:301–24.

ICH (International Conference on Harmonisation of Technical Requirements for Registration of Pharmaceuticals for Human Use): http://www.ich.org/products/guidelines/safety/article/safety-guidelines.html.

Igyarto, B.Z., Haley, K., Ortner, D. et al. 2011. Skin-resident murine dendritic cell subsets promote distinct and opposing antigen-specific T helper cell responses. *Immunity.* 35(2):260–72.

Ilkovitch, D. 2011. Role of immune-regulatory cells in skin pathology. *Journal of Leukocyte Biology.* 89(1):41–9.

INHAND. 2012. [Mecklenburg, L., Kusewitt, D., Bradley, A. et al. 2012. Proliferative and non-proliferative lesions of the rat and mouse integument. Unpublished draft].

ISO (International Organization for Standardization). 2008. http://www.iso.org/iso/home.html.

Itagaki, S., Ishii, Y., Lee. M.J. et al. 1995. Dermal histology of hairless rat derived from Wistar strain. *Experimental Animals.* 44(4):279–84.

Ito, Y., and K. Jimbow. 1987. Selective cytotoxicity of 4-S-cysteaminylphenol on follicular melanocytes of the black mouse: rational basis for its application to melanoma chemotherapy. *Cancer Research.* 47(12):3278–84.

Ito, Y., Jimbow, K., and S. Ito. 1987. Depigmentation of black guinea pig skin by topical application of cysteaminylphenol, cysteinylphenol, and related compounds. *Journal of Investigative Dermatology.* 88: 77–82.

Jacobs, A.C., Brown, P.C., Chen, C. et al. 2004. CDER photosafety guidance for industry. *Toxicologic Pathology.* 32(Suppl. 2):17–8.

Jacobs, J.J., Lehe, C., Cammans, K.D. et al. 2002. An in vitro model for detecting skin irritants: methyl green-pyronine staining of human skin explant cultures. *Toxicology in Vitro.* 16(5):581–8.

Jacobs, J.J., and R.M. Urban. 1996. More on reaction to a foreign body after hip replacement. *New England Journal of Medicine.* 335(22):1690–1.

Jacobson-Kram, D., Sistare, F.D., and A.C. Jacobs. 2004. Use of transgenic mice in carcinogenicity hazard assessment. *Toxicologic Pathology.* 32(Suppl. 1):49–52.

Jirova, D., Basketter, D., Liebsch, M. et al. 2010. Comparison of human skin irritation patch test data with in vitro skin irritation assays and animal data. *Contact Dermatitis.* 62(2):109–16.

Johnson, M.L., and R.E. Grimwood. 1994. Leukocyte colony-stimulating factors. A review of associated neutrophilic dermatoses and vasculitides. *Archives of Dermatology.* 130(1):77–81.

Kadekaro, A.L., Kavanagh R.J., Wakamatsu, K. et al. 2003. Cutaneous photobiology. The melanocyte vs. the sun: who will win the final round? *Pigment Cell Research.* 16(5):434–47.

Kao, J., Hall, J., and J.M. Holland. 1983. Quantitation of cutaneous toxicity: an in vitro approach using skin organ culture. *Toxicology and Applied Pharmacology.* 68(2):206–17.

Kao, J., Patterson, F.K., and J. Hall. 1985. Skin penetration and metabolism of topically applied chemicals in six mammalian species, including man: an in vitro study with benzo[a]pyrene and testosterone. *Toxicology and Applied Pharmacology.* 81(3 Pt 1):502–16.

Karaoui, L.R., and C. Chahine-Chakhtoura. 2009. Fatal toxic epidermal necrolysis associated with minoxidil. *Pharmacotherapy.* 29(4):460–7.

Kasraee, B. 2002. Depigmentation of brown Guinea pig skin by topical application of methimazole. *Journal of Investigative Dermatology.* 118(1):205–7.

Katagiri, T., Okubo, T., Oyobikawa, M. et al. 2001. Inhibitory action of 4-n-butylresorcinol (Recinol®) on melanogenesis and its effects on human pigmentation. *Journal of the Society of Cosmetic Chemists, Japan.* 35(1):42–9.

Kato, M., Takahashi, M., Akhand, A.A. et al. 1998. Transgenic mouse model for skin malignant melanoma. *Oncogene.* 17(14):1885–8.

Kelly, D.F. 1970. Canine cutaneous histiocytoma. A light and electron microscopic study. *Pathologia Veterinaria.* 7(1):12–27.

Khan, F.D., Roychowdhury, S., Gaspari, A.A. et al. 2006. Immune response to xenobiotics in the skin: from contact sensitivity to drug allergy. *Expert Opinion on Drug Metabolism and Toxicology.* 2(2):261–72.

Khan, K.N., Kats, A.A., Fouant, M.M. et al. 1996. Recombinant human interleukin-3 induces extramedullary hematopoiesis at subcutaneous injection sites in cynomolgus monkeys. *Toxicologic Pathology.* 24(4):391–7.

Khattri, R., Cox, T., Yasayko, S.A. et al. 2003. An essential role for Scurfin in CD4+ CD25+ T regulatory cells. *Nature Immunology*. 4(4):337–42.

Kimber, I., Basketter, D.A., Berthold, K. et al. 2001. Skin sensitization testing in potency and risk assessment. *Toxicological Sciences*. 59(2):198–208.

Kimura, T. 1996. Studies on development of hairless descendants of Mexican hairless dogs and their usefulness in dermatological science. *Experimental Animals*. 45(1):1–13.

Kimura, T., Kuroki, K., and K. Doi. 1998. Dermatotoxicity of agricultural chemicals in the dorsal skin of hairless dogs. *Toxicologic Pathology*. 26(3):442–7.

Kingston, M.E., and D. Mackey. 1986. Skin clues in the diagnosis of life-threatening infections. *Reviews of Infectious Diseases*. 8(1):1–11.

Kligman, A.M., and L.H. Kligman. 1998. A hairless mouse model for assessing the chronic toxicity of topically applied chemicals. *Food and Chemical Toxicology*. 36(9–10):867–78.

Knowles, D.P., and A.M. Hargis. 1986. Solar elastosis associated with neoplasia in two dalmations. *Veterinary Pathology*. 23(4):512–4.

Koschwanez, H.E., and E. Broadbent. 2011. The use of wound healing assessment methods in psychological studies: a review and recommendations. *British Journal of Health Psychology*. 16(Pt 1):1–32.

Kreilgaard, M., Pedersen, E.J., and J.W. Jaroszewski. 2000. NMR characterization and transdermal drug delivery potential of microemulsion systems. *Journal of Controlled Release*. 69(Dec 3):421–33.

Kronevi, T., Wahlberg, J., and B. Holmberg. 1979. Histopathology of skin, liver, and kidney after epicutaneous administration of five industrial solvents to guinea pigs. *Environmental Research*. 19(1):56–69.

Lademann, J., Richter, H., Meinke, M. et al. 2010. Which skin model is the most appropriate for the investigation of topically applied substances into the hair follicles? *Skin Pharmacology and Physiology*. 23(1):47–52.

Lafontan, M. 2012. Historical perspectives in fat cell biology: the fat cell as a model for the investigation of hormonal and metabolic pathways. *American Journal of Physiology—Cell Physiology*. Jan;302(2):C327–59.

Lambertini, L., Surin, K., Ton, T.V. et al. 2005. Analysis of p53 tumor suppressor gene, H-ras protooncogene and proliferating cell nuclear antigen (PCNA) in squamous cell carcinomas of HRA/Skh mice following exposure to 8-methoxypsoralen (8-MOP) and UVA radiation (PUVA therapy). *Toxicologic Pathology*. 33(2):292–9.

Langner, A., Wolska, H., Marzulli, F.N. et al. 1977. Dermal toxicity of 8-methoxypsoralen administered (by gavage) to hairless mice irradiated with long-wave ultraviolet light. *Journal of Investigative Dermatology*. 69(5):451–7.

Lau, D.C.W., Dhillon, B., Yan, H. et al. 2005. Adipokines: molecular links between obesity and atherosclerosis. *American Journal of Physiology—Heart and Circulatory Physiology*. 288:H2031–H2041.

Lavergne, S.N., Danhof, R.S., Volkman, E.M. et al. 2006. Association of drug-serum protein adducts and anti-drug antibodies in dogs with sulphonamide hypersensitivity: a naturally occurring model of idiosyncratic drug toxicity. *Clinical and Experimental Allergy*. 36:907–15.

Lavergne, S.N., Drescher, N.J., and L.A. Trepanier, 2008. Anti-myeloperoxidase and anti-cathepsin G antibodies in sulphonamide hypersensitivity. *Clinical and Experimental Allergy*. 38:199–207.

Le Calvez, S., Perron-Lepage, M.F., and R. Burnett. 2006. Subcutaneous microchip-associated tumours in B6C3F1 mice: a retrospective study to attempt to determine their histogenesis. *Experimental and Toxicologic Pathology*. Mar;57(4):255–65.

Liebsch, M., and H. Spielmann. 2002. Currently available in vitro methods used in the regulatory toxicology. *Toxicology Letters*. 127(1–3):127–34.

Lin, J.Y., and D.E. Fisher. 2007. Melanocyte biology and skin pigmentation. *Nature*. 445(7130):843–50.

Liu, Y., Chen, J.Y., Shang, H.T. et al. 2010. Light microscopic, electron microscopic, and immunohistochemical comparison of Bama minipig (*Sus scrofa domestica*) and human skin. *Comparative Medicine*. 60(2):142–8.

Lorenz, W., Schmal, A., Schult, H. et al. 1982. Histamine release and hypotensive reactions in dogs by solubilizing agents and fatty acids: analysis of various components in cremophor El and development of a compound with reduced toxicity. *Agents and Actions*. 12(1–2):64–80.

Louden, C., Brott, D., Katein, A. et al. 2006. Biomarkers and mechanisms of drug-induced vascular injury in non-rodents. *Toxicologic Pathology*. 34(1):19–26.

Lovell, W.W., and D.J. Sanders. 1992. Phototoxicity testing in guinea-pigs. *Food and Chemical Toxicology*. 30(2):155–60.

Lowenstine, L.J. 2003. A primer of primate pathology: lesions and nonlesions. *Toxicologic Pathology*. 31(Suppl.):92–102.

Luderschmidt, C., Bidlingmaier, F., and G. Plewig. 1982. Inhibition of sebaceous gland activity by spironolactone in Syrian hamster. *Journal of Investigative Dermatology*. 78(3):253–5.

Luger, T.A. 2002. Neuromediators—a crucial component of the skin immune system. *Journal of Dermatological Science*. 30(2):87–93.

Lumb, G., Mitchell, L., and F.A. de la Iglesia. 1985. Regression of pathologic changes induced by the long-term administration of contraceptive steroids to rodents. *Toxicologic Pathology*. 13(4):283–95.

Lynch, D., Svoboda, J., Putta, S. et al. 2007. Mouse skin models for carcinogenic hazard identification: utilities and challenges. *Toxicologic Pathology*. 35(7):853–64.

Madewell, B.R. 1981. Neoplasms in domestic animals: a review of experimental and spontaneous carcinogenesis. *Yale Journal of Biology and Medicine*. 54(2):111–25.

Madison, K.C. 2003. Barrier function of the skin: "la raison d'être" of the epidermis. *Journal of Investigative Dermatology*. Aug;121(2):231–41.

Maekawa, A., Onodera, H., Tanigawa, H. et al. 1983. Neoplastic and non-neoplastic lesions in aging Slc: Wistar rats. *Journal of Toxicological Sciences*. 8(4):279–90.

Makinen, M., Forbes, P.D., and F. Stenback. 1997. Quinolone antibacterials: a new class of photochemical carcinogens. *Journal of Photochemistry and Photobiology. B—Biology*. 37(3):182–7.

Mantzoros, C.S., Magkos, F., Brinkoetter, M. et al. 2011. Leptin in human physiology and pathophysiology. *American Journal of Physiology, Endocrinology and Metabolism*. 301(4):E567–84.

Maraschin, R., Bussi, R., Conz, A. et al. 1995. Toxicological evaluation of u-hEGF. *Toxicologic Pathology*. 23(3):356–66.

Maratea, K.A., Snyder, P.W., and G.W. Stevenson. 2006. Vascular lesions in nine Gottingen minipigs with thrombocytopenic purpura syndrome. *Veterinary Pathology*. 43(4):447–54.

Marchini, G., Lindow, S., Brismar, H. et al. 2002. The newborn infant is protected by an innate antimicrobial barrier: peptide antibiotics are present in the skin and vernix caseosa. *British Journal of Dermatology*. 147(6):1127–34.

Marrakchi, S., and H.I. Maibach. 2006. Sodium lauryl sulfate-induced irritation in the human face: regional and age-related differences. *Skin Pharmacology and Physiology*. 19(3):177–80.

Maurer, T. 1987. Phototoxicity testing—in vivo and in vitro. *Food and Chemical Toxicology*. 25(5):407–14.

McAnulty, P.A., Dayan A.D., and N.-C. Ganderup, eds. 2011. *The Minipig in Biomedical Research*. CRC Press, Boca Raton, FL.

McDonagh, A.J., and A.G. Messenger. 1994. The aetiology and pathogenesis of alopecia areata. *Journal of Dermatological Science*. 7(Suppl.):S125–35.

McDonagh, A.J., and A.G. Messenger. 1996. The pathogenesis of alopecia areata. *Dermatologic Clinics*. 14(4):661–70.

McElwee, K.J., Freyschmidt-Paul, P., Sundberg, J.P. et al. 2003a. The pathogenesis of alopecia areata in rodent models. *Journal of Investigative Dermatology. Symposium Proceedings*. 8(1):6–11.

McElwee, K.J., Silva, K., Boggess, D. et al. 2003b. Alopecia areata in C3H/HeJ mice involves leukocyte-mediated root sheath disruption in advance of overt hair loss. *Veterinary Pathology*. 40(6):643–50.

McGovern, V.J., Cochran, A.J., Van der Esch, E.P. et al. 1986. The classification of malignant melanoma, its histological reporting and registration: a revision of the 1972 Sydney classification. *Pathology*. 18(1):12–21.

McKillop, C.M., Brock, J.A., Oliver, G.J. et al. 1987. A quantitative assessment of pyrethroid-induced paraesthesia in the guinea-pig flank model. *Toxicology Letters*. 36(1):1–7.

McMillan, E.M., Stoneking, L., Burdick, S. et al. 1985. Immunophenotype of lymphoid cells in positive patch tests of allergic contact dermatitis. *Journal of Investigative Dermatology*. 84(3):229–33.

Merk, H.F. 2009. Drug skin metabolites and allergic drug reactions. *Current Opinion in Allergy and Clinical Immunology*. 9:311–25.

Merk, H.F., Sachs, B., and J. Baron. 2001. The skin: target organ in immunotoxicology of small-molecular-weight compounds. *Skin Pharmacology and Applied Skin Physiology*. 14(6):419–30.

Militzer, K., and E. Wecker. 1986. Behaviour-associated alopecia areata in mice. *Laboratory Animals*. 20(1):9–13.

Miner, J.L. 2004. The adipocyte as an endocrine cell. *Journal of Animal Science*. 82(3):935–41.

Mintz, B., Silvers, W.K., and A.J. Klein-Szanto. 1993. Histopathogenesis of malignant skin melanoma induced in genetically susceptible transgenic mice. *Proceedings of the National Academy of Sciences of the United States of America*. 90(19):8822–6.

Miyamura, Y., Coelho, S.G., Wolber, R. et al. 2007. Regulation of human skin pigmentation and responses to ultraviolet radiation. *Pigment Cell Research*. 20(1):2–13.

Moll, R., Divo, M., and L. Langbein. 2008. The human keratins: biology and pathology. *Histochemistry and Cell Biology*. 129(6):705–33.

Monteiro-Riviere, N.A., Bristol, D.G., Manning, T.O. et al. 1990. Interspecies and interregional analysis of the comparative histologic thickness and laser Doppler blood flow measurements at five cutaneous sites in nine species. *Journal of Investigative Dermatology*. 95(5):582–6.

Monteiro-Riviere, N.A., Inman, A.O., Mak., V. et al. 2001. Effect of selective lipid extraction from different body regions on epidermal barrier function. *Pharmaceutical Research*. 18(7):992–8.

Monti, D., Brini, I., Tampucci, S. et al. 2008. Skin permeation and distribution of two sunscreens: a comparison between reconstituted human skin and hairless rat skin. *Skin Pharmacology and Physiology.* 21(6):318–25.

Moore, H.L. Jr., Szczech, G.M., Rodwell., D.E. et al. 1983. Preclinical toxicology studies with acyclovir: teratologic, reproductive and neonatal tests. *Fundamental and Applied Toxicology.* 3(6):560–8.

Moore, P.F. 1986. Characterization of cytoplasmic lysozyme immunoreactivity as a histiocytic marker in normal canine tissues. *Veterinary Pathology.* 23(6):763–9.

Moskalewski, S., Terelak, B., and S. Majewski. 1988. Occurrence of large groups of mast cells in subcutaneous connective tissue in the mouse. *Archivum Immunologiae et Therapiae Experimentalis.* 36(2):141–50.

Muhammad, F., Monteiro-Riviere, N.A., and J.E. Riviere. 2005. Comparative in vivo toxicity of topical JP-8 jet fuel and its individual hydrocarbon components: identification of tridecane and tetradecane as key constituents responsible for dermal irritation. *Toxicologic Pathology.* 33(2):258–66.

Nakamura, K., and W.C. Johnson. 1968. Ultraviolet light induced connective tissue changes in rat skin: a histopathologic and histochemical study. *Journal of Investigative Dermatology.* 51:253–8.

Nakashima, N., Takahashi, K., Harada, T. et al. 1996. An epithelioid cell type of amelanotic melanoma of the pinna in a Fischer-344 rat: a case report. *Toxicologic Pathology.* 24(2):258–61.

Nasir, A. 2010a. Nanotechnology and dermatology: part I—potential of nanotechnology. *Clinics in Dermatology.* 28(4):458–66.

Nasir, A. 2010b. Nanotechnology and dermatology: part II—risks of nanotechnology. *Clinics in Dermatology.* 28(5):581–8.

National Academy of Sciences Committee for the Revision of NAS Publication 1138. 1977. *Principles and Procedures for Evaluating the Toxicity of Household Substances.* Washington, DC, National Academy of Science, pp. 23–59.

Neis, M.M., Wendel, A., Wiederholt, T. et al. 2010. Expression and induction of cytochrome p450 isoenzymes in human skin equivalents. *Skin Pharmacology and Physiology.* 23(1):29–39.

Nemecek, G.M., and A.D. Dayan. 1999. Safety evaluation of human living skin equivalents. *Toxicologic Pathology.* 27(1):101–3.

Nestle, F.O., Conrad, C., Tun-Kyi, A. et al. 2005. Plasmacytoid predendritic cells initiate psoriasis through interferon alpha production. *Journal of Experimental Medicine.* 202(1):135–43.

Ng, W., Lobach, A.R., ZHu, X., Chen, X., Liu, F., Meushi, I.G., Sharma, A., Li, J., Cai, P., Ip, J., Novalen, M., Popovic, M., Zhang, X., Tanino, T., Nakagawa, T., Li, Y., and J. Uetrecht. 2012. Animal models of idiosyncratic drug reactions. *Advances in Pharmacology.* 63:81–135.

Nickoloff, B.J. 2006. Keratinocytes regain momentum as instigators of cutaneous inflammation. *Trends in Molecular Medicine.* 12(3):102–6.

Nickoloff, B.J., and L.A. Turka. 1993. Keratinocytes: key immunocytes of the integument. *American Journal of Pathology.* 143(2):325–31.

NICNAS. 2007. Existing Chemicals Information Sheet. Sodium Lauryl Sulfate. Chemical Abstract Service (CAS) Number: 152-21-3.

NIOSH (The National Institute for Occupational Safety and Health). 2009. http://www.cdc.gov/niosh/.

Nishikawa, S., Yamashita, T., Imai, T. et al. 2010. Erratum: thesaurus for histopathological findings in publically available reports of repeated-dose oral toxicity studies in rats for 156 chemicals. *Journal of Toxicological Sciences.* 35(4):E1–8.

Nixon, G.A., Tyson, C.A., and W.C. Wertz. 1975. Interspecies comparisons of skin irritancy. *Toxicology and Applied Pharmacology.* 31(3):481–90.

Oesch, F., Fabian, E., Oesch-Bartlomowicz, B. et al. 2007. Drug-metabolizing enzymes in the skin of man, rat and pig. *Drug Metabolism Reviews.* 39:659–98.

Olson, H., Betton, G., Robinson, D. et al. 2000. Concordance of the toxicity of pharmaceuticals in humans and in animals. *Regulatory Toxicology and Pharmacology.* 32(1):56–67.

Ono, C., Yamada M., and M. Tanaka. 2003. Absorption, distribution and excretion of ^{14}C-chloroquine after single oral administration in albino and pigmented rats: binding characteristics of chloroquine-related radioactivity to melanin in-vivo. *Journal of Pharmacy and Pharmacology.* 55(12):1647–54.

Ootsuyama, A., and H. Tanooka. 1988. One hundred percent tumor induction in mouse skin after repeated beta irradiation in a limited dose range. *Radiation Research.* 115(3):488–94.

OSHA (Occupational Health and Safety Administration). 2006. http://www.osha.gov/.

Oxenhandler, R.W., Berkelhammer, J., Smith, G.D. et al. 1982. Growth and regression of cutaneous melanomas in Sinclair miniature swine. *American Journal of Pathology.* 109(3):259–69.

Paczesny, S., Braun, T.M., Levine, J.E. et al. 2010. Elafin is a biomarker of graft-versus-host disease of the skin. *Science Translational Medicine.* 2(13):13ra2.

Panteleyev, A.A., and A.M. Christiano. 2001. The Charles River "hairless" rat mutation is distinct from the hairless mouse alleles. *Comparative Medicine*. 51(1):49–55.

Panteleyev, A.A., and D.R. Bickers. 2006. Dioxin-induced chloracne—reconstructing the cellular and molecular mechanisms of a classic environmental disease. *Expimental Dermatology*. 15(9):705–30.

Parker, W.M. 1981. Autoimmune skin diseases in the dog. *Canadian Veterinary Journal*. 22(10):302–4.

Patrick, E., Maibach, H.I., and A. Burkhalter. 1985. Mechanisms of chemically induced skin irritation. I. Studies of time course, dose response, and components of inflammation in the laboratory mouse. *Toxicology and Applied Pharmacology*. 81(3 Pt 1):476–90.

Paul, C.N., Voigt, D.W., Clyne, K.E. et al. 1998. Case report: oxaprozin and fatal toxic epidermal necrolysis. *Pharmacotherapy*. 18(2):392–8.

Paus, R., and G. Cotsarelis. 1999. The biology of hair follicles. *New England Journal of Medicine*. 341(7):491–7.

Phillips, L., Steinberg, M., Maibach, H.I. et al. 1972. A comparison of rabbit and human skin response to certain irritants. *Toxicology and Applied Pharmacology*. 21(3):369–82.

Pierard, G.E. 1979. Toxic effects of metals from the environment on hair growth and structure. *Journal of Cutaneous Pathology*. 6(4):237–42.

Pilling, A.M., Harman, R.M., Jones, S.A. et al. 2002. The assessment of local tolerance, acute toxicity, and DNA biodistribution following particle-mediated delivery of a DNA vaccine to minipigs. *Toxicologic Pathology*. 30(3):298–305.

Plewig, G., and C. Luderschmidt. 1977. Hamster ear model for sebaceous glands. *The Journal of Investigative Dermatology*. 68(4):171–6.

Pollard, R.B., Robinson P., and K. Dransfield. 1998. Safety profile of nevirapine, a nonnucleoside reverse transcriptase inhibitor for the treatment of human immunodeficiency virus infection. *Clinical Therapeutics*. 20(6):1071–92.

Popovic, M., Caswell, J.L., Mannargudi, B. et al. 2006. Study of the sequence of events involved in nevirapine-induced skin rash in in brown norway rats. *Chemical Research in Toxicology*. 19:1205–14.

Popovic, M., Shenton, J.M., Chen, J., et al. 2010. Nevirapine hypersensitivity. *Handbook of Experimental Pharmacology*. 196:437–51.

Porter, R.M. 2006. The new keratin nomenclature. *Journal of Investigative Dermatology*. Nov;126(11):2366–8.

Prahalada, S., Stabinski, L.G., Chen, H.Y. et al. 1998. Pharmacological and toxicological effects of chronic porcine growth hormone administration in dogs. *Toxicologic Pathology*. 26(2):185–200.

Pritchard, J.B., French, J.E., Davis, B.J. et al. 2003. The role of transgenic mouse models in carcinogen identification. *Environmental Health Perspectives*. 111(4):444–54.

Puhvel, S.M., Sakamoto, M., Ertl, D.C. et al. 1982. Hairless mice as models for chloracne: a study of cutaneous changes induced by topical application of established chloracnegens. *Toxicology and Applied Pharmacology*. 64(3):492–503.

Quinn, A.G., Sikkink, S., and J.L. Rees. 1994. Basal cell carcinomas and squamous cell carcinomas of human skin show distinct patterns of chromosome loss. *Cancer Research*. 54(17):4756–9.

Ramot, Y., Ben-Eliahu, S., Kagan, L. et al. 2009. Subcutaneous and intraperitoneal lipogranulomas following subcutaneous injection of olive oil in Sprague–Dawley rats. *Toxicologic Pathology*. 37(7):882–6.

Ramselaar, C.G., Ruitenberg, E.J., and W. Kruizinga. 1980. Regression of induced keratoacanthomas in anagen (hair growth phase) skin grafts in mice. *Cancer Research*. 40(5):1668–73.

Randall, K.J., and J.R. Foster. 2007. The demonstration of immunohistochemical biomarkers in methyl methacrylate-embedded plucked human hair follicles. *Toxicologic Pathology*. 35(7):952–7.

Rees, J.L. 2003. Genetics of hair and skin color. *Annual Review of Genetics*. 37:67–90.

Rees, J.L. 2004. The genetics of sun sensitivity in humans. *American Journal of Human Genetics*. 75: 739–51.

Renlund, R.C., and K.P. Pritzker. 1984. Malignant fibrous histiocytoma involving the digit in a cat. *Veterinary Pathology*. 21(4):442–4.

Ricklin, M.E., Roosje, P., and A. Summerfield. 2010. Characterization of canine dendritic cells in healthy, atopic, and non-allergic inflamed skin. *Journal of Clinical Immunology*. 30(6):845–54.

Rogers, J.V., and J.N. McDougal. 2002. Improved method for in vitro assessment of dermal toxicity for volatile organic chemicals. *Toxicology Letters*. 135(1–2):125–35.

Rogers, J.V., Price, J.A., and J.N. McDougal. 2009. A review of transcriptomics in cutaneous chemical exposure. *Cutaneous and Ocular Toxicology*. 28(4):157–70.

Romani, N., Brunner, P.M., and G. Stingl. 2012. Changing views of the roles of Langerhans cells. *Journal of Investigative Dermatology*. 132:872–81.

Romani, N., Holzmann, S., Tripp, C.H. et al. 2003. Langerhans cells—dendritic cells of the epidermis. *Acta Pathologica, Microbiologica, et Immunologica Scandinavica*. 111(7–8):725–40.

Rose, E.H., Vistnes, L.M., and G.A. Ksander. 1977. The panniculus carnosus in the domestic pig. *Plastic and Reconstructive Surgery*. 59(1):94–7.

Roussel, F., and J. Dalion. 1988. Lectins as markers of endothelial cells: comparative study between human and animal cells. *Laboratory Animals*. 22(2):135–40.

Rovee, D.T., Kurowsky, C.A., and J. Labun. 1972. Local wound environment and epidermal healing. Mitotic response. *Archives of Dermatology*. 106(3):330–4.

Ruiz-Maldonado, R., and M.L. Orozco-Covarrubias. 1997. Postinflammatory hypopigmentation and hyperpigmentation. *Seminars in Cutaneous Medicine and Surgery*. 16(1):36–43.

Ryan, C.A., Hulette, B.C., and G.F. Gerberick. 2001. Approaches for the development of cell-based in vitro methods for contact sensitization. *Toxicology in Vitro*. 15(1):43–55.

Salmon, J.K., Armstrong, C.A., and J.C. Ansel. 1994. The skin as an immune organ. *Western Journal of Medicine*. 160:146–52.

Samberg, M.E., Oldenburg, S.J., and N.A. Monteiro-Riviere. 2010. Evaluation of silver nanoparticle toxicity in skin in vivo and keratinocytes in vitro. *Environmental Health Perspectives*. 118(3):407–13.

Sarmiento, U., Benson, B., Kaufman, S. et al. 1997. Morphologic and molecular changes induced by recombinant human leptin in the white and brown adipose tissues of C57BL/6 mice. *Laboratory Investigation*. 77(3):243–56.

Sasaki, M., Miyazaki, Y., and T. Takahashi. 2003. Hylan G-F 20 induces delayed foreign body inflammation in Guinea pigs and rabbits. *Toxicologic Pathology*. 31(3):321–5.

Scallan, P.J., Kettler, A.H., Levy, M.L. et al. 1988. Neutrophilic eccrine hidradenitis. Evidence implicating bleomycin as a causative agent. *Cancer*. 62(12):2532–6.

SCENIHR (Scientific Committee on Emerging and Newly Identified Health Risks). 2007. http://ec.europa.eu/health/scientific_committees/emerging/index_en.htm.

Schäkel, K., and A. Hänsel. 2011. News from dendritic cells in atopic dermatitis. *Current Opinion in Allergy and Clinical Immunology*. 11(5):445–50. Review.

Schauber, J., and R.L. Gallo. 2008. Antimicrobial peptides and the skin immune defense system. *Journal of Allergy and Clinical Immunology*. 122(2):261–6.

Schweizer, J., Loehrke, H., Hesse, B. et al. 1982. 7,12-Dimethylbenz[*a*]anthracene/12-*O*-tetradecanoyl-phorbol-13-acetate-mediated skin tumor initiation and promotion in male Sprague–Dawley rats. *Carcinogenesis*. 3(7):785–9.

Scott, D.W. 1982. Histopathologic findings in endocrine skin disorders of the dog. *Journal of the American Animal Hospital Association*. 18:173–83.

Sells, D.M., and J.P. Gibson. 1987. Carcinogenicity studies with medroxalol hydrochloride in rats and mice. *Toxicologic Pathology*. 15(4):457–67.

Semlin, L., Schafer-Korting, M., Borelli, C. et al. 2011. In vitro models for human skin disease. *Drug Discovery Today*. 16:132–9.

Shenton, J.M., Teranishi, M., Abu-Asab M. et al. 2003. Characterization of a potential animal model of an idiosyncratic drug reaction: nevirapine-induced skin rash in the rat. *Chemical Research in Toxicology*. 16:1078–89.

Shenton, J.M., Popovic, M., Chen, J. et al. 2005. Evidence of an immune-mediated mechanism for an idiosyncratic nevirapine-induced reaction in the female Brown Norway rat. *Chemical Research in Toxicology*. 18:1799–813.

Shih, B., Garsie, E., McGrouther, D., and A. Bayat. 2010. Molecular dissection of abnormal wound healing processes resulting in keloid disease. *Wound Repair and Regeneration*. 18:139–53.

Shimoda, K., Yoshida, M., Wagai, N. et al. 1993. Phototoxic lesions induced by quinolone antibacterial agents in auricular skin and retina of albino mice. *Toxicologic Pathology*. 21(6):554–61.

Shoenfeld, Y., and N. Agmon-Levin. 2011. ASIA—autoimmune/inflammatory syndrome induced by adjuvants. *Journal of Autoimmunity*. 36:4–8.

Simon, G.A., and H.I. Maibach. 2000. The pig as an experimental animal model of percutaneous permeation in man: qualitative and quantitative observations—an overview. *Skin Pharmacology and Applied Skin Physiology*. 13(5):229–34.

Singer, A.J., and R.A. Clark. 1999. Cutaneous wound healing. *New England Journal of Medicine*. 341(10):738–46.

Sistare, F.D., Thompson, K.L., Honchel, R. et al. 2002. Evaluation of the Tg.AC transgenic mouse assay for testing the human carcinogenic potential of pharmaceuticals—practical pointers, mechanistic clues, and new questions. *International Journal of Toxicology*. 21:65–79.

Smith, A.G. 1994. Important cutaneous adverse drug reactions. *Adverse Drug Reaction Bulletin*. 167:631–4.

Smith, R.S., Smith, T.J., Blieden, T.M. et al. 1997. Fibroblasts as sentinel cells. Synthesis of chemokines and regulation of inflammation. *American Journal of Pathology*. 151(2):317–22.

Solano, F., Briganti, S., Picardo, M. et al. 2006. Hypopigmenting agents: an updated review on biological, chemical and clinical aspects. *Pigment Cell Research*. 19(6):550–71.

Sommer, M.M. 1997. Spontaneous skin neoplasms in Long–Evans rats. *Toxicologic Pathology*. 25(5):506–10.

Son, W.C., Bell, D., Taylor, I., and V. Mowat. 2010. Profile of early occurring spontaneous tumors in Han Wistar rats. *Toxicologic Pathology*. 38(2):292–6.

Son, W.C., and C. Gopinath. 2004. Early occurrence of spontaneous tumors in CD-1 mice and Sprague–Dawley rats. *Toxicologic Pathology*. 32(4):371–4.

Spielmann, H., and M. Liebsch. 2001. Lessons learned from validation of in vitro toxicity test: from failure to acceptance into regulatory practice. *Toxicology in Vitro*. 15(4–5):585–90.

Steinman, R.M., Hawiger, D., and M.C. Nussenzweig. 2003. Tolerogenic dendritic cells. *Annual Review of Immunology*. 21:685–711.

Stern, R.S. 1998. Photocarcinogenicity of drugs. *Toxicology Letters*. 102–3:389–92.

Stern, R.S., Nichols, K.T., and L.H. Vakeva. 1997. Malignant melanoma in patients treated for psoriasis with methoxsalen (psoralen) and ultraviolet A radiation (PUVA). The PUVA Follow-Up Study. *New England Journal of Medicine*. 336(15):1041–5.

Stoitzner, P. 2010. The Langerhans cell controversy: are they immunostimulatory or immunoregulatory cells of the skin immune system? *Immunology and Cell Biology*. 88(4):348–50.

Storer, R.E., Sistare, F.D., Reddy, M.V. et al. 2010. An industry perspective on the utility of short-term carcinogenicity testing in transgenic mice in pharmaceutical development. *Toxicologic Pathology*. 38:51–61.

Streilein, J.W. 1989. Skin-associated lymphoid tissue. *Immunology Series*. 46:73–96.

Strid J., Tigelaar, R.E., and A.C. Hayday. 2009. Skin immune surveillance by T cells, a new order. *Seminars in Immunology*. 21(3):110–20.

Sueki, H., Gammal, C., Kudoh, K. et al. 2000. Hairless guinea pig skin: anatomical basis for studies of cutaneous biology. *European Journal of Dermatology*. 10(5):357–64.

Sundberg, J.P., Beamer, W.G., Uno, H. et al. 1999. Androgenetic alopecia: in vivo models. *Experimental and Molecular Pathology*. 67(2):118–30.

Sunderman, F.W. Jr. 1989. Carcinogenicity of metal alloys in orthopedic prostheses: clinical and experimental studies. *Fundamental and Applied Toxicology*. 13(2):205–16.

Svendsen, O. 2006. The minipig in toxicology. *Experimental and Toxicologic Pathology*. 57(5–6):335–9.

Swindle, M.M., Makin, A., Herron, A.J. et al. 2012. Swine as models in biomedical research and toxicology testing. *Veterinary Pathology*. 49(2):344–56.

Szczech, G.M., and W.E. Tucker Jr. 1985. Nail loss and footpad erosions in beagle dogs given BW 134U, a nucleoside analog. *Toxicologic Pathology*. 13(3):181–4.

Tadokoro, T., Rouzaud, F., Itami, S. et al. 2003. The inhibitory effect of androgen and sex-hormone-binding globulin on the intracellular cAMP level and tyrosinase activity of normal human melanocytes. *Pigment Cell Research*. 16:190–7.

Taguchi, S., Kuriwaki, K., Souda, M. et al. 2006. Induction of sarcomas by a single subcutaneous injection of 7,12-dimethylbenz[*a*]anthracene into neonatal male Sprague–Dawley rats: histopathological and immunohistochemical analyses. *Toxicologic Pathology*. 34(4):336–47.

Takahashi, M., Horiuchi, Y., and T. Tezuka. 2004. Presence of bactericidal/permeability-increasing protein in human and rat skin. *Experimental Dermatology*. 13(1):55–60.

Taylor, D.O., Dorn, C.R., and O.H. Luis. 1969. Morphologic and biologic characteristics of the canine cutaneous histiocytoma. *Cancer Research*. 29(1):83–92.

Tennant, R.W., Tice, R.R., and J.W. Spalding. 1998. The transgenic Tg.AC mouse model for identification of chemical carcinogens. *Toxicology Letters*. 102–3:465–71.

Therrien, J.P., Pfutzner, W., and J.C. Vogel. 2008. An approach to achieve long-term expression in skin gene therapy. *Toxicologic Pathology*. 36(1):104–11.

Tillmann, T., Kamino, K., Dasenbrock, C. et al. 1997. Subcutaneous soft tissue tumours at the site of implanted microchips in mice. *Experimental and Toxicologic Pathology*. Aug;49(3–4):197–200.

Tindall, J.P. 1985. Chloracne and chloracnegens. *Journal of the American Academy of Dermatology*. 13(4):539–58.

Tkalcevic, V.I., Cuzic, S., Parnham, M.J. et al. 2009. Differential evaluation of excisional non-occluded wound healing in db/db mice. *Toxicologic Pathology*. 37(2):183–92.

Toews, G.B., Bergstresser, P.R., and J.W. Streilein. 1980. Langerhans cells: sentinels of skin associated lymphoid tissue. *Journal of Investigative Dermatology*. 75(1):78–82.

Tokura, Y., Kobayashi, M., and K. Kabashima. 2008. Epidermal chemokines and modulation by antihistamines, antibiotics and antifungals. *Experimental Dermatology*. 17(2):81–90. Review.

Trepanier, L.A.. Danhof, R., Toll, J. et al. 2003. Clinical findings in 40 dogs with hypersensitivity associated with administration of potentiated sulfonamides. *Journal of Veterinary Internal Medicine*. 17(5):647–52.

Tsuchiya, T., Takahashi, K., Takeya, M. et al. 1993. Immunohistochemical, quantitative immunoelectron microscopic, and DNA cytofluorometric characterization of chemically induced rat malignant fibrous histiocytoma. *American Journal of Pathology*. 143(2):431–45.

Tsukahara, K., Tamatsu, Y., Sugawara, Y., and K. Shimada. 2012. Morphological study of the relationship between solar elastosis and the development of wrinkels on the forehead and lateral canthus. *Archives of Dermatology* 148:913–7.

Tucker, W.E. Jr., Krasny, H.C., de Miranda, P. et al. 1983. Preclinical toxicology studies with acyclovir: carcinogenicity bioassays and chronic toxicity tests. *Fundamental and Applied Toxicology*. 3(6):579–86.

Uetrecht, J. 2006. Role of animal models in the study of drug-induced hypersensitivity reactions. *The AAPS Journal*. 7(4):E914–21.

Valladeau, J., Clair-Moninot, V., Dezutter-Dambuyant, C. et al. 2002. Identification of mouse langerin/CD207 in Langerhans cells and some dendritic cells of lymphoid tissues. *Journal of Immunology*. 15;168(2):782–92.

van der Fits, L., Mourits, S., Voerman, J.S. et al. 2009. Imiquimod-induced psoriasis-like skin inflammation in mice is mediated via the IL-23/IL-17 axis. *Journal of Immunology*. 182(9):5836–45.

van der Laan, J.W., Brightwell, J., McAnulty, P. et al. 2010. Regulatory acceptability of the minipig in the development of pharmaceuticals, chemicals and other products. *Journal of Pharmacological and Toxicological Methods*. 62(3):184–95.

Varani, J., Perone, P., Spahlinger, D.M. et al. 2007. Human skin in organ culture and human skin cells (keratinocytes and fibroblasts) in monolayer culture for assessment of chemically induced skin damage. *Toxicologic Pathology*. 35(5):693–701.

Virtanen, I., Lehto, V.P., Lehtonen, E. et al. 1981. Expression of intermediate filaments in cultured cells. *Journal of Cell Science*. 50:45–63.

Walsh, K.M., and A.W. Gough. 1989. Hypopigmentation in dogs treated with an inhibitor of platelet aggregation. *Toxicologic Pathology*. 17(3):549–53.

Wells, M.Y., Voute, H., Bellingard, V. et al. 2010. Histomorphology and vascular lesions in dorsal rat skin used as injection sites for a subcutaneous toxicity study. *Toxicologic Pathology*. 38(2):258–66.

Wester, R.C., Mailbach, H.I., and D.A. Bucks. 1989. Paraquat poisoning by skin absorption. *Human Toxicology*. 8(3):251–2.

Westwood, F.R., Duffy, P.A., Malpass, D.A. et al. 1995. Disturbance of macrophage and monocyte function in the dog by a thromboxane receptor antagonist: ICI 185,282. *Toxicologic Pathology*. 23(3):373–84.

Wilcock, B.P., Yager, J.A., and M.C. Zink. 1986. The morphology and behavior of feline cutaneous mastocytomas. *Veterinary Pathology*. 23(3):320–4.

Williams, D.F. 2009. On the nature of biomaterials. *Biomaterials*. 30(30):5897–909.

Wilson, D.K., and P.P. Agin. 1982. Detection of skin damage in the hairless mouse: histological hints. *Journal of Histotechnology*. 5(2):87–90.

Wintroub, B.U., and R. Stern. 1985. Cutaneous drug reactions: pathogenesis and clinical classification. *Journal of the American Academy of Dermatology*. 13(2 Pt 1):167–79.

Wood, G.S., Volterra, A.S., Abel, E.A. et al. 1986. Allergic contact dermatitis: novel immunohistologic features. *Journal of Investigative Dermatology*. 87(6):688–93.

Wright, J.A., Goonetilleke, U.R., Waghe, M. et al. 1991. An immunohistochemical study of spontaneous histiocytic tumours in the rat. *Journal of Comparative Pathology*. 104(2):223–32.

Xie, J., Murone, M., Luoh, S.M. et al. 1998. Activating smoothened mutations in sporadic basal-cell carcinoma. *Nature*. 391(6662):90–2.

Xie, Y., Zhu, K.Q., Deubner, H. et al. 2007. The microvasculature in cutaneous wound healing in the female red Duroc pig is similar to that in human hypertrophic scars and different from that in the female Yorkshire pig. *Journal of Burn Care and Research*. 28(3):500–6.

Yamaguchi, Y., and V.J. Hearing. 2009. Physiological factors that regulate skin pigmentation. *Biofactors*. 35(2):193–9.

Yang, H.Y., Joris, I., Majno, G. et al. 1985. Necrosis of adipose tissue induced by sequential infections with unrelated viruses. *American Journal of Pathology*. 120(2):173–7.

Yao, F., Visovatti, S., Johnson, C.S. et al. 2001. Age and growth factors in porcine full-thickness wound healing. *Wound Repair and Regeneration*. 9(5):371–7.

Yoshitomi, K., Elwell, M.R., and G.A. Boorman. 1995. Pathology and incidence of amelanotic melanomas of the skin in F-344/N rats. *Toxicologic Pathology*. 23(1):16–25.

Yuspa, S.H. 1998. The pathogenesis of squamous cell cancer: lessons learned from studies of skin carcinogenesis. *Journal of Dermatological Science*. 17(1):1–7.

Zackheim, H.S. 1973. Tumors of the skin. In: Turusov, V.S. (ed.). *Pathology of Tumors in Laboratory Animals. Volume I—Tumors of the Rat Part 1*. International Agency for Research on Cancer, Lyon, pp. 1–21.

Zanni, M.P., Schnyder, B., von Greyerz, S. et al. 1998. Involvement of T cells in drug-induced allergies. *Trends in Pharmacological Sciences*. 19(8):308–10.

Zbinden, G. 1987. Irritancy testing under review. *Human and Experimental Toxicology*. 6:263–4.

Zhang, J., Defelice, A.F., Hanig, J.P. et al. 2010. Biomarkers of endothelial cell activation serve as potential surrogate markers for drug-induced vascular injury. *Toxicologic Pathology*. 38(6):856–71.

Zhu, K.Q., Carrougher, G.J., Gibran, N.S. et al. 2007. Review of the female Duroc/Yorkshire pig model of human fibroproliferative scarring. *Wound Repair and Regeneration*. 15:S32–S39.

20 Nervous System

Mark T. Butt, Robert Sills, and Alys Bradley

CONTENTS

20.1 INTRODUCTION

There is one nervous system, with central and peripheral components. The system extends from the brain to the intraepidermal nerve fibers and includes everything in between. All aspects of the nervous system are potential therapeutic targets and are potentially susceptible to injury by drugs, chemicals, and every novel therapy currently under development.

Some components of the nervous system are somewhat protected behind so-called barriers. Others are more wide open to exposure to environmental and administered toxins.

Between the myriad of adverse changes that can be produced in the nervous system and the anxious general public seeking ever-improving methods of treating natural, acquired, and self-induced disease states is the toxicologic pathologist.

This chapter will provide the pathologist with some of the basic information necessary to recognize and interpret the variety of lesions that might be encountered in the nervous system. For the most part, this is not a methods chapter; that information can be found in other texts (Butt 2011). However, information needed to understand how the nervous system might be affected in a unique manner is provided.

The chapter is divided into five sections: Introduction, Special Considerations, Evaluation, Non-Proliferative Lesions, and Proliferative Lesions. The first section is part philosophy/part instruction from the perspective of someone who has spent the last 20 years specializing in the evaluation of the nervous system. The second section is a collection of notable features that may help understand how various test articles might interact with the nervous system. The third section provides some information on evaluation tactics. The fourth and fifth sections, to the best extent possible, are ordered similar to the recently revised International Harmonization of Nomenclature and Diagnostic Criteria for Lesions in Rats and Mice (INHAND) document (INHAND Project 2011) on the nervous system produced by a joint initiative of the societies of toxicologic pathology from Europe (European Society of Toxicologic Pathology [ESTP]), Great Britain (British Society of Toxicologic Pathologists

[BSTP]), Japan (Japanese Society of Toxicologic Pathology [JSTP]), and North America (Society of Toxicologic Pathology [STP]), and the Society of Toxicologic Pathology's Standardized System of Nomenclature and Diagnostic Criteria Guide (McMartin et al. 1997). These documents can be considered a supplement to this chapter. Both are succinct guides (with pictures) of various microscopic changes that may be encountered in the nervous system.

It is the role of the toxicologic pathologist to make sure that a reasonable effort is made to detect nervous system changes in every study where a conclusion regarding the morphologic state of the nervous system is relevant. It is fine to examine just a few sections of brain and spinal cord, as long as the conclusions do not make the broad announcement that there are no changes in the nervous system. "Based on the tissues examined in this study, there were no detectable morphologic changes in the brain and spinal cord" would be an acceptable conclusion for such an examination, but do not be fooled into thinking a peripheral neuropathy was ruled out when the portions of the nervous system needed to make that determination were not assessed. In other words, the first step in assessing the nervous system involves a thorough protocol review to determine whether or not the necessary components have been included to actually evaluate the nervous system.

Part of the protocol assessment involves doing a literature search on the test article/therapy being evaluated. It is remarkable how much information can be obtained with an easy literature search, and even more remarkable how few pathologists perform this simple, pre-evaluation task. If you are working within the firm or agency that produced the test article, information should be readily available. But even if you are with a contract research organization, a quick review of the test article producer's website, in addition to a literature review, may reveal vital information that greatly assists the pathologist and often saves everyone time.

If information is not available for a specific test article, the toxicologic pathologist should make every attempt to learn the basic pharmacology. This information may reveal the likelihood that the test article will gain entrance into the brain (although any compound may gain access to the brain in any given animal) or possibly provide a clue as to a particular component of the nervous system that is likely to be affected. For example, a test article with N-methyl-D-aspartate (NMDA) antagonist activity may produce vacuolation or necrosis of neurons in the cingulate cortex of the rat (Fix et al. 1996). This type of compound (and many others) warrants a special investigation to detect the related neurotoxicity. A structural homology with another compound may be a very good indicator of what a particular test article could do. Conversely, structural homology with a known neurotoxicant may have absolutely no bearing on how a new test article will affect tissues. Receptors, transport mechanisms, and metabolism can be very specific and interact with even very similar molecules quite differently.

Many study sponsors like to label their test article with a moniker that means nothing to even the educated observer. If that is the case, the pathologist should make an attempt to understand the actual test article. If the sponsor or study director is adamant that the pathologist evaluate the tissues without any pre-evaluation knowledge (known colloquially as a "blinded read"), that is fine. It will simply prevent the pathologist from using all available tools and information (at least during the initial evaluation).

After the literature review, the pathologist must study the clinical signs that may have been displayed during the course of the study. As complicated and difficult as it is to evaluate, there is one great advantage to the nervous system: clinical signs can often point to a specific region of the nervous system (Bolon and O'Brien 2011). Paresis or paralysis of the hind limbs without similar signs in the thoracic limbs indicates a spinal cord lesion caudal to the T3 spinal cord segment. A head tilt to one side may indicate a lesion in the cerebrum on the same side the head is tilted toward. A loss of balance could indicate a lesion affecting the region of the nucleus of cranial nerve 8. The list of possibilities is too extensive to include in this chapter, and each case can be investigated separately, but these clinical signs can be quite helpful in making sure an important level of the nervous system is evaluated.

Various syndromes may indicate changes in a particular portion of the brain (Bolon and O'Brien 2011). For example, a combination of altered mentation with deficiencies in postural reactions could (and probably does) indicate a morphologic change in the cerebrum. Tremors and a hypermetric gait indicate a cerebellar dysfunction. Correlating the clinical signs to the sites and severity of gross and microscopic lesions is the main job of the pathologist.

Functional observational battery (FOB) (Moser 2011) assessments are a specific part of many neurotoxicity investigations. If at all possible, the data from the FOB should be thoroughly analyzed prior to the trimming of the tissues in order to include any areas of the nervous system that may ordinarily not but should be examined morphologically, on the basis of alterations from control animals or baseline values of the various FOB parameters.

Clinical pathology data should also be evaluated. Several metabolic conditions such as liver failure can cause hepatic encephalopathy that may, among other things, cause alterations in the appearance of astrocytes in the brain. Hematologic indications of anemia or infection may have impacts on brain morphology.

Bottom line: Pathology is a medical investigation. Gather all the possible information you may need to augment your morphologic evaluation. Because so little of the entire nervous system is morphologically examined in most studies, take advantage of every opportunity to make your investigation as pertinent as possible.

20.2 SPECIAL CONSIDERATIONS

20.2.1 Special Consideration #1: Applied Neuroanatomy

Anyone dealing with the nervous system should absolutely have access to one of the several fine atlases (Paxinos and Watson 1998; Saleem and Logothetis 2007) that detail the various structures of the brain. When a test article affects a specific part of the brain, such an atlas can prove to be quite valuable in assisting with identifying the correct site.

At the minimum, the pathologist should be familiar with the boundaries and location of the following sites in all species in order to provide subsites for observations in the brain:

- Cerebrum/cerebral cortex (in the brain, the term "cortex" refers to gray matter only) including olfactory bulbs (these should always be removed at necropsy in order to have accurate brain weights), frontal cortex, parietal cortex, temporal cortex, occipital cortex, cingulate cortex/gyrus, retrosplenial cortex, and the piriform cortex
- Basal nuclei (the term "ganglia" should be restricted to the peripheral portion of the nervous system), including the caudate putamen area and the globus pallidus
- Thalamus/hypothalamus
- Midbrain, including substantia nigra
- Pons region
- Cerebellum
- Medulla oblongata

Fortunately, two excellent resources now exist to assist the pathologist in examining the brain and train technical personnel in consistently trimming the brain:

- Rodent CNS Protocol, produced June 2010 by the National Institute of Environmental Health Sciences in conjunction with the National Toxicology Program, Charles River Laboratories, Experimental Pathology Laboratories, Inc. (EPL, Inc.), available from Herbert@niehs.nih.gov.
- Cynomolgus Monkey Nervous System Trimming Protocol, produced June 2010, by Pfizer, EPL, Harlan, and Consultants in Veterinary Pathology, Inc., available from info@epl-inc .com. This information is also available in Pardo et al. (2012).

More on these guides is presented below under Special Consideration #3.

The neural tube develops as the neuroectoderm proliferates, folds, and fuses, resulting in a central tube (deLahunta and Glass 2009). A column of neural crest cells forms dorsolateral to the developing tube. These neural crest cells give rise to many of the components of the peripheral nervous system, including the dorsal root ganglia, the sympathetic and parasympathetic (postganglionic) ganglia, the adrenal medulla, melanoblasts, Schwann cells (deLahunta and Glass 2009) and satellite glial cells. Some of these cells, especially the postganglionic neuron of the sympathetic nervous system and dopaminergic neurons of the pars compacta region of the substantia nigra, will stain with an immunohistochemical stain to tyrosine hydroxylase (TH), a key enzyme in the production of dopamine (neurotransmitter of many of the neurons in the pars compacta region of the substantia nigra) and norepinephrine (the neurotransmitter of the postganglionic neuron of the sympathetic nervous system). Typically, a subset of neurons in the dorsal root ganglia will also stain positively with TH (Brumovsky et al. 2006).

The ventricular system of the brain and the central canal of the spinal cord are the remnants of the inside of the tube. During development, the tube closes in a rostral and caudal direction, beginning at the level of the brain stem.

At the rostral end of the neural tube, the prosencephalon gives rise to the telencephalon (cerebrum and caudate/putamen region) and diencephalon (thalamus/hypothalamus/neurohypophysis regions). The optic vesicles grow out of the region of the diencephalon. This is important because the optic nerve (cranial nerve 2) is centrally myelinated (by oligodendrocytes) whereas the other cranial nerves are peripherally myelinated (by Schwann cells). The degree of central myelination of the optic nerve at the level of the optic disc varies somewhat between species.

The lateral ventricles are within the telencephalon; the third ventricle is the ventricular system of the diencephalon. The midbrain corresponds to the mesencephalon; the aqueduct is the ventricle. The metencephalon is divided between the pons and cerebellum. The myelencephalon forms the medulla oblongata. The fourth ventricle is associated with the metencephalon and myelencephalon.

Prior to cell proliferation and differentiation, the neuroectoderm cells span the entire thickness of the neural tube. These cells become either immature neurons or spongioblasts. The spongioblasts will later differentiate to astrocytes or oligodendrocytes. Microglial cells are derived from blood monocytes. As maturation continues, the cells arrange into three layers (deLahunta and Glass 2009): the inner layer of proliferating neuroepithelium, which later becomes a single layer of cells, the ependymal cells, which line the entire ventricle system and spinal canal; a middle layer of differentiating cells that will form the gray matter and glia; and the outer marginal layer that largely consists of neuronal processes. This arrangement of layers is best seen (in the mature animal) in the spinal cord.

For a pathologist, one important aspect of this development is the residual clusters of cells that are frequently noted in the brain adjacent to the ventricles. These cells are presumed to represent a population of resting, undifferentiated/unmigrated cells "left over" during the period of brain development. These clusters of cells are frequently misdiagnosed as areas of gliosis. Periventricular neural stem cells also occupy the periventricular region (Chojnacki et al. 2009) and may be an important therapeutic target.

Neurons of the dorsal root ganglia, sympathetic ganglia, parasympathetic ganglia, and cells of the adrenal medulla (among other structures in the body, including melanocytes) (deLahunta and Glass 2009) are derived from neural crest cells. These cells migrate away from the neural tube during early development, forming the structures listed above.

20.2.1.1 Autonomic Nervous System

Although not required by published regulatory guidelines, the autonomic components of the nervous system may require evaluation. In the laboratory animal species, the following structures are readily harvested and examined: superior/cranial cervical ganglion located in the upper neck region beneath the bifurcation of the carotid artery near the angle of the jaw, the vagosympathetic trunk (neck), the sympathetic trunk (chain of ganglia coursing bilaterally through the thoracic cavity just ventral to the vertebral column), the abdominal sympathetic ganglia (superior/cranial mesenteric ganglia surrounding the cranial mesenteric artery near the left adrenal gland), and the postganglionic parasympathetic neurons, primarily located in the outer wall of the gastrointestinal tract, but also scattered throughout other organs.

The preganglionic neurons of the sympathetic nervous system are largely within the thoracic spinal cord segments in the intermediate gray column. These neurons synapse on neurons in the sympathetic chain and other sympathetic ganglia. In these ganglia, the postganglionic neurons that utilize norepinephrine as their neurotransmitter (and hence stain for the presence of TH) innervate their effector organs.

The preganglionic neurons of the parasympathetic nervous system are within the brain (midbrain and brain stem, primarily the latter) and the sacral segments of the spinal cord. The postganglionic neurons are within the wall of their effector organs and can be evaluated during the course of the examination of those organs.

20.2.1.2 Circumventricular Organs

The circumventricular organs (CVOs) are a great source of confusion for most pathologists. Recognition and understanding of these organs are important because they are frequently confused for abnormal structures and because these structures have an incomplete blood–brain barrier (BBB) as (except for the subcommissural organ) the endothelial cells are fenestrated (Weindl and Joynt 1973). Ependymal cells covering the CVOs still provide a blood–cerebrospinal fluid (CSF) barrier. Some of the CVOs (subfornical organ and area postrema) contain neuronal cell bodies (Oldfield and McKinley 1995).

In the rat, the CVOs most commonly noted by pathologists are the organum vasculosum (bilateral/ventral/rostral wall of the third ventricle), subfornical organ (rostral/dorsal wall of the third ventricle), subcommissural organ (posterior third ventricle), median eminence (floor of the third ventricle just caudal to the optic chiasm), neurohypophysis, pineal gland, and the area postrema (dorsomedial medulla oblongata, bilateral, at the level where the fourth ventricle becomes the central canal) (Oldfield and McKinley 1995). The choroid plexus is also a CVO. The CVOs have a variety of functions that include hormonal and cytokine secretion and storage. Pathologists need to be aware that test articles that do not readily gain access to the brain may still gain access to these areas and that chemicals/drugs affecting endothelial cells may also have exaggerated effects at these sites. A description and illustration of the major CVOs can be found in Garman (2011a).

20.2.1.3 Meninges

The meninges are composed of three layers. The dura is the thick, outermost, fibrous/most collagenous layer. This is referred to in some texts as the pachymeninges. While the dura is the most structurally substantial appearing layer, the middle layer, the arachnoid, is actually the greater barrier to the egress of unwanted substances, as the cells of the arachnoid contain abundant tight junctions, effectively forming a seal. The arachnoid, along with the innermost layer, the vascular pia mater, comprise the leptomeninges.

Lesions in the dura are uncommon unless you happen to be dealing with a dura sealant or implant. Cellular infiltrates in the pia-arachnoid are quite common, even in control animals. Although direct delivery of a test article directly to the nervous system is not the focus of this chapter, placing a variety of proteins or other large molecules into the intrathecal (subarachnoid) space frequently results in some cellular infiltrates (macrophages, lymphocytes, neutrophils, eosinophils) in the pia-arachnoid. These infiltrates are often present in isolation; that is, there are no other changes suggesting tissue damage. Nomenclature is an important part of any pathology evaluation. Cellular infiltrates in the absence of tissue damage or other indicators of inflammation typically warrant a diagnosis of infiltrates, rather than, in the case of infiltrates in the meninges, a diagnosis of meningitis (unless a true meningitis is considered to be present).

The following cell types should be the focus of diagnostic interest in the nervous system. A complete description of these cell types, with excellent illustrations, can be found elsewhere (Garman 2011a).

20.2.1.3.1   Neurons

Neurons vary greatly in size, from the large motor neurons of the ventral gray columns of the spinal cord, to the large sensory neurons of the dorsal root ganglia, to the small (but abundant) neurons of the granular cell layer of the cerebellum. There are various types of neurons, mostly dependent on the nature of their connections to other neurons. For the purpose of morphometric analysis, neurons may be classified by size. For the purpose of seeking similarities between neuronal groups in the brain and elsewhere, neurons may be classified by their neurotransmitters. Neurotransmitter type is a particularly useful way of categorizing neurons because various immunohistochemical stains may allow a pathologist to identify specific populations of cells. For example, staining for choline acetyltransferase identifies cholinergic neurons that are most abundant in the basal forebrain areas (septal nuclei, diagonal band, nucleus basalis of Meynert). This population of cells is responsible for the production of acetylcholine and may be a target for therapeutics developed to treat certain neurodegenerative disorders. Staining for dopamine allows for the specific characterization of neurons in the pars compacta region of the substantia nigra and the adjacent ventral tegmental area. Knowledge of these staining patterns and the significance of the size of neurons (e.g., interneurons tend to be smaller than motor or sensory neurons) can help in the recognition of test article effects. Immunohistochemical stains for NeuN or synaptophysin label all or most neurons. This may be useful for the counting of neurons in various regions of the nervous system.

Neurons vary considerably, not just in size and neurohistochemical activity but also in the location of the cell body (soma), the length of the axon, the proximity of the dendritic zone, and the location of the telodendron or synapse area. To understand this, it helps to think of the nervous system as being composed of functional areas, which can be broadly classified as either afferent (sensory) or efferent (motor).

The large motor neurons of the ventral gray column in the spinal column are the classic bipolar neuron, with multiple dendrites and a dendritic zone close to the cell body, and a long terminal axon that courses through the ventral spinal nerve roots to a muscle (the effector site). But neuronal arrangement varies considerably. The sensory neurons of the dorsal root ganglion, for example, have their dendritic zone in the periphery (e.g., skin), communicating via the axon to the cell body in the ganglion. These neurons are unipolar, meaning that there is a single neurite (a neurite is a projection from the cell body of a neuron), the axon, which passes through the dorsal root ganglion and then into the spinal cord.

20.2.1.3.2   Astrocytes

In addition to their role in supporting endothelial cells forming the BBB, astrocytes respond to a variety of stimuli in the central nervous system (CNS). Astrocytes may form the so-called glial scars in areas of small tissue loss but tend to form a wall of cells around larger areas of cavitation (Norenberg 2005). Astrocytes become reactive (enlarged and more numerous) in response to neuronal injury, degenerative conditions, chronic edema, axonal degeneration, and a wide variety of other changes in the brain and spinal cord. As such, staining for astrocytes, generally using an immunohistochemical stain to glial fibrillary acidic protein (GFAP), an intermediate filament expressed most prominently in astrocytes, is an excellent adjunct to traditional hematoxylin and eosin (H&E) stains when examining the brain and spinal cord. Enlarged/reactive astrocytes can also be detected with H&E staining but not with the sensitivity and specificity provided by the GFAP stain. Astrocytes are the most common cells in the brain and contain numerous receptors for neurotransmitters (Agulhon et al. 2008). Astrocyte processes are in contact with most neuronal structures (cell body, axon, dendrite) and form the glial limitans, a continuous layer of astrocyte foot processes that cover the brain and spinal cord, and continue into the superficial aspects of the perivascular space surrounding blood vessels entering the meningeal surface of the brain/cord.

20.2.1.3.3   Oligodendrocytes

These are the myelinating cells of the CNS. In H&E-stained sections, oligodendrocytes often form rows in the larger white matter tracts and appear very close to or in apparent contact with neurons in the gray matter. Here, they are sometimes referred to as satellite cells, not to be mistaken for the satellite glial cells of the dorsal root and sympathetic ganglia.

Oligodendrocyte nuclei often appear to occupy blank spaces in the neuropil. This is often an artifact of immersion-fixed tissue and represents retraction of the neuropil. Oligodendrocytes can be stained with a variety of markers, including several oligodendrocyte-specific proteins and antibodies to myelin, but often the stains (in the experience of the authors) are not as robust as the GFAP stain for astrocytes.

Damage to oligodendrocytes may manifest as areas of demyelination or as splitting of myelin sheaths, which usually appears as vacuolation (later discussed in greater detail). Artifactual vacuolation is very common, especially in immersion-fixed tissue, so great caution must be exercised in making a diagnosis of vacuolation. In many cases, use of the transmission electron microscope may be required to evaluate the source of the vacuoles.

20.2.1.3.4   Microglial Cells

These cells are not derived from neuroectoderm as are the astrocytes and oligodendrocytes. Microglia are derived from blood monocytes. They migrate into the CNS and serve various functions.

Microglia respond rapidly to neuronal damage. The responses include proliferation, enlargement of individual cells, and apparent clustering in sites of neuronal cell damage. Microglia rapidly clean up cellular debris from dead neurons. The speed and efficiency of this process mean the detection of neuronal necrosis must occur in a short time frame, usually 2–7 days after necrosis.

Figure 20.1 shows the typical time frame of a microglial response to neuronal necrosis in a 1-methyl-4-phenyl-1,2,3,6-tetrahydropyridine (MPTP) mouse model of Parkinson's disease. The astrocytic response is also shown. MPTP causes necrosis of neurons in the pars compacta region of the substantia nigra of certain strains of mice and primates (including humans) and is sometimes used as a model for Parkinson's disease. The microglial response to neuronal damage tends to occur rapidly and then taper off quickly.

In addition to this response, microglia may be involved in the pathogenesis of numerous CNS disorders. Supernatants from microglial cell cultures may kill cultured neurons (Streit 2005). This toxicity may be exacerbated by the *in vitro* addition (and presumably presence *in vivo*) of endotoxin and interferon (Streit 2005).

Immunohistochemical stains for microglial cells, including staining for ionized calcium binding adaptor molecule 1 (IBA-1), can be very useful in detecting subtle areas of microglial activation, especially when combined with stains for astrocytes.

20.2.1.3.5   Ependyma

Ependymal cells are remnants of the neuroepithelial cells that formed the primordial neural tube. Ependymal cells line the ventricular system of the brain and the central canal of the spinal cord and are densely ciliated and cuboidal. The ependymal cells covering the CVOs (including the choroid plexus) tend to be more flattened with fewer cilia. Ependymal cells essentially allow free passage of the CSF to the interstitial fluid of the brain, but tight junctions between these cells form the main barrier of the blood–CSF barrier (BCSFB).

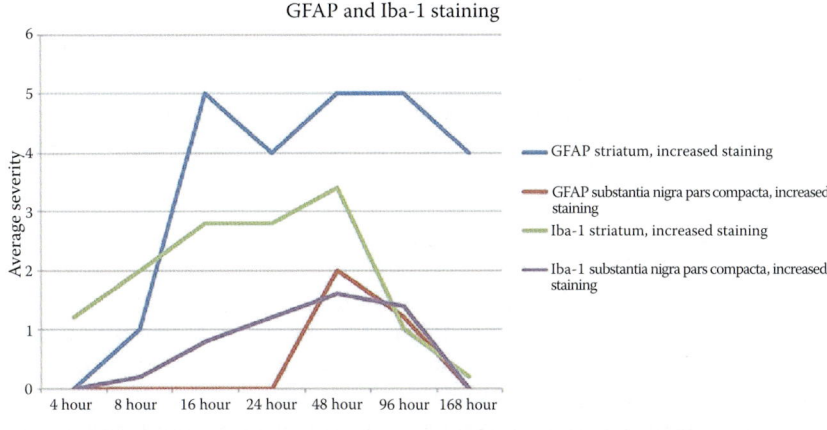

(a)

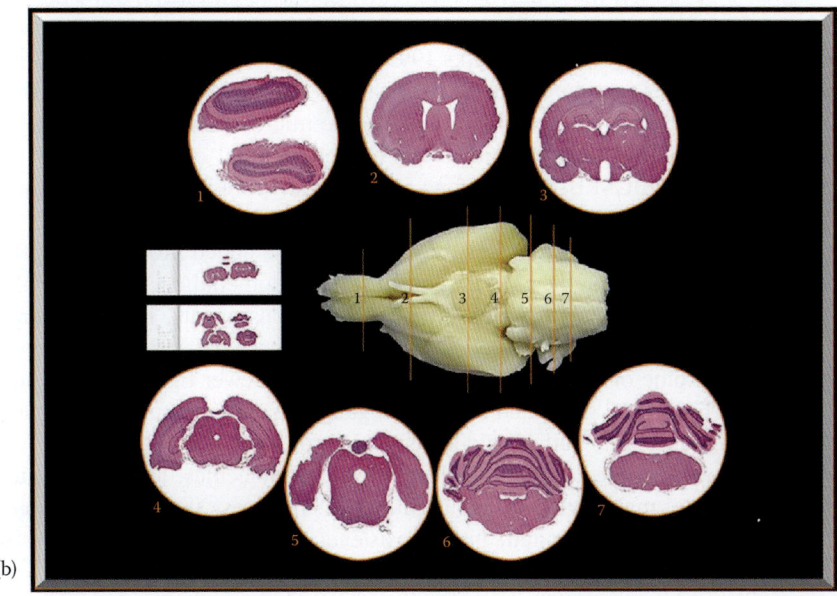

(b)

FIGURE 20.1 (a) This graph shows the glial reaction to neuronal injury in the pars compacta region of the substantia nigra and synaptic terminal disintegration in the striatum (caudate putamen area) after MPTP administration (to mice). The microglial reactions (indicated by IBA-1 staining) begin early, peak rapidly, and then quickly decrease. The astrocyte reactions (indicated by GFAP staining) begin more slowly, peak and quickly decrease in the substantia nigra, but plateau and persist in the striatum. (b) The sections produced with the trimming scheme described in the Rodent CNS Protocol produced by the National Institute of Environmental Health Sciences.

20.2.1.3.6 Schwann Cells

Schwann cells are the myelinating cells of the peripheral components of the nervous system, but Schwann cells also enclose the abundant, unmyelinated axons present outside the CNS. Schwann cells may wrap a single segment of a myelinated axon or may enclose multiple unmyelinated axons. Between the myelinated segments are gaps called the Nodes of Ranvier. The system of myelination in the peripheral nervous system allows for faster nerve conduction and increased efficiency and rate of myelin repair as compared to the CNS. Schwann cells are derived from neural crest cells.

20.2.1.3.7 Satellite Glial Cells

These cells surround neurons in ganglia in the peripheral nervous system and are also neural crest derived. They are very active functionally, performing many of the functions of the astrocyte in the brain and spinal cord. Satellite glial cells occur in the parasympathetic ganglia but are most pronounced in sympathetic and sensory (dorsal root) ganglia. These cells may be present in increased numbers in some ganglia where neurons have been lost because of exposure to a test article.

20.2.2 SPECIAL CONSIDERATION #2: THE "BARRIERS"

There are essentially three barriers that selectively isolate portions of the nervous system from exogenous and endogenous nervous system toxins. These barriers are the BBB (also known as the blood–interstitial fluid barrier), the BCSFB, and the blood–nerve barrier (BNB).

The choice of the word "barrier" is somewhat unfortunate as it tends to give sponsors, study directors, and even pathologists an undeserved sense of security with regard to the CNS safety of most test articles. In reality, these barriers are really selective gateways, allowing the mostly directional flow of various nutrients, the passage of peptides, the entrance of glucose, and the entrance of neurotransmitter precursors (Banks 1999). The primary barriers of the BBB, BCSFB, and BNB are endothelial (or ependymal) cell modifications (Vernau et al. 2011). The three major endothelial cell modifications, with features unique to the microvasculature of the nervous system, are as follows: increased tight junctions between endothelial cells (BBB and BNB) and between ependymal cells (BCSFB), no (or few) intracellular pores/fenestrations, and reduced pinocytosis.

To a lesser extent, astrocyte foot processes may provide some added protection/impediment to the passage of some substances, but the primary barrier is the endothelial/ependymal cell. Anything that can alter endothelial or ependymal cells (trauma, infectious agents, inflammation, osmotic agents, catheter or other device placement, etc.) can also alter these barriers. As previously noted, the endothelial cells of some of the CVOs are "leaky" owing to fewer tight junctions and greater numbers of fenestrae. The pineal gland and dorsal root ganglia have endothelial cells that are more permeable than their counterparts in the brain and spinal cord (Azzi et al. 1990).

Classically, lipid-soluble molecules, low-molecular-weight molecules, and some water-soluble molecules (e.g., morphine) may, owing to membrane diffusion, cross the BBB in a nonsaturable manner (Banks 1999). Although limited, pinocytosis/endocytosis may nonselectively transport nearly any substance/solute across the BBB if caught up in a receptor-mediated endocytosis (Banks 1999). Certain amino acids, vitamins, and regulatory proteins do cross the barrier. Active transport occurs for glucose, insulin, some peptides and cytokines, vitamins, and fatty acids.

Breaks in the BBB and the possibility that any given molecule (even a high-molecular-weight biologic) might somehow take advantage of a transport mechanism (either directly or by "piggybacking" on another molecule) make it theoretically possible for most substances to enter the brain. As an example, the authors have experienced, on numerous occasions, evidence of a monoclonal antibody gaining access to the brain, though such behavior would not have been expected based on what we know about the BBB.

Breaks in the barrier should always be considered as a possible mechanism for unexpected entry into the brain. There are tens of thousands of miles of blood vessels in the human brain. The chances that the BBB is entirely intact along those many miles, with all tight junctions working optimally, seem to be remote. Never automatically assume that a therapeutic, even a biologic, will not enter the brain or some other part of the nervous system.

20.2.3 SPECIAL CONSIDERATION #3: SAMPLING

If you section the kidney in the transverse or longitudinal orientation, you will likely end up with a reasonable sample to determine if there are any test article effects on the kidney. The same philosophy would seem to be applicable to the liver. Other tissues, like the lung, heart, skin, and digestive system, vary considerably and may warrant multiple sections to sufficiently characterize possible effects, but the complexity of the nervous system, and especially the tremendous variability along just about any axis of the brain, compels a somewhat involved sectioning scheme to have any hope of adequately assessing the brain in a manner sufficient to provide confidence in detecting possible test article effects. This complexity is readily apparent by studying any of the available detailed brain atlases.

To conduct a detailed examination of the brain in the rat, the most commonly used rodent species in preclinical safety studies, in a manner that attempts to capture the majority of the individual brain nuclei, it is probably necessary to examine the brain (considering transverse/coronal sections) at 0.35 mm intervals and large animal brains (dog, monkey) at approximately 1.0 to 1.25 mm intervals (Switzer 2011a). This sectioning scheme provides approximately 60 to 65 sections across the brain. While this number of sections seems shocking to most pathologists (and management), it makes sense and has proven a reliable and practical approach to guarantee that the majority of brain nuclei are examined. For example, the pars compacta region of the substantia nigra, which contains the neurons most affected in Parkinson's disease, measures approximately 2 mm (rostral to caudal) in the rat. If this is the area of greatest interest, and if multiple sections are required to make sure homologous sections between animals are available for examination, or if a stereologic investigation will be conducted, then sectioning at intervals of 0.35 mm (or less) may be necessary. Other areas that may be specifically targeted by a particular neurotoxicant may be equally small (Switzer 2011a). This level of sectioning requires (typically) embedding the entire brain and preparing a continuous series of frozen sections. While not practical for all studies, this degree of sectioning may be quite useful for ruling out neuronal necrosis in even the most specific brain nuclei.

In practice, this level of sectioning is typically reserved for directed brain investigations, especially those studies specifically designed to detect neuronal necrosis. For test articles known to be neuroactive, or known to cross the BBB, and certainly those that have been shown to cause an effect in the brain, especially if that effect includes neuronal necrosis, a directed study of the brain is advised at some time during the development cycle (Butt 2011). Staining techniques used to facilitate the detection of neuronal necrosis are discussed in Section 20.2.1.3.1.

Most preclinical safety studies are not going to include this level of sectioning. So how much is enough? Fortunately, most pathology groups now seem to embrace the concept that an increased level of brain sectioning beyond the three levels typically (formerly) performed for most studies at the National Toxicology Program (Solleveld and Boorman 1990) is warranted and considered a sound scientific practice. So while it is not possible to do too many sections of the brain, it is possible, without much increased effort or expense, to improve beyond the three sections often examined in the rat and the three or four sections often evaluated in dogs and primates. Regulatory guidelines are somewhat vague regarding how many levels of brain are enough. This topic is a chapter onto itself and is a topic of much debate among toxicologic pathologists. To keep this chapter as compact as possible, the recommendations for the sectioning and examination of the brain for routine, general preclinical toxicity studies have been provided in the form of a compact disc (CD) or manuscript by the National Institute of Environmental Health and Safety for the rodent (rat) brain and by Pardo et al. (2012) for the monkey brain (a similar approach is relevant in dogs). The information in the Pardo et al. article is also available in an interactive format as a CD. Information for ordering the CD for the rodent brain and the primate brain was provided previously in Special Consideration #1. The Rodent CNS Protocol CD describes the sectioning/examination of seven full transverse sections plus the olfactory lobes, an important but frequently unexamined area of the rodent brain. Figure 20.1b is an image from that CD and is used with the permission of the authors. This composite image shows the various levels that will be examined given the sectioning scheme. The guide also provides information on the location of key anatomic areas in those sections. The cynomolgus monkey protocol describes examination of six levels of the brain, providing for sections that will fit into a standard-sized cassette. The Pardo article should be consulted for images of the areas. This level of sectioning of the larger animal brains should be considered the absolute minimum in a preclinical safety study.

In addition to the brain, the following tissues should be harvested and examined when examining the nervous system:

- At least two levels of spinal cord (cervical and lumbar intumescence; addition of spinal cord from the C1/C2 area facilitates the detection of subtle nerve fiber degeneration in that area).
- At least two levels of dorsal root ganglia/spinal nerve roots (captured, if possible, with the transverse spinal cord sections for rodents).
- Cross and longitudinal sections of the sciatic nerve as a representative peripheral nerve.
- Other peripheral nerves if there is the possibility or suspicion of a peripheral neuropathy (based on the class or prior experience of test article). (The sural nerve is the nerve typically biopsied in humans and is a good choice for an additional peripheral nerve to examine.)
- One or more sympathetic ganglia, if there is an indication the test article may have adrenergic agonistic or antagonistic activity.
- Other areas as required by the specifics of the study and the nature of the test article.

20.2.4 SPECIAL CONSIDERATION #4: TIMING

Perhaps more so than any other organ system, the timing of evaluations of the nervous system may be critical in observing test article–related damage. This is particularly true for neuronal and microglial reactions as these may be early or transient and may or may not leave remnants that can be observed at a later time.

Conventional wisdom, especially among toxicologists and regulatory personnel but also many pathologists, suggests that if a particular test article is toxic to neurons, then daily administration of that test article for 90 days is going to produce a much more pronounced effect (lesion) as compared to giving a single dose of the test article. This conventional wisdom is (usually) wrong, although a cumulative exposure after chronic administration must always also be investigated. For many chemicals/test articles, the initial exposure defines the main toxicity event in terms of neuronal (and possibly microglial) effects. All susceptible neurons may be affected on the first exposure, and the peak time of neuronal necrosis for a wide variety of neurotoxicants is very early, in the range of 2 to 4 days after initial exposure (Switzer 2011b). Some NMDA antagonists (MK-801 is the prototype) cause early (6 to 8 h after initial exposure) neuronal vacuolation that progresses (in some neurons) to neuronal necrosis detectable 2 to 5 days after exposure (Fix et al. 1996). The neuronal effects, although somewhat widespread, primarily affect large neurons in the cingulate gyrus. The effect is subtle: only a small subset of neurons is affected. So if the brains are examined 7 days or more after initial exposure, the lesion is likely to be missed. The same scenario is true for other neurotoxicants. Neurons must be thought of as individuals, and exposure of neurons to a neurotoxicant is analogous to the exposure of a naïve, unprotected population of individuals to an infectious disease. Those that are going to get sick get sick at first exposure. Those that survive the first exposure are likely to survive subsequent exposures. You must look early to have the best chance of detecting neuronal necrosis, and the use of selective stains is an important diagnostic aid (see below).

As with neurons, microglial cells may react (i.e., acquire a reactive phenotype) early, and that reaction may subside quickly. Timing is crucial. What is noted at the end of a 90-day, 28-day, or even 14-day study may miss the change or not accurately reflect the magnitude of the initial morphologic change.

20.3 EVALUATION STRATEGY

Each pathologist will develop a unique technique for examining the nervous system. This technique will be based upon current knowledge, training, and available support. There is no wrong way to evaluate the nervous system provided an acceptable subset of tissue is evaluated at the right time and with the proper techniques.

From a pathology perspective, most morphologic evaluations are limited to light microscopic examination, often with all tissues embedded in paraffin and sections stained with H&E. Fortunately, this is often quite sufficient to provide a complete and thorough evaluation.

As noted several (but never enough) times already, the key to nervous system evaluation is to examine sufficient tissue, especially in the brain.

Many morphology-based techniques are available to augment the H&E examination.

The following guidelines provide some suggestions for the evaluation of certain anatomic structures and microscopic lesions. This is not a complete list, but is an excellent starting point.

> *Myelin/Peripheral nerve:* True demyelinating lesions may be (sometimes easily) detected with traditional H&E staining. Actual visualization of myelin surrounding peripheral nerve fibers, evaluation of the G ratio (axon diameter/total myelinated nerve fiber diameter), and determining the mechanism of subtle nerve fiber degenerations may (and usually does) require osmium postfixation, resin embedding, and toluidine blue (or other myelin) stain of nerve cross sections. Osmium postfixation even with paraffin embedding of nerve cross sections improves nerve examination (see Figure 20.6).
>
> *Unmyelinated nerve fibers:* Examination of these very small structures requires the transmission electron microscope. Although unmyelinated nerve fibers can be seen with osmium-postfixed, resin-embedded, toluidine blue–stained sections, even this preparation is not sufficient to perform morphologic or morphometric examination of unmyelinated nerve fibers.

Vacuolation in the CNS usually requires transmission electron microscopic examination to determine the location of the vacuoles. Some special stains may also assist with determining the location of vacuoles. For example, vacuoles surrounded by a rim of GFAP-positive cytoplasm suggest that the vacuoles are within astrocyte processes.

Detection of subtle neuronal necrosis may require the use of special stains (Fluoro-Jade [FJ] B; cupric silver) as noted below in Section 20.4. The advantages of some immunohistochemical techniques are presented elsewhere in this article.

Morphometrics may be the only means of detecting cell (or cell structure) losses (or gains) if the change is not sufficient to be obvious with visual inspection. For example, the loss of sensory neurons in the dorsal root ganglia may not be detectable if there is no residual damage that is still present at the time of morphologic investigation. However, using stereologic methods to do neuron counts may reveal a loss of neurons. The counting of intraepidermal nerve fibers in frozen sections of skin biopsies may be a very sensitive means of the detection of a decrease of sensory fibers in the distal extremities.

20.4 DIAGNOSTIC NEUROPATHOLOGY—NON-PROLIFERATIVE LESIONS

The next sections include lesions the toxicologic pathologist might expect to encounter in the nervous system.

In addition to this section, the reader is referred to the recently revised INHAND document regarding proliferative and non-proliferative lesions of the nervous system in rodents. The INHAND documents are a joint venture between the ESTP, the STP, the BSTP, and the JSTP. This reference is available to STP members at the following website: http://www.goreni.org/index.php.

When possible, the nomenclature used in this section will adhere to the above-referenced INHAND document.

20.4.1 NEURONS

Artifact, Dark Neuron: This is the most common "lesion" encountered by the toxicologic patholo-gist and must be distinguished from neuronal necrosis and degeneration (Figure 20.2a). Dark neurons are present in immersion-fixed brain tissue, but also occur in perfusion-fixed specimens. Dark neurons are characterized by a shrunken, dark (basophilic) nucleus and cytoplasm, often with prominent dendrites. Handling of the brain after necropsy and immersion fixation in formalin tends to exacerbate the appearance of this artifact. While large neurons seem to be affected most often, and it may be difficult to find a section of immersion-fixed brain tissue that is without dark neurons among the pyramidal cells of the cerebral cortex, any collection of neurons can be affected. This artifact seems to be most frequently misdiagnosed as a real lesion in the Purkinje cell layer of the cerebellum. This may be because these cells are organized linearly, which lends them to a thorough visual analysis. A more complete description of dark neurons can be found in Garman (2011b).

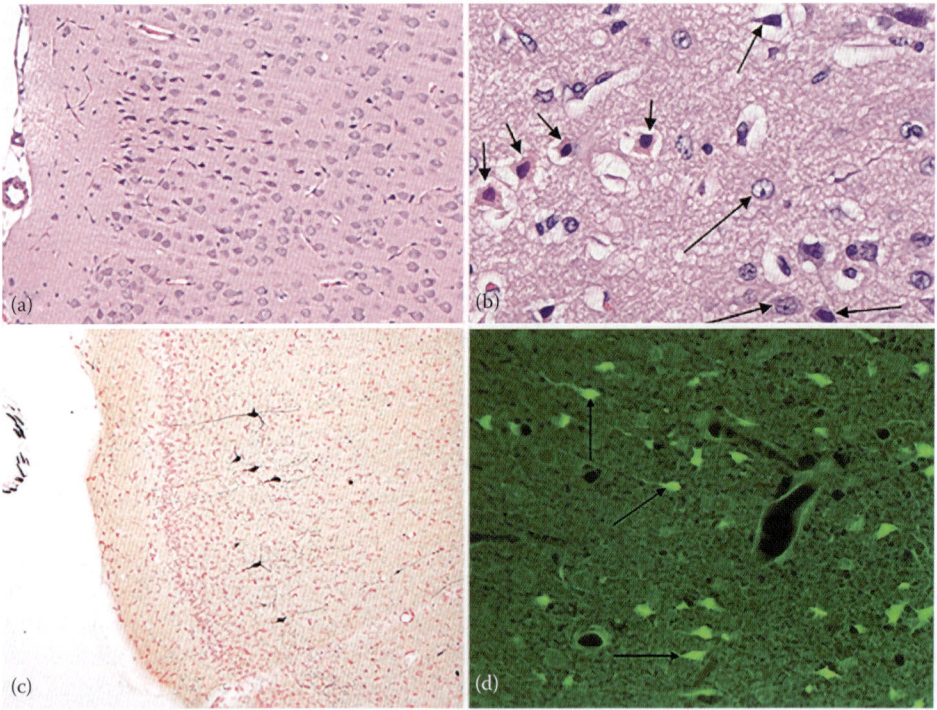

FIGURE 20.2 (a) Brain, immersion fixation, rat, H&E stain. Typical dark neurons (artifactual change) near the surface of the cerebral cortex. (b) Brain, immersion fixation, H&E stain. The short arrows point to typi-cal "red dead" neurons. Note the cell shrinkage, nuclear pyknosis, and bright pink cytoplasm. The longer arrows in the center and center/bottom show normal (appearing) neurons. The arrows at the top and bottom right indicate slightly dark neurons (artifact). (c) Brain, rat, perfusion fixation, amino cupric silver stain. The disintegrating neurons are very readily apparent, even at medium power, as black structures against a pale yellow background. The axon and dendrites of the disintegrating neurons are also visible. This stain provides for an exquisitely sensitive means of detecting disintegrating neurons and neuritis. (d) Brain, rat, perfusion fixation, FJ B stain, FITC filter. The arrows point to fluorescent neurons (there are many others in the image). This stain, while not quite as easily examined as the amino cupric silver stain, can be performed on paraffin-embedded tissue, thereby providing a means for assessing even subtle neuronal necrosis from an additional section from the same blocks used to produce the standard H&E section.

20.4.2 Neuronal Necrosis

Neuronal necrosis is usually easily identified on H&E-stained sections if necrotic cells are still present and if the necrosis is of sufficient frequency to be picked up on microscopic inspection. Upon H&E staining, the necrotic neurons appear shrunken with bright pink cytoplasm and a dark, sometimes pyknotic nucleus (Figure 20.2b). There may be some variation in appearance of necrotic neurons, as not all cells would be degenerating/dying in the exact same time frame, though the time frame may be quite narrow. In contrast, dark neurons all look the same. (Most artifacts, having occurred at the time of death/necropsy, do exist in the same time frame.)

When neuronal necrosis is subtle, the thoroughness of evaluation can be greatly enhanced by the use of a stain that is specific for this change. Such stains can increase the sensitivity of detecting necrotic neurons down to a single neuron, provided the examiner is experienced regarding the interpretation of background staining. The most common staining methodologies for identifying neuronal necrosis are amino cupric silver and FJ B or C. While the actual mechanism is not fully understood, the amino cupric silver stain is believed to label necrotic neurons and processes of necrotic neurons, including synaptic terminals, by silver particles adhering to exposed sulfide groups in amino acids that are themselves exposed because of proteolysis (Switzer 2000). This staining procedure appears to be very sensitive and accurate, with the tremendous advantage that necrotic neurons, and the processes of such neurons, are labeled black against a yellow background (Figure 20.2c). Amino cupric silver is the best means of demonstrating necrotic neurons and is the method of choice if a directed study is designed to allow for the necessary preparatory techniques. The disadvantages of using the amino cupric silver stain are as follows: animals must be fixed via perfusion fixation (always a good idea for studies desiring optimal neuropathology endpoints), cacodylate buffers are required, the brains must be sectioned frozen, and the staining technique is somewhat difficult to perform.

FJ B or C is probably the most common method (other than H&E) used to detect neuronal necrosis. This is because FJ can be used on paraffin-embedded sections, which is frequently what the pathologist has to work with or what is planned for the study. The FJ staining procedure is easy to perform. The stain labels necrotic neurons a bright green and the slides must be examined with a fluorescent microscope using a fluorescein isothiocyanate (FITC) filter or the equivalent. The recent introduction of light-emitting diode–based fluorescence (negating the need to install and focus mercury or metal halide bulbs) does make the placing of a fluorescent microscope on every pathologist's desktop a more realistic situation. Figure 20.2d shows examples of the FJ stain used to detect necrotic neurons. Because the FJ stain is so sensitive, one approach is to review the FJ-stained brain sections first and then proceed to the H&E-stained sections. This approach may allow for a somewhat more efficient review of the H&E-stained slides, since neuronal necrosis will already have been ruled in or out. As with the amino cupric silver stain, the exact molecular moiety within necrotic neurons that stains positive with FJ is unknown. The dye may be staining polyamines that accumulate after cell death or degeneration of membrane-bound molecules, or the stain may be labeling cleaved microtubule proteins (Schmued et al. 2005). Similar to the silver technique, FJ seems to consistently stain necrotic neurons produced by a wide variety of toxicants (Schmued and 2000). Unlike many fluorescent-based stains, the fluorescence on FJ-stained sections persists unless the section is exposed to intense light, such as that produced by leaving a portion of a section under a higher magnification objective (Sarkar and Schmued 2011).

In the experience of the author, the disintegrating neuronal appendages (axons, dendrites, synaptic terminals) are much easier to identify using amino cupric silver–stained sections as compared to FJ, and these processes cannot be detected by H&E. However, because most studies are performed using paraffin-embedded tissues, the FJ staining method is used more frequently and still is very sensitive in detecting even very subtle neuronal necrosis.

For the spinal cord, because the neurons are relatively compacted in a defined space, there is seldom the need for specialized neuronal necrosis stains, although even in the spinal cord, these stains enhance detection of dead neurons.

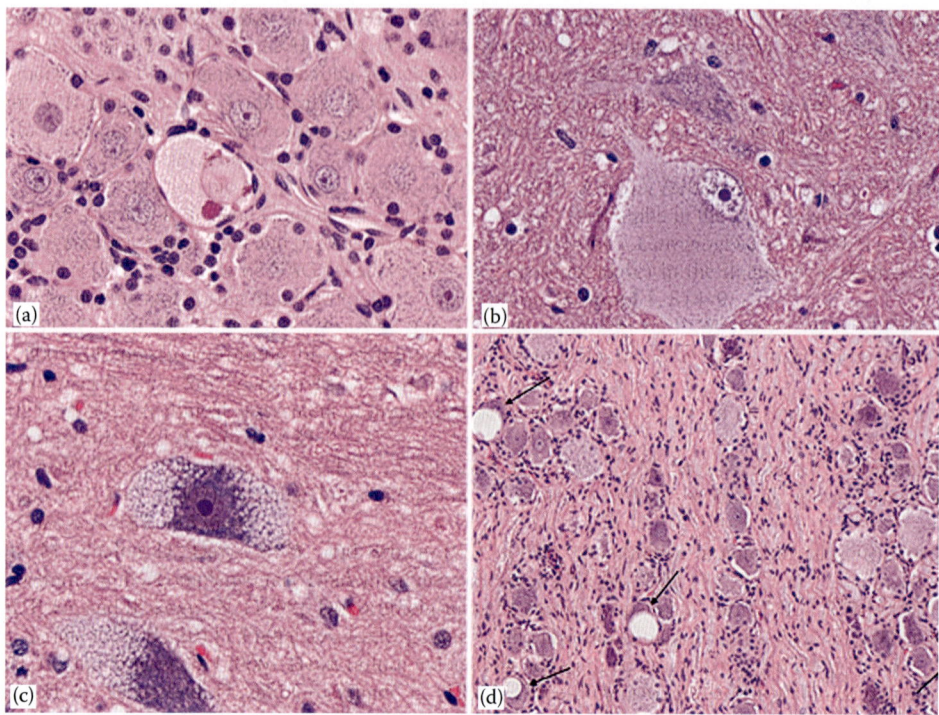

FIGURE 20.3 (a) Monkey, dorsal root ganglion, H&E stain. In the center of the image is a dead/disintegrating neuron surrounded by normal sensory neurons. These disintegrating neurons are also observed in control animals, so caution in interpreting their significance is required. In the experience of the author (Butt), the typical "red dead" neuron is very rare in peripheral nervous system ganglia. (b) Goat, spinal cord, H&E stain. The nucleus is displaced peripherally in this large motor neuron. Chromatolysis is not (typically) a precursor to a terminal event, but may be part of the evolution of the change in dorsal root ganglion neurons shown in plate a. (c) Brain, rat, H&E stain. Shown are two neurons with cytoplasm filled with well-defined vacuoles. Determining the exact location of the vacuoles usually requires TEM or specialized immunohistochemistry (or both). (d) Monkey, dorsal root ganglion, H&E stain. The arrows show sensory neurons containing one or two large, well-defined vacuoles. These vacuoles are commonly observed in control animals, so ascribing their presence to a test article should be done with caution. These vacuoles, regardless of study length, always appear the same and are not associated with detectable cell necrosis or degeneration.

In the dorsal root ganglia and in sympathetic/parasympathetic ganglia, the classic "red dead" necrotic neuron is seldom encountered. Instead, generally, neurons in this location seem to undergo a swelling and lysis that results in eventual removal of the dead cell (Figure 20.3a). This is a relatively common change often seen in control animals, so the observation of this finding requires a thorough evaluation of the concurrent control animals and a review of other studies for which slides of ganglia are available. In the experience of the author, this particular change is often missed/ignored/misinterpreted even by experienced pathologists, so the historical control data may not be useful. Chromatolysis may be a precursor to this change in peripheral nervous system ganglia neurons.

20.4.3 NEURONAL CELL LOSS

As noted previously, the window for actual detection of neuronal necrosis may be brief (Switzer and Butt 2011). If the neuronal necrosis is due to initial exposure to a particular test article (which it often is), then the actual neuronal necrosis may be missed in any study longer than 7 days in duration (i.e., in animals sacrificed more than 7 days after initial dosing). If the neuronal necrosis is missed, then the remaining lesion may be detectable as neuronal cell loss, and possibly gliosis (if a sufficient glial reaction persists).

It can be very difficult to distinguish a subtle neuronal cell loss unless the loss occurs in a population of neurons that have a readily identifiable arrangement. Two such areas in the brain are the hippocampus/dentate gyrus and the Purkinje cells. In these areas, the neurons assume a regular, linear arrangement such that the loss of even a few cells can be noted provided, of course, that these areas are included in your sectioning scheme.

There are normally gaps in the Purkinje cell layer, or at least apparent gaps. The determination as to what is a gap within biologic variation or what is a gap due to the loss of cells can be difficult. Special stains are often useful in exploring these gaps. When Purkinje cells are lost, there is generally a response by the Bergmann glial cells (astrocytes), specialized astrocytes that occupy the Purkinje cell layer. These cells become enlarged/reactive in many instances where there has been Purkinje cell necrosis. Since the identifiable astrocyte response lasts much longer than persistence of the remnants of the necrotic neurons, staining with GFAP can be quite useful in proving that a gap is due to cell loss.

In the hippocampus, staining the sections for synaptophysin can assist in establishing cell loss, though cell loss in this area is readily identifiable when related to a toxicant.

Stereologic techniques may be required to detect neuronal loss when no residual evidence of a neuronal lesion is present.

20.4.4 NEURONOPHAGIA

Literally, this is the ingestion of neurons by microglial cells and this change may be detected during the time of neuronal necrosis. This diagnosis should be limited to instances where activated microglial cells are noted in close approximation to altered neurons. Typically, this occurs as a cluster of cells, and the central remnants of the neuron is sometimes difficult to appreciate. Neuronophagia must be distinguished from the normal satellite cells (oligodendrocytes) that surround neurons (McMartin et al. 1997).

20.4.5 CHROMATOLYSIS

This is a rare change that, in the experience of the author, is most commonly seen in the motor neurons of the ventral gray column of the spinal cord and less often within the dorsal root ganglia. This change is thought to be "sublethal" and represent a response to the cell body of the neuron to repair an injury to the axon. In a chromatolytic neuron, ribosomes have detached from the rough endoplasmic reticulum, causing the loss of the normal appearance of the Nissl substance (Figure 20.3b).

20.4.6 VACUOLATION, NEURONAL

Neuronal vacuolation is a change that must be differentiated from artifactual changes that resemble vacuoles. The differentiation may be quite difficult. For neuronal vacuolation to be considered an actual change (unrelated to autolysis, fixation, or handling), there should be distinct vacuoles (Figure 20.3c) affecting individual or groups of neurons and exhibiting a notable difference from control animals. Because tissue processing can cause artifactual vacuolation, it is always necessary to process tissues across groups rather than process all controls in one batch followed by test article–treated groups in other processing runs. Neuronal vacuolation may be caused by storage diseases, dilation of various organelles, or infectious processes. The neuronal vacuoles associated with scrapie are probably the best known to veterinary pathologists. In most cases, to gain further information regarding the exact location of neuronal vacuoles, transmission electron microscopy (TEM) is useful. If TEM is used, it is important for the reviewing pathologist (or a pathologist familiar with neuropathology) to actually sit at the scope and either photograph the affected neurons or be present to direct the taking of the images. Most technical personnel are not able to differentiate between neuronal vacuoles and the many different forms of apparent vacuolation that permeate most sections of brain, especially specimens that were immersion fixed. Once the affected neurons are located, characteristics of the vacuoles should be documented with digital images or photomicrographs and noted at the time of initial observation. In other words, use the transmission electron microscope as if it is a light microscope, just with more powerful lenses. If vacuoles can be found, it should be possible (using TEM) to come up with at least a presumptive determination as to the actual intracellular location of the vacuoles, and whether the vacuoles are primarily within the neuronal cell body or the dendritic stem or in another cell type. Neuronal vacuolation may be normal in certain brain nuclei, especially those in or around the area of the hypothalamus, including the optic nucleus in dogs.

Large, smooth vacuoles are frequently noted in neurons of the dorsal root ganglion, even in control animals (Figure 20.3d). These vacuoles have been reported to be increased as a chemical (organophosphate) effect (Rogers-Corone et al. 2010). While an effect of a test article always needs to be considered, in the experience of the author, these vacuoles always appear the same (no matter the test article), are not associated with dead or degenerate neurons, and occur regularly in control animals. Stated another way, these vacuoles are most often artifacts of fixation or preparation. In any given animal, these vacuoles tend to be present in multiple dorsal root ganglia when they are present at all. The vacuoles are also regularly observed in trigeminal ganglia.

20.4.7 Neuronal Pigments

The most common pigments encountered within neurons are lipofuscin, which is golden yellow and generally associated with aging, and neuromelanin, which is most commonly noted in the hypothalamic neurons (Summers et al. 1995).

20.4.8 Neuronal Inclusions

There are several neuronal inclusions associated with infectious disease. The Negri body of rabies is a prime example. Inclusions are relatively common in cases of canine distemper and the various herpes infections. It might be possible to observe Cowdry Type A inclusions in monkeys infected with herpes viruses (including cytomegalovirus infection of immunosuppressed animals), but this would be unusual in the experience of the typical toxicologic pathologist. The toxicologic pathologist is going to encounter inclusions most often when evaluating animal models (typically transgenic models) of human disease.

Lewy bodies, characteristic of Parkinson's disease in humans, may be noted in neurons of the Lewy mouse. Like humans, the Lewy bodies stain for alpha-synuclein (Sommer et al. 2000). Unlike humans, neurodegeneration does not accompany the appearance of these inclusions. Transgenic models of Alzheimer's disease and Pick's disease (both tauopathies) may contain inclusions/intracellular structures, including neurofibrillary tangles (Alzheimer's models).

20.4.9 Neuronal Heterotopia (Ectopic Neurons)

Neuronal heterotopia refers to groups of neurons that appear normal individually but are present in an abnormal site or arrangement. Dysplasia is a term that has been used to describe this abnormality/malformation, which is believed to be due to altered migration during development, but heterotopia or ectopia appears to be more accepted. Neuronal heterotopias are well recognized in humans (Harding and Copp 2008) but rarely encountered (or perhaps just rarely recognized) in laboratory animals.

In the peripheral nervous system, ganglia are widespread and occasionally occur in unusual or unexpected places. In general, unless the pathologist is quite confident that there is an abnormality, these ganglia should be accepted as normal structures and do not warrant mention.

20.4.10 Neurons, Binucleate

Binucleate neurons (Figure 20.4) are regularly encountered in sympathetic ganglia and may be observed in the CNS (Das 1977).

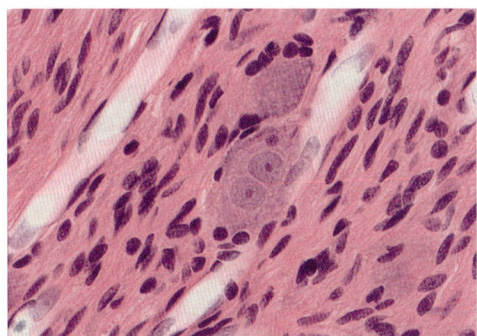

FIGURE 20.4   Monkey, sympathetic ganglion, H&E stain. If sympathetic ganglia are thoroughly searched, binucleate neurons will be found somewhat routinely in various species.

20.4.11   SATELLITOSIS

The INHAND document specifically applies this term to the proliferation of oligodendrocytes around degenerating neurons, but satellitosis has been used to describe any increase of glial cells (especially microglial cells) around neurons. It is not always possible to positively identify (with H&E-stained sections) exactly what cell type may be increased, and satellitosis is a sufficiently descriptive term to warrant a place in the diagnostic lexicon of the toxicologic pathologist. If this change appears to be test article related and not simply a response to neuronal degeneration (in which case, neuronophagia is probably the cause and a preferred diagnosis), it would be beneficial for the overall characterization of the change to use immunohistochemical stains to positively identify the cell type that is increased. Because of the relationship of this term to findings in the brain and spinal cord, satellitosis should not be used to describe a proliferation of satellite glial cells that may occur in dorsal root and sympathetic ganglia.

20.4.12   AXONAL DYSTROPHY/SPHEROIDS

Axonal dystrophy is a term used to describe swollen axons and is typically applied when a specific condition that explains a somewhat generalized effect on axons can be identified. Because "dystrophy" is a broad term, a thorough description of the microscopic appearance of the affected axons would be warranted. An alternate and usually preferred term to apply when swollen axons are noted as part of a nonspecific axonal degeneration (i.e., focal axonal swellings are a component of but not the primary change) is spheroids. Spheroids (Figure 20.5a and b) are focal swellings of axons and are encountered relatively frequently whenever axonal degeneration is also observed. The swellings vary in their pathogenesis but typically occur as an accumulation of neurofilaments and organelles. Spheroid formation is a rather nonspecific manifestation of axonal degeneration and is a common microscopic lesion. These axonal swellings appear (on H&E-stained sections) as round, eosinophilic structures and are readily observed on longitudinal and cross sections of nerves and the spinal cord.

   If a particular test article causes axonal degeneration that is consistently characterized by axonal swellings, then the term axonal dystrophy may apply. The characteristic swelling may be part of a continuum of changes, so timing after initial exposure (as with neuronal necrosis) could be critical in observing the primary morphologic change. Swelling may progress to axonal disintegration and be indistinguishable from other mechanisms of axonal degeneration.

   Spheroids are commonly noted in the cochlear nucleus of beagle dogs, including controls (Slayter et al. 1998). These spheroids are the source of frequent misinterpretation when suddenly noticed in a test article–treated animal. While a relationship to the test article should not be ruled out without investigation, it must be recognized that this is a common, spontaneous lesion in the beagle.

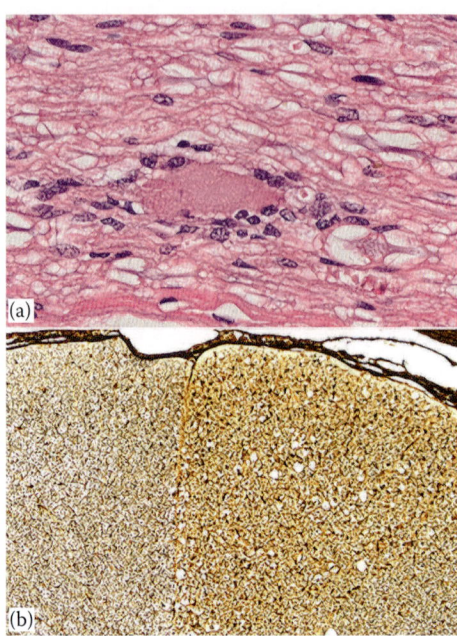

FIGURE 20.5   (a) Goat, spinal cord, H&E stain. There is a single dilated axon (spheroid). The increased cellularity is due to local hyperplasia of Schwann cells and the infiltration of macrophages. (b) Goat, spinal cord, Bielschowsky's silver stain. Numerous dark (silver positive), dilated axons are present unilaterally in the fasciculus gracilis.

20.4.13   AXONAL DEGENERATION/NERVE FIBER DEGENERATION

Axonal or nerve fiber degeneration (the nerve fiber is the axon/myelin sheath/Schwann cells) is a very common microscopic change and can be observed rather frequently (at a minimal severity) in control animals. Finding a few degenerated nerve fibers does not always indicate a test article effect. While axonal degeneration is typically the cause, this may be very difficult to verify at the light microscopic level, especially when the examination is limited to H&E staining.

Nerve fiber degeneration in either the spinal cord or peripheral nerves is typically easiest to observe in longitudinal sections, presumably because these sections are taken in parallel with the course of the nerve fiber, and therefore, there is an increased chance of seeing the degeneration. Not all nerve fiber degenerations are classic Wallerian degenerations, as it is very common to note focal swellings of myelin with an intact axon coursing through the area. These areas may be artifactual (see below, bubbles, myelin) or may represent focal swellings in the myelin sheath with possible Schwann cell (or oligodendrocyte) loss or degeneration. The term axonal degeneration should be reserved for the actual observation of axonal fragments within degenerated segments. In practice, it is usually preferred to use the term nerve fiber degeneration and then describe the various characteristics of the degeneration.

While longitudinal, H&E-stained, paraffin-embedded sections are very sensitive for detecting nerve fiber degeneration, cross sections of nerves, postfixed with osmium tetroxide, embedded in a hard plastic or resin (such as Spurr's or Epon), and stained with toluidine blue (or similar metachromatic stain) may be necessary to accurately describe the changes to the axon and myelin sheath.

It is very important to understand that, at best, myelin is poorly visualized in standard H&E-stained, paraffin-embedded sections, especially in cross sections. Use of a Luxol Fast Blue stain does improve the pathologist's ability to visualize myelin, but without osmium postfixation, the myelin sheaths do not fix sufficiently to visualize properly. Figure 20.6 compares a standard H&E-stained,

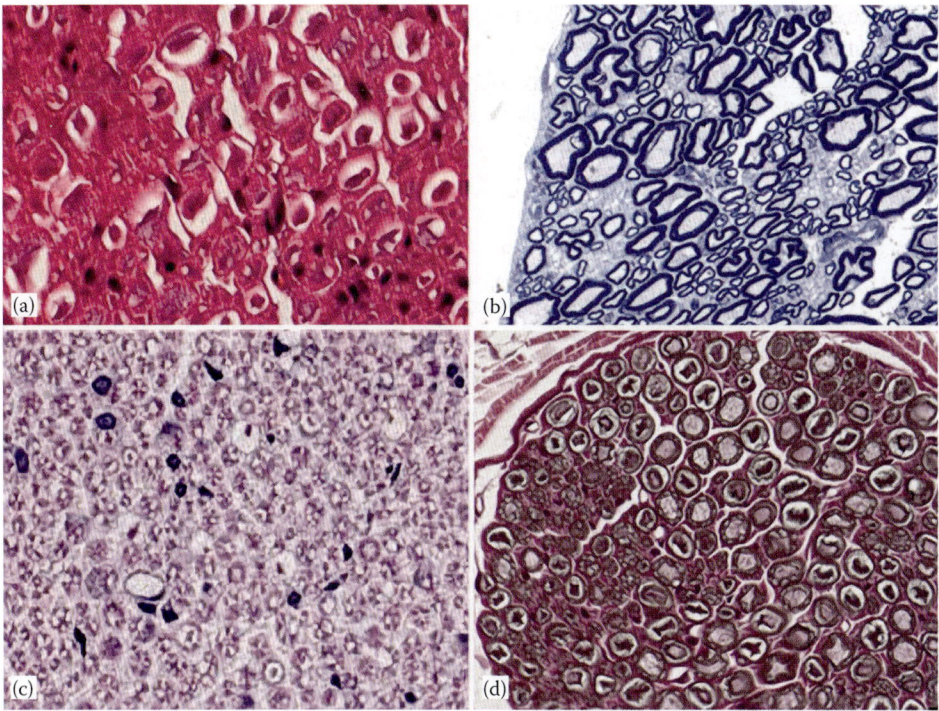

FIGURE 20.6 (a) Sciatic nerve, rat, formalin fixation, paraffin embedding, H&E stain. This image is typical of a cross section of sciatic nerve that would be examined in a preclinical toxicology study where immersion/formalin fixation and paraffin embedding are used for all tissues. (b) Sciatic nerve, rat, glutaraldehyde followed by osmium fixation, resin embedding, toluidine blue stain. This section is from a nerve fixed in 2% osmium for 1 h after glutaraldehyde fixation. Note the greatly enhanced myelin detail. A section of this quality is optimal for morphologic examination and is also suitable for morphometric examinations of nerve fiber quantity and size. (c) Sciatic nerve, rat, formalin fixation, glycol methacrylate embedding, H&E stain. Without osmium postfixation, even plastic embedding does very little to enhance myelin detail. (d) Sciatic nerve, rat, formalin followed by osmium fixation, paraffin embedding, H&E stain. Note the increased myelin detail as compared to the nerves in plates a and c. Even in paraffin sections, osmium greatly enhances a pathologist's ability to assess myelin sheaths.

paraffin-embedded cross section of nerve to nerves that have been postfixed in osmium, then embedded in either Spurr's or paraffin. The difference is striking.

20.4.14 Bubbles, Myelin

This term is sometimes used to describe focal dilations of the myelin sheath when either the axon is clearly intact or there is no evidence of axonal degeneration, such as the infiltration of macrophages (Gitter cells) into the dilated myelin sheath. This is a diagnosis that is probably best left unused. The term is included here under neurons because myelin bubbles are typically dilated myelin sheaths (or artifacts) secondary to axonal degeneration and, therefore, not a primary morphologic change.

Myelin, being primarily lipid, is prone to all manner of artifactual changes in paraffin-embedded tissues because of the exposure of the myelin to various organic solvents used for tissue processing. Even the standard fixative for preclinical studies, 10% neutral buffered formalin, causes artifactual splitting of myelin sheaths. Many artifacts of myelin could be described as "bubbles." As it is the job of the toxicologic pathologist to recognize artifacts and discount them as being relevant to a particular test article–related effect, it is preferred to use the term degeneration to describe actual abnormalities of the nerve fiber, axon, or myelin and then characterize the features of that degeneration. True bubbles in the myelin, caused by focal swellings of the myelin sheath, with or without axonal degeneration, may also be termed myelin ovoids, but this is generally going to be a feature of the broader diagnosis of nerve fiber degeneration and not a primary diagnosis. If there is a primary disorder of myelin, then demyelination or myelinopathy should be used as the diagnosis.

20.4.15 GLIAL CELLS

20.4.15.1 Gliosis, NOS (Not Otherwise Specified)

On H&E-stained sections, focal clusters of glial cells may defy definitive identification, so the term Gliosis, NOS (or just gliosis) may be used. This designation is satisfactory and likely represents clusters/accumulations of astrocytes and microglial cells lacking specific characteristics that would allow for a more specific diagnosis. If the occurrence of gliosis is frequent or appears to be related to the test article, then further staining is warranted to identify the cell type as this may provide some insight into the etiology of the change.

20.4.16 ASTROCYTES

20.4.16.1 Astrocytosis

This diagnosis is appropriate whenever there is an increase in the number and size of astrocytes, especially when in the proximity of an identified structural alteration in some component of the CNS. Reactive astrocytosis, gemistocytosis (a gemistocyte is a term for an enlarged/reactive astrocyte), and astrogliosis are synonymous terms.

Reactive astrocytes are sometimes readily apparent in H&E-stained sections, as the ability to visualize cytoplasm in an astrocyte is the main clue to the cell being diagnosed as "reactive." But staining for GFAP greatly enhances the visualization of astrocytes and provides an efficient mechanism for determining whether or not there are increased numbers of astrocytes. Figures 20.7 and 20.8a and b demonstrates the usefulness of the GFAP stain in positively identifying an astrocytic reaction.

There may be a subtle increase in numbers of glial cells (especially astrocytes) with aging, but this is seldom appreciable unless there is a causative morphologic change in the brain or spinal cord to explain the increase in cellularity.

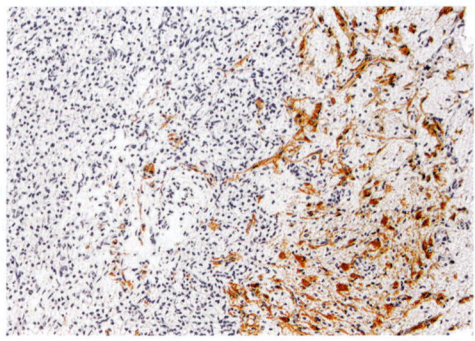

FIGURE 20.7 Rat, brain, perfusion fixation, immunohistochemical stain for GFAP/Astrocytes. The astrocytic reaction is well demonstrated with this staining procedure. The reactive astrocytes (right side of the image; stained brown) surround an area of inflammation/necrosis.

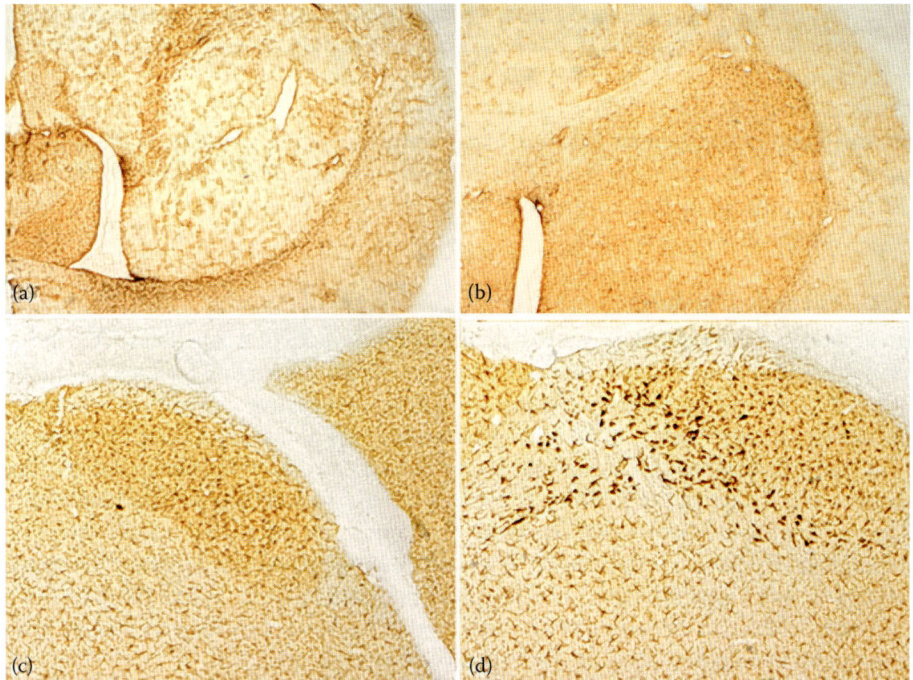

FIGURE 20.8 Mouse, brain, perfusion fixation, immunohistochemical staining for GFAP/astrocytes (a and b) and IBA-1/microglial cells (c and d). The two images at the top show a control animal (a) and an increase of GFAP staining in the area of the striatum in an MPTP-treated mouse (b). The two images at the bottom show a control animal (c) and an increase of IBA-1 staining in the area of the pars compacta region of the substantia nigra in an MPTP-treated mouse (d). H&E stains would not demonstrate these glial changes.

20.4.16.2 Alzheimer Type II Astrocytes

This term describes enlarged astrocytes with open-faced (swollen, with peripheral heterochromatin) nuclei but without a prominent increase of cytoplasm and, consequently, no increase of notable GFAP staining. These cells are usually associated with a metabolic disorder such as liver or renal failure leading to hepatic or renal encephalopathy. Alzheimer Type II astrocytes are almost exclusively observed in gray matter. Since this diagnosis confers not only a specific cellular phenotype but also a somewhat specific etiology (hyperammonemia), the term is useful diagnostically. This is a very rare diagnosis in preclinical safety studies.

20.4.16.3 Astrocyte Swelling/Vacuolation

This diagnosis is discussed below under the more general category Vacuolation (Section 20.4.19.1).

20.4.17 Microglial Cells

20.4.17.1 Microgliosis

The term microgliosis refers to the presence of reactive (enlarged and or more numerous) microglia. Focal or multifocal microgliosis frequently occurs in the nervous system in response to a variety of disorders. As previously noted, clusters of microglial cells may surround dead/degenerating neurons, presumably to phagocytose the cellular remnants. Microglial cell clusters also occur in areas of acute to subacute inflammation and may be present because of a variety of causes. Penetration of large molecules, especially proteins and even antibodies (remember, the BBB is not perfect), may elicit a microglial response. Microglial cells usually respond quickly to damage, especially to neuronal degeneration (Figures 20.8c and d), but also as a component of local inflammatory reactions.

Areas of chronic interstitial fluid accumulation, either introduced (e.g., intraparenchymal infusion into the brain) or endogenous (edema), may elicit a microglial response. If the response is in a large area, such as the corona radiata of an entire hemisphere being edematous, the microglial response may be difficult to detect with H&E but may be quite pronounced if a microglial specific immunohistochemical stain is applied.

20.4.17.2 Microglial Nodules

Because of the way most regulatory studies are designed, the toxicologic pathologist is more likely to observe microglial nodules rather than reactive microgliosis. Microglial nodules are small, focal, or multifocal clusters of microglial cells that do not appear reactive and are not associated with obvious damage. In many cases, these microglial nodules are remnants of prior (reactive) microgliosis. This is a critical point and, as with the interpretation and detection of neuronal necrosis, timing is critical. It is the job of the pathologist not only to observe and record lesions but also to offer insight as to what those lesions might represent. In many cases, microglial nodules are a remnant of an earlier focal/multifocal inflammatory response. Microglial nodules are often "written off" as being related to latent viral infections or some other potential etiology. While those causes cannot be discounted, neither can an earlier, reactive microglial response. Just because you are not seeing it, does not mean it did not occur at an earlier, unobserved time point.

20.4.18 OLIGODENDROCYTES AND SCHWANN CELLS

20.4.18.1 Myelinopathy (Demyelination, Altered Myelin/ Remyelination), Including Myelin Edema

Myelinopathy is a vague term. A more specific term (demyelination/dysmyelination) should be used, if possible, for those lesions where the primary insult appears to be a loss of myelin or alteration of myelin. Most myelin disorders, at some point, will be characterized by altered myelin with an intact/normal-appearing axon, but this may require extensive evaluation to visualize.

As noted, myelin artifacts are rampant in paraffin-embedded tissues. The most common myelin artifacts are the so-called "Buscaino bodies" or "mucocytes" as these areas sometimes appear to contain a mucinous substance. These artifacts of myelin appear as spaces or vacuoles and are very common in the cerebellar white matter, brain stem (Garman 2011a), and optic nerve. They are discussed here because, upon closer examination, these artifacts frequently have intact axons coursing through them (a silver stain can assist with identification of the axons) and are sometimes misdiagnosed as focal demyelination.

True demyelination can, of course, occur in the central or peripheral nervous system and should manifest either as a loss of myelin around intact axons or as a thinning of myelin sheaths. Demyelination is a frequent feature of nerve fiber degeneration (Figure 20.9a). In order to avoid confusion, it is recommended that if demyelination is a feature of a broader axonal degeneration, then it should be described in the narrative or comments section of the pathology report as being present in association with nerve fiber degeneration. If demyelination appears to be a primary process, then the diagnosis of demyelination or myelin degeneration should be used.

Common sense dictates that true demyelination due to administration of a test article should be a direct toxicity of Schwann cells or oligodendrocytes that manifests as focal to multifocal to generalized decreases in myelin, altered myelin formation, or altered myelin sheaths. True demyelination is rare unless a particular test article does cause necrosis/degeneration/alteration of oligodendrocytes or Schwann cells. Diphtheria toxin may cause a true demyelination owing to effects on Schwann cell myelin synthesis (Pleasure et al. 1973).

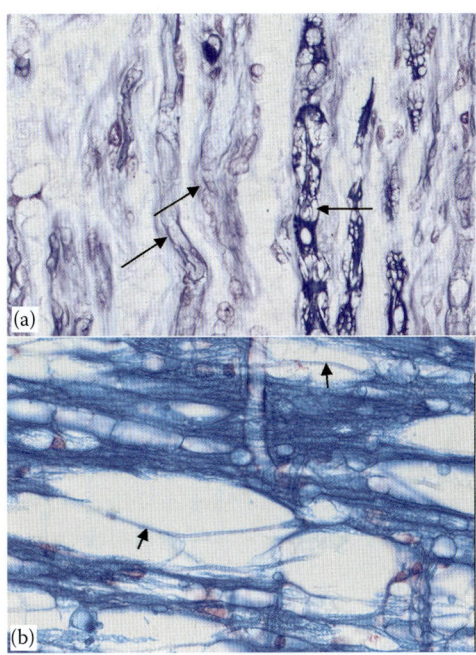

FIGURE 20.9 (a) Goat, spinal nerve root, Luxol Fast Blue stain/paraffin section. The arrow on the right shows a normally myelinated nerve fiber. The arrows on the left show nerve fibers in a stage of degeneration with decreased myelin. Decreased myelin is a common feature of general axonal degeneration and should be described as such. Primary demyelination and dysmyelination are unusual and must be differentiated from the much more common loss of myelin, which is a component of the spectrum of changes that characterize nerve fiber/axonal degeneration. (b) Rat, spinal cord, hexachlorophene toxicity, toluidine blue stain. There are large vacuoles that ultrastructurally are intramyelin separation/edema. Note the arrows, which point to intact axons traversing the large vacuoles.

Triethyl tin and hexachlorophene are two chemicals that do cause primary myelinopathies characterized by splitting of myelin sheaths. This change is also called intramyelinic edema. After hexachlorophene administration, the morphologic change is one of splitting of myelin sheaths. Figure 20.9b shows this change in a longitudinal section of spinal cord stained with Luxol Fast Blue. Note the large spaces that ultrastructurally represent separations/fluid accumulations in the myelin sheath. Many such sheaths have an intact axon coursing through the spaces. Although a very pronounced change, this must be differentiated from artifactual spaces in poorly fixed spinal cord sections.

20.4.18.2 Schwann Cell Hyperplasia

This is a common characteristic of nerve fiber degeneration. If Schwann cell hyperplasia is a prominent feature of the degeneration, it can be diagnosed separately. More often, Schwann cell hyperplasia is described as a feature of nerve fiber degeneration. Schwann cell hyperplasia can be a very prominent component of a spectrum of morphologic changes associated with the administration of some nerve growth factors.

20.4.19 MISCELLANEOUS

20.4.19.1 Vacuolation/Vacuolation White Matter

Some of this information is a bit repetitive, but because of the frequency with which the pathologist encounters vacuoles in the CNS, these are important points worth repeating.

With the exception of vacuoles that clearly occupy the cytoplasm of the neuron cell body or are within microglial cells/macrophages/pericytes, it is nearly impossible to state for certain on an H&E section the cellular or extracellular location of vacuoles/vacuolation beyond the general location (i.e., gray or white matter).

Vacuoles may occur in neuronal cell processes (dendrites/axons), glial cells (astrocyte processes; microglial processes), or myelin or lie extracellularly in the interstitial space. Vacuolation may represent a direct toxic effect, such as the vacuolation/myelin splitting that occurs with hexachlorophene administration or in lysosomal storage diseases, or they may appear as nondescript "holes" in the neuropil. The latter situation is the most common.

Vacuolation encountered by the toxicologic pathologist is typically one of three types.

The great majority of vacuolation is an artifactual change due to suboptimal fixation; this is especially true in the spinal cord white matter. This must always be differentiated from true vacuolation that may be due to, for example, intramyelinic edema. The controls should be consulted to make the determination. Along with adequate fixation, it is important to process tissues across groups, rather than process all controls in one processor run, followed by the test article–treated groups in other processor runs. Processing can have an effect on nervous system tissue, as the organic solvents are removing most of the myelin, and the pathologist never wants to be in a situation where something as simple as a processing schedule confounds the ability to make the correct diagnosis.

The diagnosis of vacuolation that is clearly associated with a particular cell type (such as neuronal vacuolation) and possibly intramyelin edema/vacuolation may be made based on evaluation of the H&E slide. However, isolating the vacuoles to a particular organelle or structure (e.g., a portion of the myelin sheath) requires the use of the transmission electron microscope. This is also true for vacuolation that occurs exclusively in white matter. To identify the actual location of the vacuoles, ultrastructural examination by the pathologist (not a technician taking photomicrographs, unless highly trained) is recommended.

If the vacuolation is clearly associated with another primary event, such as an adjacent or associated inflammation, or another process that is causing destruction of elements of the nervous system, then the vacuolation is likely a combination of interstitial fluid, swollen astrocytic processes, swollen neuronal processes, possibly vacuolated macrophages (if there is necrosis of neuropil), and other unknown elements. This type of vacuolation does not typically require additional investigation and is sometimes referred to as "rarefaction" by some pathologists. Rarefaction literally means a reduction in density and is a reasonably descriptive diagnostic term for this nonspecific vacuolated appearance of damaged neuropil. This nonspecific vacuolation typically affects gray and white matter, but mostly gray matter. However, it should be noted that if interstitial fluid accumulates, white matter is usually disproportionately affected, as fluid tends to accumulate more in white matter than in gray matter.

20.4.19.2   Infiltrates versus Inflammation

This is a critical point that involves both the art and science of toxicologic pathology. Toxicologic pathologists tend to be the most educated individuals involved in the assessment of a preclinical study. Our opinions are typically based on our training and experience. But other readers of pathology reports, including toxicologists and regulatory personnel, often lack specific medical training. Their understanding is also based on their training, experience, and perception.

We may know that a few lymphocytes in the meninges, in an animal with viral encephalitis, for example, is a highly significant event. We may even characterize the occurrence of such cells as a nonsuppurative meningitis. But to characterize a few lymphocytes in the meninges as meningitis, when the cells are just there as a low-level reaction to some unknown, insignificant event, has the tendency to cause others to overinterpret the significance of the change. Meningitis is a serious disorder; it makes the national news. So a minimal focal cellular infiltrate in the meninges of a test animal, while it could be significant, is much more likely an insignificant lesion with no relationship to the test article. Such infiltrates are occasionally observed in control animals, especially dogs and monkeys. So by convention in toxicologic pathology, inflammation is diagnosed when infiltrates of white blood cells occur in association with other indicators of tissue damage. Infiltrates, which may still be biologically significant, are diagnosed when the white blood cells are there in isolation without other indicators of tissue damage. Oddly, pathologists are quite used to this line of thinking in other tissues such as salivary glands and in many other tissues where lymphocytic infiltrates are noted in the absence of tissue damage and diagnosed as such, versus diagnosing subacute or chronic inflammation, which are normally associated with tissue damage. The same consideration should be given to the nervous system.

The INHAND document should be consulted if additional information is required concerning the distinction between inflammatory cell infiltrates versus inflammation.

20.4.19.3   Hemorrhage

As in all tissues, occasionally red blood cells outside the vascular system may be noted in the nervous system. This is most commonly observed in the meninges. While the source of hemorrhage should always be investigated, extravascular blood, usually, has an obvious source (inflammation/damage to a blood vessel).

The toxicologic pathologist may want to consider using the term microhemorrhage for describing small, focal areas of extravascular blood that may be encountered in the meninges and neuroparenchyma. It is also useful to describe the microhemorrhage using specific measurements or a scale bar on photomicrographs. Ocular micrometers or imaging programs are useful for this. It is very useful for a reviewer to know that the term "hemorrhage" refers to an area that measures 0.5 mm in diameter as opposed to a regulatory reviewer conjuring up images of massive hemorrhage in the brain. Some pathologists rarely measure microscopic changes or use photomicrographs to illustrate a change, but if such information would be useful to the reader of the pathology report, then such information should be included.

Handling and even trimming and sectioning of brain, especially those that are not well fixed, can cause artifactual hemorrhage to appear in the tissue sections. But hemorrhage can also be related to test article administration. Specifically, certain test articles that damage endothelial cells may disproportionately affect vascular-rich areas such as the choroid plexus and other CVOs (unpublished observation). Brains from found dead animals, due to autolysis, frequently have numerous areas of extravascular blood that could be incorrectly diagnosed as hemorrhage, but the change is usually an artifact.

20.4.19.4   Dilated Ventricles/Central Canal

Hydrocephalus is equivalent to dilation of portions of the ventricular system. Because the extent of this dilation tends to vary, specifying the areas of dilation is recommended. This is a somewhat common finding in all species and ventricular dilation does occur in control animals. In most cases, in control as well as test article–treated animals, the cause is not apparent.

Just about any alteration of the brain and spinal cord parenchyma can cause some degree of dilation of the ventricular system and central canal. The dilation may be active and caused by an obstruction of the flow of CSF, or be passive owing to the loss of parenchyma. Passive dilation is common with lesions that cause pronounced destruction to parenchyma, particularly in the diencephalon and telencephalon. Rats with iatrogenic ischemic strokes, usually as a result of the experimental occlusion of the internal carotid artery, frequently have ventricular dilation on the affected side and sometimes on the nonaffected side as well.

Unexpected dilated ventricles/hydrocephalus is a morphologic change that lends itself to a quick review of available historical control data, as this lesion will occasionally be noted in control animals.

20.4.19.5 Infarction

Infarction in the brain is, of course, a serious event, although in many animals where an infarct is suspected, the animals were clinically normal.

Infarction is most commonly observed in rats (and other animal models) that have had a procedure to restrict or occlude blood flow to the brain (Isayama et al. 1991; Overgaard and Meden 2000). Pathologists involved in these types of studies should familiarize themselves with 2,3,5-triphenyltetrazolium chloride staining that is used on the gross tissues to assist in infarct quantification. Studies involved with stroke models are frequently testing the ability of a particular treatment to limit damage to the parenchyma adjacent to the actual area of ischemic necrosis, the so-called penumbra region. In these animals, the area of infarction is clearly recognized, depending on the time frame (i.e., time necropsied after the ischemic insult), as a central area of nonselective necrosis, surrounded by macrophages and glial cells, mostly astrocytes.

Smaller areas, generally in the periphery of the cerebral cortex and resembling chronic infarcts, are occasionally noted in larger animal species, notably dogs and monkeys. The cause of these small lesions is not always apparent but prior trauma is suspected.

20.4.19.6 Thrombosis and Vasculitis

Thrombi are occasionally seen, usually in the meningeal vessels.

The most common vasculitis lesions are polyarteritis (Snyder et al. 1995), a.k.a. beagle pain syndrome, in beagle dogs and polyarteritis nodosa of aging male rats. Of the two, the condition in dogs seems to have a predilection for the meningeal vessels. Most of the lesions in rats are in the mesenteric arteries, but can sometimes be seen in the meninges.

These lesions have all the typical changes of fibrinoid necrosis, polymorphonuclear cellular infiltrates in the vessel wall, thickened vessel wall, and decreased lumen diameter. It is important to recognize that these conditions can occur spontaneously and to make sure this diagnosis is added to your historical control database, as the issue of whether or not vasculitis in the meninges is test article related comes up in every pathologist's career.

20.4.19.7 Mineralization

As in all tissues, mineralization can occur in areas of tissue damage/necrosis as calcium salts are deposited. Mineralization of small blood vessels in the brain, especially in primates and rodents, is a fairly common spontaneous microscopic change.

20.4.19.8 Epidermoid Cysts

Epidermoid (or squamous) cysts are seen as spontaneous lesions adjacent to the spinal cord in rats and the brain in mice. They are reported to be rare in rats (Solleveld and Boorman 1990) but, in the experience of the author (Butt), are common enough to be noted with some frequency. These cysts are reported to be more common in mice (Maronpot et al. 1999).

20.5 DIAGNOSTIC NEUROPATHOLOGY—PROLIFERATIVE LESIONS

Spontaneous hyperplastic, preneoplastic, and neoplastic findings of the brain, spinal cord, and peripheral nerves are infrequently diagnosed in preclinical toxicity studies involving the commonly used rodent strains. Most are only encountered (with any frequency) in chronic 26/52-week and 104-week carcinogenicity studies. As the terminal or early-sacrifice animals represent one time point, the true nature of some of the neoplasms with respect to malignancy cannot be clearly established. "Benign" should only be a diagnosis of morphology rather than the character of a brain tumor.

Proliferative lesions of the nervous system of rabbits, dogs, and monkeys are rarely encountered because of the typically young age of these animals on toxicity studies.

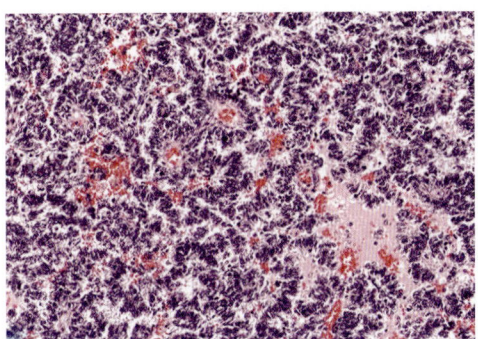

FIGURE 20.10   This is a medulloblastoma that originated in the cerebellum. The figure shows the characteristic neoplastic cells forming pseudorosettes occasionally encircling small blood vessels. Individual neoplastic cells are small, with scant cytoplasm and hyperchromatic nuclei.

20.5.1   Neuronal Neoplastic Lesions

20.5.1.1   Medulloblastoma, Malignant (Cerebellar Neuroblastoma, Primitive Neuroectodermal Tumor of Cerebellum)

Medulloblastoma is a densely cellular mass, usually within the cerebellum, composed of neuroepithelial stem cells that may exhibit neuronal differentiation. The general microscopic appearance resembles the granular cell layer of the cerebellar cortex (Figure 20.10). The cells are small, round, or elongated (carrot shaped), with scant cytoplasm and indistinct cell borders. Nuclei are round to elongated, hyperchromatic with prominent nucleoli. Formation of pseudorosettes is common in a concentric arrangement of tumor cells encircling small blood vessels or eosinophilic fibrillary material. Bizarre mitotic figures are frequent. These tumors show an invasive growth pattern, often replacing cerebellar folia, and can metastasize within the CNS via CSF-filled cavities. Specific immunohistochemical markers have not been identified for rodents. Synaptophysin and neuron-specific enolase may be useful in nonhuman primates and dogs. Human tumors demonstrate co-expression of more than one type of intermediate filament in the same neoplasm, indicating their undifferentiated, primitive neuroectodermal status. They are rarely observed in mice as a primary tumor but may be induced by direct implantation of pellets containing carcinogenic compounds into the vermis or lateral lobes of the cerebellar cortex or via transplacental and neonatal induction with the alkylating agent ethylnitrosourea (ENU). Medulloblastoma may also be induced experimentally in mice, rats, and hamsters by intracranial inoculation with various primate or human viruses (Cardesa et al. 1996; Ogawa 1989; Padgett et al. 1977; Rapp et al. 1969) or in mice by genetic engineering (Huse and Holland 2009).

20.5.2   Glial Cell Neoplastic Lesions

Glial cell tumors are believed to arise from neoplastic radial glia cells (RGCs). RGCs are mitotically active, multipotent progenitor cells that give rise to neurons, astrocytes, oligodendrocytes, and ependymal cells. These neoplasms may expand along CSF-filled spaces into the spinal cord, but metastasis outside the nervous system has not been reported in laboratory animals. Animals affected by all tumor types show the same spectrum of clinical signs consistent with an intracranial mass, including torticollis, abnormal gait, posterior apresis, loss of balance, loss of grip reflex, and head tilt.

20.5.3 ASTROCYTOMA, MALIGNANT (GLIOMA, ASTROCYTIC)

These are poorly demarcated tumors, usually of modest size, confined to one major area of the CNS (low grade) or extensive, multicentric, or diffuse lesions with no discernible boundaries spreading over two or more major areas of the CNS (high grade) (Figure 20.11a). Even large tumors seldom cause clinical signs before the end of a 104-week rat study. They show variable cellularity and may infiltrate the meninges and ependyma. The neoplastic cells show uniform or anaplastic features, including round or fusiform nuclei, a variable amount of eosinophilic cytoplasm, and indistinct cell borders. In larger tumors, there may also be foci of hemorrhage and necrosis, with palisading of neoplastic astrocytes around necrotic foci. Neoplastic cells appearing as perineuronal satellitosis and perivascular cuffing may be present at the periphery of the neoplasm. Reactive astrocytes (gemistocytes positive for GFAP) may be present.

Neoplastic astrocytes often spread into Virchow–Robin spaces along radiating blood vessels.

TEM and Ramon y Cajal's gold sublimate staining reveal the presence of glial filaments in the perikaryon and processes of neoplastic astrocytes.

Astrocytomas from humans and domestic animals commonly express GFAP and are labeled by phosphotungstic acid hematoxylin (PTAH) stain. Spontaneous neoplastic astrocytes in the rat and mouse brain generally lack GFAP reactivity but may stain positively for lysozyme, PTAH, and vimentin (Pruimboom-Brees et al. 2004). In ENU-induced gliomas in rats, most astrocytomas were negative for GFAP and Leu-7 but positive for S-100 and (usually) vimentin (Raju et al. 1990; Zook et al. 2000) The exact cell of origin for many tumors with the appearance of a classic astrocytoma in rats is somewhat controversial (partially to the lack of GFAP staining).

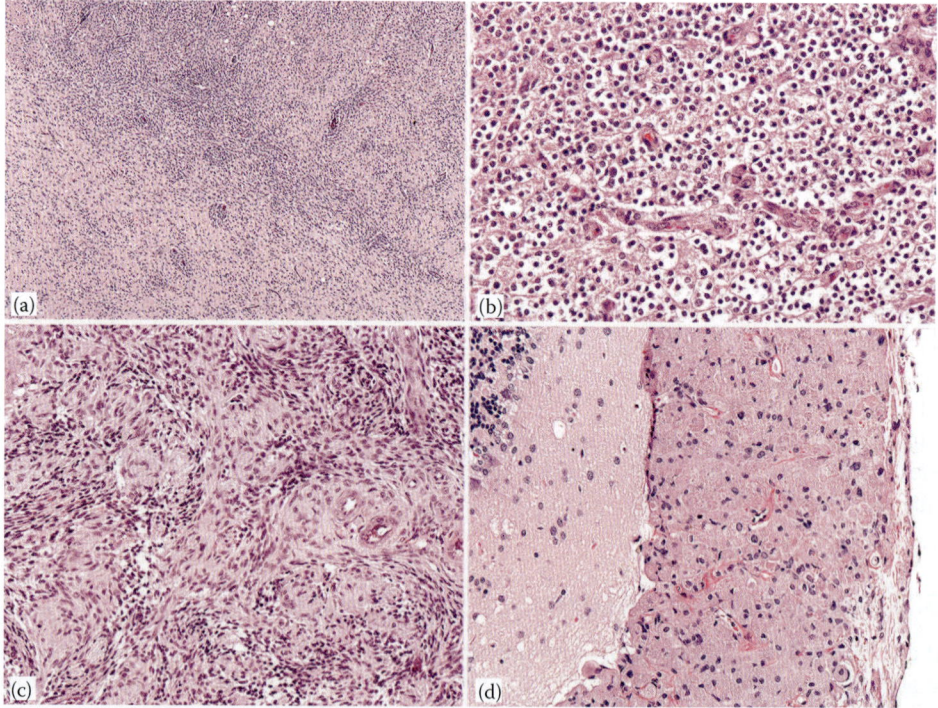

FIGURE 20.11 (a) This malignant astrocytoma lacks discernible boundaries and displays extensive infiltration of the adjacent neuropil. (b) Oligodendroglioma with sheets of neoplastic cells characterized by round, central, hyperchromatic nuclei; clear cytoplasm (perinuclear halo); and distinct cell boundaries. Note the characteristic "honeycomb" pattern. (c) Schwannoma characterized by palisading spindle cells with elongated hyperchromatic nuclei and eosinophilic cytoplasm. (d) Granular cell tumor of the meninges over the cerebellum: note the characteristic abundant cytoplasm and variably well-defined cell borders.

20.5.4 Glioma, Mixed, Malignant (Oligoastroglioma)

Low-grade tumors have well-defined borders and are confined to one major area of the CNS. High-grade tumors have an indistinct border and are typically present in multiple areas of the brain and spinal cord. The mass consists of a sheet of neoplastic oligodendrocytes and astrocytes in variable proportions, with each cell type constituting at least 20% of the neoplasm and in one of two arrangements: cell types intermingled or separate large cell regions adjacent to one another and each containing predominantly a single cell type. In the high-grade tumors, cellular atypia and pleomorphism are widespread, and astrocytic or oligodendrocytic differentiation may not be obvious in some areas. Occasional tumor giant cells, generally of astrocytic lineage, are present. Foci of necrosis, marked vascular proliferation, edema, and hemorrhage may occur. Vascular endothelial cell hypertrophy and hyperplasia may be present.

Experimental studies have indicated that gliomas in adult rats are initially composed of either differentiated astrocytes or oligodendrocytes. The cellular composition becomes mixed and anaplastic as the neoplasms increase in size. The malignant mixed (anaplastic) glioma in rodents shares some histological features with the human lesion designated glioblastoma multiforme (GBM). Some pathologists consider a diagnosis of GBM specific to human neuro-oncology and do not use the term in diagnosing neoplasms in the rat.

20.5.5 Oligodendroglioma, Malignant

These are rare tumors that usually occur in the ventrolateral cerebrum and involve the thalamus, basal nuclei, hypothalamus, and corpus callosum (Figure 20.11b). Low-grade tumors are confined to one major area of the CNS, whereas high-grade tumors extend throughout multiple areas of the brain or spinal cord. The tumors are composed of sheets, rows, or nests of small, neoplastic cells with round, central, hyperchromatic nuclei, clear to lightly stained cytoplasm (perinuclear halo), and distinct cell borders. The cytoplasm of the neoplastic oligodendrocytes accumulates acid mucopolysaccharides and therefore stains with Alcian blue while being virtually resistant to the usual histopathology stains such as eosin. The pronounced clear perinuclear halo is a common artifact of delayed fixation and results in the classic "honeycomb" or "fried-egg" pattern. Sheets of neoplastic cells are intersected by fibrovascular stroma and mucopolysaccharide-rich edema fluid (Janisch and Schreiber 1994). Early tumors show satellitosis around cortical neurons and small blood vessels. Other glial cells, such as astrocytes and transitional cell forms between oligodendrocytes and astrocytes, may be present in varying numbers. Prominent microvascular proliferation with atypical capillary endothelial hyperplasia ("garlands") can be extensive, especially at the periphery of the neoplasm.

Neoplastic cells in low-grade tumors are uniform. The high-grade malignant tumors exhibit focal or diffuse anaplasia as evidenced by increased cellularity, pronounced cellular atypia, pleomorphism, nuclear polymorphism, prominent proliferation of glomeruloid vessels at the tumor margins, increased mitotic index, necrosis, and meningeal infiltration. Necrosis with cystic changes and hemorrhage with hemosiderosis may be present.

Some oligodendrogliomas may contain a considerable population of astrocytes that are reactive rather than neoplastic. The GFAP immunohistochemical stain can be used in rodents to distinguish reactive astrocytes (GFAP positive) from neoplastic astrocytes (GFAP negative). Neoplastic oligodendrocytes stain positively for galactose cerebroside and carbonic anhydrase C. Positive immunostaining for myelin basic protein has been reported in human and rat tumors and may be of use to confirm a diagnosis in the mouse. Some human oligodendrogliomas express S-100 and Leu-7, but this pattern is not specific for oligodendrogliomas. In ENU-induced gliomas in rats, most oligodendrogliomas are Leu-7 positive but are negative for GFAP and usually S-100; neoplastic cells are generally vimentin negative but may be focally positive (Zook et al. 2000). Anaplastic tumors lose positivity for Leu-7 and alcianophilia (Janisch and Schreiber 1994). Oligodendrocyte transcription factor-1 is a potential oligodendrocyte marker in humans. Oligodendrogliomas are the most common, chemically induced tumor in the rat (Janisch and Schreiber 1994).

20.5.6 Schwann Cell Neoplasms

Schwannomas begin as foci of hypercellularity within a nerve. Schwann cell neoplasms may arise in the cranial vault, adjacent to large peripheral nerves and nerve plexi, or within soft tissues.

20.5.6.1 Schwannoma (Neurilemmoma, Neurinoma)

These are expansive, compressing lesions located near a peripheral nerve or nerve plexus, commonly growing without producing clinical signs (Figure 20.11c). Benign tumors are usually encapsulated. Malignant schwannomas are unencapsulated lesions, although still commonly asymptomatic unless compression and invasion of adjacent tissues are present. As with many neoplasms, features indicative of potential malignancy include a high mitotic rate, cellular or mitotic atypia, and locally invasive growth or metastasis. Two basic patterns are characteristically observed:

> *Antoni A pattern:* Schwann cells are elongated with indistinct cell borders and form nuclear palisades (i.e., cell nuclei arranged in parallel bands). Adjacent palisades and the intervening cytoplasm of adjacent cells form "Verocay bodies," in which the nuclear palisades form parallel rows separated by homogeneous, anuclear, eosinophilic intercellular material.
> *Antoni B pattern:* There are sparsely cellular regions, with a clear matrix sometimes containing cystic cavities.

One pattern may predominate over another pattern. Antoni A and B patterns are not always apparent in a given neoplasm. Several tumor variants are also defined by their morphologic characteristics: cellular variant composed mainly of cellular Antoni A tissue, with no Verocay bodies; granular cell variant with cytoplasmic granules comparable to those in granular cell tumors of the meninges; melanotic variant containing melanosomes; and plexiform variant in which a multinodular pattern, presumably involving the various branches of a nerve plexus, predominates.

Schwann cell differentiation can be confirmed using positive immunohistochemistry for S-100, proteolipid protein, or peripheral myelin protein 22 kDa, or by demonstration of convoluted cytoplasmic processes lined by a continuous basal lamina as observed by TEM. In the rat, characteristic lesions occur in the heart (endocardial schwannoma, schwannomatosis, cardiac neurilemmoma), near the ear pinna, inside the eye (intraocular) and orbit, and in the mandibular salivary gland. The incidence is quite low in all strains tested (Novilla et al. 1991).

Schwannomas may be induced in rats by direct-acting alkylating agents such as N-nitrosoethylurea or methylmethane sulfonate, which act as transplacental carcinogens. Schwannomas have also been induced in rats after postnatal exposure to 7,12-dimethylbenz[α]anthracene or N-nitrosomethylurea. Malignant schwannomas have been described in double transgenic mice expressing simian virus 40 large tumor antigen and prokaryotic β-galactosidase (LacZ) under the control of the MBP promoter (Jensen et al. 1993). Genetically engineered mouse models of neurofibromatosis, with manipulation of genes NF1 or NF2, induce peripheral nerve sheaths tumors, including schwannomas (Stemmer-Rachamimov et al. 2004). Malignant melanotic schwannomas can be induced in hamsters by injection of unsymmetrical dimethylhydrazine or 1,1-dimethyl-hydrazine (Ernst and Mohr 1988).

20.5.7 Hamartoma, Lipomatous (Lipoma)

Lipomatous hamartomas, occasionally observed in the brains of rodents, are composed of single or multiple, well-demarcated foci of mature, well-differentiated, white adipose cells containing a single, large fat droplet (Budka 1974). Small lipocytic infiltrates are classified as lipomatous hamartomas based on occurrence at an aberrant site. They are predominantly located in the midline or ventricles of the brain associated with meninges or choroid plexus. This lesion is not a neoplasm, but its biological behavior is that of a space-occupying benign tumor. Lipomatous hamartomas have been described in C57BL and C3H/HeJ mice (Adkison and Sundberg 1991). It has been reported in rats only once (Brander and Perentes 1995). In man, this lesion is thought to be caused by neural tube closure defects during embryogenesis (Fitz 1982).

20.5.8 Granular Cell Tumors

The most common meningeal neoplasms in the rat, occurring much less frequently in mice, are granular cell tumors (Figure 20.11d). They are considered to be of neural crest origin. They may occur in the cerebrum and cerebellum as solitary, pink to yellow growths that are well demarcated from the surrounding brain tissue. In some cases, they may be diffuse and extend along blood vessels and into the brain parenchyma (Solleveld and Boorman 1990). Microscopically, benign granular cell tumors are composed of a monomorphic population of polygonal cells with central to eccentric, round to oval nuclei. The cytoplasm contains abundant eosinophilic granules that stain positive with periodic acid–Schiff (Krinke et al. 2000). Less common are smaller cells with oval hyperchromatic nuclei and scant granular cytoplasm. Malignant granular cell tumors are generally more compressive and invasive and consist of multiple micronodular clusters of neoplastic cells. Mitotic figures are rarely observed.

20.5.9 Meningioma

Meningiomas may be seen in the mouse or rat as plaques of meningeal thickenings on the dorsal or dorsolateral surfaces of the cerebrum, optic nerves, or spinal cord. Microscopically, benign meningiomas are classified as fibroblastic or meningothelial (Gopinath 1986; Mitsumori et al. 1987). Fibroblastic meningiomas are characterized by closely packed spindle cells with pale, eosinophilic, fibrillar cytoplasm forming irregular, interwoven bundles containing varying amounts of collagen separating individual cells. Meningothelial meningiomas are characterized by sheets or lobules of large epithelioid cells, with abundant eosinophilic cytoplasm. Mitotic figures are rare. Malignant meningiomas (meningeal sarcomas) are invasive with extensive infiltration of atypical and pleomorphic neoplastic cells into the brain parenchyma and along blood vessels. They can be classified as fibrous, spondyloid, or undifferentiated. Mitotic figures are frequently seen and sometimes bizarre in appearance. Generally, benign meningiomas are more common than the malignant forms. Meningioangiomatosis must be differentiated from malignant meningiomas. This is a benign proliferation of cells within the meninges where there is perivascular penetration but no other indications of malignancy, such as atypia, pleomorphism, or high mitotic rates (Balme et al. 2008).

20.5.10 Choroid Plexus Tumors

Choroid plexus tumors are rare in rats and mice. These tumors occur in the ventricles of the brain that are lined by choroid plexus epithelium. Choroid plexus papillomas are characterized by papillary projections that are formed by a single layer of cuboidal to columnar epithelial cells with abundant eosinophilic cytoplasm. Choroid plexus carcinomas invade the adjacent brain parenchyma and are characterized by pseudostratification of the epithelium that is atypical and pleomorphic. Mitotic figures are generally present (Solleveld et al. 1991).

20.5.11 Ependymoma

Ependymomas are rare in rats and mice and are located near the ventricles and aqueduct of the brain and the central canal of the spinal cord (Gopinath 1986; Radovsky and Mahler 1999). Benign ependymomas are characterized by polygonal cells that have round to oval, hyperchromatic nuclei and indistinct borders that are arranged in rows and rosettes around empty lumens. Pseudorosettes surrounding blood vessels may be present. Subcellular organelles including cilia and associated basal bodies (blepharoplasts) are common and are consistent with well-differentiated ependymal cells.

Malignant ependymomas invade the neuropil adjacent to the ventricular system. Cellular atypia, pleomorphism, and mitotic figures are common.

20.5.12 MALIGNANT RETICULOSIS

Malignant reticulosis is more often seen in the rat than in the mouse and is characterized by diffuse infiltrates of a mixture of lymphoid to histiocytic-type cells with pleomorphic nuclei. Prominent perivascular and periventricular infiltrates often extend along the leptomeninges. The stroma contains abundant reticulin and collagen fibers (Solleveld and Boorman 1990; Solleveld et al. 1991). Synonyms for malignant reticulosis include lymphoreticulosis, microgliomatosis, and primary malignant histiocytoma of the brain. The mixed cell morphology, growth pattern, and prominent perivascular infiltrates are important criteria for distinguishing malignant reticulosis from gliomas and lymphomas.

REFERENCES

Adkison, D. L., and J. P. Sundberg. 1991. "Lipomatous" hamartomas and choristomas in inbred laboratory mice. *Vet Pathol* 28:305–312.

Agulhon, C., J. Petravicz, A. McMullen et al. 2008. What is the role of astrocyte calcium in neurophysiology? *Neuron* 59:932–946.

Azzi, G., J. Bernaudin, C. Bouchaud et al. 1990. Permeability of the normal rat brain, spinal cord and dorsal root ganglia microcirculations to immunoglobulins G. *Biol Cell* 68:31–36.

Balme, E., D. R. Roth, and E. Perentes. 2008. Cerebral meningioangiomatosis in a CD-1 mouse: a case report and comparison with humans and dogs. *Exp Toxicol Pathol* 60:247–251.

Banks, W. A. 1999. Physiology and pathology of the blood–brain barrier: implications for microbial pathogenesis, drug delivery and neurodegenerative disorders. *J Neurovirol* 5:538–555.

Bolon, B. and D. O'Brien. 2011. Localizing neuropathological lesions using neurological findings. In *Fundamental Neuropathology for Pathologists and Toxicologists: Principles and Techniques*, ed. B. Bolon and M. Butt, 89–104. Hoboken, NJ: J. Wiley and Sons, Inc.

Brander, P., and E. Perentes. 1995. Intracranial lipoma in a laboratory rat. *Vet Pathol* 32:65–67.

Brumovsky, P., M. J. Villar, and T. Hokfelt. 2006. Tyrosine hydroxylase is expressed in a subpopulation of small dorsal root ganglion neurons in the adult mouse. *Exp Neurol* 200:153–165.

Budka, H. 1974. Intracranial lipomatous hamartomas (intracranial "lipoma"). A study of 13 cases including combination with medulloblastoma, colloid and epidermoid cysts, angiomatosis and other malformations. *Acta Neuropathol (Berl)* 28:205–222.

Butt, M. 2011. Evaluation of the adult nervous system in preclinical studies. In *Fundamental Neuropathology for Pathologists and Toxicologists: Principles and Techniques*, ed. B. Bolon and M. Butt, 321–338. Hoboken, NJ: J. Wiley and Sons, Inc.

Cardesa, A., G. M. ZuRhein, F. F. Cruz-Sanchez et al. 1996. Tumours of the nervous system. In *Pathology of Tumours in Laboratory Animals, Volume III: Tumours of the Hamster*, ed. V. S. Turusov and U. Mohr, 427–465. IARC Scientific Publication No. 126 Lyon.

Chojnacki, A. K., G. K. Mak, and S. Weiss. 2009. Identity crisis for adult periventricular neural stem cells: subventricular zone astrocytes, ependymal cells or both? *Nat Rev Neurosci* 10:153–156.

Das, G. 1977. Binucleated neurons in the central nervous system of laboratory animals. *Cell Mol Life Sci* 33:1179–1180.

deLahunta, A., and E. Glass. 2009. *Veterinary Neuroanatomy and Clinical Neurology*. 29–53. St. Louis, MO: Saunders Elsevier.

Ernst, H., and U. Mohr. 1988. Malignant melanotic schwannomas induced by 1,1-dimethylhydrazine, European Hamster. In *Monographs on Pathology of Laboratory Animals. Nervous System*, ed. T. C. Jones, G. C. Hard, and U. Mohr, 160–164. Berlin: Springer-Verlag.

Fitz, C. R. 1982. Midline anomalies of the brain and spine. *Radiol Clin North Am* 20:95–104.

Fix, A. S., J. F. Ross, S. R. Stitzel et al. 1996. Integrated evaluation of central nervous system lesions: stains for neurons, astrocytes, and microglia reveal the spatial and temporal features of MK-801-induced neuronal necrosis in the rat cerebral cortex. *Toxicol Pathol* 24:291–304.

Garman, R. 2011a. Histology of the central nervous system. *Toxicol Pathol* 39:22–35.

Garman, R. 2011b. Common histologic artifacts in nervous system tissues. In *Fundamental Neuropathology for Pathologists and Toxicologists: Principles and Techniques*, ed. B. Bolon and M. Butt, 191–202. Hoboken, NJ: J. Wiley and Sons, Inc.

Gopinath, C. 1986. Spontaneous brain tumours in Sprague–Dawley rats. *Food Chem Toxicol* 24:113–120.

Harding, B., and A. Copp. 2008. Malformations. In *Greenfield's Neuropathology, 8th edition*, ed. S. Love, D. Louis, and D. Ellison, 424–425. London: Edward Arnold Ltd.

Huse, J. T., and E. C. Holland. 2009. Genetically engineered mouse models of brain cancer and the promise of preclinical testing. *Brain Pathol* 19:132–143.

INHAND Project. 2011. Nervous System. http://www.goreni.org/index.php.

Isayama, K., L. H. Pitts, and M. C. Nishimura. 1991. Evaluation of 2,3,5-triphenyltetrazolium chloride staining to delineate rat brain infracts. *Stroke* 22:1394–1398.

Janisch, W., and D. Schreiber. 1994. Neoplasms of the central and peripheral nervous system in laboratory animals. In *Pathology of Neoplasia and Preneoplasia in Rodents. EULEP Colour Atlas*, ed. P. Bannasch and W. Gossner, 125–141. Stuttgart, Germany: Schattauer.

Jensen, N.A., M. L. Rodriguez, J. S. Garvey et al. 1993. Transgenic mouse model for neurocristopathy: schwannomas and facial bone tumors. *Proc Natl Acad Sci USA* 90:3192–3196.

Krinke, G. J., W. Kaufmann, A. T. Mahrous et al. 2000. Morphologic characterization of spontaneous nervous system tumors in mice and rats. *Toxicol Pathol* 28:178–192.

Maronpot, R., G. Boorman, and B. Baul. 1999. *Pathology of the Mouse*. 453–456. St. Louis, MO: Cache River Press.

McMartin, D. N., J. L. O'Donoghue, R. Morrissey et al. 1997. Non-proliferative lesions of the nervous system in rats, NS-1. In *Guides for Toxicologic Pathology*. Washington, DC: STP/ARP/AFIP. https://www.toxpath.org/ssdnc/NervousNonprolifRat.pdf.

Mitsumori, K., R. R. Maronpot, and G. A. Boorman. 1987. Spontaneous tumors of the meninges in rats. *Vet Pathol* 24:50–58.

Moser, V. 2011. Behavioral model systems for evaluating neuropathology. In *Fundamental Neuropathology for Pathologists and Toxicologists: Principles and Techniques*, ed. B. Bolon and M. Butt, 105–114. Hoboken, NJ: J. Wiley and Sons, Inc.

Norenberg, M. 2005. The reactive astrocytes. In *The Role of Glia in Neurotoxicity, 2nd edition*, ed. M. Aschner and L. Costa. Washington, DC: CRC Press.

Novilla, M. N., G. E. Sandusky, D. M. Hoover et al. 1991. A retrospective survey of endocardial proliferative lesions in rats. *Vet Pathol* 28:156–165.

Ogawa, K. 1989. Embryonal neuroepithelial tumors induced by human adenovirus type 12 in rodents. 2. Tumor induction in the central nervous system. *Acta Neuropathol* 78:232–244.

Oldfield, B. J., and M. J. McKinley. 1995. Circumventricular organs. In *The Rat Nervous System*, ed. G. Paxinos, 391–404. San Diego: Academic Press.

Overgaard, K., and P. Meden. 2000. Influence of different fixation procedures on the quantification of infarction and oedema in a rat model of stroke. *Neuropathol Appl Neurobiol* 26:243–250.

Padgett, B. L., D. L. Walker, G. M. ZuRhein et al. 1977. Differential neurooncogenicity of strains of JC virus, a human polyoma virus, in newborn Syrian hamsters. *Cancer Res* 37:718–720.

Pardo, I. D., R. H. Garman, K. Weber et al. 2012. Technical guide for nervous system sampling of the cynomolgus monkey for general toxicity studies. *Toxicol Pathol*. 40:624–636.

Paxinos, G., and C. Watson. 1998. *The Rat Brain in Stereotaxic Coordinates, 4th edition*. San Diego: Academic Press.

Pleasure, D., B. Feldmann, and D. Prockop. 1973. Diphtheria toxin inhibits the synthesis of myelin proteolipid and basic proteins by peripheral nerve in vitro. *J Neurochem* 20:81–90.

Pruimboom-Brees, I. M., D. J. Brees, A. C. Shen et al. 2004. Malignant astrocytoma with binucleated granular cells in a Sprague–Dawley rat. *Vet Pathol* 41:287–290.

Radovsky, A., and J. F. Mahler. 1999. Nervous system. In *Pathology of the Mouse. Reference and Atlas*, ed. R. Maronpot, G. Boorman, and B. Gaul, 460–461. St. Louis, MO: Cache River Press.

Raju, N. R., M. J. Yaeger, D. L. Okazaki et al. 1990. Immunohistochemical characterization of rat central and peripheral nerve tumors induced by ethylnitrosourea. *Toxicol Pathol* 18:18–23.

Rapp, F., S. Pauluzzi, T. A. Waltz et al. 1969. Induction of brain tumors in newborn hamsters by simian adenovirus SA7. *Cancer Res* 29:1173–1178.

Rogers-Corone, T., M. Burgess, J. Hinckley et al. 2010. Vacuolation of sensory ganglion neuron cytoplasm in rats with long-term organophosphates. *Toxicol Pathol* 38:554–559.

Saleem, K. S., and N. K. Logothetis. 2007. *A Combined MRI and Histology Atlas of the Rhesus Monkey Brain in Stereotaxic Coordinates*. San Diego: Academic Press.

Sarkar, S., and L. Schmued. 2011. Fluoro-Jade dyes: fluorochromes for the histochemical localization of degenerating neurons. In *Fundamental Neuropathology for Pathologists and Toxicologists: Principles and Techniques*, ed. B. Bolon and M. Butt, 171–180. Hoboken, NJ: J. Wiley and Sons, Inc.

Schmued, L., and K. Hopkins. 2000. Fluoro-Jade: novel fluorochromes for detecting toxicant induced neuronal degeneration. *Toxicol Pathol* 18:91–99.

Schmued, L., C. Stowers, A. Scalle et al. 2005. Fluoro-Jade results in ultra high resolution and contrast labeling of degenerating neurons. *J Brain Res* 1035:24–32.

Slayter, M., B. Summers, and R. Meade. 1998. Axonal spheroids in the cochlear nucleus of normal beagle dogs. *Vet Pathol* 35:150–153.

Snyder, P., E. Kazacos, J. Scot-Moncrieff et al. 1995. Pathologic features of naturally occurring juvenile polyarteritis in beagle dogs. *Vet Pathol* 32:337–345.

Solleveld, H., and G. Boorman. 1990. Brain. In *Pathology of the Fischer Rat Reference and Atlas*, ed. G. Boorman, S. Eustis, M. Elwell, and W. MacKenzie. San Diego: Academic Press.

Solleveld, H. A., E. J. Gorgacz, and A. Koestner. 1991. Central nervous system neoplasms in the rat. In *Guides for Toxicologic Pathology*. Washington, DC: STP/ARP/AFIP.

Sommer, B., S. Barbieri, K. Hofele et al. 2000. Mouse models of alpha-synucleinopathy and Lewy pathology. *Exp Gerontol* 35:1289–1403.

Stemmer-Rachamimov, A. O., D. N. Louis, G. P. Nielsen et al. 2004. Comparative pathology of nerve sheath tumors in mouse models and humans. *Cancer Res* 64:3718–3724.

Streit, W. 2005. The role of microglia in neurotoxicity. In *The Role of Glia in Neurotoxicity, 2nd edition*, ed. M. Aschner and L. Cota, 29–40. Washington, DC: CRC Press.

Summers, B., J. Cummings, and A. deLahunta. 1995. *Veterinary Neuropathology*. 7. St. Louis, MO: Mosby.

Switzer, R. 2000. Application of silver degeneration stains. *Toxicol Pathol* 28:70–83.

Switzer, R. 2011a. Recommended neuroanatomical sampling practices for comprehensive brain evaluation in nonclinical safety studies. *Toxicol Pathol* 39:73–84.

Switzer, R. 2011b. Fundamentals of neurotoxicity detection. In *Fundamental Neuropathology for Pathologists and Toxicologists: Principles and Techniques*, ed. B. Bolon and M. Butt, 139–158. Hoboken, NJ: J. Wiley and Sons, Inc.

Switzer, R., and M. Butt. 2011. Histological markers of neurotoxicity (nonfluorescent). In *Fundamental Neuropathology for Pathologists and Toxicologists: Principles and Techniques*, ed. B. Bolon and M. Butt, 181–190. Hoboken, NJ: J. Wiley and Sons, Inc.

Vernau, W., K. M. Vernau, and B. Bolon. 2011. Cerebrospinal fluid analysis in toxicological neuropathology. In *Fundamental Neuropathology for Pathologists and Toxicologists: Principles and Techniques*, ed. B. Bolon and M. Butt, 271–284. Hoboken, NJ: J. Wiley and Sons, Inc.

Weindl, A., and R. Joynt. 1973. Barrier properties of the subcommissural organ. *Arch Neurol* 29:16–22.

Zook, B. C., S. J. Simmens, and R. V. Jones. 2000. Evaluation of ENU-induced gliomas in rats: nomenclature, immunochemistry, and malignancy. *Toxicol Pathol* 28:193–201.

21 Special Senses: Eye and Ear

James A. Render, Kenneth A. Schafer,
and Richard A. Altschuler

CONTENTS

21.1 EYE

21.1.1 INTRODUCTION

Ophthalmic toxicology is a broad topic that involves *in silico*, *in vitro*, and *in vivo* preclinical testing as a method of predicting potential clinical toxicity (Hockwin et al. 1991; Somps et al. 2009). Routine ophthalmic examination involves direct ophthalmoscopy, indirect ophthalmoscopy, and slit lamp biomicroscopy, which can detect the exact location of ocular changes (Bistner and Riis 1984; Kuiper et al. 1997; Munger 2002). To ensure a microscopic correlate, the pathologist must be aware of the route of ocular exposure and clinical ophthalmic findings at necropsy, trimming, and microscopic examination. Treatment-related findings need to be differentiated from artifacts, spontaneous changes, and iatrogenic findings, so histologic sections of good quality with proper orientation and minimal tissue artifacts are essential (Dubielzig et al. 2010; Short 2008, Whiteley and Peiffer 2002).

21.1.2 EXTRAOCULAR TISSUES

Extraocular tissues include the superior and inferior eyelids (separated by the palpebral fissure), nictitating membrane with lacrimal nictitans gland, and other orbital contents, such as extraocular muscles, connective tissue, glands, and vascular structures (Samuelson 2007). Eyelids have an outer cutaneous surface and an inner surface (palpebral conjunctiva) with openings of meibomian glands at the margins. The conjunctiva of the eyelids and the nictitating membrane contain conjunctiva-associated lymphoid tissue (CALT) (Knop and Knop 2000). Spontaneous alterations of the eyelids include congenital, inflammatory, and neoplastic changes. Examples of congenital findings include entropion and incomplete formation of the palpebral fissure (Hubert et al. 1999). Spontaneous inflammation of the eyelid may involve the meibomian glands inciting a granulomatous response. Since the lipid secretion of meibomian glands forms the outer layer of the precorneal tear film, a decrease in secretion may lead to inadequate hydration of the outer cornea. Neoplasms may arise from any of the structures in the eyelid and have been reviewed (Ackerman et al. 1998).

Toxicity of the eyelids often involve the meibomian glands and include dilatation of ducts, hyperplasia of ductular epithelium, hypersecretion, reduced secretion, and granulomatous inflammation (Bryce et al. 2001; Grant 1986; Jester et al. 1989; Kremer et al. 1994; Lambert and Smith 1988; Ohnishi and Kohno 1979). Additional treatment-related findings include lengthening of eyelashes from topical administration of prostaglandin analogues (Johnstone and Albert 2002).

The extraocular muscles consist of four rectus muscles, two oblique muscles, and, in some species, the retractor bulbi (Samuelson 2007). Toxicity involving the extraocular muscle is infrequent, but prolonged light exposure may result in myofiber degeneration and inflammation in albino rats (O'Steen et al. 1978).

Changes may occur in other orbital structures. Any increase in the size of the intraorbital contents results in anterior displacement of the globe (proptosis or exophthalmos). This ocular finding is often secondary to orbital inflammation, edema, or neoplasia, but has been associated with systemic administration of compounds, such as acetonitrile (Grant 1986). Orbital fascia consists of periorbita, Tenon's capsule, and fascial sheaths of extraocular muscles and may be a site of compound (or chemical) exposure. The mouse and rat have a retro-orbital sinus and retro-orbital plexus, respectively, that are used for venipuncture. The dog has the zygomatic salivary gland in the posterior orbit (Samuelson 2007). Rodents have an orbital harderian gland and the rabbit has a Harder's gland (Krinke et al. 1994; Prince 1964; Sakai 1981). The secretion of the harderian gland contains porphyrins that may be photosensitizers in ultraviolet light and the lumina may contain brown accretions that accumulate with age.

Spontaneous findings of the harderian gland include inflammatory cell infiltrates and chromodacryorrhea, a nonspecific secretion ("red tears") caused by stress, necrosis, inflammation, or administration of cholinergic drugs (Harkness and Ridgeway 1980). Necrosis, edema, inflammation, and squamous metaplasia may be caused by sialodacryoadenitis virus in young rodents, retrobulbar trauma from venipuncture, and prolonged exposure to high-intensity light (Figure 21.1a) (Heywood 1973; Kurisu et al. 1996; McGee and Maronpot 1979; O'Steen et al. 1978; Strum and Shear 1982). Decreased secretion may occur after administration of a drug (e.g., atropine sulfate) (Iwai et al. 2000).

Hyperplasia of the harderian gland occurs in aged rodents (Ackerman et al. 1998; Haseman et al. 1998; Krinke et al. 2001). The finding may occur in association with degeneration, inflammation, and ductular squamous metaplasia and may be the result of toxicity (Mohr 1994). For example, chronic administration of aflatoxin to hamsters results in proliferative changes of the harderian gland (Herrold 1969).

The Harder's gland is a large bilobed gland located in the orbit of rabbits and is composed of white and pink lobes. The white lobe has smaller lumina and stains more intensely, whereas the pink lobe has larger lumina and contains larger lipid droplets. Common microscopic findings of the Harder's gland include variability of luminal size, infiltrates of lymphoplasmacytic cells, and focal areas of atrophy.

Most large laboratory animals have a relatively small main lacrimal gland located in the anterior, superior, and temporal aspect of the orbit, but other lacrimal glands may be present. Rodents have intraorbital and extraorbital lacrimal glands that normally have a degree of cytomegaly, karyomegaly, and nuclear pseudoinclusions (Sullivan et al. 2009). Spontaneous alterations of the lacrimal gland include lymphoplasmacytic cell infiltrates, focal glandular hyperplasia, degeneration,

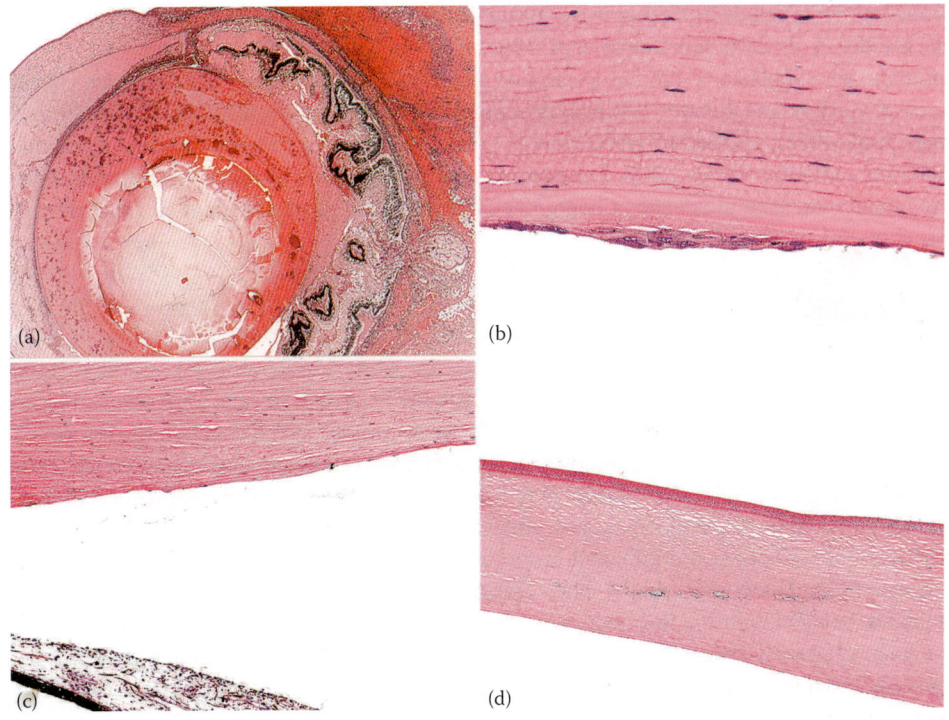

FIGURE 21.1 (a) Hematoxylin and eosin, 2.5× objective. Extensive ocular findings (plasmoid aqueous and vitreous, cataract, serous retinal detachment and retinal degeneration, orbital hemorrhage, and necrosis) in a mouse owing to retrobulbar venipuncture. (b) Hematoxylin and eosin, 40× objective. Focal corneal endothelial hypertrophy and hyperplasia in a dog in response to a device in the anterior chamber. (c) Hematoxylin and eosin, 10× objective. Attenuation of corneal endothelium of a monkey owing to a device in the anterior chamber. (d) Hematoxylin and eosin, 5× objective. Linear track of a transcorneal injection in a dog with deposits of birefringent crystalline material from the powdery "lubricant" used.

necrosis, hypertrophy, atrophy, inflammation, pigment accumulations, and ductal squamous hyperplasia (Elwell and Boorman 1990; Greaves 2007; Mohr 1994). Hyperplasia of the lacrimal gland may occur spontaneously or experimentally, and harderianization (harderian metaplasia) can be observed in the exorbital lacrimal gland of rats, especially males (Haseman et al. 1998; Krinke et al. 2001; Yoshitomi and Boorman 1990). Pigmentation of the lacrimal glands has been observed after administration of various compounds, including a brown-black discoloration in dogs after administration of practolol (Tanaka et al. 1983). Lacrimal gland acini are sensitive to radiation, and treatment-related changes in lacrimal glands may include degeneration, decreased secretion, or dacryorrhea (Gazda et al. 1992). Chronic inflammation of the lacrimal glands leads to atrophy, replacement by fibrous connective tissue, and lymphoplasmacytic infiltrates that may lead to decreased tear production and changes in the cornea and conjunctiva (i.e., keratoconjunctivitis sicca [KCS]). For example, administration of 5-aminosalicylic acid in dogs may lead to KCS (Barnett and Joseph 1988). The Schirmer tear test can be used in the detection and monitoring of KCS in large animals (Kuiper et al. 1997).

The nictitating membrane is a fold of conjunctiva that contains a plate of cartilage surrounded by a lacrimal nictitans gland. The membrane is located at the medial angle of the palpebral fissure of rabbits, dogs, and minipigs, but absent in rodents and nonhuman primates (Samuelson 2007). The nictitans gland contributes to the tear production, and decreased secretions may result in KCS.

The lacrimal fluid is drained via puncta in the medial eyelid margins into canaliculi, which open into the lacrimal sac and eventually into the nasolacrimal duct. Treatment-related alterations of the nasolacrimal duct include epithelial hyperplasia, inflammation, or blockage after the placement of stents (Breider et al. 1996; Greenman et al. 1995; Wilhelm et al. 2006).

Spontaneous neoplasia of the harderian and lacrimal glands occur in aged rodents (Ackerman et al. 1998; Carlton and Render 1991b; Haseman et al. 1998; Jones et al. 1991; Krinke et al. 2001; Sheldon et al. 1983). Harderian gland tumors can be induced in rodents by various carcinogens and ionizing radiation (Grant 1986). For example, chronic administration of 1,2,3-trichloropropane resulted in an increased incidence of benign neoplasms of the harderian gland of mice (Irwin et al. 1995).

21.1.3 CORNEA

The cornea is composed of a precorneal tear film, an outer, non-keratinized stratified squamous epithelial layer, an anterior limiting membrane (Bowman's layer), stroma, Descemet's membrane, and corneal endothelium (Hockwin et al. 1991; Samuelson 2007). The function of the cornea is to transmit and refract light, so transparency is dependent upon relative stromal dehydration (deturgescence) and a lack of vessels. The nutrient supply for the cornea consists of the precorneal tear film, limbal scleral vessels, and aqueous humor. Intact corneal epithelium is hydrophobic and varies in thickness but consists of several distinct layers of cells and abruptly changes to bulbar conjunctiva at the corneoscleral junction (limbus). The corneal epithelium is well innervated with pain receptors and may be replaced within a few days.

Bowman's layer is a superficial, dense, acellular anterior limiting membrane that is present in humans and nonhuman primates (Merindano et al. 2002). This structure is not a membrane but composed of collagen fibers.

The corneal stroma of the common laboratory animals is composed of thin collagen fibers arranged in a lattice pattern, along with a few fibroblasts (keratocytes). The stroma is lined internally by Descemet's membrane, a thin, uniform layer produced by corneal endothelial cells, and terminates peripherally at the pectinate ligament.

The corneal endothelium is a single layer of flat, hexagonal, mesenchymal cells joined apically by tight junctions and have a Na/K ATP-dependent pump in the cell membrane to maintain stromal deturgescence (Baroody et al. 1987; Doughty 1994; Joyce 2003). Endothelial cell density is variable among species and within the cornea (less dense in the superior cornea than in the inferior cornea). Endothelial cells decrease in number with age. Humans, nonhuman primates, and cats have little or no regenerative capacity and undergo repair by cell sliding (migration) and individual cell enlargement. Dogs have some regenerative capacity, but repair is still mostly due to cell sliding (Figure 21.1b). The endothelial cells of rabbits can divide and form multinucleated cells. Trauma to the corneal endothelium may allow proliferation of keratocytes with the formation of a fibrous membrane on the inner surface of the cornea (retrocorneal membrane) (Sherrard and Rycroft 1967).

The cornea is routinely examined by direct ophthalmoscopy and slit lamp biomicroscopy, but other techniques include measurement of innervation (esthesiometry), stromal thickness (pachymetry), corneal endothelial density (specular microscopy), tear quantity (Schirmer tear test), and *in vivo* confocal microscopy (Böhnke and Masters 1999; Kuiper et al. 1997; Messmer 2008; Ollivier et al. 2007). Slit lamp biomicroscopy allows for a magnified view of structures of the anterior segment and a cross-sectional view of the cornea. As a result, this sensitive technique is frequently used in assessing topical irritation.

Irritation of drugs or ocular medical devices (following guidelines provided by the International Organization for Standardization, Genève, Switzerland) to the outer cornea can be assessed by the modified Draize ocular irritation scoring method (Hackett and McDonald 1991; Maurer et al. 1998, 2001; Wilhelmus 2001). This *in vivo* method is used to evaluate the potential ocular irritation of a topical compound or medical device in albino rabbits and has been used less in recent years as *in vitro* and *ex vivo* substitutes are used (Curren et al. 2000; Sina et al. 1995; Whiteley and Peiffer

2002). The *in vivo* irritation test may be accompanied by use of a fluorescein stain to check for breaks in the epithelial layer (Schmidt 1971).

KCS is characterized by keratinization, epidermalization, pigmentation, fibrosis, neovascularization, and mononuclear or mixed cellular inflammation of the superficial cornea. The cause may be a lack of lacrimal secretion, a lack of blinking (lagophthalmos), or a lack of corneal sensation (Kast 1991; Roerig et al. 1980). A lack of tear production may be due to inflammation of the lacrimal gland or administration of certain pharmacological compounds (e.g., local anesthetics). Decreases or alterations in tear production may also occur with a reduction in meibomian gland secretions (Funk and Landes 2005; Pyrah et al. 2001). Decreased secretion from the meibomian glands may also result in KCS.

Nonspecific changes in the corneal epithelium include hyperplasia, goblet cell metaplasia, and keratinization. Corneal hyperplasia may be focal, diffuse, or nodular, and is generally not considered to be a preneoplastic finding, but may be a compound-induced finding (Reindel et al. 2001). Spontaneous proliferative corneal changes have been reviewed (Ackerman et al. 1998; Geiss and Yoshitomi 1999).

Spontaneous opacities may occur in all laboratory animal species, especially in rats (Carlton and Render 1991a; Peiffer et al. 1994; Taradach and Greaves 1984; Tucker 1997; Van Winkle and Balk 1986). Causes of clinical corneal opacification include stromal edema and the presence of deposits. Edema is a nonspecific alteration characterized by increased thickness of the stroma due to increased interstitial fluid that disrupts the regular arrangement of the stromal collagen. The finding may be accompanied by inflammation and neovascularization, and causes may vary but include compound-induced toxicity (Lock et al. 2006).

Corneal deposits often consist of mineral. Some deposits are a feature of corneal dystrophy, but others may be due to other causes (Peiffer et al. 1994; Taradach et al. 1981). Corneal dystrophy is a spontaneous, noninflammatory, bilateral corneal change that occurs in several laboratory animals (Moore et al. 1987; Port and Dodd 1983; Shibuya et al. 2001). Microscopically, the finding consists of mineralized deposits along the corneal epithelial basement membrane (Bruner et al. 1992; Carlton and Render 1991a; Hoffman et al. 1983; Losco and Troup 1988). Mineralized deposits in the cornea adjacent to the palpebral fissure are referred to clinically as band keratopathy.

The presence of blood may result in a reddish color, and an influx of melanocytes or melanin results in brown to black discoloration. The cornea may acquire pigmentation that is associated with the administration of compounds (e.g., minocycline) (Morrow and Abbott 1998).

Corneal inflammation first occurs at the limbus and extends into the corneal epithelium and stroma, often along with blood vessels. The cause may be the result of injury, infection, dust, photosensitization, or toxicity (Fraunfelder et al. 2008; Kuno et al. 1991; Taradach and Greaves 1984; Taradach et al. 1981; Whiteley and Peiffer 2002; Zarfoss et al. 2007).

Neovascularization is the formation of blood vessels in a normally avascular corneal stroma and may be associated with stromal edema and inflammation (Klintworth and Burger 1983). New blood vessels are often more permeable, leak fluid, and may enhance stromal migration of inflammatory cells. Occasionally in rabbits, individual limbal blood vessels may spontaneously extend a short distance into the peripheral cornea. Neovascularization may also occur after topical administration of compounds (e.g., EP4-prostaglandin E2 agonists) (Aguirre et al. 2009). Once vessels are present, they often persist as nonperfused ghost vessels.

Corneal lipidosis is a spontaneous or compound-induced finding characterized by cholesterol clefts in the corneal stroma, with or without infiltrates of large, pale, foamy macrophages. The condition has been reported in the dog, guinea pig, Watanabe heritable hyperlipidemic rabbit, and rabbits fed high-fat diets (Garibaldi and Goad 1988; Sebesteny et al. 1985; Spangler et al. 1982; Williams and Sullivan 2010).

Administration of cationic amphiphilic drugs in humans and animals can produce corneal phospholipidosis characterized by lipid deposits in lysosomes of the corneal epithelium and keratocytes

(Drenkhahn et al. 1983; Fraunfelder et al. 2008). In humans, phospholipidosis may be reversible with little or no visual impairment (Davidson and Rennie 1986).

Changes in Descemet's membrane include tears (stria), anterior bulging due to deep corneal ulcer (descemetocele), thickening with age, and duplication or irregularity due to changes in the adjacent corneal endothelium (Kafarnik et al. 2009). Additionally, Descemet's membrane may extend onto structures of the filtration angle (descemetization) or retain material from transcorneal injections.

Corneal endothelial cells help maintain clarity of the cornea, and loss of corneal endothelial cells results in corneal edema. Corneal endothelial cells may be physically removed by intracameral medical devices or by administration of compounds (e.g., 5-fluorouracil) (Figure 21.1c) (Grant 1986). Damage to the endothelium may be due to administration of phototoxic chemicals or changes in ionic concentration, bicarbonate levels, pH, and tonicity of the local environment (Hull et al. 1984).

Iatrogenic corneal findings include incisions, suture material, and needle tracks (Figure 21.1d). Complications of corneal incisions include inflammatory cell infiltration, disorganization of the collagen lamellae, cell necrosis, collagenolysis, deposition of foreign material, formation of epithelial inclusion cysts, downgrowth of corneal epithelium into the incision, loss of corneal endothelium, retrocorneal membrane, adherence of the iris to the cornea (anterior synechia), entrapment of the iris into a corneal incision (Figure 21.2a), or bulging of the iris into a corneal defect (staphyloma) (Dubielzig et al. 2010).

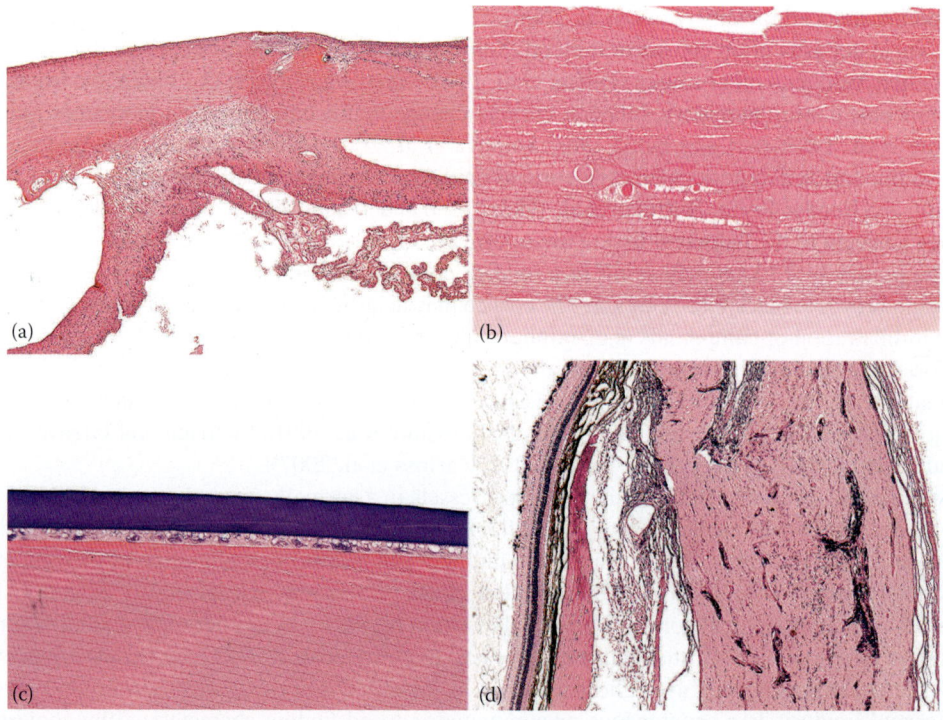

FIGURE 21.2 (a) Hematoxylin and eosin, 10× objective. Entrapment of the iris within a corneal surgical incision in a monkey. (b) Hematoxylin and eosin, 60× objective. Artifactual changes (swelling and fragmentation of lens fibers, globule formation, and fluid accumulation) in the lens of a monkey due fixation with a fixative containing glacial acetic acid. (c) Hematoxylin and eosin, 40× objective. Diffuse basophilia of anterior lens capsule of a rabbit after an intravitreal injection of a synthetic oligonucleotide that preferentially accumulates in the lens capsule. (d) Hematoxylin and eosin, 5× objective. Macrophages with basophilic contents lining the ILM of the retina and vessels within the optic nerve after an intravitreal injection.

21.1.4   Conjunctiva

Bulbar conjunctiva extends from the limbus to cover the episclera and then becomes palpebral conjunctiva on the inner surface of the eyelids (Hockwin et al. 1991; Samuelson 2007). Conjunctiva also covers the third eyelid and is composed of a single row of epithelial cells that are squamous in appearance near the palpebral margins but contains goblet cells in areas less exposed. Rats and mice do not normally have lymphoid follicles in the conjunctiva, but CALT occurs in non-rodents (Chodosh et al. 1998; Knop and Knop 2000). Heterophils are often present in the palpebral conjunctiva of rabbit.

Conjunctival inflammation may occur in laboratory animals as a spontaneous change. When acute, it is characterized grossly by congestion and edema (chemosis) (Taradach and Greaves 1984). Chronic conjunctival inflammation is characterized by increased numbers of goblet cells, epithelial hyperplasia, increased prominence of CALT, and perivascular infiltrates of inflammatory cells. Sequelae of conjunctival inflammation include increased density of goblet cells, epidermalization, and keratinization of the conjunctival epithelium. Causes of the conjunctival inflammation include infectious agents, as well as topical administration of compounds or chemicals (e.g., ricin) (Strocchi et al. 2005).

Miscellaneous conjunctival alterations include amyloidosis, squamous cell metaplasia, epithelial neoplasia, microgranuloma, and pseudopterygium (Ackerman et al. 1998). Conjunctival microgranulomas often occur when lipid-containing substances are deposited beneath the bulbar conjunctiva, and pseudopterygium is a flap of bulbar conjunctiva that extends over the cornea (Dubielzig et al. 2010). It occurs spontaneously in rabbits and is not associated with irritation or inflammation but may grow back after removal.

21.1.5   Sclera and Episclera

The sclera is an outer supportive tunic of the globe composed of collagenous connective tissue and covered anteriorly by the episclera (Hockwin et al. 1991; Samuelson 2007). The episclera is a vascularized layer between the bulbar conjunctiva that contains lymphoplasmacytic cell infiltrates in a response to superficial corneal irritation. Alterations of the sclera are often secondary to primary findings in other ocular structures or may occur spontaneously, such as osseous or cartilaginous metaplasia of aging rats. The sclera may also contain iatrogenic injection tracks, incisions, or sutures (Short 2008; Yoshitomi and Boorman 1990).

21.1.6   Uvea

The uvea is the vascular tunic of the globe and includes the iris, ciliary body, and choroid (Hockwin et al. 1991; Samuelson 2007). Vessels in the iridal stroma serve as a part of the blood–eye barrier and since the anterior surface of the iris does not contain epithelium or a basement membrane, breakdown of this barrier allows fibrin and protein (aqueous flare), blood (hyphema), and inflammatory cells, especially polymorphonuclear cells (hypopyon), to enter the anterior chamber (Szalay et al. 1975). Macrophages may adhere to the corneal endothelium (keratic precipitates).

The ciliary body consists of an anterior portion (pars plicata) with ciliary processes and ciliary muscles and a flat posterior portion (pars plana) that is often the entry site for intravitreal injections. In the rabbit, ciliary processes attach to the posterior aspect of the iris (iridal processes). Ciliary muscles are well developed in the nonhuman primate but absent in the rat and mouse. At the ora ciliaris retinae or ora serrata (humans and nonhuman primates), there is an abrupt transition to retina and choroid.

Aqueous humor is continuously produced by the ciliary processes. It forms in the posterior chamber, flows through the pupil, enters the anterior chamber, and exits through the filtration angle. The filtration angle contains a porous pectinate ligament extending from the root of the iris to the termination of Descemet's membrane. Aqueous flows through spaces of the uveal and corneoscleral meshwork and into the angular aqueous plexus or canal of Schlemm (humans and nonhuman primates). Any blockage in this continuous flow of aqueous humor causes intraocular pressure (IOP) to rise.

The majority of the choroid is composed of the substantia propria, which contains vessels and melanocytes. Areas devoid of pigmentation may occur as a spontaneous change in nonhuman primates (Kobayashi and Kohshima 2001). A potential space exists between the outermost portion of the choroid (suprachoroid) and the sclera. This space may be used in the treatment of the posterior segment (Short 2008). The innermost layer of the choroid is the choriocapillaris, and the basal lamina of the endothelial cells forms a membrane with the basal lamina of the retinal pigment epithelium (RPE) (Bruch's membrane).

The tapetum lucidum is a specialized layer in the inner choroid of certain laboratory animals, but not pigs, rodents, rabbits, and nonhuman primates (Samuelson 2007). The tapetum lucidum is mostly in the superior half of the ocular fundus and, in the dog, is composed of specialized epithelium (tapetum cellulosum) with the purpose of reflecting light to aid vision in low ambient light. The epithelial cells have intracytoplasmic, reflective, crystalline rods (tapetal rods) rich in zinc. The cells are arranged in multiple layers, centrally tapering to a single cell thickness at the periphery, and the RPE overlying the tapetum lucidum is nonpigmented. Funduscopically, the tapetum lucidum is hyperreflective when the overlying sensory retina is thinned (usually the outer retina) and may be hyporeflective in appearance when it is a target of toxicity (e.g., β-adrenergic blocking agents) (Schiavo et al. 1984).

Intraocular inflammation often involves the uvea and needs to be prevented or minimized quickly in order to prevent permanent damage to the specialized structures of the eye. Ocular immunity plays an important role in this process and has been reviewed by Biros (2007). Features include a blood–eye barrier, absence of lymphatics, and maintenance of a unique immunoprivileged site as a result of anterior chamber–associated immune deviation. This involves an inability to initiate a delayed-type immune response to an intraocular antigen. Potentially toxic compounds are prevented from reaching the interior of the globe by the blood–eye barrier consisting of a vascular portion (vessels of the iris and sensory retina) and an epithelial portion (ciliary epithelium and the RPE). Vessels are lined by endothelial cells with tight junctions and a complete basement membrane. In the retina, Müller cells also contribute to the barrier (Rapoport 1997).

The iris can be examined for morphological changes by direct ophthalmoscopy and slit lamp biomicroscopy. The function of the iris can be assessed by testing the pupillary light response and measuring the diameter of the pupil (Murray and Loughnane 1981). The filtration angle can be examined by gonioscopy and the IOP may be examined by tonometry (Ollivier et al. 2007). Tonometry measurements and sensitivity vary among species (Hockwin et al. 1991; Kuiper et al. 1997; Loget 1995; Munger 2002). The choroid, especially the area of the tapetum lucidum, may be examined through a transparent retina by direct and indirect ophthalmoscopy (Ollivier et al. 2007).

Compound-induced morphological changes of the uvea of laboratory animals include edema, inflammation, degeneration, abnormal pigmentation, cytoplasmic vacuolation, cellular necrosis, or changes in the IOP. These changes must be differentiated from spontaneous findings that include congenital, traumatic, inflammatory, degenerative, metaplastic or proliferative processes (Hubert et al. 1999; Taradach and Greaves 1984). For example, colchicine, naphthol, and urethane cause edema, inflammation, or degeneration of the ciliary body, while naphthalene causes degeneration of the ciliary body and the choroid (Grant 1986). Heterotopic bone (osseous choristoma or osseous metaplasia) occurs as a spontaneous finding within the ciliary body of guinea pigs (Williams and Sullivan 2010).

Increased or decreased pigmentation may occur after administration of compounds (Hockwin et al. 1991). Darkening of the iris occurs in cynomolgus monkeys after topical administration of the prostaglandin F2a analogues (Lindquist et al. 1999). Increased pigmentation may be due to increased melanin synthesis or the proliferation of melanin-containing cells as noted in the iris of hooded rats treated with urethane (Roe et al. 1963).

Cytoplasmic vacuolation may occur in the epithelium of the iris, ciliary body, or both as a result of many causes. Administration of disobutamide to dogs causes phospholipidosis that is characterized by vacuolation of the cells of the iris (Koizumi et al. 1986). Diffuse cytoplasmic vacuolation of the iridal and ciliary epithelium occurred in rabbits treated with 6-aminonicotinamide (Render and Carlton 1991a).

Uveal inflammation may be a manifestation of toxicity. For example, ciliary inflammation occurs after administration of cyclophosphamide to rats and uveal inflammation occurs after intravenous infusion of a dopaminergic compound to dogs (Kerry et al. 1993; Levine 1991). Inflammation associated with toxicity must be differentiated from spontaneous inflammation. Rats and mice may develop spontaneous anterior uveal inflammation (Taradach and Greaves 1984). Infiltration of mononuclear cells into the ciliary body and choroid in nonhuman primates is a common spontaneous finding (Sinha et al. 2006). Inflammation may include ciliary edema, aqueous flare, hypopyon, hyphema, uveal depigmentation, and clinical tapetal discoloration, which may occur with choroidal inflammation and fibrosis or adhesions (anterior or posterior synechia) that occur as sequelae (Dubielzig et al. 2010). Inflammation may occur with intracameral or intravitreal injections or the implantation of medical devices, and intravitreal injections may result in prolapse of the vitreous (Short 2008).

Toxicity involving the tapetum lucidum is occasionally observed in the dog, and since humans do not have this ocular structure, compound-related tapetal findings may not be relevant to humans (Heywood 1974; Hockwin et al. 1991). In an attempt to determine relevancy, atapetal beagles, which have tapetal cells but lack intracytoplasmic rodlets, are sometimes used (Bellhorn et al. 1975; Heywood 1972). For example, administration of imidazoquinaline to normal beagles results in tapetal and retinal changes, but atapetal beagles have no retinal changes (Schiavo 1972). The principal toxicity-related finding involving the tapetum lucidum is degeneration (Haggerty et al. 2007; Heywood et al. 1976). Tapetal cells appear dull, discolored, or mottled, funduscopically. Microscopically, inflammation, edema, hemorrhage, or retinal detachment will be present (Hockwin et al. 1991; Rubin 1974).

Toxicity involving the tapetum lucidum of beagles may be subdivided into zinc chelators and non-chelators. Since tapetal cells contain a high concentration of zinc, administration of zinc chelators, such as hydroxypyridinethione, to dogs causes tapetal and choroidal necrosis and edema with secondary effects involving the retina (Delahunt et al. 1962; Gopinath et al. 1987; Moe et al. 1960; Rubin 1974). Non-chelators, such as pyridinethione, also cause tapetal edema and degeneration, retinal edema, and retinal detachment in dogs (Cloyd et al. 1978). These changes were specific for the tapetum since no changes were observed in nonhuman primates, rats, rabbits, or atapetal beagles (Grant 1986). Other non-chelators cause phospholipidosis, which can cause alterations in the appearance of the tapetum lucidum.

Many spontaneous uveal findings are congenital and detected during pre-study ocular examinations, including persistent pupillary membrane and posterior coloboma (Bellhorn 1974; Heywood 1973; Hubert et al. 1994; Kuno et al. 1991; Rubin 1974; Taradach and Greaves 1984; Taradach et al. 1981). Other uveal findings may be associated with toxicity and include thickened ciliary epithelial basement membranes of dogs after administration of an anticholinesterase pesticide and silver deposits on basement membranes and within uveal pigmented epithelial cells after systemic administration of silver lactate to rats (Grant 1986).

Spontaneous uveal neoplasia rarely occurs in laboratory animals, and when it occurs in mice, it is generally malignant (Ackerman et al. 1998; Albert et al. 1982; Ernst et al. 1991; Everitt and Shadduck 1991; Geiss and Yoshitomi 1999; Krinke et al. 2001; Mohr 1994; Owen and Duprat 1991).

21.1.7 Intraocular Pressure

Aqueous humor is constantly being produced by the ciliary body and, generally, most exits the globe through the filtration angle. The IOP can be measured using rebound or applanation tonometry (Pereira et al. 2011). Mechanisms for drug-related causes of decreased IOP include increased uveoscleral outflow, interference with aqueous formation in the ciliary body, and damage to the ciliary body (Grant 1986; Lutjen-Drecoll and Tamm 1988). The IOP is increased after administration of compounds that cause pupillary dilatation, which causes the anterior chamber to be shallow and the filtration angle to be narrow (Hadjikoutis et al. 2005). Grant (1986) reviewed several causes of increased IOP, including subconjunctival injections of certain chemicals, intracameral injections of particulate or viscous solutions slowing aqueous outflow by causing obstruction, or intraocular inflammation and destruction of endothelial cells lining the trabecular meshwork.

Prolonged increases in IOP may lead to permanent structural changes of glaucoma characterized by enlargement of the globe (buphthalmos or buphthalmia), diffuse bluish corneal opacity (edema), breaks in Descemet's membrane (stria), thinning of the uvea and sclera, luxation of the lens, ciliary atrophy, and thinning of the inner retina. Retinal ganglion cells are lost first (inner retinal degeneration), followed by losses of neurons in the inner nuclear layer (INL). As the globe becomes stretched, the sensory retina may become detached, contributing to degeneration of photoreceptor cells (outer retinal degeneration). The optic disc becomes cupped, especially in rabbits because of their poorly developed lamina cribrosa. Enlargement of the globe may interfere with adequate hydration of the cornea resulting in secondary KCS (Rubin 1974; Suckow and Douglas 1997).

Glaucoma may be due to maldevelopment within the filtration angle (goniodysgenesis) or acquired obstruction of aqueous outflow. With goniodysgenesis, the root of the iris is located adjacent to the peripheral margin of Descemet's membrane, and there may be splitting and extension of Descemet's membrane onto structures around the pectinate ligament (i.e., descemetization). Examples of primary glaucoma include an inherited condition in New Zealand white rabbits and open-angle glaucoma in beagles (Gad 2007; Gelatt et al. 1998).

Secondary glaucoma may be associated with inflammation, neoplasia, neovascularization, or lens luxation (Dubielzig et al. 2010). Rodents develop glaucoma after inflammation in the anterior segment, particularly if adhesions lead to anterior synechia. Older DBA/2J (D2) mice develop secondary glaucoma from dispersion of melanin pigment (John et al. 1998).

21.1.8 LENS

The anatomy of the lens is well documented in the literature (Hockwin et al. 1991; Samuelson 2007). Basically, the lens is surrounded by a capsule that is divided into anterior and posterior aspects. A single cell layer of lenticular epithelium is located beneath the anterior capsule. Lenticular epithelial cells constantly divide in the proliferative zone, move to the equator, and elongate in the region of the nuclear bow to constantly form lens fibers. The lens fibers elongate and meet at the anterior and posterior suture lines. Lens fibers are constantly moving inward toward the nucleus, resulting in continuous compression of the lens nucleus and eventually hardening (nuclear sclerosis) in aged animals. The anterior lens epithelium continues to deposit basement membrane so that the anterior capsule thickens as an animal ages.

The lens is normally transparent, a feature that is dependent upon adequate nutrition from the aqueous humor and, to a lesser extent, the vitreous (Gum et al. 2007). The lens epithelium maintains critical levels of dehydration for transparency by a Na/K ATPase pump, and anaerobic glycolysis is the main energy source. Approximately 35% of the lens is composed of proteins, including soluble proteins called crystallins. These proteins decrease with age while insoluble proteins (albuminoids) increase with age.

The main alteration of the lens is loss of transparency (opacification). Although some refer to any clinical opacity of the lens as a cataract, others reserve the term "cataract" for those lenticular opacities that are permanent. Findings in the lens, including cataract, should be identified as to their location and can be identified by use of direct microscopy, slit lamp biomicroscopy, and Scheimpflug imaging (Hockwin et al. 1991; Somps et al. 2009).

Various types of spontaneous opacities have been described in laboratory animals, and these findings need to be differentiated from treatment-related findings (Balazs et al. 1970). Congenital opacities are generally detected during pre-study examinations, and other lenticular opacities are inherited (Heywood 1971; Peiffer 1991b). Reversible opacification of the lens may be induced by compounds or may be associated with cold temperature, anoxia, asphyxia, dehydration, and stress (Fraunfelder and Burns 1970). Examples of reversible changes include prominent suture lines from lens fiber swelling, minimal swelling of individual lens fibers without degenerative changes, and cold cataracts in rodents and other animals. The cold cataract is characterized by clinically reversible opaque lenses in the absence of microscopic findings. There are several compounds (e.g., triparanol) that cause reversible lenticular opacification of the rodent lens (Rathbun et al. 1973).

Irreversible microscopic changes that are likely to correlate with a clinical opacity include bladder cells, clefts, vacuoles, liquefaction, lens fiber fragmentation, Morgagnian globule formation, mineralization, and collapse of the lens capsule. Some of these changes (pooling of fluid, swelling of lenticular fibers, and globule formation) may be caused by fixation, especially in nonhuman primate lenses with fixatives containing acetic acid. These artifactual changes may be observed in nonhuman primate lenses (Figure 21.2b). Additional morphological changes in the lens associated with cataract include migration of lenticular cells along the posterior capsule, excessive proliferation of lenticular epithelial cells, and fibrous metaplasia (Dubielzig et al. 2010).

Changes in the lens capsule include rupture and abnormal staining. Intraocular surgery or intravitreal injections can result in inadvertent rupture of the capsule. Infrequently, intravitreal injections of a therapeutic agent (e.g., oligonucleotides) may diffuse into the lens capsule and produce abnormal staining microscopically, without clinical findings (Figure 21.2c). The thin posterior capsule is susceptible to rupture from trauma, or in rabbits owing to an infection with *Encephalitozoon cuniculi* (Giordano et al. 2005).

Changes in lenticular epithelial cells associated with toxicity may occur but need to be differentiated from spontaneous changes (Balazs and Rubin 1971). For example, hyperplasia of lenticular epithelial cells may be associated with toxicity, but may also be a spontaneous finding in aged rats. Administration of 4-diethylaminoethoxy-α-ethyl-benzhydrol to rats causes secondary lenticular epithelial proliferation, followed by lenticular fiber degeneration. Perturbation of cell division may occur after exposure to ionizing radiation, administration of antimitotic anticancer agents, or the administration of certain compounds (e.g., busulfan) (Grant 1986; Turton and Hooson 1998). Lens epithelium irradiated by UVB light undergoes apoptosis and hyperplasia.

Among the laboratory animal species, lenticular opacities are most frequent in rodents but can occur in any species (Balazs et al. 1970; Bellhorn 1973, 1974; Geiss and Yoshitomi 1999; Heywood 1973; Heywood et al. 1976; Loget 1995; Taradach and Greaves 1984). Many compounds can cause cataract formation in animals (Grant 1986; Render and Carlton 1991c; Whiteley and Peiffer 2002). Some factors contributing to cataractogenesis include aging, disrupted metabolism, nutritional deficiency, exposure to oxygen radicals, x-rays, microwaves, gamma radiation, and UVA or UVB light (Gehring 1971; Grant 1986; Peiffer 1991a; Render and Carlton 1991b; Wegener 1995). Cataractogenesis associated with aging is thought to be the net result of oxidative stress (Geiss and Yoshitomi 1999; Taylor et al. 1995; Wegener 1995). Cataract may result from high concentrations of galactose, xylose, or glucose within the lens (Grant 1986; Turton and Hooson 1998). These sugars are converted to sugar alcohols that become trapped in the lens, accumulate, and result in osmotic swelling. Cataract may be produced after administration of compounds (e.g., alloxan or streptozotocin) and xenobiotics may cause cataract by a variety of mechanisms (Gajdosík et al. 1999; Geiss and Yoshitomi 1999; Grant 1986; Rubin 1974; Turton and Hooson 1998). Drugs, such as acetaminophen, cause cataract through oxidative stress mechanisms. Buthionine sulfoximine causes osmotic swelling of lenticular fibers. Naphthalene causes an inhibition of enzymes or disruption in protein metabolism. Compounds such as triparanol cause disruption of lipid metabolism and compounds such as busulfan produce radiomimetic cataracts. There may not always be a correlation between findings in animals and those in humans. Administration of some compounds, such as glucocorticoids, cause cataract in humans, but this is difficult to replicate in animals.

21.1.9 Vitreous Body

Primary vitreous refers to the embryonic hyaloid vascular system that normally regresses after the eye is fully developed, but may persist on the posterior lens capsule (posterior polar opacity), or as a vascular remnant extending from the optic disc. The presence of embryonic vascular remnants is more common in rats, but also occurs in other species, and causes vitreous hemorrhage (Heywood 1973; Hubert et al. 1999; Kuno et al. 1991; Rubin 1974; Taradach et al. 1981).

Secondary vitreous is neuroectodermal in origin and refers to the vitreous body in fully developed eyes. The transparent vitreous body fills the vitreous chamber and helps maintain the shape of the globe, transmits light to the retina, and maintains the normal position of the retina (Hockwin et al. 1991; Samuelson 2007). The vitreous body is composed mostly of water, but also contains hyaluronic acid, histiocytes (hyalocytes), complex carbohydrates, and collagen fibrils that join the retinal inner limiting membrane (ILM). The gel-to-liquid ratio of the vitreous body varies among species and age (Samuelson 2007). The vitreous body is a storage site for retinal metabolites and protects the lens and retina from toxic compounds. Hyaluronic acid not only provides viscoelasticity but also acts as a barrier to the diffusion of macromolecules. Processes leading to decreased hyaluronic acid and vitreal liquefaction will affect the nutrient supply, waste removal, and drug delivery to the lens and retina.

Vitreal alterations are detected by direct or indirect ophthalmoscopy and may be spontaneous, iatrogenic, or due to toxicity (Hockwin et al. 1991). In most species, liquefaction (syneresis) occurs with aging, and separation of the vitreous body from the retinal ILM may result in retinal tears and detachment (Samuelson 2007). Other spontaneous changes include the presence of multiple, small white opacities (asteroid hyalosis) in dogs and fibrosis and calcification in rodents (Haggerty et al. 2007; Heywood et al. 1976; Taradach and Greaves 1984). Vascularization of the vitreous body may occur as a result of a defect in the ILM or as a part of experimental neovascularization.

Most iatrogenic findings in the vitreous body are due to intravitreal injections or implantations of medical devices to treat the retina. Findings include inflammatory cell infiltration, increased plasma in the vitreous resulting in a more intense stain with eosin (plasmoid vitreous), hemorrhage, liquefaction, and displacement, which may lead to retinal detachment (Short 2008; Taradach and Greaves 1984). Intravitreal injections may result in vitreous prolapse through the injection tracks or retinal toxicity from the injected compound (e.g., ketorolac tromethamine in rabbits) (Komarowska et al. 2009). Intravitreal macrophages may engulf injected material and the optic nerve is one route of clearance of intravitreal injected drugs, so macrophages that have migrated into the vitreous after intravitreal injections may move into the optic nerve (Figure 21.2d).

21.1.10 Retina and Optic Nerve

Retinal structures are generally similar among laboratory animals and well documented in the literature (Hockwin et al. 1991; Samuelson 2007). Basically, the retina consists of the inner transparent sensory (neurosensory) retina and the outer pigmented RPE separated by a potential space (subretinal space). The sensory retina is only attached at two locations (the ora ciliaris retina and the optic disc), allowing for separation of the sensory retina (retinal detachment). Axons of retinal ganglion cells converge to form the optic nerve, and the peripheral retina abruptly becomes the ciliary body at the ora ciliaris retina (ora serrata in humans and nonhuman primates).

The function, morphology, and pathology of the RPE has been reviewed (Mecklenburg and Schraermeyer 2007; Whiteley and Peiffer 2002). Apical villi of the RPE envelop the photoreceptor outer segments but are separated by the interphotoreceptor matrix. During the disk-shedding process, the RPE engulfs and degrades the photoreceptor cell outer segments. Disc shedding may be measured as a function of the RPE (LaVail 1976). Some breakdown products are recycled, but lipofuscin may accumulate as a result of oxidation of polyunsaturated fatty acids as a part of the aging process. Unlike other laboratory animals, lipid bodies normally occur in the RPE of rabbits (Prince 1964).

The lateral surface of RPE cells contributes to the blood–eye barrier, and the basilar surface of the RPE forms a basal lamina that combines with the basal lamina of choriocapillaris endothelial cells (Bruch's membrane). The basilar surface of the RPE has a convoluted appearance owing to spaces that can be expanded as an artifact during perfusion fixation.

Outer segments of the photoreceptors are composed of numerous stacked membranes, and inner segments contain numerous organelles. The nuclei of photoreceptors are located in the outer nuclear layer (ONL) and synapse with neurons from the INL. The ONL is generally thicker than the INL, and if it is less than or equal to the thickness of the INL, photoreceptor degeneration should be considered. Neurons with cell bodies in the INL synapse with neurons from the ganglion cell layer (GCL) containing cell bodies of various types of ganglion cells and amacrine cells. Axons of ganglion cells form the nerve fiber layer, which is thicker closer to the optic disc. Additional cells in the sensory retina include Müller cells, astrocytes, and glial cells. Macroglial cells occur in the INL of rabbits (Prince 1964). Müller cells are regarded as specialized retinal astrocytes that extend processes to the vitreal interface to form the ILM and toward the inner segments of photoreceptors to form the outer limiting membrane.

The retina is one of the most metabolically active tissues in the body. The inner retina (cells with nuclei in the GCL and the INL) get nutrients from retinal vessels, but photoreceptors receive nutrients from the choriocapillaris. Retinal vessels also contribute to the formation of the blood–eye (blood-retina) barrier.

The primary methods for clinically evaluating the retina for toxicity are indirect ophthalmoscopy (fundoscopy) and flash electroretinogram, although clinical evaluation may also involve fluorescein angiography, confocal scanning laser tomography, ultrasonography, and optical coherence tomography (Dietrich 2007; Hockwin et al. 1991; Munger 2002; Rubin 1974). Flash electroretinography is a sensitive and objective assessment of retinal function of laboratory animals and human patients and is used as a biomarker for retinal degeneration (Narfström et al. 2002; Rosolen et al. 2005).

The appearance of the ocular fundus of laboratory animals is well documented (Rubin 1974). Examination involves the retinal vessels, the area centralis (rabbit, dog), the macula (humans and nonhuman primates), the choroid (choroidal vessels in albino animals and the tapetum lucidum in the dog), and the optic disc. There are different patterns of retinal vessels for animals, but most of the commonly used laboratory animals (except rabbit and guinea pig) and humans have a holangiotic pattern (Prince 1964). The area centralis is a localized area of increased cone photoreceptors that is located temporal and slightly superior to the optic disc in dogs but inferior to the optic disc in rabbits (visual streak) (Hebel 1976; McIlwain 1996; Oyster et al. 1981). This area of the retina has similarities to the macula in nonhuman primates, which is located temporal and slightly superior to the optic disc.

Retinal changes induced by toxicity must be differentiated from spontaneous background findings, including those associated with senile, genetic, or light-induced retinopathy. For some compounds, the only manifestation of toxicity may be an increase in the incidence of onset of a spontaneous finding (Taradach and Greaves 1984); thus, knowledge of spontaneously occurring findings is important.

Retinal findings generally involve retinal vessels, photoreceptor cells, or ganglion cells. Changes in the retinal vasculature associated with toxicity include necrosis, vascular proliferation, microaneurysms, thickening, or calcification, which may lead to retinal hemorrhage or edema. Retinal hemorrhage associated with toxicity must be differentiated from other causes such as coagulopathies, retinal hypertension, vascular disease, ocular trauma, or chest compression during handling of rats (Hubert et al. 1994). Retinal vascular changes may be evaluated clinically by vascular angiography and microscopically by trypsin digestion of the retina (Fischer and Slatter 2007). Examples of vascular toxicity include vascular proliferation within the subretinal space owing to urethane anesthesia and retinal edema resulting from administration of naphthalene to rabbits (Rubin 1974).

Alterations involving photoreceptors include dysplasia, dystrophy, and degeneration. The term "retinal dysplasia" is used to describe focal or multifocal disorganization of the sensory retina owing to faulty development and is usually characterized by retinal rosettes, abnormal alignment of photoreceptor cells, and possible degeneration. Spontaneous retinal dysplasia occurs in many laboratory animals, especially rats and rabbits (Rubin 1974). In the rat, retinal dysplasia generally consists of unilateral, linear areas of thinning or loss of the outer layers of the sensory retina, with occasional direct abutment of the INL to the choroid or sclera (Hubert et al. 1994; Kuno et al. 1991; Lin and Essner 1987; Schardein et al. 1975; Taradach and Greaves 1984; Taradach et al. 1981). The finding may occur more frequently in males with an increased incidence with age. One example is referred to as linear retinopathy (Figure 21.3a). Retinal dysplasia may also occur as a finding associated with toxicity (e.g., cytosine in rat pups) (Percy and Danylchuk 1977).

Retinal dystrophy is a condition that generally affects photoreceptors, the RPE, or both and varies in time of onset and progression in severity. The condition is inherited in nonhuman primates, rats, and several strains of mice, including several mutant and transgenic mouse strains (Aguirre et al. 1998; Drager and Hubel 1978; Heywood 1974; Hubert et al. 1999; Lai et al. 1975; Matuk 1991; Pittler and Baehr 1991; Rubin 1974; Taradach and Greaves 1984; Von Sallman and Grimes 1972).

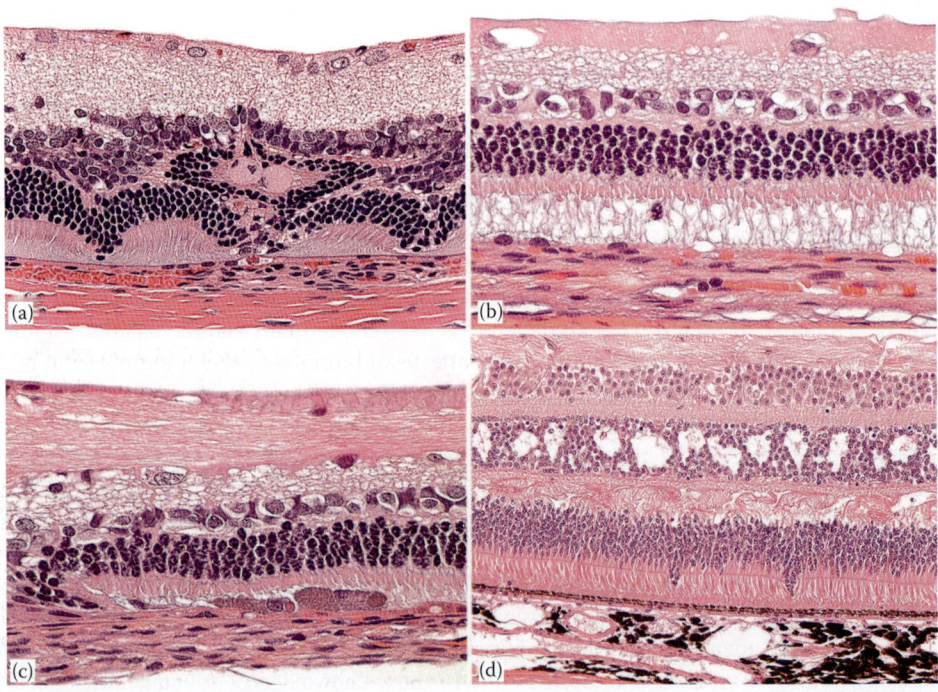

FIGURE 21.3   (a) Hematoxylin and eosin, 60× objective. Multifocal loss of inner and outer segments of photoreceptors in a Sprague–Dawley rat consistent with the spontaneous condition linear retinopathy. Distorted appearance of the retina in the center of the image is a result of a tangential cut through the retina. (b) Hematoxylin and eosin, 60× objective. Photoreceptor nucleus spontaneously displaced into the layer of inner and outer segments in the retina of a rabbit. (c) Hematoxylin and eosin, 60× objective. Spontaneous hypertrophy of the RPE adjacent to the optic nerve of a rabbit with accumulation of lysozymes and lipofuscin. (d) Hematoxylin and eosin, 20× objective. Retinal changes (spaces within the INL and multifocal extension of photoreceptor nuclei into a layer of inner and outer segments) after intravitreal injection of test article in a monkey.

Degeneration of photoreceptor cells of laboratory animals may be spontaneous (e.g., aging or from light exposure) or the result of toxicity. Retinal degeneration due to aging is characterized by a gradual decrease in the number of photoreceptors, especially rods, and thinning of the ONL, which is clearly evident by 2 years in the rat (Geiss and Yoshitomi 1999; Heywood 1974; Hockwin et al. 1991; Lai et al. 1978, 1979; Lin and Essner 1987; Taradach and Greaves 1984; Tucker 1997; Weisse et al. 1974). For all laboratory animals and humans, the gradual loss of photoreceptors with aging includes the displacement of photoreceptor nuclei into the inner and outer segment layers (Figure 21.3b) (Lai 1980; Lai et al. 1982). Displaced photoreceptor nuclei are generally low in number, especially in the central retina, and contain a normal density of chromatin. They are more frequently observed in the periphery or posterior pole. Displaced nuclei are more frequently observed in the retina of very young rats, older rats, and rats exposed to high ambient light intensities or in globes with ocular disease. The nuclei are observed with or without degeneration of adjacent photoreceptors.

Since the peripheral retina is thinner than the central retina, degeneration associated with aging is more noticeable in this region and may begin with changes in the RPE. Changes typical of senile peripheral retinal degeneration include retinal thinning with a loss of nuclei in the ONL and INL, fusion of the nuclear layers, displacement of photoreceptor nuclei into the inner and outer segment layers, hypertrophy of the RPE, and possibly migration of RPE cells or macrophages into the sensory retina (Lai et al. 1978, 1982; O'Steen et al. 1974; Rubin 1974; Taradach and Greaves 1984; Weisse et al. 1974).

Light-induced photoreceptor degeneration has been reported in rats, mice, nonhuman primates, rabbits, and minipigs (Bellhorn 1980; Dureau et al. 1996; Greenman et al. 1982; Hockwin et al. 1991; Hubert et al. 1999; Kuwabara and Gorn 1968; Lai et al. 1978; LaVail 1980; La Vail et al. 1987; Lawill 1973; Noell et al. 1966; Organisaciak and Winkler 1994; O'Steen et al. 1972; Peiffer and Porter 1991; Perez and Perentes 1994; Tso 1973; Tso and Woodford 1983; Weisse et al. 1974). Pigmentation of the uvea, especially the iris, of non-albino animals protects the retina from light damage by absorbing light. In rats, females have a tendency to be more affected than males, and sensitivity may vary with strain. Mice appear to be quite sensitive to increased light intensity, and sensitivity varies with uveal pigmentation. Exposure to light contributes to the natural aging process of the retina, especially for albino animals, but short-term exposure to high levels of light intensity or long-term exposure of normal light and dark cycles may cause photoreceptor degeneration. This is especially true for rodents on the top of a cage rack in comparison to animals on the bottom of the cage rack. Other factors that influence the development of light-induced retinopathy include wavelength, duration of exposure, length of time for dark adaptation, age of initial exposure, maturity of the retina, body temperature, albinism, decreased prior daily light exposure, changes in light/ dark cycle length, and diet, including a deficiency or excess of vitamin A or deficiency of vitamin E or taurine. In general, light-induced retinal degeneration is more prominent in the central retina, and rods are more sensitive than cones. Alterations include a decrease in the thickness of the ONL, disorganization and thinning of the layers of outer segments and inner segments, and possibly the increase in displaced photoreceptor nuclei.

A common background finding occurring in many laboratory mammals, especially dogs and nonhuman primates, is peripheral cystoid retinal degeneration (Dubielzig et al. 2010; Rubin 1974). This finding, which increases in prevalence with age, is noted in the superior nasal quadrant of dogs as early as 8 weeks, and in the peripheral temporal retina of nonhuman primates. The finding should be distinguished from splitting of the retinal layers (retinoschisis).

A change associated with aging observed in the retina of nonhuman primates is hyaline deposits beneath the RPE (drusen-like bodies) (Hope et al. 1992; Ishibashi et al. 1986). These structures consist of subretinal concretions on Bruch's membrane.

Retinal fold is a focal detachment of the sensory retina, and spontaneous retinal folds have been reported in many species of laboratory animals, especially in young animals (Hockwin et al. 1991; Hubert et al. 1999; Kuno et al. 1991; Rubin 1974). Microscopically, retinal folds affect the outer layers of the retina and are differentiated from artifacts by an association with preretinal traction membranes or subretinal deposits, hemorrhage, or aggregates of RPE cells (Gartner and Henkind 1981; Rubin 1974).

Spontaneous retinal detachment is uncommon in laboratory animals and may be associated with preretinal traction membranes, retinal holes or tears, the presence of fluid or hemorrhage within the subretinal space, and buphthalmos associated with glaucoma (Dubielzig et al. 2010; Rubin 1974). Traction membranes may develop secondarily to changes in the vitreous body from neovascular disease or intraocular surgery. Serous retinal detachment may develop secondarily to hypertension or choroidal edema that may be associated with compound administration (e.g., pyrithione or diethylthiocarbazone) (Grant 1986). With true retinal detachment, the RPE cells are often hypertrophied and individualized, and with time, retinal detachment will result in photoreceptor degeneration.

A common morphological change in the RPE is hypertrophy. Hypertrophic RPE cells may occur as a single row of uniform, diffusely enlarged cells without retinal detachment, a single row of individualized cells with retinal detachment, or a focal cluster of cells usually containing granular cytoplasm and possibly lipofuscin (Figure 21.3c). The latter form of hypertrophy is a common spontaneous change in rabbits, especially around the optic disc, but may be present in other locations (Render and Schafer, personal communication). Since the RPE engulfs and degrades photoreceptor outer segments, lipofuscin may accumulate with age or with toxicity, (e.g., lead toxicity) (Mecklenburg and Schraermyer 2007). The RPE may undergo other morphological changes, such as loss of cellular polarity, loss of apical villi, and depigmentation. These findings occur in response to injury. RPE cells may also undergo hyperplasia, with or without metaplasia, in response to stimuli including injuries, chronic inflammation, and long-standing retinal detachment with traction.

Compounds that bind to melanin are often examined to determine if they will cause retinal toxicity, but binding to melanin by a compound does not automatically mean that there will be toxicity (Dayhaw-Barker 2002; Leblanc et al. 1998). There may be no effect or there may be a protective effect (Hockwin et al. 1991). For example, administration of vigabatrin resulted in retinal findings in albino Sprague–Dawley rats, but not in pigmented Lister-Hooded rats (Butler et al. 1987). In contrast, retinal degeneration in rats exposed to fenthion was more severe in pigmented rats (Imai et al. 1983).

Changes in the sensory retina and the RPE associated with various drug and chemical toxicities have previously been reviewed (Frame and Carlton 1991; Grant 1986; Kuiper et al. 1997; Marmor and Wolfensberger 1998; Mecklenburg and Schraermyer 2007; Whiteley and Peiffer 2002). The site and severity of toxicity within the retina may vary because of the high degree of subspecialization among neurons of the different retinal layers, and determining the primary cell type affected by a toxin on the basis of morphological appearance may be difficult (Bouldin et al. 1984). For example, spaces may occur within the INL after treatment and the exact pathogenesis is not always known (Figure 21.3d).

The most common finding in the retina associated with toxicity is degeneration.

Retinal degeneration is a nonspecific term used to describe apoptosis, necrosis, atrophy, or vacuolation of retinal tissue and needs to be defined, if used. In general, toxicities causing retinal degeneration affect the inner retina, principally the ganglion cells, or affect the outer retina, principally the photoreceptors or RPE. Degenerative changes of photoreceptors include shortening of the outer segments, a finding that may be reversible if the photoreceptors remain viable. With time, photoreceptor degeneration may be characterized by disorganization or thinning of the layer of photoreceptor inner and outer segments and thinning of the ONL. Funduscopically, photoreceptor degeneration may be manifested as tapetal hyperreflectivity in the dog and cat. Microscopically, photoreceptor degeneration resulting from toxicity may appear similar to spontaneous photoreceptor degeneration.

Vacuolation is one of the changes that can occur in various cells in the retina. For example, hexachlorophene causes vacuolation of the photoreceptors (Frame and Carlton 1991). Cationic amphiphilic drugs result in phospholipidosis with an accumulation of membranous whorls in the RPE as a result of an interference with enzymatic degradation of phospholipids (Drenkhahn and Lüllmann-Rauch 1978; Lüllmann and Lüllmann-Rauch 1981). Certain cell types may be specifically affected by cationic amphiphilic drugs. For example, chloroquine mainly affects neurons and Müller cells, while triparanol affects the RPE and Müller cells. The RPE is particularly at risk because of its role in phagocytosis and processing of large amounts of membranous material from rod outer segments. Lysosomal inclusions containing concentric lamellae accumulate in the RPE in animals given intra-vitreal injections of gentamycin and accumulate if degradation is impaired.

Causes of degeneration of the RPE include aging, sensory retinal detachment, and toxicity (e.g., aminophenoxyalkanes) (Mecklenburg and Schraermyer 2007). Toxicity and degeneration of the RPE and photoreceptors is not necessarily due to binding of drugs to melanin in the RPE; therefore, binding of drugs to melanin is not predictive of toxicity (Leblanc et al. 1998).

Alterations involving the sensory retina consist of vascular changes, degeneration of ganglion cells, photoreceptors or other neurons, and reactions by glial cells. Some compounds, such as tri-methyltin, may produce alterations in more than one type of retinal cell (Grant 1986; Whiteley and Peiffer 2002). Müller cells may undergo cytoplasmic vacuolation and necrosis owing to D,L-α-aminoadipic acid toxicity (Pedersen and Karlsen 1979).

Numerous compounds affect the RPE, and some will cause an alteration in the blood–retinal barrier. Toxicologic alterations in the RPE may be concurrent with alterations in photoreceptors or cause secondary degenerative changes in the photoreceptors (Mecklenburg and Schraermyer 2007).

The predicative value of retinal findings in laboratory animals due to ocular toxicity may vary between rodent and non-rodent species and between animals and humans (Heywood 1985). For example, enrofloxacin is an antimicrobial agent that has interspecies differences in sensitivity to retinal toxicity (Gelatt et al. 2001). Retinal lesions in animals may be difficult to correlate to reti-nal lesions in humans. Some drugs (e.g., ethambutol and vigabatrin) that cause retinal lesions in laboratory animals do not appear to cause retinal changes in humans (Butler et al. 1987; Heng et al. 1999).

Photoreceptor degeneration is associated with various drug and chemical toxicities (Frame and Carlton 1991; Grant 1986). Mechanisms of chemically induced retinal degeneration vary with com-pound and species. Some toxicities have a direct effect on a retinal cell while other compounds have an indirect effect, for example, affecting the endothelial cells of the choriocapillaris.

Initial degenerative changes affecting photoreceptors may be a shortening of outer segments, which can be a reversible change as long as the photoreceptors are still viable. Generally, this acute phase of photoreceptor degeneration is not detected microscopically, but more advanced changes may be detected including shortening, fragmentation, and disorganization of the outer segments with outward migration of photoreceptor cell nuclei, phagocytosis of photoreceptor debris by the RPE, and thinning of the ONL from a loss of photoreceptor nuclei.

Ganglion cell degeneration may occur directly owing to toxicity, secondary to glaucoma, or as a spontaneous condition. A helpful way of detecting a loss of ganglion cells is an examination of a cross section of retrobulbar optic nerve for degeneration of ganglion cell axons. Ganglion cell toxicity may be species specific as far as susceptibility. For example, methanol toxicity occurs in humans and nonhuman primates, but not in the rabbit or dog (Rubin 1974). Toxicities involving ganglion cells occur with several compounds (Heng et al. 1999; Parhad et al. 1986). Doxorubicin causes an inhibition of slow transport resulting in neurofilamentous axonal swelling and necrosis (Parhad et al. 1986). Glutamate causes neuronal depolarization resulting in an influx of ions that causes cell swelling and necrosis of ganglion cells, with possible vacuolation in the plexiform layers of rodents (Lucas and Newhouse 1957). Overstimulation of a glutamate receptor may also result in a loss of ganglion cells and has been implicated in toxicity associated with retinal ischemia. Ethambutol toxicity, which is mediated through an excitotoxic pathway, is characterized by axonal swellings within the optic nerves of rats and visual disturbances in human patients (Heng et al. 1999). Toxicities involving ganglion cells may also involve other types of retinal cells. For example, chloroquine toxicity affects ganglion cells, photoreceptors, and the RPE in humans and animals by intracellular accumulation of membranous phospholipid inclusions. This change may be irreversible after cessation of administration, and susceptibility to toxicity may vary among laboratory animals (Davidson and Rennie 1986; Grant 1986). Ganglion cell loss because of toxicity must be differentiated from potential spontaneous conditions, such as idiopathic bilateral optic neuropathy in rhesus and cynomolgus monkeys (Fortune et al. 2005; Leedle et al. 2008). In this condition, ganglion cells are lost in the macular region, resulting in a loss of axons in the temporal aspect of both optic nerves.

Ganglion cell axons converge to form the optic disc and the optic nerve, which is composed of retinal ganglion cell axons, glial cells, and pia mater septae (Samuelson 2007). The optic disc has a slight peripheral elevation and central depression (physiologic cup), which is prominent in rabbits. Clinically, the optic disc can be evaluated funduscopically for size, clarity, and color, and optic disc blood flow can be measured by laser Doppler flowmetry (Rubin 1974).

Alterations in the optic nerve of laboratory animals include spontaneous and toxicologic changes. Spontaneous changes that are congenital may be detected during the pre-study examination and other changes may be detected in additional funduscopic examinations. Degeneration of the optic nerve and the optic tracts may be unilateral or bilateral with a loss of axons and gliosis. Idiopathic bilateral optic neuropathy has been reported in rhesus and cynomolgus monkeys (Fortune et al. 2005; Leedle et al. 2008). Degeneration of the optic nerve is generally characterized by a loss of ganglion cells in the retina and includes conditions such as glaucoma, which results in ganglion cell loss and cupping of the optic disc (Dubielzig et al. 2010). Optic nerve axons decrease with age in animals, while the number of astrocytes and glial membranes increases (Cavallotti et al. 2001).

Toxic optic neuropathy has been reported with numerous compounds in humans and laboratory animals (Grant 1986; McCaa 1985). Alterations may include axonal swelling, with or without demyelination, loss of axons, reactive gliosis, and vascular endothelial proliferation.

Optic neuritis is an ophthalmic term that often has no microscopic correlate, but may represent mild edema. Papilledema is edema of the optic disc and is characterized by bulging of the optic disc into the vitreous chamber. The finding may or may not be accompanied by destruction of axons or myelin. Optic disc swelling may be due to edema or neurofilament accumulation, and papilledema may be a manifestation of ocular toxicity (e.g., salicylanilide) (Brown et al. 1972). Spontaneous neoplasia of the optic nerve and retina is rare in laboratory animals but reported in the optic nerve of rats. Treatment-related neoplasms have been induced by administration of nickel-containing compounds (Ackerman et al. 1998; Albert et al. 1982; Shadduck and Everitt 1991; Yoshitomi and Boorman 1990).

21.2 EAR

21.2.1 External Ear

The ear consists of three parts: the external ear, middle ear, and inner ear (Banks 1993). The external ear consists of the pinna (auricle) and the external ear canal (external auditory meatus), which ends medially at the external surface of the tympanic membrane. The structures of the external ear are supported by auricular cartilage, and the secretions from the sebaceous and ceruminous glands contribute to the formation of cerumen. In rodents, Zymbal's gland is a sebaceous gland located anterior and ventral to the external ear canal. Pathologic changes of the external ear can involve the skin or specific structures of the external ear (Kelemen 1978). Inflammation of the external auditory canal is usually not an issue in toxicologic studies unless clinical signs, such as shaking of the head or ear scratching, are observed. When inflammation does occur, it is characterized by thickening of the wall of the external auditory canal from edema, and the presence of a tan or brown crusty exudate within the canal (Gad 2007). The cause may be ear mites (e.g., *Psoroptes cuniculi* in rabbits or *Otodectes cynotis* in dogs). Auricular chondritis is a spontaneous condition reported in several strains of rats that appears as nodular or diffuse thickening of the pinna by granulomatous inflammation of fibrochondrous to chondroosseous tissue (Chiu 1991; Kitagaki et al. 2003). Differential diagnoses include chondrolysis and neoplasms.

Ductal cysts and neoplasms of Zymbal's gland may occur as a spontaneous finding in aged rats (Greaves 2007). Malignant neoplasms of the auditory sebaceous gland have been induced by a variety of chemical carcinogens in the rat and by the ingestion of benzene in the mouse (Huff et al. 1988; Maltoni et al. 1988).

21.2.2 MIDDLE EAR

The middle ear contains an air-filled space within the temporal bone (tympanic cavity) delineated laterally by the tympanic membrane at the end of the external auditory meatus and medially by the inner ear. The Eustachian (auditory) tube extends anteriorly from the tympanic cavity to connect with the nasal pharynx, and the mucous membranes lining these structures are similar. The auditory tube allows for equilibration of sound pressure to the air-filled middle ear space, provides drainage of fluids, but may also be a route of infection for the middle ear. The inner aspect of the tympanic membrane is covered by a mucous membrane of the middle ear, and the outer aspect is covered by mucosa of the external auditory meatus.

The middle ear contains a chain of three small bones (ossicles). The malleus is attached to the tympanic membrane and articulates with the incus (Figure 21.4a). The incus articulates with the stapes and the footplate is attached to the membranous oval window of the cochlea. Muscles of the middle ear include the tensor tympani (attached to the malleus) and the stapedius (attached to the stapes), and contraction of the muscles restricts movement of the ossicles and reduces transmission of sound.

Examination of the middle ear begins with a gross inspection under a dissection microscope, including physical manipulation of the ossicles as a test of their mobility. Mobility of the ossicles can be reduced by buildup of fluid or an exudate in the tympanic cavity or by osseous fixation of the articulations (Figure 21.4b and c). Otosclerosis is the osseous fixation of the stapes with the oval window and is the most common cause of middle ear dysfunction in adult patients. The ossicles can also become brittle and break from clinical conditions, such as osteogenesis imperfecta or inflammatory exudate in the middle ear.

Cholesteatoma may occur with blockage of the auditory tube and consists of firm nodules of a keratinized stratified squamous epithelium with rete peg formation overlying connective tissue. Cholesteatoma has been reported in many species and can be induced experimentally by applying irritants or surgically ligating the external ear canal (Hottendorf 1991; McGinn et al. 1982; Steinbach and Grüninger 1980). The finding must be differentiated from chronic granulation tissue and squamous cell carcinoma, a condition reported in aged gerbils (Rowe et al. 1974).

Infections of the middle ear occur in laboratory animals, especially guinea pigs; therefore, it is important to check for evidence of previous or current infections before animals are included in a toxicity study. Changes include a thickening of the otic capsule, increased thickness of the mucosal lining of the middle ear, mucosal gland formation, fibrosis, and osteosclerosis. An infection in the middle ear may spread to the inner ear, resulting in loss of sensory cells and hearing loss. Treatment of middle ear infections should be done with care since many drugs used as treatments may also have ototoxic properties. Compounds may reach the tympanic cavity after systemic administration or by inserting a needle through the tympanic membrane and directly depositing the compound.

Decreased middle ear function will be manifested as a reduction in hearing. Hearing loss may result from lesions in the middle ear (conductive hearing loss) or from lesions affecting the sensory cells in the inner ear (sensorineural hearing loss). Hearing loss can be detected by behavioral and physiological tests. Behavioral tests include the pinna reflex (movement of the pinna after a loud noise) and the acoustic startle reflex (movement, usually jumping, in response to a loud unexpected sound). A physiological test used to measure hearing in animals and people is the auditory brain stem response (ABR). In general, middle ear lesions are more likely to raise the hearing thresholds in low and middle ranges of frequencies, while most ototoxic drugs affecting the inner ear are more likely to raise thresholds at higher frequencies.

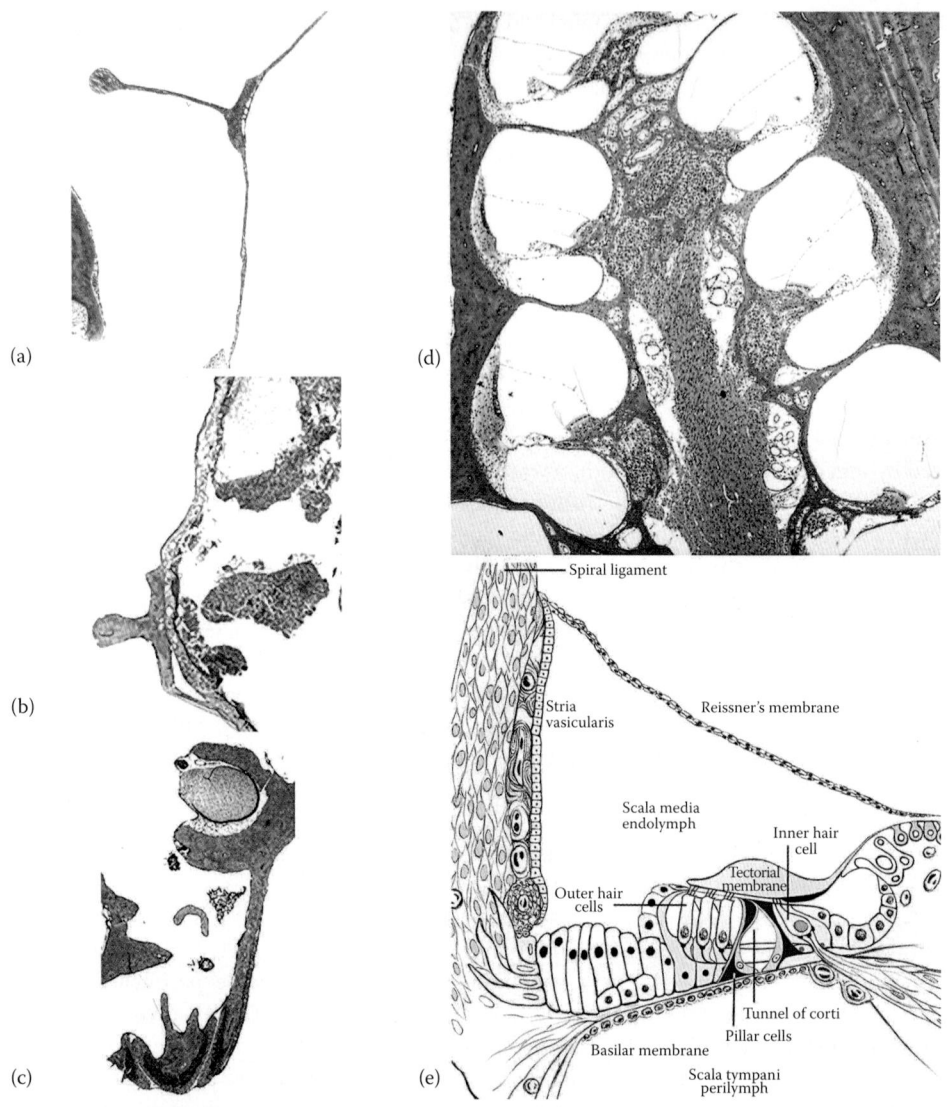

FIGURE 21.4 (a–c) Plastic sections through the middle ear: (a) normal tympanic membrane; (b) tympanic membrane with reactive cells and material in the middle ear; (c) reactive cells by the footplate of the stapes. (d) Paramodiolar plastic section through the inner ear of a guinea pig at a low magnification to illustrate several turns of the spiral cochlea. (e) Schematic of a cross-sectional profile through the cochlear spiral showing cellular components around the scala media. The cells of stria vascularis make up the lateral margin on the left. The osseous spiral lamina and basilar membrane are the lower margin with the organ of Corti overlying them and the tectorial membrane overlying the organ of Corti. The organ of Corti has a tunnel formed by inner and outer pillar cells, with three rows of outer hair cells lateral to the tunnel (left in the schematic) and one row of inner hair cells medial to the tunnel. Outer phalangeal cells (Deiters cells) cup outer hair cells at their bases and inner phalangeal cells surround outer hair cells.

21.2.3 Inner Ear: Auditory System

The inner ear is located in the petrous portion of the temporal bone, medial to the middle ear, and consists of an auditory (cochlea) and a vestibular component (vestibule and semicircular canals). Reviews of cochlear histology provide more detail than this chapter can provide (Forge et al. 2011; Hawkins 1973; Raphael and Altschuler 2003; Santi 2001). The cochlea has a spiraling shape. The number of turns in this spiral varies among species, ranging from 2 1/2 turns in most nonhuman primates, the rat, and the mouse to 4 1/4 turns in guinea pig and chinchilla (Figure 21.4d). The cochlea has two different fluid components: an inner membranous tube (scala media) filled with endolymph and an outer fluid space containing perilymph that is divided into two compartments (scala vestibuli and scala tympani), which are joined at their apical ends by the helicotrema. Endolymph is similar to intracellular fluid, while perilymph is similar to cerebrospinal fluid (CSF) and has a connection to CSF through the cochlear aqueduct. Differences in the ionic composition between endolymph and perilymph create the endocochlear potential, which is critical to the auditory transduction process. Vibration of the footplate of the stapes causes movement of the oval window and perilymph in the scala vestibuli, which causes movement of perilymph in the scala tympani and, eventually, movement of the round window. These fluid compartments of the cochlea spiral around a centrally located core (the modiolus) that contains cell bodies of the auditory nerve (spiral ganglion) and their central projections directed toward the brain stem (the auditory nerve).

The scala media has a triangular shape in cross section with a membranous spiral lamina (basilar membrane), a lateral periosteal spiral ligament with the stria vascularis, and an upper membrane (Reissner's membrane) (Figure 21.4e). The hair cells and several different types of supporting cells form the organ of Corti that lies on the basilar membrane. The hair cells are most often implicated in auditory disorders or trauma from stresses such as drugs and noise. Perilymph of the scala tympani can diffuse through the basilar membrane and fill the tunnel of Corti with cortilymph. The pear-shaped inner hair cells are arranged in a single row along the cochlear spiral. Hair cells are so named because they have many modified microvilli (stereocilia) projecting from their apex into the endolymph of the scala media. There are usually three rows of stereocilia, each at a different height. There are also three or four rows of cylinder-shaped outer hair cells. Outer hair cells have three rows of stereocilia graded in height and are more specialized than the inner hair cell. The lateral wall of the outer hair cell is surrounded by cortilymph in the spaces of Nuel. In mammals, there is no regeneration of hair cells after loss, but mammalian vestibular hair cells may regenerate to some extent (Forge et al. 2011).

Certain types of supporting cells make physical contact with the hair cells. The apical portions of these supporting cells and the hair cells make junctional complexes, including tight junctions, which form the barrier between the endolymph of the scala media and the perilymph of the scala tympani. Maintenance of this barrier is critical because intermixing of fluids can alter the structure and function of the cochlear cells. These supporting cells are part of an active process that reacts to trauma or toxicity of the hair cells by forming "scars" that maintain the fluid barrier. The presence of scars is a critical marker of hair cell loss.

Supporting cells can be differentiated from the sensory hair cells by several markers, including antibodies to cytokeratins and connexins, which are not expressed in hair cells.

Other cochlear structures include Reissner's membrane, the tectorial membrane, and the stria vascularis. The latter structure is responsible for secreting endolymph and regulating ion movement in generating the endocochlear potential. Transduction in the cochlea is detailed in a review (Hudspeth 2005). Movement of the fluid through the scala media in a manner that is frequency specific, causing movement of the stereocilia of the hair cells. Every frequency can be mapped to a specific location along the cochlear spiral, and this has been established for many species to be used as animal models (Eldredge et al. 1981; Greenwood 1961; Müller et al. 2005, web site of Dr. Santi: http://mousecochlea.ccgb.umn.edu/digcyto_java.php).

Disruption of critical elements in the transduction process by noise or test article may cause hearing loss. There must be an endocochlear potential that is maintained by the stria vascularis. The stereocilia of hair cells must be stiff and their links intact. The hair cells must be present and functional, and the auditory nerve terminals at the inner hair cell base must be present and intact.

Outer hair cells are the most sensitive to disorders of the inner ear including noise, ototoxins, aging, and trauma. Hearing loss in the range of 10–50 dB is usually attributed to loss or dysfunction of the outer hair cells. The movement of outer hair cells sets up an "emission" that can be easily measured with an external recording device in the ear canal ("otoacoustic emissions"), providing a quick way to assess outer hair cell function and potential toxicity.

There are certain techniques used to examine the structures of the inner ear for evidence of toxicity (Forge et al. 2011; Schuknecht 1974). Most postmortem assessments of cochlear tissues involve fixation of the cochlear tissues, usually with aldehydes. If only the tissues associated with the fluid spaces (organ of Corti, stria vascularis) will be assessed, then a local intrascalar infusion of fixative into the scala tympani through the round window is possible. An exit needs to be created either at the oval window or with a hole in the bone to allow fluids to escape. If the auditory nerve and spiral ganglion cells will also be assessed, then vascular fixation followed by an intrascalar infusion is preferred. In either case, the connection between inner hair cells and the auditory nerve is very sensitive to the fixation process, and swelling and bursting of the afferent terminals at the inner hair cell bases are a common fixation artifact. Whole mounts of the cochlear spiral (surface preparations) are useful for assessing cells of the organ of Corti. This requires removal of the otic capsule, lateral wall with stria vascularis, and the tectorial and Reissner's membranes with dissection of the organ of Corti into segments (Fex and Altschuler 1986). The number of segments depends on the number of turns (more segments for guinea pigs and fewer segments for rats and mice). The surface preparations can then be processed for scanning electron microscopy or stained and processed for brightfield examination using differential interference contrast or fluorescence microscopy. While scanning electron microscopy was once the method of choice, the most common approach now is staining a component or components of hair cells, supporting cells, or both with a fluorescent chromophore for phalloidin and viewing under epifluorescent optics or with laser scanning or two-photon confocal microscopes (Figure 21.5a and b). With this approach, it is possible to screen the presence or absence of hair cells along the entire cochlear spiral and map their presence or absence by position from apex to base, producing what is called a cytocochleogram (Figure 21.5c). Different frequencies can be placed on the cytocochleogram chart, on the basis of chartings of frequency place already in the literature (Greenwood 1961; Müller et al. 2005, web site of Dr. Santi: http://mousecochlea.ccgb.umn.edu/digcyto_java.php).

Assessment of cochlear tissues can also be done via light and electron microscopy by embedding the temporal bones in plastic. At the light microscopic level, paramodiolar sections can provide assessments of multiple cochlear elements through all turns (Figure 21.4d). Transmission electron microscopy can be used to focus on specific elements, such as synapses and stereocilia elements. The choice of fixative depends on the method of examination, such as immunostaining or *in situ* hybridization (O'Malley et al. 2009). Paraformaldehyde or formalin is often used for light microscopy and mixed aldehydes (paraformaldehyde and glutaraldehyde) are common fixatives for transmission electron microscopy. Fixation can be accomplished with just local intrascalar infusion or with vascular perfusion followed by local intrascalar infusion. The latter step is necessary if quality preservation of the spiral ganglion neurons (SGNs) and modiolar tissues is desired. The synapse between inner hair cells and type I SGN is very sensitive to fixation artifact, and swelling and bursting of type I SGN peripheral process terminal at the inner hair cell bases are common. Decalcification or removal of the otic capsule is necessary before sectioning. Common quantitative assessments from sections include SGN counts and densities, measurement of strial thickness, and inner and outer hair cell assessments. Immunostaining in cryostat and paraffin sections is commonly used to differentiate cochlear cell types and assess specific changes. These methods may be supplemented by use of explant cultures of inner ears of chickens and evaluating the lateral line of fish (Chiu et al. 2008; Mangiardi et al. 2004: Ton and Parng 2005).

Hair cells, particularly the outer hair cells, are commonly lost as a consequence of a variety of stresses to the cochlea, including ototoxic drugs, noise overstimulation, diseases, genetic disorders, and aging, and in mammals, the loss is permanent. A scattered loss of outer hair cells can be expected in the organ of Corti of control laboratory animals and in humans with normal hearing. This loss is most often in the basal half of the cochlea, and in the first row of outer hair cells. The most apical cochlea also commonly has confined regions where outer hair cells are absent; however,

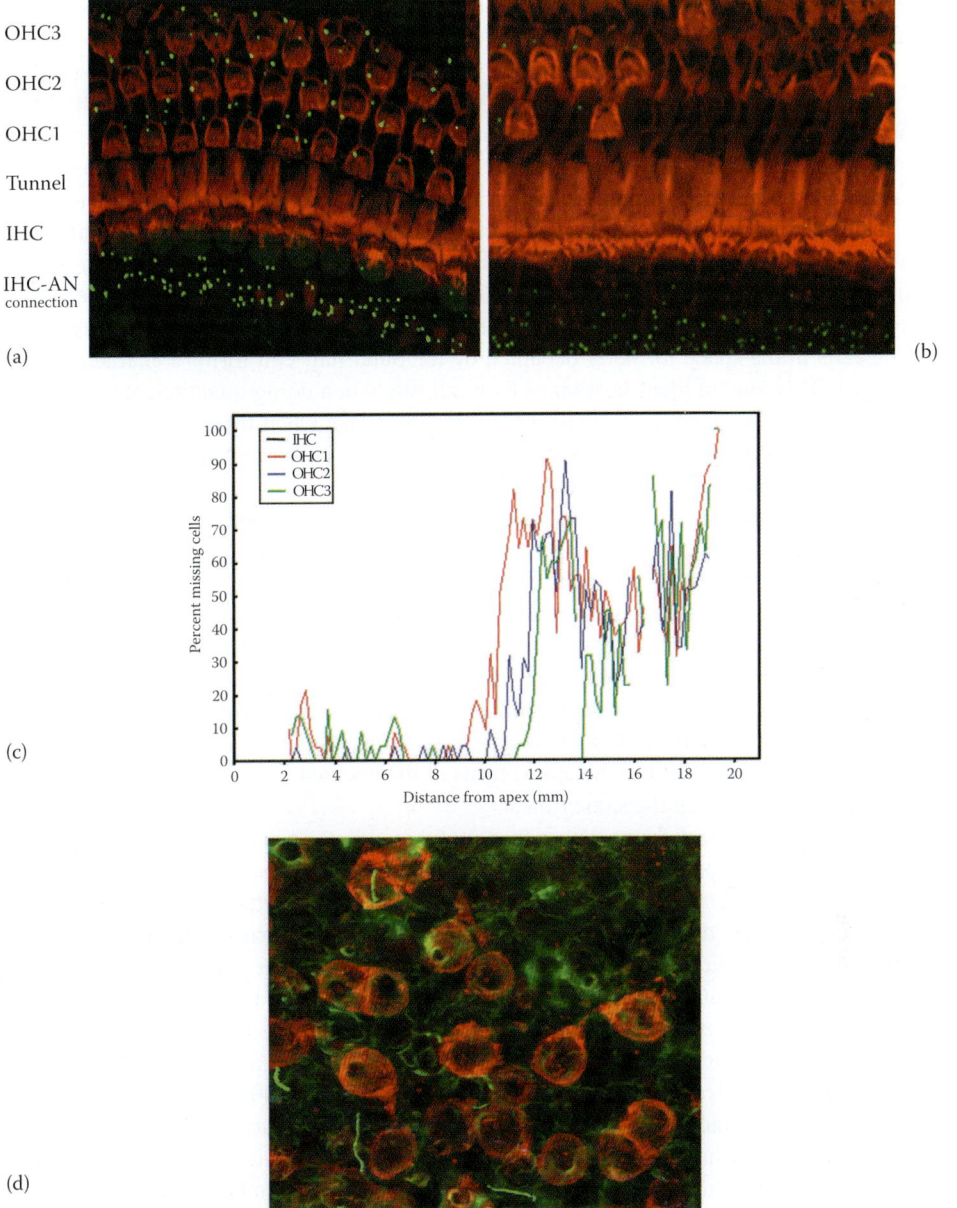

FIGURE 21.5 (a) Surface preparation of the organ of Corti of mouse stained with phalloidin (red wavelength) and CTBP2 immunostaining (green wavelength) viewed with laser scanning confocal microscope. (b) Surface preparation of the organ of Corti of mouse stained with phalloidin (red wavelength) and CTBP2 immunostaining (green wavelength) viewed with laser scanning confocal microscope. Notice the loss of some outer hair cells. (c) Cytocochleogram from a guinea pig treated systemically with the ototoxic aminoglycoside antibiotic gentamycin, showing loss of outer hair cells in the basal cochlea. (d) Surface preparation from a mouse sacculus with phalloidin labeling the filamentous actin in hair cells and supporting cells and with calretinin immunostaining of calyces at the bases of type I vestibular hair cells.

this is a consequence of disorganization of the outer hair cells in this most apical region rather than being initially present and then lost.

Scar formation in the cochlea is a response of the supporting cells to the loss of traumatized sensory hair cells (Bohne 1976; Raphael and Altschuler 1991, 1992). Supporting cells swell and fill in the spaces of Nuel, so that they are now touching the lateral wall of the outer hair cell. Loss of the spaces of Nuel is the earliest sign of scar formation (type 1 scar). The upper portions of the neighboring supporting cells then push into the upper area where the outer hair cells reside below the cuticular plate and then envelop it. The apices of the supporting cells form junctional complexes and maintain the barrier between the endolymph of the scala media and the perilymph of the scala tympani, thus maintaining the endocochlear potential and cochlear function. When the type 1 scar is viewed from above with a fluorescent filamentous actin label (phalloidin), the convergence of the supporting cells in the space formerly occupied by the outer hair cell forms a characteristic actin-labeled bridge. This aids in identification of hair cell loss when doing quantitative assessments for a cytocochleogram. The type 1 scar will remain in this phase when there is only moderate outer hair cell loss, but it progresses to other phases when many hair cells are lost in the same region, and particularly if inner hair cells are also lost.

In type 2 scar formation, the phalangeal cells have either transformed or been replaced by other more lateral supporting cells and appear as several rows of cells with a squamous epithelial appearance. Pillar cells may transform or may be replaced by layers of epithelium, particularly when inner hair cells are also traumatized and encapsulated by neighboring supporting cells. Type 2 scars may completely occupy the location of the organ of Corti and may be retained, or may progress toward forming a type 3 scar, which is a single layer of epithelium over the basilar membrane and osseous spiral lamina. A large stress may cause a significant loss of hair cells, which may cause scar formation and immediately progress to type 2 or type 3 scarring. There may be times when an earlier phase of scar formation is found in the apical turns of the cochlea, and a later phase of scar formation in the basal turns, both at the same time.

There are many classes of drugs that induce ototoxic effects in cochlear and vestibular epithelium, including aminoglycoside antibiotics, the diuretic ethacrynic acid, quinine, salicylates, and the anticancer drug cisplatin (Forge et al. 2011; McCormik and Nuttal 1976; Rybak et al. 2008; Sergi et al. 2003). Often, drug ototoxicity is a consequence of ototoxins inducing reactive oxygen species (ROS) or free radical formation, particularly in cells of the organ of Corti. Increased ROS formation occurs across multiple cochlear cell types, and the level of increase does not always correlate with the resulting toxicity. Both hair cells and supporting cells may have increases in ROS; however, hair cells are more likely to have a toxic effect. Many cochlear cell types have cytochemical changes after aminoglycoside treatment (Imamura and Adams 2003).

It is important to characterize the pattern of hair cell damage, since different insults may have different patterns or may have similar patterns (Forge et al. 2011). Outer hair cells are usually most sensitive to ototoxicity, with inner hair cells becoming affected only at higher doses of an ototoxin. There is also an ototoxicity gradient among outer hair cells, with outer hair cells in the basal cochlea and in the first row being the most sensitive and most commonly lost. The initial loss of outer hair cells in the basal cochlea may also be observed with aging, genetic mutation, or excessive noise (Steel and Kros 2001; Wang et al. 2002; Wright et al. 1987). There is evidence that outer hair cells, particularly in the basal cochlea, have decreases in some common endogenous antioxidant pathways, which might explain their increased sensitivity (Sha et al. 2001). A few drugs affect the inner hair cells more than the outer hair cells (e.g., carboplatin in chinchillas) (Wang et al. 2003).

Cells in the stria vascularis and fibroblasts of the lateral wall can also be affected by aminoglycosides and other ototoxic drugs (Rybak 2007; Rybak et al. 2008; Schacht and Hawkins 2006; Van Ruijven et al. 2005). Cisplatin causes changes in the stria vascularis, with initial effects on the marginal cells (bulging), as well as edema of vascular spaces with shrinkage in the volume of intermediate and marginal cell zones with time. Cisplatin also directly affects SGN but is not toxic to vestibular structures. The stria vascularis may be affected by drugs that affect blood flow such as furosemide. Findings associated with toxicity include swelling of vessels in the stria vascularis, some damage to cellular elements, and loss of endocochlear potential, suggesting loss of stria vascularis function. Organometals, solvents (e.g., toluene and styrene), and quinine may induce or potentiate ototoxicity.

There are multiple factors that may influence sensitivity to ototoxic drugs, including genetic influences, efficacy of antioxidant pathways, and other endogenous protective mechanisms (Rybak et al. 2008). Sensitivity to ototoxins can change during cochlear development and maturation, and susceptibility also varies among animal species. For example, there are periods of increased susceptibility to aminoglycoside ototoxicity, as well as periods of decreased susceptibility. There is conflicting literature about differences in the susceptibility to aminoglycoside and cisplatin ototoxicity by albino versus pigmented strains of laboratory animal.

Noise overstimulation is the most common cause of acquired hearing loss and may potentiate ototoxicity (Engström et al. 1970; Forge et al. 2011; Henderson et al. 2008). At moderate levels of noise, outer hair cell function can be compromised by effects on stereocilia as well as lateral wall and intracellular pathways; however, the outer hair cell can recover and function will return. This leads to a temporary loss of hearing, with a period in which thresholds for hearing are elevated, called a temporary threshold shift (Nordmann et al. 2000). Noise can also induce a loss of hair cells by different mechanisms, depending on the type and level of the noise. Loss of hair cells leads to a permanent elevation of thresholds for hearing, termed a permanent threshold shift. Noise overstimulation leads to excessive levels of ROS and, as with ototoxins, excessive levels of ROS can induce loss through apoptotic pathways. Noise can also induce a physical damage to the sensory cells, resulting in necrosis. The amount of noise necessary to cause sensory cell loss varies among species and is related to a combination of the intensity of sound and the length of time it is applied, where less time is needed for cell loss associated with higher intensity. The position of damage from noise is related to its frequency, with the greatest effect in the region of the cochlear spiral processing that frequency, with hair cells being the most sensitive, especially the outer hair cells. A broad band of noise across multiple frequencies will result in more damage to outer hair cells of the basal cochlear and first row outer hair cells.

Other factors can increase sensitivity to noise such as age and genetic factors influencing efficacy of endogenous protective pathways (Kujawa and Liberman 2006; Makary et al. 2011). Animals with infections or with a less than optimal diet can have increased ototoxicity from aminoglycosides (Rybak et al. 2008).

Over-release of the excitatory amino acid transmitter glutamate from inner hair bases at their synapse with type I SGN can cause swelling and bursting of the auditory nerve peripheral processes from excitotoxic mechanisms. Such over-release will occur from noise overstimulation but can also be a consequence of trauma or stress from ototoxins, vascular disturbances, or disruption of cochlear homeostasis. Drugs that cause vascular changes can disrupt the connections between inner hair cells and the auditory nerve. Excitotoxicity can be caused by infusion of compounds into cochlear fluids, causing changes in the pH, osmolarity, or composition of the fluids. Excitotoxic swelling and bursting can occur during fixation of the cochlea since vascular supply is interrupted before fixation occurs; hence, fixation must be rapid. The fixative must be adjusted for proper pH and osmolarity.

Disruption of the connection between the inner hair cells and the auditory nerve may be permanently lost (Kujawa and Liberman 2009; Lin et al. 2011; Makary et al. 2011). A moderate noise that does not result in loss of sensory cells can still result in a 30% loss in the connections between inner hair cell and the auditory nerve. While synapses between the inner hair cells and the auditory nerve are not typically assessed in ototoxicity studies, this may be considered, since connections may be lost even if hair cells are not lost. The identification of pre-synaptic ribbons can be used as a marker for the connections since there is one ribbon per synapse and the ribbons move away from the synapses and disappear shortly after the connection is lost.

In addition to ototoxicity, hearing loss can be genetic in origin or a consequence of infectious disease. When studying ototoxicity, it is important to choose strains of laboratory animals that do not carry mutations that may cause deafness. For example, significant genetic hearing loss occurs at 3 months of age in C57 Black 6 Mice with the AHL locus (Yoshida and Liberman 1999).

Intermediate cells of the stria vascularis are derived from wandering melanocytes and normally contain melanin granules. Most albino animals have amelanotic intermediate cells. There is conflicting literature as to whether the amount of melanin in the stria vascularis influences susceptibility to noise and ototoxins. Therefore, in strains of animals with variability in skin or coat color, or pigmentation and patterning, it is important to ensure that there are similarities in coats among groups.

Assessment of otopathology is often matched with the assessment of cochlear function. The simplest test in many animal models is snapping fingers and looking for movement of the animal's ears ("Preyer's reflex"). This test is only sensitive to large hearing deficits and will not be reliable in all animal species. The most common assessment is the ABR. The frequencies at which there is hearing loss can be determined, in addition to differentiating between only outer hair cell loss and the loss of outer and inner hair cells. The extent of inner and outer hair cell loss and changes in ABR are based on threshold shifts. Differentiation hair cell loss (sensory) and auditory nerve dysfunction (neural) can also be determined (Liberman and Beil 1979). Outer hair cell function can also be tested by examining otoacoustic emissions. The acoustic startle reflex can be used to test hearing thresholds, gap detection, pre-pulse inhibition, and tinnitus. Further testing of the auditory nerve can be done by measuring round window noise and ensemble spontaneous activity of the auditory nerve or by placing electrodes into the nerve and recording compound action potentials.

21.2.4   INNER EAR: VESTIBULAR SYSTEM

The vestibular portion of the inner ear is located in the petrous portion of the temporal bone, with a continuation of both the membranous and bony labyrinth arising from the basal portion of the cochlea. The vestibular portion of the inner ear has two divisions: the vestibule, which is closest to the cochlea, and three semicircular canals. Portions of the horizontal or lateral semicircular canal can often be viewed from the middle ear. The superior or anterior semicircular canal is in a more superior or anterior location and the inferior or posterior semicircular canal is in an inferior or posterior location. Each of the three semicircular canals has a swelling close to one of its bases (ampulla) that contains sensorineural epithelium (crista), and ducts of the three semicircular canals empty into the vestibule that contains two swellings with neuroepithelium (maculae). The one closest to the cochlea is the sacculus, while that closest to the semicircular canals is the utricle.

The neuroepithelial regions of the vestibular periphery contain hair cells and supporting cells. There are two types of hair cells, the pear-shaped type I hair cells and the cylinder-shaped type II hair cells. Both function as primary receptors for the vestibular pathways. There are supporting cells that have junctional complexes with their neighbors forming a barrier between endolymph and perilymph. More peripheral in location is a specialized epithelium containing "dark cells," which are responsible for secreting and maintaining the endolymph and the endolymphatic potential.

The hair cells of the semicircular canals are oriented so that their tallest row faces the same direction. The stereocilia are embedded in an overlying gelatinous mass (cupula). Angular movement of the head results in movement of the endolymph in the opposite direction. The movement of the endolymph moves the cupula, and all the hair cell stereocilia will then move in this same direction. Stereocilia are oriented so that movement of the cupula will be in an excitatory direction on one side of the head and in an inhibitory direction on the other side.

The semicircular canals are most sensitive to angular acceleration and deceleration and have a large involvement in vestibular reflexes, particularly vestibular–ocular reflexes that move the eyes to keep them fixed on a target.

The neurosensory epithelium of the sacculus and utricle maculae is flat. The stereocilia of type I and type II hair cells of the utricle and sacculus are embedded in a gelatinous mass (otolith). The otolith contains calcium carbonate and calcite crystals (otoconia). These add weight to the otolith and allow sensitivity to gravity. The hair cells in the macula have several rows of stereocilia arranged in a specific orientation. Movement of the endolymph fluid in the sacculus is induced by linear acceleration or deceleration and also influenced by gravity, even when the head is at rest.

Morphological assessment of the utricle, sacculus, and semicircular canals is similar to the methods used for assessment of the cochlea. The choice of fixative will depend on the method (light microscopy, immunostaining, or transmission electron microcopy) that will be used. Fixation can be vascular, followed by local infusion (through the round window), or just local. Whole mounts or surface preparations of the macular of sacculus or utricle or the crista ampullaris of semicircular canals are the common methods if the focus is on vestibular sensorineural epithelium. Immunostaining of surface preparations with antibodies that differentiate cell types or connections is often applied to whole mounts (Figure 21.5d). Phalloidin is used to label the filamentous actin in hair cells and supporting cells and allows assessment of potential hair cell loss. Calretinin or tenascin is used to label the calyces at the base of type I hair cells. Whole mounts can also be processed for laser scanning confocal microscopy.

Morphological findings that involve vestibular structures result in clinical signs as head tilt and circling and are collectively referred to as vestibular syndrome (Frith et al. 2007; Gad 2007). The condition occurs spontaneously, especially in mice and guinea pigs. In mice, the condition may be caused by bacterial infections, central nervous system lesions, or necrotizing arteritis. The etiology of arteritis is unknown, but in some strains, it may be immune mediated (Andrews et al. 1994). Suppurative inflammation involving the middle ear of guinea pigs and rabbits may be detected clinically by head tilt, wry neck, torticollis, incoordination, and circling behavior (Gad 2007). The most common cause is a bacterial agent, and findings may involve vestibular structures, auditory structures, or both (Boot and Walvoort 1986). An inherited degenerative condition occurs in the waltzer strain of guinea pig characterized by a tendency to "waltz" or whirl without eliciting a nystagmus response (Gad 2007).

The vestibular hair cells are sensitive and most often lost in vestibular disorders, but vestibular hair cells in mammals have some regenerative capacity to recover from some moderate levels of trauma (Forge et al. 1993).

Many of the same classes of compounds that cause loss of hair cells in the cochlea will also cause loss of hair cells in the vestibular neurosensory epithelium, including aminoglycoside antibiotics. Some aminoglycosides cause more cochlear than vestibular ototoxicity (e.g., kanamycin) and other aminoglycosides cause more vestibular than cochlear ototoxicity, such as gentamycin. Type I hair cells are more sensitive to aminoglycoside ototoxicity than type II hair cells. Effects are also seen on otolith structures and otoconia, suggesting effects on epithelial cells responsible for its secretion and maintenance. With loss of hair cells, there is eventually loss of afferent terminals and Scarpa's ganglion cells (Rybak et al. 2008).

A vestibular disorder can often be noticed in animals by animal circling, but abnormalities of the semicircular canals can be determined by testing for the vestibular–ocular reflex, the movement of the eyes in response to angular rotation of the head. Most animal models require more complex testing and often involve swimming tests.

REFERENCES

Ackerman, L.J., Yoshitomi, K., Fix, A.S., and Render, J.A. 1998. Proliferative lesions of the eye in rats. OSS. In: *Guides for Toxicologic Pathology*. STP/ARP/AFIP, Washington, DC.

Aguirre, G.D., Ray, J., and Stramm, L.E. 1998. Diseases of the retinal pigment epithelium–photoreceptor complex in non-rodent animal models. In: *The Retinal Pigment Epithelium* (M.F. Marmor, T.J. Wolfensberger, eds.), Oxford University Press, Oxford.

Aguirre, S.A., Huang, W., Prasanna, G., and Jessen, B. 2009. Corneal neovascularization and occular irritancy responses in dogs following topical administration of an EP-4 prostaglandin E2 agonist. *Toxicol Pathol* 37:911–920.

Albert, D.M., Gonder, J.R., Papale, J., Craft, J.L., Dohlman, H.R., Reid, M.C., and Sunderman, F.W. 1982. Induction of ocular neoplasms in Fischer rats by intraocular injection of nickel subsulfide. *Invest Ophthalmol Vis Sci* 22:768–782.

Andrews, A.G., Dysko, R.C., Spilman, S.C., Kunkel, R.G., Brammer, D.W., and Johnson, K.J. 1994. Immune complex vasculitis with secondary ulcerative dermatitis in aged C57BL/6NNia mice. *Vet Pathol* 31:293–300.

Balazs, T., Ohtake, S., and Noble, J.F. 1970. Spontaneous lenticular changes in the rat. *Lab Anim Care* 20:215–219.

Balazs, T., and Rubin, L. 1971. A note on the lens in aging Sprague–Dawley rats. *Lab Anim Sci* 21:267–268.

Banks, W.J. 1993. Eye and ear. In: *Applied Veterinary Histology*. 3rd ed. Mosby Year Book, St. Louis, pp. 469–495.

Barnett, K.C., and Joseph, E.C. 1988. Keratoconjunctivitis sicca in the dog following 5-aminosalicylic acid administration. *Hum Toxicol* 6:377–383.

Baroody, R.A., Bito, L.Z., DeRousseau, C.J., and Kaufman, P.L. 1987. Ocular development and aging. 1. Corneal endothelial changes in cats and in free-ranging and caged rhesus monkeys. *Exp Eye Res* 45:607–622.

Bellhorn, R.W. 1973. A survey of ocular findings in 16 to 24 month old Beagles. *J Am Vet Med Assoc* 162:139–141.

Bellhorn, R.W. 1974. A survey of ocular finding in eight to ten-month-old Beagles. *J Am Vet Med Assoc* 164:1114–1116.

Bellhorn, R.W. 1980. Lighting in the animal environment. *Lab Anim Sci* 30:440–450.

Bellhorn, R.W., Bellhorn, M.B., Swarm, R.L., and Impellizzeri, C.W. 1975. Hereditary tapetal abnormality in the beagle. *Ophthalmic Res* 7:250–260.

Biros, D.J. 2007. Ocular immunity. In: *Veterinary Ophthalmology*. 4th ed. (K. Gelatt, ed.), Blackwell Publishing, Ames, pp. 223–235.

Bistner, S.I., and Riis, R.C. 1984. Ophthalmological study. 4940 beagles examined 1974–1981. Beagle Dog Breeding Colony, Marshall Research Animals, North Rose, NY. Unpublished observations. In: Spontaneous lesions in laboratory animals: incidence in relation to age (C. Taradach and P. Greaves, eds.), *CRC Crit Rev Toxicol* 12:121–147.

Bohne, B.A. 1976. Healing of the noise-damaged inner ear. In: *Haring and Davis: Essays Honoring Hallowell Davis* (S.K. Hirsh, D.H. Eldredge, I.J. Hirsh, and S.R. Siverman, eds.), Washington University Press, St. Louis, pp. 85–96.

Böhnke, M., and Masters, B.R. 1999. Confocal microscopy of the cornea. *Progress Retinal Eye Res* 18:553–628.

Boot, R., and Walvoort, H.C. 1986. Otitis media in guinea pigs: pathology and bacteriology. *Lab Anim* 20:242–248.

Bouldin, T.W., Goines, N.D., Krigman, M.R. 1984. Trimethyltin retinopathy. Relationship of subcellular response to neuronal subspecialization. *J Neuropathol Exp Neurol* 43:162–174.

Breider, M.A., Bleavins, M.R., Reindel, J.F., Gough, A.W., and de la Iglesia, F. 1996. Cellular hyperplasia in rats following continuous intravenous infusion of recombinant human epidermal growth factor. *Vet Pathol* 33:184–194.

Brown, W.R., Rubin, L., Hite, M., and Zwickery, R.E. 1972. Experimental papilledema in the dog induced by salicylanilide. *Toxicol Appl Pharmacol* 21:532–541.

Bruner, R.H., Keller, W.F., Stitzel, K.A., Sauers, L.J., Reer, P.J., Long, P.H., Bruce, R.D., and Alden, C.L. 1992. Spontaneous corneal dystrophy and generalized basement membrane changes in Fischer-344 rats. *Toxicol Pathol* 20:357–366.

Bryce, F., Iverson, F., Andrews, P., Barker, M., Cherry, W., Mueller, R., Pulido, O., Hayward, S., Fernie, S., and Arnold, D.L. 2001. Effects elicited by toxaphene in the cynomolgus monkey (*Macaca fascicularis*): a pilot study. *Food Chem Toxicol* 39:1243–1251.

Butler, W.H., Ford, G.P., and Newberne, J.W. 1987. A study of the effects of vigabatrin on the central nervous system and of Sprague–Dawley and Lister–Hooded rats. *Toxicol Pathol* 15:143–148.

Carlton, W.W., and Render, J.A. 1991a. Calcification of the cornea. In: *Monographs on Pathology of Laboratory Animals: Eye and Ear* (T.C. Jones, U. Mohr, and R.D. Hunt, eds.), Springer-Verlag, Berlin, pp. 16–20.

Carlton, W.W., Render, J.A. 1991b. Adenoma and adenocarcinoma, Harderian gland, mouse, rat, and hamster. In: *Monographs on Pathology of Laboratory Animals: Eye and Ear* (T.C. Jones, U. Mohr, and R.D. Hunt, eds.), Springer-Verlag, Berlin, pp. 133–137.

Cavallotti, D., Cavallotti, C., Pescosolido, N., Iannetti, G.D., and Pacella, E. 2001. A morphometric study of age changes in the rat optic nerve. *Ophthalmologica* 215:366–371.

Chiu, L.L., Cunningham, L.L., Raible, D.W., Rubel, E.W., and Ou, H.C. 2008. Using the zebrafish lateral line to screen for ototoxicity. *J Assoc Res Otolaryngol* 9:178–190.

Chiu, T. 1991. Auricular chondritis, rat. In: *Monographs on Pathology of Laboratory Animals: Eye and Ear* (T.C. Jones, U. Mohr, R.D. Hunt, eds.), Springer-Verlag, Berlin, pp. 149–155.

Chodosh, J., Nordquist, R.E., and Kennedy, R.C. 1998. Comparative anatomy of mammalian conjunctival lymphoid tissue: a putative mucosal immune site. *Dev Comp Immunol* 22:621–630.

Cloyd, C.G., Wyman, M., Shadduck, J.A., Winrow, M.J., and Johnson, G.R. 1978. Ocular toxicity studies with zinc pyridinethione. *Toxicol Appl Pharmacol* 45:771–782.

Curren, D.R., Evans, M.G., Raabe, H., Ruppalt, R.R., and Harbell, J. 2000. Correlation of histopathology, opacity, and permeability of bovine corneas exposed in vitro to known ocular irritants. *Vet Pathol* 37:557.

Davidson, S.I., and Rennie, I.G. 1986. Ocular toxicity from systemic drug therapy. An overview of clinically important adverse reactions. *Med Toxicol* 1:217–224.

Dayhaw-Barker, P. 2002. Retinal pigment epithelium melanin and ocular toxicity. *Int J Toxicol* 21:451–454.

Delahunt, C.S., Stebbins, R.B., Anderson, J., and Bailey, J. 1962. The cause of blindness in dogs given hydrox-ylpyridinethione. *Toxicol Appl Pharmacol* 4:286–291.

Dietrich, U.M. 2007. Ophthalmic examination and diagnostics. Part 3: diagnostic ultrasonography. In: *Veterinary Ophthalmology*. 4th ed. (K.N. Gelatt, ed.), Blackwell Publishing Professional, Philadelphia, pp. 507–535.

Doughty, M.J. 1994. The cornea and corneal endothelium in the aged rabbit. *Optom Vis Sci* 71:809–818.

Drager, U.C., and Hubel, D.H. 1978. Studies of visual function and its decay in mice with hereditary retinal degeneration. *J Comp Neurol* 180:85–114.

Drenkhahn, D., Jacobi, B., and Lüllmann-Rauch, R. 1983. Corneal lipidosis in rats treated with amphiphilic cationic drugs. *Arzneimittelforschung* 33:827–831.

Drenkhahn, D., and Lüllmann-Rauch, R. 1978. Drug-induced retinal lipidosis: differential susceptibilities of pigment epithelium and neuroretina toward several amphiphilic cationic drugs. *Exp Mol Pathol* 28:360–371.

Dubielzig, R.R., Ketring, K.L., McLellan, G.J., and Albert, D.M. 2010. *Veterinary Ocular Pathology: A Comparative Review*. Saunders Elsevier, Edinburgh.

Dureau, P., Jeanny, J.-C., Clerc, B., Dufier, J.-L., and Courtois, Y. 1996. Long term light-induced retinal degeneration in the miniature pig. *Mol Vis* 2:1–14.

Eldredge, D.H., Miller, J.D., and Bohne, B.A. 1981. A frequency-position map for the chinchilla cochlea. *J Acoust Soc Am* 69:1091–1095.

Elwell, M.R., and Boorman, G.A. 1990. Tumours of the Harderian gland. In: *Pathology of Tumours in Laboratory Animals. Vol. I. Tumours of the Rat*. 2nd ed. (V.S. Turusov and U. Mohr, eds.), IARC Scientific Publications No. 99, Lyon, pp. 79–88.

Engström, H., Ades, H.W., and Bredberg, G. 1970. Normal structure of the organ of Corti and the effect of noise-induced cochlear damage. In: *Sensorineural Hearing Loss*. Ciba Found Symposium, pp. 127–156.

Ernst, H., Rittinghausen, S., and Mohr, U. 1991. Melanoma of the eye, mouse. In: *Monographs on Pathology of Laboratory Animals: Eye and Ear* (T.C. Jones, U. Mohr, and R.D. Hunt, eds.), Springer-Verlag, Berlin, pp. 44–47.

Everitt, J.I., and Shadduck, J.A. 1991. Melanoma of the uvea, rat. In: *Monographs on Pathology of Laboratory Animals: Eye and Ear* (T.C. Jones, U. Mohr, and R.D. Hunt, eds.), Springer-Verlag, Berlin, pp. 40–43.

Fex, J., and Altschuler, R.A. 1986. Neurotransmitter-related immunocytochemistry of the organ of Corti. *Hear Res* 22:249–263.

Fischer, M.W., and Slatter, D.H. 2007. Preparation and orientation of canine retinal vasculature. A modified trypsin digestion technique. *Austr J Ophthalmol* 6:46–50.

Forge, A., Li, L., Corwin, J.T., and Nevill, G. 1993. Ultrastructural evidence for hair cell regeneration in the mammalian inner ear. *Science* 259:1616–1619.

Forge, A., Taylor, R., and Bolon, B. 2011. Toxicological neuropathology of the ear. In: *Fundamental Neuropathology for Pathologists and Toxicologists: Principles and Techniques* (B. Bolon and M.T. Butt, eds.), John Wiley & Sons, Inc., Hoboken, NJ, pp. 413–428.

Fortune, B., Wang, L., Bui, B.V., Burgoyne, C.F., and Cioffi, G.A. 2005. Idiopathic bilateral optic atrophy in the rhesus macaque. *Invest Ophthalmol Visual Sci* 46:3943–3956.

Frame, S.R., and Carlton, W.W. 1991. Toxic retinopathy: rat, mouse and hamster. In: *Monographs on Pathology of Laboratory Animals: Eye and Ear* (T.C. Jones, U. Mohr, and R.D. Hunt, eds.), Springer-Verlag, Berlin, pp. 116–124.

Fraunfelder, F.T., and Burns, R.P. 1970. Acute reversible lens opacity: caused by drugs, cold anoxia, asphyxia, stress, death and dehydration. *Exp Eye Res* 10:19–30.

Fraunfelder, F.T., Fraunfelder, F.W., and Chambers, W.A. 2008. *Clinical Ocular Toxicology*. Saunders Elsevier, Philadelphia.

Frith, C.H., Goodman, D.G., and Boysen, B.G. 2007. The mouse: pathology. In: *Animal Models in Toxicology* (S.C. Gad, ed.), CRC Press, Taylor and Francis Group, Boca Raton, pp. 72–121.

Funk, J., and Landes, C. 2005. Histopathologic findings after treatment with different oxidosqualene cyclases (OSC) inhibitors in hamsters and dogs. *Exp Toxicol Pathol* 57:29–38.

Gad, S.C. 2007. *Animal Models in Toxicology.* 2nd ed. CRC Press, Taylor and Francis Group, Boca Raton, pp. 113–114, 211, 389–390, 471–473, and 640–644.

Gajdosík, A., Gajdosík, A., Gajdosíková, A., Stefek, M., Nararová, J., and Hozová, R. 1999. Streptozotocin-induced experimental diabetes in male Wistar rats. *Gen Physiol Biophys* 18:54–62.

Garibaldi, B.A., and Goad, M.E.P. 1988. Lipid keratopathy in the Watanabe (WHHL) rabbit. *Vet Pathol* 25:173–174.

Gartner, S., and Henkind, P. 1981. Lange's folds: a meaningful ocular artifact. *J Ophthalmol* 88:1307–1310.

Gazda, M.J., Schultheiss, T.E., Stephens, L.C., Ang, K.K., and Peters, L.J. 1992. The relationship between apoptosis and atrophy in irradiated lacrimal gland. *Int J Radiat Oncol Biol Phys* 24:693–697.

Gehring, P.J. 1971. The cataractogenic activity of chemical agents. *CRC Crit Rev Toxicol* 1:93–118.

Geiss, V., and Yoshitomi, K. 1999. Eyes. In: *Pathology of the Mouse* (R.R. Maronpot, G.A. Boorman, B.W. Gaul, eds.), Cache River Press, Saint Louis, pp. 471–490.

Gelatt, K.N., Brooks, D.E., and Samuelson, D.A. 1998. Comparative glaucomatology I: the spontaneous glaucomas. *J Glaucoma* 7:187–201.

Gelatt, K.N., van der Woerdt, A., Ketring, K.L., Anrew, E.E., Brooks, D.E., Biros, D.J., Denis, H.M., and Cutler, T.J. 2001. Enrofloxacin-associated retinal degeneration in cats. *Vet Ophthalmol* 4: 99–106.

Giordano, C., Weigt, A., Vercelli, A., Rondena, M., Gril, G., and Giudice, C. 2005. Immunohistochemical identification of *Encephalitozoon cuniculi* in phacoclastic uveitis in four rabbits. *Vet Ophthalmol* 8:271–275.

Gopinath, C., Prentice, D.E., and Lewis, D.J. 1987. *Atlas of Experimental Toxicological Pathology, Vol. 13, The Eye and Ear*, MTP Press, Lancaster, pp. 145–155.

Grant, W.M. 1986. *Toxicology of the Eye.* 3rd ed. Charles C. Thomas, Springfield.

Greaves, P. 2007. *Histopathology of Preclinical Toxicity Studies.* 3rd ed. Academic Press, New York, pp. 883–933.

Greenman, D.L., Bryant, P., Kodell, R.L., and Shelldon, W. 1982. Influence of cage shelf on retinal atrophy in mice. *Lab Anim Sci* 32:353–356.

Greenman, D.L., Cronin, G.M., Dahlgren, R., Allen, R., and Allaben, W. 1995. Chronic feeding study of pyrilamine in Fischer 344 rats. *Fundam Appl Toxicol* 25:1–8.

Greenwood, D.D. 1961. Critical bandwidth and frequency coordinates of the basilar membrane. *J Acoust Soc Am* 33:1344–1356.

Gum, G.G., Gelatt, K.N., and Esson, D.W. 2007. Physiology of the eye. In: *Veterinary Ophthalmology.* 4th ed. (K. Gelatt, ed.), Blackwell Publishing, Ames, pp. 149–182.

Hackett, R.B., and McDonald, T.O. 1991. Eye irritation. In: *Advances in Modern Toxicology: Dermatotoxicology.* 4th ed. (F. Marzulli and H. Maibach, eds.), Hemisphere Publishing Corp., Washington, DC, pp. 749–815.

Hadjikoutis, S., Morgan, J.E., Wild, J.M., and Smith, P.E.M. 2005. Ocular complications of neurological therapy. *Eur J Neurol* 12:499–507.

Haggerty, G.C., Peckman, J.C., Thomassen, R.W., and Gad, S.C. 2007. The dog. In: *Animal Models in Toxicology.* 2nd ed. (S.C. Gad, ed.), CRC Taylor and Francis Group, Boca Raton, pp. 563–662.

Harkness, J.E., and Ridgeway, M.D. 1980. Chromodacryorrhea in laboratory rats (*Rattus norvegicus*): etiologic considerations. *Lab Anim Sci* 30:841–844.

Haseman, J.K., Hailey, J.R., and Morris, R.W. 1998. Spontaneous neoplasm incidence in Fischer 344 rats and B6C3F1 mice in two-year carcinogenicity studies: a National Toxicology Program update. *Toxicol Pathol* 26:428–441.

Hawkins, J.E. 1973. Comparative otopathology: aging, noise, and ototoxic drugs. *Adv Oto-Rhino-Laryngol* 20:124–141.

Hebel, R. 1976. Distribution of retinal ganglion cells in five mammalian species (pig, sheep, ox, horse, dog). *Arch Embryol* 150:45–51.

Henderson, D., Hu, B., and Bielefeld, E. 2008. Patterns and mechanisms in noise-induced cochlear pathology. In: *Auditory Trauma, Protection and Repair* (J. Schacht, A.N. Pepper, and R.R. Fray, eds.), Springer-Verlag, Berlin, pp. 195–218.

Heng, J.E., Vorwerk, C.K., Lessell, E., Zurakowski, D., Levin, L.A., and Dreyer, E.B. 1999. Ethambutol is toxic to retinal ganglion cells via an excitotoxic pathway. *Invest Ophthalmol Vis Sci* 40:190–196.

Herrold, K.M. 1969. Aflatoxin induced lesions in Syrian hamsters. *Br J Cancer* 23:655–660.

Heywood, R. 1971. Developmental changes in the lens of the young beagle dog. *Vet Rec* 88:411–414.

Heywood, R. 1972. An anomaly of the ocular fundus of the beagle dog. *J Small Anim Pract* 13:213–215.

Heywood, R. 1973. Some clinical observations on the eyes of Sprague–Dawley rats. *Lab Anim* 7:19–27.

Heywood, R. 1974. Drug-induced retinopathies in the beagle dog. *Br Vet J* 130:564–569.

Heywood, R. 1985. Clinical and laboratory assessment of visual dysfunction. In: *Toxicology of the Eye, Ear and Other Special Sense Organs* (A.C. Hayes, ed.), Raven, New York, pp. 61–77.

Heywood, R., Hepworth, P.L., and Van Abbe, N.J. 1976. Age changes in the eyes of the beagle dog. *J Small Anim Pract* 17:171–177.

Hockwin, O., Green, K., and Rubin, L. 1991. *Manual of Ototoxicity Testing of Drugs*. Gustav Fischer Verlag, Stuttgart, pp. 255–317.

Hoffman, E.W., Yang, J.E., Waggie, K.S., Durham, J.B., Burge, J.R., and Walker, S.E. 1983. Band keratopathy in MRL/I and MRL/n mice. *Arthritis Rheum* 26:645–652.

Hope, G.M., Dawson, W.W., Engel, H.M., Ulshafer, R.J., Kessler, M.J., and Sherwood, M.B. 1992. A primate model for age related macular drusen. *Br J Ophthalmol* 76:11–16.

Hottendorf, G.H. 1991. Cholesteatoma, aural, gerbil. In: *Monographs on Pathology of Laboratory Animals: Eye and Ear* (T.C. Jones, U. Mohr, and R.D. Hunt, eds.), Springer-Verlag, Berlin, pp. 156–158.

Hubert, M.F., Gerin, G., and Durand-Cavagna, G. 1999. Spontaneous lesions in young Swiss mice. *Lab Anim Sci* 49:232–240.

Hubert, M-F., Gillet, J.P., and Durand-Cavagna, G. 1994. Spontaneous retinal changes in Sprague–Dawley rats. *Lab Anim Sci* 44:561–567.

Hudspeth, A.J. 2005. How the ear's works work: mechanical transduction and amplification by hair cells. *C R Biol* 328:155–162.

Huff, J.E., Eastin, W., Roycroft, J., Eustis, S.L., and Haseman, J.K. 1988. Carcinogenesis studies of benzene, methyl benzene, and dimethyl benzenes. *Ann NY Acad Sci* 534:427–441.

Hull, D.S., Green, K., and Laughter, L. 1984. Cornea endothelial rose bengal photosensitization: effect on permeability, sodium flux, and ultrastructure. *Invest Ophthalmol Vis Sci* 25:455–460.

Imai, H., Miyata, M., Uga, S., and Ishikawa, S. 1983. Retinal degeneration in rats exposed to an organophosphate pesticide (fenthion). *Environ Res* 30:453–465.

Imamura, S., and Adams, J.C. 2003. Changes in cytochemistry of sensory and nonsensory cells in gentamicin-treated cochleas. *J Assoc Otolaryngol* 4:196–218.

Irwin, R.D., Haseman, J.K., and Eustis, S.L. 1995. 1,2,3-Trichloropropane: a multisite carcinogen in rats and mice. *Toxicol Sci* 25:241–252.

Ishibashi, T., Sorgente, N., Patterson, R., and Ryan, S.J. 1986. Pathogenesis of drusen in the primate. *Invest Ophthalmol Vis Sci* 27:184–193.

Iwai, H., Tagawa, Y., Hayasaka, I., Yanai, T., and Masegi, T. 2000. Effects of atropine sulfate on rat Harderian glands: correlation between morphologic changes and porphyrin levels. *J Toxicol Sci* 25:151–159.

Jester, J.V., Nicolaides, N., Kiss-Pavvolgyi, I., and Smith, R.E. 1989. Meibomian gland dysfunction: II. The role of keratinization in a rabbit model of MGD. *Invest Ophthalmol Vis Sci* 30:936–945.

John, S.W.M.J., Smith, R.S., Savinova, O., Hawes, N.L., Chang, B., Turnbull, D., Davidsson, M., Roderick, T.H., and Heckenlively, J.R. 1998. Essential iris atrophy, pigment dispersion and glaucoma in DBA/2J mice. *Invest Ophthalmol Vis Sci* 39:951–962.

Johnstone, M.A., and Albert, D.M. 2002. Prostaglandin-induced hair growth. *Surv Ophthalmol* 47(Suppl 1): S185–202.

Jones, T.C., Mohr, U., and Hunt, R.D. 1991. *Monographs on Pathology of Laboratory Animals: Eye and Ear*. Springer-Verlag, Berlin, pp. 143–149.

Joyce, N.C. 2003. Proliferative capacity of the corneal endothelium. *Prog Retin Eye Res* 22:359–389.

Kafarnik, C., Murphy, C.J., and Dubielzig, R.R. 2009. Canine duplication of Descemet's membrane. *Vet Pathol* 46:464–473.

Kast, A. 1991. Keratoconjunctivitis sicca and sequelae, mouse and rat. In: *Monographs on Pathology of Laboratory Animals: Eye and Ear* (T.C. Jones, U. Mohr, and R.D. Hunt, eds.), Springer-Verlag, Berlin, pp. 29–37.

Kelemen, G. 1978. Diseases of the ear. In: *Pathology of Laboratory Animals. Vol. I.* (K. Benirshke, F.M. Garner, and T.C. Jones, eds.), Springer, Berlin, pp. 628–629.

Kerry, P.J., Wakefield, I.D., and Evans, J.G. 1993. Ocular changes induced in the Beagle dog by intravenous infusion of a novel dopaminergic compound, FPL 65447. *Toxicol Pathol* 21:274–282.

Kitagaki, M., Suwa, T., Yanagi, M., and Shiratori, K. 2003. Auricular chondritis in young ear-tagged Crj:CD(SD) IGS rats. *Lab Anim* 37:249–253.

Klintworth, G.K., and Burger, P.C. 1983. Neovascularization of the cornea: current concepts of its pathogenesis. *Int Ophthalmol Clin* 23:27–39.

Knop, E., and Knop, N. 2000. Conjunctiva-associated lymphoid tissue in the human eye. *Invest Ophthalmol Vis Sci* 41:1270–1279.

Kobayashi, H., and Kohshima, S. 2001. Unique morphology of the human eye and its adaptive meaning: comparative studies on external morphology of the primate eye. *J Hum Evol* 40:419–435.

Koizumi, H., Watanabe, M., Numata, H., Sakai, T., and Morishita, H. 1986. Species differences in vacuolation of the choroid plexus induced by the piperidine-ring drug disobutamide in the rat, dog, and monkey. *Toxicol Appl Pharmacol* 84:125–148.

Komarowska, I., Heilweil, G., Rosenfeld, P.J., Perlman, I., and Loewenstein, A. 2009. Retinal toxicity of commercially available intravitreal ketorolac in albino rabbits. *Retina* 29:98–105.

Kremer, I., Gaton, D.D., David, M., Gaton, E., and Shapiro, A. 1994. Toxic effects of systemic retinoids on meibomian glands. *Ophthalmol Res* 26:124–128.

Krinke, A.L., Schaetti, Ph., and Krinke, G.J. 1994. Changes in the major ocular glands. In: *Pathobiology of the Aging Rat. Vol. 2* (U. Mohr, D.L. Dungworth, and C.C. Capen, eds.), ILSI Press, Washington, DC.

Krinke, G., Fix, A., Jacobs, M., Render, J., and Weisse, I. 2001. Eye and Harderian gland. In: *International Classification of Rodent Tumors. The Mouse.* (U. Mohr, ed.), Springer-Verlag, Heidelberg, pp. 347–359.

Kuiper, B., Boevé, M.H., Jansen, T., Roelofs-van Emden, M.E., Thuring, J.W.G.M., and Wijnands, M.V.W. 1997. Ophthalmologic examination in systemic toxicity studies: an overview. *Lab Anim* 31: 177–183.

Kujawa, S.G., and Liberman, M.C. 2006. Acceleration of age-related hearing loss by early noise exposure: evidence of a misspent youth. *J Neurosci* 26:2115–2123.

Kujawa, S.G., and Liberman, M.C. 2009. Adding insult to injury: cochlear nerve degeneration after "temporary" noise-induced hearing loss. *J Neurosci* 29:1477–1485.

Kuno, H., Usui, T., Eydelloth, R.S., and Wolf, E.D. 1991. Spontaneous ophthalmic lesions in young Sprague–Dawley rats. *J Vet Med Sci* 53:607–614.

Kurisu, K., Sawamoto, O., Watanabe, H., and Ito, A. 1996. Sequential changes in the Harderian gland of rats exposed to high intensity light. *Lab Anim Sci* 46:71–76.

Kuwabara, T., and Gorn, G.A. 1968. Retinal damage by visible light: an electron microscopic study. *Arch Ophthalmol* 79:69–78.

Lai, Y.-L. 1980. Outward movement of photoreceptor cells in normal rat retina. *Invest Ophthalmol Vis Sci* 19:849–856.

Lai, Y.-L., Jacoby, R.O., and Jonas, A.M. 1978. Age-related and light associated retinal changes in Fischer rats. *Invest Ophthalmol Vis Sci* 17:634–638.

Lai, Y.-L., Jacoby, R.O., Jonas, A.M., and Papermaster, D.S. 1975. A new form of hereditary retinal degeneration in Wag/Rij rats. *Invest Ophthalmol* 14:62–67.

Lai, Y.-L., Jacoby, R.O., and Yao, P.C. 1979. Animal model: peripheral degeneration in rats. *Am J Pathol* 97:449–452.

Lai, Y.-L., Masuda, K., Mangum, M.D., Lug, R., Macrae, D.W., Fletcher, G., and Liu, Y.-P. 1982. Subretinal displacement of photoreceptor nuclei in human retina. *Exp Eye Res* 34:219–228.

Lambert, R.W., and Smith, R.E. 1988. Pathogenesis of blepharoconjunctivitis complicating 13-*cis*-retinoic acid (Isoretinoin) therapy in a laboratory model. *Invest Opthalmol Vis Sci* 29:1559–1564.

LaVail, M.M. 1976. Rod outer segment disk shedding in rat retina: relationship to cyclic lighting. *Science* 194:1071–1074.

LaVail, M.M. 1980. Eye pigmentation and constant light damage in the rat retina. In: *The Effects of Constant Light on the Visual Processes* (T.P. Williams and B. Baker, eds.), Plenum Press, New York, pp. 357–387.

LaVail, M.M., Gorrin, G.M., and Repaci, M.A. 1987. Strain differences in sensitivity to light-induced photoreceptor degeneration in albino mice. *Curr Eye Res* 6:825–834.

Lawill, T. 1973. Effects of prolonged exposure of rabbit retina to low-intensity light. *Invest Ophthalmol Vis Sci* 12:45–51.

Leblanc, B., Jezequel, S., Davies, T., Hanton, G., and Taradach, C. 1998. Binding of drugs to eye melanin is not predictive of ocular toxicity. *Reg Toxicol Pharmacol* 28:124–132.

Leedle, R., Dubielzig, R., and Christian, B. 2008. Bilateral optic atrophy in cynomolgus monkeys. *Vet Pathol* 45:781.

Levine, S. 1991. Cyclitis produced by cyclophosphamide, rat. In: *Monographs on Pathology of Laboratory Animals: Eye and Ear* (T.C. Jones, U. Mohr, and R.D. Hunt, eds.), Springer-Verlag, Berlin, pp. 38–39.

Liberman, M.C., and Beil, D.G. 1979. Hair cell condition and auditory nerve response in normal and noise-damaged cochleas. *Acta Otolaryngol* 88:161–176.

Lin, H.W., Furman, A.C., Kujawa, S.G., and Liberman, M.C. 2011. Primary degeneration in the guinea pig cochlea after reversible noise-induced threshold shift. *J Assoc Res Otolaryngol* 12:605–616.

Lin, W.L., and Essner, E. 1987. An electron microscopic study of retinal degeneration in Sprague–Dawley rats. *Lab Anim Sci* 37:180–186.

Lindquist, N.G., Larsson, B.S., and Stjernschantz, J. 1999. Increased pigmentation of iridal melanocytes in primates induced by a prostaglandin analogue. *Exp Eye Res* 69:431–436.

Lock, E.A., Gaskin, P., Ellis, M., Provan, W.M., and Smith, L.L. 2006. Tyrosinemia produced by 2-(2-nitro-4-fluoromethylbenzoyl)-cyclohexane-1,3-dione (NTBC) in experimental animals and its relationship to corneal injury. *Toxicol Appl Pharmacol* 215:9–16.

Loget, O. 1995. Spontaneous ocular findings and esthesiometry/tonometry measurement in the Göttingen mini-pig (conventional and microbiologically defined). *Ocular Toxicol* 351–362.

Losco, P.E., and Troup, C.M. 1988. Corneal dystrophy in Fischer 344. *Lab Anim Sci* 38:702–710.

Lucas, D.R., and Newhouse, J.P. 1957. Toxic effects of sodium l-glutamate on the inner layers of the retina *Arch Ophthalmol* 58:193–201.

Lüllmann, H., and Lüllmann-Rauch, R. 1981. Tamoxifen-induced generalized lipidosis in rats subchronically treated with high doses. *Toxicol Appl Pharmacol* 61:138–146.

Lutjen-Drecoll, E., and Tamm, E. 1988. Morphological study of the anterior segment of cynomolgus monkey eyes following treatment with prostaglandin F2c. *Exp Eye Res* 47:761–769.

Makary, C.A., Shin, J., Kujawa, S.G., Liberman, M.C., and Merchant, S.N. 2011. Age-related primary cochlear neuronal degeneration in human temporal bones. *J Assoc Res Otolaryngol* 12:711–717.

Maltoni, C., Conti, B., Perino, G., and DiMaio, V. 1988. Further evidence of benzene carcinogenicity. Results on Wistar rats and Swiss mice treated by ingestion. *Ann NY Acad Sci* 534:412–426.

Mangiardi, D.A., McLaughlin-Williamson, K., May, K.E., Messana, E.P., Mountain, D.C., and Cotanche, D.A. 2004. Progression of hair cell ejection and molecular markers of apoptosis in the avian cochlea following gentamicin treatment. *J Comp Neurol* 475:1–18.

Marmor, M.F., and Wolfensberger, T.J. 1998. *The Retinal Pigment Epithelium: Function and Disease*. Oxford University Press, Oxford.

Matuk, Y. 1991. Inherited retinal degeneration, RCS rat. In: *Monographs on Pathology of Laboratory Animals: Eye and Ear* (T.C. Jones, U. Mohr, and R.D. Hunt, eds.), Springer-Verlag, Berlin, pp. 92–100.

Maurer, J.K., Molai, A., Parker, R.D., Li. L., Carr, G.J., Petroll, W.M., Cavanagh, H.D., and Jester, J.V. 2001. Pathology of ocular irritation with bleaching agents in the rabbit low-volume eye test. *Toxicol Pathol* 29:308–319.

Maurer, J.K., Parker, R.D., and Carr, G.J. 1998. Ocular irritation: microscopic changes occurring over time in a rat with surfactants of known irritancy. *Toxicol Pathol* 26:217–225.

McCaa, C.S. 1985. Anatomy, physiology and toxicology of the eye. In: *Toxicology of the Eye, Ear and Other Special Sense Organs* (A.C. Hayes, ed.), Raven, New York, pp. 1–15.

McCormik, J.G., and Nuttal, A.L. 1976. Auditory research. In: *The Biology of the Guinea Pig* (J. Wagner and P.J. Manning, eds.), Academic Press, New York, pp. 281–303.

McGee, M.A., and Maronpot, R.R. 1979. Harderian gland dacryoadenitis in rats resulting from orbital bleeding. *Lab Anim Sci* 29:639–641.

McGinn, M.D., Chole, R.A., and Henry, K.D. 1982. Cholesteatoma, experimental induction in the Mongolian gerbil, *Meriones unguiculatus*. *Acta Otolaryngol* 93:61–67.

McIlwain, J.T. 1996. *An Introduction to the Biology of Vision*, Cambridge University Press, Cambridge, pp. 87–88.

Mecklenburg, L., and Schraermeyer, U. 2007. An overview on the toxic morphological changes in the retinal pigment epithelium after systemic compound administration. *Toxicol Pathol* 35:252–267.

Merindano, M.D., Costa, J., Canals, M., Potau, J.M., and Ruano, D. 2002. A comparative study of Bowman's layer in some mammals: relationships with other constituent corneal structures. *Eur J Anat* 6:133–139.

Messmer, E.M. 2008. Confocal microscopy: when is it helpful to diagnose corneal and conjunctival disease? *Exp Rev Ophthalmol* 3:177–192.

Moe, R.A., Kirpan, J., and Linegar, C.R. 1960. Toxicology of hydroxypyridinethione. *Toxicol Appl Pharmacol* 2:156–170.

Mohr, U. 1994. *International Classification of Rodent Tumours. Part I—The Rat. 7. Central Nervous System; Heart; Eye; Mesothelium*. World Health Organization, International Agency for Research on Cancer, Lyon, pp. 34–51.

Moore, C.P., Dubielzig, R., and Glaza, S.M. 1987. Anterior corneal dystrophy of American Dutch belted rabbits: biomicroscopic and histopathologic findings. *Vet Pathol* 24:28–33.

Morrow, G.L., and Abbott, R.L. 1998. Minocycline-induced scleral, dental, and dermal pigmentation. *Am J Ophthalmol* 125:396–397.

Müller, M., von Hünerbein, K., Hoidis, S., and Smolders, J.W. 2005. A physiological place-frequency map of the cochlea in the CBA/J mouse. *Hear Res* 202:63–73.

Munger, R.J. 2002. Veterinary ophthalmology in laboratory animal studies. *Vet Ophthalmol* 5:167–175.

Murray, R.B., and Loughnane, M.H. 1981. Infrared video pupillometry: a method used to measure the pupillary effects of drugs in small laboratory animals in real time. *J Neurosci Methods* 3:365–375.

Narfström, K., Ekesten, B., Rosolen, S.E., Spiess, B.M., Percicot, C.L., and Ofri, R. 2002. Guidelines for clinical electroretinography in the dog. *Doc Ophthalmol* 105:83–92.

Noell, W.K., Walker, V.S., Kang, B.S., and Berman, S. 1966. Retinal damage by light in rats. *Invest Ophthalmol* 5:450–473.

Nordmann, A.S., Bohne, B.A., and Harding, G.W. 2000. Histopathological differences between temporary and permanent threshold shift. *Hear Res* 139:13–30.

Ohnishi, Y., and Kohno, T. 1979. Polychlorinated biphenyls poisoning in monkey eye. *Invest Ophthalmol Vis Sci* 18:981–984.

Ollivier, F.J., Plummer, C.E., and Barrie, K.P. 2007. Ophthalmic examination and diagnostics. Part 1: the eye examination and diagnostic procedures. In: *Veterinary Ophthalmology*. 4th ed. (K. Gelatt, ed.), Blackwell, Ames, pp. 438–483.

O'Malley, J.T., Merchant, S.N., Burgess, B.J., Jones, D.D., and Adams, J.C. 2009. Effects of fixative and embedding medium on morphology and immunostaining of the cochlea. *Audiol Neurootol* 14:78–87.

Organisaciak, D.T., and Winkler, B.S. 1994. Retinal light damage: practical and theoretical considerations. In: *Progress in Retinal Research, Volume 13* (G. Chader and N. Osborne, eds.), Pergamon Press, New York, pp. 1–29.

O'Steen, W.K., Anderson, K.V., and Shear, C.R. 1974. Photoreceptor degeneration in albino rats: dependency on age. *Invest Ophthalmol* 13:334–339.

O'Steen, W.K., Kraeer, S.L., and Shear, C.R. 1978. Extraocular muscle and Harderian gland degeneration and regeneration after exposure of rats to continuous fluorescent illumination. *Invest Ophthalmol Vis Sci* 17:847–856.

O'Steen, W.K., Shear, C.R., and Anderson, K.V. 1972. Retinal damage after prolonged exposure to visible light. A light and electron microscopic study. *Am J Anat* 134:5–21.

Owen, R.A., and Duprat, P. 1991. Leiomyoma of the iris, Sprague–Dawley rat. In: *Monographs on Pathology of Laboratory Animals: Eye and Ear* (T.C. Jones, U. Mohr, and R.D. Hunt, eds.), Springer-Verlag, Berlin, pp. 47–49.

Oyster, C.W., Takahashi, E.S., and Hurst, D.C. 1981. Density, soma size, and regional distribution of rabbit retinal ganglion cells. *J Neurosci* 1:1331–1346.

Parhad, I.M., Griffin, J.W., and Miller, N.R. 1986. Optic disc swelling in IDPN treated experimental animals. *Comp Pathol Bull AFIP* 18:2–3.

Pedersen, O.O., and Karlsen, R.L. 1979. Destruction of Müller cells in the adult rat by intravitreal injection of D,L-alpha-aminoadipic acid. An electron microscopic study. *Exp Eye Res* 28:569–575.

Peiffer, R.L., Pohm-Thorsen, L., and Corcoran, K. 1994. Models in ophthalmology and vision research. In: *The Biology of the Laboratory Rabbit*. 2nd ed. (P.J. Manning, D.H. Ringler, and C.E. Newcomer, eds.), Academic Press, New York, pp. 410–433.

Peiffer, R.L., and Porter, D.P. 1991. Light-induced retinal degeneration, rat. In: *Monographs on Pathology of Laboratory Animals: Eye and Ear* (T.C. Jones, U. Mohr, and R.D. Hunt, eds.), Springer-Verlag, Berlin, pp. 82–87.

Peiffer, R.P. 1991a. Radiation-induced cataracts, mouse and rat. In: *Monographs on Pathology of Laboratory Animals: Eye and Ear* (T.C. Jones, U. Mohr, and R.D. Hunt, eds.), Springer-Verlag, Berlin, pp. 73–81.

Peiffer, R.P. 1991b. Inherited cataracts, mouse. In: *Monographs on Pathology of Laboratory Animals: Eye and Ear* (T.C. Jones, U. Mohr, and R.D. Hunt, eds.), Springer-Verlag, Berlin, pp. 55–60.

Percy, D.H., and Danylchuk, K.D. 1977. Experimental retinal dysplasia due to cytosine arabinoside. *Invest Ophthalmol Vis Sci* 16:353–364.

Pereira, F.Q., Bercht, B.S., Soares, M.G., da Mota, G.B., and Pigatto, J.A.T. 2011. Comparison of a rebound and an application tonometer for measuring intraocular pressure in normal rabbits. *Vet Ophthalmol* 14:321–326.

Perez, J., and Perentes, E. 1994. Light-induced retinopathy in the albino-rat in long-term studies—an immunohistochemical and quantitative approach. *Exp Toxicol Pathol* 46:229–235.

Pittler, S.J., and Baehr, W. 1991. Identification of a nonsense mutation in the rod photoreceptor cGMP phosphodiesterase beta-subunit gene of the rd mouse. *Proc Natl Acad Sci USA* 88:8322–8326.

Port, C.D., and Dodd, D.C. 1983. Two cases of corneal epithelial dystrophy in rabbits. *Lab Anim Sci* 33:587–588.

Prince, J.H. 1964. *The Rabbit in Eye Research*. Charles C. Thomas, Publisher, Springfield.

Pyrah, I.T., Kalinowski, A., Jackson, D., Davies, W., Davis, S., Aldridge, A., and Greaves, P. 2001. Toxicologic lesions associated with two related inhibitors of oxidosqualene cyclase in the dog and mouse. *Toxicol Pathol* 29:174–179.

Raphael, Y., and Altschuler, R.A. 1991. Scar formation after drug-induced cochlear insult. *Hear Res* 51:173–183.

Raphael, Y., and Altschuler, R.A. 1992. Early microfilament reorganization in injured auditory epithelia. *Exp Neurol* 115:32–36.

Raphael, Y., and Altschuler, R.A. 2003. Structure and innervation of the cochlea. *Brain Res Bull* 60:397–422.

Rapoport, S.I. 1997. Osmotic opening of blood–brain and blood–ocular barriers. *Exp Eye Res* 25(Suppl):499–509.

Rathbun, W.B., Harris, J.E., Vagstad, G., and Gruber, L. 1973. The reversal of triparanol-induced cataract in the rat. IV. Reduced sulfhydryl groups in soluble protein and glutathione. *Invest Ophthalmol* 12: 388–390.

Reindel, J.F., Gough, A.W., Pilcher, G.D., Bobrowski, W.F., Sobocinski, G.P., and de la Iglesia, F.A. 2001. Systemic proliferative changes and clinical signs in cynomolgus monkeys administered a recombinant derivative of human epidermal growth factor. *Toxicol Pathol* 29:159–173.

Render, J.A., and Carlton, W.W. 1991a. Toxic effects of 6-aminonicatinomide, uvea, rabbit. In: *Monographs on Pathology of Laboratory Animals: Eye and Ear* (T.C. Jones, U. Mohr, and R.D. Hunt, eds.), Springer-Verlag, Berlin, pp. 50–54.

Render, J.A., and Carlton, W.W. 1991b. Cataract due to tryptophan deficiency, rat. In: *Monographs on Pathology of Laboratory Animals: Eye and Ear* (T.C. Jones, U. Mohr, and R.D. Hunt, eds.) Springer-Verlag, Berlin, pp. 61–63.

Render, J.A., and Carlton, W.W. 1991c. Induced cataracts, lens, rat. In: *Monographs on Pathology of Laboratory Animals: Eye and Ear* (T.C. Jones, U. Mohr, and R.D. Hunt, eds.), Springer-Verlag, Berlin, pp. 63–73.

Roe, F.J., Millican, D., and Mallett, J.M. 1963. Induction of melanotic lesions of the iris in rats by urethane given during the neonatal period. *Nature* 199:1201–1202.

Roerig, D.L., Hasegawa, A.T., Harris, G.J., Lynch, K.L., and Wang, R.I.H. 1980. Occurrence of corneal opacities in rats after acute administration of 1-α-acetylmethadol. *Toxicol Appl Pharmacol* 56:155–163.

Rosolen, S.G., Rigaudiére, F., Le Gargasson, J.-F., and Brigell, M.G. 2005. Recommendations for a toxicological screening ERG procedure in laboratory animals. *Doc Ophthalmol* 110:57–66.

Rowe, S.E., Simmons, J.R., Ringler, D.H., and Lay, D.M. 1974. Spontaneous neoplasms in aging Gerbillinae. A summary of forty-four neoplasms. *Vet Pathol* 11:28–51.

Rubin, L.F. 1974. *Atlas of Veterinary Ophthalmoscopy*. Lea & Febiger, Philadelphia.

Rybak, L.P. 2007. Mechanisms of cisplatin ototoxicity and progress in otoprotection. *Curr Opin Otolaryngol Head Neck Surg* 15:364–369.

Rybak, L.P., Talaska, A.E., and Schacht, J. 2008. Drug-induced hearing loss. In: *Auditory Trauma, Protection and Repair* (J. Schacht, A.N. Pepper, R.R. Fay, eds.), Springer-Verlag, pp. 219–256.

Sakai, Y. 1981. The mammalian Harderian gland: morphology, biochemistry and physiology. *Arch Histol Jpn* 44:299–333.

Samuelson, D.A. 2007. Ophthalmic anatomy. In: *Veterinary Ophthalmology*. 4th ed. (K. Gelatt, ed.), Blackwell, Ames, pp. 37–148.

Santi, P.A. 2001. Cochlear microanatomy and ultrastructure. In: *Physiology of the Ear* (A.F. Jahn and J. Santos Sacchi, eds.), Singular Publishing, New York, pp. 173–200.

Schacht, J., and Hawkins, J.E. 2006. Sketches of otohistory. Part 11: ototoxicity: drug-induced hearing loss. *Audiol Neurootol* 11:1–6.

Schardein, J.L., Lucas, J.A., and Fitsgerald, J.E. 1975. Retinal dystrophy in Sprague–Dawley rats. *Lab Anim Sci* 25:323–326.

Schiavo, D.M. 1972. Retinopathy from administration of an imidazo quinazoline to beagles. *Toxicol Appl Pharmacol* 23:782–783.

Schiavo, D.M., Sinha, D.P., Black, H.E., Arthaud, L., Massa, T., Murphy, B.F., Szot, R.J., and Schwartz, E. 1984. Tapetal changes in beagle dogs. I. Ocular changes after oral administration of a beta-adrenergic blocking agent—SCH 19927. *Toxicol Appl Pharmacol* 72:187–194.

Schmidt, R.E. 1971. Ophthalmic lesions in non-human primates. *Vet Pathol* 8:28–36.

Schuknecht, H.F. 1974. *Pathology of the Ear*. Harvard University Press, Cambridge.

Sebesteny, A., Sheraidah, G.A., Trevan, D.J., Alexander, R.A., and Ahmed, A.I. 1985. Lipid keratopathy and atheromatosis in an SPF laboratory rabbit colony attributable to diet. *Lab Anim* 19:180–188.

Sergi, B., Ferrararesi, A., Troiani, D., Paludetti, G., and Fetoni, A. 2003. Cisplatin ototoxicity in the guinea pig: vestibular and cochlear damage. *Hear Res* 182:56–64.

Sha, S.H., Taylor, R., Forge, A., and Schacht, J. 2001. Differently vulnerability of basal and apical hair cells is based on intrinsic susceptibility to free radicals. *Hear Res* 155:1–8.

Shadduck, J.A., and Everitt, J.I. 1991. Retinoblastoma, experimental, rat and hamster. In: *Monographs on Pathology of Laboratory Animals: Eye and Ear* (T.C. Jones, U. Mohr, and R.D. Hunt, eds.), Springer-Verlag, Berlin, pp. 114–116.

Sheldon, W.G., Curtis, M., Kodell, R.L., and Weed, L. 1983. Primary Harderian gland neoplasms in mice. *J Natl Cancer Inst* 71:61–68.

Sherrard, E.S., and Rycroft, P.V. 1967. Retrocorneal membranes: I. Their origin and structure. *Brit J Ophthalmol* 51:379–381.

Shibuya, K., Sugimoto, K., and Satou, K. 2001. Spontaneous ocular lesions in aged Crj: CD(SD)IGS rats. *Anim Eye Res* 20:15–19.

Shively, J.N., and Epling, G.P. 1970. Fine structure of the canine eye: cornea. *Am J Vet Res* 31:713–722.

Short, B. 2008. Safety evaluation of ocular drug delivery formulations and practical considerations. *Toxicol Pathol* 36:49–62.

Sina, J.F., Galer, D.M., Sussman, R.G., Gautheron, P.D., Sargent, E.V., Leong, B., Shah, P.V., Curren, R.D., and Miller, K. 1995. A collaborative evaluation of seven alternatives to the Draize eye irritation test using pharmaceutical intermediates. *Fund Appl Toxicol* 26:20–31.

Sinha, D.P., Cartwright, M.E., and Johnson, R.C. 2006. Incidental mononuclear cell infiltrate in the uvea of cynomolgus monkeys. *Toxicol Pathol* 34:148–151.

Somps, C.J., Greene, N., Render, J.A., Aleo, M.D., Forner, J.H., Dykens, J.A., and Phillips, G. 2009. A current practice for predicting ocular toxicity of systemically delivered drugs. *Cut Ocular Toxicol* 28:1–18.

Spangler, W.L., Waring, G.O., and Morrin, L.A. 1982. Oval lipid corneal opacities in Beagles. *Vet Pathol* 19:150–159.

Steinbach, E., and Grüninger, G. 1980. Experimental production of cholesteatoma in rabbits by using non-irritants (skin tolerants). *J Laryngol Otol* 94:269–279.

Steel, K.P., and Kros, C.J. 2001. A genetic approach to understanding auditory function. *Nat Genet* 27:143–149.

Strocchi, P., Dozza, B., Pecorella, I., Fresina, M., Campos, E., and Stirpe, F. 2005. Lesions caused by ricin applied to rabbit eyes. *Invest Ophthalmol Vis Sci* 46:1113–1116.

Strum, J.M., and Shear, C.R. 1982. Constant light exposure induces damage and squamous metaplasia in Harderian glands of albino mice. *Tissue Cell* 14:149–161.

Suckow, M.A., and Douglas, F.A. 1997. *The Laboratory Rabbit*, CRC Press LLC, Boca Raton, FL, p. 51.

Sullivan, D.A., Jensen, R.V. Suzuki, T., and Richards, S.M. 2009. Do sex steroids exert sex-specific and/or opposite effects on gene expression in lacrimal and meibomian glands? *Mol Vis* 15:1553–1572.

Szalay, J., Nunziata, B., and Henkind, P. 1975. Permeability of iridal blood vessels. *Exp Eye Res* 21:531–543.

Tanaka, N., Ohkawa, T., Hiyama, T., and Nakajima, A. 1983. Evaluation of the ocular toxicity of two beta blocking drugs, cartolol and practolol, in beagle dogs. *J Pharmacol Exp Ther* 224:424–430.

Taradach, C., and Greaves, P. 1984. Spontaneous lesions in laboratory animals: incidence in relation to age. *CRC Crit Rev Toxicol* 12:121–147.

Taradach, C., Régnier, B., and Perraud, J. 1981. Eye lesions in Sprague–Dawley rats: type and incidence in relation to age. *Lab Anim* 15:285–287.

Taylor, A., Lipman, R.D., Jahngen-Hodge, J., Palmer, V., Smith, D., Padhye, N., Dallal, G.E., Cyr, D.E., Laxman, E., Shepard, P., Morrow, F., Salomon, R., Perrone, G., Asmundsson, G., Meydani, M., Blumberg, J., Mune, M., Harrison, D.E., Archer, J.R., and Shigenaga, M. 1995. Dietary calorie restriction in the Emory mouse: effects of lifespan, eye lens cataract prevalence and progression, levels of ascorbate, glutathione, glucose, and glycohemoglobin, tail collagen breaktime, DNA and RNA oxidation, skin integrity, fecundity, and cancer. *Mech Ageing Dev* 791:33–35.

Ton, C., and Parng, C. 2005. The use of zebrafish for assessing ototoxic and otoprotective agents. *Hear Res* 208:79–88.

Tso, M.O.M. 1973. Photic maculopathy in rhesus monkeys: a light and electron microscopy study. *Invest Ophthalmol Vis Sci* 12:17–34.

Tso, M.O.M., and Woodford, B.J. 1983. Effect of photic injury on the retinal tissues. *Ophthalmology* 90:952–963.

Tucker, M.J. 1997. Special sense organs and associated tissues. In: *Diseases of the Wistar Rat*. Taylor and Francis, London, pp. 237–247.

Turton, J., and Hooson, J. 1998. The eye. In: *Target Organ Pathology, Organs of Special Sense*. Taylor and Francis, London, pp. 451–466.

Van Ruijven, M.W., de Groot, J.C., Klis, S.F., and Smoorenburg, G.F. 2005. The cochlear targets of cisplatin: an electrophysiological and morphological time-sequence study. *Hear Res* 205:241–248.

Van Winkle, T.J., and Balk, M.W. 1986. Spontaneous corneal opacities in laboratory mice. *Lab Anim Sci* 36:248–255.

Von Sallman, L., and Grimes, P. 1972. Spontaneous retinal degeneration in mature Osborne–Mendel rats. *Archiv Ophthalmol* 88:404–411.

Wang, Y., Ding, D., and Salvi, R.J. 2003. Carboplatin-induced early cochlear lesion in chinchillas. *Hear Res* 181:65–72.

Wang, Y., Hirose, K., and Liberman, M. 2002. Dynamics of noise-induced cellular injury and repair in the mouse cochlea. *J Assoc Res Otolaryngol* 3:248–268.

Wegener, A.R. 1995. In vivo studies on the effect of UV-radiation on the eye lens in animals. *Doc Ophthalmol* 88:221–232.

Weisse, I., Stötzer, H., and Seitz, R. 1974. Age and light-dependent changes in the rat eye. *Virchows Archiv A Pathol Anat Histopathol* 362:145–156.

Whiteley, H.E., and Peiffer, R.L. 2002. The eye. In: *Handbook of Toxicologic Pathology*. 2nd ed., Vol. 2, Academic Press, Salt Lake City, pp. 539–584.

Wilhelm, K.E., Grabolle, B., Urbach, H., Tolba, R., Schild, H., and Paulsen, F. 2006. Evaluation of polyurethane nasolacrimal duct stents: in vivo studies in New Zealand rabbits. *Cardiovasc Intervent Radiol* 29:846–853.

Wilhelmus, K.R. 2001. The Draize eye test. *Survey Ophthalmol* 45:493–515.

Williams, D., and Sullivan, A. 2010. Ocular diseases in the guinea pig (*Cavia porcellus*): a survey of 1000 animals. *Vet Ophthalmol* 13:54–62.

Wright, A., Davis, A., Bredberg, G., Ulehlova, L., and Spencer, H. 1987. Hair cell distributions in the normal human cochlea. *Acta Otolaryngol Suppl* 444:1–48.

Yoshida, N., and Liberman, M.C. 1999. Stereociliary anomaly in guinea pig: effects of hair bundle rotation on cochlear sensitivity. *Hear Res* 131:29–38.

Yoshitomi, K., and Boorman, G.A. 1990. Eye and associated glands. In: *Pathology of the Fischer Rat* (G.A. Boorman, S.L. Eustis, M.R. Elwell, C.A. Montgomery Jr., and W.F. Mackenzie, eds.), Academic Press, San Diego, pp. 239–259.

Zarfoss, M., Bentley, E., Milovancev, M., Schmiedt, C., Dubielzig, R., and McAnulty, J. 2007. Histopathologic evidence of capecitabine corneal toxicity in dogs. *Vet Pathol* 44:700–702.

Index

Page numbers followed by f and t indicate figures and tables, respectively.

A

AA amyloid, 438
Abdominal cavity, 102
Aberrant crypt foci (ACF), 265f, 266
ABR; *see* Auditory brain stem response (ABR)
Absorption, 59, 60, 62, 65, 66, 66f
    intestinal, and secretion, 266–268, 267f
    pH-dependent, 67
    xenobiotic, 267
AC; *see* Adenylyl cyclase (AC)
Acetaminophen, 68
Acetylcholine, 271
Achlorhydria, 286
Acid blockers, potassium-competitive, 287
Acinar cells, 351
    apoptosis of, 351
    focal lesions, 355
    immunohistochemical stains of, 347
Acinar epithelium
    protein markers of, 348
    vacuolation of, 348, 350
    of Xbp1 gene, 352
ACTH; *see* Adrenocorticotropic hormone (ACTH)
Activated partial thromboplastin time (APTT), 154
Active splenic hematopoiesis (extramedullary
    hematopoiesis), 486
Acute kidney injury (AKI), 426
    assessment of, 426–427
    macroscopic observations, 427
    urine biomarkers, 428–429
Acute myelocytic leukemias, 507
Acyl-coenzyme A:cholesterol acyltransferase (ACAT),
    687
Adenocarcinomas, 276, 277f, 288, 298, 390, 473
    mucinous, 298–299
Adenohypophyseal cells, 659
Adenomas, 276, 287, 289f, 382, 467
Adenomatous polyposis coli (APC), 264
Adenomyosis, 792
    development of, 790, 791
Adenosquamous carcinomas, 383
Adenylyl cyclase (AC), 625
Adipose aggregates, 461–462
Ad libitum diet, 601
ADMET (absorption, distribution, metabolism, excretion,
    toxicity), 88
Adnexa, 846
    neoplastic skin changes
        benign hair follicle tumor, 880
        sebaceous cell adenoma, 880
        sebaceous cell carcinoma, 880
        sebaceous cell hyperplasia, 879

non-neoplastic skin changes, dermatotoxicity,
    pathologic findings, 871–873
Adrenal cortex, 680
    carcinomas of, 689
    diffuse hyperplasia of, 689
    toxicity studies, 683
    ultrastructural evaluation of, 687
Adrenal cortical vacuolation, 232
Adrenal corticosteroids, 680
Adrenal gland, 679
    female mouse, 684f
Adrenal hormone assessment, 163
Adrenal steroidogenesis
    cholesterol, 681
Adrenocortical hypertrophy, 686
Adrenocortical toxicity, 686
Adrenocorticotropic hormone (ACTH), 657, 680, 838
    hypersecretion, chronic, 680
    steroid production, 681
Adrenocorticotropic hormone stimulation tests, 163
Age-related atrophy, 533
Aglomerular pronephros, 426
Agnogenic myeloid metaplasia, 510
Ahr nuclear translocator (Arnt), 72
Airways
    inflammation, 385
    mucins, 373
    neoplastic changes, 389–390
    surfactant, 374
    wall remodeling, 389
Alanine aminotransferase (ALT), 135, 154, 155, 320
Albino rabbit, 850
Albumin, 159, 160, 427
Alcian blue (AB) stain, 300f
Alcohol fixation, 105
Aldehyde fixatives, 105
Aldosterone formation, 682
Aldosterone synthetase, 681
ALK5, immunohistochemical analysis, 610
Alkaline phosphatase (ALP), 135, 156
Alkaline tide, 263
Allergic cutaneous drug reactions, 862
Allopurinol, 507
Alloxan, 698
Alpha glutathione-s-transferase (αGST), 428
Alpha-2U-globulin nephropathy, 426
Alveolar edema, 401
Alveolar hemorrhage, 402
Alveolar macrophage (AM), 373
    cytoplasmic neutral lipid droplets, 391f
Alzheimer's disease, 912
Ameloblastic (ameloblastoma-like) epithelium, 582
Ameloblastic odontomas, 582